The Complete Mental Health Directory

2014/2015

Ninth Edition

The Complete Mental Health Directory

A Comprehensive
Source Book for
Professionals and Individuals

A Sedgwick Press Book

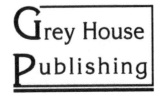

Grey House
Publishing

PUBLISHER: Leslie Mackenzie
EDITOR: Richard Gottlieb
EDITORIAL DIRECTOR: Laura Mars

PRODUCTION MANAGER, COMPOSITION: Kristen Thatcher
MARKETING DIRECTOR: Jessica Moody

Grey House Publishing, Inc.
4919 Route 22
Amenia, NY 12501
518.789.8700
FAX 518.789.0545
www.greyhouse.com
E-MAIL: books@greyhouse.com

While every effort has been made to ensure the reliability of the information presented in this publication, Grey House Publishing neither guarantees the accuracy of the data contained herein nor assumes any responsibility for errors, omissions or discrepancies. Grey House accepts no payment for listing; inclusions in the publication of any organization, agency, institution, publication, service or individual does not imply endorsement of the editors or publisher.

Errors brought to the attention of the publisher and verified to the satisfaction of the publisher will be corrected in future editions.

First edition printed 1999
Ninth edition printed 2014

Biennial
Spine title: The complete mental health directory
    v. ; 27.5
"A comprehensive source book for individuals and professionals"
Includes indexes
ISSN: 1538-0556

1. Mental health services – United States – Directories.

RA790.6.C625
362 – dc21
ISBN: 978-1-61925-269-1

2001-233121

Table of Contents

Introduction
Adolescent Health Highlight: Mental Health Disorders
New Trends in Mental Health Treatment
Bill of Rights for Children's Mental Health Disorders and Their Families
Disorders by Diagnostic Category
User's Guide

SECTION ONE: Disorders

Each disorder chapter includes a detailed description and some or all of the following categories: *Associations & Agencies; Books; Periodicals & Pamphlets; Research Centers; Support Groups & Hot Lines; Video & Audio; Web sites.* See *Diagnostic Categories* in the front matter for a complete list of disorders covered.

SECTION TWO: Associations & Organizations

SECTION THREE: Government Agencies

SECTION FOUR: Professional & Support Services

Introduction

This is the ninth edition of *The Complete Mental Health Directory*. This unique reference directory provides comprehensive coverage of 21 broad mental health disorder categories, from Adjustment Disorders to Tic Disorders. Within these categories are nearly 100 specific disorders, including Obsessive Compulsive Disorder, Asperger's Syndrome, Bipolar Disorder, Postpartum Depression, Schizophrenia, Somatization Disorder, Paraphilias and many more.

A repeated winner of the **Annual National Health Information Awards** by the Health Information Resource Center for "the Nation's best consumer health programs and materials," this edition provides information on topics that more and more Americans find themselves dealing with, including Post Traumatic Stress Disorder, Eating Disorders, and Sleep Disorders, as well as individual chapters on Pediatric and Adolescent Issues, and Suicide, which sometimes results from specific mental disorders.

Coverage of the nearly 100 disorders includes clear, concise descriptions, with current diagnoses and treatment methods. Users will find a variety of disorder-specific resources, including Associations, Books, Periodicals, Research Centers, and Support Groups. In addition to disorder-specific resources, *The Complete Mental Health Directory* includes Professional Services, Publishers, Facilities, Clinical Management and Pharmaceutical Companies.

In addition to more than 4,500 listings, *The Complete Mental Health Directory* begins with three informative articles:
> Adolescent Health Highlight: Mental Health Disorders
> New Trends in Mental Health Treatment
> Bill of Rights for Children's Mental Health Disorders and Their Families

Praise for previous edition:

"This is a sourcebook for people suffering from mental illnesses, connecting them with appropriate resources . . . and for practitioners to help them discover the vast number of resources . . . The editors succeed in opening up this wide array of materials to those who need them. This will be a helpful addition to public, academic, and medical libraries. . . . Even in this digital age, a print directory may still be the quickest and easiest way to get at the kinds of information this book provides."

4 Star Review, Doody's Review Service

"...certain times and situations call for a print resource, especially in the field of mental health services. Having one in hand is helpful. ... [The] section ... on professional services includes a wealth of resources. Summing up: Recommended. All levels."

Choice Magazine

SECTION ONE: Disorders

This section consists of 21 chapters dealing with broad categories of mental health issues from Adjustment Disorders to Tic Disorders. Each chapter begins with a description, written in clear, accessible language and includes symptoms, prevalence and treatment options. These descriptions include information on specific syndromes within a general category, such as Social Anxiety Disorder within the Anxiety Disorders chapter. Following the descriptions are specific resources relevant to the disorder, including Associations, Books, Government Agencies, Periodicals, Pamphlets, Support Groups, Hot Lines, Resource Centers, Audio & Video Tapes, and Web Sites.

SECTIONS TWO & THREE: Associations, Organizations, Government Agencies

More than 1,000 National Associations, and Federal and State Agencies are profiled in these sections that offer general mental health services and support for patients and their families.

SECTION FOUR: Professional Support & Services
This section provides resources that support the many different professionals in the mental heath field. Included are specific chapters on Accreditation and Quality Assurance, Associations, Books, Conferences and Meetings, Periodicals, Training and Recruitment, Audio & Video tapes, Web sites, and Workbooks and Manuals.

SECTION FIVE: Publishers
This section lists major publishers of books and magazines that focus on health care or mental health issues. This material is suitable for both professionals in the mental health industry, as well as patients and their network community.

SECTION SIX: Facilities
This section lists major facilities and hospitals, arranged by states that provide treatment for persons with mental health disorders.

SECTION SEVEN: Clinical Management
Here you will find products and services that support the Clinical Management aspect of the mental health industry, including Directories and Databases, Management Companies, and Information Services that provide patient and medical data, as well as marketing information.

SECTION EIGHT: Pharmaceutical Companies
This section offers information on the pharmaceutical companies that manufacture drugs to treat mental health disorders. Several companies and many drugs have been added to this edition. This data is presented in two ways: First, alphabetically by company name, including address, phone, fax, web site, and a list of specific drugs manufactured. Second, alphabetically by name of drug, including the disorder it is typically prescribed for, and reference to the company or companies that manufacture it.

INDEXES: Disorder Index lists entries by disorders and disorder categories. **Entry Index** is an alphabetical list of all entries. **Geographic Index** lists entries by state.

This information in this revised edition is crucial for those suffering from a mental condition and their support network, including professionals who diagnose and treat mental disorders. It combines, in a single volume, disorder descriptions written in clear, layman's terms, and a wide variety of resources. Here's where you'll find where to go and who to ask – for the most diagnosed mental health disorders in the country.

For even easier access, *The Complete Mental Health Directory* is available in our online database platform, http://gold.greyhouse.com. Subscribers have access to all of this health information, and can search by geographic area, disorder, contacts, keyword and so much more. With this new, online database, locating mental health resources has never been faster or easier.

Publication # 2013-1

January 2013

Mental Health Disorders

By David Murphey, Ph.D., Megan Barry, B.A., and Brigitte Vaughn, M.S.

Mental disorders are diagnosable conditions characterized by changes in thinking, mood, or behavior (or some combination of these) that can cause a person to feel stressed out and impair his or her ability to function. These disorders are common in adolescence. This *Adolescent Health Highlight* presents the warning signs of mental disorders; describes the types of mental disorders and their prevalence and trends; discusses the consequences and risk of mental disorders; presents treatment options and barriers to accessing mental health care; and provides mental health resources.

The definition and complexities of mental disorders

Medical science increasingly recognizes the vital link between a person's physical health and his or her mental/emotional health. Mind and body are connected as one, each affected by the other, and both are influenced by a person's genetic inheritance, environment, and experience. Just as the absence of disease does not adequately define physical health, mental health consists of more than the absence of mental disorders. Mental health is best seen as falling along a continuum, which fluctuates over time, and across individuals, as well as within a single individual.[3]

As defined in this *Highlight*, mental disorders are diagnosable conditions characterized by changes in thinking, mood, or behavior (or some combination of these) that are associated with distress or impaired functioning.[4] As with symptoms of physical illness, symptoms of mental disorders occur on a spectrum from mild to severe. People with mental disorders, however, often have to bear the special burden of the societal stigma associated with their condition. This burden sometimes prevents people from acknowledging their illness and from seeking support and effective treatment for it. Just as with physical health, failure to address symptoms early on can have serious negative consequences.

What are the warning signs of mental disorders?

It is important to make a clear distinction between the normal ups and downs of mood and outlook, and diagnosable mental disorders. Everyone, especially many adolescents, experiences mood swings—from feeling blue, to expressing giddy excitement, to being anxious or irritable. Adolescents are biologically prone to have more of these mood swings because of the hormonal changes associated with this period in life, coupled with the fact that their brains are still developing.[6,8] Many adolescents can worry that they're "losing it," when, in reality, these mood swings may be normal occurrences.[6,10]

Fast Facts

1. Mental disorders in adolescence are common: An estimated one in five adolescents has a diagnosable disorder.[1]

2. Adolescence is the time when many mental disorders first arise. More than half of all mental disorders and problems with substance abuse (such as binge drinking and illegal drug use) begin by age 14.[2]

3. The most prevalent mental disorder experienced among adolescents is depression,[4] with more than one in four high school students found to have at least mild symptoms of this condition.[5]

4. Adolescents with mental disorders are at increased risk of getting caught up in harmful behaviors, such as substance abuse and unprotected sexual activity.[1,6,7]

5. Many effective treatments exist for mental disorders, most involving some combination of psychotherapy and medication.[9]

6. The majority of adolescents with mental disorders do not seek out or receive treatment, a consequence of various barriers to care, including the fear of being stigmatized by peers and others.[4]

However, when psychological symptoms cause major emotional distress, or interfere substantially with daily life and social interactions over a period of time, professional evaluation is warranted, just as it is with any serious illness. Not all mental disorders among adolescents have obvious, reliable symptoms, but parents, teachers, and others should be alert to some warning signs that an adolescent may be in trouble. These signs include persistent irritability, anger, or social withdrawal, as well as major changes in appetite or sleep.[11,12]

What are the types of mental disorders, and which are the most common among adolescents?

Mental health professionals use various classifications to identify the diverse range of mental disorders. Many adolescent mental disorders fall under the broad categories of mood disorders (e.g., depression and bipolar disorder); behavioral disorders (e.g., various acting-out behaviors, including aggression, destruction of property, and some problems of attention and hyperactivity); and anxiety disorders (including social anxiety disorder, obsessive-compulsive disorder (OCD), post-traumatic stress disorder, and phobias).[4,13] Many adolescents with mental disorders have symptoms indicative of more than one disorder.[3]

FIGURE 1: Percentage of students in grades 9-12 who reported symptoms of depression*, by gender, 2011

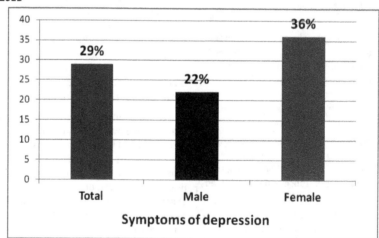

* Symtoms of depression in this survey are an affirmative response to the statement "reported feeling sad or hopeless almost every day for two weeks or longer during the past year."

Source: Centers for Disease Control and Prevention. (2012). Youth Risk Behavior Surveillance Survey- United States, 2011. Surveillance summaries: MMWR 2012; 61 (No SS-4) .

Adolescence is a time when many mental disorders first arise; in fact, more than half of all mental disorders and problems with substance abuse (such as binge drinking and illegal drug use) begin by age 14, and three-quarters of these difficulties begin by age 24.[2] Accurate estimates of the number of adolescents who have diagnosable mental disorders are difficult to come by, for several reasons: many adolescents are reluctant to disclose these disorders; definitions of disorders vary; and most diagnoses rely on clinical judgment rather than on biological markers (such as a blood test).[14] However, available data suggest that 20 percent of adolescents have a diagnosable mental disorder.[1] Depression is the single most common type reported by adolescents, though it is often

29 percent of high school students in grades 9-12 reported feeling sad or hopeless almost every day for two weeks or longer during the past year— a red flag for possible clinical depression.

accompanied by other mental disorders.[4] In 2011, more than one in four (29 percent) high school students in grades 9-12 who participated in a national school-based survey reported feeling sad or hopeless almost every day for two weeks or longer during the past year—a red flag for possible clinical depression (see Figure 1).[15]

Another survey that collected information from adolescents between the ages of 12 and 17 found that in 2008, about one in 12 (8 percent) reported experiencing a major depressive episode during the past year (see Figure 2).[16] These estimates have not changed much over the past five to 10 years.[5] A slightly lower percentage of adolescents (3 percent) met the criteria for conduct disorders.[4] Adolescents with conduct disorders are extremely uncooperative, are persistent in defying societal rules and authority figures, and are often severely angry, aggressive, and destructive.[17]

FIGURE 2: Percentage of adolescents with selected mental disorders*

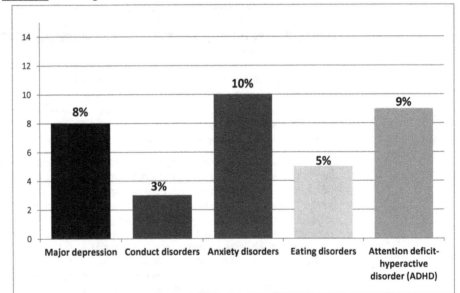

These data are from different reporting years: major depression, 2008; anxiety disorders, 1999; conduct disorders, 1995; and eating disorders and ADHD, 2005. Estimates are based on adolescents' self-reports of symptoms, not clinical diagnoses, except for ADHD, where estimates are based parent's reporting that a professional had given that diagnosis.

Sources: Substance Abuse and Mental Health Services Administration. (2009). Results from the 2008 National Survey on Drug Use and Health: National Findings (Office of Applied Studies, NSDUH Series H-36, HHS Publication No. SMA 09-4434). Rockville, MD. Knopf, D. et al. (2008). The mental health of adolescents: A national profile, 2008. National Adolescent Health Information Center.

An estimated 10 percent of adolescents have anxiety disorders, the most common of which are OCD, post-traumatic stress disorder, and phobias.

An estimated 10 percent of adolescents reported symptoms of an anxiety disorder.[4] Among the more common anxiety disorders are OCD, social anxiety disorder, post-traumatic stress disorder (PTSD), and phobias. OCD is characterized by recurrent and persistent thoughts, images, or impulses (obsessions) that are unwanted, and/or repetitive behaviors or rituals (compulsions) that cause distress.[18] PTSD can develop after a person has seen or lived through a dangerous or frightening event. This disorder is characterized by flashbacks or bad dreams, emotional numbness, and/or intense guilt or worry, among other symptoms.[19] Phobias are intense, irrational fears of things or circumstances that pose little or no actual danger. Facing, or even the thought of facing, the feared object or situation can spur panic attacks or severe anxiety.[13] Panic disorders (a type of anxiety disorder characterized by a racing heartbeat, shortness of breath, and other pronounced physical symptoms) affect around one percent of adolescents.[20]

About five percent of adolescents report symptoms of an eating disorder.[4] Less common are autism spectrum disorders (a diverse category of conditions, typically marked by severe impairments in social and communication skills).[21]

Some estimates put the prevalence of ADHD as high as nine percent among 12- to 17-year-olds.

Adolescents with attention deficit-hyperactivity disorder (ADHD) have difficulty paying attention, controlling impulses, and staying organized.[12] Some estimates put the prevalence of the disorder as high as nine percent among 12- to 17-year-olds.[4] Adolescent males are more likely than are females to have ever been diagnosed with ADHD.[4] However, biases may exist in the identification of young people with ADHD, including lower rates of diagnosis among Hispanic children[22] and higher rates for those who are young for their grade.[23]

What are some of the consequences of mental disorders?

Mental disorders take a toll on adolescents, their parents, and friends, and contribute significantly to health care costs. The consequences can be short- or long-term. Indeed, most mental disorders diagnosed among adults began during adolescence, although other mental disorders experienced by adolescents may diminish by early adulthood if they are treated.[4,9]

Substance abuse disorders frequently go hand in hand with mental disorders.[4] In addition, mental disorders are often associated with other negative emotional and behavioral patterns in adolescence—including impaired relationships, lower academic performance, a higher risk of unprotected sex and teen pregnancy, and increased involvement with the juvenile justice system. However, many adolescents who experience these issues do not have a mental disorder, and many youth with mental disorders do not have these problems.[1,6,7] The single most disturbing potential consequence of adolescent mental disorders is suicide—the third leading cause of death among 10- to 24-year-olds in the United States. Although suicide can have multiple causes, 90 percent of adolescents who commit suicide had a diagnosable mental disorder, and up to 60 percent of them were suffering from depression at the time of their death.[24]

The single most disturbing potential consequence of adolescent mental disorders is suicide—the third leading cause of death among 10- to 24-year-olds in the United States.

How do risks of mental disorders vary across adolescents?

Adolescent males generally are more likely than are their female peers to be diagnosed with behavioral problems, including conduct disorders, ADHD, and autism spectrum disorders.[4,25] Adolescent females are more commonly diagnosed with depression and eating disorders than are males.[4,26] Adolescents whose parents have lower levels of education (e.g., no college degree) have more risk of having a mental disorder than do adolescents whose parents have higher levels of education. Adolescents whose parents are divorced are also more likely to have mental disorders than are adolescents whose parents are married or cohabiting.[27] Other groups of adolescents particularly at risk for mental disorders include those involved in bullying (either as victims or perpetrators), those who have experienced sexual or physical abuse, and those whose parents have a history of mental disorders.[24,28] Among ethnic groups, Hispanic and black adolescent females have a higher risk of depressive symptoms than do adolescent females from other racial/ethnic groups.[15]

How can mental disorders be treated?

As in other arenas of health, early intervention or prevention can be an effective way to address potential mental disorders before they reach the stage requiring treatment. Although not all mental disorders are accompanied by early warning signs, people who interact with and care about adolescents should be alert to marked changes in mood or behavior that may suggest problems. At the same time, concerned adults can help adolescents maintain positive mental health by providing caring, supportive relationships, encouraging healthy behaviors, and teaching effective strategies for coping with stress.[29]

Most mental disorders are treatable, although what works for particular individuals may vary. Often a combination of psychosocial therapy (personal or group counseling with a psychotherapist) and medication is effective. For many types of disorders (e.g., depression and OCD), cognitive-behavioral therapies and medications have been shown to be effective in many cases.[7] Cognitive-behavioral therapies seek to help people modify negative or irrational thoughts and to replace dysfunctional behaviors with more rational ones. For other types of disorders (such as ADHD), behavioral parent training and classroom management techniques may be effective.[9] When psychiatric medications are prescribed, they are typically administered in combination with other treatment approaches, such as individual psychotherapy, group therapy, or family therapy. In general, experts agree that medication should not be the only treatment followed, and that any treatment plan should be supervised by a clinician with specific training in adolescent mental health.[9]

Other strategies have also been used successfully with particular mental disorders. For depression, some evidence shows that increased physical exercise may provide some benefits.[30] For conduct disorders, promising results have been found when the young person with the disorder is treated, together with his or her family and community, using a "systems" approach. The systems approach attempts to address multiple problem behaviors that the adolescent is exhibiting by providing multiple types of services, such as education, child protection, juvenile justice, and mental health services.[7] In other words, systems approaches involve coordinating services from different providers and are tailored to meet the needs of the individual adolescent.

Some families may choose unconventional therapies (sometimes referred to as complementary or alternative medicine) as a way to treat physical and mental disorders. Examples of these include diet modifications, such as eliminating sugar, or foods with dyes and additives; herbal or vitamin supplements; and music or dance therapy. Although these practices have become more widespread in recent years, particularly for autism spectrum disorders, they have not met the same rigorous standards of evidence as more traditional treatments, and consumers should be skeptical of dramatic or poorly substantiated claims for effectiveness.[31] Talking to a trained clinician is key in determining the proper treatment for any mental disorder.

How do adolescents access mental health services, and what are barriers to care?

Parents, other family members, and friends can all play roles in encouraging adolescents who are experiencing emotional distress to seek help. Mental health services for adolescents are provided by a mix of specialists (psychiatrists, psychologists, social workers, and others) in the public and private sectors. In general, this system of diverse providers is crisis-oriented and designed for treating people with diagnosed mental disorders (particularly as reflected in reimbursement policies.) The system is less structured to address prevention and health promotion, early identification of difficulties, and timely, effective treatment.[14,32]

School health centers are often helpful in identifying the mental health care needs of adolescents, partly because adolescents spend much of their time in school, and partly because these clinics are accessible to students in low-income and underserved racial and ethnic minority groups, who are more likely to be without health insurance.[14,33] However, few school mental health professionals are able to provide intensive care on their own.[14] Primary care providers (pediatricians and others) are often the gatekeepers for identifying mental disorders in adolescents. However, these providers may lack the time in their practices—as well as the specific expertise—to identify and manage these disorders. Moreover, efforts to coordinate care between primary care providers and mental health professionals vary considerably in their effectiveness.

Studies have found that most children and adolescents with mental disorders (between 60 and 90 percent) do not seek out or receive the services that they need.[4] The societal stigma associated with mental disorders may help explain why many adolescents do not seek treatment. Also, parents, school officials, and medical providers often miss opportunities to address the prevention and early identification of mental disorders. Additional barriers include services that are poorly coordinated (e.g., among schools, primary health care providers, and social services agencies); a lack of health insurance (although most adolescents are insured); restrictions by insurers on coverage for certain services; and a shortage of providers with specific expertise in adolescent mental health.[14]

Implications for preventing risky adolescent behaviors

Young people with mental disorders, in general, are more vulnerable to involvement in risky activities that jeopardize their health and well-being than are young people in the larger adolescent population.[1,6] Suicide attempts and self-injury are the most dire of these threats, but other troublesome behaviors warrant scrutiny as well. For example, adolescents with depression are also more likely than are their nondepressed peers to engage in substance abuse and early sexual activity;[5] and adolescents with conduct disorders are more likely to engage in early sexual activity, early drug and alcohol use, interpersonal violence, and delinquency.[12] Thus, prevention—in addition to early diagnosis and treatment of mental disorders—is essential for reducing many other serious problem behaviors.[29]

Strategies and approaches to reduce mental health disorders among adolescents

The National Prevention Strategy is a comprehensive plan designed the government's National Prevention Council to help improve the health of Americans at every stage of life. Its mental health recommendations include:

- Promoting early identification of mental health needs and access to quality services. Clinicians are key to identifying mental health needs, so integrating mental health care into traditional health care settings and social service, community, and school settings is important, especially for adolescents who have experienced trauma.

- Reducing the stigma associated with mental health services. Doing so will improve access to and use of the effective mental health treatment that is available.[34]

The U.S. Preventive Services Task Force recommends that adolescents (ages 12-18) be screened for major depressive disorder (MDD) when there are appropriate services available for accurate diagnosis, psychotherapy, and follow-up.[35]

Resources

The Child Trends DataBank includes brief summaries of well-being indicators, including several that are related to mental disorders and mental health:

The Child Trends DataBank includes brief summaries of well-being indicators, including several that are related to mental disorders and mental health.

- Attention Deficit-Hyperactivity Disorder (ADHD): http://childtrendsdatabank.org/?q=76
- Adolescents Who Feel Sad or Hopeless: http://childtrendsdatabank.org/?q=node/126
- Autism Spectrum Disorders: http://childtrendsdatabank.org/?q=node/372
- Bullying: http://childtrendsdatabank.org/?q=node/370
- Disordered Eating: Symptoms of Bulimia: http://childtrendsdatabank.org/?q=node/123
- Suicidal Teens: http://childtrendsdatabank.org/?q=node/128
- Teen Homicide, Suicide, and Firearm Deaths: http://childtrendsdatabank.org/?q=node/124

The Childs Trends LINKS (Lifecourse Interventions to Nurture Kids Successfully) database summarizes evaluations of out-of-school time programs that work (or not) to enhance children's development. The LINKS Database is user-friendly and directed especially to policy makers, program providers, and funders.

- Programs related to anxiety disorders/symptoms, conduct/disruptive disorders, and eating disorders can be found by selecting those boxes under mental health.

- Evaluations of programs proven to work (or not) for reducing depression/depressive symptoms, suicidal thoughts or behaviors, anxiety/anxious symptoms, and post-traumatic stress disorder, in addition to other mental health behaviors, are summarized in the fact sheet What works to prevent or reduce internalizing problems or social-emotional difficulties in adolescents: Lessons from experimental evaluations of social interventions.

- Evaluations of programs proven to work (or not) for reducing ADHD are summarized in a fact sheet What works for acting-out (externalizing) behavior: Lessons from experimental evaluations of social interventions.

Other selected resources include:

- The National Institute of Mental Health (NIMH) provides a number of resources, including fact sheets on brain development and mental disorders in adolescence (http://www.nimh.nih.gov/health/topics/child-and-adolescent-mental-health/index.shtml).

The National Institute of Mental Health provides a number of resources, including fact sheets on brain development and mental disorders in adolescence.

- The Centers for Disease Control and Prevention (CDC) has information about mental health changes in early adolescence (http://www.cdc.gov/ncbddd/child/earlyadolescence.htm) and middle or older adolescence (http://www.cdc.gov/ncbddd/child/middleadolescence15-17.htm), as well as a number of resources on suicide prevention (http://www.cdc.gov/ViolencePrevention/suicide/).

- The Substance Abuse and Mental Health Services Administration (SAMHSA) provides the Mental Health Services Locator, an online, map-based program people can use to find facilities in their vicinity (http://store.samhsa.gov/mhlocator). SAMSHA also maintains an online library of free publications and resources, with more than 200 documents focused on adolescent behavioral health issues (http://store.samhsa.gov/home). In addition, SAMHSA supports the Suicide Prevention Resource Center (http://www.sprc.org), which helps organizations and individuals to develop suicide prevention programs, interventions, and policies.

- Healthcare.gov provides prevention goals and guidelines for several key indicators of adolescent mental health, including screenings for depression and decreasing the rate of suicide attempts (http://www.healthcare.gov/center/councils/nphpphc/strategy/report.pdf).

In addition, health professionals, educators, and others can direct adolescents and their families to a number of federal resources.

- GirlsHealth.gov, from the Office on Women's Health, offers tip sheets about adolescents and their feelings, including "How to know if your 'blues' are depression" (http://girlshealth.gov/feelings/).
- Adolescents (or anyone) in suicidal crisis or emotional distress can call the National Suicide Prevention Lifeline at 1-800-273-TALK; calls made to this 24-hour hotline are routed to the caller's nearest crisis center.

Adolescents (or anyone) in suicidal crisis or emotional distress can call the National Suicide Prevention Lifeline at 1-800-273-TALK.

Acknowledgements

The authors would like to thank Jennifer Manlove, Lina Guzman, and Marci McCoy-Roth at Child Trends for their careful review of and helpful comments on this brief.

Editor: Harriet J. Scarupa

References

[1] Schwarz, S. W. (2009). *Adolescent mental health in the United States: Facts for Policymakers* Retrieved November 9, 2012, from http://nccp.org/publications/pdf/text_878.pdf

[2] Kessler, R. C., Berglund, P., Demler, O., Jin, R., Merikangas, K. R., & Walters, E. E. (2005). Lifetime prevalence and age-of-onset distributions of DSM-IV disorders in the National Comorbidity Survey Replication. *Archives of General Psychiatry, 62*(6), 593–602.

[3] U.S. Department of Health and Human Services. (1999). *Mental health: A report of the Surgeon General*. Retrieved November 9, 2012, from http://www.surgeongeneral.gov/library/mentalhealth/home.html

[4] Knopf, D. K., Park, J., & Mulye, T. P. (2008). *The mental health of adolescents: A national profile, 2008* Retrieved November 9, 2012, from http://nahic.ucsf.edu/downloads/MentalHealthBrief.pdf

[5] Child Trends. (2010). *Child Trends Databank: Adolescents who feel sad or hopeless*. Retrieved November 9, 2012, from http://www.childtrendsdatabank.org/alphalist?q=node/126

[6] Kapphahn, C. J., Morreale, M. C., Rickert, V. I., & Walker, L. R. (2006). Financing mental health services: A position paper of the Society for Adolescent Medicine. *Journal of Adolescent Health, 39*, 456-458.

[7] Grisso, T. (2008). Adolescent offenders with mental disorders. *Future of Children, 18*(2), 143-164.

[8] Casey, B. J., Jones, R. M., & Hare, T. A. (2008). The adolescent brain. *Annals of the New York Academy of Science, 1124*, 111-126.

[9] National Institute of Mental Health. (2009). *Treatment of children with mental illness: Frequently asked questions about the treatment of mental illness in children*. Retrieved November 9, 2012, from http://www.nimh.nih.gov/health/publications/treatment-of-children-with-mental-illness-fact-sheet/nimh-treatment-children-mental-illness-faq.pdf

[10] Arnett, J. J. (1999). Adolescent storm and stress, reconsidered. *American Psychologist, 54*, 317-326.

[11] American Academy of Child and Adolescent Psychiatry. (2008). *Facts for Families: The depressed child*: National Institute of Mental Health. from http://www.aacap.org/galleries/FactsForFamilies/04_the_depressed_child.pdf

[12] Burland, J. (2001). *Parents and teachers as allies: Recognizing early-onset mental illness in children and adolescents*. Arlington, VA: National Alliance for the Mentally Ill.

[13] U.S. Department of Health and Human Services, & National Institutes of Health. *Anxiety disorders*. Retrieved November 9, 2012, from http://www.nimh.nih.gov/health/publications/anxiety-disorders/nimhanxiety.pdf

[14] Committee on Adolescent Health Care Services and Models of Care for Treatment Prevention and Healthy Development, National Research Council, & Institute of Medicine. (2009). *Adolescent health services: Missing opportunities*. Washington, DC: National Academies Press. Retrieved November 9, 2012, from http://www.nap.edu/catalog.php?record_id=12063

[15] Centers for Disease Control and Prevention. (2012). Youth Risk Behavior Surveillance-United States, 2011. *Morbidity and Mortality Weekly Report, 61*(4).

[16] Substance Abuse and Mental Health Services Administration Center for Behavioral Health Statistics and Quality. (2011). *The NSDUH Report: Major Depressive Episode and Treatment among Adolescents: 2009*. Rockville, MD. Retrieved November 9, 2012, from http://www.oas.samhsa.gov/2k11/009/AdolescentDepression.htm

[17] Substance Abuse and Mental Health Services Administration Center for Mental Health Services. (2006). *Helping children and youth with conduct disorder and oppositional defiant disorder: Systems of care*. Washington, D.C.

[18] American Academy of Child & Adolescent Psychiatry. (2001). *Facts for Families: Obsessive-compulsive disorder in children and adolescents* Retrieved November 9, 2011, from http://www.aacap.org/galleries/FactsForFamilies/60_obsessive_compulsive_disorder_in_children_and_adolescents.pdf

[19] U.S. Department of Health and Human Services, National Institutes of Health, & National Institutes of Mental Health. *NIMH fact sheet: Post-Traumatic Stress Disorder research*. Retrieved November 9, 2012, from http://nimh.nih.gov/health/publications/post-traumatic-stress-disorder-research-fact-sheet/post-traumatic-stress-disorder-research-fact-sheet.pdf

[20] Diler, R. S. (2003). Panic disorder in children and adolescents. *Yonsei Medical Journal* Retrieved November 9, 2012, from http://www.eymj.org/Synapse/Data/PDFData/0069YMJ/ymj-44-174.pdf

[21] Lord, C., & Bishop, S. L. (2010). Autism spectrum disorders. *Social Policy Report, 24*(2), 1-27. Retrieved November 9, 2012, from http://www.srcd.org/index.php?option=com_content&task=view&id=232&Itemid=550

[22] Leigh, W. A., & Wheatley, A. L. (2009). *Trends in child health, 1997-2006: Assessing racial/ethnic disparities in diagnoses of ADHD/ADD and of learning disability.* Washington, DC: Joint Center for Political and Economic Studies.

[23] Elder, T. E. (2010). The importance of relative standards in ADHD diagnoses: Evidence based on exact birth dates. *Journal of Health Economics, 29*, 641-656.

[24] National Center for Mental Health Checkups at Columbia University. (2010). *Youth suicide and prevention. TeenScreen.* Retrieved November 9, 2012, from http://www.teenscreen.org/images/stories/PDF/YouthSuicideandPrevention.pdf

[25] McMorrow, S., & Howell, E. (2010). *State mental health systems for children: A review of the literature and available data sources,* from http://www.urban.org/UploadedPDF/412207-state-mental.pdf

[26] Rosen, D. S., & The Committee on Adolescence. (2010). Clinical report identification and management of eating disorders in children and adolescence. *Pediatrics, 126*(6), 1240-1253.

[27] Merikangas, K. R., He, J., Burstein, M., Swanson, S. A., Avenevoli, S., Cui, L., et al. (2010). Lifetime prevalence of mental disorders in U.S. adolescents: Results from the National Comorbidity Survey replication-Adolescent Supplement (NCS-A). *Journal of the American Academy of Child and Adolescent Psychiatry, 49*(10), 980-989.

[28] Keller, M. C. (2008). The evolutionary persistence of genes that increase mental disorders risk. *Association for Psychological Science, 17*(6), 395-399.

[29] National Academy of Sciences. (2009). *Preventing mental, emotional, and behavioral disorders among young people: Progress and possibilities. Report Brief for Researchers.* Retrieved December 18, 2012, from http://www.bocyf.org/prevention_researchers_brief.pdf

[30] National Alliance on Mental Illness. (2009). *Children and adolescents and depression. Fact Sheet.* Retrieved November 9, 2012, from http://www.nami.org/Content/NavigationMenu/Mental_Illnesses/Depression/children_and_adolescents.pdf

[31] Myers, S. M., Johnson, C. P., & The Council on Children With Disabilities. (2007). Management of children with autism spectrum disorders. *Pediatrics, 120*(5), 1162-1182.

[32] National Institute for Health Care Management. (2009). *Strategies to support the integration of mental health into pediatric primary care.* Retrieved November 9, 2012, from http://nihcm.org/pdf/PediatricMH-FINAL.pdf

[33] U.S. Census Bureau. (2010). *Current Population Survey, 2010 Annual Social and Economic Supplement.* Retrieved November 9, 2012, from http://www.census.gov/hhes/www/cpstables/032010/health/h08_000.htm

[34] National Prevention Council. (2011). *National Prevention Strategy.* Washington, DC: U.S. Department of Health and Human Services, Office of the Surgeon General. Retrieved December 6, 2012, from http://www.healthcare.gov/prevention/nphpphc/strategy/report.pdf

[35] U.S. Preventive Services Task Force. (2009). *Major depressive disorder in children and adolescents.* Retrieved December 6, 2012, from http://www.uspreventiveservicestaskforce.org/uspstf/uspschdepr.htm

nami

New Trends in Mental Health Treatment

By Sara Battista, NAMI Communications Intern

Despite the unprecedented number of people living with mental illness in the U.S., only about one-third of those in need of treatment will ever seek professional help. Although traditional psychotherapy is undoubtedly effective for many, some mental health professionals are actively searching for new treatment methods in order to make mental health care more accessible for the general public. Ultimately, they argue that alternative forms of treatment other than psychotherapy are necessary if the medical community hopes to see a decline in the prevalence and affliction of mental illness in the U.S.

In an article from January 2011 published in *Perspectives of Psychological Science,* Dr. Alan Kazdin and Dr. Stacey Blase suggested that in order to relieve the burden of mental illness, the medical community needs to come up with more effective models of treatment delivery that are more practical and accessible for the majority of those in need.

The authors argued that every day obstacles including a lack of access to facilities or practitioners, ethnic and cultural barriers and transportation prevent too many people from receiving treatment. Since the one-on-one model of psychotherapy can be limiting due to time, geographical and financial constraints, the authors recommended a transition to the many other treatment methods in order to more efficiently help a larger portion of individuals. Technology, diet and exercise and support groups were among their many suggestions for new models of treatment that they believed in combination, would reduce the burden of mental illness in the U.S. Since the publication of their cogent arguments in 2011, many new, innovative forms of treatment have revolutionized the world of therapy, bringing the mental health community closer to their goal of providing accessible care for all Americans.

Technology

With millions of Americans surfing the Internet on a daily basis, technological advances are a practical way to provide people living with mental illness with helpful resources. To begin with, the Internet makes connecting with health care professionals accessible from the home or office. Web-based interventions can be accessed through chat-rooms, email, and video chat via webcam. The use of open forums like NAMI's discussion groups also allow people who share common experiences with mental illness to connect online— a tool proven invaluable by the copious amount of research confirming the positive impact of social connection on psychological wellbeing. These technological developments not only broaden the portion of the population with access to therapeutic intervention, but also likely increase the possibility that clients will continue treatment.

The use of smart phones also offers users access to hundreds of virtual treatment resources. For example, an app called the CBTReferee utilizes methods adapted from cognitive behavioral therapy (CBT), which is a highly effective treatment for a variety of mental illnesses including depression and anxiety disorders. Rather than the traditional method of carrying around a notepad, the app allows users to log their thoughts as they occur in order to monitor flawed thinking. Once thoughts are logged, users are able to evaluate what is untrue, unrealistic or unfair about each thought process.

Another popular therapeutic app called BellyBio Interactive Breathing asks users to place their smartphones on their stomach as it guides them through a deep breathing exercise useful in fighting anxiety and stress. This free app monitors breathing patterns while simultaneously generating peaceful music and light in synch with the deep abdominal breathing movements. BellyBio is especially useful for those living with anxiety disorders looking for effective relaxation tools.

Nutrition

Numerous scientific studies have confirmed the correlation between physical and mental health. Although maintaining a healthy physical lifestyle alone may not provide sufficient treatment for mental disorders, there are specifics habits one can easily implement into any schedule that have strong benefits for mental health maintenance.

The University of Maryland Medical Center reports that regular intake of omega-3 fatty acids can be beneficial in the treatment and prevention of a range of mental illnesses including depression, schizophrenia, bipolar disorder and attention deficit hyperactivity disorder (ADHD). Research suggests that children with ADHD may have a deficiency in omega-3 fatty acids, proposing that consuming foods rich in omega-3 fatty acids may be beneficial for managing behavioral symptoms. Likewise, taking omega-3 supplements in addition to medication may improve the symptoms of depression. Also notable is the protective effect of omega-3 fatty acids against Alzheimer's disease and dementia, as research suggests that increasing intake reduces the risk of cognitive decline.

In addition to dietary adjustments, other useful physical health tips include regularly practicing meditation and yoga, both of which have been proven to have a therapeutic effect.

Meditation

A comprehensive study published in 2012 in *Scientific Review of Mental Health Practices* examined over 250 published studies on meditation, investigating 45 years of research on a diverse range of meditation techniques and how they influenced both mental and physical health. Results from the study make a strong case for the value of meditation, as the vast majority of findings support the effectiveness of meditation practices in cultivating positive psychological health.

Current research continues to promote the benefits of practicing meditation. For example, an article published in *Evidence-Based Complementary and Alternative Medicine* in 2013 investigated the effects of a six-week focused meditation training program on emotion and attention regulation in undergraduate students. Findings from this study revealed that the students who participated in the meditation training presented a greater reduction of negative emotion interference, along with a significant reduction in anxiety levels and an increase in concentrated attention, as compared to the students who did not meditate. Notably, the frequency of meditation was significant, as an increase in the frequency of practice led to improved emotional regulation. Results from this study suggest that meditation is a practical and effective treatment option for college students, who are at a higher risk of experiencing mental health issues.

Yoga

A new study published this August in *Complementary Therapies in Medicine* analyzed the effects of yoga practice and the health characteristics of individuals who practice yoga. Responses from 1,045 surveys of participants between the ages of 19 and 87 showed a consensus that yoga led to improvements in the following areas: energy (84.5 percent), happiness (86.5 percent), social relationships (67 percent), sleep (68.5 percent), and weight (57.3 percent), Not surprisingly, the more participants practiced yoga, the higher their odds of reporting that yoga improved their mental and physical health.

NAMI's Hearts and Minds initiative is an example of an educational program that promotes mind and body health practices for individuals who live with mental illness. Under the "Mindfulness" section on NAMI's Hearts and Minds website, users can find expert advice on how to implement holistic methods that complement medication and therapy in order to provide additional support during the recovery process. Practices covered include basic meditation, guided imagery, yoga and Tai Chi, and creative outlets such as writing, art, music and dance.

Support Groups

Self-help tools such as books, the media and support groups can effectively reach countless individuals at a low cost. Support groups have been shown to have a therapeutic effect, as they foster connections between people who can relate to one another through their shared experiences with mental illness. Often, the experience of feeling understood and accepted by others helps people to feel less isolated. The ability to openly communicate about frustrations and challenges associated with mental illness is emotionally beneficially, while also giving group members the opportunity share effective techniques for managing symptoms.

Support groups such as NAMI Connection, a weekly recovery support group for people living with mental illness, connects people who are facing similar challenges and attempting to overcome their shared adversities. Such support groups allow people to learn from each other's experiences, share coping strategies and offer each other encouragement and understanding.

While authors Kazdin and Blase raise some valuable points about the importance of improving the accessibility of mental health care for the general public, they still acknowledge the value of individual therapy. Rather than arguing against the effectiveness of psychotherapy, the authors emphasize the importance of finding new ways to expand upon traditional therapy in order to reduce the prevalence of mental illness.

Likewise, the authors also do not advise the independent use of any of their suggestions as a singular replacement for treatment. Rather, they suggest that collaboration between these disciplines and many others could better accommodate the large number of people living with mental illness. In fact, the authors are still open to exploring many other fields in the search for effective treatment options, as they said in their article, "Our illustrations are to advocate for partnerships rather than to limit who those partners might be." While their suggestions are a good starting point, more research is still needed on applied intervention methods as they work towards the goal of decreasing mental health problems in the U.S.

National Alliance on Mental Illness
page printed from **http://www.nami.org/**
(800) 950-NAMI; info@nami.org
©2014

Bill of Rights for Children's Mental Health Disorders and their Families

The children's mental health coalition has created a Bill of Rights for Children with Mental Health Disorders and their Families. The coalition includes the American Academy of Child and Adolescent Psychiatry (AACAP), the Autism Society of America (ASA), the Child and Adolescent Bipolar Foundation (CABF), Children and Adults with Attention-Deficit Hyperactivity Disorder (CHADD), the Federation of Families for Children's Mental Health (FFCMH), Mental Health America (MHA), and the National Alliance on Mental Illness (NAMI).

The Bill of Rights was created because of the inconsistency of accessible mental healthcare services throughout the country. It states:

1. Treatment must be family-driven and child-focused. Families and youth, (when appropriate), must have a primary decision-making role in their treatment.

2. Children should receive care in home and community-based settings as close to home as possible.

3. Mental health services are an integral part of a child's overall healthcare. Insurance companies must not discriminate against children with mental illnesses by imposing financial burdens and barriers to treatment, such as differential deductibles, co-pays, annual or lifetime caps, or arbitrary limits on access to medically necessary inpatient and/or outpatient services.

4. Children should receive care from highly-qualified professionals who are acting in the best interest of the child and family, with appropriate informed consent.

5. Parents and children are entitled to as much information as possible about the risks and benefits of all treatment options, including anticipated outcomes.

6. Children receiving medications for mental disorders should be monitored appropriately to optimize the benefit and reduce any risks or potential side effects which may be associated with such treatments.

7. Children and their families should have access to a comprehensive continuum of care, based on their needs, including a full range of psychosocial, behavioral, pharmacological, and educational services, regardless of the cost.

8. Children should receive treatment within a coordinated system of care where all agencies (e.g., health, mental health, child welfare, juvenile justice, and schools, etc.) delivering services work together to support recovery and optimize treatment outcome.

9. Children and families are entitled to an increased investment in high-quality research on the origin, diagnosis, and treatment of childhood disorders.

10. Children and families need and deserve access to mental health professionals with appropriate training and experience. Primary care professionals providing mental health services must have access to consultation and referral resources from qualified mental health professionals.

http://www.acap.org/cs/root/resources_for_families/patient_bill_of_rights

Disorders by Diagnostic Category

Adjustment Disorders

Alcohol and Substance Abuse & Dependence

Anxiety Disorders
Agoraphobia
General Anxiety Disorder
Obsessive Compulsive Disorder
Panic Disorder
Phobias
Post Traumatic Stress Disorder
Social Anxiety

Cognitive Disorders
Delirium
Dementia, i.e. Alzheimer's Disease
Amnestic Disorder

Dissociative Disorders
Depersonalization Disorder
Dissociative Amnesia
Dissociative Fugue
Dissociative Identity Disorder

Eating Disorders
Anorexia Nervosa
Bulimia Nervosa

Impulse Control Disorders
Kleptomania
Pathological Gambling
Pyromania
Trichotillomania

Mental Disorders Usually Diagnosed in Childhood or Adolescence
Attention Deficit/Hyperactivity Disorder (ADHD)
Autism Spectrum Disorder
Asperger's Syndrome
Autistic Disorder
Conduct Disorder
Tic Disorders
Chronic Motor or Vocal Tic Disorder
Transient Tic Disorder
Tourette's Syndrome

Mood Disorders
Bipolar Depression
Depression
Dythymic Disorder
Major Depression
Postpartum Depression
Premenstruam Dysphoric Disorder

Personality Disorders
Antisocial Personality Disorder
Avoidant Personality Disorder
Borderline Personality Disorder
Dependent Personality Disorder
Histrionic Personality Disorder
Narcissistic Personality Disorder
Obsessive-Compulsive Personality Disorder
Paranoid Personality Disorder
Schizoid Personality Disorder
Schizotypal Personality Disorder

Psychotic Disorders
Brief Psychotic Disorder
Delusional Disorders
Schizoaffective Disorder
Schizophrenia

Psychosomatic Disorder
Hypochondria
Factitious Disorder
Malingering Disorder
Somatization Disorder

Sexual/Gender Identification Disorders
Sexual Desire Disorder
Sexual Arousal Disorder
Orgasmic Disorder Sympton
Sexual Pain Disorder
Paraphilias (Perversions)
Exhibitionism
Fetishism
Frotteurism
Pedophilia
Sexual Masochism
Sexual Sadism
Transvestic Fetishism
Voyeurism

Sleep Disorders
Primary Insomnia
Primary Hypersomnia
Narcolepsy
Breathing-related Sleep Disorder
Circadian Rhythm Sleep Disorder
Substance Abuse Induced Sleep Disorder
Nightmare Disorder
Sleep Terror Disorder

User's Guide

Below is a sample listing illustrating the kind of information that is or might be included in an Association entry, with additional fields that apply to publication and trade show listings. Each numbered item of information is described in the paragraphs on the User's Key.

1. **12345**

2. **Association for People with Mental Illness**
3. 29 Simmons Street
    Philadelphia, PA 15201

        4. 234-555-1111
        5. 234-555-1112
        6. 800-555-1113
        7. TDD: 234-555-1114
        8. info@association-mh.com
        9. www.association-mh.com

10. William Lancaster, Executive Director
    Monty Spitz, Marketing Manager
    Kathleen Morrison, Medical Consultant

11. Association for Mental Health is funded by the Mental Health Community Support Program. The purpose of the association is to share information about services, providers, and ways to cope with mental illnesses. Available services include referrals, professional seminars, support gourps, and a variety of publications.

12. 1 M *Members*

13. *Founded*: 1984

14. Bi-monthly

15. $59.00

16. 110,000

User's Key

1. **Record Number:** Entries are listed alphabetically within each category and numbered sequentially. The entry numbers, rather than the page numbers, are used in the indexes to refer to listings.

2. **Title:** Formal name of association or publication. Where names are completely capitalized, the listing will appear at the beginning of the section. If listing is a publication or trade show, the publisher or sponsoring organization will appear below the title.

3. **Address:** Location or permanent address of the association.

4. **Phone Number:** The listed phone number is usually for the main office of the association, but may also be for the sales, marketing, or public relations office as provided.

5. **Fax Number:** This is listed when provided by the association.

6. **Toll-Free Number:** This is listed when provided by the association.

7. **TDD:** This is listed when provided by the association. It refers to Telephone Device for the Deaf.

8. **E-mail:** This is listed when provided by the association.

9. **Web Site:** This is listed when provided by the association and is also referred to as a URL address.

10. **Key Executives:** Lists key contacts of the association, publication or sponsoring organization.

11. **Description:** This paragraph contains a brief description of the association, their purpose and services.

12. **Members:** Total number of association members.

13. **Founded:** Year association was founded.

14. **Frequency:** If listing is a publication.

15. **Subscription Price:** If listing is a publication.

16. **Circulation:** If listing is a publication.

Adjustment Disorders

Introduction

The experience of stress in life is inevitable and begins in utero. When we are faced with a painful event or situation, we do our best to cope, get through it, and move on. How we cope and how long it takes vary according to the stressful situation and the resources the individual brings to it. In most situations, we respond appropriately to the stressful event or situation and show an adaptive response.

Adjustment Disorders are maladaptive reactions to a stressful event or situation. The adjustment is to a real event or situation (e.g., the breaking up of a relationship, being laid off), and the disorder signifies that the reaction is more extreme than would be warranted considering the stressor, or it keeps the individual from functioning as usual.

SYMPTOMS

• The development of emotional or behavioral symptoms is in response to an identifiable stressor except bereavement within three months of the appearance of the stressor;
• The emotions or behaviors are significant either because the distress is more extreme than would normally be caused by the stressor, or because the emotions or behaviors are clearly impairing the person's social, school, or work functioning;
• If the symptoms persist for less than six months after the stressor ends, the disorder is considered acute; if symptoms persist for longer than six months, the disorder is considered to be chronic.
• Adjustment Disorders are divided into several subtypes:

• **Depressed Mood** - predominant mood is depression, with symptoms such as tearfulness, hopelessness, sadness, sleep disturbances;
• **Anxiety** - predominant symptoms are edginess, nervousness, worry, or in children, fears of separation from important attachment figures;
• **Anxiety and Depressed Mood** - chief manifestations are a combination of depression and anxiety;
• **Disturbance of Conduct** - predominant symptoms are conduct which involves either a violation of other people's rights (e.g., reckless driving, fighting), or the violation of social norms and rules.

ASSOCIATED FEATURES

Many commonplace events can be stressful (e.g., first day of impending surgical procedure), the onset of the disturbance is usually immediate but may not last more than six months after the stressor ends. If the stressor or its consequences continue (such as a long-term illness), the Adjustment Disorder may also continue. Whatever the nature of the event, it caused the person to feel overwhelmed. A person may be reacting to one or many stressors; the stressor may affect one person or the whole family. The more severe the stressor, the more likely that an Adjustment Disorder will develop. If a person is already vulnerable, e.g., is suffering from a disability including a mental disorder, an Adjustment Disorder is more likely.

The diagnosis of an Adjustment Disorder is called a residual category, meaning that other possible diagnoses must be ruled out first. For example, symptoms that are part of a personality disorder and become worse under stress are not usually considered to be Adjustment Disorders unless they are new types of symptoms for the individual.

There are three questions to consider in diagnosing Adjustment Disorder: How out-of-proportion is the response to the stressor? How long does it go on? To what extent does it impair the person's ability to function in social, workplace, and school settings?

The emotional response may show itself in excessive worry and edginess, excessive sadness and hopelessness or a combination of these. There may also be changes in behavior in response to the stressful event or situation, with the person violating other people's rights or breaking agreed-upon rules and regulations. The emotional response and the changes in behavior persist, even after the stressful event or circumstances have ended. Finally, the response significantly affects the person's normal functioning in social, school or work settings.

Adjustment Disorders increase the risk of suicidal behavior and completed suicide, and they also complicate the course of other medical conditions (for example, patients may not take their medication, eat properly, etc).

PREVALENCE

Men and women of all ages, as well as children, can suffer from this disorder. In outpatient mental health centers the diagnosis of Adjustment Disorder is made in five to twenty percent of patients.

TREATMENT OPTIONS

Anyone who is experiencing one or more stressful events or circumstances, and feels overwhelmed or markedly distressed and cannot function normally, should seek help. A psychiatrist or other mental health professional should make an evaluation including a referral for physical examination if necessary. Treatment prescribed is often psychotherapy and, depending on the circumstances, can include individual, couple, or family therapy. Medication is sometimes prescribed for a few weeks or months. In most instances long-term therapy will not be necessary and the person can expect marked improvement within 8 to 12 sessions.

Associations & Agencies

2 **Alive Alone**
1112 Champaign Drive
PO Box 182
Van Wert, OH 45891-2569
419-238-7879
E-mail: alivalon@bright.net
www.alivealone.org

Kay Bevington, Founder
Rodney Bevington, Founder
Sam Brewster, Webmaster

Alive Alone is an organization for the education and charitable purposes to benefit bereaved parents, whose only child or all children are deceased, by providing a self-help network and publications to promote communication and healing, to assist in resolving their grief, and a means to reinvest their lives for a positive future.

Year Founded: 1988

3 At Health
7829 Center Boulveard South East
Suite 226
Snoqualmie, WA 98065
425-292-0329
888-284-3258
Fax: 623-322-0498
E-mail: support@athealth.com
www.athealth.com

Providing trustworthy online information, tools, and training that enhance the ability of practitioners to furnish high quality, personalized care to those they serve. For the meantl health consumer, find practitioners, treatment center, learn about disorders and conditions, and about medications being used, news and resources.

4 Center For Mental Health Services
SAMSHA's National Mental Health Information Center
1 Choke Cherry Road
Room 6-1057
Rockville, MD 20857
240-276-1310
877-726-4727
Fax: 240-276-1320
TDD: 800-487-4889
E-mail: info@mentalhealth.org
www.beta.samhsa.gov/about-us/who-we-are/offices-center

Michael E Etzinger, B.S.M.E, , M.B., SAMHSA Executive Officer, Director
Paolo Del Vecchio, M.S.W, Director, Center for Mental Health
Deborah Baldwin, M.P.A, Acting Director, Consumer Affairs
Elizabeth Lopez, Ph.D, Acting Deputy Director

Information about resources, technical assistance, research, training, networks, and other federal clearing houses, and fact sheets and materials.

Year Founded: 1992

5 Center for Loss in Multiple Birth (CLIMB), Inc.
PO Box 91377
Anchorage, AK 99509-1377
907-222-5321
E-mail: climb@pobox.alaska.net
www.climb-support.org

Jean Kollantai, Founder
Berney Richert, Webmaster

Providing parent-to-parent support for all who have experienced the death of one or more of twins or higher multiple birth children at any time from conception through birth, infancy and early childhood. Also assisting extended families, caregivers, twins and multiples organizations and others who are seeking to understand and support the needs of parents with a multiple birth loss.

Year Founded: 1987

6 Center for Mental Health Services (CMHS)
1 Choke Cherry Road
Room 6-1057
Rockville, MD 20857
240-276-1310
877-726-4727
Fax: 240-276-1320
TDD: 800-487-4889
E-mail: info@mentalhealth.org
www.beta.samhsa.gov/about-us/who-we-are/offices-center

Michael E Etzinger, B.S.M.E., M.B., SAMHSA Executive Officer, Directorr
Paolo Del Vecchio, M.S.W, Director, Center for Mental Healt
Deborah Baldwin, M.P.A, Acting Director, Consumer Affairs
Elizabeth Lopez, Ph.D, Acting Deputy Director

CMHS leads Federal efforts to treat mental illnesses by promoting mental health and by preventing the development or worsening of mental illness when possible. Congress created CMHS to bring new hope to adults who have serious mental illnesses and to children with serious emotional disorders. CMHS provides information about mental health via a toll-free the web site, and more than 600 publications. Developed for users of mental health services and their families, the general public, policy makers, providers, and the media.

Year Founded: 1992

7 Empty Cradle
30520 Rancho California Road
Suite 107-63
Temecula, CA 92591
619-595-3887
E-mail: support@emptycradle.org
www.emptycradle.org

A nonprofit support group for San Diego and Riverside County area parents who have experienced the loss of a baby through early pregnancy loss, stillbirth or infant death. Goal is to offer bereaved families support by means of a resource parent network, through monthly meetings, written material and partnership with the health care community.

Year Founded: 1982

8 First Candle
1314 Bedford Avenue
Suite 210
Baltimore, MD 21208-6605
410-415-6628
800-221-7437
E-mail: info@firstcandle.org
www.www.healthynewbornnetwork.org/partner/first-candle

Susan Gerber Berning, Chief Executive Officer
Gina Dyson, Chief Financial Officer
Akesha Scott, MA, Marketing Manager
Lori Simmons, MS, Bereavement Specialist

First Candle is one of the nation's leading nonprofit organizations dedicated to safe pregnancies and the survival of babies through the first years of life. Current priority is to eliminated Stillbirth, Sudden Infance Death Syndrome (SIDS) and other Suddent Unexpected Infant Deaths (SUID) with programs of research, education and advocacy. Helping babies survive and thrive.

9 Grief Recovery After a Substance Passing (GRASP)
42-335 Washington Street
Suite F175
Palm Desert, CA 92211
760-262-8612
E-mail: denisecullen@broken-no-more.org
www.grasphelp.org

Gary Cullen, Vice President and Chief Financi
Denise Cullen, MSW, LCSW, Executive Director

GRASP was founded to help provide sources of help, compassion and most of all, understanding, for families or individuals who have had a loved one die as a result of substance abuse or addiction.

Year Founded: 1996

10   M.I.S.S. Foundation/Center for Loss & Trauma
77 East Thomas Road
Suite 221
Phoeniz, AZ 85012
602-279-6477
888-455-6477
Fax: 629-979-1001
E-mail: info@missfoundation.org
www.missfoundation.org

Dr Joanne Cacciatore PhD FT LMSW, Founder And
Chairman
Kelli Montgomery, Executive Director
Jeff Bell, Vice President
Sandie Edie, Secretary, Ex officio

Offers emergency and on-going support for families suffering from the loss of a child. Provides information, referrals, phone support, newsletter, pen pals, literature, advocacy and online chat room support. Information on local group development.

Year Founded: 1995

11   National Association for the Dually Diagnosed (NADD)
132 Fair Street
Kingston, NY 12401-4802
845-331-4336
800-331-5362
Fax: 845-331-4569
E-mail: info@thenadd.org
www.thenadd.org

Donna McNELIS, PhD, President
Robert J Fletcher DSW, Chief Executive Officer
Dan Baker, PhD, Vice President
Julia Pearce, Secretary

Nonprofit organization designed to promote interest of professional and parent development with resources for individuals who have the coexistence of mental illness and mental retardation. Provides conferences, educational services and training materials to professionals, parents, concerned citizens and service organizations.

Year Founded: 1983

12   National Mental Health Consumers' Self-Help Clearinghouse
1211 Chestnut Street
Suite 1100
Philadelphia, PA 19107-4103
215-751-1810
800-553-4539
Fax: 215-636-6312
E-mail: info@mhselfhelp.org
www.mhselfhelp.org

Joseph Rogers, Executive Director/ Founder
Susan Rogers, Director
Britani Nestel, Program Specialist
Christa Burkett, Technical Assistance Coordinator

The nation's first national consumer technical assistance center, playing a major role in the development of the mental health consumer movement. The movement strives for dignity, respect, and opportunity for those with mental illnesses. Helps consumers organize coalitions, establish self-help groups and other consumer-driven services, advocate for mental health reform, and fight the stigma and discrimination associated with mental illnesses.

Year Founded: 1986

13   National Organization of Parents of Murdered Children
4960 Ridge Avenue
Suite 2
Cincinnati, OH 45202-2129
513-721-5683
888-818-7662
Fax: 513-345-4489
E-mail: natlpomc@aol.com
www.pomc.org

Howard S Klerk Jr., President
Dan Levey, National Executive Director
Terrie Jacoby, Vice President
Martha Lasher-Warner, Secretary

Provides self help groups to support persons who survived the violent death of someone close, as they seek to recover. Newsletter, and court accompaniment also provided in many areas. Offers guidelines for starting local chapters. Parole Block Program and Second Option Service also available.

Year Founded: 1978

14   National Youth Network
42165 Turqueries Avenue
Palm Desert, CA 92211
877-496-2463
E-mail: info@nationalyouth.com
www.nationalyouth.com

Since 1990, The National Youth Network, initially known as The Western Youth Network, has been helping parents and professionals alikein providing education and information regarding programs and services for underachieving youth suffering with adjustment disorders.

Year Founded: 1990

15   Survivors of Loved Ones' Suicides (SOLOS)
8310 Ewing Halsell Drive
San Antonio, TX 78229
800-273-8255
E-mail: solossanantonio@gmail.com
www.www.solossa.org

Tony Mata, SOLOS Facilitator
Angie Navarette, SOLOS Facilitator

Offers various e-mail support groups for persons affected by suicide. Groups include: survivors of a loved one's suicide, parents of attempters, medical/crisis response professionals, parents, spouses, siblings, gay/lesbians, men, grandparents, teens and children who have lost someone to suicide. Also groups for persons affected by murder-suicides, post-partum depression suicides, and facilitators of suicide support groups.

Year Founded: 1987

16   The Center for Family Support
2811 Zulette Avenue
Bronx, NY 10461
718-518-1500
Fax: 718-518-8200
E-mail: eberg@cfsny.org
www.cfsny.org

Steven Vernikoff, Executive Director
Virgil Seepersad, Director of Finance
Eileen Berg, Director of Quality Assurance
Barbara Greenwald, Associate Executive, Director

The Center for Family Support is committed to providing support and assistance to individuals with developmental and related disabilities, and to the family members who care for them.

Year Founded: 1954

17   UNITE, Inc.
1068 West Baltimore Pike
C/o Riddle Hospital
Media, PA 19063
610-296-2411
888-488-6483
E-mail: administrator@unitegriefsupport.org
www.unitegriefsupport.org

Barbara Bond-Moury, Board Chairperson
Don Porreca, President
Karen Powers, Vice President of Fundraising
John Flanagan, Treasurer

A non-profit organization providing grief support following the loss of a baby, including miscarriage, ectopic pregnancy, stillbirth and infant death to parents in the Philadelphia area. Offers grief support groups, literature, educational programs, training workshops, group development assistance, and referral assistance.

Year Founded: 1975

Books

18   Don't Despair on Thursdays: the Children's Grief-Management Book
ADD WareHouse
300 NorthWest 70th Avenue
Suite 102
Plantation, FL 33317-2360
954-792-8100
800-233-9273
Fax: 954-792-8545
E-mail: websales@addwarehouse.com
www.addwarehouse.com

David Melton, Illustrator
Nancy R. Thatch, Editor
Adolph Moser, Author

Children are sure to be comforted by the friendly manner and sensitivity that this book imparts as it explains the grief process to children and helps them understand that grieving is a normal response. For children ages 4-10. *$12.72*

61 pages Year Founded: 1996 ISBN 0-933849-60-5

19   Don't Feed the Monster on Tuesdays: The Children's Self-Esteem Book
ADD WareHouse
300 NorthWest 70th Avenue
Suite 102
Plantation, FL 33317-2360

954-792-8100
800-233-9273
Fax: 954-792-8545
E-mail: websales@addwarehouse.com
www.addwarehouse.com

Adolph Moser, Author

Helps kids understand negative self-talk by picturing a nasty green monster who lives in your head and says mean things. With colorful cartoons and kid-friendly language, the book offers explanations for those bad feelings and ways to overcome them. *$18.95*

55 pages Year Founded: 1991 ISBN 0-933849-38-9

20   Drug Therapy and Adjustment Disorders
Mason Crest Publishers
450 Parkway Drive
Suite D
Broomall, PA 19008-4017
610-543-6200
866-627-2665
Fax: 610-543-3878
www.masoncrest.com

Sherry Bonice, Author
Michelle Luke, Mktg Dir & Public Relations
Louis Cohen, Principal & Creative Director
Sherry Bonnice, Author

Part of the Series: Psychiatric Disorders: Drugs & Psychology for the Mind and Body. Learn about the antidepressants and antianxiety drugs available to treat adjustment disorders. *$24.95*

128 pages Year Founded: 2004 ISBN 1-590845-60-8

21   Preventing Maladjustment from Infancy Through Adolescence
Sage Publications
2455 Teller Road
Thousand Oaks, CA 91320-2234
805-499-0721
800-818-7243
Fax: 800-583-2665
E-mail: info@sagepub.com
www.sagepub.com

Annette U Rickel, Author
Larue Allen, Author
Tracey A Ozmina, EVP, Chief Opersting Officer
Chris Hickok, SVP, Chief Financial Officer

The book begins with a historical overview of prevention research, essential concepts and research practices for identifying populations at risk, and other types of intervention programs. *$83.22*

160 pages Year Founded: 1987 ISBN 0-803928-68-8

22   Stress Response Syndromes: Personality Styles and Interventions
The Rowman & Littlefield Publishing Group
4501 Forbes Blvd
Suite 200
Lanham, MD 20706
301-459-3366
Fax: 301-429-5746
E-mail: customercare@rowman.com
www.rowman.com/RLPublishers

Mardi J Horowitz, Author
George Franzak, Chief Financial Officer

Karin Cholak, Senior Marketing Manager
Kimberly Lyons, Senior Marketing Manager

Incorporation of the most recent advances in the understanding and treatment of stress response syndromes to date. Describes the general characteristics, including signs and symptoms, and elaborates on treatment techniques that integrate cognitive and dynamic approaches. Fourth Edition *$61.00*

451 pages Year Founded: 2001 ISBN 0-765703-13-0

23 Transition from School to Post-School Life for Individuals with Disabilities: Assessment from an Educational and School Psychological Perspective
Charles C Thomas Publisher Ltd.
2600 South First Street
Springfield, IL 62704
217-789-8980
800-258-8980
Fax: 217-789-9130
E-mail: books@ccthomas.com
www.ccthomas.com

Edward M. Levinson, Editor

Designed to assist professionals in developing and implementing transition services for students with disabilities. Specifically, this book focuses on the importance of assessment in transition planning and targets the various domains that should be included in any achool-to-work transition assessment. advocates a transdisciplinary school-based approach to transition assessment that involves not only school-based professionals in the assessment process but community agency representatives as well. Available in paperback for $41.95. *$131.47*

285 pages Year Founded: 1927 ISBN 0-398074-80-1

24 Treatment of Stress Response Syndromes
American Psychiatric Publishing, Inc.
1000 Wilson Boulevard
Suite 1825
Arlington, VA 22209-3901
703-907-7322
800-368-5777
Fax: 703-907-1091
E-mail: appi@psych.org
www.appi.org

Mardi J Horowitz, M.D., Author
Ron McMillen, Chief Executive Officer
John McDuffie, Editorial Director

A comprehensive clinical guide to treating patients with disorders related to loss, trauma and terror. Author Mardi J Horowitz, MD, is the clinical researcher who is largely responsible for modern concepts of posttraumatic stress disorder (PTSD). In this book he reveals the latest strategies for treating PTSD and expands the coverage to include several related diagnoses. *$37.95*

136 pages Year Founded: 2003 ISBN 1-585621-07-1

25 When A Friend Dies: A Book for Teens About Grieving & Healing
Free Spirit Publishing Inc.
217 Fifth Avenue North
Suite 200
Minneapolis, MN 55401-1299
612-338-2068
800-737-7323

Fax: 866-419-5199
www.freespirit.com

Marilyn E Gootman Ed.D, Author
Marilyn E Gootman, Author

The death of a friend is a wrenching event for anyone at any age. Teenagers especially need help coping. This compassionate book answers questions grieving teens often have, like 'How should I be acting?''Is it wrong to go to parties and have fun?' and 'What if I can't handle my grief on my own?' The author has seen her children suffer from the death of a friend, and she knows what teens go through. Also recommended for parents and teachers of teens who have experienced a painful loss. *$4.77*

128 pages Year Founded: 1983 ISBN 0-915793-66-0

Periodicals & Pamphlets

26 A Journey Together
Bereaved Parents of the USA
PO Box 622
St Peters, MO 63376
443-865-9666
800-273-8255
E-mail: jbgoodrich@sbcglobal.net
www.bereavedparentsusa.org

Richard Berman, Editor
Lee Ann Hutson, Vice President, Web Liason
Linda Fehrman, Secretary
John Goodrich, National Contact

The newsletter contains articles of interest to the bereaved about grief. It also has book reviews and information about upcoming Grief Gatherings and other support groups.

4 per year

27 Journal of Mental Health Research
NADD Press
132 Fair Street
Kingston, NY 12401-4802
845-331-4336
800-331-5362
Fax: 845-334-4569
E-mail: info@thenadd.org
www.thenadd.org

Donna McNELIS, PhD, President
Robert J Fletcher DSW, Chief Executive Officer
Dan Baker, PhD, Vice President
Julia Pearce, Secretary

Bi-monthly publication designed to promote interest of professional and parent development with resources for individuals who have the coexistence of mental illness and mental retardation.

4 per year Year Founded: 1983

28 The NADD Bulletin
NADD Press
132 Fair Street
Kingston, NY 12401-4802
845-331-4336
800-331-5362
Fax: 845-334-4569
E-mail: info@thenadd.org
www.thenadd.org

Donna McNELIS, PhD, President
Robert J Fletcher DSW, Chief Executive Officer

Dan Baker, PhD, Vice President
Julia Pearce, Secretary

Bi-monthly publication designed to promote interest of professional and parent development with resources for individuals who have the coexistence of mental illness and mental retardation.

6 per year Year Founded: 1983

Support Groups & Hot Lines

29 Bereaved Parents of the USA
PO Box 622
St Peters, MO 63376
708-748-7866
800-273-8255
E-mail: jbgoodrich@sbcglobal.net
www.bereavedparentsusa.org

Lee Ann Hutson, President
Jodi Norman, Vice President
Delain Johnson, Secretary
Bill Lagemann, Treasurer

BP/USA is a national non-profit self-help group that offers support, understanding, compassion and hope especially to the newly bereaved, whether they are granparents, parents or siblings.

30 Compassionate Friends, Inc
1000 Jorie Boulevard
Suite 140
Oak Brook, IL 60523
630-990-0010
877-969-0010
Fax: 630-990-0246
E-mail: nationaloffice@compassionatefriends.org
www.compassionatefriends.org

Patrick O'Donnell, President
Lisa Corrao, Chief Operating Officer
Georgia Cockerham, Vice President
Alan Pederson, Interim Executive Director

Bereavement support for families grieving the death of a child of any age regardless of cause.

Year Founded: 1978

31 Friends for Survival, Inc.
PO Box 214463
Sacramento, CA 95821
916-392-0664
800-646-7322
E-mail: ffs@truevine.net
www.friendsforsurvival.org

A national non-profit outreach organization open to those who have lost family or friends by suicide, and also to professionals who work with those who have been touched by a suicide tragedy. Dedicated to providing a variety of peer support services that comfort those in grief, encourage healing and growth, foster the development of skills to cope with a loss and educate the entire community regarding the impact of suicide.

32 National Share Office
42 Jackson Street
Saint Charles, MO 63301-3468
636-947-6164
800-821-6819
Fax: 636-947-7486

E-mail: info@nationalshare.org
www.www.nationalshare.org

Michael Margherio, President
Gary Wellman, Vice President
Matthew Hans, Secretary
Megan Rowekamp, CPA, Treasurer

Pregnancy and infant loss support.

Year Founded: 1977

33 Parents of Murdered Children, Inc.
4960 Ridge Avenue
Suite 2
Cincinnati, OH 45209
513-721-5683
888-818-7662
Fax: 513-345-4489
E-mail: natlpomc@aol.com
www.pomc.com

Howard S Klerk Jr, President
Dan Levey, National Executive Director
Terrie Jacoby, Vice President
Carole DiAddezio, Treasurer

For the families and friends of those who have died by violence. Provides the on-going emotional support needed to help parents and other survivors facilitate the reconstruction of a new life and to promote a healthy resolution. Not only does POMC help survivors deal with their acute grief but also helps with the criminal justice system.

Year Founded: 1978

34 Rainbows
1007 Church Street
Suite 408
Evanston, IL 60201
847-952-1770
800-266-3206
Fax: 847-952-1774
E-mail: info@rainbows.org
www.rainbows.org

Anthony Taglia, Chair
Bob Thomas, Executive Director and CEO
Burt Heatherly, CFO
Bill Olbrisch, National Community Outreach Dir.

Rainbows is an international, non-profit organization that fosters emotional healing among children grieving a loss from a life-altering crisis. Rainbows believes that grieving youth deserve supporting, loving listeners as they struggle with their feelings. Available to participants of all races and religions. Serves as an advocate for youth who face life-altering crises.

Year Founded: 1983

35 Survivors of Loved Ones' Suicides (SOLOS)
PO Box 592
Dumfries, VA 22026-592
703-580-8958
E-mail: solos@1000deaths.com
www.1000deaths.com

For the families and friends who have suffered the suicide loss of a loved one.

Video & Audio

36 Effective Learning Systems, Inc.
5108 W 74th
St #390160
Minneapolis, MN 55439
239-948-1660
800-966-0443
Fax: 239-948-1664
E-mail: info@efflearn.com
www.effectivelearning.com

Robert E Griswold, President/ Founder
Deirdre M Griswold, VP

The mission of Effective Learning Systems is to develop and distribute the most effective programs- incorporating the most powerful, scientifically sound techniques- to help as many people as possible learn to use the power of their mind to achieve their goals and realize significant, positive changes in their lives. Audio tapes for self-help.

Year Founded: 1972

Web Sites

37 AtHealth.Com
At Health

Providing trustworthy online information, tools, and training that enhance the ability of practitioners to furnish high quality, personalized care to those they serve. For mental health consumers, find practitioners, treatment centers, learn about disorders and medications, news and resources.

38 forums.grieving.com
Death and Dying Grief Support

Information on grief and loss.

39 www.alivealone.org
Alive Alone

An organization for the education and charitable purposes to benefit bereaved parents, whose only child or all children are deceased, by providing a self-help network and publications to promote communication and healing, to assist in resolving their grief, and a means to reinvest their lives for a positive future.

40 www.bereavedparentsusa.org
Bereaved Parents of the USA (BP/USA)

Self-help group that offers support, understanding, compassion and hope especially to the newly bereaved be they bereaved parents, grandparents or siblings struggling to rebuild their lives after the death of their children, grandchildren or siblings.

41 www.cfsny.org
Center for Family Support

Provides services and programs for individuals living with developmental and related disabilities, and for the families that care for them at home.

42 www.climb-support.org
Center for Loss in Multiple Birth (CLIMB), Inc.

Support by and for parents who have experienced the death of one or more of their twins or higher multiples during pregnance, birth, in infancy, or childhood. Newsletter, information on specialized topics, pen pals, phone support.

43 www.compassionatefriends.org
The Compassionate Friends

Organization for those having lost a child.

44 www.counselingforloss.com
Counseling for Loss and Life Changes, Inc.

Offers individual and family counseling services for grieving people.

45 www.cyberpsych.org
CyberPsych

CyberPsych presents information about psychoanalysis, psychotherapy and topics like anxiety disorders, substance abuse, homophobia, and traumas. It hosts mental health organizations and individuals with content of interest to the public and professional communities. There is also a free therapist finder service.

46 www.divorceasfriends.com
Bill Ferguson's How to Divorce as Friends

Articles, Resources, and Support to help minimize conflict in divorce situations.

47 www.divorcecentral.com
Divorce Central

Offers helpful advice and suggestions on what to expect emotionally, and how to deal with the emotional effects of divorce.

48 www.divorceinfo.com
Divorce Information

Simply written and covers all the issues.

49 www.divorcemag.com
Divorce Magazine

The printed magazine's commercial site.

50 www.divorcesupport.com
Divorce Support

Covers all aspects of divorce.

51 www.emptycradle.org
Empty Cradle

A peer support group for parents who have experienced the loss of baby due to early pregnancy loss, stillbirth or infant death.

52 www.firstcandle.org
First Candle

For those who have suffered the loss of an infant through SIDS.

53 www.friendsforsurvival.org
Friends for Survival

Assisting anyone who has suffered the loss of a loved one through suicide death.

54 www.grasphelp.org
Grief Recovery After A Substance Passing

Support and advocacy group for parents who have suffered the death of a child due to substance abuse. Provides opportunity for parents to share theri grief and experiences without shame or recrimination. They will provide information and suggestions for those wanting to start a similar group elsewhere.

55 www.griefnet.org
GriefNet

Internet community of persons dealing with grief, death, and major loss.

56 www.mhselfhelp.org
National Mental Health Consumers' Self-Help Clearinghouse

Encouraging the development and growth of consumer self-help groups.

57 www.misschildren.org
Mothers in Sympathy and Support (MISS) Foundation

Provides immediate and ongoing support to grieving families, empowerment through community volunteerism opportunities, public policy and legislative education, and programs to reduce infant and toddler death through research and education.

58 www.nationalshare.org
National SHARE Office

Pregnancy and infant loss support.

59 www.planetpsych.com
PlanetPsych

Learn about disorders, their treatments and other topics in psychology. Articles are listed under the related topic areas. Ask a therapist a question for free, or view the directory of professionals in your area. If you are a therapist sign up for the directory. Current features, self-help, interactive, and newsletter archives.

60 www.pomc.com
National Organization of Parents Of Murdered Children, Inc.

Help for anyone who has suffered the loss of a murdered child.

61 www.psychcentral.com
Psych Central

Personalized one-stop index for psychology, support, and mental health issues, resources, and people on the Internet.

62 www.psycom.net/depression.central.grief.html
Grief and Bereavement

Helpful information for those grieving from the loss of a loved one.

63 www.rainbows.org
Rainbows

Group for grieving parents and children.

64 www.relationshipjourney.com
The Relationship Learning Center

Marriage and relationship counseling and information.

65 www.safecrossingsfoundation.org
Safe Crossings Foundation

For children facing a loved one's death.

66 www.spig.clara.net/guidline.htm
Shared Parenting Information Group (SPIG)

Useful information that helps to decrease the stress associated with separation.

67 www.thenadd.org
National Association for The Dually Diagnosed: NADD

An association for persons with developmental disabilities and mental health needs.

68 www.unitegriefsupport.org
UNITE, Inc.

Grief support after miscarriage, stillbirth and infant death.

69 www.widownet.org
WidowNet

Online information and self-help resource for, and by, widows and widowers. Topics covered include grief, bereavement, recovery, and other information helpful to people who have suffered the death of a spouse or life partner.

Directories & Databases

70 After School and More
Resources for Children with Special Needs
116 E 16th Street
5th Floor
New York, NY 10003-2164
212-677-4650
Fax: 212-254-4070
E-mail: info@resourcenyc.org
www.resourcesnyc.org

Rachel Howard, Executive Director
Stephen Stern, Director , Finance and Administr
Todd Dorman, Director, Communications and Out
Helen Murphy, Director, Program and Fund Devel

The most complete directory of after school programs for children with disabilities and special needs in the metropolitan New York area focusing on weekend and holiday programs. *$25.00*

ISBN 0-967836-57-3

Alcohol/Substance Abuse & Dependence

Introduction

Substance abuse and addictive disorders are among the most destructive mental disorders in America today, contributing to a host of medical and social problems and to widespread individual suffering. Alcohol, a drug that is widely available and socially approved, is the most abused of all substances, and alcohol addiction is a pervasive mental disorder. Like all addictive disorders, alcohol addiction is characterized by repeated use despite repeated adverse consequences, and by physical and psychological craving.

Alcohol addiction can be treated, but successful recovery is dependent on acceptance by the patient that he or she has an illness; lack of this acceptance is often the greatest stumbling block to treatment.

Relapse is common for several reasons: lack of acceptance of the diagnosis; genetic vulnerability; and social factors. Successful treatment very often requires involvement by the patient in some form of self-help group, such as Alcoholics Anonymous or another 12-step program. The great majority of motivated individuals with these disorders can recover, but it often requires three or more separate episodes of treatment to more or less permanently prevent relapse and lead to recovery.

Scientific understanding of how alcohol works on the body and the brain, and the underlying physiology of addiction, has advanced remarkably in recent years. With the help of brain imaging and other techniques, we can now see that these disorders are associated with structural changes in the brain.

The substances referred to in this section include: amphetamines; marijuana; cocaine (and its purer derivative, crack); hallucinogens, such as LSD; inhalants, such as butane gas or cleaning fluid; opioids, such as morphine, heroin, or codeine; and benzodiazepines like Valium and Xanax. Caffeine and nicotine, both of which have the potential for abuse and dependence, are not included. The United States Food and Drug Administration has proposed adding nicotine to the list of addictive substances they monitor.

SYMPTOMS

Alcohol and Substance Abuse Symptoms:
• Repeated use resulting in inability to fulfill fundamental obligations at work, school, or home, e.g., repeated absences, poor work performance, family neglect;
• Repeated use, resulting in dangerous situation, e.g., driving or operating a machine while impaired;
• Repeated alcohol and substance-related legal problems, e.g., arrests for disorderly conduct;
• Continued use despite persistent social or interpersonal problems worsened by the effects of substance abuse.

Alcohol and Substance Dependence Problems:
• Alcohol or substance is often taken in greater amounts or for a longer period than intended;
• Repeated wish or unsuccessful attempts to control use;
• A great deal of time is taken to get and use alcohol or substance or to recover from its effects;
• Important social, work, or recreational activities are missed because of use;
• Use continues in spite of the person knowing about the persistent psychological or physical problems it causes, e.g., depression induced by cocaine or continued drinking.

Tolerance:
• Need for increased amounts of alcohol or the substance to achieve desired effect;
• Diminished effects with continued use of the same amount of alcohol or substance;
• Alcohol abuse can occur without tolerance, as in binge drinking, a particular problem for young people on college campuses and elsewhere.

Withdrawal:
• Characteristic withdrawal syndrome, prolonged taking and then stopping/reducing alcohol or substance causing physical and mental symptoms;
• Same or a related substance is taken to avoid/alleviate the withdrawal symptoms.

ASSOCIATED FEATURES

Frequently, alcohol abuse and dependence occur together with dependence on other substances, and alcohol may be used to counteract the ill effects of these substances. Depression, anxiety, and sleep disorders are common in alcohol dependence.

Typically, accidents, injuries and suicide accompany alcohol dependence, and it is estimated that half of all traffic accidents involve alcoholic intoxication. Absenteeism, low work productivity and injuries on the job are often caused by alcohol dependence. Alcohol is also the most common cause of preventable birth defects, including fetal alcohol syndrome, according to the American Psychiatric Association.

Women and men tend to have different drinking patterns. Society is more tolerant of male drunkeness than of female; women tend to drink alone and in secret and are more susceptible to medical complications of alcoholism. Alcohol abuse severely damages organ systems including the brain, the liver, the heart, and the digestive tract.

Genetics has a considerable influence on a person's propensity for substance abuse disorders, and such disorders are associated with significant changes in the brain. These changes underscore the fact that alcohol and substance abuse problems are medical diseases, not failure of character. At the same time, those suffering from these disorders have an obligation to seek and utilize treatment and to ensure that their disorders do not cause injury to others.

Many individuals with substance or alcohol-use disorders take more than one substance and suffer from other mental symptoms and disorders as well. Individuals with a wide variety of mental disorders sometimes abuse drugs as an attempt to medicate themselves. Forty-seven percent of people with Schizophrenia have drug abuse/disorders. People with Antisocial Personality Disorder often abuse substances, including amphetamines such as cocaine. Substance-related disorders can also lead to other mental disorders. Use of the synthetic hallucinogen Ecstasy is associated with acute and paranoid psychoses, and the prolonged use of cocaine (a stimulant) can lead to paranoid psychosis with violent behavior. Substance use and the effects on an individual's employment and relationships, as well as legal difficulties, can precipitate anxiety and mood disorders. Intravenous substance abuse is associated with a high risk of HIV infections and other medical complications.

Chronic drug and alcohol abuse can lead to difficulty in memory and problem solving, and impaired sexual functioning.

Childhood sexual abuse is strongly associated with substance dependence and with a number of other mental symptoms and disorders.

PREVALENCE

Alcohol dependence and abuse are among the most prevalent mental disorders in the general population. One community study in the US found that about eight percent of the adult population had alcohol dependence and about five percent had alcohol abuse at some time in their lives. Approximately six percent had alcohol dependence or abuse during the preceding year.

There are large cultural differences in attitudes toward substances. In some cultures, mood altering drugs, including alcohol, are well accepted; in others they are strictly forbidden.

Those between the ages of 18 and 24 have a high prevalence for abuse of all substances. Early adolescent drug and alcohol use is associated with a slight but significant decline in intellectual abilities. Substance related disorders are more common among males than females. The lifetime prevalence of use of any drugs (aside from alcohol) in the US is 11.9 percent; in males it is twice as high as in females. About thirteen percent of the general population is estimated to use cannabis (marijuana); about seven to nine percent of 18 to 25 year-olds have used amphetamines at least once; eight to 15.5 percent of 26 to 34 year-olds have used hallucinogens like LSD at least once. Inhalants have been used at least once by five percent of the population. Inhalants are used mainly by boys between eight and 19 years old, and especially by 13 to 15 year-olds.Diagnosis and treatment of alcohol dependence has improved as understanding of the physiology of addiction has advanced. But successful treatment still relies on acceptance by the patient that he or she has an illness, as well as support from other people who have gone through the same process. For this reason, medical treatment is most often successful when it is accompanied by involvement in a support group, for both the patient and family members; these may include Alcoholics Anonymous (AA) and Al-Anon, 12-step spiritual programs that have gained popluarity over the years. Local groups can be found in every community and are listed in the phone book and on the Internet. Recently, similar groups have formed that do not emphasize spirituality, as these do, but rely on group support for sobriety.

There is a growing controversy over the need for people who have had an alcohol problem to abstain completely from alcohol for the rest of their lives, one of the central beliefs of AA. Some researchers and clinicians are arguing that is is possible for some former alcoholics to resume controlled drinking. AA, in the past, has discouraged members from using psychotropic medications; this is often counterproductive. Many alcohol treatment programs have been developed with men's needs and personalities in

mind. Successful programs for women are far less confrontational that men's programs and include arrangements for child care. There are far too few of these programs. There is a tendency for women's alcohol and substance abuse disorders to be addressed punitively rather than therapeutically. Women who are pregnant and/or are mothers may be disciplined to seek treatment if they risk imprisonment and loss of child custody - outcomes that don't help them or their children.

Treatment for alcoholism has been hospital-based in the past, but has increasingly moved to the outpatient setting. New treatment protocols and medications allow for outpatient detoxification/withdrawal in many cases. There is a considerable dispute about the need for inpatient care, which may not be covered by health insurance. Much depends upon the nature of the individual's support system. Hospital treatment is necessary for withdrawal when alcohol use has been heavy and steady. Delirium tremens, a consequence of very heavy drinking, can be fatal.

Medical treatment of alcohol dependence may include Anabuse, a drug that makes an individual violently ill if alcohol is used. Group or hospital-based treatment may also be useful, and psychotherapy can help the patient more effectively deal with underlying conflicts and interpersonal problems.

Denial of illness and ambivalence about abstinence can make treatment difficult. A patient's cravings can be overwhelmingly intense, and the individual's social circle is often composed of other substance abusers, making it hard for the individual to maintain relationships while becoming or remaining abstinent - the goal of treatmen

TREATMENT OPTIONS

t. A wide range of intervention may be needed, including a general assessment of the drug abuse, and evaluation of medical, social, and psychological problems. It is best to involve partner/family/friends to help the person gain new understanding of the problem and to make the general assessment complete. An explicit treatment plan should be worked out with the person (and partner/family/friends if appropriate) with concrete goals for which the person takes responsibility, which should include not only stopping substance abuse, but dealing with associated problems concerning health, personal relationships and work.

Associations & Agencies

72 **AMERSA The Association for Medical and Research in Substance Abuse**
201 Hillsdale Road
Suite 102
Cranston, RI 02920
401-243-8460
Fax: 877-418-8769
E-mail: admin@amersa.org
www.amersa.org

Daniel Alford, MD, MPH, President
J Paul Seale, MD, Vice President
Lauren Matukaitis Broyles, PhD, Secretary
David C Lewis, MD, Emeritus-Director

AMERSA founded in1976, is a mutidisciplinary organization of health care professionals dedicated to improving education in the care of individuals with substance abuse problems.

Year Founded: 1975

73 Adult Children of Alcoholics World Service Organization, Inc.
PO Box 3216
Torrance, CA 90510-USA
592-595-7831
E-mail: info@adultchildren.org
www.adultchildren.org

Adult Children of Alcoholica is a 12 Step, 12 Tradition program of women and men who grew up in an alcoholic or otherwise dysfunctional home. They meet with each other in a mutually respectful, safe environment and acknowledge their common experiences. They discover how childhood affected them in the past and in the present.

74 Alcoholics Anonymous (AA): Worldwide
475 Riverside Drive at West 120th Street
11th Floor
New York, NY 10115
212-870-3400
Fax: 212-870-3003
E-mail: tf@aa.org
www.aa.org

Bill W, Founder

A fellowship of men and women who share their experience, strength and hope with each other that they may solve their common problem and help others to recover from alcoholism.

Year Founded: 1975

75 American Academy of Addiction Psychiatry (AAAP)
400 Massasoit Avenue
Suite 307
East Providence, RI 02914
401-524-3076
Fax: 401-272-0922
E-mail: information@aaap.org
www.www.aaap.org

Laurence Westreich, MD, President
Frances R. Levin, MD, Immediate Past-President
John A. Renner, Jr., MD, President-Elect

The annual meeting provides the latest scientific developments in Addiction Psychiatry and Addiction Medicine to physicians and allied health professionals who treat patients with substance use and mental health disorders. The meeting is structured to encourage interaction among clinicians from various disciplines, approaches, and settings.

76 American Council on Alcoholism
1000 East Indian School Road
Suite B
Phoenix, AZ 85014-4810
800-527-5344
E-mail: info@aca-usa.com
www.www.aca-usa.com

Lloyd R Vacovsky, Chairman
Jeff Becker, Vice Chairman
Rebecca Honeycutt Adler, Treasurer
Yvonne Theodre, Secretary

ACA is dedicated to educating the public about the effects of alcohol, alcoholism, alcohol abuse & the need for prompt, effective, readily-available & affordable alcoholism treatment.

77 American Public Human Services Association
1133 19th Street, NorthWing
Suite 400
Washington, DC 20036-3623
202-682-0100
Fax: 202-289-6555
E-mail: jfriedman@aphsa.org
www.aphsa.org

Reggie Bicha, President
Tracy Wareing, Executive Director
Nicole Lobban, Human Resources Director
Uma Ahluwalia, Treasurer

APHSA pursues excellence in health and human services by supporting state and local agencies, informing policymakers, and working with partners to drive innovative, integrated and efficient solutions in policy and practice.

Year Founded: 1930

78 American Society of Addiction Medicine
4601 North Park Avenue
Upper Arcade, Suite 101
Chevy Chase, MD 20815-4520
301-656-3920
Fax: 301-656-3815
E-mail: email@asam.org
www.asam.org

Stuart Gitlow, MD, MPH, MBA, FAPA, President
Penny S Mills, MBA, Executive Vice President/CEO
Carolyn C Lanham, CAE, Chief Operating Officer
Lori Koran, MD, FACP, FASAM, Treasurer

ASAM's core purpose is the improve the care and treatment of people with the disease of addiction and advance the practice of Addiction Medicine.

79 Career Assessment & Planning Services
Goodwill Industries-Suncoast
10596 Gandy Boulevard
St. Petersburg, FL 33702
727-523-1512
888-279-1988
E-mail: gw.marketing@goodwill-suncoast.com
www.goodwill-suncoast.org

Oscar J Horton, Chairman
R. Lee Waits, President and CEO Emeritus
Deborah A. Passerini, President, Board Officer
Martin W Gladysz, Senior Vice Chairman

Provide a comprehensive assessment to help physically, emotionally or developmentally disabled persons develop a plan for employment. In addition to making employment and training recommendations, Goodwill identifies community resources that could improve the quality of life for those who are unprepared for immediate placement in employment.

Year Founded: 1954

80 Center for Mental Health Services (CMHS)
1 Choke Cherry Road
Room 6-1057
Rockville, MD 20857
240-276-1310
877-726-4727
Fax: 240-276-1320
TDD: 800-487-4889

E-mail: info@mentalhealth.org
www.beta.samhsa.gov/about-us/who-we-are/offices-center
Michael E Etzinger, B.S.M.E, , M.B., SAMHSA Executive Officer, Director
Paolo Del Vecchio, M.S.W, Director, Center for Mental Healt
Deborah Baldwin, M.P.A, Acting Director, Consumer Affairs
Elizabeth Lopez, Ph.D, Acting Deputy Director

CMHS leads Federal efforts to treat mental illnesses by promoting mental health and by preventing the development or worsening of mental illness when possible. Congress created CMHS to bring new hope to adults who have serious mental illnesses and to children with serious emotional disorders. CMHS provides information about mental health via a toll-free the web site, and more than 600 publications. Developed for users of mental health services and their families, the general public, policy makers, providers, and the media.

Year Founded: 1992

81   Centre for addiction and Mental Health
1001 Queen Street West
30-60 White Squirrel Way
Toronto, ON M6J 1-4
416-595-6111
800-463-6273
E-mail: info@camh.ca
www.www.camh.ca/en/hospital/Pages/home.aspx

Bud Purves, Board Chair
Dr Catherine Zahn, President and CEO, CAMH
Darrell Gregerson, President and CEO for CAMH Found
Dr Benoit Mulsant, Physician-in-Chief

The Centre for Addiction and Mental Health is one of the largest menatl health and addiction teaching hospitals nationwide. CAMH combines clinical care, research, education, policy development, and health promotion to help transform the lives of people affected by mental health and addiction issues.

82   Community Anti-Drug Coalition of America
625 Slaters Lane
Suite 300
Alexandria, VA 22314
703-706-0560
800-543-2322
Fax: 703-706-0565
E-mail: info@cadca.org
www.cadca.org

Arthur T Dean, Chairman, CEO
Mitchell Anderson, Vice President, Chief Financial
Neil Austrian, Vice Chairman
Kareemah Abdullah, Director, NCADCI and VP

Since 1992, CADCA has been training local grassroots groups, known as community anti-drug coalitions, in effective problem solving strategies, teaching them how to assess thier local substance abuse related problems and develop a comprehensive plan to address them. Today CADCA is oneof the nation's leading drug abuse prevention organozation, representing the interests of more than 5,000 community anti-ddrug coalitions in the country

Year Founded: 1992

83   Grief Recovery After Substance Passing (GRASP)
42-335 Washington Street
Suite F 175
Palm Desert, CA 92211
760-262-8612
E-mail: denisecullen@broken-no-more.org
www.grasphelp.org

Gary Cullen, Vice President & CFO
Denise Cullen, Executive Director
Denise Angela Cullen, MSW, LCSW, Administrator

GRASP was founded to help provide sources of help, compassion and most of all, understanding, for families or individuals who have had a loved one die as a result of substance abuse or addiction.

Year Founded: 2002

84   Mental Health America
2000 N. Beauregard Street
6th Floor
Alexandria, VA 22311
703-684-7722
800-969-6642
Fax: 703-684-5968
E-mail: infoctr@mentalhealthamerica.net
www.mentalhealthamerica.net

Ann Boughtin, Chair
David Shern PhD, Interim President and CEO
Dianne Felton, Chief Operating Officer
Mike Turner, Vice President of Development

Formerly known as the National Mental Health Association, dedicated to promoting mental health, preventing mental and substance use conditions and achievving victory over mental illnesses and addictions through advocacy, education, research and service.

85   NAADAC, The Association for Addiction Professionals
1001 North Fairfax Street
Suite 201
Alexandria, VA 22314-1587
703-741-7686
800-548-0497
Fax: 703-741-7698
E-mail: naadac@naadac.org
www.naadac.org

Robert C Richards, MA, NCAC II, CA, NAADAC President
Ron Pritchard, CSAC, CAS, Mid-Atlantic Regional Vice Presi
John Lisy, LICDC, OCPS II, LIS, Treasurer
Thurston S Smith, CCS, NCACI, ICADC, Secretary

Represents the professional interests of more than 75000 addiction counselors, educators and other addiction-focused health care professionals in the United States, Canada and abroad. Members are addiction counselors, educators and other addiction-focused health care professionals, who specialize in addiction prevention, treatment, recovery support and education. The premier global organization of addiction focused professionals who enhance the health and recovery of individuals, families and communities.

Year Founded: 1974

86 NAATP National Association of Addiction Treatment Providers
11380 Prosperity Farms Road
Suite 209A
Palm Beach Gardens, FL 33410
561-429-4527
Fax: 561-429-4650
E-mail: info@naatp.org
www.naatp.org

Michael E Walsh, MS, CAP, BRI I, President and Chief Executive Of
James B Moore, Executive Director
Scott Munson, Executive Director
Dwayne Beason, President

NAATP provides leadership, advocacy, training and other mamber support services to assure the continued availability and highest quality of addiction treatment nationwide.

Year Founded: 1978

87 National Alliance on Mental Illness
3803 North Fairfax Drive
Suite 100
Arlington, VA 22203
703-524-7600
800-950-6264
Fax: 703-524-9094
E-mail: info@nami.org
www.nami.org

Keris Jan Myrick, MBA, MS, PhD., President
Mary Giliberti, J.D, Executive Director
Jim Payne, J.D, First Vice President
David Levy, Chief Financial Officer

Year Founded: 1969

88 National Association of State Alcohol/Drug Abuse Directors
1025 Connecticut Avenue North West
Suite 605
Washington, DC 20036-5430
202-293-0090
Fax: 202-293-1250
E-mail: dcoffice@nasadad.org
www.nasadad.org

Rob Morrison, Executive Director
Hollis McMullen, Finance Director
Rick Harwood, Deputy Executive Director/Direct
Eric Campbell, Administrative Assistant

NASADAD's basic purpose is to foster and support the development of effective alcohol and other drug abuse prevention and treatment programs throughout every state. NASADAD serves as a focal point for the examination of alcohol and other drug related issues of common interest to both other national organizations and federal agencies.

Year Founded: 1971

89 National Coalition for the Homeless
2201 P Street, NorthWest
Washington, DC 20037-1033
202-462-4822
Fax: 202-462-4823
E-mail: info@nationalhomeless.org
www.nationalhomeless.org

Jerry Jones, Executive Director
Michael Stoops, Director of Community Organising

Megan Hustings, Director of Operations
Barbara Anderson, Secretary

NCH strives on dealing with the issue of alcoholics and drug users as not a stereotype but an illness. NCH helps with dealing with issue of treatment, counseling, and support to overcome the the addiction itself and helping people regain their lives back.

Year Founded: 1981

90 National Council for Behavioral Health
1701 K Street NorthWest
Suite 400
Washington, DC 20006
202-684-7457
Fax: 202-684-7472
E-mail: communications@thenationalcouncil.org
www.www.thenationalcouncil.org

Jeffrey Waiter, Chair
Linda Rosenberg, President and CEO
Jeannie Campbell, Executive VP and COO
Bruce Pelleu, VP, Finance and Administration an

The unifying voice of America's behavioral health organizations. Serves the nation's most vulnerable citizens-more than 6 million adults and children with mental illnesses and addiction disorders

91 National Council on Alcoholism and Drug Dependence
217 Broadway
Suite 712
New York, NY 10007
212-269-7797
800-622-2255
Fax: 212-269-7510
E-mail: national@ncadd.org
www.ncadd.org

William H Foster, PhD, President/CEO
Leah Brook, Affiliate Relations Director
Jayne Restivo, Director of Development
Jill Price, Business Manager

Fights the stigma and the disease of alcoholism and other drug addictions. Founded by Marty Mann, the first woman to find long-term sobriety in Alcoholics Anonymous, NCADD provides education, information, intervention and treatment through offices in New York and Washington, and a nationwide network of Affiliates. Founded in 1944.

Year Founded: 1944

92 National Institute on Alcohol Abuse and Alcoholism
5635 Fishers Lane
MSC 9304
Bethesda, MD 20892-1
301-443-3860
Fax: 301-443-8774
E-mail: niaaaweb-r@exchange.nih.gov
www.niaaa.nih.gov

George Koob, PhD, Director
Kenneth R. Warren, Ph.D., Deputy Director

NIAAA provides leadership in the national effort to reduce alcohol-related problems by conducting and supportin research in a wide range of scientific areas including genetics, neuroscience, epidemiology, health risks and benefits of alcohol consumption, prevention, and treatment. Also collaborates with other research institutes and other agencies or organizations engaged in alcohol-related work, and translating research findings to health care providers, researchers, policymakers and the general public.

93 National Mental Health Consumers' Self-Help Clearinghouse

1211 Chestnut Street
Suite 1100
Philadelphia, PA 19107-4103
215-751-1810
800-553-4539
Fax: 215-636-6312
E-mail: info@mhselfhelp.org
www.mhselfhelp.org

Joseph Rogers, Executive Director/ Founder
Susan Rogers, Director
Britani Nestel, Program Specialist
Christa Burkett, Technical Assistance Coordinator

The nation's first national consumer technical assistance center, striving for dignity, respect, and opportunity for those with mental illnesses.

Year Founded: 1986

94 National Organization on Fetal Alcohol Syndrome

1200 Eton Court, NorthWest
3rd Floor
Washington, DC 20007-3239
202-785-4585
800-66 -OFAS
Fax: 202-466-6456
E-mail: information@nofas.org
www.nofas.org

Kate Boyce, Chairman
Tom Donaldson, President
Kathleen Tavenner Mitchell, MHS, Vice President and National Spok
Katelyn Reitz, Director of Development

Helping children and families by fighting the leading known cause of mental retardation and birth defects. Dedicated to eliminating birth defects caused by alcohol consumption during pregnancy and to improving the quality of life for those affected individuals and families.

Year Founded: 1990

95 Research Society on Alcoholism

7801 North Lamar Boulevard
Suite D-89
Austin, TX 78752-1038
512-454-0022
Fax: 512-454-0812
E-mail: rsastaff@sbcglobal.net
www.rsoa.org

Laura Nagy, PhD, President
Tamara Phillips, PhD, Vice President
Debra Sharp, Director
Michael Miles, MD, PhD, Treasurer

The Research Society on Alcoholism was established in 1976 to assist and encourage the application research to the solution of problems related to alcoholism. RSA serves as a meeting ground for scientists working in all fields of alcoholism and alcohol-related problems. The Society, through its emphasis on research, has served as the interdisciplinary crossroads for the understanding of the causes and potential cures for alcoholism.

Year Founded: 1976

96 SAMHSA's Fetal Alcohol Spectrum Disorders Center for Excellence (FASD)

2101 Gaither Road
Suite 600
Rockville, MD 20850
866-786-7327
E-mail: fasdcenter1@ngc.com
www.fasdcenter.samhsa.gov

Patricia Getty, Contact

Focus on exploring innovative service delivery strategies, developing comprehensive systems of care for FASD prevention and treatment, training staff, families and individuals with an FASD, and preventing alcohol use among women of childbearing age. The mission of the FASD Center for Excellence is to facilitate the development and improvement of prevention and treatment, and care systems in the United States by providing national leadership and facilitating collaboration in the field.

Year Founded: 2001

97 SAMHSA's National Mental Health Information Center

1 Choke Cherry Rd.
Rockville, MD 20857
240-221-4021
877-786-4727
Fax: 240-221-4295
TDD: 866-889-2647
www.store.samhsa.gov

98 Section for Psychiatric and Substance Abuse Services (SPSPAS)

155 North Wacker Drive
Chicago, IL 60606-4425
312-422-3000
800-424-4301
Fax: 312-422-4796
www.aha.org/about/membership/constituency/psych/

James H Hinton, Chairman
Richard J Umbdenstock, President and CEO
Richard J Pollack, Executive VP, Advocacy and Public
Lisa Allen, Senior VP, Chief Human Resources

A membership section that represents over 1, 300 behavioral health providers and professionals who are members of the American Hospital Association (AHA). The purpose of this section is to promote and enhance the understanding and importance of behavioral health care through AHA policy, advocacy, and service efforts specific to psychiatric and substance abuse service providers.

99 Substance Abuse & Mental Health Services Administration of the US Dept of Health and Human Services (SAMHSA)

1 Choke Cherry Road
Rockville, MD 20857
240-276-2000
877-726-4727
TDD: 800-487-4889
TTY: 800-487-4889
www.samhsa.gov

Daryl W Kade, MA, SAMHSA Chief Financial Officer a
Michael E Etzinger, BSME, MBA, SAMHSA Executive Officer and Dir

Paolo Del Vecchio, MSW, Director, CMHS
Francis M Harding, Director, CSAP

SAMHSA's mission is to reduce the impact of substance abuse and mental illness on America's communities. The Agency was established by Congress to target effectively substance abuse and mental health services to the people most in need and to translate research in these areas more effectively and more rapidly into the general health care system. SAMHSA has demonstrated that prevention works, treatment is effective, and people recover from mental and substance use disorders. Behavioral health services improve health statuse and reduce health care costs to society. The Agency's programs are carried out through: the Center for Mental Health Services (CMHS); The Centers for Substance Abuse Prevention and Treatment (CSAP/T); and the Office of Applied Studies.

Year Founded: 1992

100 Substance Abuse and Mental Health Services Administration (SAMHSA)
1 Choke Cherry Road
Rockville, MD 20857
877-726-4727
Fax: 240-221-4292
TDD: 800-487-4889
TTY: 800-487-4889
E-mail: SAMHSAInfo@samhsa.hhs.gov
www.samhsa.gov

Daryl W Kade, MA, SAMHSA Chief Financial Officer a
Michael E Etzinger, BSME, MBA, SAMHSA Executive Officer and Dir
Paolo Del Vecchio, MSW, Director, CMHS
Francis M Harding, Director, CSAP

Mission is to reduce the impact of substance abuse and mental illness on America's communities. To accomplish its work SAMHSA administers a combination of competitive, formula, and block grant programs and data collection activities.

Year Founded: 1992

101 The Center for Family Support
2811 Zulette Avenue
Bronx, NY 10461
718-518-1500
Fax: 718-518-8200
E-mail: svernikoff@cfsny.org
www.cfsny.org

Steven Vernikoff, Executive Director
Virgil Seepersad, Director of Finance
Eileen Berg, Director of Quality Assurance
Barbara Greenwald, Associate Executive, Director

The Center for Family Support, Inc. (CFS) is a non-profit human service agency that provides individualized support services and programs for individuals living with developmental disabilities, and for the families that care for them.

Year Founded: 1954

Books

102 Woman's Journal: Helping Women Recover - Special Edition for Use in the Criminal Justice
Jossey-Bass / Wiley & Sons
111 River Street
Hoboken, NJ 07030-5774

201-748-6000
Fax: 201-748-6088
E-mail: info@wiley.com
www.wiley.com

Stephanie S Covington, Author
Elias E Cousens, EVP, Chief Financial Officer
William J Arlington, Sr. Vice President HR
Gary M Rinck, SVP, General Counsel

Includes important new evidence-based data and new proven techniques for her unique and exclusive program, as well as new ways to treat trauma and substance abuse, new principles for gender responsive strategies with women offenders, and a new module on sexuality and women's recovery. The latest, and most up-to-date theory and practice for this very focused but substantial field of treatment. It contains exercises for use in group sessions, summaries of information presented from the facilitator's guide, and reflection questions and activities for use after group sessions. *$30.00*

156 pages Year Founded: 2008 ISBN 0-787988-71-5

103 A Woman's Journal: Helping Women Recover - Special Edition for Use in the Criminal Justice System, Revised
Jossey-Bass / Wiley & Sons
111 River Street
Hoboken, NJ 07030-5774
201-748-6000
Fax: 201-748-6088
E-mail: info@wiley.com
www.wiley.com

Stephanie S Covington, Author
Ellis E Cousens, EVP, Chief Financial Officer
William J Arlington, Sr Vice President HR
Gary M Rinck, SVP, General Counsel

Designed to meet the unique needs of substance-abusing women. Created for use with women's groups in a variety of correctional settings. Offers mental health professionals, corrections personnel, and program administrators the tools they need to implement this highly effective program. *$30.00*

156 pages Year Founded: 2008 ISBN 0-787988-71-5

104 Addiction Workbook: A Step by Step Guide to Quitting Alcohol and Drugs
NewHarbinger Publications
5674 Shattuck Avenue
Oakland, CA 94609-1662
510-652-0215
800-748-6273
Fax: 800-652-1613
E-mail: customerservice@newharbinger.com
www.newharbinger.com

Patrick Fanning, Author

This comprehensive workbook explains the facts about addiction and provides simple, step by step directions for working through the stages of the quitting process. *$18.95*

160 pages Year Founded: 1973 ISBN 1-572240-43-1

105 Addiction: Why Can't They Just Stop?
Rodale Books
733 Third Avenue
New York, NY 10017-3293

212-697-2040
Fax: 212-682-2237
www.rodale.com

John Hoffman, Editor
Susan Froemke, Editor

Addiction offers a comprehensive and provocative look at the impact of chemical dependency on addicts, their loved ones, society, and the economy.

256 pages ISBN 1-594867-15-1

106 Alcohol & Other Drugs: Health Facts
ETR Associates
4 Carbonero Way
Scotts Valley, CA 95066-4200
831-438-4060
800-321-4407
Fax: 800-435-8433
E-mail: Support@etr..freshdesk.com
www.pub.etr.org

Lucas Stang, Author
Nora J Krantzler, Author
William M Kane, Author
Maria Quackenbush, Author

Offers clear, concise background information on alcohol and other drugs, and provides assessment of the impact on youth. Also, discusses risk and protective factors, current trends, and prevention strategies. *$17.00*

151 pages Year Founded: 1981

107 Alcohol and the Community
Cambridge University Press
32 Avenue of the Americas
New York, NY 10013-2473
212-337-5000
800-872-7423
E-mail: newyork@cambrigde.org
www.www.cambridge.org

Harold H Holder, Author

The authors challenge the current implicit models used in alcohol problem prevention and demonstrate an ecological perspective of the community as a complex adaptive system composed of interacting subsystems. This volume represents a new and sensible approach to the prevention of alcohol dependence and alcohol-related problems. *$110.00*

200 pages Year Founded: 1584 ISBN 0-521591-87-2

108 Alcoholism Sourcebook
Omnigraphics
155 West Congress
Suite 200
Detroit, MI 48226
313-961-1340
800-234-1340
Fax: 313-961-1383
E-mail: contact@omnigraphics.com
www.omnigraphics.com

Joyce Brennfleck Shannon, Author
Peter Ruffner, Co-Founder

Omnigraphics is the publisher of the Health Reference Series, a growing consumer health information resource with more than 100 volumes in print. Each title in the series features an easy to understand format, nontechnical language, comprehensive indexing, and resources for further information. Material in each book has been collected from a wide

range of government agencies, professional associations, periodicals, and other sources. *$78.00*

610 pages Year Founded: 1985 ISBN 0-780803-25-6

109 American Psychiatric Association Practice Guideline for the Treatment of Patients With Substance Use Disorders
American Psychiatric Publishing, Inc.
1000 Wilson Boulevard
Suite 1825
Arlington, VA 22209-3901
703-907-7322
800-368-5777
Fax: 703-907-1091
E-mail: appi@psych.org
www.appi.org

Robert E Hales MD, Editor-in-Chief
Saul Levin, M.D., M.P.A., CEO and Medical Director
John McDuffie, Editorial Director
Laura W Roberts, M.D., Deputy Editor

Offers guidance to psychiatrists caring for patients with substance use disorders. Includes treatment for alcohol, cocaine and opioids addiction. *$29.50*

126 pages ISBN 0-890423-03-2

110 Broken: My Story of Addiction and Redemption
The Viking Press, Penguin Publishers
375 Hudson Street
New York, NY 10014-3657
212-366-2372
Fax: 212-366-2933
E-mail: ecommerce@us.penguingroup.com
www.www.us.penguingroup.com

William Cope Moyers, Author
Coram Williams, Chief Financial Officer
David Shanks, Chief Executive Officer

Broken tells the story of what happened between then and now-from growing up the privileged son of Bill Moyers to his descent into alcholism and drug addiction, his numerous stabs at getting clean, his many relapses, and how he managed to survive. *$5.43*

384 pages Year Founded: 1936 ISBN 0-143112-45-7

111 Clinical Supervision in Alcohol and Drug Abuse Counseling: Principles, Models, Methods
Jossey-Bass
111 River Street
Hoboken, NJ 07030-5774
201-748-6000
Fax: 201-748-6088
E-mail: info@wiley.com
www.as.wiley.com/WileyCDA/

David J. Powell, Author
Archie Brodsky, Author
William J Arlington, Sr Vice President HR
Edward Melando, VP, Corporate Controller

Firmly grounded in both theory and practice, this book offers methods of supervisory contracting, observation, case presentation, modeling, intervention, and evaluation. Ethical and legal concerns are also addressed. *$25.95*

448 pages Year Founded: 1998 ISBN 0-787973-77-7

112 Concerned Intervention: When Your Loved One Won't Quit Alcohol or Drugs
NewHarbinger Publications
5674 Shattuck Avenue
Oakland, CA 94609-1662
510-652-0215
800-748-6273
Fax: 800-652-1613
E-mail: customerservice@newharbinger.com
www.newharbinger.com

John O'Neill, Author
Pat O'Neill, Author

Practical guide to group intervention techniques with lessons from experiences of families seeking counseling and treatment. *$13.95*

190 pages Year Founded: 1973 ISBN 1-879237-37-7

113 Concise Guide to Treatment of Alcoholism and Addictions
American Psychiatric Publishing, Inc.
1000 Wilson Boulevard
Suite 1825
Arlington, VA 22209-3901
703-907-7322
800-368-5777
Fax: 703-907-1091
E-mail: appi@psych.org
www.appi.org

Avram H Mack, M.D, Author
Amy L Harrington, M.D, Author
Richard J Frances, M.D, Author
Rebecca D Rinehart, Publisher

Presents information on available treatment options for alcoholism and addictions, substance abuse in the workplace and laboratory testing. *$29.95*

172 pages ISBN 0-880483-26-1

114 Drug Abuse Sourcebook
Omnigraphics
155 West Congress
Suite 200
Detroit, MI 48226
313-961-1340
800-234-1340
Fax: 313-961-1383
E-mail: contact@omnigraphics.com
www.omnigraphics.com

Laura Larsen, Author
Peter Ruffner, Co-Founder

Basic consumer health information about the abuse of cocaine, club drugs, hallucinogens, heroin, inhalants, marijuana, and other illicit substances, prescription medications, and over-the-counter medicines: along with facts about addiction and related health effects, drug abuse treatment and recover, drug testing, prevention programs, glossaries of drug-related terms, and directories of resources for more information. *$95.00*

640 pages Year Founded: 1985 ISBN 0-780810-79-2

115 Dynamics of Addiction
Hazelden
15251 Pleasant Valley Road
PO Box 11
Center City, MN 55012-0176
651-213-4200
800-328-9000
E-mail: info@hazelden.org
www.www.hazelden.org

George A Mann, Author
Marvin Sappala MD, Chief Medical Officer
Nick Motu, Publisher, VP of Marketing
Mark Sheets, Executive Director

Offers practical advice on how to raise balanced kids who can stand on their own feet, resist unhealthy peer pressures, and still be accepted by others. *$2.50*

16 pages Year Founded: 1987 ISBN 0-935908-38-2

116 Eye Opener
Hazelden
PO Box 11
Center City, MN 55012-0011
651-213-4200
800-328-9000
Fax: 651-213-4793
E-mail: info@hazelden.org
www.hazelden.org

Mark Mishek, President and CEO, Hazeldon Betty
James A Blaha, VP Finance, Administration/CFO
Marvin D Seppala, MD, Chief Medical Officer
Mark Sheets, Execurive Director, Regional serv

Popular meditations on A.A. philosophy, written for every day of the year. This effective tool has been a recovery-basic for over 30 years. *$13.95*

384 pages Year Founded: 1949 ISBN 0-894860-23-2

117 Fetal Alcohol Syndrome, Fetal Alcohol Effects: Strategies for Professionals
Hazelden
15251 Pleasant Valley Road
PO Box 176
Center City, MN 55012-176
651-213-4000
800-328-9000
Fax: 651-213-4590
E-mail: customersupport@hazelden.org
www.hazelden.org

Diane Malbin, Author
Mark Sheets, Executive Director
Marvin Seppala MD, Chief Medical Officer
Nick Motu, Publisher, VP of Marketing

If you're a chemical dependency counselor or work with women in pregnancy planning or self-care, this resource is filled with facts to help you better meet your clients needs. *$5.25*

43 pages Year Founded: 1996 ISBN 0-894869-51-5

118 Getting Beyond Sobriety: Clinical Approaches to Long-Term Recovery
Jossey-Bass / Wiley & Sons
111 River Street
Hoboken, NJ 07030-5790
201-748-5774
Fax: 201-748-6088
E-mail: custserv@wiley.com
www.wiley.com

Michael Craig Clemmens, Author
Ellis E Cousens, EVP, Chief Financial Officer
William J Arlington, Sr Vice President HR
Edward J Melando, VP, Corporate Controller

This method will lead to a change in behavior within the individual, while developing and expanding connection with others. *$ 42.50*

198 pages Year Founded: 1997 ISBN 0-787908-40-1

119 Getting Hooked: Rationality and Addiction
Cambridge University Press
32 Avenue of the Americas
New York, NY 10013-2473
212-337-5000
E-mail: newyork@cambrigde.org
www.www.cambridge.org

John Elster, Editor
Ole Jorgen Skog, Editor
Richard Fisher, Managing Director
Andrew Gilfillan, Managing Director

The essays in this volume offer thorough and up-to-date discussion on the relationship between addiction and rationality. Includes contributions from philosophers, psychiatrists, neurobiologists, sociologists and economists. Offers the neurophysiology of addiction, examination of the Becker theory of rational addiction, an argument for a visceral theory of addiction, a discussion of compulsive gambling as a form of addiction, discussions of George Ainslie's theory of hyperbolic discounting, analyses of social causes and policy implications and an investigation into relapse. *$75.00*

300 pages Year Founded: 1584 ISBN 0-521640-08-3

120 Handbook of the Medical Consequences of Alcohol and Drug Abuse (Contemporary Issues in Neuropharmacology)
Routledge, Taylor & Francis Group
8th Floor, 711 3rd Avenue
New York, NY 10017
212-563-7800
800-634-7064
Fax: 212-563-2269
E-mail: orders@taylorandfrancis.com
www.www.routledge.com

Dr William Francis, Founder
Richard Taylor, Founder
John Brick, Author

Describes the most current research on the acute and chronic effects of alcohol, stimulants, inhalents, marijuana, and opiates on human organ systems and behavior. Also provides in-depth explanations of the mechanisms by which these psychoactive drugs exert their biobehavioral effects as well as current thinking about- and definitions of- abuse, dependence, and alcohol/drug use.

354 pages Year Founded: 2003 ISBN 0-789018-63-2

121 Inside Recovery: How the Twelve Step Program Can Work for You
The Rosen Publishing Group
29 East 21st Street
New York, NY 10010-6209
212-777-3017
800-237-9932
Fax: 888-436-4643
E-mail: info@rosenpublishing.com
www.rosenpublishing.com

Susan Banfield, Author

Describes the practices and principles of twelve-step programs, how they can be used in dealing with such problems as alcoholism and drug addiction, and how to get involved in them. *$25.25*

64 pages Year Founded: 1950 ISBN 0-823926-34-6

122 Inside a Support Group: Help for Teenage Children of Alcoholics
Rosen Publishing Group
29 East 21st Street
New York, NY 10010-6209
212-777-3017
800-237-9932
Fax: 888-436-4643
E-mail: info@rosenpub.com
www.rosenpublishing.com

Margi Trapani, Author

Gives teens an inside look at Alateen, an organization designed to help teens cope with a loved one's addiction to alcohol. *$25.25*

64 pages Year Founded: 1950 ISBN 0-823925-08-7

123 Kicking Addictive Habits Once & for All: A Relapse Prevention Guide, Revised
Jossey-Bass / Wiley & Sons
111 River Street
Hoboken, NJ 07030-5774
201-748-6000
800-956-7739
Fax: 201-748-6088
E-mail: info@wiley.com
www.wiley.com

Dennis C Daley, Author
Ellis E Cousens, EVP, Chief Financial Officer
William J Arlington, Sr Vice President HR
Edward J Melando, VP, Corporate Controller

All aspects of changing bad habits and developing a balanced lifestyle are addressed in the book. *$26.00*

224 pages Year Founded: 1997 ISBN 0-787940-68-3

124 LSD: Still With Us After All These Years: Based on the National Institute of Drug Abuse Studies on the Resurgence of Contemporary LSD Use
Jossey-Bass / Wiley & Sons
111 River Street
Hoboken, NJ 07030-5774
201-748-6000
Fax: 201-748-6088
E-mail: info@wiley.com
www.wiley.com

Leigh A Henderson, Author
William J Glass, Author
William J Arlington, Sr Vice President HR
Edward J Melando, VP, Corporate Controller

Offers an insightful look at LSD use and provides an essential resource for parents, counselors, and educators. The book examines why young people are using LSD- its appeal, experience, and where kids are getting. Solidly researched and dispassionately written, this book weaves current studies and anecdotes with recent statistics to create a vivid, complete, and credible picture of contemporary LSD use. *$ 24.00*

176 pages Year Founded: 1998 ISBN 0-787943-79-7

125 Let's Talk Facts About Substance Abuse & Addiction
American Psychiatric Publishing, Inc.
1000 Wilson Boulevard
Suite 1825
Arlington, VA 22209-3901
703-907-7322
800-368-5777
Fax: 703-907-1091
E-mail: appi@psych.org
www.appi.org

Robert E Hales MD, Editor-in-Chief
Saul Levin, M.D., M.P.A., CEO and Medical Director
John McDuffie, Editorial Director
Laura W Roberts, M.D., Deputy Editor

Straight talk about a difficult subject. *$26.95*

126 Living Skills Recovery Workbook
Elsevier Science, Health Science Division
10900 Euclid Avenue
Cleveland, OH 44106-7169
212-368-0808
Fax: 212-268-2295
E-mail: custserv@elsevier.com
www.www.centerforebp.case.edu

Pat Precin, MS OTR/L, Author
Bill Godfrey, Chief Information Officer
Michael Hansen, Chief Executive Officer
Gavin Howe, Executive Vice President

Provides clinicians with the tools necessary to help patients with dual diagnoses acquire basic living skills. Focusing on stress management, time management, activities of daily living, and social skills training, each living skill is taught in relation to how it aids in recovery and relapse prevention for each patient's individual lifestyle and pattern of addiction. Book is now printed as ordered. *$39.95*

197 pages Year Founded: 1999 ISBN 0-750671-18-7

127 Living Sober I
Jossey-Bass / Wiley & Sons
111 River Street
Hoboken, NJ 07030-5790
201-748-8677
Fax: 201-748-2665
www.wiley.com

Dr Dennis Daley, Presenter
Ellis E Cousens, EVP, Chief Financial Officer
William J Arlington, Sr Vice President, HR
Edward J Melando, VP, Corporate Controller

Emphasizes the specific coping skills essential to a client's recovery. *$495.00*

87 pages Year Founded: 1999

128 Living Sober II
Jossey-Bass / Wiley & Sons
111 River Street
Hoboken, NJ 07030-5774
201-748-6000
Fax: 201-748-6088
E-mail: info@wiley.com
www.wiley.com

Dennis C Daley, Author
Ellis E Cousens, EVP, Chief Financial Officer
William J Arlington, Sr Vice President HR
Edward J Melando, VP, Corporate Controller

Emphasizes the specific coping skills essential to a client's recovery.

27 pages

129 Motivating Behavior Changes Among Illicit-Drug Abusers: Research on Contingency Management Interventions
American Psychological Association
750 First Street, NorthEast
Washington, DC 20002-4242
202-336-5500
800-374-2721
Fax: 202-336-5518
TDD: 202-336-6123
TTY: 202-336-6123
www.www.apa.org

Stephen T Higgins, Editor
Kenneth Silverman, Editor
Stephen T Higgins, Author
Kenneth Silverman, Author

Scientifically based method focused on the use of incentives to change behavior. Research in multiple applications of contingency management techniques. Test case of effective utilization of the method in treating illicit-drug abusers. *$39.95*

399 pages Year Founded: 1999 ISBN 1-557985-70-7

130 Motivational Interviewing: Preparing People to Change Addictive Behavior
Guilford Press
72 Spring Street
New York, NY 10012-4068
800-365-7006
Fax: 212-966-6708
E-mail: info@guilford.com
www.www.guilford.com

William R. Miller, Ph.D., Author
Stephen Rollnick, Ph.D., Author

Explains how to work through ambivalence to facilitate change, presents detailed guidelines for using the authors' approach with a variety of clinical populations, and reflect on the process of learning MI. Chapters contributed by other leading experts address such special topics as MI and the stages-of-change model; using the approach with groups, couples, and adolescents; and applications to general medical care, health promotion, and criminal justice settings. *$42.00*

348 pages Year Founded: 1973 ISBN 0-898624-69-X

131 New Treaments for Chemical Addictions
American Psychiatric Publishing, Inc.
1000 Wilson Boulevard
Suite 1825
Arlington, VA 22209-3901
703-907-7322
800-368-5777
Fax: 703-907-1091
E-mail: appi@psych.org
www.appi.org

Robert E Hales MD, Editor-in-Chief
Ron McMillen, Chief Executive Officer
John McDuffie, Editorial Director
Rebecca Rinehart, Publisher

Examines new approaches for an old problem. *$37.50*

248 pages ISBN 0-880488-38-7

132 Points for Parents Perplexed about Drugs
Hazelden
PO Box 11
Center City, MN 55012-0011
651-213-4000
800-257-7810
Fax: 651-213-4793
E-mail: info@hazelden.org
www.hazelden.org

David C Hancock, Author
Mark Sheets, Executive Director
Marvin Seppala MD, Chief Medical Officer
Nick Motu, Publisher, VP of Marketing

Clear guidelines help teachers, parents, family members and others recognize, evaluate, and deal with adolescent drug abuse. Excellent support for family counseling programs. *$3.25*

15 pages Year Founded: 1949 ISBN 0-894861-40-9

133 Relapse Prevention for Addictive Behaviours: A Manual for Therapists
Blackwell Publishing
Commerce Place
350 Main Street
Malden, MA 02148-5020
781-388-8200
Fax: 781-388-8210
www.www.blackwellpublishing.com

Wendy Wallace, Co-Author
Jane Pullin, Co-Author
F. Keaney, Co-Author
Richard D. T. Farmer, Co-Author

Applies cognitive-behavioral strategies and lifestyle procedures to treat people with addiction problems. *$43.95*

224 pages Year Founded: 1991 ISBN 0-632024-84-4

134 Rethinking Substance Abuse: What the Science Shows, and What We Should Do about It
The Guilford Press
72 Spring Street
New York, NY 10012-4019
800-365-7006
Fax: 212-966-6708
E-mail: info@guilford.com
www.www.guilford.com

William R. Miller Ph.D., Editor
Kathleen M. Carroll Ph.D., Editor

This state-of-the-art book brings together leading experts to describe what treatment and prevention would look like if it were based on the best science available. The volume incorporates developmental, neurobiological, genetic, behavioral, and social-environmental perspectives. Tightly edited chapters summarize current thinking on the nature and causes of alcohol and other drug problems; discuss what works at the individual, family, and societal levels; and offer robust principles for developing more effective treatments and services.

320 pages Year Founded: 1973 ISBN 1-572302-31-3

135 Sex, Drugs, Gambling & Chocolate: A Workbook for Overcoming Addictions
Impact Publishers
PO Box 6016
Atascadero, CA 93423-6016
805-466-5917
800-246-7228
Fax: 805-466-5919
E-mail: info@impactpublishers.com
www.impactpublishers.com

Robert Dr A.Thomas, Horvath
Author Emmons PhD, Founder

This workbook is loaded with practical suggestions and will appeal to anyone who has unsuccessfully sought to overcome a serious addiction or habit using more traditional (i.e. 12 step) treatment approaches. The workbook approach is straightforward and adaptable to a variety of addictive behaviors. The information presented is not hostile towards, or totally incompatible with other approaches to addiction, but is primarily intended for those who want a scientifically proven, rational approach to behavior change. *$15.95*

240 pages Year Founded: 1970 ISBN 1-886230-55-2

136 Sober Siblings: How to Help Your Alcoholic Brother or Sister-and Not Lose Yourself
Da Capo Press
250 West 57th Street
15th Floor
New York, NY 10107
212-340-8100
E-mail: intlorders@perseusbooks.com
www.www.perseusbooksgroup.com/perseus/home.jsp

Patricia Olsen, Author
Petros Levounis, Author

An empowering, practical guide to help the brothers and sisters of alcoholics-by a journalist and sibling of two alcoholics, and an addiction specialist *$16.00*

243 pages Year Founded: 2008 ISBN 1-600940-55-2

137 Substance Abuse Treatment and the Stages of Change: Selecting and Planning Interventions
The Guilford Press
72 Spring Street
New York, NY 10012-4019
800-365-7006
Fax: 212-966-6708
E-mail: info@guilford.com

Gerard J. Connors, Co-Author
Dennis M. Donovan, Co-Author
Carlo C. DiClemente, Co-Author

Synthesizes the latest theory and research on the process of addictive behavior change, helping the clinician more effectively conceptualize and address the needs of particular clients. It offers concrete guidance for tailoring interventions to clients with varying levels of motivation or readiness to change, describing what works- and what doesn't- at different points in the recovery process. Ideal for practicing clinicians, the book is also an invaluable text for graduate-level courses.

274 pages Year Founded: 2004 ISBN 1-593850-97-2

138 Substance Abuse: Information for School Counselors, Social Workers, Therapists, and Counselors
Allyn & Bacon
800-922-0579
www.www.pearsoned.co.uk/Imprints/AllynBacon/

Gary L. Fisher, Author
Thomas C. Harrison, Author

This text provides updated coverage and practical clinical examples to reflect the rapid changes in the field of addiction. In a reader-friendly style, the authors present balanced coverage of various treatment models as well as objective discussions dealing with the controversies in this field. The text covers topics spanning the entire field- pharmacology, assessment and diagnosis, treatment, recovery, prevention, children, families, and other addictions- providing students with a broad view of the AOD field aswell as the pervasiveness of the problem in all areas of behavioral health and general fields.

384 pages Year Founded: 2004 ISBN 0-205403-36-0

139 Teach & Reach: Tobacco, Alcohol & Other Drug Prevention
ETR Associates
4 Carbonero Way
Scotts Valley, CA 95066-4200
831-438-4060
Fax: 831-438-4284
www.www.etr.org

Peggy Flynn, Project Director
Nicole Ellen Jones, Board Member
Dr. Douglas Kirby, Advisory Board
Marcia Quackenbush, Author

Empowers students to build commitment to stay tobacco, alcohol and drug free; look to peer norms to support healthy, responsible choices; enhance protective factors that prevent tobacco, alcohol and other drug use; and learn skills that can keep them free of tobacco, alcohol and other drug use. For youth in grades 7-12. *$22.00*

Year Founded: 2004 ISBN 1-560716-98-3

140 Teen Guide to Staying Sober (Drug Abuse Prevention Library)
Rosen Publishing
29 East 21st Street
New York, NY 10010-6209
212-777-3017
800-237-9932
Fax: 888-436-4643
E-mail: info@rosenpub.com
www.rosenpublishing.com

Christina Chiu, Author

Discusses the social and physical effects of alcohol, the reasons teenagers drink, the problems caused by teenage alcoholism, and possible preventive measures and treatments. *$25.25*

64 pages Year Founded: 1950 ISBN 0-823927-65-2

141 The Meaning of Addiction: An Unconventional View
Jossey-Bass / Wiley & Sons
111 River Street
Hoboken, NJ 07030-5774
201-748-6000
Fax: 201-748-6088

E-mail: info@wiley.com
www.wiley.com

Stanton Peele, Author
Ellis E Cousens, EVP, Chief Financial Officer
William J Arlington, Sr Vice President HR
Edward J Melando, VP, Corporate Controller

A controversial and persuasive analysis of addiction. This compelling and controversial book challenges the widely accepted belief that alcohol and drug addiction have a genetic or biological basis. The so-called disease theory suggests that a substance or activity can cause the addict to lose control of his behavior. Stanton Peele demonstrates how this notion fails to make sense of scientific observations. *$34.00*

224 pages Year Founded: 1998 ISBN 0-787943-82-0

142 The Mother's Survival Guide to Recovery: All About Alcohol, Drugs & Babies
NewHarbinger Publications
5674 Shattuck Avenue
Oakland, CA 94609-1662
510-652-0215
800-748-6273
Fax: 800-652-1613
E-mail: customerservice@newharbinger.com
www.newharbinger.com

Laurie L Tanner, Author

Seeking to help women surmount the grief of using whilst pregnant, and tap into the strength that their addictions have buried, this text is aimed at women of all backgrounds. It explains what addiction is, helps to decide whether they are addicts, and where to get help. For women in addiction, this offers an alternative to the loneliness, desolation and rejection of their lives. *$12.95*

138 pages Year Founded: 1973 ISBN 1-572240-49-0

143 The Science of Addiction: From Neurobiology to Treatment
W.W. Norton
500 Fifth Avenue
New York, NY 10110
212-354-5500
800-233-4830
Fax: 212-869-0856
www.books.wwnorton.com

Carlton K Erickson, Author

Presents a comprehensive overview of the rolse that brain function and genetics play in addiction.

312 pages Year Founded: 1923 ISBN 0-393704-63-7

144 The Science of Prevention: Methodological Advances from Alcohol and Substance Research
American Psychological Association
750 First Street, NorthEast
Washington, DC 20002-4242
202-336-5500
800-374-2721
Fax: 202-336-5518
TDD: 202-336-6123
TTY: 202-336-6123
www.www.apa.org

Kendel J Bryant, Editor
Michael Windle, Editor
Stephen G West, Editor

The editors and contributors explore the implications of prospective longitudinal research that measures risk and protective factors, and illustrates developmental trajectories and the sequence of abuse. They look at intervention research with an eye toward how certain components may interact with individual and environmental factors and offer many concrete suggestions for improving methodological quality. *$39.95*

458 pages Year Founded: 1997 ISBN 1-557984-39-5

145 The Selfish Brain: Learning from Addiction
Hazelden
PO Box 11
Center City, MN 55012-0011
651-213-4200
800-328-9000
Fax: 651-213-4793
E-mail: info@hazelden.org
www.hazelden.org

Robert L Dupont, MD, Author
Mark Sheets, Executive Director
Marvin Seppala MD, Chief Medical Officer
Nick Motu, Publisher, VP Of Marketing

Helps clients or loved ones face addiction and recovery by exploring the biological, historical and cultural aspects of addiction and its destructiveness. *$18.95*

544 pages Year Founded: 1949 ISBN 1-568383-63-0

146 The Seven Points of Alcoholics Anonymous
Hazelden
PO Box 11
Center City, MN 55012-0011
651-213-4200
800-328-9000
Fax: 651-213-4793
E-mail: info@hazelden.org
www.hazelden.org

Richmond Walker, Author
Mark Sheets, Executive Director
Marvin Seppala MD, Chief Medical Director
Nick Motu, Publisher, VP of Marketing

This book is the summation of Walker's knowledge on the practice and fundamentals of 12 Step recovery. Topics include an overview and history of A.A., the nature of alcoholism and recovery, the 12 Step way and fellowship, surrender, character defects, amends, living One Day at a Time, and sharing. *$9.85*

112 pages Year Founded: 1949 ISBN 1-592850-50-2

147 The Twelve-Step Facilitation Handbook: A Systematic Approach to Early Recovery from Alcoholism and Addiction
Hazelden Publishing
PO Box 11
Center City, MN 55012-0011
651-213-4200
800-257-7810
E-mail: customersupport@hazelden.org
www.www.hazelden.org

Joseph Nowinski, Author
Stuart Baker, Author

Marvin Seppala MD, Chief Medical Director
Nick Motu, Publisher, VP of Marketing

This book provides clinicians with the tools they need to encourage chemically dependent clients to take advantage of the healing power of twelve-step programs. *$24.95*

248 pages Year Founded: 2003 ISBN 1-592850-96-0

148 Treating Alcoholism (Jossey-Bass Library of Current Clinical Technique)
Jossey-Bass Publishers
111 River Street
Hoboken, NJ 07030-5774
201-748-6000
Fax: 201-748-6088
E-mail: info@wiley.com
www.as.wiley.com/WileyCDA/

Stephanie Brown, Editor
Irvin D Yalom, General Editor
William J Arlington, Sr Vice President HR
Edward J Melando, VP, Corporate Controller

In this comprehensive book, editor Stephanie Brown presents a model of alcoholism treatment to help readers guide alcoholics and their families on the path to long-term recovery. Experts in the field give skills to address the myriad problems associated with alcoholism by providing up-to-date information and illustrative case examples. This book, filled with a wealth of information, will help set specific therapeutic techniques for working with alcoholics and the families of alcoholics in a clinical setting. *$40.00*

448 pages Year Founded: 1997 ISBN 0-787938-76-9

149 Twenty-Four Hours a Day
Hazelden
PO Box 11
Center City, MN 55012-0011
651-213-4200
800-257-7810
Fax: 651-213-4793
E-mail: info@hazelden.org
www.hazelden.org

Mark Mishek, President and CEO, Hazeldon Betty
James A Blaha, VP Finance, Administration/CFO
Marvin D Seppala, MD, Chief Medical Officer
Mark Sheets, Execurive Director, Regional serv

Daily meditation in this classic book helps clients develop a solid foundation in a spiritual program, learn to relate the Twelve Steps to their everyday lives and accomplish their treatment and aftercare goals. Includes 366 daily meditations with special consideration and extra encouragement given during holidays. Helps clients find the power to stay sober each day and not to take that first drink. *$14.95*

400 pages Year Founded: 1949 ISBN 0-894868-34-9

150 When Parents Have Problems: A Book for Teens and Older Children Who Have a Disturbed or Difficult Parent
Charles C Thomas Publisher Ltd.
2600 South First Street
Springfield, IL 62704
217-789-8980
800-258-8980
Fax: 217-789-9130
E-mail: books@ccthomas.com
www.ccthomas.com

Susan B Miller, Author
PhD Miller, Author

Numerous books have been written for adults who grew up coping with troubled and difficult parents. This newly revised second edition expands the information in the previous edition by updating current knowledge that provides a thorough overview for children who are coping with difficult and/or troubled parents. Two chapters have been added. The first addresses parents who have difficult personalities. The second new chapter addresses parents in poverty. Additional topics discuss mistreatment, selfishness, when parents are in pain, when parents cause pain, powerhouse feelings, troubled parents and ordinary teen life. An excellent resource for therapists, counselor, and others who work with children and teenagers. *$19.95*

105 pages Year Founded: 1927 ISBN 0-398087-13-5

151 You Can Free Yourself from Alcohol and Drugs; How to Work a Program That Keeps You in Charge
NewHarbinger Publications
5674 Shattuck Avenue
Oakland, CA 94609-1662
510-652-0215
800-748-6273
Fax: 800-652-1613
E-mail: customerservice@newharbinger.com
www.newharbinger.com

Doug Althauser, Author

An alternative approach that removes the traditional reliance on a higher power. This ten-goal programme respects the individual beliefs of addicts and alcoholics while still requiring them to change their lifestyle from one of dependence to recovery. *$13.95*

192 pages Year Founded: 1973 ISBN 1-572241-18-7

Periodicals & Pamphlets

152 About Alcohol
ETR Associates
4 Carbonero Way
Scotts Valley, CA 95066-4200
831-438-4060
800-321-4407
Fax: 831-438-4284
E-mail: support@etr.freshdesk.com
www.etr.org

David Kitchen, MBA, Chief Financial Officer
Talita Sanders, BS, Director, Human Resources
Coleen Cantwell, MPH, Director, Business Development Pl
Matt McDowell, BS, Director, Marketing

What it is, why it's dangerous, and its negative effects on the body and in prenatal development. Title #079.

153 About Crack Cocaine
ETR Associates
4 Carbonero Way
Scotts Valley, CA 95066-4200
831-438-4060
800-321-4407
Fax: 831-438-4284
E-mail: customerservice@etr.org
www.etr.org

Mary Nelson, President

Describes what crack cocaine is and why it's dangerous and lists the effects on the body. *$16.00*

154 About Drug Addiction
ETR Associates
4 Carbonero Way
Scotts Valley, CA 95066-4200
831-438-4060
800-321-4407
Fax: 831-438-4284
E-mail: support@etr.freshdesk.com
www.etr.org

David Kitchen, MBA, Chief Financial Officer
Talita Sanders, BS, Director, Human Resources
Coleen Cantwell, MPH, Director, Business Development Pl
Matt McDowell, BS, Director, Marketing

Includes answers to commonly asked questions about drug addiction, a 13'x 17' wall chart presents the stages of addiction and recovery, covers denial, withdrawal and relapse. *$18.00*

155 Alateen Talk
Al-Anon Family Group Headquarters
1600 Corporate Landing Parkway
Virginia Beach, VA 23454-5617
757-563-1600
888-425-2666
Fax: 757-563-1655
E-mail: wso@al-anon.org
www.al-anon.alateen.org

Alateen members from all over the world share their experience, strength, and hope through the written words of Alateen Talk. Their sharings relate to their personal lives, how their Alateen group is functioning, and ways in which to carry the Alateen message to young people who are still suffering from someone else's drinking. *$7.50*

4 pages 4 per year ISSN 1054-1411

156 Alcohol ABC's
ETR Associates
4 Carbonero Way
Scotts Valley, CA 95066-4200
831-438-4060
800-321-4407
Fax: 831-438-4284
E-mail: customerservice@etr.org
www.etr.org

PALS , Author

Presents the consequenes of drinking and explains the difference between use and abuse in a straightforward, matter-of-fact way. Title #R712.

157 Alcohol Issues Insights
Beer Marketer's Insights
49 East Maple Avenue
Suffern, NY 10901-5507
845-507-0040
Fax: 845-507-0041
E-mail: eric@beerinsights.com
www.beerinsights.com

Eric Shepard, Editor

Newsletter that provides information on the use and misuses of alcohol. Covers such topics as misrepresentation in the media, minimum age requirements, advertising bans, deterrence of drunk driving, and the effects of tax increases on alcoholic beverage consumption. *$375.00*

4 pages 12 per year ISSN 1067-3105

158 Alcohol Self-Test
ETR Associates
4 Carbonero Way
Scotts Valley, CA 95066-4200
831-438-4060
800-321-4407
Fax: 831-438-4284
E-mail: support@etr.freshdesk.com
www.etr.org

David Kitchen, MBA, Chief Financial Officer
Talita Sanders, BS, Director, Human Resources
Coleen Cantwell, MPH, Director, Business Development Pl
Matt McDowell, BS, Director, Marketing

Thought provoking questions include: What do I know about alcohol? How safely do I drink? When and why do I drink? Title #H259.

159 Alcohol: Incredible Facts
ETR Associates
4 Carbonero Way
Scotts Valley, CA 95066-4200
831-438-4060
800-321-4407
Fax: 831-438-4284
E-mail: support@etr.freshdesk.com
www.etr.org

David Kitchen, MBA, Chief Financial Officer
Talita Sanders, BS, Director, Human Resources
Coleen Cantwell, MPH, Director, Business Development Pl
Matt McDowell, BS, Director, Marketing

Strange but true facts to trigger discussion about alcohol use, social consequences, and risks involved. Title #R719.

160 Alcoholism: A Merry-Go-Round Named Denial
Hazelden
PO Box 11
Center City, MN 55012-0011
651-213-4200
800-257-7810
Fax: 651-213-4793
E-mail: info@hazelden.org
www.hazelden.org

Joseph L Kellerman, Author

Revised and expanded for today's recovering person, family, and concerned others, this classic piece defines the roles of the alcoholic and those who are close to the alcoholic. This new version includes easier-to-understand, more accessible language and expanded descriptions of The Enabler, The Victim, and The Provoker roles. Also includes a section on the disease in adolescents and seniors- increasing its value to everyone touched by substance abuse. *$3.50*

20 pages Year Founded: 1949 ISBN 0-894860-22-4

161 Alcoholism: A Treatable Disease
Hazelden
PO Box 11
Center City, MN 55012-0011
651-213-4200
800-257-7810

E-mail: info@hazelden.org
www.hazelden.org

A hard look at the disease of chemical dependence, the confusion and delusion that go with it, intervention and a hopeful conclusion - alcoholism is treatable. *$2.95*

20 pages Year Founded: 1978 ISBN 0-935908-37-4

162 American Journal on Addictions
American Academy of Addiction Psychiatry
400 Massasoit Avenue
Suite 307, 2nd Floor
Easy Providence, RI 02914
401-524-3076
Fax: 401-272-0922
E-mail: aja@aaap.org
www.www.aaap.org

Ismene L Petrakis, MD, Chair, Area Director
Laurence M Westreich MD, President
Thomas R Kosten, MD, Editor-in-Chief, AJA
Shelly F Greenfield, MD, MPH, Vice President

Covers a wide variety of topics ranging from codependence to genetics, epidemiology to dual diagnostics, etiology to neuroscience, and much more. Features of the journal, all written by experts in the field, include special overview articles, clinical or basic research papers, clinical updates, and book reviews within the area of addictions.

ISSN 1055-0496

163 Binge Drinking: Am I At Risk?
ETR Associates
4 Carbonero Way
Scotts Valley, CA 95066-4200
831-438-4060
800-321-4407
Fax: 831-438-4284
E-mail: support@etr.freshdesk.com
www.etr.org

David Kitchen, MBA, Chief Financial Officer
Talita Sanders, BS, Director, Human Resources
Coleen Cantwell, MPH, Director, Business Development Pl
Matt McDowell, BS, Director, Marketing

Easy-to-follow checklists help students decide if they have a problem with binge drinking, make a plan, and get help. Title #R018.

164 Crossing the Thin Line: Between Social Drinking and Alcoholism
Hazelden
PO Box 11
Center City, MN 55012-0011
651-213-4200
800-257-7810
Fax: 651-213-4793
E-mail: info@hazelden.org
www.hazelden.org

Terence Williams, Author
Mark Sheets, Executive Director
Marvin Seppala MD, Chief Medical Officer
Nick Motu, Publisher, VP of Marketing

This pamphlet encourages people to look at their own drinking habits to decide if they are crossing the very thin line between social drinking and alcoholism. An excellent resource for anyone who has wondered about his or her own drinking habits. *$2.95*

20 pages Year Founded: 1949 ISBN 0-894860-77-1

165   Designer Drugs
ETR Associates
4 Carbonero Way
Scotts Valley, CA 95066-4200
831-438-4060
800-321-4407
Fax: 831-438-4284
E-mail: customerservice@etr.org
www.etr.org

M Foster Olive, Author

Traces the evolution of designer drugs like China White and MDMA, explains how addiction works and suggests why designer drugs are so addictive. *$16.00*

112 pages

166   Drinking Facts
ETR Associates
4 Carbonero Way
Scotts Valley, CA 95066-4200
831-438-4060
800-321-4407
Fax: 831-438-4284
E-mail: support@etr.freshdesk.com
www.etr.org

David Kitchen, MBA, Chief Financial Officer
Talita Sanders, BS, Director, Human Resources
Coleen Cantwell, MPH, Director, Business Development Pl
Matt McDowell, BS, Director, Marketing

Addresses changing attitudes about drinking, and examines the basic facts of alcohol. Shows how to avoid risky situations, explains about the blood alcohol levels, and offers tips for curbing consumption. Title #R843

167   Drug Dependence, Alcohol Abuse and Alcoholism
Elsevier Publishing
1600 John F Kennedy Boulevard
Suite 1800
Philadelphia, PA 19103-2879
314-872-8370
800-542-2522
Fax: 314-432-1380
E-mail: usbkinfo@elsevier.com
www.elsevier.com

Erik Engstrom, CEO

This journal aims to provide its readers with a swift, yet complete, current awareness service. Careful selection of relevent abstracts (and other bibliographic data) from the latest issues of 4, 000 leading international biomedical journals. The journal covers all aspects of the abuse of drugs, alcohol and organic solvents and includes material relating to experimental pharmacology of addiction, although, in general, experimental pharmacology of narcotics is not covered.

Year Founded: 1880 ISSN 0925-5958

168   Drug Facts Pamphlet
ETR Associates
4 Carbonero Way
Scotts Valley, CA 95066-4200
831-438-4060
800-321-4407
Fax: 831-435-8433
E-mail: support@etr.freshdesk.com
www.etr.org

David Kitchen, MBA, Chief Financial Officer
Talita Sanders, BS, Director, Human Resources
Coleen Cantwell, MPH, Director, Business Development Pl
Matt McDowell, BS, Director, Marketing

Overview of 11 of the most commonly abused drugs includes: Description of drug, short-term effects and long-term effects. *$18.00*

169   Drug and Alcohol Dependence An International Journal on Biomedical an Psychosocial Approaches
Customer Support Services
1600 John F Kennedy Boulevard
Suite 1800
Philadelphia, PA 19103-2879
212-633-3730
800-654-2452
Fax: 212-633-3680
www.elsevier.com

Eric C. Strain, Editor-in-Chief
Andraya Dolbee, Editorial Office Manager

An international journal devoted to publishing original research, scholarly reviews, commentaries, and policy analyses in the area of drug, alcohol and tobacco use and dependence. Articles range from studies of the chemistry of substances of abuse, their actions at molecular and cellular sites, in vitro and in vivo investigations of their biochemical, pharacological and behavioural actions, laboratory-based and clinical research in humans, substance abuse treatment and prevention research, and studies employing methods from epidemiology, sociology, and economics.

15 per year Year Founded: 1880 ISSN 0376-8716

170   DrugLink
Facts and Comparisons
Red Lion Lane
Trefoil House
Hemel Hempstead, UK HP3 9-E
192-326-0733
800-223-0554
Fax: 192-327-1781
www.www.druglink.co.uk

Rosemary Farmer, Chairman
John Pins, VP of Finance
Denise Basow MD, VP, General Manager, Editor
David Del Toro, VP, General Manager

DrugLink is an eight-page newsletter that provides abstracts of drug-related articles from various journals. DrugLink allows health care professionals to stay up-to-date on hot topics without having to subscribe to multiple publications. *$52.95*

8 pages Year Founded: 1984 ISBN 1-089559-0 -

171   Drugs: Talking With Your Teen
ETR Associates
4 Carbonero Way
Scotts Valley, CA 95066-4200
831-438-4060
800-321-4407
Fax: 831-435-8433
E-mail: support@etr.freshdesk.com
www.etr.org

David Kitchen, MBA, Chief Financial Officer
Talita Sanders, BS, Director, Human Resources

Coleen Cantwell, MPH, Director, Business Development Pl
Matt McDowell, BS, Director, Marketing

Suggestions for effective communication include: avoid scare tatics, clarify family rules, other alternative for drug use. *$ 16.00*

172 Getting Involved in AA
Hazelden
PO Box 11
Center City, MN 55012-0011
651-213-4200
800-328-9000
Fax: 651-213-4793
E-mail: info@hazelden.org
www.hazelden.org

Bob W, Author
Mark Sheets, Executive Director
Marvin Seppala MD, Chief Medical Officer
Nick Motu, Publisher, VP of Marketing

Shares the experiences of many members in joining AA and answers questions readers may have. The author's message is that your entry to AA can go smoothly. *$3.50*

32 pages Year Founded: 1949 ISBN 0-894861-36-0

173 Getting Started in AA
Hazelden
PO Box 11
Center City, MN 55012-0011
651-213-4200
800-328-9000
Fax: 651-213-4793
E-mail: info@hazelden.org
www.hazelden.org

Hamilton B, Author

The tradition and wisdom associated with the Twelve Step AA program has been captured in this comprehensive guide. Practical suggestions for staying sober; summaries of AA principles, concepts, and slogans; and a historical overview help the reader understand the spirit of the program. *$13.95*

232 pages Year Founded: 1949 ISBN 1-568380-91-7

174 Getting What You Want From Drinking
ETR Associates
4 Carbonero Way
Scotts Valley, CA 95066-4200
831-438-4060
800-321-4407
Fax: 831-438-3618
E-mail: support@etr.freshdesk.com
www.etr.org

David Kitchen, MBA, Chief Financial Officer
Talita Sanders, BS, Director, Human Resources
Coleen Cantwell, MPH, Director, Business Development Pl
Matt McDowell, BS, Director, Marketing

Practical ideas for drinking more safely, preventing hangovers, weight gain, and injuries; blood alcohol chart shows the effect of alcohol on the mind and body. Title #H220.

175 Hazelden Voice
Hazelden Foundation
PO Box 11
Center City, MN 55012-0011
612-213-4200
800-257-7810

Fax: 651-213-4793
E-mail: info@hazelden.org
www.hazelden.org

Mark Mishek, President and CEO, Hazeldon Betty
James A Blaha, VP Finance, Administration/CFO
Marvin D Seppala, MD, Chief Medical Officer
Mark Sheets, Execurive Director, Regional serv

Reports on Hazelden activities and programs, and discusses developments and issues in chemical dependency treatment and prevention. Carries notices of professional education opportunities, reviews of resources in the field, and a calendar of events.

Year Founded: 1949

176 I Can't Be an Alcoholic Because...
Hazelden
PO Box 11
Center City, MN 55012-0011
651-213-4200
800-328-9000
Fax: 651-213-4793
E-mail: info@hazelden.org
www.hazelden.org

David C Hancock, Author
Mark Sheets, Executive Director
Marvin Seppala MD, Chief Medical Officer
Nick Motu, Publisher, VP of Marketing

This pamphlet describes fallacies and misconceptions about alcoholism and includes facts and figures about alcohol, its use, and its abuse. Available in Spanish. *$1.95*

20 pages Year Founded: 1949 ISBN 0-894861-58-1

177 ICPA Reporter
ICPADD
12501 Old Columbia Pike
Silver Spring, MD 20904-6601
301-680-6719
Fax: 301-680-6707
www.www.icpa.ca

Ed Wozniak, Executive Director
Tineke De Waele, Executive Director Designee
Cassandra Johnson, Business Manager
Koert Swierstra, Office of the President

Reports on activities of the Commission worldwide, which seeks to prevent alcoholism and drug dependency. Recurring features include a calendar of events and notices of publications available.

4 pages 4 per year

178 Journal of Substance Abuse Treatment
Elsevier Publishing
1600 John F Kennedy Boulevard
Suite 1800
Philadelphia, PA 19103-2879
314-872-8370
800-545-2522
Fax: 314-432-1380
E-mail: custserv@elsevier.com
www.elsevier.com

Mark P. McGovern, Editor-in-Chief

Features original research, systematic reviews and reports on meta-analyses and, with editorial approval, special articles on the assessment and treatment of substance use and addictive disorders, including alcohol, illicit and prescription drugs, and nicotine.

Year Founded: 1880 ISSN 0740-5472

179 NIDA Notes
National Institute of Drug Abuse (NIDA)
6001 Executive Boulevard
Room 5213, MSC 9561
Bethesda, MD 20892-9561
301-443-1124
Fax: 301-443-7397
E-mail: information@lists.nida.nih.gov
www.drugabuse.gov

Beverly Jackson, Manager
Beverly Jackson, Public Information Director

Covers the areas of drug abuse treatment and prevention research, epidemiology, neuroscience and behavioral research, health services research and AIDS. Seeks to report on advances in the field, identify resources, promote an exchange of information, and improve communications among clinicians, researchers, administrators, and policymakers. Recurring features include synopses of research advances and projects, NIDA news, news of legislative and regulatory developments, and announcements.

180 Real World Drinking
ETR Associates
4 Carbonero Way
Scotts Valley, CA 95066-4200
800-321-4407
Fax: 831-438-3618
E-mail: customerservice@etr.org
www.etr.org

Mary Nelson, President

Credible young people talk about benefits of not drinking and risks of drinking. Title #R746.

181 Teens and Drinking
ETR Associates
4 Carbonero Way
Scotts Valley, CA 95066-4200
800-321-4407
Fax: 831-438-3618
E-mail: customerservice@etr.org
www.etr.org

Mary Nelson, President

Includes common sense messages about drinking, binge drinking, and important things to know about drinking. Title #R717.

182 The Chalice
Calix Society
PO Box 9085
St Paul, MN 55109-9969
651-773-3117
800-398-0524
www.calixsociety.org

William J Montroy, Founder

Directed toward Catholic and non-Catholic alcoholics who are maintaining their sobriety through affiliation with and participation in Alcoholics Anonymous. Emphasizes the virtue of total abstinence, through contributed stories regarding spiritual and physical recovery. Recurring features include statistics, book announcements, and research. *$15.00*

4-6 pages 24 per year

183 The Prevention Researcher
Integrated Research Services
66 Club Road
Suite 370
Eugene, OR 97401-2464
541-683-9278
800-929-2955
Fax: 541-683-2621
E-mail: info@tpronline.org
www.www.tpronline.org

Steven Ungerleider PhD, Advisory Board
Gerald Mader PhD, Advisory Board
Juan Jerry Lopez MSW, Advisory Board

A quarterly journal that provides professionals with practical, relevant research for their work with youth. Each issue features a single topic focused on successful adolescent development. Articles are written by authors who lead in their respective fields and whose research covers the latest findings on significant issues facing today's youth. *$20.00*

12-16 pages 4 per year   ISSN 1086-4385

184 When Someone You Care About Abuses Drugs and Alcohol: When to Act, What to Say
Hazelden
PO Box 11
Center City, MN 55012-0011
651-213-4200
800-328-9000
Fax: 651-213-4793
E-mail: info@hazelden.org
www.hazelden.org

Mark Mishek, President and CEO, Hazeldon Betty
James A Blaha, VP Finance, Administration/CFO
Marvin D Seppala, MD, Chief Medical Officer
Mark Sheets, Execurive Director, Regional serv

Assists concerned family members and friends in determining their options for helping someone abusing alcohol and/or drugs. Addictive behavior is described, with clear guidelines for how and when to respond to the abuser's behavior. Throughout, the personal responsibility of concerned family and friends is reinforced, with suggestions for examining our motives for intervening. *$2.95*

20 pages Year Founded: 1949 ISBN 1-592855-29-6

185 Why Haven't I Been Able to Help?
Hazelden
15251 Pleasant Valley Road
PO Box 176
Center City, MN 55012-176
651-213-4200
800-257-7810
Fax: 651-213-4590
E-mail: customersupport@hazelden.org
www.hazelden.org

Mark Mishek, President, CEO
Mark Sheets, Executive Director
Marvin Seppala MD, Chief Medical Officer
Nick Motu, Publisher, VP of Marketing

Explains how the spouse also gets trapped by the disease, and discusses how the disease progresses within the alcoholic. Ends on a note of hope by briefly indicating how the alcoholic, the spouse, and other family members can escape the trap of alcoholism. *$2.50*

18 pages ISBN 0-935908-40-4

186 Your Brain on Drugs
Hazelden
PO Box 11
Center City, MN 55012-0011
651-213-4200
800-257-7810
E-mail: info@hazelden.org
www.www.hazelden.org

John O'Neill, L.C.D.C., Author
Carlton Erickson, Author
Nick Motu, Publisher, VP of Marketing
Marvin Seppala MD, Chief Medical Officer

This pamphlet explains the effects of alcohol and other drugs on the brain. Illustrations, activities, and exercises help to reinforce easy-to-read text. *$3.50*

32 pages Year Founded: 1996 ISBN 1-568389-04-3

Research Centers

187 UAMS Psychiatric Research Institute
4224 Shuffield Drive
Little Rock, AR 72205
501-526-8100
Fax: 501-660-7542
E-mail: kramerteresal@uams.edu
www.www.psychiatry.uams.edu

Combining research, education and clinical services into one facility, PRI offers inpatiend and outpatient services, with 40 psychiatric beds, therapy options, and specialized treatment for specific disorders, including: addictive eating, anxiety, deppressive and post-traumatic stress disorders. Research focuses on evidence-based care takes into consideration the education of future medical personnel while relying on research scientists to provide innovative forms of treatment. PRI includes the Center for Addiction Research as well as a methadone clinic.

Support Groups & Hot Lines

188 Adult Children of Alcoholics
PO Box 3216
Torrance, CA 90510-3216
562-595-7831
E-mail: info@adultchildren.org
www.adultchildren.org

An anonymous Twelve Step, Twelve Tradition program of women and men who grew up in an alcoholic or otherwise dysfunctional homes.

189 Al-Anon Family Group National Referral Hotline
1600 Corporate Landing Parkway
Virginia Beach, VA 23454-5617
757-563-1600
Fax: 757-563-1655
E-mail: wso@al-anon.org
www.al-anon.alateen.org

Al-Anon is a mutual support group of peers who share their experience in applying the Al-Anon principles to problems related to the effects of a problem drinker in their lives. It is not group therapy and is not led by a counselor or therapist; This support network complements and supports professional treatment.

190 Alateen and Al-Anon Family Groups
1600 Corporate Landing Parkway
Virginia Beach, VA 23454-5617
757-563-1600
888-425-2666
Fax: 757-563-1655
E-mail: wso@al-anon.org
www.al-anon.alateen.org/sitemap.html

Mary Ann Keller, Director Members Services

A fellowship of men, women, children and adult children affected by another persons drinking.

191 Alcoholics Anonymous (AA): World Services
475 Riverside Drive at West 120th St.
11th Floor
New York, NY 10115
212-870-3400
www.aa.org

For men and women who share the common problems of alcoholism.

192 Chemically Dependent Anonymous
PO Box 423
Severna Park, MD 21146
888-232-4673
E-mail: publicinfo@cdaweb.org
www.www.cdaweb.org

A 12-step fellowship for anyone seeking freedom from drug and alcohol addiction. The basis of the program is abstinence from all mood-changing and mind-altering chemicals, including street-type drugs, alcohol and unnecessary medication.

193 Cocaine Anonymous
21720 S. Wilmington Ave
Suite 304
Long Beach, CA 90810-1641
310-559-5833
Fax: 310-559-2554
E-mail: cawso@ca.org
www.ca.org

Fellowship of men and women who share their experience, stength and hope with each other in hope that they may solve their common problem and help others recover from their addiction.

194 Infoline
United Way of Connecticut
1344 Silas Deane Highway
Rocky Hill, CT 06067-1350
860-571-7500
800-203-1234
Fax: 860-571-7525
TTY: 800-671-0737
www.ctunitedway.org

Richard Porth, CEO

Infoline is a free, confidential, help-by-telephone service for information, referral, and crisis intervention. Trained professionals help callers find information, discover options or deal with a crisis by locating hundreds of services in their area on many different issues, from substance abuse to elder needs to suicide to volunteering in your community. Infoline is certified by the American Association of Suicidology. Operates 24 hours a day, everyday. Multilingual caseworkers are available. For Child Care Infoline, call 1-800-505-1000.

195 Join Together Online
352 Park Avenue South
9th Floor
New York, NY 10010
212-922-1560
855-378-4373
Fax: 212-922-1570
E-mail: info@jointogether.org
www.www.drugfree.org/join-together

Patricia F Russo, Chairman
Stephen J Pasierb, President, CEO
Robert Caruso, CFO
Paul Healy, Chief Development Officer

Join Together is a collaboration of the Boston University School of Public Health and The Partnership at Drugfree.org, dedicated to advancing effective drug and alcohol policy, prevention and treatment.

196 MADD-Mothers Against Drunk Drivers
511 E John Carpenter Freeway
Suite 700
Irving, TX 75062-8187
877-275-6233
Fax: 214-869-2206
www.www.madd.org

Jan Withers, National President
Debbie Weir, CEO

Mission is to stop drunk driving, support the victims of this violent crime and prevent underage drinking. MADD's work has saved nearly 300, 000 lives and counting.

Year Founded: 1980

197 Marijuana Anonymous
PO Box 7807
Torrance, CA 90504-9207
800-766-6779
E-mail: office@marijuana-anonymous.org
www.marijuana-anonymous.org

A fellowship of men and women who share experience, strength and hope with each other to solve common problem and help others to recover from marijuana addiction.

198 Nar-Anon Family Groups
22527 Crenshaw Blvd
Suite 200B
Torrance, CA 90505
310-534-8188
800-477-6291
Fax: 310-534-8688
E-mail: wso@naranon.org
www.nar-anon.org

Cathy Khaledi, Executive Director

Twelve-step program for families and friends of addicts.

199 Narcotics Anonymous
PO Box 9999
Van Nuys, CA 91409-9099
818-773-9999
Fax: 818-700-0700
www.na.org

For narcotic addicts: Peer support for recovered addicts.

200 Pathways to Promise
5400 Arsenal Street
Saint Louis, MO 63139-1403

Fax: 314-516-8405
E-mail: info@pathways2promise.org
www.pathways2promise.org

An interfaith cooperative of many faith groups, providing assistance and a resource center which offers liturgical and educational materials, program models, caring ministry with people experiencing a mental illness and their families.

201 Rational Recovery
PO Box 800
Lotus, CA 95651-800
530-621-2667
www.rational.org

Jack Trimpey, President

Exclusive, worldwide source of counseling, guidance and direct instruction on self-recovery from addiction to alcohol and other drugs through planned, permanent abstinence.

Year Founded: 1986

202 SADD: Students Against Destructive Decisions
255 Main Street
Marlborough, MA 01752-5505
508-481-3568
877-723-3462
Fax: 508-481-5759
E-mail: info@sadd.org
www.sadd.org

Danna Mauch, PhD, Chairman
Penny Wells, President and CEO
Susan Scarola, Treasurer
James E Champagne, Secretary/Clerk

SADD's mission is to provide students with the best prevention tools possible to deal with the issues of underage drinking, other drug use, risky and impaired driving, and other destructive decisions.

Year Founded: 1981

203 SMART-Self Management and Recovery Training
7304 Mentor Avenue
Suite F
Mentor, OH 44060-5463
440-951-5357
866-951-5357
Fax: 440-951-5358
E-mail: info@smartrecovery.org
www.smartrecovery.org

Shari Allwood, Executive Director

The leading self-empowering addiction recovery support group. Participants learn tools for addiction recovery based on the latest scientific research and participate in a world-wide community which includes free, self-empowering, science-based mutual help groups.

Video & Audio

204 Alcohol Abuse Dying For A Drink
Educational Video Network
1401 19th Street
Huntsville, TX 77340
936-295-5767
800-762-0060
Fax: 936-294-0233

E-mail: info at evn.org
www.www.evndirect.com

A video explaining alcohol abuse and its consequenses.
$59.95

Year Founded: 2004 ISBN 1-589501-48-9

205 Alcohol and Sex: Prescription for Poor Decision Making
ETR Associates
4 Carbonero Way
Scotts Valley, CA 95066-4200
831-438-4060
800-321-4407
Fax: 800-435-8433
E-mail: customerservice@etr.org
www.etr.org

Pamela Anderson, PhD, Senior Research Associate
Eric Blanke, BS, Director, Solutions
Nancy Calvin, CES, Administrative Specialist
Shannon Campe, BA, Research Associate III

Explains how alcohol use can interfere with healthy decisions about sex and intimacy, as well as describing the effects of alcohol on the brain. Also, includes information about the date rape drug, how alcohol affects relationships, and includes a Teacher Resource Book. *$139.95*

206 Alcohol and You
Educational Video Network
1401 19th Street
Huntsville, TX 77340
936-295-5767
800-762-0060
Fax: 936-294-0233
E-mail: info at evn.org
www.www.evndirect.com

A video explaining alcohol abuse and its consequenses.
$49.95

Year Founded: 2001 ISBN 1-588451-32-7

207 Alcohol and the Brain
Educational Video Network
1401 19th Street
Huntsville, TX 77340
936-295-5767
800-762-0060
Fax: 936-294-0233
E-mail: info at evn.org
www.www.evndirect.com

A video explaining alcohol abuse and its consequenses.
$79.95

Year Founded: 2004 ISBN 1-589501-32-7

208 Alcohol: the Substance, the Addiction, the Solution
Hazelden
15251 Pleasant Valley Road
PO Box 11
Center City, MN 55012-0011
651-213-4200
800-328-9000
Fax: 651-213-4793
E-mail: info@hazelden.org
www.hazelden.org

Mark Mishek, President and CEO
James A. Blaha, Vice President Finance and Admin

Ann Bray, General Counsel and Vice Preside
Sharon Birnbaum, Corporate Director of Human Reso

Weaves dramatic personal stories of recovery from alcoholism with essential facts about alcohol itself. Emphasizes the impact of using and abusing alcohol in conjunction with other drugs. Educates about the dangers of this legally sanctioned drug, including the myth of safer versions such as wine and beer. *$149.00*

Year Founded: 1949

209 Binge Drinking
ETR Associates
4 Carbonero Way
Scotts Valley, CA 95066-4200
831-438-4060
800-321-4407
Fax: 831-438-3618
E-mail: customerservice@etr.org
www.etr.org

Pamela Anderson, PhD, Senior Research Associate
Eric Blanke, BS, Director, Solutions
Nancy Calvin, CES, Administrative Specialist
Shannon Campe, BA, Research Associate III

Explains the physiological and psychological effects of alcohol, covers the warning signs for alcohol poisoning and procedures to take to save someone, and delivers a no-nonsense message about why binge drinking is dangerous. Describes the catastrophic realities that can result from party behavior, such as car crashes, falls, bad decisions and acquaintance rape. *$139.95*

210 Cocaine & Crack: Back from the Abyss
Hazelden
15251 Pleasant Valley Road
PO Box 11
Center City, MN 55012-0011
651-213-4200
800-257-7810
Fax: 651-213-4793
E-mail: info@hazelden.org
www.hazelden.org

Mark Mishek, President and CEO
James A. Blaha, Vice President Finance and Admin
Ann Bray, General Counsel and Vice Preside
Sharon Birnbaum, Corporate Director of Human Reso

Provides clients in correctional, educational, and treatment settings an understanding of the history, pharamacology, and medical impact of cocaine/crack use through personal stories of addiction and recovery. Reveals proven methods for overcoming addiction and discusses the best ways to maintain recovery. 46 minutes. *$149.00*

Year Founded: 1949 ISBN 1-592852-97-1

211 Cross Addiction: The Back Door to Relapse
Hazelden
15251 Pleasant Valley Road
PO Box 11
Center City, MN 55012-0011
651-213-4200
800-328-9000
Fax: 651-213-4793
E-mail: info@hazelden.org
www.hazelden.org

Mark Mishek, President and CEO
James A. Blaha, Vice President Finance and Admin

Ann Bray, General Counsel and Vice Preside
Sharon Birnbaum, Corporate Director of Human Reso

Firsthand testimony from recovering alcoholics and addicts, chemicl dependency professionals, and a medical doctor dispel the myth that there is any such thing as a safe substance for people in recovery. *$225.00*

Year Founded: 1949

212 Disease of Alcoholism Video
Hazelden
15251 Pleasant Valley Road
PO Box 11
Center City, MN 55012-0011
651-213-4200
800-328-9000
Fax: 651-213-4793
E-mail: info@hazelden.org
www.hazelden.org

Mark Mishek, President and CEO
James A. Blaha, Vice President Finance and Admin
Ann Bray, General Counsel and Vice Preside
Sharon Birnbaum, Corporate Director of Human Reso

This video is used daily in treatment, corporations, and schools. Dr. Ohlms discusses startling and convincing information on the genetic and physiological aspects of alcohol addiction. *$395.00*

Year Founded: 1949

213 Effective Learning Systems, Inc.
5108 W 74th Street
#390160
Minneapolis, MN 55439
239-948-1660
800-966-0443
www.www.effectivelearning.com

Bob Griswold, Founder
Deirdre M Griswold, VP

Audio tapes for stress management, deep relaxation, anger control, peace of mind, insomnia, weight and smoking, self-image and self-esteem, positive thinking, health and healing. Since 1972, Effective Learning Systems has helped millions of people take charge of their lives and make positive changes. Over 75 titles available, each with a money-back guarantee. Price range $12-$14.

Year Founded: 1972

214 Fetal Alcohol Syndrome and Effect
Hazelden
15251 Pleasant Valley Road
PO Box 11
Center City, MN 55012-0011
651-213-4200
800-328-9000
Fax: 651-213-4793
E-mail: info@hazelden.org
www.hazelden.org

Mark Mishek, President and CEO
James A. Blaha, Vice President Finance and Admin
Ann Bray, General Counsel and Vice Preside
Sharon Birnbaum, Corporate Director of Human Reso

If you're a chemical dependency counselor or work with women in pregnancy planning or self-care, this resource is filled with facts to help you better meet your clients needs. *$225.00*

Year Founded: 1949

215 Fetal Alcohol Syndrome and Effect, Stories of Help and Hope
Hazelden
15251 Pleasant Valley Road
PO Box 11
Center City, MN 55012-0011
651-213-4200
800-328-9000
Fax: 651-213-4793
E-mail: info@hazelden.org
www.hazelden.org

Mark Mishek, President and CEO
James A. Blaha, Vice President Finance and Admin
Ann Bray, General Counsel and Vice Preside
Sharon Birnbaum, Corporate Director of Human Reso

Provides clients with a factual defintion of the medical diagonosis of fetal alcohol syndrome and its effects, including how children are diagnosed and the positive prognosis possible for these children. *$225.00*

Year Founded: 1949

216 Heroin: What Am I Going To Do?
Hazelden
15251 Pleasant Valley Road
PO Box 11
Center City, MN 55012-0011
651-213-4200
800-328-9000
Fax: 651-213-4793
E-mail: info@hazelden.org
www.hazelden.org

Mark Mishek, President and CEO
James A. Blaha, Vice President Finance and Admin
Ann Bray, General Counsel and Vice Preside
Sharon Birnbaum, Corporate Director of Human Reso

Shares powerful stories and keen insights from recovering heroin addicts and the rewards of clean living. Teaches clients how to use honesty, surrender and responsibility as the power tools for a successful recovery. Deglamorizes heroin use, with a portrait of drug's inevitable degration of the mind, body and spirit. 30 minutes. *$225.00*

Year Founded: 1949

217 I'll Quit Tomorrow
Hazelden
15251 Pleasant Valley Road
PO Box 11
Center City, MN 55012-0011
651-213-4200
800-328-9000
Fax: 651-213-4793
E-mail: info@hazelden.org
www.hazelden.org

Mark Mishek, President and CEO
James A. Blaha, Vice President Finance and Admin
Ann Bray, General Counsel and Vice Preside
Sharon Birnbaum, Corporate Director of Human Reso

Show clients the progressive nature of alcoholism through one of the most powerful films ever made about this disease. This three-part video series and facilitator's guide use a dramatic personal story to provide a clear and thorough introduction to the disease concept of alcoholism, enabling the intervention process, treatment and the hope of healing and recovery. *$300.00*

Year Founded: 1949

218 Marijuana: Escape to Nowhere
Hazelden
15251 Pleasant Valley Road
PO Box 11
Center City, MN 55012-176
651-213-4200
800-328-9000
Fax: 651-213-4793
E-mail: info@hazelden.org
www.hazelden.org

Mark Mishek, President and CEO
James A. Blaha, Vice President Finance and Admin
Ann Bray, General Counsel and Vice Preside
Sharon Birnbaum, Corporate Director of Human Reso

Challenges myths about marijuana by clearly stating that marijuana is addictive and use results in physical, emotional and spiritual consequences. Explains to clients in simple language the pharmacology of today's more potent marijuana and shares the hope and healing of recovery. 30 minutes. *$225.00*

Year Founded: 1949

219 Medical Aspects of Chemical Dependency
Active Parenting Publishers
Hazelden
15251 Pleasant Valley Road
PO Box 11
Center City, MN 55012-0011
651-213-4200
800-328-9000
Fax: 651-213-4793
E-mail: info@hazelden.org
www.hazelden.org

Mark Mishek, President and CEO
James A. Blaha, Vice President Finance and Admin
Ann Bray, General Counsel and Vice Preside
Sharon Birnbaum, Corporate Director of Human Reso

This curriculum helps professionals educate clients in treatment and other settings about medical effects of chemical use and abuse. The program includes a video that explains body and brain changes that can occur when using alcohol or other drugs, a workbook that helps clients apply the information from the video to their own situations, a handbook that provides in-depth information on addiction, brain chemistry and the physiological effects of chemical dependency and a pamphlet that answers critical questions clients have about the medical effects of chemical dependency. Available to purchase separately. Program value packages available. *$225.00*

Year Founded: 1949

220 Methamphetamine: Decide to Live Prevention Video
Hazelden
15251 Pleasant Valley Road
PO Box 11
Center City, MN 55012-0011
651-213-4200
800-328-9000
Fax: 651-213-4793
E-mail: info@hazelden.org
www.hazelden.org

Mark Mishek, President and CEO
James A. Blaha, Vice President Finance and Admin

Ann Bray, General Counsel and Vice Preside
Sharon Birnbaum, Corporate Director of Human Reso

Methamphetamine: Decide to Live presents the latest information on the devastating consequences of meth addiction and the struggles and rewards of recovery. Facts, medical aspects, personal stories, and insights on the recovery process illuminate the path to healing. The video is divided into two parts and is 38 minutes long. *$225.00*

Year Founded: 1949

221 Prescription Drugs: Recovery from the Hidden Addiction
Hazelden
15251 Pleasant Valley Road
PO Box 11
Center City, MN 55012-0011
651-213-4200
800-328-9000
Fax: 651-213-4793
E-mail: info@hazelden.org
www.hazelden.org

Mark Mishek, President and CEO
James A. Blaha, Vice President Finance and Admin
Ann Bray, General Counsel and Vice Preside
Sharon Birnbaum, Corporate Director of Human Reso

Combines essential facts about prescription drugs with vivid personal stories of addiction and recovery. Classifies prescription medications and gives the corresponding street forms. Offers solutions to problems unique to prescription drugs, addresses the particular needs of older adults and elaborates on the dangers of cross-addiction. 31 minutes. *$225.00*

Year Founded: 1949

222 Reality Check: Marijuana Prevention Video
Hazelden
15251 Pleasant Valley Road
PO Box 11
Center City, MN 55012-0011
651-213-4200
800-328-9000
Fax: 651-213-4793
E-mail: info@hazelden.org
www.hazelden.org

Mark Mishek, President and CEO
James A. Blaha, Vice President Finance and Admin
Ann Bray, General Counsel and Vice Preside
Sharon Birnbaum, Corporate Director of Human Reso

This video creates a strong message for kids about the dangers of marijuana use. A combination of humor, animated graphics, testimonials and music deliver the facts on the pharmacology of marijuana and both it's short and long use consequences. Suitable for kids grades 7-12.
15 minute video. *$225.00*

Year Founded: 1949

223 SmokeFree TV: A Nicotine Prevention Video
Hazelden
15251 Pleasant Valley Road
PO Box 11
Center City, MN 55012-0011
651-213-4200
800-328-9000
Fax: 651-213-4793

E-mail: info@hazelden.org
www.hazelden.org

Mark Mishek, President and CEO
James A. Blaha, Vice President Finance and Admin
Ann Bray, General Counsel and Vice Preside
Sharon Birnbaum, Corporate Director of Human Reso

Key facts, consequences of use and refusal skills guide children in understanding why they should avoid nicotine. Animated graphics, stories, humor, and music appeal to young people. Pharmacology of nicotine, its consequences and ways to refuse it are also explored. 15 minute video. *$225.00*

Year Founded: 1949

224   Straight Talk About Substance Use and Violence
ADD WareHouse
300 NW 70th Avenue
Suite 102
Plantation, FL 33317-2360
954-792-8100
800-233-9273
Fax: 954-792-8545
E-mail: websales@addwarehouse.com
www.addwarehouse.com

Mark Mishek, President and CEO
James A. Blaha, Vice President Finance and Admin
Ann Bray, General Counsel and Vice Preside
Sharon Birnbaum, Corporate Director of Human Reso

Substance abuse and violence prevention begins with this three video program featuring the frank testimonials of 19 teens with significant chemical dependency issues who range in age from 13 to 22. In the starkest terms they discuss their most personal issues: substance abuse, sexual abuse, physical abuse, suicide attempts, violent acting out, depression, and abusive relationships. Includes 95 page discussion guide and three 30 minute videos. *$259.00*

Year Founded: 1990

225   What Should I Tell My Child About Drinking?
NADD-National Council on Alcoholism and Drug Dependence, Inc.
217 Broadway
Suite 712
New York, NY 10007-3128
212-269-7797
800-622-2255
Fax: 212-269-7510
E-mail: national@ncadd.org
www.www.ncadd.org

Greg Muth, Chairman
William H. Foster, PhD, President and Chief Executive Of
Leah Brock, Director of Affiliate Relations
Jayne Restivo, Director of Development

Offers a series of teachable moments for different age groups that provide parents a structured opportunity to discuss alcohol with their children *$59.99*

12 pages Year Founded: 1944

Web Sites

226   www.aa.org
AA-Alcoholics Anonymous

Group sharing their experience, strength and hope with each other to recover from alcoholism.

227   www.addictionresourceguide.com
Addiction Resource Guide

A comprehensive directory of addiction treatment facilities online.

228   www.adultchildren.org
Adult Children of Alcoholics World Services Organization, Inc.

12 step and 12 tradition program for adults raised in an environment including alcohol or other dysfunctions.

229   www.al-anon.alateen.org
Al-Anon/Alateen

Program for relatives and friends of persons with alcohol problems.

230   www.alcoholism.about.com
The Alcoholism Home Page

Information about addictive drug use, behaviors, and alcoholism.

231   www.cfsny.org
Center for Family Support

Providing care givers with all aspects of service needed.

232   www.doitnow.org
The Do It Now Foundation

Copies of brochures on drugs, alcohol, smoking, drugs and kids, and street drugs.

233   www.drugabuse.gov
National Institute on Drug Abuse

Many publications useful for patients. Research Reports, summaries about chemicals and treatments.

234   www.drugabuse.gov/drugpages
Commonly Abused Drugs: Street Names for Drugs of Abuse

Current names, periods of detection, medical uses.

235   www.drugfree.org/join-together
Join Together

Alcohol and substance abuse information, legislative alerts, new and updates.

236   www.higheredcenter.org
National Clearinghouse for Alcohol & Drug Information

One-stop resource for information about abuse prevention and addiction treatment.

237   www.jacsweb.org
Jewish Alcoholics Chemically Dependent Persons

Ten articles dealing with denial and ignorance.

238 www.lifering.org
LifeRing

Offers nonreligious approach with links to groups.

239 www.madd.org
MADD-Mothers Against Drunk Driving

A crusade to stop alcohol consumption, and underage drinking.

240 www.mentalhealth.com
Internet Mental Health

On-line information and a virtual encyclopedia related to mental disorders, possible causes and treatments. News, articles, on-line diagnostic programs and related links. Designed to improve understanding, diagnosis and treatment of mental illness throughout the world. Awarded the Top Site Award and the NetPsych Cutting Edge Site Award.

241 www.mhselfhelp.org
National Mental Health Consumers Self-Help Clearinghouse

Encourages the development and growth of consumer self-help groups.

242 www.naadac.org
The Association for Addiction Professionals

NAADAC is the premier global organization of addiction focused professionals who enhance the health and recovery of individuals, families and communities. NAADAC's mission is to lead, unify and empower addiction focused professionals to achieve excellence through education, advocacy, knowledge, standards of practice, ethics, professional development and research.

243 www.niaaa.nih.gov
National Institute on Alcohol Abuse & Alcoholism

Supports research nationwide on alcohol abuse and alcoholism.

244 www.nofas.org
National Organization on Fetal Alcohol Syndrome

Develops and implements innovative prevention and education strategies assessing fetal alcohol syndrome.

245 www.psychcentral.com
Psych Central

Personalized one-stop index for psychology, support, and mental health issues, resources, and people on the Internet.

246 www.sadd.org
SADD-Students Against Destructive Decisions

Peer leadership organization dedicated to preventing destructive decisions.

247 www.samhsa.gov
Substance Abuse and Mental Health Services Administration

Provides links to government resources related to substance abuse and mental health.

248 www.sapacap.com
American Council on Alcohol Problems

Referrals to DWI classes and treatment centers.

249 www.smartrecovery.org
Self Help for Substance Abuse & Addiction

Four-Point program includes maintaining motivation, coping with urges, managing feelings and behavior, balancing momentary/enduring satisfactions.

250 www.soulselfhelp.on.ca/coda.html
Souls Self Help Central

Discusses self-help, mental health, issues of co-dependency.

251 www.store.samhsa.gov
SAMHSA's National Mental Health Info Center

Information about resources, technical assistance, research, training, networks, and other federal clearing houses, and fact sheets and materials.

252 www.thenationalcouncil.org
National Council for Commuity Behavioral Healthcare

A network for sharing information and provding assistance among those working in the healthcare management field.

253 www.well.com
Web of Addictions

Links to fact sheets from trustworthy sources.

Directories & Databases

254 **National Directory of Drug and Alcohol Abuse Treatment Programs**
SAMHSA
1 Choke Cherry Road
Rockville, MD 20857
877-SAM-SA 7
www.store.samhsa.gov

Directory of substance abuse treatment programs for use by persons seeking treatment and by professionals. Lists facility name, address, telephone number and services offered. Updated annually. Searchable on-line version on web site. CD-ROM

Anxiety Disorders

Introduction

It is perfectly normal to feel worried or nervous sometimes, especially if there is an obvious reason: a loved one is late coming home; a pending yearly evaluation meeting at work; an important social event is looming. Even when you are nervous or anxious with good cause, you continue performing life's functions adequately. Indeed, some anxiety is not only normal, it is necessary, helping us to avoid trouble and danger - like preparing for a test in school, or making sure your child is safely buckled into a car. But if you can't rid yourself of your worry, you worry all the time, and about everything. If people close to you comment that you seem bothered and unlike yourself, or if your nervousness is affecting your relationships and your work, it is time to seek help. Sometimes a person who suffers from persistent anxiety turns to alcohol or other drugs in an effort to seek relief.

Different kinds of Anxiety Disorders have been identified. Several of the most prevalent are discussed in detail below. Treatment is tailored to the particular disorder and has become more effective as a result.

SYMPTOMS

Agoraphobia
• Usually involves fears connected with being outside the home and alone;
• Anxiety about being in places or situations from which it is difficult or embarrassing to escape (e.g., in the middle seat of a row in a theatre) or in which help may not be immediately available (as in an airplane);
• Such situations are avoided or endured with distress and fear of having a panic attack;
• The anxiety significantly interferes with the individual's ability to participate normally in work, domestic, and/or recreational activities.

Social Anxiety Disorder
• Fear of being humiliated or embarrassed in a social situation with strangers or where other people are watching;
• Being in the situation causes intense anxiety, sometimes with panic attacks;
• Realizing that the fear is irrational;
• Unlike simple shyness, the fear leads to avoidance of important or uncomplicated social situations and interferes with the ability to function at work or with friends.

General Anxiety Disorder
• Excessive worry and anxiety on most days for at least six months about several events or activities such as work or school performance;
• Difficulty in controlling the worry;
• The anxiety is connected with at least three of the following: restlessness/feeling on edge; being easily tired; difficulty concentrating; irritability; muscle tension; difficulty falling/staying asleep or restless sleep;
• The anxiety or physical symptoms seriously affect the person's social life, work life, or other important areas.

Phobias
• Persistent, unreasonable, and exaggerated fear of the presence or anticipated presence of a particular object or situation (e.g., snake, flying in an airplane; blood);
• The presence of such an object or situation triggers immediate anxiety which may be a panic attack;
• Knowledge that the fear is exaggerated and unreasonable;
• The phobic situation is either avoided or experienced with extreme distress;
• The avoidance, fearful anticipation, and distress seriously affects the person's normal routine, work and social activities, and relationships.

Panic Disorder
A panic attack is a period of intense fear in which four or more of the following symptoms escalate suddenly, reaching a peak within ten minutes, after which they diminish:
• Palpitations and pounding;
• Rapid heart beat;
• Sweating;
• Trembling or shaking;
• Shortness of breath;
• Feeling of choking;
• Chest pain;
• Nausea;
• Feeling dizzy or faint;
• Feelings of unreality or detachment;
• Fear of losing control or going crazy;
• Fear of dying;
• Numbness or tingling;
• Chills or hot flashes.

Obsessive Compulsive Disorder (OCD)
Individuals with OCD have overwhelming obsessions and/or compulsions. Obsessions are repeated, intrusive, unwanted thoughts that cause distressing emotions such as anxiety or anguish; a compulsion is a ceaseless urge to do something to lessen the anxiety caused by the obsession.
• Recurrent and persistent thoughts, impulses or images that are experienced as intrusive and inapororiate and that cause marked anxiety or distress;
• Thoughts and worries are not simply excessive worries about eal-life problems, but can be inflated misinterpretations of actions and words of others;
• Repetitive behaviors that the person feels driven to perform in response to an obsession, or according to rules that must be applied rigidly;
• The person recognizes that the obsessions or compulsions are unreasonable;
• The obsessions or compulsions cause marked distress, are time consuming, or significantly interfere with the person's normal routine, occupational or academic functioning, or usual social activities.

ASSOCIATED FEATURES

Anxiety can be acute and intense such as the fear of imminent death in a panic attack or it can be experienced as the state of chronic nagging worry in Generalized Anxiety Disorder. Whatever its intensity or frequency, it persists over time. One of the hallmarks of Anxiety Disorders is that the person is unable to control the anxiety, even when he or she knows it is exaggerated and unreasonable, as in Obsessive Compulsive Disorder. To other people, the person may seem edgy, irritable, to have unexpected outbursts of anger, or to be consumed by an unreasonable fear. For the anxious person, the problem takes up time and effort and becomes a major preoccupation. The OCD affected persona can further that time and expenditure of energy in creating a ritual to manage the obsession, such as performing an action a specific number of times in a particular manner. People with PTSD can go to lengths to avoid trigger situations, seriously disrupting normal life.

In addition to the psychological effects (and entangled with them) are the physical effects, that is, a frequent or constant state of physical arousal and tension. This can lead to gastrointestinal upset, headaches, and cardiovascular disease. Using alcohol or drugs to resolve the problem is common but ineffective and dangerous. Anxiety Disorders negatively affect all aspects of life-family, work, and friends.

PREVALENCE

Anxiety Disorders are the most common psychiatric disorders in the U.S. Anxiety Disorders are approximately twice as common in women as in men.

Obsessive Compulsive Disorder usually begins in adolescence or early adulthood, but may begin in childhood. In males the onset is earlier (between 6 and 15 years old) than for women (between 20 and 29), though it is equally common in both.

PTSD can occur at any point in any person's life, and more often occur in women and children than in men. One might imagine that a person would become resistant to the effects of repeated traumas, but in fact each traumatic event furthers the individual's vulnerability over future events.

TREATMENT OPTIONS

It is very important to have a full evaluation so that a proper diagnosis can be made. In general, people should have a primary care evaluation as part of the diagnostic process for all disorders, so as to rule out a general medical condition that could be causing the signs and symptoms. For example, hyperthyroidism can cause anxiety problems; hypothyroidism can look like depression. Self medication with alcohol, tranquilizers, or other drugs is dangerous and can lead to serious drug abuse. Many people who abuse drugs are suffering from an underlying Anxiety Disorder. Treatment will vary depending on which of the Anxiety Disorders is diagnosed. Medications, psychotherapy or both will be prescribed. Some psychotherapies which have proven helpful in certain cases are cognitive-behavioral therapies, including exposure therapy, and eye movement desensitisation reprogramming (EMDR). Benzodiazepines, or minor tranquillizers, can be useful for the acute treatment of anxiety symptoms; care must be taken, because these medications have addictive potential. Selective Serotonin Reuptake Inhibitors, or SSRIs, which were originally developed as Antidepressants, have proved to be effective in several Anxiety Disorders and are now the mainstays of treatment. Since new drugs are frequently introduced, and already approved medications given new therapeutic indications by the USDA, it is wise to consult an expert or recent expert reference before making a treatment decision.

Patients with OCD may benefit from behavioral therapy and/or a variety of medications. Particularly effective is exposure and response prevention therapy, in which a therapist carefully exposes the patient to situations that cause anxiety and provoke the obsessive compulsive behavior. Slowly the patient learns to decrease and eventually end the ritualistic behaviors.

With the PTSD patient, SSRI's are useful in conjunction with behavioral therapies and EMDR. These therapies allow the patient to recognize the thought process that results in the traumatic stress conditions, and over time, learn to experience certain stimuli without distress. Sufferers of PTSD will also benefit from support groups and confidence and esteem building exercises.

It is important to note that suddenly stopping an SSRI can cause rebound symptoms including sleeplessness, headaches, and irritability. Medications should be tapered under the care of a physician.

Associations & Agencies

256 A.I.M. Agoraphics in Motion
PO Box 725363
Berkley, MI 48072
248-547-0400
E-mail: anny@ameritech.net
www.www.aimforrecovery.com

James Fortune, President
Robert Diedrich, Vice President
Jonathan Gogoleski, Treasurer
Mary Ann Gogoleski, SWT Director

AIM is a nationwide, nonprofit, support group organization, committed to the support and recovery of those suffering with anxiety disorders, and their families.
Year Founded: 1983

257 Anxiety and Depression Association of America
8701 Georgia Avenue
Suite 412
Silver Spring, MD 20910-3643
240-485-1001
Fax: 240-485-1035
www.adaa.org

Mark H Pollack, MD, President
Alies Muskin, Executive Director
Murray Stein, MD, MPH, Treasurer
Cindy J Aaronson, MSW, PhD, Secretary

A national non profit organization dedicated exclusively to promoting the prevention, treatment, and cure of anxiety disorders and improving the lives of all people touched by these disorders.
Year Founded: 1980

258 Anxiety and Phobia Treatment Center
White Plains Hospital Center
41 East Post Road
White Plains, NY 10601
914-681-1038
E-mail: jchessa@wphospital.org
www.www.phobia-anxiety.org

Fredric Neuman, M.D., Director
Martin Seif, Ph.D, Associate Director
Judy Lake Chessa, L.M.S.W, Coordinator

Treatment groups for individuals suffering from phobias. Deals with fears through contextual therapy, a treatment and study of the phobia in the actual setting in which the phobic reactions occur.
Year Founded: 1971

259 Association of Traumatic Stress Specialists
500 Old Buncombe Road
500 Old Buncombe Road
Greenville, SC 29617

864-294-4337
Fax: 864-294-4384
E-mail: admin@atss.info
www.atss.info

Chrys Harris, PhD., CTS, President
Bill Mc Dermott, C.Psych, CTS, Vice President
Linda Hood, B.A., CTSS, Secretary
Diane Travers, LCSW, CTS, Chair of Certification Board

Helps the traumatized through international service, education and professional development

260 Career Assessment & Planning Services
Goodwill Industries-Suncoast
10596 Gandy Boulevard
PO Box 14456
St. Petersburg, FL 33702
727-523-1512
888-279-1988
Fax: 727-563-9300
E-mail: gw.marketing@goodwill-suncoast.com
www.goodwill-suncoast.org

Oscar J Horton, Chairman
R. Lee Waits, President and CEO Emeritus
Deborah A. Passerini, President, Board Officer
Martin W Gladysz, Senior Vice Chairman

Provides a comprehensive assessment, which can predict current and future employment and potential adjustment factors for physically, emotionally, or developmentally disabled persons who may be unemployed or underemployed. Assessments evaluate interests, aptitudes, academic achievements, and physical abilities (including dexterity and coordination) through coordinated testing, interviewing and behavioral observations.

Year Founded: 1954

261 Center for Mental Health Services (CMHS)
1 Choke Cherry Road
Room 6-1057
Rockville, MD 20857
240-276-1310
877-726-4727
Fax: 240-276-1320
TDD: 800-487-4889
E-mail: info@mentalhealth.org
www.beta.samhsa.gov/about-us/who-we-are/offices-center

Michael E Etzinger, B.S.M.E, , M.B., SAMHSA Executive Officer, Director
Paolo Del Vecchio, M.S.W, Director, Center for Mental Healt
Deborah Baldwin, M.P.A, Acting Director, Consumer Affairs
Elizabeth Lopez, Ph.D, Acting Deputy Director

CMHS leads Federal efforts to treat mental illnesses by promoting mental health and by preventing the development or worsening of mental illness when possible. Congress created CMHS to bring new hope to adults who have serious mental illnesses and to children with serious emotional disorders. CMHS provides information about mental health via a toll-free the web site, and more than 600 publications. Developed for users of mental health services and their families, the general public, policy makers, providers, and the media.

Year Founded: 1992

262 Freedom From Fear
308 Seaview Avenue
Staten Island, NY 10305-2246
718-351-1717
Fax: 718-667-8893
E-mail: help@freedomfromfear.org
www.freedomfromfear.org

Irwin Freeman, President
Mary Guardino, Founder, Executive Director
Mark Sisti, PhD, 1st Vice President
Jonathan W Stewart, MD, Treasurer

The mission of Freedom From Fear is to aid and counsel individuals and their families who suffer from anxiety and depressive illness.

Year Founded: 1984

263 International Critical Incident Stress Foundation
3290 Pine Orchard Lane
Suite 106
Ellicott City, MD 21042-2254
410-750-9600
Fax: 410-750-9601
E-mail: info@icisf.org
www.icisf.org

Becky Stroll, LCSW, CTS, Chair of the Board
Donald Howell, Executive Director
Richard Barton, Chief Executive Officer
Lisa Joubert, Director of Finance

A nonprofit, open membership foundation dedicated to the prevention and mitigation of disabling stress by education, training and support services for all emergency service professionals.

264 International Obsessive Compulsive Disorder Foundation
18 Tremont Street
Suite 903
Boston, MA 02196
617-973-5801
Fax: 617-973-5803
E-mail: info@iocdf.org
www.ocfoundation.org

Denise Egan Stack LMHC, President
Jeff Szymanski, PhD, Executive Director
Susan B Dailey, Vice President
Michael J Stack, CFA, Treasurer

For sufferers of obsessive-compulsive disorder and their families and friends. To educate the public and professional communities about OCD and related disorders; to provide assistance to individuals with OCD and related disorders, their family and friends, and to support research into the causes and effective treatments.

Year Founded: 1986

265 International Society for Traumatic Stress Studies
111 Deer Lake Road
Suite 100
Deerfield, IL 60015-1591
847-480-9028
Fax: 847-480-9282
E-mail: istss@istss.org
www.www.istss.org/Home.htm

Nancy Kassam-Adams, PhD, President
Meaghan O'Donnell, PhD, Vice President
Rick Koepke, Executive Director
Grete A Dyb, MD, PhD, Treasurer

Provides a forum for sharing research, clinical strategies, public policy concerns and theoretical formulation on trauma in the US and worldwide. Dedicated to discovery and dissemination of knowledge and to the stimulation of policy, program and services.

Year Founded: 1985

266 Mental Health America
2000 North Beauregard Street
6th Floor
Alexandria, VA 22311
703-684-7722
800-969-6642
Fax: 703-684-5968
E-mail: info@mentalhealthamerica.net
www.www.mentalhealthamerica.net

Ann Boughtin, Chair
David L Shern, Ph.D., Interim President and CEO
Dianne Felton, Chief Operating Officer
Mike Turner, VP of Development

MHA is the leading advocacy agency addressing the full spectrum of mental and substance use conditions and their effects nationwide. MHA's actions inform, support, and enable mental wellness and recovery from mental illness including anxiety and post traumatic stress disorder.

267 NAPCSE National Association of Parents with Children in Special Education
3642 E Sunnydale Drive
Chandler Heights, AZ 85142
800-754-4421
Fax: 800-424-0371
E-mail: contact@napcse.org
www.www.napcse.org

Dr George Giuliani, President
Dr Roger Pierangelo, Vice President

The NAPCSE is dedicated to ensuring that all children and adolescents with special needs and anxiety receive the best education possible. NAPCSE serves the interest of the parents with children in special education programs by giving them numerous resources within the field of special education. By having an association that they can truly call their own, parents with children in special education now have an association that is completely devoted to their needs.

268 National Alliance on Mental Illness
3803 North Fairfax Drive
Suite 100
Arlington, VA 22203-3080
703-524-7600
800-950-6264
Fax: 703-524-9094
E-mail: helpline@nami.org
www.nami.org

Keris Jan Myrick, MBA, MS, PhD., President
Mary Giliberti, J.D, Executive Director
Jim Payne, J.D, First Vice President
David Levy, Chief Financial Officer

Year Founded: 1969

269 National Anxiety Foundation
3135 Custer Drive
Lexington, KY 40517-4001
859-272-7166
www.www.lexington-on-line.com

Stephen Cox MD, President
Linda Vernon Blair, Vice President
C. Todd Strecker, Secretary, Treasurer

To alleviate suffering and to save lives by educating the public about anxiety disorders.

270 National Association for the Dually Diagnosed (NADD)
132 Fair Street
Kingston, NY 12401
845-331-4336
800-331-5362
Fax: 845-331-4569
E-mail: info@thenadd.org
www.thenadd.org

Donna McNELIS, PhD, President
Robert J Fletcher DSW, Chief Executive Officer
Dan Baker, PhD, Vice President
Julia Pearce, Secretary

Nonprofit organization designed to promote interest of professional and parent development with resources for individuals who have the coexistence of mental illness and mental retardation. Provides conferences, educational services and training materials to professionals, parents, concerned citizens and service organizations.

Year Founded: 1983

271 National Council Community Behavioral Health
1701 K Street NW
Suite 400
Washington, DC 20006
202-684-7457
Fax: 202-386-9391
E-mail: communications@thenationalcouncil.org
www.www.thenationalcouncil.org

Jeffrey Walter, Chair
Linda Rosenberg, MSW, President & CEO
Jeannie Campbell, Executive VP and Chief Operating
David Ptaszek, LCSW, Vice Chair

The National Council Community Behavioral Health organization works hard to give nearly 6 million adults, children and families with mental illnesses and addiction disorders a chance to recover and lead productive and successful lives.

272 National Mental Health Consumers' Self-Help Clearinghouse
1211 Chestnut Street
Suite 1100
Philadelphia, PA 19107-4103
215-751-1810
800-553-4539
Fax: 215-636-6312
E-mail: info@mhselfhelp.org
www.mhselfhelp.org

Joseph Rogers, Executive Director/ Founder
Susan Rogers, Director
Britani Nestel, Program Specialist
Christa Burkett, Technical Assistance Coordinator

A national consumer technical assistance center that has played a major role in the development of the mental health consumer movement.

Year Founded: 1986

273 SAMHSA's National Mental Health Information Center
PO Box 42557
Washington, DC 20015-557
240-221-4021
800-789-2647
Fax: 240-221-4295
TDD: 866-889-2647
www.mentalhealth.samhsa.gov

274 Territorial Apprehensiveness (TERRAP) Programs
14 Wood Lake Square
Houston, TX 77063-3207
713-266-5111
800-274-6242
Fax: 337-474-2782
E-mail: Lisavcano@gmail.com
www.terraphouston.com

Lisa V Cano, LCSW, Owner, Clinical Director

Developed by Dr. Arthur Hardy in the 1950's, Territorial Apprehensiveness Programs are designed to assist in the treatment of territorial, social and generalized anxieties.

Year Founded: 1981

275 The Center for Family Support
2811 Zulette Avenue
Bronx, NY 10461
718-518-1500
Fax: 718-518-8200
E-mail: svernikoff@cfsny.org
www.cfsny.org

Steven Vernikoff, Executive Director
Virgil Seepersad, Director of Finance
Eileen Berg, Director of Quality Assurance
Barbara Greenwald, Associate Executive, Director

The Center for Family Support is committed to providing support and assistance to individuals with developmental and related disabilities, and to the family members who care for them.

Year Founded: 1954

276 The Selective Mutism Foundation Inc.
PO Box 13133
Attention: Carolyn Miller
Sissonville, WV 25360-0133
E-mail: info@selectivemutismfoundation.org
www.selectivemutismfoundation.org

Sue Newman, Co-Founder/Director
Carolyn Miller, Co-Founder/Director
Diane Pombier, Treasurer

Promote further research, advocacy, social acceptance, and the understanding of Selective Mutism as a debilitating disorder

Year Founded: 1991

Books

277 100 Q&A About Panic Disorder
Jones and Bartlett Publishers
5 Wall Street
Burlington, MA 01803
978-443-5000
800-832-0034
Fax: 978-443-8000
E-mail: info@jblearning.com
www.jblearning.com

Carol Berman, MD, Author
Ty Field, Chief Executive Officer
James Homer, President
Alison Pendergast, Chief Marketing Officer

$22.95

136 pages Year Founded: 1983 ISBN 9-780763-77-6

278 Acceptance and Commitment Therapy for Anxiety Disorders
NewHarbinger Publications
5674 Shattuck Avenue
Oakland, CA 94609-1662
510-652-0215
800-748-6273
Fax: 800-652-1613
E-mail: customerservice@newharbinger.com
www.newharbinger.com

Georg H Eifert, PhD, Author
John P Forsyth, PhD, Author
Steven C Hayes, PhD, Author

The first step-by-step professional book that teaches how to apply and integrate acceptance and mindfulness for treatment with anxiety disorders. $59.95

304 pages Year Founded: 1973 ISBN 1-572244-27-5

279 After the Crash: Assessment and Treatment of Motor Vehicle Accident Survivors
American Psychological Publishing
750 First Street, NorthEast
Washington, DC 20002-4242
202-336-5500
800-374-2721
Fax: 202-336-5518
TDD: 202-336-6123
TTY: 202-336-6123
www.apa.org

Edward B Blanchard, PhD, ABPP, Author
Edward J Hickling, PsyD, Author
Suzanne Bennett-Johnson, PhD, President

In this timely second edition, written in a clear and lucid style and illustrated by a wealth of charts, guides, case studies, and clinical advice, the authors report on new, international research and provide updates on their own long-standing research protocols within the groundbreaking Alabny MVA Project. $29.95

475 pages Year Founded: 1892 ISBN 1-591470-70-6

280 Aging and Post Traumatic Stress Disorder
American Psychiatric Publishing, Inc.
1000 Wilson Boulevard
Suite 1825
Arlington, VA 22209-3901
703-907-7322
800-368-5777

Fax: 703-907-1091
E-mail: appi@psych.org
www.appi.org

Robert E Hales MD, Editor-in-Chief
Saul Levin, M.D., M.P.A., CEO and Medical Director
John McDuffie, Editorial Director
Laura W Roberts, M.D., Deputy Editor

Provides both literature reviews and data about animal and clinical studies and training for important current concepts of aging, the stress response and the interaction between them. *$85.00*

280 pages ISBN 0-880485-13-5

281 **An End to Panic: Breakthrough Techniques for Overcoming Panic Disorder**
NewHarbinger Publications
5674 Shattuck Avenue
Oakland, CA 94609-1662
510-652-0215
800-748-6273
Fax: 800-652-1613
E-mail: customerservice@newharbinger.com
www.newharbinger.com

Elke Zuercher-White, PhD, Author
Elke Zuercher-White, Author

A state of the art treatment program covers breathing re-training, taking charge of fear fueling thoughts, overcoming the fear of physical symptoms, coping with phobic situations, avoiding relapse, and living in the here and now. *$24.95*

232 pages Year Founded: 1973 ISBN 1-572241-13-8

282 **Anxiety & Phobia Workbook**
NewHarbinger Publications
5674 Shattuck Avenue
Oakland, CA 94609-1662
510-652-0215
800-748-6273
Fax: 800-652-1613
E-mail: customerservice@newharbinger.com
www.newharbinger.com

Edmund J. Bourne, PhD, Author

This comprehensive guide is recommended to those struggling with anxiety disorders. Includes step by step instructions for the crucial cognitive - behavioral techniques that have given real help to hundreds of thousands of readers struggling with anxiety disorders. *$24.95*

496 pages Year Founded: 1973 ISBN 1-572248-91-5

283 **Anxiety Cure: Eight Step-Program for Getting Well**
John Wiley & Sons
605 3rd Avenue
New York, NY 10158-180
212-850-6301
E-mail: info@wiley.com

Stephen M Smith, Pres., Chief Executive Officer
Ellis E Cousens, EVP, CFO, Operations Officer
William J Arlington, Senior Vice President of HR
Edward J Melando, VP, Corporate Controller

Anxiety disorders are the most common type of emotional trouble and among the most treatable. Dupont provides a practical guide featuring a step-by-step program for curing the six kinds of anxiety. *$14.95*

256 pages ISBN 0-471247-01-4

284 **Anxiety Disorders**
Cambridge University Press
40 W 20th Street
New York, NY 10011-4211
212-924-3900
800-872-7423
Fax: 212-691-3239
E-mail: marketing@cup.org
www.cup.org

Stephen Bourne, Chief Press Executive / Director

This comprehensive text covers all the anxiety disorders found in the latest DSM and ICD classifications. Provides detailed information about seven principal disorders, including anxiety in the medically ill. For each disorder, the book covers diagnosis criteria, epidemiology, etiology and pathogenesis, clinical features, natural history and different diagnosis. Describes treatment approaches, both psychological and pharmacological. *$105.00*

394 pages ISBN 0-521515-57-3

285 **Anxiety and Its Disorders**
Guilford Press
72 Spring Street
New York, NY 10012-4068
212-431-9800
800-365-7006
Fax: 212-966-6708
E-mail: info@guilford.com

Bob Matloff, President
David H Barlow, Author

Incorporating recent advances from cognitive science and neurobiology on the mechanisms of anxiety and using emotion theory as basic theoretical framework. Ties theory and research of emerging clinical knowledge to create a new model of anxiety with profound implications for treatment. *$76.50*

704 pages ISBN 1-572304-30-8

286 **Anxiety, Phobias, and Panic**
Grand Central Publishing
322 South Enterprise Blvd
Lebanon, IN 46052
800-759-0190
www.www.hachettebookgroup.com

Reneau Z Peurifoy, Author
Kenneth Michaels, EVP, Chief Operating Officer
Chris Barba, EVP, Sales and Marketing
Sophie Cottrell, VP, Communications Director

Congratulations! You are about to start a journey along the path to freedom.

400 pages Year Founded: 1837 ISBN 0-446692-77-9

287 **Anxiety, Phobias, and Panic: Step-By-Step Program for Regaining Control of Your Life**
Time Warner Books
3 Center Plaza
Boston, MA 02108-2084
800-759-0190
Fax: 800-331-1664
E-mail: sales@aoltwbg.com
www.twbookmark.com

Reneau Z Peurifoy, Author

Helps you identify stress and reduce stress anxiety, recognize and change distorted mental habits, stop thinking and acting like a victim, eliminate the excessive need for approval, make anger your friend and ally, stand up for yourself and feel good about yourself, and conquer your fears and take charge of your life. *$11.00*

384 pages ISBN 0-446670-53-7

288 Beyond Anxiety and Phobia
NewHarbinger Publications
5674 Shattuck Avenue
Oakland, CA 94609-1662
510-652-0215
800-748-6273
Fax: 800-652-1613
E-mail: customerservice@newharbinger.com
www.newharbinger.com

Edmund J. Bourne, PhD, Author

Helping people try to get beyond anxiety and their phobia. *$24.95*

264 pages Year Founded: 1973 ISBN 1-572242-29-9

289 Biology of Anxiety Disorders
American Psychiatric Publishing, Inc.
1000 Wilson Boulevard
Suite 1825
Arlington, VA 22209-3901
703-907-7322
800-368-5777
Fax: 703-907-1091
E-mail: appi@psych.org
www.appi.org

Rudolf Hoehn-Saric, M.D, Editor
Daniel R McLeod, Ph.D, Editor
John McDuffie, Editorial Director

Provides the most recent data on the neurobiology and pathophysiology af anxiety from a variety of perspectives. *$32.00*

280 pages Year Founded: 1993 ISBN 0-880484-76-4

290 Boy Who Couldn't Stop Washing
Penguin Group
375 Hudson Street
New York, NY 10014-3672
212-366-2000
800-631-8571
Fax: 212-366-2933
E-mail: online@penguinputnam.com

John Makinson, Chairman, CEO
Coram Williams, Chief Financial Officer
David Shanks, CEO
Judith Rapoport, Author

The Boy Who Wouldn't Stop Washing: Experience and Treatment of Obsessive-Compulsive Disorder. A comprehensive treatment of obsessive-compulsive disorder that summarizes evidence that the disorder is neurobiological. It also describes the effect of medication combined with behavioral therapy. *$7.99*

304 pages Year Founded: 1991 ISBN 0-451172-02-7

291 Brain Lock: Free Yourself from Obsessive Compulsive Behavior
Harper Collins
10 E 53rd Street
New York, NY 10022-5299
212-207-7000

Brian Murray, Group President
Jeffrey M Schwartz, Author

A simple four-step method for overcoming OCD that is so effective, it's now used in academic treatment centers throughout the world. Proved by brain-imaging tests to actually alter the brain's chemistry, this method dosen't rely on psychopharmaceuticals but cognitive self-therapy and behavior modification to develop new patterns of response. Offers real-life stories of actual patients. Paperback. *$14.99*

256 pages Year Founded: 1997 ISBN 0-060987-11-1

292 Childhood Obsessive Compulsive Disorder
Sage Publications
2455 Teller Road
Thousand Oaks, CA 91320-2234
805-499-0721
800-818-7243
Fax: 800-583-2665
E-mail: info@sagepub.com
www.sagepub.com

Greta Francis, Author
Rod A Gragg, Author
Stephen Bar, Managing Director
Ziyad Marar, Deputy Managing Director

Childhood Obsessive Compulsive Disorder: Developmental Clinical Psychology and Psychiatry. *$62.00*

120 pages Year Founded: 1996 ISBN 0-803959-22-2

293 Comorbidity of Mood and Anxiety Disorders
American Psychiatric Publishing, Inc.
1000 Wilson Boulevard
Suite 1825
Arlington, VA 22209-3901
703-907-7322
800-368-5777
Fax: 703-907-1091
E-mail: appi@psych.org
www.appi.org

Jack D Maser, Ph.D., Editor
C. Robert Cloninger, M.D., Editor
John McDuffie, Editorial Director
Jack Maser PhD, Author

Presents a systematic examination of the concurrence of different symptoms and syndromes in patients with anxiety or mood disorders. *$147.00*

888 pages Year Founded: 1990 ISBN 0-880483-24-5

294 Compulsive Acts: A Psychiatrist's Tales of Rituals and Obsessions
University of California Press
2120 Berkeley Way
Berkeley, CA 94704-1012
510-642-4247
Fax: 510-643-7127
www.ucpress.edu

Elias Aboujaoude, Author
Alison Mudditt, Director
Elias Aboujaude, Author

The author tells stories inspired by memorable patients he has treated, taking readers from his initial contact through the stages of the doctor-patient relationship. Stories include a man who can't let anyone get within a certain distance of his nose, two kleptomaniacs, an Internet addict who chooses virtual life over real life, a professor with a dangerous gambling habit, and others with equally debilitating compulsive conditions. *$29.95*

192 pages Year Founded: 2008 ISSN 978-0520255678ISBN 0-520255-67-4

295 Concise Guide to Anxiety Disorders
American Psychiatric Publishing, Inc.
1000 Wilson Boulevard
Suite 1825
Arlington, VA 22209-3901
703-907-7322
800-368-5777
Fax: 703-907-1091
E-mail: appi@psych.org
www.appi.org

Eric Hollander, M.D., Author
Daphne Simeon, M.D, Author
John McDuffie, Editorial Director
Eric Hollander, MD, Author

Concise Guide to Anxiety Disorders summarizes the latest research and translates it into practical treatment strategies for the best clinical outcomes. Designed for daily use in the clinical setting, it serves as an instant library of current information, quick to access and easy to understand. Every clinician who diagnoses and treats patients with anxiety disorders-including psychiatrists, residents and medical students, psychologists, and mental health professionals-will find this book invaluable for making informed treatment decisions. *$53.00*

272 pages Year Founded: 2003 ISBN 1-585620-80-7

296 Consumer's Guide to Psychiatric Drugs
NewHarbinger Publications
5674 Shattuck Avenue
Oakland, CA 94609-1662
510-652-0215
800-748-6273
Fax: 800-652-1613
E-mail: customerservice@newharbinger.com
www.newharbinger.com

Mary C. Talaga, Author
John D. Preston, Author
John H. O'Neal, Author

Helps consumers understand what treatment options are available and what side effects to expect. Covers possible interactions with other drugs, medical conditions and other concerns. Explains how each drug works, and offers detailed information about treatments for depression, bipolar disorder, anxiety and sleep disorders, as well as other conditions. *$16.95*

340 pages Year Founded: 1973 ISBN 1-572241-11-X

297 Coping with Anxiety
NewHarbinger Publications
5674 Shattuck Avenue
Oakland, CA 94609-1662
510-652-0215
800-748-6273
Fax: 800-652-1613
E-mail: customerservice@newharbinger.com
www.newharbinger.com

Edmund J. Bourne, PhD, Author
Lorna Garano, Author

Ten simple steps, proven to help relieve anxiety. *$ 14.95*

176 pages Year Founded: 1973 ISBN 1-572243-20-1

298 Coping with Post-Traumatic Stress Disorder
Rosen Publishing Group
29 East 21st Street
New York, NY 10010-6209
212-777-3017
800-237-9932
Fax: 888-436-4643
E-mail: info@rosenpub.com
www.rosenpublishing.com

Carolyn Simpson, Author
Dwain Simpson, Author

$33.25

176 pages Year Founded: 1950 ISBN 0-823934-56-X

299 Coping with Social Anxiety: The Definitive Guide to Effective Treatment Options
Holt Paperbacks
175 Fifth Avenue
New York, NY 10010-7703
646-307-5151
Fax: 212-633-0748
E-mail: customerservice@mpsvirginia.com
www.us.macmillan.com

Eric Hollander, Author
Nickolas Bakalar, Author

An essential guide for the 5.3 million American sufferers of social anxiety from a leading psychiatrist and researcher. *$17.00*

256 pages Year Founded: 2005 ISBN 0-805075-82-8

300 Coping with Trauma: A Guide to Self Understanding
8730 Georgia Avenue
Suite 600
Silver Spring, MD 20910-3643
240-485-1001
E-mail: AnxDis@adaa.org
www.adaa.org

Alies Muskin, Manager
Michelle Alonso, Communications/Membership

301 Don't Panic: Taking Control of Anxiety Attacks
Anxiety Disorders Association of America
8701 Georgia Avenue
Suite 412
Silver Spring, MD 20910-3643
240-485-1001
Fax: 240-485-1035
E-mail: AnxDis@adaa.org
www.adaa.org

Mark H Pollack, MD, President
Alies Muskin, Executive Director
Murray Stein, MD, MPH, Treasurer
Cindy J Aaronson, MSW, PhD, Secretary

Book on overcoming panic and anxiety.

Year Founded: 2009

302 **Drug Therapy and Anxiety Disorders**
Mason Crest Publishers
450 Parkway Drive
Suite D
Broomall, PA 19008-4017
610-543-6200
866-627-2665
Fax: 610-543-3878
E-mail: dtaylor@masoncrest.com
www.masoncrest.com

Shirley Brinkerhoff, Author
Dan Hilferty, President
Michelle Luke, Director of Marketing
Michael Toglia, Special Sales

This volume provides readers with a clear introduction to anxiety disorders. Numerous case studies give insight into the world of mental disorders and helps readers understand the symptoms and treatments of this disorder, which includes: generalized anxiety disorder, social phobia, specific phobia, obsessive-compulsive disorder (covered more extensively in a separate column), post-traumatic stress disorder, and panic disorder.

128 pages ISBN 1-590845-61-7

303 **Drug Therapy and Obsessive-Compulsive Disorder**
Mason Crest Publishers
450 Parkway Drive
Suite D
Broomall, PA 19008-4017
610-543-6200
866-627-2665
Fax: 610-543-3878
E-mail: dtaylor@masoncrest.com
www.masoncrest.com

Shirley Brinkerhoff, Author
Dan Hilferty, President
Michelle Luke, Director of Marketing
Michael Toglia, Special Sales

This volume provides readers with a clear and understandable introduction to obsessive-compulsive disorder (OCD). Numerous case studies are included, which give insight into the world of those who experience this disorder; these anecdotes also help readers understand the symptoms and treatments of this disease. Famous historical figures who suffered from OCD, such as Samuel Johnson (1709-1784) and Howard Hughes (1905-1975) are mentioned as well.

128 pages ISBN 1-590845-69-2

304 **Dying of Embarrassment: Help for Social Anxiety and Social Phobia**
NewHarbinger Publications
5674 Shattuck Avenue
Oakland, CA 94609-1662
510-652-0215
800-748-6273
Fax: 800-652-1613
E-mail: customerservice@newharbinger.com
www.newharbinger.com

Barbara G Markway, Author
C Alec Pollard, Author
Teresa Flynn, Author
Cheryl N Carmin, Author

Clear, supportive instructions for assessing your fears, improving or developing new social skills, and changing self defeating thinking patterns. *$13.95*

208 pages Year Founded: 1973 ISBN 1-879237-23-7

305 **Effecive Treatments for PTSD: Practice Guidelines from the International Society for Traumatic Stress Studies**
The Guilford Press
72 Spring Street
New York, NY 10012-4019
212-431-9800
800-365-7006
Fax: 212-966-6708
E-mail: info@guilford.com

Bob Matloff, President
Edna Foa, Author
Terence Keane, Author
Matthew Friedman, Author

The treatment guidelines presented in this book were developed under the auspices of the PTSD Treatment Guidelines Task Force established by the Board of Directors. *$38.25*

658 pages Year Founded: 2010 ISBN 1-609181-49-9

306 **Effective Treatments for PTSD**
Guilford Press
72 Spring Street
New York, NY 10012-4068
212-431-9800
800-365-7006
Fax: 212-966-6708
E-mail: info@guilford.com

Bob Matloff, President

Represents the collaborative work of experts across a range of theoretical orientations and professional backgrounds. Addresses general treatment considerations and methodological issues, reviews and evaluates the salient literature on treatment approaches for children, adolescents and adults. *$44.00*

379 pages ISBN 1-572305-84-3

307 **Emotions Anonymous Book**
Emotions Anonymous International Service Center
PO Box 4245
Saint Paul, MN 55104-0245
651-647-9712
Fax: 651-647-1593
E-mail: info@EmotionsAnonymous.org
www.EmotionsAnonymous.org

Karen Mead, Executive Director

The Big Book of EA: A fellowship of men and women who share their experience, strength and hope with each other, that they may solve their common problem and help others recover from emotional illness. *$15.00*

261 pages ISBN 0-960735-65-5

308 **Encyclopedia of Phobias, Fears, and Anxieties**
Facts on File
132 West 31st Street
17th Floor
New York, NY 10001-3406
212-613-2800
800-322-8755
E-mail: custserv@factsonfile.com

Ronald M Doctor, PhD, Author
Ada Kahn, PhD, Author
Christine Adame, Author

Providing the basic information on common phobias and anxieties, some 2000 entries explain the nature of anxiety disorders, panic attacks, specific phobias, and obsessive-complusive disorders. *$75.00*

592 pages Year Founded: 2000 ISBN 0-816039-89-5

309 Flying Without Fear
NewHarbinger Publications
5674 Shattuck Avenue
Oakland, CA 94609-1662
510-652-0215
800-748-6273
Fax: 800-652-1613
E-mail: customerservice@newharbinger.com
www.newharbinger.com

Duane Brown, Author
Duane Brown, Author

Program to confront fears of flying and guides you through first takeoff and later flights. *$16.95*

184 pages Year Founded: 1973 ISBN 1-572240-42-3

310 Free from Fears: New Help for Anxiety, Panic and Agoraphobia
Anxiety Disorders Association of America
8730 Georgia Avenue
Suite 600
Silver Spring, MD 20910-3643
240-485-1001
E-mail: AnxDis@adaa.org
www.adaa.org

Alies Muskin, Manager
Michelle Alonso, Communications/Membership

Book shows you how to recognize the avoidance trap, combat fears, and modify your behavior for a lasting cure.

311 Freeing Your Child from Anxiety: Powerful, Practical Solutions to Overcome Your Child's Fears, Worries, and Phobias
Broadway Books
1745 Broadway
New York, NY 10019-4368
212-662-0231
E-mail: bwaypub@randomhouse.com

Sherif Isak, Owner
Tamar E Chansky, PhD, Author

From the children: When I was little my mom worked the graveyard shift at the hospital. *$13.99*

320 pages Year Founded: 2008 ISBN 0-307485-11-3

312 Freeing Your Child from Obsessive-Compulsive Disorder: A Powerful, Practical Program for Parents of Children and Adolescents
Three Rivers Publishing
1745 Broadway
New York, NY 10019
212-782-9000
Fax: 212-940-7408
E-mail: crownpublicity@randomhouse.com
www.crownpublishing.com

Tamar Chansky, PhD, Author

Creates a clear road map to understanding and overcoming OCD based on her successful practice treating hundreds of children and teenages with this disorder. *$11.99*

368 pages Year Founded: 2011 ISBN 0-307794-44-4

313 Funny, You Don't Look Crazy: Life With Obsessive Compulsive Disorder
Dilligaf Publishing
64 Court Street
Ellsworth, ME 04605
207-667-5031

An honest look at people who live with Obsessive Compulsive Disorder and those who love them.

128 pages Year Founded: 1994 ISBN 0-963907-00-X

314 Getting Control: Overcoming Your Obsessions and Compulsions
Penguin Putnam
375 Hudson Street
New York, NY 10014-3672
212-366-2000
800-227-9604
Fax: 212-366-2933

David Shanks, CEO
Lee Baer, Author

Updated guide to treating OCD based on clinically proven techniques of behavior therapy. Offers a step-by-step program including assessing symptoms, setting realistic goals and creating specific therapeutic exercises. *$16.00*

272 pages Year Founded: 2000 ISBN 0-452281-77-6

315 Handbook of PTSD: Science and Practice
The Guilford Press
72 Spring Street
New York, NY 10012-4019
212-431-9800
800-365-7006
Fax: 212-966-6708
E-mail: info@guilford.com

Bob Matloff, President
Seymour Weingarten, Editor-in-Chief
Matthew Friedman, Author

Unparalleled in its breadth and depth, this state-of-the-art handbook reviews the latest scientific advances in understanding trauma and PTSD. *$42.50*

592 pages Year Founded: 2010 ISBN 1-609181-74-1

316 Haunted by Combat: Understanding PTSD in War Veterans
Rowman & Littlefield Publishers
4501 Forbes Boulevard
Suite 200
Lanham, MD 20706
301-459-3366
301-459-5748
Fax: 301-429-5748
www.rowman.com

Daryl S Paulson, Author
Stanley Krippner, Author
Jeff Harris, Vice President of Credit
Mike Cornell, Vice President of Operations

Across history, the condition has been called soldier's heart, shell shock, or combat fatigue. *$18.99*

226 pages Year Founded: 2010 ISBN 1-442203-91-4

317 Healing Fear: New Approaches to Overcoming Anxiety
NewHarbinger Publications
5674 Shattuck Avenue
Oakland, CA 94609-1662
510-652-0215
800-748-6273
Fax: 800-652-1613
E-mail: customerservice@newharbinger.com
www.newharbinger.com

Edmund Bourne, PhD, Author

Covers a wide range of healing strategies that help you learn how to relinquish control, discover a unique purpose that is bigger than your particular fears, and find ways to restructure your work and home environments to make them more congruent with the real you. *$ 16.95*

398 pages   Year Founded: 1973 ISBN 1-572241-16-0

318 How to Help Your Loved One Recover from Agoraphobia
Anxiety Disorders Association of America
8730 Georgia Avenue
Suite 600
Silver Spring, MD 20910-3643
240-485-1001
E-mail: AnxDis@adaa.org
www.adaa.org

Alies Muskin, Manager
Michelle Alonso, Communications/Membership

Book is helpful for sufferer and family members to understand what a sufferer is going through. *$45.00*

256 pages

319 I Can't Get Over It: Handbook for Trauma Survivors
NewHarbinger Publications
5674 Shattuck Avenue
Oakland, CA 94609
510-652-0215
800-748-6273
Fax: 800-652-1613
E-mail: customerservice@newharbinger.com
www.newharbinger.com

Aphrodite T Matsakis, PhD, Author

Guides readers through the healing process of recovering from Post Traumatic Stress Disorder. From the emotional experience to the process of healing, this book is written for survivors of all types of trauma including war, sexual abuse, crime, family violence, rape and natural catastrophes. *$16.95*

416 pages   Year Founded: 1973 ISBN 1-572240-58-X

320 Imp of the Mind: Exploring the Silent Epidemic of Obsessive Bad Thoughts
Penguin Putnam
375 Hudson Street
New York, NY 10014-3672
212-366-2000
800-227-9604
Fax: 212-366-2933

David Shanks, CEO
Lee Baer, Author

Draws on new advances to explore the causes of obsessive thoughts, and the difference between harmless and dangerous bad thoughts. *$15.00*

176 pages   Year Founded: 2002 ISBN 0-525945-62-8

321 Integrative Treatment of Anxiety Disorders
American Psychiatric Publishing, Inc.
1000 Wilson Boulevard
Suite 1825
Arlington, VA 22209-3901
703-907-7322
800-368-5777
Fax: 703-907-1091
E-mail: appi@psych.org
www.appi.org

James M Ellison, M.D., M.P.H., Editor
Ron McMillen, Chief Executive Officer
John McDuffie, Editorial Director

An overview of the spectrum of anxiety disorders, and reviews the treatment alternatives. *$67.00*

349 pages   Year Founded: 1996 ISBN 0-880487-15-1

322 It's Not All In Your Head: Now Women Can Discover the Real Causes of their Most Misdiagnosed Health Problems
Anxiety Disorders Association of America
8730 Georgia Avenue
Suite 600
Silver Spring, MD 20910-3643
240-485-1001
E-mail: AnxDis@adaa.org
www.adaa.org

Susan Swedo, MD, Author
Henreitta Leonard, MD, Author

This book will present you with information about when, how and from whom to seek treatment.

336 pages

323 Let's Talk Facts About Obsessive Compulsive Disorder
American Psychiatric Publishing, Inc.
1000 Wilson Boulevard
Suite 1825
Arlington, VA 22209-3901
703-907-7322
800-368-5777
Fax: 703-907-1091
E-mail: appi@psych.org
www.appi.org

Robert E Hales MD, Editor-in-Chief
Ron McMillen, Chief Executive Officer
John McDuffie, Editorial Director

$49.00

6 pages   Year Founded: 2006 ISBN 0-890423-87-5

324 Managing Social Anxiety: A Cognitive Behavioral Therapy Approach Client Workbook
Oxford University Press
2001 Evans Road
Carry, NC 27513-2010
919-677-0977
800-445-9714

Fax: 919-677-2673
E-mail: custserv.us@oup.com

Debra Hope, Author
Richard Heimberg, Author
Cynthia Turk, Author

This is a client workbook for those in treatment or considering treatment for social anxiety. *$39.95*

Year Founded: 2010 ISBN 0-195336-68-2

325 Managing Traumatic Stress Risk: A Proactive Approach
Charles C Thomas Publisher Ltd.
2600 South First Street
Springfield, IL 62794-9265
217-789-8980
800-258-8980
Fax: 217-789-9130
www.ccthomas.com

This volume represents the first systematic review of critical incident and disaster hazards, the contextual factors that influence risk, and their implications for traumatic stress risk management. It provides the hazard assessment and risk analysis information which, combined with information on resilience, facilitates the systematic analysis of traumatic stress risk and proactive and methodical development of mitigation and risk reduction strategies. This book is also available in paperback for $41.95. *$61.95*

258 pages Year Founded: 2004 ISBN 0-398075-17-4

326 Master Your Panic and Take Back Your Life: Twelve Treatment Sessions to Overcome High Anxiety
Impact Publishers
PO Box 6016
Atascadero, CA 93423-6016
805-466-5917
800-246-7228
Fax: 805-466-5919
E-mail: info@impactpublishers.com
www.impactpublishers.com

Denise F Beckfield, PhD, Author

Practical, self empowering book on overcoming agoraphobia and debilitating panic attacks is now completely revised and expanded to include the latest information and research findings on relaxation, breathing, medication and other treatments. *$17.95*

304 pages Year Founded: 1970 ISBN 1-886230-47-7

327 Mastery of Your Anxiety and Panic: Workbook
Oxford University Press
2001 Evans Road
Cary, NC 27513-2010
919-677-0977
800-445-9714
Fax: 919-677-2673
E-mail: custserv.us@oup.com

David H Barlow, Author
Michelle G Craske, Author

If you are prone to panic attacks and constantly worry about when the next attack may come, you may suffer from panic disorder and/or agoraphobia. Though panic disorder seems irrational and uncontrollable, it has been proven that a treatment like the one outlined in this book can help you take control of your life. *$31.95*

Year Founded: 2006 ISBN 0-195311-35-3

328 OCD Workbook: Your Guide to Breaking Free From Obsessive-Compulsive Disorder
NewHarbinger Publications
5674 Shattuck Avenue
Oakland, CA 94609-1662
510-652-0215
800-748-6273
Fax: 800-652-1613
E-mail: customerservice@newharbinger.com
www.newharbinger.com

Bruce M Hyman, PhD, LCSW, Author
Cherlene Pedrick, RN, Author

Offers the latest information about the neurobiological causes of obsessive-compulsive disorder(OCD), new developments in medication and other treatment options for the disorder, and a new chapter outlining cutting-edge daily coping strategies for sufferers. *$24.95*

352 pages Year Founded: 1973 ISBN 1-572249-21-9

329 OCD in Children and Adolescents: A Cognitive-Behavioral Treatment Manual
Guilford Press
72 Spring Street
New York, NY 10012-4068
212-431-9800
800-365-7006
Fax: 212-966-6708
E-mail: info@guilford.com

Bob Matloff, President
John S March, Author
Karen Mulle, Author

Written for clinicians, the book includes tips for parents, and treatment guidelines. The cognitive - behavioral approach to OCD has been problematic for many to understand because patients with symptoms of increased anxiety are told that their treatment initially involves further increases in their anxiety levels. The authors provide this in a modified and developmentally appropriate approach. *$39.00*

298 pages Year Founded: 1998 ISBN 1-572302-42-6

330 Obsessive Compulsive Anonymous
Obsessive Compulsive Anonymous
PO Box 215
New Hyde Park, NY 11040-0910
516-739-0662
E-mail: west24th@aol.com
www.obsessivecompulsiveanonymous.com

Literature for the OCA program. *$19.00*

ISBN 0-962806-62-5

331 Obsessive-Compulsive Disorder Casebook
American Psychiatric Publishing, Inc.
1000 Wilson Boulevard
Suite 1825
Arlington, VA 22209-3901
703-907-7322
800-368-5777
Fax: 703-907-1091
E-mail: appi@psych.org
www.appi.org

John H Greist, M.D., Editor
James W Jefferson, M.D., Editor
John McDuffie, Editorial Director

Presents 60 case histories of OCD with a discussion by the author and editors regarding their opinion on each diagnosis. *$39.95*

220 pages ISBN 0-880487-29-1

332 Obsessive-Compulsive Disorder Spectrum
American Psychiatric Publishing, Inc.
1000 Wilson Boulevard
Suite 1825
Arlington, VA 22209-3901
703-907-7322
800-368-5777
Fax: 703-907-1091
E-mail: appi@psych.org
www.appi.org

Jose A Yaryura-Tobias, M.D., Author
Fugen A Neziroglu, Ph.D., Author
John McDuffie, Editorial Director

Comprehensive examination of OCD, related disorders and treatment regimens. *$68.50*

344 pages ISBN 0-880487-07-0

333 Obsessive-Compulsive Disorder in Children and Adolescents: A Guide
Madison Institute of Medicine
7617 Mineral Point Road
Suite 300
Madison, WI 53717-1623
608-827-2470
E-mail: mim@miminc.org
www.factsforhealth.org

Hugh F Johnston, Author
J.Jay Fruehling, Author
J. Jay Frueling, MA, Author

The guide is a comprehensive introduction to obsessive-compulsive disorder for parents who are learning about the illness. Discusses treating symptoms by a combination of behavioral therapy and medication and describes various drugs that can be used with children and adolescents in terms of their effects on brain functioning, symptom control, and side-effects. The book is attuned to the difficulties families of OCD children face. *$5.95*

66 pages ISBN 1-890802-28-X

334 Obsessive-Compulsive Disorder in Children and Adolescents
American Psychiatric Publishing, Inc.
1000 Wilson Boulevard
Suite 1825
Arlington, VA 22209-3901
703-907-7322
800-368-5777
Fax: 703-907-1091
E-mail: appi@psych.org
www.appi.org

Judith L Rapoport, M.D., Editor
Ron McMillen, Chief Executive Officer
John McDuffie, Editorial Director

Examines the early development of obsessive - compulsive disorder and describes effective treatments. *$47.50*

368 pages ISBN 0-880482-82-6

335 Obsessive-Compulsive Disorder: Theory, Research and Treatment
Guilford Press
72 Spring Street
New York, NY 10012-4068
212-431-9800
800-365-7006
Fax: 212-966-6708
E-mail: info@guilford.com

Bob Matloff, President
Richard Swinson, Author
Martin Antony, Author
S Rachman, Author

Part I: Psychopathology and Theoretical Perspectives; Part II: Assessment and Treatment; Part III: Obsessive Compulsive Spectrum Disorders; Appendix: List of Resources. *$38.25*

478 pages Year Founded: 2001 ISBN 1-572307-32-0

336 Obsessive-Compulsive Disorders: A Complete Guide to Getting Well and Staying Well
Oxford University Press
2001 Evans Road
Cary, NC 27513-2010
919-677-0977
800-445-9714
Fax: 919-677-2673
E-mail: custserv.us@oup.com

In defining obsessive-compulsive disorders (OCDs), our language creates problems, because it treats the terms 'obsessive' and 'compulsion' very loosely. *$39.95*

Year Founded: 2000 ISBN 0-195140-92-3

337 Obsessive-Compulsive Disorders: Practical Management
Elsevier
PO Box 28430
Saint Louis, MO 63146-930
314-453-7010
800-460-3110
Fax: 314-453-7095
www.elsevier.com

Michael A Jenike, MD, Author
Lee Baer, PhD, Author
Wiliam E Minichiello, EdD, Author

Topics include the clinical picture, illnesses relation to obsessive-compulsive disorder, spectrum disorders, patient and clinical management and pathophysiology and assessment. *$73.00*

886 pages Year Founded: 1998 ISBN 0-815138-40-7

338 Obsessive-Compulsive Disorders: The Latest Assessment and Treatment Strategies
Jones & Bartlett
5 Wall Street
Burlington, MA 01803
978-443-5000
800-832-0034
Fax: 978-443-8000
E-mail: info@jblearning.com
www.jblearning.com

Gail Steketee, PhD, Author
Teresa Pigott, MD, Author

Previously considered a rare mental condition, obsessive compulsive disorder (OCD) now appears to be a hidden epidemic with over 6.5 million sufferers. *$40.95*

104 pages Year Founded: 1983 ISBN 1-887537-28-5

339 Obsessive-Compulsive Related Disorders
American Psychiatric Publishing, Inc.
1000 Wilson Boulevard
Suite 1825
Arlington, VA 22209-3901
703-907-7322
800-368-5777
Fax: 703-907-1091
E-mail: appi@psych.org
www.appi.org

Eric Hollander, M.D., Editor
Ron McMillen, Chief Executive Officer
John McDuffie, Editorial Director

Discusses the way compulsivity and impulsivity are understood, diagnosed and treated. *$22.50*

304 pages Year Founded: 1992 ISBN 0-880484-02-0

340 Over and Over Again: Understanding Obsessive-Compulsive Disorder
Jossey-Bass/Wiley
111 River Street
Hoboken, NJ 07030-5773
201-748-6000
Fax: 201-748-6088
E-mail: custserv@wiley.com
www.wiley.com

Fugen Neziroglu, Author
Jose A Yarvura-Tobias, Author

This sensitive and insightful book, the result of the author's years of research and experimentation, is a much needed survival manual for OCD sufferers and the families and friends who share their pain. *$35.00*

240 pages Year Founded: 1997 ISBN 0-787908-76-8

341 Overcoming Anxiety, Depression, and Other Mental Health Disorders in Children and Adults
Interdesciplinary Council on Development and Learning Disorders
4938 Hampden Lane
Suite 800
Bethesda, MD 20814
301-656-2667
E-mail: info@icdl.com
www.icdl.com

Dr Stanley I Greenspan, Author

Reveals strategies for family members as well as professionals from different disciplines to help both children and adults. The most common mental health disorders, including anxiety, depression, obsessive-compulsive patterns, ADD/ADHD, borderline states, and others, are discussed literally with a new set of eyeglasses

168 pages ISBN 0-976775-88-3

342 Overcoming Obsessive-Compulsive Disorder: Client Manual: A Behavioral and Cognitive Protocol for the Treatment of OCD
NewHarbinger Publications
5674 Shattuck Avenue
Oakland, CA 94609
800-748-6273
Fax: 800-652-1613
E-mail: customerservice@newharbinger.com
www.newharbinger.com

Matthew McKay PhD, Founder/Author
Gail Steketee PhD, Author

This protocol outlines a fourteen-session treatment for individual adults diagnosed with obsessive-compulsive disorder. This protocol is based on imagined exposure, in vivo exposure, response prevention and avoidance reduction. Copyright 1998 *$29.95*

104 pages Year Founded: 1973 ISBN 1-572241-29-9

343 Panic Disorder and Agoraphobia: A Guide
Madison Institute of Medicine
7617 Mineral Point Road
Suite 300
Madison, WI 53717-1623
608-827-2470
E-mail: mim@miminc.org
www.factsforhealth.org

John H. Greist, Author
James W Jefferson, MD, Author

Learn about the causes of panic disorder and agoraphobia and how patients can overcome these disabling disorders with medications and behavior therapy in this booklet written by leading experts on the subject. *$5.95*

69 pages Year Founded: 2004

344 Panic Disorder: Critical Analysis
Guilford Press
72 Spring Street
New York, NY 10012-4068
212-431-9800
800-365-7006
Fax: 212-966-6708
E-mail: info@guilford.com

Bob Matloff, President
Richard McNally, Author

Provides a comprehensive, integrative exploration of panic disorder. Discusses the phenomenology of the disorder, with extensive reviews of the epidemiology, biological aspects and psychopharmacalogic treatments, followed by detailed explorations of psychological aspects, including predictability and controllability and psychological treatments including cognitive behavioral techniques. *$38.00*

276 pages Year Founded: 1994 ISBN 0-898622-63-8

345 Pharmacotherapy for Mood, Anxiety and Cognitive Disorders
American Psychiatric Publishing, Inc.
1000 Wilson Boulevard
Suite 1825
Arlington, VA 22209-3901
703-907-7322
800-368-5777
Fax: 703-907-1091
E-mail: appi@psych.org
www.appi.org

Uriel Halbreich, M.D., Editor
Stuart A Montgomery, M.D., Editor
John McDuffie, Editorial Director

Takes a critical look at the different medications available for treating mood, anxiety and cognitive disorders. Also, it takes a look at their relevance to pathobiology and the underlying mechanisms, and the limitations. *$99.00*

832 pages Year Founded: 2000 ISBN 0-880488-85-9

346 Phobic and Obsessive-Compulsive Disorders: Theory, Research, and Practice
Kluwer Academic/Plenum Publishers
233 Spring Street
New York, NY 10013-1522
212-242-1490
www.kluweracademicpublishers.com

Paul M.G. Emmelkamp, Author

$24.95

366 pages Year Founded: 1992 ISBN 0-306410-44-3

347 Post-Traumatic Stress Disorder: Assessment, Differential Diagnosis, and Forensic Evaluation
Professional Resource Press
PO Box 3197
Sarasota, FL 34230-3197
941-343-9601
800-443-3364
Fax: 941-343-9201
E-mail: orders@prpress.com
www.prpress.com

Carroll L Meek, Author, Editor

A concise yet thorough examination of PTSD. An excellent resource for psychologists, psychiatrists, and lawyers involved in litigation concerning PTSD. *$26.95*

264 pages Year Founded: 1990 ISBN 0-943158-35-4

348 Posttraumatic Stress Disorder in Litigation: Guidelines for Forensic Assessment
American Psychiatric Publishing, Inc.
1000 Wilson Boulevard
Suite 1825
Arlington, VA 22209-3901
703-907-7322
800-368-5777
Fax: 703-907-1091
E-mail: appi@psych.org
www.appi.org

Robert I Simon, M.D., Editor
Ron McMillen, Chief Executive Officer
John McDuffie, Editorial Director

This essential collection by 13 leading US experts sheds important new light on forensic guidelines for effective assessment and diagnosis and determination of disability, serving both plaintiffs and defendants in litigation involving PTSD claims. Mental health and legal professionals, third-party payers, and interested laypersons will welcome this balanced approach to a complex and difficult field. *$44.95*

272 pages Year Founded: 2003 ISBN 1-585620-66-1

349 Psychiatric Treatment of Victims and Survivors of Sexual Trauma: A Neuro-Bio-Psychological Approach
Charles C Thomas Publisher Ltd.
2600 South First Street
Springfield, IL 62704
217-789-8980
800-258-8980
Fax: 217-789-9130
E-mail: books@ccthomas.com
www.ccthomas.com

Jamshid A Marvasti, MD, Author

Psychological trauma is a multifaceted phenomenon with extensive involvement of biochemical and neurological changes. This book originated on the basis of clinical observations and the authors believe that trauma is the region in which psych and soma meet each other and integrate, becoming a single entity. The authors attempt to integrate the psychosocial and bio-neuro-endocrine aspects of human experience, including trauma. *$53.95*

234 pages Year Founded: 1927 ISBN 0-398074-60-7

350 Psychological Trauma
American Psychiatric Publishing, Inc.
1000 Wilson Boulevard
Suite 1825
Arlington, VA 22209-3901
703-907-7322
800-368-5777
Fax: 703-907-1091
E-mail: appi@psych.org
www.appi.org

Rachel Yehuda, Ph.D., Editor
Ron McMillen, Chief Executive Officer
John McDuffie, Editorial Director

Epidemiology of trauma and post-traumatic stress disorder. Evaluation, neuroimaging, neuroendocrinology and pharmacology. *$29.00*

236 pages Year Founded: 1998 ISBN 0-880488-37-9

351 Real Illness: Obsessive-Compulsive Disorder
National Institute of Mental Health
6001 Executive Boulevard
Room 8184
Bethesda, MD 20892-1
301-443-4513
866-615-6464
TTY: 301-443-8431
E-mail: nimhinfo@nih.gov

Do you have disturbing thoughts and behaviors you know don't make sense but that you can't seem to control? This easy brochure explains how to get help.

9 pages

352 Rebuilding Shattered Lives: Responsible Treatment of Complex Post-Traumatic and Dissociative Disorders
John Wiley & Sons
111 River Street
Hoboken, NJ 07030-5774
201-748-6000
800-225-5945
Fax: 201-748-6088
E-mail: info@wiley.com
www.wiley.com

James A Chu, Author

Essential for anyone working in the field of trauma therapy. Part I discusses recent findings about child abuse, the changes in attitudes toward child abuse over the last two decades and the nature of traumatic memory. Part II is an overview of principles of trauma treatment, including symptom control, establishment of boundaries and therapist self - care. Part III covers special topics, such as dissociative identity disorder, controversies, hospitalization and acute care. *$73.95*

271 pages Year Founded: 1998 ISBN 0-471247-32-4

353 Relaxation & Stress Reduction Workbook
NewHarbinger Publications
5674 Shattuck Avenue
Oakland, CA 94609-1662
510-652-0215
800-748-6273
Fax: 800-652-1613
E-mail: customerservice@newharbinger.com
www.newharbinger.com

Martha Davis, Author
Elizabeth Robbins Eshelman, Author
Matthew McKay, Author

Step by step instructions cover progressive muscle relaxation, meditation, autogenics, visualization, thought stopping, refuting irrational ideas, coping skills training, job stress management, and much more. *$17.95*

392 pages Year Founded: 1973 ISBN 1-879237-82-2

354 Rewind, Replay, Repeat: A Memoir of Obsessive-Compulsive Disorder
Hazelden Publishing & Educational Services
PO Box 11
Center City, MN 55012-0011
651-213-4200
800-257-7810
Fax: 651-213-4793
E-mail: info@hazelden.org
www.hazelden.org

Jeff Bell, Author

The revealing story of one man's struggle with obsessive-compulsive disorder (OCD) and his hard-won recovery. Readers will learn what OCD feels like from the inside, and how healing from such a devastating condition is possible through therapy, determination, and the support of loved ones.

368 pages Year Founded: 1949 ISBN 1-592853-71-4

355 School Personnel
Obsessive-Compulsive Foundation
18 Tremont Street
Suite 903
Boston, MA 02196
617-973-5801
Fax: 617-973-5803
E-mail: info@iocdf.org
www.ocfoundation.org

Denise Egan Stack LMHC, President
Jeff Szymanski, PhD, Executive Director
Susan B Dailey, Vice President
Michael J Stack, CFA, Treasurer

School Personnel: A Critical Link in the Identification, Treatment and Management of OCD in Children and Adolescents. Recognizing OCD in the school setting, current

treatments, the role of school personnel in identification, assessment, and educational interventions, are thoroughly covered in this brief, but informative booklet especially targeted to educators and guidance counselors. *$4.00*

19 pages Year Founded: 1986 ISBN B-0006QK-6V-6

356 Shy Children, Phobic Adults: Nature and Treatment of Social Phobia
American Psychological Association
750 First Street, NorthEast
Washington, DC 20002-4242
202-336-5500
800-374-2721
Fax: 202-336-5518
TDD: 202-336-6123
TTY: 202-336-6123
www.www.apa.org

Deborah C. Beidel, PhD, ABPP, Author
Sameuel M. Turner, PhD, Author

Recent advances in the understanding of social phobia. Isolates the controversies that have yet to be resolved. Provides a clear description of effective treatments now available.

398 pages Year Founded: 1998 ISBN 1-557984-61-1

357 Social Anxiety Disorder: A Guide
Madison Institute of Medicine
7617 Mineral Point Road
Suite 300
Madison, WI 53717-1623
608-827-2470
E-mail: mim@miminc.org
www.factsforhealth.org

John H. Greist, Author
James W Jefferson, MD, Author
David J. Katzelnick, MD, Author

Do you fear public speaking or do you avoid social situations because you worry you may do something embarassing or humiliating? Learn how social anxiety disorder, also known as social phobia, is diagnosed and treated in this thorough publication written by leading experts on the subject. *$5.95*

67 pages Year Founded: 2007

358 Stop Obsessing: How to Overcome Your Obsessions and Compulsions
Anxiety Disorders Association of America
8701 Georgia Avenue
Suite 412
Silver Spring, MD 20910-3643
240-485-1001
E-mail: AnxDis@adaa.org
www.adaa.org

Edna Foa, Author
Reid Wilson, Author

Book provides knowledgeable descriptions of the steps, the challenges, and the value of self - treatment.

Year Founded: 1980

359 Stress Response Syndromes: Personality Styles and Interventions
Jason Aronson-Rowman & Littlefield Publishers
200 Park Avenue South
Suite 1109
New York, NY 10003-1512
212-529-3888
E-mail: custerv@rowman.com
www.rowmanlittlefield.com

Mardi J Horowitz, Author

Incorporation of the most recent advances in the understanding and treatment of stress response syndromes to date. Describes the general characteristics, including signs and symptoms, and elaborates on treatment techniques that integrate cognitive and dynamic approaches. *$43.00*

451 pages ISBN 0-765703-13-0

360 Stress-Related Disorders Sourcebook
Omnigraphics
155 West Congress
Suite 200
Detroit, MI 48226
313-961-1340
800-234-1340
Fax: 313-961-1383
E-mail: contact@omnigraphics.com
www.omnigraphics.com

Amy L. Sutton, Author

Omnigraphics is the publisher of the Health Reference Series, a growing consumer health information resource with more than 100 volumes in print. Each title in the series features an easy to understand format, nontechnical language, comprehensive indexing and resources for further information. Material in each book has been collected from a wide range of government agencies, professional associations, periodicals, and other sources. *$85.00*

621 pages Year Founded: 1985 ISBN 0-780805-60-7

361 Take Charge: Handling a Crisis and Moving Forward
American Institute for Preventive Medicine
30445 Northwestern Highway
Suite 350
Farmington Hills, MI 48334-3107
248-539-1800
800-345-2476
Fax: 248-539-1808
E-mail: aipm@healthy.net
www.HealthyLife.com

Don R Powell, PhD, President/CEO
Elaine Frank, M.Ed, R.D, Vice President
Jeanette Karwan, Director, Product Development

Take Charge helps people effectively live their lives after September 11th. This full color booklet provides just the right amount of information to effectively address the many concerns people have today. It will help people to be prepared for any kind of disaster, be it a terrorist attack, fire or flood. *$4.25*

32 pages Year Founded: 1983

362 Ten Simple Solutions To Panic
NewHarbinger Publications
5674 Shattuck Avenue
Oakland, CA 94609-1662

510-652-0215
800-748-6273
Fax: 800-652-1613
E-mail: customerservice@newharbinger.com
www.newharbinger.com

Randi E McCabe, PhD., Author
Martin Antony, PhD., Author

Provides readers who have at one time or another experienced unexplainable, intense mental and physical attacks over time. *$11.95*

152 pages Year Founded: 1973 ISBN 1-572243-25-2

363 Textbook of Anxiety Disorders
American Psychiatric Publishing, Inc.
1000 Wilson Boulevard
Suite 1825
Arlington, VA 22209-3901
703-907-7322
800-368-5777
Fax: 703-907-1091
E-mail: appi@psych.org
www.appi.org

Dan J Stein, M.D., Ph.D., Editor
Eric Hollander, M.D., Editor
Barbara O Rothbaum, Ph.D., A.B.P, Editor

US and international experts cover every major anxiety disorder, compare it with animal behavior and the similarities in the brain that exist, how disorders can relate to age specific groups, and covers the latest developments in understanding and treating these disorders. *$77.00*

822 pages Year Founded: 2010 ISBN 0-880488-29-8

364 The 10 Best-Ever Anxiety Management Techniques: Understanding How Your Brain Makes You Anxious and What You Can Do to Change It
W.W. Norton & Company, Inc.
500 Fifth Avenue
New York, NY 10110
212-354-5500
800-233-4830
Fax: 212-869-0856
www.books.wwnorton.com

Margaret Wehrenberg, Author

A strategy-filled handbook to understand, manage, and conquer your own your own stress. *$18.95*

256 pages Year Founded: 1923 ISBN 0-393705-56-0

365 The Agoraphobia Workbook
NewHarbinger Publications
5674 Shattuck Avenue
Oakland, CA 94609-1662
510-652-0215
800-748-6273
Fax: 800-652-1613
E-mail: customerservice@newharbinger.com
www.newharbinger.com

C Allen Pollard, PhD, Author
Elke Zuercher-White, Author

Self-help resource to help readers overcome the disorder in all its forms *$19.95*

192 pages Year Founded: 1973 ISBN 1-572243-23-6

366   The American Psychiatric Publishing Textbook of Anxiety Disorders
American Psychiatric Publishing, Inc.
1000 Wilson Boulevard
Suite 1825
Arlington, VA 22209-3901
703-907-7322
800-368-5777
Fax: 703-907-1091
E-mail: appi@psych.org
www.appi.org

Dan J Stein, M.D., Ph.D., Editor
Eric Hollander, M.D., Editor
Barbara O Rothbaum, Ph.D., A.B.P, Editor

Gives a detailed look at the history, classification, preclinical models, concepts and combined treatment of anxiety disorders. *$92.00*

822 pages   Year Founded: 2010 ISBN 0-880488-29-8

367   The Anxiety & Phobia Workbook, 5th Edition
NewHarbinger Publications
5674 Shattuck Avenue
Oakland, CA 94609-1662
510-652-0215
800-748-6273
Fax: 800-652-1613
E-mail: customerservice@newharbinger.com
www.newharbinger.com

Edmund J. Bourne, PhD, Author

Research conducted by the National Institute of Mental Health has shown that anxiety disorders are the number one mental health problem among American women and.
$24.95

496 pages   Year Founded: 1973 ISBN 1-572244-13-5

368   The Imp of the Mind: Exploring the Silent Epidemic of Obsessive Bad Thoughts
Plume
375 Hudson Street
New York, NY 10014-3657
212-366-2372
Fax: 212-366-2933
E-mail: ecommerce@us.penguingroup.com
www.www.us.penguingroup.com

Lee Baer, PhD, Author

Dr. Lee Baer combines the latest research with his own extensive experience in treating this widespread syndrome. Drawing on information ranging from new advances in brain technology to pervasive social taboos, Dr. Baer explores the root causes of bad thoughts, why they can spiral out of control, and how to recognize the crucial difference between harmless and dangerous bad thoughts. *$12.99*

176 pages   Year Founded: 1936 ISSN 978-0452283077ISBN 0-452283-07-8

369   The Worry Control Workbook
NewHarbinger Publications
5674 Shattuck Avenue
Oakland, CA 94609-1662
510-652-0215
800-748-6273
Fax: 800-652-1613
E-mail: customerservice@newharbinger.com
www.newharbinger.com

Mary Ellen Copeland, Author

Self help program that shares experiences of people who have developed ways to overcome chronic worry. Step by step format helps identify areas likely to reoccur and develop new skills. *$15.95*

266 pages   ISBN 1-572241-20-9

370   Tormenting Thoughts and Secret Rituals: The Hidden Epidemic of Obsessive-Compulsive Disorder
Random House
1745 Broadway
3rd Floor
New York, NY 10019-4343
212-782-9000
Fax: 212-302-7985
E-mail: ecustomerservice@randomhouse.com
www.randomhouse.com

Ian Osborn, MD, Author

Discusses the various forms Obsessive-Compulsive Disorder (OCD) takes and, using the most common focuses of obsession, presents detailed cases whose objects are filth, harm, lust, and blasphemy. He explains how the disorder is currently diagnosed and how it differs from addiction, worrying, and preoccupation. He summarizes the recent findings in the areas of brain biology, neuroimaging and genetics that show OCD to be a distinct chemical disorder of the brain. *$14.95*

336 pages   Year Founded: 1999 ISBN 0-440508-47-9

371   Traumatic Stress: Effects of Overwhelming Experience on Mind, Body and Society
Guilford Press
72 Spring Street
New York, NY 10012-4068
212-431-9800
800-365-7006
Fax: 212-966-6708
E-mail: info@guilford.com

Besell van der Kolk, Author
Alexander McFarlane, Author

The current state of research and clinical knowledge on traumatic stress and its treatment. Contributions from leading authorities summarize knowledge emerging. Addresses the uncertainties and controversies that confront the field of traumatic stress, including the complexity of posttraumatic adaptations and the unproven effectiveness of some approaches to prevention and treatment. *$42.50*

596 pages   Year Founded: 2006 ISBN 1-572300-88-4

372   Triumph Over Fear: A Book of Help and Hope for People with Anxiety, Panic Attacks, and Phobias
Bantam Dell Publishing Group
1745 Broadway
New York, NY 10019
212-782-9000
E-mail: ecustomerservice@randomhouse.com
www.randomhouse.com

Jerilynn Ross, Author

Resource and guide for both lay and professional readers. *$16.00*

320 pages   Year Founded: 1995 ISSN 9780553081329ISBN 0-553081-32-2

373 Trust After Trauma: A Guide to Relationships for Survivors and Those Who Love Them
NewHarbinger Publications
5674 Shattuck Avenue
Oakland, CA 94609-1662
510-652-0215
800-748-6273
Fax: 800-652-1613
E-mail: customerservice@newharbinger.com
www.newharbinger.com

Aphrodite Matsakis, PhD, Author

Survivors guided through process of strengthening existing bonds, building new ones, and ending cycles of withdrawal and isolation. *$24.95*

352 pages Year Founded: 1973 ISBN 1-572241-01-2

374 Understanding Post Traumatic Stress Disorder and Addiction
Sidran Institute
200 E Joppa Road
Suite 207
Baltimore, MD 21286-3107
410-825-8888
888-825-8249
Fax: 410-337-0747
E-mail: sidran@sidran.org
www.sidran.org

Katie Evans, Author

This booklet discusses PTSD, how to recognize it and how to begin a dual recovery program from chemical dependency and PTSD. The workbook includes information to enhance your understanding of PTSD, activities to help identify the symptoms of dual disorders, a self evaulation of your recovery process and ways to handle situations that may trigger PTSD. *$7.20*

48 pages

375 What to Do When You Worry Too Much: A Kid's Guide to Overcoming Anxiety
American Psychological Association
750 First Street, NorthEast
Washington, DC 20002-4242
202-336-5500
800-374-2721
Fax: 202-336-5518
TTY: 202-336-6123
www.apa.org

Dawn Huebner, PhD, Author
Bonnie Matthews, Illustrator

Interactive self-help book designed to guide 6-12 year olds and thier parents through the techniques most often used in the treatments of generalized anxiety. *$9.38*

88 pages Year Founded: 1892 ISBN 1-591473-14-4

376 What to Do When You're Scared and Worried: A Guide for Kids
Free Spirit Publishing
217 Fifth Avenue North
Suite 200
Minneapolis, MN 55401-1299
612-338-2068
800-735-7323
Fax: 866-419-5199
www.freespirit.com

James J Christ, Author

This book is all about fears and worries: things that everyone deals with at some point in thier lives.

128 pages Year Founded: 1983

377 When Once Is Not Enough: Help for Obsessive Compulsives
NewHarbinger Publications
5674 Shattuck Avenue
Oakland, CA 94609-1662
510-652-0215
800-748-6273
Fax: 800-652-1613
E-mail: customerservice@newharbinger.com
www.newharbinger.com

Gail Steketee, Author
Kerrin White, Author

How to recognize and confront fears, using simple rituals, positive coping strategies and handling complications. *$14.95*

229 pages Year Founded: 1973 ISBN 0-934986-87-8

378 When Perfect Isn't Good Enough: Strategies for Coping with Perfectionism
NewHarbinger Publications
5674 Shattuck Avenue
Oakland, CA 94609-1662
510-652-0215
800-748-6273
Fax: 800-652-1613
E-mail: customerservice@newharbinger.com
www.newharbinger.com

Martin Antony, PhD, Author
Richard P Swinson, MD, FRCPC, FRCP, Author

This step by step guide explores the nature of perfectionism and offers a series of exercises to help you challenge unrealistic expectations and work on the specific situations in your life where perfectionism is a problem. *$14.95*

312 pages Year Founded: 1973 ISBN 1-572241-24-1

379 Who Gets PTSD? Issues of Posttraumatic Stress Vulnerability
Charles C Thomas Publisher Ltd.
2600 South First Street
Springfield, IL 62704
217-789-8980
800-258-8980
Fax: 217-789-9130
E-mail: books@ccthomas.com
www.ccthomas.com

John M. Violanti, Author, Editor
Douglas Paton, Editor

Major topics in the text include: assessing psychological distress and physiological vulnerability in police officers, personal, organizational, and contextual influences in stress vulnerability; differences in vulnerability to posttraumatic deprivation: gender differences in police work , stress and trauma, trauma types, etc. *$ 46.95*

216 pages Year Founded: 1927 ISBN 3-980761-89-

Periodicals & Pamphlets

380 101 Stress Busters
ETR Associates
4 Carbonero Way
Scotts Valley, CA 95066-4200
831-438-4060
800-321-4407
Fax: 831-438-3618
E-mail: support@etr.freshdesk.com
www.etr.org

David Kitchen, MBA, Chief Financial Officer
Talita Sanders, BS, Director, Human Resources
Coleen Cantwell, MPH, Director, Business Development Pl
Matt McDowell, BS, Director, Marketing

These 101 stress busters were written by students to help
fellow students relieve stress: tell a joke, laugh out loud,
beat a pillow to smitherines. *$16.00*

381 Anxiety Disorders
National Institute of Mental Health
6001 Executive Boulevard
Rockville, MD 20852
301-443-4513
866-615-6464
TTY: 301-443-8431
E-mail: nimhinfo@nih.gov
www.www.nimh.nih.gov/

Thomas Insel MD, Director
Phillip Sun Wang, Deputy Director
Marlene Guzman, Senior Advisor to the Director
Mayada Akil, Senior Advisor

A detailed booklet that describes the symptoms, causes, and
treatments of the major anxiety disorders, with information
on getting help and coping.

22 pages

382 Anxiety Disorders Fact Sheet
**Center for Mental Health Services: Knowledge
Exchange Network**
3803 North Fairfax Drive
Suite 100
Arlington, VA 22203
703-524-7600
800-950-6264
Fax: 703-524-9094
TDD: 866-889-2647
E-mail: ken@mentalhealth.org
www.www.nami.org

This fact sheet presents basic information on the symptoms,
formal diagnosis, and treatment for generalized anxiety disorder, panic disorders, phobias, and post-traumatic stress
disorder.

3 pages Year Founded: 1979

383 Anxiety Disorders in Children and Adolescents
**Center for Mental Health Services: Knowledge
Exchange Network**
1 Choke Cherry Road
Rockville, MD 20015
800-789-2647
Fax: 240-747-5470
TDD: 866-889-2647
E-mail: ken@mentalhealth.org
www.mentalhealth.samhsa.gov/

Tracy L Morris, Editor
John S March, Editor

This fact sheet defines anxiety disorders, identifies warning
signs, discusses risk factors, describes types of help available, and suggests what parents or other caregivers can do.

395 pages

384 Facts About Anxiety Disorders
National Institute of Mental Health
6001 Executive Boulevard
Rockville, MD 20852
301-443-4513
866-615-6464
TTY: 301-443-8431
E-mail: nimhinfo@nih.gov
www.www.nimh.nih.gov/

Series of fact sheets that provide overviews and descriptions of generalized anxiety disorder, obsessive-compulsive
disorder, panic disorder, post-traumatic stress disorder, social phobia, and the Anxiety Disorders Education Program.

**385 Families Can Help Children Cope with Fear,
Anxiety**
PO Box 42490
Washington, DC 20015
800-789-2647
Fax: 301-984-8796
TDD: 866-889-2647
www.mentalhealth.org

2 pages

386 Five Smart Steps to Less Stress
ETR Associates
4 Carbonero Way
Scotts Valley, CA 95066-4200
831-438-4060
800-321-4407
Fax: 831-438-3618
E-mail: support@etr.freshdesk.com
www.etr.org

David Kitchen, MBA, Chief Financial Officer
Talita Sanders, BS, Director, Human Resources
Coleen Cantwell, MPH, Director, Business Development Pl
Matt McDowell, BS, Director, Marketing

Steps to managing stress include: know what stresses you,
manage your stress, take care of your body, take care of
your feelings, ask for help. *$16.00*

387 Five Ways to Stop Stress
ETR Associates
4 Carbonero Way
Scotts Valley, CA 95066-4200
831-438-4060
800-321-4407
Fax: 831-438-3618
E-mail: support@etr.freshdesk.com
www.etr.org

David Kitchen, MBA, Chief Financial Officer
Talita Sanders, BS, Director, Human Resources
Coleen Cantwell, MPH, Director, Business Development Pl
Matt McDowell, BS, Director, Marketing

An easy to read pamphlet that discusses how to recognize
the signs of stress, explains the big and little changes that
can produce stress and the different causes of stress.
$18.00

388 Getting What You Want From Stress
ETR Associates
4 Carbonero Way
Scotts Valley, CA 95066-4200
831-438-4060
800-321-4407
Fax: 831-438-3618
E-mail: customerservice@etr.org
www.etr.org

Mary Nelson, President

Includes signs of stress, some stress can be healthy, and when to change, when to adapt. *$18.00*

389 Helping Children and Adolescents Cope with Violence and Disasters
National Institute of Mental Health
6001 Executive Boulevard
Room 8184
Rockville, MD 20852
301-443-4513
866-615-6464
TTY: 301-443-8431
E-mail: nimhinfo@nih.gov
www.www.nimh.nih.gov/

A booklet that describes what parents can do to help children and adolescents cope with violence and disasters.

390 Journal of Anxiety Disorders
Elsevier Publishing
1600 John F Kennedy Boulevard
Suite 1800
Philadelphia, PA 19103-2879
212-989-5800
800-325-4177
Fax: 212-633-3820
E-mail: custserv.ehs@elsevier.com
www.www.journals.elsevier.com/journal-of-anxiety-disor

Deborah Beidel, Author

Interdisciplinary journal that publishes research papers dealing with all aspects of anxiety disorders for all age groups (child, adolescent, adult and geriatrics). *$195.00*

8 per year Year Founded: 2012 ISSN 0887-6185

391 Let's Talk Facts About Panic Disorder
American Psychiatric Publishing, Inc.
1000 Wilson Boulevard
Suite 1825
Arlington, VA 22209-3901
703-907-7322
800-368-5777
Fax: 703-907-1091
E-mail: appi@psych.org
www.appi.org

Robert E Hales MD, Editor-in-Chief
Ron McMillen, Chief Executive Officer
John McDuffie, Editorial Director

Contains an overview of the illness, its symptoms, and the illness's effect on family and friends. A biliography and list of resources make them ideal for libraries or patient education. *$29.95*

6 pages Year Founded: 2006 ISBN 0-890423-57-1

392 Let's Talk Facts About Post-Traumatic Stress Disorder
American Psychiatric Publishing, Inc.
1000 Wilson Boulevard
Suite 1825
Arlington, VA 22209-3901
703-907-7322
800-368-5777
Fax: 703-907-1091
E-mail: appi@psych.org
www.appi.org

Robert E Hales MD, Editor-in-Chief
Ron McMillen, Chief Executive Officer
John McDuffie, Editorial Director

$12.50

8 pages Year Founded: 2005 ISBN 0-890423-63-6

393 OCD Newsletter
18 Tremont Street
Suite 903
Boston, MA 02196
617-973-5801
Fax: 617-973-5803
E-mail: info@iocdf.org
www.ocfoundation.org

Denise Egan Stack LMHC, President
Jeff Szymanski, PhD, Executive Director
Susan B Dailey, Vice President
Michael J Stack, CFA, Treasurer

A source of news, entertainment, and inspiration to individuals with OCD, their loved ones, and to OCD professionals and researchers.

8-12 pages Year Founded: 1986

394 Panic Attacks
ETR Associates
4 Carbonero Way
Scotts Valley, CA 95066-4200
831-438-4060
800-321-4407
Fax: 831-438-3618
E-mail: support@etr.freshdesk.com
www.etr.org

David Kitchen, MBA, Chief Financial Officer
Talita Sanders, BS, Director, Human Resources
Coleen Cantwell, MPH, Director, Business Development Pl
Matt McDowell, BS, Director, Marketing

Describes causes of panic attacks, including genetics, stress, and drug use; prevention and treatment, and how to stop a panic attack in its tracks. *$16.00*

395 Real Illness: Panic Disorder
National Institute of Mental Health
6001 Executive Boulevard
Room 8184
Bethesda, MD 20892
301-443-4513
866-615-6464
TTY: 301-443-8431
E-mail: nimhinfo@nih.gov

Do you often have feelings of sudden fear that don't make sense? If so, you may have panic disorder. Read this pamplet of simple information about getting help.

9 pages

396 Real Illness: Post-Traumatic Stress Disorder
6001 Executive Boulevard
Room 8184
Bethesda, MD 20892
301-443-4513
866-615-6464
TTY: 301-443-8431
E-mail: nimhinfo@nih.gov
9 pages

397 Stress
ETR Associates
4 Carbonero Way
Scotts Valley, CA 95066-4200
831-438-4060
800-321-4407
Fax: 831-438-3618
E-mail: customerservice@etr.org
www.etr.org

Mary Nelson, President

Includes common changes that cause stress, symptoms of stress, and effects on feelings, actions and physical health.

398 Stress Incredible Facts
ETR Associates
4 Carbonero Way
Scotts Valley, CA 95066-4200
831-438-4060
800-321-4407
Fax: 831-438-3618
E-mail: support@etr.freshdesk.com
www.etr.org

David Kitchen, MBA, Chief Financial Officer
Talita Sanders, BS, Director, Human Resources
Coleen Cantwell, MPH, Director, Business Development Pl
Matt McDowell, BS, Director, Marketing

Strange-but-true facts to trigger discussion about how stress affects the body, how to use it and long-term risks.

399 Stress in Hard Times
ETR Associates
4 Carbonero Way
Scotts Valley, CA 95066-4200
831-438-4060
800-321-4407
Fax: 831-438-3618
E-mail: customerservice@etr.org
www.etr.org

Mary Nelson, President

Discusses stress caused by troubling world events, describes short and long term symptoms, and suggests ways to cope. *$ 16.00*

400 Teen Stress!
ETR Associates
4 Carbonero Way
Scotts Valley, CA 95066-4200
831-438-4060
800-321-4407
Fax: 831-438-3618
E-mail: support@etr.freshdesk.com
www.etr.org

David Kitchen, MBA, Chief Financial Officer
Talita Sanders, BS, Director, Human Resources

Coleen Cantwell, MPH, Director, Business Development Pl
Matt McDowell, BS, Director, Marketing

Explains what stress is, outlines the causes and effects and offers ideas for handling stress. *$16.00*

Research Centers

401 UAMS Psychiatric Research Institute
4224 Shuffield Drive
Little Rock, AR 72205
501-526-8100
Fax: 501-660-7542
E-mail: kramerteresal@uams.edu
www.www.psychiatry.uams.edu

John Fortney PhD, Director
Geoff Curran PhD, Associate Director
Keith Berner MD, Clinical Faculty

Combining research, education and clinical services into one facility, PRI offers inpatiend and outpatient services, with 40 psychiatric beds, therapy options, and specialized treatment for specific disorders, including: addictive eating, anxiety, deppressive and post-traumatic stress disorders. Research focuses on evidence-based care takes into consideration the education of future medical personnel while relying on research scientists to provide innovative forms of treatment. PRI includes the Center for Addiction Research as well as a methadone clinic.

Support Groups & Hot Lines

402 Agoraphobics Building Independent Lives
2008 Bremo Road
Suite #101
Richmond, VA 23226
804-257-5591
866-400-6428
Fax: 804-447-7786
E-mail: info@mhav.org
www.mhav.org

Joanne Whitley, President
Ali Faruk, Vice President & Public Policy C
Anne Edgerton, Executive Director
Sarah Rudden, Project Coordinator

A nonprofit organization for people dealing with anxiety and panic disorders, incorporated in the State of Virginia. It has support groups nationwide.

403 Emotions Anonymous International Service Center
PO Box 4245
Saint Paul, MN 55104-0245
651-647-9712
Fax: 651-647-1593
E-mail: info@EmotionsAnonymous.org
www.EmotionsAnonymous.org

Karen Mead, Executive Director

Fellowship of men and women who share their experience, strength and hope with each other, that they may solve their common problem and help others recover from emotional illness.

404 International OCD Foundation
18 Tremont Street
Suite 903
Boston, MA 02108

617-973-5801
Fax: 617-973-5803
E-mail: info@ocfoundation.org
www.ocfoundation.org

Denise Egan Stack LMHC, President
Susan B. Dailey, Vice President
Michael J. Stack CFA, Treasurer
Diane Davey RN, Secretary

An international not-for-profit organization made up of people with Obsessive Compulsive Disorder and related disorders, as well as their families, friends, professionals and others.

Year Founded: 1986

405 **Obsessive-Compulsive Anonymous**
PO Box 215
New Hyde Park, NY 11040
516-739-0662
Fax: 212-768-4679
E-mail: west24th@aol.com
www.obsessivecompulsiveanonymous.com

Is a fellowship of people who share their Experience, Strength, and Hope with each other that they may solve their common problem and help others to recover from OCD.

406 **Recovery International**
105 W. Adams St.
Suite 2940
Chicago, IL 60603
312-337-5661
866-221-0302
Fax: 312-726-4446
E-mail: info@recoveryinternational.org
www.www.recoveryinternational.org

John Rosenheim, 1st Vice Chair
Rudolph Pruden, Chair/Acting Treasurer

The mission of Abraham Low Self-Help Systems is to use the cognitive-behavioral peer-to-peer, self-help training system developed by Abraham Low, MD, to help individuals gain skills to lead more peaceful and productive lives.

Year Founded: 1937

Video & Audio

407 **Anxiety Disorders**
American Counseling Association
5999 Stevenson Avenue
Alexandria, VA 22304-3304
703-823-9800
800-347-6647
Fax: 703-823-0252
TDD: 703-823-6862
E-mail: webmaster@counseling.org
www.counseling.org

Cirecie A. West-Olatunji, President
Richard Yep, Executive Director
Thelma Daley, Treasurer

Increase your awareness of anxiety disorders, their symptoms, and effective treatments. Learn the effect these disorders can have on life and how treatment can change the quality of life for people presently suffering from these disorders. Includes 6 audiotapes and a study guide. *$140.00*

Year Founded: 1952

408 **DSM-IV-TR**
American Psychiatric Publishing, Inc.
1000 Wilson Boulevard
Suite 1825
Arlington, VA 22209-3901
703-907-7322
800-368-5777
Fax: 703-907-1091
E-mail: appi@psych.org
www.appi.org

Cathryn A Galanter, M.D, Editor
Peter S Jensen, M.D, Editor
John McDuffie, Editorial Director

Series of three clinical programs that reveals additions and changes for mood, psychotic and anxiety disorders. Each video focuses on a different level of disorder as well as giving three 10 minute interviews. Approximately 60 minutes. *$57.00*

744 pages Year Founded: 2009 ISBN 0-880488-98-0

409 **Dealing With Social Anxiety**
Educational Video Network
1401 19th Street
Huntsville, TX 77340
936-295-5767
800-762-0060
Fax: 936-294-0233
E-mail: info at evn.org
www.www.evndirect.com

A video to learn and understand social anxiety. *$89.95*

Year Founded: 2002 ISBN 1-589501-48-9

410 **Driving Far from Home**
NewHarbinger Publications
5674 Shattuck Avenue
Oakland, CA 94609-1662
510-652-0215
800-748-6273
Fax: 800-652-1613
E-mail: customerservice@newharbinger.com
www.newharbinger.com

Edmund J. Bourne, Author

120 minute videotape that reduces fear associated with leaving the safety of your home base. *$15.95*

Year Founded: 1973 ISBN 1-572240-14-8

411 **Effective Learning Systems, Inc.**
5108 W 74th Street
#390160
Minneapolis, MN 55439
952-943-1660
800-966-0443
E-mail: info@efflearn.com
www.www.effectivelearning.com

Bob Griswold, Founder
Deirdre M Griswold, VP

Audio tapes for stress management, deep relaxation, anger control, peace of mind, insomnia, weight and smoking, self-image and self-esteem, positive thinking, health and healing. Since 1972, Effective Learning Systems has helped millions of people take charge of their lives and make positive changes.

Year Founded: 1972

412 **Hope and Solutions for OCD**
International OCD Foundation
18 Tremont Street
Suite 903
Boston, MA 02108
617-973-5801
Fax: 617-973-5803
E-mail: info@ocfoundation.org
www.ocfoundation.org

Denise Egan Stack LMHC, President
Susan B. Dailey, Vice President
Michael J. Stack CFA, Treasurer
Diane Davey RN, Secretary

Finally, a video series about obsessive compulsive disorder. With some straight forward solutions, answers, and advice for individuals who have OCD, their families, their doctors, and school personnel. The Awareness Foundation for OCD & Related Disorders had produced this highly useful, informative, and inspirational series to help guide those with OCD towards confidence, recovery, and hope. *$89.95*

Year Founded: 1986

413 **Legacy of Childhood Trauma: Not Always Who They Seem**
Research Press
Dept 12 W
PO Box 9177
Champaign, IL 61826-9177
217-352-3273
800-519-2707
Fax: 217-352-1221
E-mail: rp@researchpress.com
www.researchpress.com

This powerful video focuses on the connection between so-called delinquent youth, and the experience of childhood trauma such as emotional, sexual, or physical abuse. Four young adults, survivors of childhood trauma, candidly discuss their troubled childhood and teenage years and reveal how, with the help of caring adults, they were able to salvage their lives. They offer valuable guidelines and insights on working with adolescents who have experienced childhood trauma. *$ 195.00*

414 **Touching Tree**
Obsessive-Compulsive Foundation
18 Tremont Street
Suite 903
Boston, MA 02108
617-973-5801
Fax: 617-973-5803
E-mail: info@ocfoundation.org
www.ocfoundation.org

Denise Egan Stack LMHC, President
Susan B. Dailey, Vice President
Michael J. Stack CFA, Treasurer
Diane Davey RN, Secretary

This video will foster awareness of early onset obsessive-compulsive disorder (OCD) and demonstrate the symptoms and current therapies that are most successful. Typical ritualistic compulsions of children and adolescents such as touching, hand washing, counting, etc. are explained. *$49.95*

Year Founded: 1986

415 **Treating Trauma Disorders Effectively**
Colin A Ross Institute for Psychological Trauma
1701 Gateway
Suite 349
Richardson, TX 75080-3546
972-918-9588
Fax: 972-918-9069
E-mail: rossinst@rossinst.com
www.rossinst.com

Dr Colin A Ross, MD, Founder, President
Melissa Caldwell, Manager

A training video that gives a comprehensive overview of clinical interventions with trauma patients. The video teaches advanced techniques for treating Dissociative Identity Disorder, Post Traumatic Stress Disorder, & trauma related Depression, Anxiety, Addictions, and Borderline Personality Disorder. The video's teaching modalities consist of case examples, with dramatic reenactments, and narrator discussion by Colin Ross, M.D. The teaching methods used clearly demonstrate effective therapeutic techniques that are backed by years of experience and research. *$85.00*

Year Founded: 1995

416 **Understanding Mental Illness**
Educational Video Network
1401 19th Street
Huntsville, TX 77340
936-295-5767
800-762-0060
Fax: 936-294-0233
E-mail: info at evn.org
www.www.evndirect.com

A video to learn and understand mental illness and how it affects you. *$79.95*

Year Founded: 2004 ISBN 1-589501-48-9

417 **Understanding and Treating the Hereditary Psychiatric Spectrum Disorders**
Hope Press
PO Box 188
Duarte, CA 91009-188
818-303-0644
800-209-9182
Fax: 818-358-3520
E-mail: dcomings@earthlink.net
www.hopepress.com

David E Comings MD, Presenter

Learn with ten hours of audio tapes from a two day seminar given in May 1997 by David E Comings MD. Tapes cover: ADHD, Tourette Syndrome, Obsessive-Compulsive Disorder, Conduct Disorder, Oppositional Defiant Disorder, Autism and other Hereditary Psychiatric Spectrum Disorders. Eight audio tapes. *$75.00*

Year Founded: 1997

Web Sites

418 **www.apa.org/practice/traumaticstress.html**
American Psychological Association

Provides tips for recovering from disasters and other traumatic events.

419 **www.bcm.tmc.edu/civitas/caregivers.htm**
Caregivers Series

Sophisticated articles describing the effects of childhood trauma on brain development and relationships.

420 **www.cyberpsych.org**
CyberPsych

Presents information about psychoanalysis, psychotherapy and special topics such as anxiety disorders, the problematic use of alcohol, homophobia, and the traumatic effects of racism. Explains in detail what anxiety it is how it is treated and the symptoms associated with anxiety.

421 **www.goodwill-suncoast.org**
Career Assessment & Planning Services

A comprehensive assessment for the developmentally disabled persons who may be unemployed or underemployed.

422 **www.guidetopsychology.com**
A Guide To Psychology & Its Practice

Free information on various types of psychology.

423 **www.healthanxiety.org**
Anxiety and Phobia Treatment Center

Treatment groups for individuals suffering from phobias.

424 **www.healthyminds.org**
Anxiety Disorders

American Psychiatric Association publication diagnostic criteria and treatment.

425 **www.icisf.org**
International Critical Incident Stress Foundation

A nonprofit, open membership foundation dedicated to the prevention and mitigation of disabling stress by education, training and support services for all emergency service professionals. Continuing education and training in emergency mental health services for psychologists, psychiatrists, social workers and licensed professional counselors.

426 **www.lexington-on-line.com**
Panic Disorder

Explains development and treatment of panic disorder.

427 **www.mayoclinic.com**
Mayo Clinic

Provides information on obsessive-compulsive disorder and anxiety.

428 **www.mentalhealth.Samhsa.Gov**
Center for Mental Health Services Knowledge Exchange Network

Information about resources, technical assistance, research, training, networks and other federal clearinghouses.

429 **www.mentalhealth.com**
Internet Mental Health

On-line information and a virtual encyclopedia related to mental disorders, possible causes and treatments. News, articles, on-line diagnostic programs and related links. Designed to improve understanding, diagnosis and treatment of mental illness throughout the world. Awarded the Top Site Award and the NetPsych Cutting Edge Site Award.

430 **www.nami.org**
National Alliance on Mental Illness

From its inception in 1979, NAMI has been dedicated to improving the lives of individuals and families affected by mental illness.

431 **www.ncptsd.org**
National Center for PTSD

Aims to advance the clinical care and social welfare of U.S. Veterans through research, education and training on PTSD and stress-related disorders

432 **www.nimh.nih.gov/anxiety/anxiety/ocd**
National Institute of Health

Information on anxiety disorders and OCD.

433 **www.nimh.nih.gov/publicat/ocdmenu.cfm**
Obsessive-Compulsive Disorder

Introductory handout with treatment recommendations.

434 **www.npadnews.com**
National Panic/Anxiety Disorder Newsletter

This resource was founded by Phil Darren who collects and collates information of recovered anxiety disorder sufferers who want to distribute some of the lessons that they learned with a view to helping others.

435 **www.ocdhope.com/gdlines.htm**
Guidelines for Families Coping with OCD

436 **www.ocfoundation.org**
Obsessive-Compulsive Foundation

An international not-for-profit organization composed of people with obsessive compulsive disorder and related disorders, their families, friends, professionals and other concerned individuals.

437 **www.panicattacks.com.au**
Anxiety Panic Hub

Information, resources and support.

438 **www.panicdisorder.about.com**
Agoraphobia: For Friends/Family

439 **www.planetpsych.com**
Planetpsych.com

Learn about disorders, their treatments and other topics in psychology. Articles are listed under the related topic areas. Ask a therapist a question for free, or view the directory of professionals in your area. If you are a therapist sign up for the directory. Current features, self-help, interactive, and newsletter archives.

440 **www.psychcentral.com**
Psych Central

Personalized one-stop index for psychology, support, and mental health issues, resources, and people on the Internet.

441 **www.ptsdalliance.org**
Post Traumatic Stress Disorder Alliance

Website of the Post Traumatic Stress Disorder Alliance.

442 **www.selectivemutismfoundation.org**
Selective Mutism Foundation

Promotes awareness and understanding for individuals and
families affected by mutism.

443 **www.selfhelpmagazine.com/articles/stress**
Meditation, Guided Fantasies, and Other Stress
Reducers

Meditative and stress reduction resources for eyes, ears,
minds, and hearts.

444 **www.sidran.org**
Sidran Institute, Traumatic Stress Education &
Advocacy

Helps people understand, recover from, and treat traumatic
stress (including PTSD), dissociative disorders, and
co-occuring issues, such as addictions, self injury, and
suicidality.

445 **www.sidran.org/trauma.html**
Trauma Resource Area

Resources and Articles on Dissociative Experiences Scale
and Dissociative Identity Disorder, PsychTrauma Glossary
and Traumatic Memories.

446 **www.terraphouston.com**
Territorial Apprehensiveness Programs (TERRAP)

Shirley Riff, Director

Formed to disseminate information concerning the recognition, causes and treatment of anxieties, fears and phobias.

447 **www.thenadd.org**
NADD: National Association for the Dually
Diagnosed

Promotes interest of professional and parent development
with resources for individuals who have coexistence of
mental illness and mental retardation.

448 **www.trauma-pages.com**
David Baldwin's Trauma Information Pages

Focus primarily on emotional trauma and traumatic stress,
including PTSD (Post-traumatic Stress Disorder) and dissociation, whether following individual traumatic experi-
ence(s) or a large-scale disaster.

ADHD

Introduction

Attention-Deficit/Hyperactivity Disorder (AD/HD) includes (1) a pervasive pattern of inattention, and (2) difficulty in controlling impulses including the impulse to be constantly on the move. Since many chilren are inattentive, impulsive, and rambunctious at times, it is important to note that the diagnosis in not made unless these behaviors are more severe than is typical for a person at a comparable developmental level. The symptoms must appear before age seven.

The problems of hyperactivity show themselves in constant movement, especially among younger children. Preschool children with hyperactivity cannot sit still, even for quiet activities that usually absorb children of the same age, are always on the move and run rather than walk. In older children the intensity of the hyperactivity is reduced but fidgeting, getting up during meals or homework, and excessive talking continue.

People with Attention-Deficit/Hyperactivity Disorder have great difficulty controlling all their impulses, not just the craving for movement and stimulation. They have little sense of time (five minutes seems like hours), and waiting for something is intolerable. Thus, they are impatient, interrupt, make comments out of turn, grab objects from others, clown around, and cause trouble at home, in school, work, and in social settings.

The consequences of ADHD can be severe. From a young age, people with Attention-Deficit/Hyperactivity Disorder tend to experience failure repeatedly, including rejection by peers, resulting in low self-esteem and sometimes more serious problems.

SYMPTOMS

1. Inattention, as compared with others at the same developmental level
• Often fails to attend to details, or makes careless mistakes in schoolwork, work or other activities;
• Often finds it difficult to maintain attention in tasks or play activities;
• Often does not seem to listen when spoken to;
• Often doesn't follow through on instructions and doesn't finish schoolwork, chores, or tasks;
• Often has difficulty organizing tasks or activities;
• Often avoids tasks that demand sustained mental effort, such as schoolwork or homework;
• Often loses things needed for tasks or activities, such as toys and school assignments;
• Often is easily distracted;
• Often is forgetful in daily activities.

2. Hyperactivity, as compared with others at the same developmental level
• Often fidgets with hands or feet, or squirms in chair;
• Often leaves seat in classroom or other situations where remaining seated is expected;
• Often runs or climbs about in situations in which it is inappropriate (among adolescents or adults, this may be a feeling of restlessness);
• Often has difficulty playing or handling leisure activities quietly;
• Often is on the go, moving excessively;

• Often talks excessively.
• Often blurts out answers impulsively before questions are finished;
• Often has difficulty waiting in turn;
• Often intrudes impulsively on others' games, activities or conversations.

Parts of this description may apply to all or most children at times, but behaving in this way nearly all the time wreaks havoc on the child and family. Three distinctions are made in the diagnosis:

Attention-Deficit/Hyperactivity Disorder, Combined Type if six or more items from List (1) and six or more from List (2) are applicable;

Attention-Deficit/Hyperactivity Disorder, Predominantly Inattentive Type if six or more items from List (1) only are applicable;

Attention-Deficit/Hyperactivity Disorder, Predominantly Hyperactive-Impulsive Type if six or more items from List (2) only are applicable.

ASSOCIATED FEATURES

Certain behaviors often go along with Attention-Deficity/Hyperactivity Disorder. The person is often frustrated and angry, exhibiting outbursts of temper and bossiness. To others, the lack of application and inability to finish tasks may look like laziness or irresponsibility. Other conditions may also be associated with the disorder, including Hyperthyroidism (an overactive thyroid). There may be a higher prevalence of anxiety, depression, and learning disorders among people with AD/HD.

A careful assessment and diagnosis by a professional familiar with AD/HD are essential, especially since some of the typical AD/HD behaviors may resemble those of other disorders. Family, school, and other possible problems must be taken into account and addressed. This is a lifelong disorder, though sometimes attenuated in adulthood.

The diagnosis is especially difficult to establish in young children, e.g., at the toddler and preschool level, because behavior that is typical at that age is similar to the symptoms of AD/HD. Children at that age may be extremely active but not develop the disorder.

PREVALENCE

AD/HD occurs in various cultures. It is much more frequent in males than females, with male to female ratios at 4:1 in the general population, and 9:1 in clinic populations. The prevalence among school-age children is from three percent to five percent.

There is emerging literature concerning adult AD/HD, and evidence that some adults can benefit from the same treatments used for children.

TREATMENT OPTIONS

Treatment should be based on an understanding that Attention-Deficit/Hyperactivity Disorder is not intentional, and punishment is not a cure.

The person with AD/HD has great need for external motivation, consistency, and structure. This should be provided by a professional who is familiar with the disorder. For a school-aged child, it is important to enlist the help of the school in designing a treatment plan which should include concrete steps aimed at developing specific competencies (e.g., handling time, sequencing, problem-solving, and social interaction).

Medication is often prescribed but should not be the only treatment. Newer preparations of medications, such as Concerta, offer once or twice a day dosing, so that children do not need to take medication during the school day. Since this condition affects all members of the family, the family needs help in providing consistency and structure, and in changing the role of the person with AD/HD as the family member who always gets into trouble.

Current treatments can have a positive impact and, in some cases, transform behaviors so that a formerly chaotic life becomes one over which the person has much greater control and more frequent experience of success.

Associations & Agencies

450 Attention Deficit Disorder Association
PO Box 7557
Wilmington, DE 19803-9997
800-939-1019
Fax: 800-939-1019
E-mail: info@add.org
www.www.add.org

Evelyn Polk Green, MS.Ed, President
Linda Roggli, PCC, Vice President
Paul S Galonsky, MPA, Public Policy Chair
Linda Walker, Workplace Committee Chair

Provides children, adolescents and adults with ADD information, support groups, publications, videos, and referrals. Also, generates hope, awareness, empowerment and connections worldwide.

451 Center For Mental Health Services
1 Choke Cherry Road
Room 6-1057
Rockville, MD 20857
240-276-1310
877-726-4727
Fax: 240-276-1320
TDD: 800-487-4889
TTY: 800-487-4889
E-mail: info@mentalhealth.org
www.beta.samhsa.gov/about-us/who-we-are/offices-center

Michael E Etzinger, B.S.M.E, , M.B., SAMHSA Executive Officer, Director
Paolo Del Vecchio, M.S.W, Director, Center for Mental Health
Deborah Baldwin, M.P.A, Acting Director, Consumer Affairs
Elizabeth Lopez, Ph.D, Acting Deputy Director

CMHS leads Federal efforts to treat mental illnesses by promoting mental health and by preventing the development or worsening of mental illness when possible. Congress created CMHS to bring new hope to adults who have serious mental illnesses and to children with serious emotional disorders. CMHS pursues its mission by helping states improve and increase the quality and range of their treatment, rehabilitation, and support services for people with mental illnesses, their families, and communities.

Year Founded: 1992

452 Center for Mental Health Services (CMHS)
1 Choke Cherry Road
Room 6-1057
Rockville, MD 20857
240-276-1310
877-726-4727
Fax: 240-276-1320
TDD: 800-487-4889
E-mail: info@mentalhealth.org
www.beta.samhsa.gov/about-us/who-we-are/offices-center

Michael E Etzinger, B.S.M.E, , M.B., SAMHSA Executive Officer, Director
Paolo Del Vecchio, M.S.W, Director, Center for Mental Health
Deborah Baldwin, M.P.A, Acting Director, Consumer Affairs
Elizabeth Lopez, Ph.D, Acting Deputy Director

CMHS leads Federal efforts to treat mental illnesses by promoting mental health and by preventing the development or worsening of mental illness when possible. Congress created CMHS to bring new hope to adults who have serious mental illnesses and to children with serious emotional disorders. CMHS provides information about mental health via a toll-free the web site, and more than 600 publications. Developed for users of mental health services and their families, the general public, policy makers, providers, and the media.

Year Founded: 1992

453 Children and Adults with AD/HD (CHADD)
4601 Presidents Drive
Suite 300
Lanham, MD 20706
301-306-7070
800-233-4050
Fax: 301-306-7090
www.chadd.org

Barbara S Hawkins, BA, President
Ruth Hughes, PhD, Chief Executive Officer
M Jeffry Spahr, MBA, JD, Secretary
Michael MacKay, Treasurer

National nonprofit organization representing children and adults with attention deficit/hyperactivity disorder (AD/HD). Available on Facebook and Twitter.

Year Founded: 1987

454 Learning Disabilities Association of America
4156 Library Road
Pittsburgh, PA 15234-1349
412-341-1515
Fax: 412-344-0224
E-mail: info@LDAAmerica.org
www.ldaamerica.org

Patricia H Latham, President
Mary Clare Reynolds, Executive Director
B.J Wiemer, First Vice President
Ed Schlitt, Second Vice President

Educating individuals with learning disabilities and their parents about the nature of the disability and inform them of their rights, encourages research in neuro-physiological and psychological aspects of learning disabilities.

Year Founded: 1964

455 National Alliance on Mental Illness
3803 North Fairfax Drive
Suite 100
Arlington, VA 22203
703-524-7600
888-999-6264
Fax: 703-524-9094
E-mail: helpline@nami.org
www.nami.org

Keris Jan Myrick, MBA, MS, PhD., President
Mary Giliberti, J.D, Executive Director
Jim Payne, J.D, First Vice President
David Levy, Chief Financial Officer

The nation's largest grassroots mental health organization dedicated to building better lives for the millions of Americans affected by mental illness. NAMI advocates for access to services, treatment, supports and research and is steadfast in its commitment to raising awareness and building a community of hope for all of those in need.

Year Founded: 1969

456 National Association for the Dually Diagnosed (NADD)
132 Fair Street
Kingston, NY 12401-4802
845-331-4336
800-331-5362
Fax: 845-331-4569
E-mail: info@thenadd.org
www.thenadd.org

Donna McNELIS, PhD, President
Robert J Fletcher DSW, Chief Executive Officer
Dan Baker, PhD, Vice President
Julia Pearce, Secretary

Nonprofit organization designed to promote interest of professional and parent development with resources for individuals who have the coexistence of mental illness and mental retardation. Provides conferences, educational services and training materials to professionals, parents, concerned citizens and service organizations.

Year Founded: 1983

457 National Center for Learning Disabilities
361 Park Avenue South
Suite 1401
New York, NY 10016
212-545-7510
888-575-7373
Fax: 212-545-9565
E-mail: info@ncld.org
www.www.ncld.org

Frederic M Poses, Chairman of the Board
James H Wendorf, Executive Director
Mary Kalikow, Vice Chair
John R Langeler, Treasurer

The National Center for Learning Disabilities (NCLD) ensures sucess for all individuals with learning disabilities in school, at work and in life. They connect connect paretns and others with resources, guidelines and support so they can advocate effectively for their children.

Year Founded: 1977

458 National Dissemination Center for Children with Disabilities (NICHCY)
1825 Connecticut Ave NW
Suite 700
Washington, DC 20009
800-695-0285
Fax: 202-884-8441
TTY: 202-884-8200
E-mail: nichcy@fhi360.org
www.nichcy.org

NICHCY is the center that provides information to the nation on: disabilities in children and youth; programs and services for infants, children, and youth with disabilities; IDEA, the nation's special education law; and research-based information on effective practices for children with disabilities.

459 National Mental Health Consumers' Self-Help Clearinghouse
1211 Chestnut Street
Suite 1100
Philadelphia, PA 19107-4103
215-751-1810
800-553-4539
Fax: 215-636-6312
E-mail: info@mhselfhelp.org
www.mhselfhelp.org

Joseph Rogers, Executive Director/ Founder
Susan Rogers, Director
Britani Nestel, Program Specialist
Christa Burkett, Technical Assistance Coordinator

The latest information on mental health and consumer/survivor issues. Includes updates on important issues, linking readers to new sources, funding opportunities and the most recent developments in the consumer movement. Also find conference announcements and job postings from across the nation.

Year Founded: 1986

460 National Resource Center on ADHD
A Program of CHADD
4601 Presidents Drive
Suite 300
Lanham, MD 20706
800-233-4050
E-mail: info@help4adhd.org
www.www.help4adhd.org

Timothy J MacGeorge, MSW, Director

The National Resource Center was established in 2002 to be the national clearinghouse for the latest evidence-based information on ADHD. The NRC provides comprehensive information and support to individuals with ADHD, their families and friends, and the professionals involved in their lives.

461 PACER Center
8161 Normandale Blvd
Bllomington, MN 55437
952-838-9000
888-248-0822
Fax: 952-838-0199
TTY: 952-838-0190
E-mail: info@pacer.org
www.www.pacer.org

Paula F Goldberg, Executive Director, Co-Founder
Paul Luehr, President

Alison Bakken, Vice-President
Jessica Broyles, Treasurer

PACER provides information, training, and assistance to parents of children and young adults with disabilities; physical, learning, cognitive, emotional, and health. Its mission is to improve and expand opportunities that enhance the quality of life for children and youth with disabilitiesand their families.

Year Founded: 1976

462 SAMHSA's National Mental Health Information Center
PO Box 42557
Washington, DC 20015-557
240-221-4021
800-789-2647
Fax: 240-221-4295
TDD: 866-889-2647
www.mentalhealth.org

A Kathryn Power MEd, Director
Edward B Searle, Deputy Director

463 The Center For Family Support
2811 Zulette Avenue
Bronx, NY 10461
718-518-1500
Fax: 718-518-8200
E-mail: svernikoff@cfsny.org
www.cfsny.org

Steven Vernikoff, Executive Director
Virgil Seepersad, Director of Finance
Eileen Berg, Director of Quality Assurance
Barbara Greenwald, Associate Executive, Director

An agency that continues to develop new programs to serve families and individuals with their care needs. They offer services throughout the New York City region including: New Jersey, Long Island and the Lower Hudson Valley.

Year Founded: 1954

464 The National Federation of Families for Children's Mental Health
9605 Medical Center Drive
Suite 208
Rockville, MD 20850
240-403-1901
Fax: 240-403-1909
E-mail: ffcmh@ffcmh.org
www.www.ffcmh.org

Sandra Spencer, Executive Director
Lizzette Albright, Finance Director
Lynda Gargan, Senior Managing Director
Nicole Marshall, Projects and Logistics Manager

The National Federation of Families Childrens Mental Health provides advocacy at the national level for the rights of children and youth with emotional, behaviorah and mental health challenges and their families. They provide leadership and technical assistance to a nation-wide network of family run organizations that deal with illnesses such as ADHD.

Year Founded: 1989

465 A Birds-Eye View of Life with ADD and ADHD: Advice from Young Survivors
Cherish the Children
PO Box 189
Cedar Bluff, AL 35959-189
Fax: 256-779-5203
E-mail: chirs@chrisdendy.com
www.www.chrisdendy.com/bev.htm

Chris A Zeigler Dendy, Author
Alex Zeigler, Author

Written expressly for teenagers, preteens, and young adults, by teenagers and a young adult who are struggling with ADD or ADHD. This survival guide offers factual information and practical advice in words and examples that young people can easily understand and put into practice. Written with humor and compassion, A Bird's Eye View offers down-to-earth tips for coping with a variety of issues: disorganization, forgetfulness, always being late, sleep problems, memorization, procrastination, restlessness, medication, writing essays, and algebra. This book is meant to be helpful yet still interesting to read.

466 ADD & Learning Disabilities: Reality, Myths, & Controversial Treatments
Bantam Doubleday Dell Publishing
1745 Broadway
New York, NY 10019-4343
212-782-9000

Barbara Ingersoll, Author
Sam Goldstein, PhD., Author

For parents of children with learning disabilities and attention deficit disorder - and for educational and medical professionals who encounter these children - two experts in the field have devised a handbook to help identify the very best treatments. *$10.36*

256 pages ISBN 0-385469-31-4

467 ADD & Romance: Finding Fulfillment in Love, Sex, & Relationships
ADD WareHouse
300 NW 70th Avenue
Suite 102
Plantation, FL 33317-2360
954-792-8100
800-233-9273
Fax: 954-792-8545
E-mail: sales@addwarehouse.com
www.addwarehouse.com

Jonathan Halverstadt, Author
Daniel Amen, Author

Licensed therapist Jonathan Scott Halverstadt looks at how attention deficit disorder can damage romantic relationships when partners do not take time, or do not know how, to address this unique problem. The book aims to give people with A.D.D. and their partners the tools they need to build and sustain a more satisfying and fulfilling relationship. *$12.95*

230 pages Year Founded: 1998 ISBN 0-878332-09-X

468 ADD Kaleidoscope: The Many Faces of Adult Attention Deficit Disorder
Hope Press 91009-188
Fax: 818-358-3520
E-mail: dcomings@earthlink.net
www.hopepress.com

Joan Andrews, Author
Denise E. Davis, Author

A comprehensive presentation of all aspects of attention deficit disorder in adults. While often thought of as a child-hood disorder, ADD symptoms usually continue into adult-hood where they can cause a wide range of problems with personal interactions, work performance, attitude towards one's employer, and interactions with spouses and children. *$24.95*

293 pages ISBN 1-878267-03-5

469 ADD Success Stories: Guide to Fulfillment for Families with Attention Deficit Disorder
ADD WareHouse
300 NorthWest 70th Avenue
Suite 102
Plantation, FL 33317-2360
954-792-8944
800-233-9273
Fax: 954-792-8545
E-mail: websales@addwarehouse.com
www.addwarehouse.com

Thom Hartmann, Author
John J. Ratey, Author

Real-life stories of people with ADD who achieved success in school, at work, in marriages and relationships. Thou-sands of interviews and histories as well as new research show children and adults from all walks of life how to reach the next-step, a fulfilling, successful life with ADD. Discover which occupations are best for people with ADD. *$12.00*

288 pages Year Founded: 1995 ISBN 1-887424-03-2

470 ADD in the Workplace: Choices, Changes and Challenges
ADD WareHouse
300 NW 70th Avenue
Suite 102
Plantation, FL 33317-2360
954-792-8944
800-233-9273
Fax: 954-792-8545
E-mail: sales@addwarehouse.com
www.addwarehouse.com

Kathleen Nadeau, Author

This book contains information that seeks to help adults move from resignation to determination in forging a path to success. Whether this means finding an ADD-friendly en-vironment, requesting reasonable workplace accommoda-tions, or creating a freelance nich, this book will point out the right directions. *$24.00*

256 pages Year Founded: 1997 ISBN 0-876308-47-7

471 ADD/ADHD Checklist: an Easy Reference for Parents & Teachers
ADD WareHouse
300 NorthWest 70th Avenue
Suite 102
Plantation, FL 33317-2360
954-792-8944
800-233-9273
Fax: 954-792-8545
E-mail: websales@addwarehouse.com
www.addwarehouse.com

Harvey C Parker, Owner

Written by a nationally known educator with two decades of experience in working with ADD/ADHD students. For fast, reliable information about attention deficit disorder, parents and teachers need only to refer to The ADD/ADHD Checklist. *$12.00*

272 pages Year Founded: 2002

472 ADHD Monitoring System
ADD WareHouse
300 NorthWest 70th Avenue
Suite 102
Plantation, FL 33317-2360
954-792-8944
800-233-9273
Fax: 954-792-8545
E-mail: websales@addwarehouse.com
www.addwarehouse.com

Harvey C Parker, Owner

Provides a simple, cost effective way to carefully monitor how well a student with ADHD is doing at school. Parents and teachers will be able to easily track behavior, academic performance, quality of student classwork and homework. Contains monitoring forms along with instructions for use. *$8.95*

473 ADHD Parenting Handbook: Practical Advice for Parents
Taylor Trade Publishing
5360 Manhattan Circle
Suite 100
Boulder, CO 80303-4249
303-543-7835
Fax: 303-543-0043
E-mail: rrinehart@rowman.com
www.rowman.com/taylortrade

Colleen Alexander Roberts, Author

Practical advice for parents from parents, and proven tech-niques for raising hyperactive children without losing your temper.

224 pages Year Founded: 1994 ISBN 0-878338-62-4

474 ADHD Survival Guide for Parents and Teachers
Hope Press
PO Box 188
Duarte, CA 91009-188
818-303-0644
800-321-4039
Fax: 626-358-3520
E-mail: dcomings@earthlink.net
www.hopepress.com

Richard A. Lougy, MFT, Author
David K. Rosenthal, MD, Author

Fills an important need expressed by parents, teachers, and other caretakers of ADHD children who have asked for clear, practical, and easily understood strategies to deal with ADHD children.

Year Founded: 2002 ISBN 1-878267-43-4

475 ADHD and Teens: Parent's Guide to Making it Through the Tough Years
ADD WareHouse
300 NorthWest 70th Avenue
Suite 102
Plantation, FL 33317-2360
954-792-8944
800-233-9273
Fax: 954-792-8545
E-mail: websales@addwarehouse.com
www.addwarehouse.com

Colleen Alexander Roberts, Author

A manual of practical advice to help parents cope with the problems that can arise during these years. A crash course is offered on parenting styles that really work with teens with ADHD and how these styles allow the teen to safely move from dependence to independence. *$13.00*

199 pages Year Founded: 1995 ISBN 0-878338-99-3

476 ADHD and the Nature of Self-Control
Guilford Press
72 Spring Street
New York, NY 10012
212-431-9800
800-365-7006
Fax: 212-966-6708
E-mail: info@guilford.com
www.guilford.com

Russell A. Barkley, PhD, Author

Provides a radical shift of perspective on ADHD, arguing that the disorder is a developmental problem of self control and that an attention deficit is a secondary characteristic. Combines neuropsychological research and the theory on the executive functions, illustrating how normally functioning individuals are able to bring behavior under the control of time and orient their actions toward the future. *$46.00*

410 pages Year Founded: 1973 ISBN 1-572302-50-X

477 ADHD in the Young Child: Driven to Redirection: A Guide for Parents and Teachers of Young Children with ADHD
ADD WareHouse
300 NW 70th Avenue
Suite 102
Plantation, FL 33317-2360
954-792-8944
800-233-9273
Fax: 954-792-8545
E-mail: sales@addwarehouse.com
www.addwarehouse.com

Cathy Reimers PhD, Author
Bruce A. Brunger, Author

The authors sensitively and effectively describe what life is like living with a young child with ADHD. With the help of over 75 cartoon illustrations they provide practical solutions to common problems found at home, in school and elsewhere. *$18.95*

202 pages Year Founded: 1999 ISBN 1-886941-32-7

478 ADHD: A Complete and Authoritative Guide
American Academy Of Pediatrics
141 Northwest Point Boulevard
Elk Grove Village, IL 60007-1098
847-434-4000
800-433-9016

Fax: 847-434-8000
www.aap.org

Sherill Tippins, Editor
Michael I. Reiff MD, FAAP, Editor-in-Chief

Based on the American Academy of Pediatrics' own clinical practice guidelines for ADHD and written in clear, accessible language, ths book answers the common question: How is ADHD diagnosed? What are today's best treatment options? and Will my child outgrow ADHD?

355 pages Year Founded: 2004 ISBN 1-581101-21-X

479 Adventures in Fast Forward: Life, Love and Work for the ADD Adult
ADD WareHouse
300 NW 70th Avenue
Suite 102
Plantation, FL 33317-2360
954-792-8944
800-233-9273
Fax: 954-792-8545
E-mail: sales@addwarehouse.com
www.addwarehouse.com

Kathleen G. Nadeu, Author

For all adults with ADD, this book is designed to be a practical guide for day-to-day life. No matter where you are in the scenario - curious about ADD, just diagnosed or experiencing particular problems, this book will give you effective strategies to help anticipate and negotiate the challenges that come with the condition. Filled with important tools and tactics for self-care and success. *$23.00*

224 pages Year Founded: 1996 ISBN 0-876308-00-0

480 All About Attention Deficit Disorder: Revised Edition
ADD WareHouse
300 NW 70th Avenue
Suite 102
Plantation, FL 33317-2360
954-792-8944
800-233-9273
Fax: 954-792-8545
E-mail: sales@addwarehouse.com
www.addwarehouse.com

Harvey C Parker, Owner

A practical and comprehensive manual for parents and teachers interested in understanding the facts about ADD. Chapters on home management, the 1-2-3 Magic discipline method, facts about medication management and practical ideas for teachers to use in managing learning and classroom behavior. *$13.00*

165 pages

481 All Kinds of Minds
ADD WareHouse
300 NW 70th Avenue
Suite 102
Plantation, FL 33317-2360
954-792-8944
800-233-9273
Fax: 954-792-8545
E-mail: sales@addwarehouse.com
www.addwarehouse.com

Dr. Mel Levine, Author

Young students with learning disorders- children in primary and elementary grades -can now gain insight into the difficulties they face in school. This book helps all children understand and respect all kinds of minds and can encourage children with learning disorders to maintain their motivation and keep from developing behavior problems stemming from their learning disorders. *$38.00*

283 pages

482 Answers to Distraction
ADD WareHouse
300 NorthWest 70th Avenue
Suite 102
Plantation, FL 33317-2360
954-792-8944
800-233-9273
Fax: 954-792-8545
E-mail: websales@addwarehouse.com
www.addwarehouse.com

Edward M. Hallowell, Author
John J. Ratey, Author

A user's guide to ADD presented in a question and answer format ideal for parents of children and adolescents with ADD, adults with ADD and teachers who work with students who have ADD. *$13.00*

334 pages Year Founded: 1996 ISBN 0-553378-21-X

483 Attention Deficit Disorder and Learning Disabilities: Reality, Myths, and Controversial Treatments
Bantam Doubleday Dell Publishing
1745 Broadway
10th Floor
New York, NY 10019-4343
E-mail: ddaypub@randomhouse.com
www.www.randomhouse.com

Barbara D. Ingersoll, Author
Sam Goldstein, Author

Discusses ADHD and learning disabilities as well as their effective treatments. Warns against nutritional and other alternative treatments. *$12.95*

256 pages Year Founded: 1993 ISBN 0-385469-31-4

484 Attention Deficit Hyperactivity Disorder in Children: A Medication Guide
Madison Institute of Medicine
7617 Mineral Point Road
Suite 300
Madison, WI 53717-1623
608-827-2470
E-mail: mim@miminc.org
www.factsforhealth.org

Hugh F. Johnston, Author
J. Jay Fruehling, Author

Written for parents, this explains the various medications used commonly to treat ADHD/ADD. It includes a review of the symptoms of ADHD, medication therapy, commonly asked questions, and side effects of medications. *$5.95*

41 pages

485 Attention Deficits and Hyperactivity in Children: Developmental Clinical Psychology and Psychiatry
Sage Publications
2455 Teller Road
Thousand Oaks, CA 91320-2234
800-818-7243
Fax: 800-583-2665
E-mail: info@sagepub.com
www.sagepub.com

Stephen P. Hinshaw, Author

Provides background information and evaluates key debates and questions that remain unanswered about ADHD. Includes what tools can be used to gain optimal information about this disorder and which factors predict subsequent functioning in adolescence and adulthood. Advances, challenges and unresolved problems in diverse but relevant areas are analyzed and placed in context. Paperback also available. *$43.95*

161 pages Year Founded: 1993 ISBN 0-803951-96-5

486 Attention-Deficit Hyperactivity Disorder in Adults: A Guide
Madison Institute of Medicine
6515 Grand Teton Plaza
Suite 100
Madison, WI 53719
608-827-2470
Fax: 608-827-2444
E-mail: mim@miminc.org
www.factsforhealth.org

Hugh F. Johnston, MD, Author

This guide provides an overview of adult ADHD and how it is treated with medications and other treatment approaches. *$5.95*

58 pages Year Founded: 2002

487 Beyond Ritalin
ADD WareHouse
300 NorthWest 70th Avenue
Suite 102
Plantation, FL 33317-2360
954-792-8944
800-233-9273
Fax: 954-792-8545
E-mail: websales@addwarehouse.com
www.addwarehouse.com

Stephen W. Garber, PhD, Author

Beyond Ritalin: Facts About Medication and Other Strategies for Helping Children, Adolescents and Adults with Attention Deficit Disorders. The authors respond to concerns all parents and individuals have about using medication to treat disorders such as ADHD, explain the importance of a treatment program for those with this condition and discuss fads and fallacies in current treatments. *$13.50*

272 pages Year Founded: 1996 ISBN 0-060977-25-6

488 Conduct Disorders in Children and Adolescents
American Psychiatric Publishing, Inc.
1000 Wilson Boulevard
Suite 1825
Arlington, VA 22209-3901
703-907-7322
800-368-5777
Fax: 703-907-1091

E-mail: appi@psych.org
www.appi.org

G Pirooz Sholevar, M.D., Editor
Ron McMillen, Chief Executive Officer
John McDuffie, Editorial Director

Examines the phenomenology, etiology, and diagnosis of conduct disorders, and describes therapeutic and preventive interventions. Includes the range of treatments now availaable, including individual, family, group, and behavior therapy; hospitalization; and residential treatment. *$52.00*

414 pages Year Founded: 1995 ISBN 0-880485-17-5

489 Consumer's Guide to Psychiatric Drugs
NewHarbinger Publications
5674 Shattuck Avenue
Oakland, CA 94609-1662
510-652-0215
800-748-6273
Fax: 800-652-1613
E-mail: customerservice@newharbinger.com
www.newharbinger.com

Mary C. Talaga, Author
John D. Preston, Author
John H. O'Neal, Author

The authors explain how each drug works, tell readers what to expect in terms of side-effects, interaction with other drugs and medical condition, and other concerns, and offer detailed information about treatments for depression, bipolar disorder, anxiety and sleep disorders, and a comprehensive range of other conditions. *$16.95*

340 pages Year Founded: 1973 ISBN 1-572241-11-X

490 Daredevils and Daydreamers: New Perspectives on Attention Deficit/Hyperactivity Disorder
ADD WareHouse
300 NW 70th Avenue
Suite 102
Plantation, FL 33317-2360
954-792-8100
800-233-9273
Fax: 954-792-8545
E-mail: sales@addwarehouse.com
www.addwarehouse.com

Barbara Ingersoll, Author

From obtaining a good diagnosis through the most recent, cutting edge medical and psychological solutions offered, Ingersoll's examples and research have an immediacy missing from the other books in the field. In addition, the othor tackles a number of peripheral issues other books ignore such as the problem of the ADHD child in adoptive families, divorced families and step-families, and she handles real-world issues (like soiling and bed-wetting) that others disregard. *$11.00*

256 pages Year Founded: 1997 ISBN 0-385487-57-6

491 Distant Drums, Different Drummers: A Guide for Young People with ADHD
ADD WareHouse
300 NorthWest 70th Avenue
Suite 102
Plantation, FL 33317-2360
954-792-8944
800-233-9273
Fax: 954-792-8545

E-mail: websales@addwarehouse.com
www.addwarehouse.com

Barbara D. Ingersoll, Author

This book presents a positive perspective of ADHD - one that stresses the value of individual differences. Written for children and adolescents struggling with ADHD, it offers young readers the opportunity to see themselves in a positive light and motivates them to face challenging problems. Ages 8-14. *$16.00*

48 pages Year Founded: 1995 ISBN 0-964854-80-6

492 Don't Give Up Kid
ADD WareHouse
300 NW 70th Avenue
Suite 102
Plantation, FL 33317-2360
954-792-8944
800-233-9273
Fax: 954-792-8545
E-mail: sales@addwarehouse.com
www.addwarehouse.com

Jeanne Gehret, Author
M.A. Gehret, Author
Sandra A. Depauw, Illustrator

Alex, the hero of this book, is one of two million children in the US who have learning disabilities. This book gives children with reading problems and learning disabilities a clear understanding of their difficulties and the necessary courage to learn to live with them. Ages 5-12. *$13.00*

40 pages Year Founded: 1996 ISBN 1-884281-10-9

493 Down and Dirty Guide to Adult Attention Deficit Disorder
ADD WareHouse
300 NorthWest 70th Avenue
Suite 102
Plantation, FL 33317-2360
954-792-8944
800-233-9273
Fax: 954-792-8545
E-mail: websales@addwarehouse.com
www.addwarehouse.com

Harvey C Parker, Owner

A book about ADD that is immensely entertaining, informative and uncomplicated. Describes concepts essential to understanding how this disorder is best identified and treated. You'll find a refreshing absence of jargon and an abundance of common sense, practical advice and healthy skepticism. *$17.00*

194 pages

494 Driven to Distraction: Recognizing and Coping with Attention Deficit Disorder from Childhood through Adulthood
ADD WareHouse
300 NorthWest 70th Avenue
Suite 102
Plantation, FL 33317-2360
954-792-8944
800-233-9273
Fax: 954-792-8545
E-mail: websales@addwarehouse.com
www.addwarehouse.com

Harvey C Parker, Owner
John J Ratey MD

Through vivid stories of the experiences of their patients (both adults and children), this books shows the varied forms ADD takes - from the hyperactive search for high stimulation to the floating inattention of daydreaming - and the transforming impact of precise diagnosis and treatment. The authors explain when and how medication can be helpful, and since both authors have ADD, their advice on effective behavior-modification techniques is enriched by their own experience. Also available on audiotape for $16.00. *$13.00*

319 pages Year Founded: 1995

495 Drug Therapy and Childhood & Adolescent Disorders
Mason Crest Publishers
450 Parkway Drive
Suite D
Broomall, PA 19008-4017
610-543-6200
866-627-2665
Fax: 610-543-3878
E-mail: dtaylor@masoncrest.com
www.masoncrest.com

Shirley Brinkerhoff, Author
Dan Hilferty, President
Michelle Luke, Director, Marketing
Michael Toglia, Special Sales

This book provides readers with an easy-to-understand introduction to this topic. Numerous case sstudies and examples give insight in the four disorders first diagnosed in childhood and adolescence that can be treated with psychiatric drugs, and helps readers understand the symptoms and treatments of these disorders. The disorders included in this volume are: mental retardation, pervasive developmental disorders, attention-deficit and disruptive behavior disorders and tic disorders.

128 pages ISBN 1-590845-63-3

496 Eagle Eyes: A Child's View of Attention Deficit Disorder
ADD WareHouse
300 NorthWest 70th Avenue
Suite 102
Plantation, FL 33317-2360
954-792-8944
800-233-9273
Fax: 954-792-8545
E-mail: websales@addwarehouse.com
www.addwarehouse.com

Harvey C Parker, Owner

This book helps readers of all ages understand ADD and gives practical suggestions for organization, social cues and self calming. Expressive illustrations enhance the book and encourage reluctant readers. Ages 5-12. *$13.00*

30 pages

497 Eukee the Jumpy, Jumpy Elephant
ADD WareHouse
300 NorthWest 70th Avenue
Suite 102
Plantation, FL 33317-2360
954-792-8944
800-233-9273

Fax: 954-792-8545
E-mail: websales@addwarehouse.com
www.addwarehouse.com

Harvey C Parker, Owner
Esther Trevino

A story about a bright young elephant who is not like all the other elephants. Eukee moves through the jungle like a tornado, unable to pay attention to the other elephants. He begins to feel sad, but gets help after a visit to the doctor who explains why Eukee is so jumpy and hyperactive. With love, support and help, Eukee learns ways to help himself and gain renewed self-esteem. Ideal for ages 3-8. *$15.00*

22 pages Year Founded: 1995

498 Facing AD/HD: A Survival Guide for Parents
Research Press
Dept 24 W
PO Box 9177
Champaign, IL 61826-9177
217-352-3273
800-519-2707
Fax: 217-352-1221
E-mail: rp@researchpress.com
www.researchpress.com

Janet Morris, Author
Robert W Parkinson, Founder

Provides parents with the skills they need to help minimize the everyday struggles and frustrations associated with AD/HD. The book addresses structure, routines, setting goals, using charts, persistency with consistency, teamwork, treatment options, medication and more. *$ 14.95*

232 pages ISBN 0-878223-81-9

499 First Star I See
ADD WareHouse
300 NW 70th Avenue
Suite 102
Plantation, FL 33317-2360
954-792-8944
800-233-9273
Fax: 954-792-8545
E-mail: sales@addwarehouse.com
www.addwarehouse.com

Harvey C Parker, Owner

This entertaining and funny look at ADD without hyperactivity is a must-read for middle grade girls with ADD, their teachers and parents. *$11.00*

150 pages

500 Gene Bomb
Hope Press
PO Box 188
Duarte, CA 91009-188
818-303-0644
800-321-4039
Fax: 626-358-3520
E-mail: dcomings@earthlink.net
www.hopepress.com

David E Comings, Author

Gene Bomb: Does Higher Education and Advanced Technology Accelerate the Selection of Genes for Learning Disorders, Addictive and Disruptive Behaviors? Explores the hypothesis that autism, learning disorders, alcoholism, drug abuse, depression, attention deficit disorder, and other disruptive behavioral disorders are increaseing in frequency because of an increasing selection, in the 20th century, for the genes associated with these conditions. *$29.95*

304 pages ISBN 1-878267-38-8

501 Give Your ADD Teen a Chance: A Guide for Parents of Teenagers with Attention Deficit Disorder
ADD WareHouse
300 NorthWest 70th Avenue
Suite 102
Plantation, FL 33317-2360
954-792-8944
800-233-9273
Fax: 954-792-8545
E-mail: websales@addwarehouse.com
www.addwarehouse.com

Harvey C Parker, Owner

Parenting teenagers is never easy, especially if your teen suffers from ADD. This book provides parents with expert help by showing them how to determine which issues are caused by 'normal' teenager development and which are caused by ADD. *$15.00*

299 pages

502 Grandma's Pet Wildebeest Ate My Homework
ADD WareHouse
300 NW 70th Avenue
Suite 102
Plantation, FL 33317-2360
954-792-8944
800-233-9273
Fax: 954-792-8545
E-mail: sales@addwarehouse.com
www.addwarehouse.com

Harvey C Parker, Owner

Parents and teachers dealing with hyperactive or daydreaming kids will find this book outstanding. As an ADHD adult himself, Quinn draws upon his own experience, making use of straightforward, creative behavioral management techniques, along with a keen sense of humor. A highly informative and enlightened book. *$16.95*

272 pages

503 Healing ADD: Simple Exercises That Will Change Your Daily Life
ADD WareHouse
300 NW 70th Avenue
Suite 102
Plantation, FL 33317-2360
954-792-8944
800-233-9273
Fax: 954-792-8545
E-mail: sales@addwarehouse.com
www.addwarehouse.com

Harvey C Parker, Owner

Presents simple methods involving visualization and positive thinking that can be readily picked up by adults and taught to children with ADD. *$10.00*

178 pages

504 Help 4 ADD@High School
ADD WareHouse
300 NorthWest 70th Avenue
Suite 102
Plantation, FL 33317-2360
954-792-8944
800-233-9273
Fax: 954-792-8545
E-mail: websales@addwarehouse.com
www.addwarehouse.com

Harvey C Parker, Owner

This new book was written for teenagers with ADHD. Designed like a web site, it has short, easy-to-read information packed sections which tell you what you need to know about how to get your life together - for yourself, not for your parents or your teachers. Includes tips on studying, ways your high school can help you succeed, tips on getting along better at home, on dating, exercise and much more. *$19.95*

119 pages

505 HomeTOVA: Attention Screening Test
ADD WareHouse
300 NW 70th Avenue
Suite 102
Plantation, FL 33317-2360
954-792-8944
800-233-9273
Fax: 954-792-8545
E-mail: sales@addwarehouse.com
www.addwarehouse.com

Harvey C Parker, Owner

Screen yourself or your child (ages 4 to 80 plus) for attention problems. After a simple installation on your home computer (Windows 95/98 OS only), the Home TOVA program runs with use of a mouse. Takes 21.6 minutes and measures how fast, accurate and consistent a person is in responding to squares flashing on a screen. Each program is limited to two administrators. *$29.95*

506 How to Do Homework without Throwing Up
ADD WareHouse
300 NorthWest 70th Avenue
Suite 102
Plantation, FL 33317-2360
954-792-8944
800-233-9273
Fax: 954-792-8545
E-mail: websales@addwarehouse.com
www.addwarehouse.com

Harvey C Parker, Owner

Cartoons and witty insights teach important truths about homework and strategies for getting it done. Learn how to make a homework schedule, when to do the hardest homework, where to do homework, the benefits of homework and more. Useful in motivating students with ADD. For ages 8-13. *$9.00*

67 pages

507 Hyperactive Child, Adolescent, and Adult
Oxford University Press
198 Madison Avenue
New York, NY 10016-4341
212-726-6400
800-451-7556

Michael Cunningham, Manager

Discusses symptoms and treatment of ADD/ADHD in children and adults with practical suggestions for the management of children. *$27.00*

172 pages ISBN 0-195042-91-3

508 Hyperactive Children Grown Up: ADHD in Children, Adolescents, and Adults
Guilford Press
72 Spring Street
New York, NY 10012-4068
212-431-9800
800-365-7006
Fax: 212-966-6708
E-mail: info@guilford.com

Bob Matloff, President
Seymour Weingarten, Editor-in-Chief

Explores what happens to hyperactive children when they grow to adulthood. Based on the McGill prospective studies, which spans more than 30 years, the volume reports findings on the etiology, treatment and outcome of attention deficits and hyperactivity at all stages of development. Paperback also available. *$44.95*

473 pages ISBN 0-898620-39-2

509 I'm Somebody, Too!
ADD WareHouse
300 NorthWest 70th Avenue
Suite 102
Plantation, FL 33317-2360
954-792-8944
800-233-9273
Fax: 954-792-8545
E-mail: websales@addwarehouse.com
www.addwarehouse.com

Harvey C Parker, Owner

Because it is written for an older, non-ADD audience, this book explains ADD in depth and explains methods to handle the feelings that often result from having a family member with ADD. For children ages 9 and older. *$13.00*

159 pages

510 Is Your Child Hyperactive? Inattentive? Impulsive? Distractible?
ADD WareHouse
300 NorthWest 70th Avenue
Suite 102
Plantation, FL 33317-2360
954-792-8944
800-233-9273
Fax: 954-792-8545
E-mail: websales@addwarehouse.com
www.addwarehouse.com

Harvey C Parker, Owner

Written with compassion and hope, this parent guide prepares you for the process of determining if your child has ADD and guides you in your dealings with educators, doctors and other professionals. *$13.00*

256 pages Year Founded: 1995

511 Learning to Slow Down and Pay Attention
ADD WareHouse
300 NorthWest 70th Avenue
Suite 102
Plantation, FL 33317-2360
954-792-8944
800-233-9273
Fax: 954-792-8545
E-mail: websales@addwarehouse.com
www.addwarehouse.com

Harvey C Parker, Owner

Written for children to read, and illustrated with charming cartoons and activity pages, the book helps children identify problems and explains how their parents, teachers and doctors can help. For children 6-14. *$10.00*

96 pages

512 Living with Attention Deficit Disorder: Workbook for Adults with ADD
NewHarbinger Publications
5674 Shattuck Avenue
Oakland, CA 94609-1662
510-652-0215
800-748-6273
Fax: 800-652-1613
E-mail: customerservice@newharbinger.com
www.newharbinger.com

M Susan Roberts, Author
Gerald J Jansen, Author

Includes strategies for handling common problems at work and school, dealing with intimate relationships, and finding support. *$17.95*

165 pages Year Founded: 1973 ISBN 1-572240-63-6

513 Medications for Attention Disorders and Related Medical Problems: Comprehensive Handbook
ADD WareHouse
300 NW 70th Avenue
Suite 102
Plantation, FL 33317-2360
954-792-8944
800-233-9273
Fax: 954-792-8545
E-mail: sales@addwarehouse.com
www.addwarehouse.com

Harvey C Parker, Owner

ADHD and ADD are medical conditions and often medical intervention is regarded by most experts as an essential component of the multimodal program for the treatment of these disorders. This text presents a comprehensive look at medications and their use in attention disorders. *$37.00*

420 pages

514 Meeting the ADD Challenge: A Practical Guide for Teachers
Research Press
PO Box-7886
Champaign, IL 61826
217-352-3273
800-519-2707
Fax: 217-352-1221
E-mail: rp@researchpress.com
www.researchpress.com

Dr Michael J Asher, Author
Dr Steven B Gordon, Author

Information on the needs and treatment of children and adolescents with ADD. The book addresses the defining characteristics of ADD, common treatment approaches, myths about ADD, matching intervention to student, use of behavior rating scales and checklists, evaluating interventions, regular versus special class placement, helping students regulate their own behavior and more. Includes case examples. *$21.95*

196 pages Year Founded: 1968 ISBN 0-878223-45-2

515 Misunderstood Child: Understanding and Coping with Your Child's Learning Disabilities
ADD WareHouse
300 NW 70th Avenue
Suite 102
Plantation, FL 33317-2360
954-792-8944
800-233-9273
Fax: 954-792-8545
E-mail: sales@addwarehouse.com
www.addwarehouse.com

Harvey C Parker, Owner

In this revised and updated edition you will find promising treatment options for children, adolescents and adults with learning disabilities, discussion of ADHD, pros and cons of using medication, revision to federal and state laws covering discrimination and educational rights, new approaches for those of college age and older. *$15.00*

403 pages

516 My Brother's a World Class Pain: Sibling's Guide to ADHD
ADD WareHouse
300 NorthWest 70th Avenue
Suite 102
Plantation, FL 33317-2360
954-792-8944
800-233-9273
Fax: 954-792-8545
E-mail: websales@addwarehouse.com
www.addwarehouse.com

Harvey C Parker, Owner

While they frequently bear the brunt of the ADHD child's impulsiveness and distractibility, siblings usually are not afforded opportunities to understand the nature of the problem and to have their own feelings and thoughts addressed. This story shows brothers and sisters how they can play an important role in the family's quest for change. *$12.00*

34 pages Year Founded: 1992

517 Put Yourself in Their Shoes: Understanding Teenagers with Attention Deficit Hyperactivity Disorder
ADD WareHouse
300 NorthWest 70th Avenue
Suite 102
Plantation, FL 33317-2360
954-792-8944
800-233-9273
Fax: 954-792-8545
E-mail: websales@addwarehouse.com
www.addwarehouse.com

Harvey C Parker, Owner

Contains up-to-date information on how ADHD affects the lives of adolescents at home, in school, in the workplace and in social relationships. Chapters discuss how to get a good assessment, controversial treatments and medications for ADHD, building positive communication at home, problem-solving strategies to resolve family conflict, ADHD and the military, study strategies to improve learning, ADHD and delinquency, two hundred educational accommodations for ADHD teens and more. *$19.00*

229 pages Year Founded: 1999

518 RYAN: A Mother's Story of Her Hyperactive/Tourette Syndrome Child
Hope Press
PO Box 188
Duarte, CA 91009-188
818-303-0644
800-321-4039
Fax: 626-358-3520
E-mail: dcomings@earthlink.net
www.hopepress.com

Susan Hughes, Author

A moving and informative story of how a mother struggled with the many behavioral problems presented by her son with Tourette syndrome, ADHD and oppositional defiant disorder. *$9.95*

153 pages ISBN 1-878267-25-6

519 Shelley, The Hyperative Turtle
ADD WareHouse
300 NorthWest 70th Avenue
Suite 102
Plantation, FL 33317-2360
954-792-8944
800-233-9273
Fax: 954-792-8545
E-mail: websales@addwarehouse.com
www.addwarehouse.com

Harvey C Parker, Owner

The story of a bright young turtle who's not like all the other turtles. Shelley moves like a rocket and is unable to sit still for even the shortest periods of time. Because he and the other turtles are unable to understand why he is so wiggly and squirmy, Shelley begins to feel naughty and out of place. But after a visit to the doctor, Shelley learns what 'hyperactive' means and that it is necessary to take special medicine to control that wiggly feeling. Ideal for ages 3-7. *$14.00*

20 pages Year Founded: 1990

520 Sometimes I Drive My Mom Crazy, But I Know She's Crazy About Me
ADD WareHouse
300 NorthWest 70th Avenue
Suite 102
Plantation, FL 33317-2360
954-792-8944
800-233-9273
Fax: 954-792-8545
E-mail: websales@addwarehouse.com
www.addwarehouse.com

Harvey C Parker, Owner

This warm and humorous story of a young boy with ADHD addresses the many difficult and frustrating issues kids like him confront every day - from sitting still in the classroom, to remaining calm, to feeling 'different' from other children. This book is an amusing look at how a youngster with ADHD can develop a sense of self-worth through better understanding of this disorder. Ages 6-12. *$16.00*

124 pages Year Founded: 1990

521 Stuck on Fast Forward: Youth with Attention Deficit/Hyperactivity Disorder
Mason Crest Publishers
450 Parkway Drive
Suite D
Broomall, PA 19008-4017
610-543-6200
866-627-2665
Fax: 610-543-3878
E-mail: dtaylor@masoncrest.com
www.masoncrest.com

Shirley Brinkerhoff, Author
Dan Hilferty, President
Michelle Luke, Director, Marketing
Michael Toglia, Special Sales

Provides a comprehensive, yet easy to understand, overview of attention deficit/hyperactivity disorder. ADHD is an increasingly common diagnosis for school-aged and preschool children today, as parents, educators, and medical professionals struggle to deal with children who often don't sit still, don't pay attention, or act impulsively and even inappropriately. The debate over diagnosis and treatment of such symptoms is intense, and Stuck on Fast Forward explores all sides of the issue.

128 pages ISBN 1-590847-28-8

522 Succeeding in College with Attention Deficit Disorders: Issues and Strategies for Students, Counselors and Educators
ADD WareHouse
300 NorthWest 70th Avenue
Suite 102
Plantation, FL 33317-2360
954-792-8944
800-233-9273
Fax: 954-792-8545
E-mail: websales@addwarehouse.com
www.addwarehouse.com

Harvey C Parker, Owner

Written for college students, their couselors and educators. Based on the real life experiances of adults who were interviewed as part of a research study, this book offers a vivid picture of how college students with ADD can cope and find success in school. *$18.00*

189 pages Year Founded: 1990

523 Survival Guide for College Students with ADD or LD
ADD WareHouse
300 NorthWest 70th Avenue
Suite 102
Plantation, FL 33317-2360
954-792-8944
800-233-9273
Fax: 954-792-8545
E-mail: websales@addwarehouse.com
www.addwarehouse.com

Harvey C Parker, Owner

A useful guide for high school or college students diagnosed with attention deficit disorder or learning disabilities. Provides the information needed to survive and thrive in a college setting. Full of practical suggestions and tips from an experienced specialist in the field and from college students who also suffer from these difficulties. *$10.00*

56 pages Year Founded: 1990

524 Survival Strategies for Parenting Your ADD Child
Underwood Books
PO Box 1919
Nevada City, CA 95959
Fax: 530-274-7179
E-mail: contact@underwoodbooks.com
www.underwoodbooks.com

George T Lynn, Author

Survival Strategies for Parenting Your ADD Child: Dealing with Obsessions, Compulsions, Depression, Explosive Behavior and Rage. Provides parents with methods which can heal the fractures and pain that occur in families with troubled children. *$12.95*

240 pages ISBN 1-887424-19-9

525 Taking Charge of ADHD: Complete, Authoritative Guide for Parents
ADD WareHouse
300 NorthWest 70th Avenue
Suite 102
Plantation, FL 33317-2360
954-792-8944
800-233-9273
Fax: 954-792-8545
E-mail: websales@addwarehouse.com
www.addwarehouse.com

Harvey C Parker, Owner

Written for parents who are ready to take charge of their child's life. Strong on advocacy and parental empowerment, this book provides step-by-step methods for managing a child with ADHD in a variety of everyday situations, gives information on medications and discusses numerous techniques for enhancing a child's school performance. *$18.00*

294 pages Year Founded: 1990

526 Teenagers with ADD and ADHD: A Guide for Parents and Professionals
Woodbine House
6510 Bells Mill Road
Bethesda, MD 20817-1636
301-897-3570
800-843-7323
Fax: 301-897-5838
E-mail: info@woodbinehouse.com
www.woodbinehouse.com

Chris A Zeigler Dendy, MS, Author

The newly updated and expanded guide to raising a teenager with an attention deficit disorder is more comprehensive than ever. Thousands more parents can rely on Dendy's compassionately presented expertise based on the latest research and decades of her experience as a parent, teacher, school psychologist, and mental health counselor.

418 pages Year Founded: 1985

527 Teenagers with ADD: A Parent's Guide
Woodbine House
6510 Bells Mill Road
Bethesda, MD 20817-1636
301-897-3570
800-843-7323
Fax: 301-897-5838
E-mail: info@woodbinehouse.com
www.woodbinehouse.com

Chris A Zeigler Dendy, MS, Author

Double-column book full of information, suggestions and case studies. Lively, upbeat, comprehensive and well targeted to the problems parents face with ADD teenagers. *$18.95*

370 pages Year Founded: 1985 ISBN 0-933149-69-7

528 The AD/HD Forms Book: Identification, Measurement, and Intervention
Research Press
PO Box-7886
Champaign, IL 61826
217-352-3273
800-519-2707
Fax: 217-352-1221
E-mail: rp@researchpress.com
www.researchpress.com

Dr Michael J Asher, Author
Dr. Steven B Gordon, Author

A collection of intervention procedures and over 30 reproducible forms and checklists for use with any AD/HD program for children or adolescents. Each item is prefaced by a brief description of its purpose and use. The AD/HD Forms Book helps educators, mental health professionals and parents translate their knowledge into action. *$ 25.95*

117 pages Year Founded: 1968 ISBN 0-878223-78-9

529 The ADD Hyperactivity Handbook for Schools: Effective Strategies for Identifying and Teaching ADD Students in Elementary and Secondary Schools
ADD WareHouse
300 NorthWest 70th Avenue
Suite 102
Plantation, FL 33317-2360
954-792-8944
800-233-9273
Fax: 954-792-8545
E-mail: websales@addwarehouse.com
www.addwarehouse.com

Harvey C. Parker, Author

Written in a practical, easy-to-read style, this handbook for educators who need to effectively assist children with ADD offers proven techniques teachers can use in elementary and secondary school classrooms to help students and families overcome the challenges of ADD. This text is also useful for school psychologists, guidance personnel, student education specialists, and administrators. *$29.00*

330 pages Year Founded: 1990 ISBN 0-962162-92-2

530 Understanding Girls with Attention Deficit Hyperactivity Disorder
ADD WareHouse
300 NorthWest 70th Avenue
Suite 102
Plantation, FL 33317-2360
954-792-8944
800-233-9273
Fax: 954-792-8545
E-mail: websales@addwarehouse.com
www.addwarehouse.com

Harvey C Parker, Owner

Symptoms of ADHD are often overlooked or misunderstood in girls who are often diagnosed much later, and their ADHD symptoms may go untreated. This groundbreaking book reveals how ADHD affects girls from preschool through high school years. Gender differences are discussed along with issues related to school success, medication treatment, family relationships and susceptibility to other disorders such as anxiety, depression and learning problems. *$19.95*

291 pages Year Founded: 1990

531 Voices From Fatherhood: Fathers, Sons and ADHD
ADD WareHouse
300 NorthWest 70th Avenue
Suite 102
Plantation, FL 33317-2360
954-792-8944
800-233-9273
Fax: 954-792-8545
E-mail: websales@addwarehouse.com
www.addwarehouse.com

Harvey C Parker, Owner
Patricia O Quinn MD

Written to specifically help fathers navigate the complex world of parenting and ADHD, this book helps fathers enhance and deepen their relationships with their sons while providing them with strategies for guiding their sons. *$20.00*

184 pages Year Founded: 1990

532 What Makes Ryan Tick?
Hope Press
PO Box 188
Duarte, CA 91009-188
818-303-0644
800-321-4039
Fax: 626-358-3520
E-mail: dcomings@earthlink.net
www.hopepress.com

Susan Hughes, Author

What Makes Ryan Tick? A Family's Triumph over Tourette's Syndrome and Attention Deficit Hyperactivity Disorder. A moving and informative story how a mother struggled with the many behavioral problems presented by her son with Tourettes syndrome, ADHD and oppositional defiant disorder. *$15.95*

303 pages ISBN 1-878267-35-3

533 Women with Attention Deficit Disorder
ADD WareHouse
300 NorthWest 70th Avenue
Suite 102
Plantation, FL 33317-2360
954-792-8944
800-233-9273
Fax: 954-792-8545
E-mail: websales@addwarehouse.com
www.addwarehouse.com

Harvey C Parker, Owner

Combines real-life histories, treatment experiences and recent clinical research to highlight the special challenges facing women with Attention Deficit Disorder. After describing what to look for and what to look out for in treatment and counseling, this book outlines empowering steps that women living with ADD may use to change their lives. Also available on audiotape. 3 hours on 2 cassettes for $20.00. *$12.00*

354 pages Year Founded: 1990

534 You Mean I'm Not Lazy, Stupid or Crazy?
ADD WareHouse
300 NorthWest 70th Avenue
Suite 102
Plantation, FL 33317-2360
954-792-8944
800-233-9273
Fax: 954-792-8545
E-mail: websales@addwarehouse.com
www.addwarehouse.com

Harvey C Parker, Owner
Peggy Ramundo

This book is the first written by ADD adults for ADD adults. A comprehensive guide, it provides accurate information, practical how-to's and moral support. Readers will also get information on unique differences in ADD adults, the impact on their lives, treatment options available for adults, up-to-date research findings and much more. Also available on audiotape. *$14.00*

460 pages Year Founded: 1990

Periodicals & Pamphlets

535 ADDitude Magazine
ADD Warehouse
300 NW 70th Avenue
Suite 102
Plantation, FL 33317-2360
954-792-8944
800-233-9273
Fax: 954-792-8545
E-mail: sales@addwarehouse.com
www.addwarehouse.com

Harvey C Parker, Owner

Provides valuable resource information for professionals-teachers, healthcare providers, employers and others-who interact with AD/HD people everyday. *$19.97*

536 Attention-Deficit/Hyperactivity Disorder in Children and Adolescents
Center for Mental Health Services: Knowledge Exchange Network
PO Box 42557
Washington, DC 20015-557
800-789-2647
Fax: 301-984-8796
TDD: 866-889-2647
E-mail: ken@mentalhealth.org
www.mentalhealth.samhsa.gov/publications/

This fact sheet defines attention-deficit/hyperactivity disorder, describes the warning signs, discusses types of help available, and suggests what parents or other caregivers can do.

3 pages Year Founded: 1997

537 Learning Disabilities: A Multidisciplinary Journal
Learning Disabilities Association of America
4156 Library Road
Pittsburgh, PA 15234-1349
412-341-1515
Fax: 412-344-0224
E-mail: info@LDAAmerica.org
www.ldaamerica.org

Steven C Russell, PhD, Editor
Heather Nicklow, Accounting Manager
Sharon Tanner, Membership and Development
Maureen Swanson, Healthy Children Project

The most current research designed for professionals in the field of LD. *$60.00*

Year Founded: 1964

538 Treatment of Children with Mental Disorders
National Institute of Mental Health
6001 Executive Boulevard
Room 8184
Bethesda, MD 20892-9663
301-443-4513
866-615-6464
TTY: 301-443-8431
E-mail: nimhinfo@nih.gov
www.www.nimh.nih.gov/

Francis S Collins MD, PhD, Director
James M Anderson, MD, PhD, Director
Robin L Kawazoe, Deputy Director

A short booklet that contains questions and answers about therapy for children with mental disorders. Includes a chart of mental disorders and medications used.

Support Groups & Hot Lines

539 Children and Adults with AD/HD (CHADD)
4601 Presidents Drive
Suite 300
Lanham, MD 20706
301-306-7070
800-233-4050
Fax: 301-306-7090
www.chadd.org

Barbara S. Hawkins, BA, President
Ruth Hughes, PhD, CEO
Susan Buningh, MRE, Executive Editor
Trish White, Director of Membership and Affil

Non-profit organization serving individuals with AD/HD and their families. Over 16, 000 members in 200 local chapters throughout the United States. Chapters offer support for individuals, parents, teachers, professionals, and others. Available on Facebook and Twitter.

Video & Audio

540 ADHD & LD: Powerful Teaching Strategies & Accomodations
ADD Warehouse
300 NW 70the Avenue
Suite 102
Plantation, FL 33317-2360
954-792-8100
800-233-9273
Fax: 954-792-8545

E-mail: websales@addwarehouse.com
www.addwarehouse.com

Sandra Rief, Author

Provides instructional strategies for engaging attention and active participation, classroom management and behavioral interventions, gives academic strategies and accomodations, and collaborates teaming for success. 45 minutes. *$129.00*

Year Founded: 1990

541 ADHD-Inclusive Instruction & Collaborative Practices
ADD Warehouse
300 NW 70th Avenue
Suite 102
Plantation, FL 33317-2360
954-792-8100
800-233-9273
Fax: 954-792-8545
E-mail: websales@addwarehouse.com
www.addwarehouse.com

Sandra Rief, Author

Describes classroom modifications, teaching strategies, and interventions that can be used to maximize learning and ensure that all students achieve success. 38 minutes. *$99.00*

Year Founded: 1990 ISBN 1-887943-04-8

542 ADHD: What Can We Do?
ADD WareHouse
300 NW 70th Avenue
Suite 102
Plantation, FL 33317-2360
954-792-8100
800-233-9273
Fax: 954-792-8545
E-mail: websales@addwarehouse.com
www.addwarehouse.com

Russell A. Barkley, Author

Can serve as a companion to ADHD: What Do We Know?, this video focuses on the most effective ways to manage ADHD, both in the home and in the classroom. Scenes depict the use of behavior management at home and accommodations and interventions in the classroom which have proven to be effective in the treatment of ADHD. Thirty five minutes. *$95.00*

Year Founded: 1990 ISBN 0-898629-72-1

543 ADHD: What Do We Know?
ADD WareHouse
300 NW 70th Avenue
Suite 102
Plantation, FL 33317-2360
954-792-8100
800-233-9273
Fax: 954-792-8545
E-mail: websales@addwarehouse.com
www.addwarehouse.com

Russell A. Barkley, Author

This video provides an overview of the disorder and introduces the viewer to three young people who have ADHD. Discusses how ADHD affects the lives of the children and adults, causes of the disorder, associated problems, outcome in adulthood and provides vivid illustrations of how individuals with ADHD function at home, at school and on the job. Thirty five minutes. *$95.00*

Year Founded: 1990 ISBN 0-898629-71-3

544 Adults with Attention Deficit Disorder: ADD Isn't Just Kids Stuff
ADD WareHouse
300 NW 70th Avenue
Suite 102
Plantation, FL 33317-2360
954-792-8100
800-233-9273
Fax: 954-792-8545
E-mail: websales@addwarehouse.com
www.addwarehouse.com

Harvey C Parker, Owner

Explains this often misunderstood condition and the effects it has on one's work, home and social life. With the help of a panel of six adults, four ADD adults and two of their spouses, the book addresses the most common concerns of adults with ADD and provides information that will help families who are experiencing difficulties. 86 minutes. *$47.00*

Year Founded: 1990

545 Educating Inattentive Children
ADD WareHouse
300 NW 70th Avenue
Suite 102
Plantation, FL 33317-2360
954-792-8100
800-233-9273
Fax: 954-792-8545
E-mail: websales@addwarehouse.com
www.addwarehouse.com

Samuel Goldstein, Ph.D., Author
Michael Goldstein, M.D., Author

This two-hour video is ideal for in-service to regular and special educators concerning problems experienced by inattentive elementary and secondary students. Provides educators with information necessary to indentify and evaluate classroom problems caused by inattention and a well-defined set of practical guidelines to help educate children with ADD. *$49.00*

Year Founded: 1990

546 Medication for ADHD
ADD WareHouse
300 NW 70th Avenue
Suite 102
Plantation, FL 33317-2360
954-792-8100
800-233-9273
Fax: 954-792-8545
E-mail: websales@addwarehouse.com
www.addwarehouse.com

Dr. Andrew Adesman, Author

This comprehensive DVD addresses the critical questions regarding the use of medication in the treatment of ADD or ADHD. Allows those involved with ADHD to make well-informed and constructive decisions that may deeply change someone's life. *$39.95*

Year Founded: 1990 ISBN 1-889140-18-X

547 **New Look at ADHD: Inhibition, Time and Self Control**
Guilford Press
72 Spring Street
New York, NY 10012-4068
212-431-9800
800-365-7006
Fax: 212-966-6708
E-mail: info@guilford.com

Bob Matloff, President
Seymour Weingarten, Editor-in-Chief

This video provides an accessible introduction to Russell A Barkley's influential theory of the nature and origins of ADHD. The program brings to life the conceptual framework delineated in Barkley's other books. Discusses concrete ways that our new understanding of the disorder might facilitate more effective clinical interventions. This lucid, state of the art program is ideal viewing for clinicians, students and inservice trainees, parents of children with ADHD and adults with the disorder. 30 minutes. *$95.00*

Year Founded: 2000 ISBN 1-572304-97-9

548 **Outside In: A Look at Adults with Attention Deficit Disorder**
ADD Warehouse
300 NW 70th Avenue
Suite 102
Plantation, FL 33317-2360
954-792-8100
800-233-9273
Fax: 954-792-8545
E-mail: websales@addwarehouse.com
www.addwarehouse.com

Ted Kay, Director

Documentary film about adults with ADD and their journeys and the strategies they used to succeed. 29 minutes *$27.95*

Year Founded: 1990

549 **Understanding Mental Illness**
Educational Video Network
1401 19th Street
Huntsville, TX 77340
936-295-5767
800-762-0060
Fax: 936-294-0233
E-mail: info at evn.org
www.www.evndirect.com

A video to learn and understand mental illness and how it affects you. *$79.95*

Year Founded: 2004 ISBN 1-589501-48-9

550 **Understanding and Treating the Hereditary Psychiatric Spectrum Disorders**
Hope Press
10 Mill Road
Duarte, CA 91010
626-622-4978
800-209-9182
Fax: 626-358-3520
E-mail: dcomings@earthlink.net
www.hopepress.com

Books cover: ADHD, Tourette Syndrome, Obsessive-Compulsive Disorder, Conduct Disorder, Oppositional Defiant Disorder, Autism and other Hereditary Psychiatric Spectrum Disorders. *$75.00*

Year Founded: 1997

551 **Understanding the Defiant Child**
Guilford Press
72 Spring Street
New York, NY 10012-4068
212-431-9800
800-365-7006
Fax: 212-966-6708
E-mail: info@guilford.com

Bob Matloff, President
Seymour Weingarten, Editor-in-Chief

Presents information on Oppositional Defiant Disorder and Conduct Disorder with scenes of family interactions, showing the nature and causes of these disorders and what can and should be done about it. Thirty five minutes with a manual that contains more information. 30 minutes. *$95.00*

Year Founded: 1997 ISBN 1-572301-66-X

552 **Why Won't My Child Pay Attention?**
ADD WareHouse
300 NW 70th Avenue
Suite 102
Plantation, FL 33317-2360
954-792-8100
800-233-9273
Fax: 954-792-8545
E-mail: websales@addwarehouse.com
www.addwarehouse.com

Sam Goldstein, PhD, Author

Provides an easy-to-follow explanation concerning the effect ADD has on children at school, home and in the community. Provides guidelines to help parents and professionals successfully and happily manage the problems these behaviors can cause. 76 minutes. *$38.00*

Year Founded: 1990

Web Sites

553 **www.CHADD.org**
Children/Adults with Attention Deficit/Hyperactivity Disorder

554 **www.LD-ADD.com**
Attention Deficit Disorder and Parenting Site

555 **www.aap.org**
American Academy of Pediatrics Practice Guidelines on ADHD

Site serves the purpose of giving the public guidelines for diagnosing and evaluating children with possible ADHD.

556 **www.add.about.com**
Attention Deficit Disorder

Hundreds of sites.

557 **www.add.org**
Attention Deficit Disorder Association

Provides information, resources and networking to adults with ADHD and to the professionals who work with them.

558 www.additudemag.com
Happy Healthy Lifestyle Magazine for People with ADD

559 www.addvance.com
Answers to Your Questions About ADD

provides answers to questions about ADD, ADHD for families and individuals at every stage of life from preschool through retirement years.

560 www.adhdnews.com/Advocate.htm
Advocating for Your Child

561 www.adhdnews.com/sped.htm
Special Education Rights and Responsibilities

Writing IEP's and TIEPS. Pursuing special education services.

562 www.babycenter.com/rcindex.html
BabyCenter

563 www.cfsny.org
Center for Family Support

Devoted to the physical well-being and development of the retarded child and the sound mental health of parents.

564 www.cyberpsych.org
CyberPsych

Hosts the American Psychoanalyists Foundation, American Association of Suicideology, Society for the Exploration of Psychotherapy Intergration, and Anxiety Disorders Association of America. Also subcategories of the anxiety disorders, as well as general information, including panic disorder, phobias, obsessive compulsive disorder (OCD), social phobia, generalized anxiety disorder, post traumatic stress disorder, and phobias of childhood. Book reviews and links to web pages sharing the topics.

565 www.nami.org
National Alliance on Mental Illness

From its inception in 1979, NAMI has been dedicated to improving the lives of individuals and families affected by mental illness.

566 www.nichcy.org
National Information Center for Children and Youth with Disabilities

Excellent information in English and Spanish.

567 www.nimh.nih.gov/publicat/adhd.cfm
Attention Deficit Hyperactivity Disorder

Thirty page booklet.

568 www.oneaddplace.com
One ADD Place

569 www.planetpsych.com
Planetpsych.com

Learn about disorders, their treatments and other topics in psychology. Articles are listed under the related topic areas. Ask a therapist a question for free, or view the directory of professionals in your area. If you are a therapist sign up for the directory. Current features, self-help, interactive, and newsletter archives.

570 www.psychcentral.com
Psych Central

Personalized one-stop index for psychology, support, and mental health issues, resources, and people on the Internet.

571 www.thenadd.org
National Association for the Dually Diagnosed

Nonprofit organization to promote interests of professional and parent development with resources for individuals who have coexistence of mental illness and mental retardation.

Autism Spectrum Disorders

Introduction

Autism Spectrum Disorders are a distinct group of neurological conditions characterized by impairment in language and communication skills; two of the most common are Autistic Disorder and Asperger's Syndrome.

Autistic Disorder is a pervasive developmental disorder whose main symptoms are a marked lack of interest in connecting, interacting, or communicating with others. People with this disorder cannot share something of interest with other people, rarely make eye contact with others, avoid physical contact, show little facial expression, and do not make friends. Autistic Disorder is a profound, lifelong condition associated with wide ranging and severe disabilities, including behavior problems, such as hyperactivity, obsessive compulsive behavior, self injury, and tics. Although present before age three, the disorder may not be apparent until later, although parents often sense that there is something wrong because of their child's marked lack of interest in social interaction. Very young children with autism not only show no desire for affection and cuddling, but show actual aversion to it. There is no socially directed smiling or facial responsiveness, and no responsiveness to the voices of parents and siblings. As a result, parents may sometimes worry that their child is deaf. Later, the child may be more willing to interact socially, but the quality of interaction is unusual, usually inappropriately intrusive with little understanding of social rules and boundaries. The autistic child seems not to have the abilities and desires that would make it possible for him or her to become a social being. Instead, the child seems locked up in an alien interior world, which is both incomprehensible and inaccessible to parents, siblings and others.

Asperger's Syndrome (AS) is named for Austrian pediatrician Hans Asperger, who in 1944, observed four children who had normal intelligence, but lacked nonverbal communication skills; additionally they did not demonstrate empathy with their peers, and were physically clumsy. Dr. Asperger called the condition 'Autistic psychopathy' and described it as a personality disorder marked by social isolation.

Twin and family studies have shown a genetic predisposition to AS and other ADs. Several genes, but not one specific gene, have recently been identified as associated with autism. Some researchers have proposed that the disorder may stem from abnormalities during critical stages of fetal development, including defects in the genes that control and regulate normal brain growth and growth patterns.

There is no standardized screening tool available to diagnose Asperger's Syndrome. Most doctors rely on the presence of a core group of behaviors to diagnose the syndrome.

SYMPTOMS

Autism: Impairment in the Quality of Social Interaction
- Gross lack of nonverbal behavior (e.g., eye contact, facial expression, body postures, and gestures), which gives meaning to social interaction and social behavior;
- Failure to make friends in age-appropriate ways;
- Lack of spontaneously seeking to share interests or achievements with others (e.g., not showing things to others, not pointing to, or bringing interesting objects to others);
- Lack of social or emotional give and take (e.g., not joining in social play or simple games with others);
- Notable lack of awareness of others. Oblivious of other children (including siblings), of their excitement, distress, or needs.

Autism: Marked Impairment in the Quality of Communication
- Delay in, or lack of, spoken language development. Those who speak cannot initiate or sustain comunication with others;
- Lack of spontaneous make-believe or imitative play common among young children;
- When speech does develop, it may be abnormal and monotonous;
- Repetitive use of language.

Autism: Restricted Repetitive Patterns or Behavior
- Restricted range of interests often fixed on one subject and its facts (e.g., baseball);
- A great deal of exact repetition in play, (e.g., lining up play objects in the same way again and again);
- Resistance and distress if anything in the environment is changed, (e.g., a chair moved to a different place);
- Insistence on following certain rules and routines (e.g., walking to school by the same route each day);
- Repeated body movements (e.g., body rocking, hand clapping);
- Persistent preoccupation with details or parts of objects (e.g., buttons).

Asperger's Syndrome in Contrast to Autism:
Asperger's Syndrome causes two types of symptoms: problems with social interactions and stereotyped, repetitive patterns of behavior. Individuals with AS have limited interests and are preoccupied with a particular subject to the exclusion of other activities. Some other characteristics are:
- Repetitive routines or rituals;
- Peculiarities in speech and language, such as speaking in an overly formal manner or in a monotone, or taking figures of speech literally;
- Socially and emotionally inappropriate behavior and the inability to interact successfully with peers;
- Problems with non-verbal communication, including the restricted use of gestures, limited or inappropriate facial expressions, or a peculiar, stiff gaze;
- Clumsy and uncoordinated motor movements.

ASSOCIATED FEATURES

Autism seems to bring with it an increased risk of other disorders. Seventy-five percent of autistic children have cognitive deficits, and twenty-five percent have cognitive abilities at or above average. Twenty-five percent of individuals with autism also have seizure disorders. The development of intellectual skills is usually uneven. An autistic child may be able to read extremely early, but not be able to comprehend what he or she reads. Other symptoms include hyperactivity, short attention span, impulsivity, aggressiveness, and self injury, such as head banging, hair pulling, and arm biting (particularly in young children). There may be unusual responses to stimuli: less than normal sensitivity to pain but extreme sensitivity to sounds or to being touched. There may be abnormalities in emotional expression, giggling or weeping for no apparent reason, and little or no emotional reaction when one would be expected. Similar abnormal responses may be shown in relation to fear; an absence of fear in response to real danger, but great fearfulness in the presence of harmless objects.

In adolescence or adulthood, people with Autistic Disorder who have the capacity for insight may become depressed when they realize how seriously impaired they are. Autistic Disorder sometimes follows medical and obstetrical problems, such as encephalitis, anoxia (absence of oxygen) during birth, and maternal rubella during pregnancy.There is some evidence of genetic transmission. The disorder is not caused by inappropriate parenting or by routine immunizations.

The person with Asperger's may not develop age-appropriate relationships or attempt to share interests or pleasures with others. He or she may be unable to reciprocate others' feelings, have difficulty using gestures or facial expressions, be extremely preoccupied with a very narrow area of interest, insist upon very rigid routines, make repetitive movements, and focus on parts of objects rather than the objects as a whole.

Asperger's Syndrome does not interfere with the development of language or thinking. However, its symptoms interfere with the individual's social or occupational functioning.

PREVALENCE

By definition, Autistic Disorder is present before age three. There are two to five cases of the disorder per 10, 000 births. Rates of autism are four to five times greater among males than females. Females with Autistic Disorder are more likely to be severely retarded than are males with Autistic Disorder. Follow-up studies suggest that only a small percentage of people with Autistic Disorder live independent adult lives. Even the highest functioning adults continue to have problems in social interaction and communication, together with greatly restricted interests and activities. The siblings of people with the disorder are at increased risk.

After years of controversy, there is a growing consensus that the incidence and prevalence of autism spectrum disorders has increased significantly in recent years. The reason(s) for the increase are not clear.

The incidence of Asperger's Syndrome is estimated to be two out of every 10, 000 children. Boys are three to four times more likely than girls to have the disorder. Although diagnosed mainly in children, it is being increasingly diagnosed in adults with other mental health conditions such as depression, obsessive-compulsive disorder, and attention-deficit/hyperactivity disorder.

TREATMENT OPTIONS

It is difficult or unusual to be able to eradicate all the symptoms of Autistic Disorder, but there are many intervention and education programs which help to improve functioning. It is extremely important, however, that a proper assessment and diagnosis be made. Since the disturbance in behavior is so wide ranging, this can require an array of professional skills - psychological, languauge development, neuropsychological, and medical. Such a multiple assessment establishes the presence or absence of other disorders, the level of intellectual functioning,

together with individual strengths and weaknesses, and the child's capacity for social and personal self-sufficiency. Since the symptoms of Autistic Disorder vary widely, a proper assessment is the foundation for designing and planning an individually tailored intervention program.

The autistic person may benefit from a combination of educational and behavioral interventions, which may reduce many of the behavioral disturbances, and improve the quality of life for the person and his or her family. In some cases, medication may also be prescribed. The diagnosis of Autistic Disorder can be a shattering experience for any family. The outcome of the diagnosis is open-ended and uncertain and includes a lifetime of care. Every member of the family is affected and it is vital to work with and support them.

Some new, inensive, multi-dimensional treatments are promising, but few people have access to them at this time.

Treatment for Asperger's Syndrome address the core symptoms of the disorder: poor communication skills; obsessive or repetitive routines; and physical clumsiness. No single treatment works best, but the program would include social skills training, cognitive behavioral therapy, medication, occupational/physical therapy, and parent training and support.

Associations & Agencies

573 Achieve Beyond
7000 Austin Street
Suite 200
Forest Hills, NY 11375
718-762-7633
Fax: 212-679-7867
E-mail: info@achievebeyondusa.com
www.www.achievebeyondusa.com

Dr Trudy Font-Padron, PhD, Founder, Executive Director
Julie Matuza, Chief Executive Officer
Robert Padron, MBA, Executive Director

Achieve Beyond is dedicated to provide quality English and Bilingual evaluations and therapeutic and education services to children ages 0-21 years suffering from imapriments due to ADHD and other illnesses. They use a family centered and multilingual approach to ensure parents that their child's development needs are met in a nurturing and supportive environment.

Year Founded: 1995

574 Asperger Autism Spectrum Education Network
9 Aspen Circle
Edison, NJ 08820-2832
732-321-0880
E-mail: info@aspennj.org
www.aspennj.org

Lori Shery, President
Rich Meleo, Vice President
Elizabeth Yamashita, Vice President
Ann Hiller, Secretary

A non-profit organization which provides families and individuals whose lives are affected by Autism Spectrum Disorders with education about the issues surrounding the disorders; support in knowing that they are not alone, and in helping individuals achieve their maximum potential; advocacy in areas of appropriate educational programs, medical research funding, adult issues and increased public awareness and understanding.

575 Asperger's Association of New England (AANE)
51 Water Street
Suite 206
Watertown, MA 02472-4411
617-393-3824
866-597-AANE
Fax: 617-393-3827
E-mail: info@aane.org
www.aane.org

Shannah Varon, MBA, President
Anne Marie Gross, B.A, Vice President
Jayne Burke, Secretary
Doug Rainville, Treasurer

Fosters awareness, respect, acceptance and support for individuals with AS and related conditions and their families. AANE offers a full array of educational events for people with an interest in Asperger's Syndrome.

Year Founded: 1996

576 Autism Network International
PO Box 35448
Syracuse, NY 13235-5448
E-mail: jisincla@syr.edu
www.ani.ac

Jim Sinclair, Owner, Coordinater
James Bordner, Co-Owner

ANI is an organization run by autistic people, for autistic people. We offer education, peer advocacy, and peer support.

577 Autism Research Foundation
72 East Concord Street
Room No-1014
Boston, MA 02118-2526
617-414-7012
Fax: 617-414-7207
E-mail: tarf@ladders.org
www.theautismresearchfoundation.org

Courtney LaPorte, Executive Director
Dr Margaret Bauman, Founding Diretor
Grace Bourey, Executive Assistant
Kelly Landrigan, Communications Coordinator

A nonprofit, tax-exempt organization dedicated to researching the neurological underpinnings of autism and other related developmental brain disorders. Seeking to rapidly expand and accelerate research into the pervasive developmental disorders.

Year Founded: 1990

578 Autism Research Institute
4182 Adams Avenue
San Diego, CA 92116-2599
619-281-7165
866-366-3361
Fax: 619-563-6840
www.autism.com

Stephen M Edelson, PhD, Executive Director
Jane Johnson, Managing Director
Valerie Paradiz , PhD, Director, ARI Autistic Global Ins
Rebecca McKenney, Office Manager

Provides information on Autism and Asperger's Syndrome.

Year Founded: 1976

579 Autism Society
4340 East-West Highway
Suite 350
Bethesda, MD 20814
301-657-0881
800-328-8476
Fax: 301-657-0869
E-mail: info#autism-society.org
www.autism-society.org

James Ball, Ed D, BCBA-D, Executive Chair
Scott Badesch, President & CEO
John Dabrowski, Chief Financial Officer
Lars Perner, PhD, Secretary

Promotes lifelong access and opportunities for persons within the autism spectrum and their families, to be fully included, participating members of their communities through advocacy, public awareness, education and research related to autism. Hosts a national conference, publishes a magazine, engages in public policy activities at local, state and federal levels, and provides information and referral services via phone and email. The Autism Society consists of a nationwide network of local chapters.

Year Founded: 1965

580 Autism Speaks
1 East 33rd Street
4th Floor
New York, NY 10016
212-252-8584
Fax: 212-252-8676
E-mail: familyservices@autismspeaks.org
www.www.autismspeaks.org

Liz Feld, President
Jennifer Bizub, Chief Human Resources Officer
Alec M Elbert, Chief Strategy and Development O
Jamitha Fields, Vice President - Community Affai

Autism Speaks was founded in 2005. Autism Speaks has grown into the nation's largest autism science and advocacy organization, dedicated to funding research into the causes, prevention, treatments and a cure for autism; increasing awareness of autismspectrum disorders; and advocating for the needs of individuals with autism and their families.

581 Autistic Services
4444 Bryant Stratton Way
Williamsville, NY 14221-6013
716-631-5777
888-288-4764
Fax: 716-565-0671
E-mail: tpanzarella@autism-services-inc.org
www.autisticservices.org

Thomas Mazur, President
Veronica Federiconi, Executive Director
John Lordi, PhD, Vice President
Matthew Shriver, Treasurer

Agency exclusively dedicated to serving the unique lifelong needs of individuals with autism. Also a regional resource for parents, school districts, physicians and other professionals.

582 Brain Resources and Information Network (BRAIN)
PO Box 5801
Bethesda, MD 20824-5801
301-496-5751
800-352-9424
Fax: 301-402-2186
TTY: 301-468-5981
E-mail: braininfo@ninds.nih.gov
www.ninds.nih.gov

Denise Dorsey, Chief Administrative Officer
Peter Soltys, Chief Information Officer
Story C Landis, PhD, Director
Marian Emr, Director, Office of Communication

The mission of NINDS is to reduce the burden of neurological disease - a burden borne by every age group, by every segment of society, by people all over the world.

Year Founded: 1950

583 Center for Mental Health Services (CMHS)
1 Choke Cherry Road
Room 6-1057
Rockville, MD 20857
240-276-1310
877-726-4727
Fax: 240-276-1320
TDD: 800-487-4889
E-mail: info@mentalhealth.org
www.beta.samhsa.gov/about-us/who-we-are/offices-center

Michael E Etzinger, B.S.M.E, , M.B., SAMHSA Executive Officer, Director
Paolo Del Vecchio, M.S.W, Director, Center for Mental Healt
Deborah Baldwin, M.P.A, Acting Director, Consumer Affairs
Elizabeth Lopez, Ph.D, Acting Deputy Director

CMHS leads Federal efforts to treat mental illnesses by promoting mental health and by preventing the development or worsening of mental illness when possible. Congress created CMHS to bring new hope to adults who have serious mental illnesses and to children with serious emotional disorders. CMHS provides information about mental health via a toll-free the web site, and more than 600 publications. Developed for users of mental health services and their families, the general public, policy makers, providers, and the media.

Year Founded: 1992

584 Community Services for Autistic Adults and Children
8615 East Village Avenue
Montgomery Village, MD 20886-4316
240-912-2220
Fax: 301-926-9384
TTY: 800-735-2258
E-mail: iparegol@csaac.org
www.www.csaac.org/

Ian Paregol, Executive Director
Marcee Smith, Ph.D., Assistant Executive Director of
Donald Rodrick, M.S., Chief Financial Officer
Eva Chung, Chief Human Resources Officer

Enables individuals to achieve to their highest potential and contribute as confident members in their community, instead of living in institutions.

Year Founded: 1979

585 FACES Autism Services
220D Twin Dolphin Drive
Redwood City, CA 94065
650-622-9601
Fax: 650-367-1565
E-mail: info@facesforkids.org
www.www.facesforkids.org

Karen Kennan, Exec Director Childrens Services
Matt Tritto, M.S., Clinical Director
Catherine Norrid, Director, Administration
Kelly Montague, M.S., BCBA, Case Consultant

FACES enables children with autism to reach their full potential by providing a resource for early intervention services based upon the science of Applied Behavior Analysis, k-12 school and parent consultation, and community education.

586 Families for Early Autism Treatment
PO Box 255722
Sacramento, CA 95865-5722
916-303-7405
Fax: 916-303-7405
E-mail: feat@feat.org
www.feat.org

A nonprofit organization of parents and professionals, designed to help families with children who are diagnosed with autism or pervasive developmental disorder.

Year Founded: 1993

587 Generation Rescue
13636 Ventura Boulevard
Suite 259
Sherman Oaks, CA 91423
877-982-8847
E-mail: info@generation rescue.org
www.www.generationrescue.org

Candace McDonald, Executive Director
J B Handley, Co-Founder
Lisa Handley, Co-Founder
Deirdre Imus, National Advocate

Generation Rescue is dedicated to recovery for children with autism spectrum disordersby providing guidance and supoort for medical treatmentto directly improve the child's quality of life for all families in need.

Year Founded: 2005

588 Indiana Resource Center for Autism (IRCA)
1905 North Range Road
Bloomington, IN 47408-2601
812-855-6508
800-825-4733
Fax: 812-855-9630
TTY: 812-855-9396
E-mail: prattc@indiana.edu
www.www.iidc.indiana.edu/index.php?pageId=32

Cathy Pratt, PhD, BCBA-D, Center Director
David Mank, PhD, Director, Indiana Institute On Di
Doug Ryner, IT Director
Harriet L Figg, Business Manager/Fiscal Officer

Conducts outreach training and consultations, engage in research, develop and disseminate information on behalf of individuals across the autism spectrum, Aspergers syndrome, and other pervasive developmental disorders. Provides communities, organizations, agencies and families with the knowledge and skills to support children and adults in typical early intervention, school, community work and home.

589 National Alliance on Mental Illness

3803 North Fairfax Drive
Suite 100
Arlington, VA 22203-3080
703-524-7600
800-950-6264
Fax: 703-524-9094
E-mail: helpline@nami.org
www.nami.org

Keris Jan Myrick, MBA, MS, PhD., President
Mary Giliberti, J.D, Executive Director
Jim Payne, J.D, First Vice President
David Levy, Chief Financial Officer

Nation's leading self-help organization for all those affected by severe brain disorders. Mission is to bring consumers and families with similar experiences together to share information about services, care providers, and ways to cope with the challenges of schizophrenia, manic depression, and other serious mental illnesses.

Year Founded: 1969

590 National Association for the Dually Diagnosed (NADD)

132 Fair Street
Kingston, NY 12401-4802
845-331-4336
800-331-5362
Fax: 845-331-4569
E-mail: info@thenadd.org
www.thenadd.org

Donna McNELIS, PhD, President
Robert J Fletcher DSW, Chief Executive Officer
Dan Baker, PhD, Vice President
Julia Pearce, Secretary

Nonprofit organization designed to promote interest of professional and parent development with resources for individuals who have the coexistence of mental illness and mental retardation. Provides conferences, educational services and training materials to professionals, parents, concerned citizens and service organizations.

Year Founded: 1983

591 National Autism Center

41 Pacella Park Drive
Randolph, MA 02368
877-313-3833
Fax: 781-440-0401
E-mail: info@nationalautismcenter.org
www.www.nationalautismcenter.org

Lauren C Solotar, Ph.D., ABPP, President
Hanna Rue, Ph.D., BCBA-D, Executive Director
Deidre L Donaldson, Ph.D., Chief Clinical Officer
Marisa L Morelos, Psy.D., ASD Clinic Director

The National Autism Center is for the promotion of evidence based practice. It is dedicated to serving children and adolescents with Autism Spectrum Disorder(ASD) by providing reliable information, promotign best practices, and offering comprehensive resources to families, practitioners, and communities.

592 National Institute of Mental Health
National Institutes of Health

6001 Executive Blvd
Room 6200, MSC 9663
Bethesda, MD 20892-9663
301-443-4513
866-615-6464
TTY: 301-443-8431
E-mail: nimhinfo@nih.gov
www.www.nimh.nih.go

Francis S Collins, MD, PhD, Nih Director
Lawrence Tabak, DDS, PhD, Deputy Director
Kathy L Hudson, PhD, Deputy Dir For Science

Provides information and support on Autism and Asperger's Syndrome.

593 National Institute on Deafness and Other Communication Disorders Information Clearinghouse

31 Center Drive
MSC 2320
Bethesda, MD 20892-2320
301-496-7243
800-241-1044
Fax: 301-402-0018
TTY: 800-241-1055
E-mail: nidcinfo@nidcd.nih.gov
www.www.nidcd.nih.gov

Mark Rotariu, Chief, Financial management Branc
Timothy J Wheeles, Executive Officer and Chief
James F Battey, Jr MD, PhD, Director
Judith A Cooper, PhD, Deputy Director

Support and services for individuals with Autism and Asperger's Syndrome.

Year Founded: 1988

594 National Mental Health Consumers' Self-Help Clearinghouse

1211 Chestnut Street
Suite 1100
Philadelphia, PA 19107-4103
215-751-1810
800-553-4539
Fax: 215-636-6312
E-mail: info@mhselfhelp.org
www.mhselfhelp.org

Joseph Rogers, Executive Director/ Founder
Susan Rogers, Director
Britani Nestel, Program Specialist
Christa Burkett, Technical Assistance Coordinator

A national consumer technical assistance center that has played a major role in the development of the mental health consumer movement.

Year Founded: 1986

595 New England Center for Children

33 Turnpike Road
Southborough, MA 01772-2108
508-481-1015
Fax: 508-485-3421
E-mail: info@necc.org
www.necc.org

Lisel Macenka, Chair of the Board
L Vincent Strully, Jr, President, Chief Executive Office

Katherine E Foster, Med, Executive Vice President, Chief O
RoseAnn Lovely, MBA, Chief Development Officer, Treasu

Serving students between the ages of 3 and 22 diagnosed with autism, learning disabilities, language delays, mental retardation, behavior disorders and related disabilities; educational curriculum encompasses both the teaching of functional life skills.

Year Founded: 1975

596 The Center for Family Support
2811 Zulette Avenue
Bronx, NY 10461
718-518-1500
Fax: 718-518-8200
www.cfsny.org

Steven Vernikoff, Executive Director
Virgil Seepersad, Director of Finance
Eileen Berg, Director of Quality Assurance
Barbara Greenwald, Associate Executive, Director

An agency that continues to develop new programs to serve families and individuals with their care needs. They offer services throughout the New York City region including: New Jersey, Long Island and the Lower Hudson Valley.

Year Founded: 1954

Books

597 A Book: A Collection of Writings from the Advocate
Autism Society of North Carolina Bookstore
4182 Adams Avenue
San Diego, CA 92116
919-743-0204
866-366-3361
Fax: 919-743-0208
www.www.autism.com

Beth Sposato, Author
Paul Wendler, Chief Financial Officer
David Laxton, Director, Communications
Kay Walker, Director, Development

A collection of articles and writings from the Advocate, the national newsletter of the Autism Society of America.
$12.00

93 pages Year Founded: 1967

598 A Parent's Guide to Asperger Syndrome and High-Functioning Autism
Guilford Press
72 Spring Street
New York, NY 10012
212-431-9800
800-365-7006
Fax: 212-966-6708
E-mail: info@guilford.com
www.guilford.com

Sally Ozonoff, Author
Geraldine Dawson, Author
James McPartland, Author

How to Meet the Challenges and Help Your Child Thrive. Covers definitions, diagnsosis, causes and treatments as well as living with AS-HFA, channeling a child's strengths, and dealing with home and social world and life as an adult. *$18.95*

278 pages Year Founded: 1973 ISBN 1-572305-31-2

599 Activities for Developing Pre-Skill Concepts in Children with Autism
Autism Society of North Carolina Bookstore
505 Oberlin Road
Suite 230
Raleigh, NC 27605-1345
919-743-0204
800-442-2762
Fax: 919-743-0208
www.www.autismsociety-nc.org

Toni Flowers, Author
Paul Wendler, Chief Financial Officer
David Laxton, Director, Communications
Kay Walker, Director, Development

Chapters include auditory development, concept development, social development and visual-motor integration.
$34.00

217 pages

600 Adults with Autism
Cambridge University Press
32 Avenue of the Americas
New York, NY 10013-2473
212-337-5000
E-mail: newyork@cambrigde.org
www.www.cambridge.org

Hugh Morgan, Author
Andrew Chandler, Chief Financial Officer
Richard Fisher, Managing Director
Andrew Gilfilan, Managing Director, Europe

Provides pratical help and guidance specifically for those caring for the growing recognized population of adults with autism. *$ 50.00*

312 pages Year Founded: 1534 ISBN 0-521456-83-5

601 Are You Alone on Purpose?
Autism Society of North Carolina Bookstore
505 Oberlin Road
Suite 230
Raleigh, NC 27605-1345
919-743-0204
800-442-2762
Fax: 919-743-0208
www.www.autismsociety-nc.org

Nancy Werlin, Author
Paul Wendler, Chief Financial Officer
David Laxton, Director, Communications
Kay Walker, Director, Development

This is the story of Alison, the twin sister of an autistic boy, who develops a friendship with a boy who has become paralyzed. Alison's feelings of isolation from her family and brother are discussed as she develops a true friendship.
$14.95

211 pages

602 Aspects of Autism: Biological Research
Autism Society of North Carolina Bookstore
505 Oberlin Road
Suite 230
Raleigh, NC 27605-1345
919-743-0204
800-442-2762
Fax: 919-743-0208
www.www.autismsociety-nc.org

Lorba Wing, Author
Paul Wendler, Chief Financial Officer
David Laxton, Director, Communications
Kay Walker, Director, Development

Reviews the evidence for a physical cause of autism and the roles of genetics, magnesium and vitamin B6. *$15.00*

120 pages

603 Asperger Syndrome: A Practical Guide for Teachers
ADD WareHouse
300 NorthWest 70th Avenue
Suite 102
Plantation, FL 33317-2360
954-792-8944
800-233-9273
Fax: 954-792-8545
E-mail: websales@addwarehouse.com
www.addwarehouse.com

Harvey C Parker, Owner

A clear and concise guide to effective classroom practice for teachers and support assistants working with children with Asperger Syndrome in school. The authors explain characteristics of children with Asperger Syndrome, discusses methods of assessment and offers practical strategies for effective classroom interventions. *$24.95*

90 pages Year Founded: 1990

604 Asperger's Syndrome: A Guide for Parents and Professionals
ADD WareHouse
300 NorthWest 70th Avenue
Suite 102
Plantation, FL 33317-2360
954-792-8944
800-233-9273
Fax: 954-792-8545
E-mail: websales@addwarehouse.com
www.addwarehouse.com

Harvey C Parker, Owner

Providing a description and analysis of the unusual characteristics of Asperger's syndrome, with strategies to reduce those that are most conspicuous or debilitating. This guide brings together the most relevant and useful information on all aspects of the syndrome, from language and social behavior to motor clumsiness. *$18.95*

223 pages Year Founded: 1990

605 Autism
Autism Society of North Carolina Bookstore
505 Oberlin Road
Suite 230
Raleigh, NC 27605-1345
919-743-0204
800-442-2762
Fax: 919-743-0208
www.www.autismsociety-nc.org

Heather Bargett Veague, PhD, Author
Christine Collins, PhD, Editor
David Laxton, Director, Communications
Kay Walker, Directord, Development

In a question-and-answer format, the authors respond to questions about autism asked by countless parents and family members of children and youths with autism. *$26.00*

606 Autism & Asperger Syndrome
Cambridge University Press
32 Avenue of the Americas
New York, NY 10013-2473
212-337-5000
800-872-7423
Fax: 212-691-3239
E-mail: newyork@cambrigde.org
www.www.cambridge.org

Uta Frith, Editor
Andrew Chandler, Chief Financial Officer
Richard Fisher, Managing Director
Andrew Gilfillan, Managidn Director, Europe

Six clinician-researchers present aspects of Asperger Syndrome, one form of autism. Research summaries are enlivened by case studies. *$24.00*

257 pages Year Founded: 1534

607 Autism & Sensing: The Unlost Instinct
Jessica Kingsley Publishers
400 Market Street
Suite 400
Philadelphia, PA 19106-2614
215-922-1161
866-416-1078
Fax: 215-922-1474
E-mail: hello.usa@jkp.com
www.jkp.com

Donna Williams, Author
Dee Brigham, Company Secretary, Director
Jemima Kingsley, Director
Octavia Kingsley, Production Director

Available in paperback. *$26.95*

200 pages Year Founded: 1987 ISBN 1-853026-12-3

608 Autism Bibliography
TASH
29 W Susquehanna Avenue
Suite 210
Baltimore, MD 21204-5218
410-828-8274
Fax: 410-828-6706
E-mail: info@tash.org
www.tash.org

Sobfey , Author
Jean Trainor, Vice President
Barbara Loescher, Treasurer

Three hundred recent references to publications on autism along with brief abstracts. *$9.00*

609 Autism Spectrum
Autism Society of North Carolina Bookstore
505 Oberlin Road
Suite 230
Raleigh, NC 27605-1345
919-743-0204
800-442-2762
Fax: 919-743-0208
www.www.autismsociety-nc.org

Chantal Sicile-Kira, Author
Paul Wendler, Chief Financial Officer
David Laxton, Director, Communications
Kay Walker, Director, Development

An excellent publication for new parents and professionals. *$28.95*

360 pages

610 **Autism Spectrum Disorders: The Complete Guid to Understanding Autism, Asperger's Syndrome, Pervasive Developmental Disorder, and Other ASDs**
Penguin Group (USA)
375 Hudson Street
New York, NY 10014-3672
212-366-2000
Fax: 212-366-2933
www.www.penguin.com

John Makinson, Chief Executive Officer
Coram Willimas, Chief Financial Officer
David Shanks, Chief Executive Officer

Twelve years ago, we were in the local doctor's office in a small village in England, where we had just moved.

611 **Autism Treatment Guide**
Autism Society of North Carolina Bookstore
505 Oberlin Road
Suite 230
Raleigh, NC 27605-1345
919-743-0204
800-442-2762
Fax: 919-743-0208
www.www.autismsociety-nc.org

Elizabeth K Gerlach, Author
Paul Wendler, Chief Financial Officer
David Laxton, Director, Communications
Kay Walker, Director, Development

A comprehensive book covering treatments and methods used to help individuals with autism. *$12.75*

157 pages

612 **Autism and Pervasive Developmental Disorders**
Cambridge University Press
32 Avenue of the Americas
New York, NY 10013-2473
212-337-5000
Fax: 212-691-3239
E-mail: newyork@cambrigde.org
www.www.cambridge.org

Fred R Volkmar, Editor
Andrew Chandler, Chief Financial Officer
Richard Fisher, Managing Director
Andrew Gilfillan, Managing Director, Europe

Featuring contributions from leading authorities in the clinical and social sciences, this volume reflects recent progress in the understanding of autism and related conditions, and offers an international perspective on the present state of the discipline. Chapters cover current approaches to definition and diagnosis; prevalence and planning for service delivery; cognitive, genetic and neurobiological features and pathophysiological mechanisms. *$75.00*

356 pages Year Founded: 1534 ISBN 0-521553-86-5

613 **Autism: An Inside-Out Approach An Innovative Look at the Mechanics of Autism and its Developmental Cousins**
Jessica Kingsley Publishers
400 Market Street
Suite 400
Philadelphia, PA 19106-2614

215-922-1161
866-416-1078
Fax: 215-922-1474
E-mail: hello.usa@jkp.com
www.jkp.com

Donna Williams, Author
Dee Brigham, Company Secretary, Director
Jemima Kingsley, Director
Octavia Kingsley, Production Director

Written by an autistic person for people with autism and related disorders, carers, and the professionals who work with them, is a practical handbook to understanding, living with and working with autism. *$23.95*

336 pages Year Founded: 1987 ISBN 1-853023-87-6

614 **Autism: An Introduction to Psychological Theory**
Harvard University Press
79 Garden Street
Cambridge, MA 02138-1400
617-495-2600
Fax: 617-495-5898
E-mail: CONTACT_HUP@harvard.edu
www.www.hup.harvard.edu

Francesca Happe, Author

Provides a concise overview of current psychological theory and research that synthesizes the established work on the biological foundations, cognitive characteristics, and behavioral manifestations of this disorder. *$32.00*

160 pages Year Founded: 1913 ISBN 0-674053-12-5

615 **Autism: Explaining the Enigma**
Autism Society of North Carolina Bookstore
505 Oberlin Road
Suite 230
Raleigh, NC 27605-1345
919-743-0204
800-442-2762
Fax: 919-743-0208
www.www.autismsociety-nc.org

Uta Frith, Author
Paul Wendler, Chief Financial Officer
David Laxton, Director, Communications
Kay Walker, Director, Development

Explains the nature of autism. *$27.95*

264 pages

616 **Autism: From Tragedy to Triumph**
Branden Publishing Company
PO Box 812094
Wellesley, MA 02482-13
Fax: 781-790-1056
E-mail: branden@branden.com
www.www.brandenbooks.com

Julia Crowder, Author
Carol Johnson, Author

A new book that deals with the Lovaas method and includes a foreward by Dr. Ivar Lovaas. The book is broken down into two parts, the long road to diagnosis and then treatment. *$12.95*

187 pages Year Founded: 1998 ISBN 0-828319-65-0

617 Autism: Identification, Education and Treatment
Autism Society of North Carolina Bookstore
505 Oberlin Road
Suite 230
Raleigh, NC 27605-1345
919-743-0204
800-442-2762
Fax: 919-743-0208
www.www.autismsociety-nc.org

Dianne Zager, Author
Psul Wendler, Chief Financial Officer
David Laxton, Director, Communications
Kay Walker, Director, Development

Chapters include medical treatments, early intervention and communication and development in autism. *$36.00*

392 pages

618 Autism: Nature, Diagnosis and Treatment
Guilford Press
72 Spring Street
Department 4E
New York, NY 10012-4019
212-431-9800
800-365-7006
Fax: 212-966-6708
E-mail: exam@guilford.com

Geraldine Dawson, Author

Foremost experts explore new perspectives on the nature and treatment of autism. Covering theory, research and the development of hypotheses and models, this book provides a balance between depth and breadth by focusing on questions most central to the field. For each question, an expert examines theoretical issues as well as empirical findings to offer new directions and testable hypotheses for future research. *$51.00*

417 pages ISBN 0-898627-24-9

619 Autism: Strategies for Change
Groden Center
86 Mount Hope Avenue
Providence, RI 02906-1648
401-274-6310
Fax: 401-421-3280
E-mail: grodencenter@grodencenter.org
www.grodencenter.org

Gerald Groden, Editor
M Grace Baron, Editor

A comprehensive approach to the education and treatment of children with autism and related disorders. Clinicians, parents, and students of autism who are, or want to be advocates for change will find in this book a blueprint, and much detail, on how to bring change about. This applies at the level of program planning and management as well as of clinical or education practice. *$21.95*

350 pages Year Founded: 1976

620 Autistic Adults at Bittersweet Farms
Haworth Press
10 Alice Street
Binghamton, NY 13904-1503
607-722-5857
800-429-6784
Fax: 607-722-1424

E-mail: getinfo@haworthpressinc.com
www.haworthpress.com

Norman Giddan, Author
Jane J Giddan, Author

A touching view of an inspirational residential care program for autistic adolescents and adults. *$17.95*

226 pages ISBN 1-560240-57-1

621 Avoiding Unfortunate Situations
Autism Society of North Carolina Bookstore
505 Oberlin Road
Suite 230
Raleigh, NC 27605-1345
919-743-0204
800-442-2762
Fax: 919-743-0208
E-mail: info@autismsociety-nc.org
www.www.autismsociety-nc.org

Dennis Debbaudt, Author
Ellen Kerfoot, Editor
David Laxton, Director, Communications
Kay Walker, Director, Development

A collection of tips and information from and about people with autism and other developmental disabilities. *$5.00*

18 pages Year Founded: 1970

622 Beyond Gentle Teaching
Autism Society of North Carolina Bookstore
505 Oberlin Road
Suite 230
Raleigh, NC 27605-1345
919-743-0204
800-442-2762
Fax: 919-743-0208
www.www.autismsociety-nc.org

John J McGee, Author
Frank J Menolascino, Author
David Laxton, Director, Communications
Kay Walker, Director, Development

A nonaversive approach to helping those in need. *$35.00*

233 pages

623 Biology of the Autistic Syndromes
Autism Society of North Carolina Bookstore
505 Oberlin Road
Suite 230
Raleigh, NC 27605-1345
919-743-0204
800-442-2762
Fax: 919-743-0208
www.www.autismsociety-nc.org

Christopher Gillberg, Author
Mary Coleman, Author
David Laxton, Director, Communications
Kay Walker, Director, Development

A revision of the original, classic text in the light of new developments and current knowledge. This book covers the epidemiological, genetic, biochemical, immunological and neuropsychological literature on autism. *$74.95*

300 pages

624 Camps 2009-2010
Resources for Children with Special Needs
116 E 16th Street
5th Floor
New York, NY 10003-2164
212-677-4650
Fax: 212-254-4070
E-mail: info@resourcenyc.org
www.resourcesnyc.org

Rachel Howard, Executive Director
Vicky Garwood Burton, Executive, Development Assistant
Hilda Melendez, Family, Community Educator

The guide includes a dozen new camps and updates on more than 300 camps and programs that provide a wide range of summer activities for children with emotional, developmental, learning and physical disabilities, health issues and other special needs. Day camps in the New York metro area are included as well as sleepaway camps in the Northeast. *$25.00*

133 pages Year Founded: 2009 ISBN 0-967836-57-3

625 Children with Autism: A Developmental Perspective
Harvard University Press
79 Garden Street
Cambridge, MA 02138-1400
617-495-2600
Fax: 617-495-5898
E-mail: CONTACT_HUP@harvard.edu
www.www.hup.harvard.edu

Marian Sigman, Author
Lisa Capps, Author

Views autism through the lens of developmental psychpathology, a discipline grounded in the belief that studies of normal and abnormal development can inform and enhance one another.

284 pages Year Founded: 1913

626 Children with Autism: Parents' Guide
Woodbine House
6510 Bells Mill Road
Bethesda, MD 20817-1636
301-897-3570
800-843-7323
Fax: 301-897-5838
E-mail: info@woodbinehouse.com
www.woodbinehouse.com

Michael D. Powers, Editor

Recommended as the first book parents should read, this completely revised volume offers information and a complete introduction to autism, while easing the family's fears and concerns as they adjust and cope with their child's disorder. *$14.95*

456 pages ISBN 1-890627-04-6

627 Communication Unbound: How Facilitated Communication Is Challenging Views
Baker & Taylor International
2709 Water Ridge Parkway
Charlotte, NC 28217-4596
704-357-3500
800-775-1800
www.btol.com

Tom Morgan, Chairman, CEO
Arnie Wright, President, COO

Jeff Leonard, Chief Financial Officer
George Coe, Pres of Library Education

Addresses the ways in which we receive persons with autism in our society, our community and our lives. *$18.95*

240 pages

628 Diagnosis and Treatment of Autism
Autism Society of North Carolina Bookstore
505 Oberlin Road
Suite 230
Raleigh, NC 27605-1345
919-743-0204
800-442-2762
Fax: 919-743-0208
www.www.autismsociety-nc.org

Christopher Gillberg, Editor
Paul Wendler, Chief Financial Officer
David Laxton, Director, Communications
Kay Walker, Director, Development

Various chapters written by professionals working with autistic children and adults. *$110.00*

629 Facilitated Communication and Technology Guide
Autism Society of North Carolina Bookstore
505 Oberlin Road
Suite 230
Raleigh, NC 27605-1345
919-743-0204
800-442-2762
Fax: 919-743-0208
www.www.autismsociety-nc.org

Carol Lee Berger, Author
Paul Wendler, Chief Financial Officer
David Laxton, Director, Communications
Kay Walker, Director, Development

Chapters include technology and facilitated communication, augmentative and alternative communication, spelling boards, speech synthesizers and software. *$20.00*

630 Fighting for Darla: Challenges for Family Care & Professional Responsibility
Baker & Taylor International
2709 Water Ridge Parkway
Charlotte, NC 28217-4596
704-357-3500
800-775-1800
www.btol.com

Follows the story of Darla, a pregnant adolescent with autism. *$18.95*

176 pages ISBN 0-807733-56-3

631 Fragile Success - Ten Autistic Children, Childhood to Adulthood
Autism Society of North Carolina Bookstore
505 Oberlin Road
Suite 230
Raleigh, NC 27605-1345
919-743-0204
800-442-2762
Fax: 919-743-0208
www.www.autismsociety-nc.org

Virgina Walker Sperry, Author
Paul Wendler, Chief Financial Officer

David Laxton, Director, Communications
Kay Walker, Director, Development

A book about the lives of autistic children, whom the author has followed from their early years at the Elizabeth Ives School in New Haven, CT, through to adulthood.
$24.95

304 pages

632 Handbook of Autism and Pervasive Developmental Disorders
ADD WareHouse
300 NW 70th Avenue
Suite 102
Plantation, FL 33317-2360
954-792-8944
800-233-9273
Fax: 954-792-8545
E-mail: sales@addwarehouse.com
www.addwarehouse.com

Harvey C Parker, Owner

A comprehensive view of all information presently available about autism and other pervasive developmental disorders, drawing on findings and clinical experience from a number of related disciplines psychiatry, psychology, neurobiology and pediatrics. *$95.00*

1092 pages

633 Helping People with Autism Manage Their Behavior
Autism Society of North Carolina Bookstore
505 Oberlin Road
Suite 230
Raleigh, NC 27605-1345
919-743-0204
800-442-2762
Fax: 919-743-0208
www.www.autismsociety-nc.org

Nancy J Darylmple, Author
Paul Wendler, Chief Financial Officer
David Laxton, Director, Communications
Kay Walker, Director, Development

Covers the broad topic of helping people with autism manage their behavior. *$7.00*

634 Hidden Child: The Linwood Method for Reaching the Autistic Child
Woodbine House
6510 Bells Mill Road
Bethesda, MD 20817-1636
301-897-3570
800-843-7323
Fax: 301-897-5838
E-mail: info@woodbinehouse.com
www.woodbinehouse.com

Jeanne Simons, Author
Sabine Oishi, Author

Chronicle of the Linwood Children's Center's successful treatment program for autistic children. *$14.95*

251 pages Year Founded: 1985 ISBN 0-933149-06-9

635 How to Teach Autistic & Severely Handicapped Children
Autism Society of North Carolina Bookstore
505 Oberlin Road
Suite 230
Raleigh, NC 27605-1345
919-743-0204
800-442-2762
Fax: 919-743-0208
www.www. autismsociety-nc.com

Laura Schreibman, Author
Robert L Koegel, Author
David Laxton, Director, Communications
Kay Walker, Director, Development

Book provides procedures for effectively assessing and teaching autistic and other severely handicapped children. *$9.00*

636 I'm Not Autistic on the Typewriter
TASH
2013 H Street NW
Suite 715
Washington, D. 20006
202-540-9020
Fax: 202-540-9019
E-mail: info@tash.org
www.tash.org

Barbara Trader, Executive Director
Jonathan Riethmaier, Advocacy Communications Manager
Edwin Canizalez, Events and Training Manager
Jenny Stonemeier, Education Policy Director

An introduction to the facilitated communication training method. *$25.00*

637 Inner Life of Children with Special Needs
Taylor & Francis
325 Chestnut Street
Philadelphia, PA 19106-2614
215-625-8900
Fax: 215-625-2940
www.taylorandfrancis.com

Ved Prakash Varma, Editor

210 pages

638 Joey and Sam
Autism Society of North Carolina Bookstore
505 Oberlin Road
Suite 230
Raleigh, NC 27605-1345
919-743-0204
800-442-2762
Fax: 919-743-0208
www.www.autismsociety-nc.org

IIIana Katz, Author
M.D.Ritvo Edward, Author
David Laxton, Director, Communications
Kay Walker, Director, Development

A beautifully illustrated storybook for children, focusing on a family with two sons, one of whom suffers from autism.
$16.95

1 pages

639 Keys to Parenting the Child with Autism
Autism Society of North Carolina Bookstore
505 Oberlin Road
Suite 230
Raleigh, NC 27605-1345
919-743-0204
800-442-2762
Fax: 919-743-0208
www.www.autismsociety-nc.org

Marlene Targ Brill, Med, Author
Paul Wendler, Chief Financial Officer
David Laxton, Director, Communications
Kay Walker, Director, Development

This book explains what autism is and how it is diagnosed. *$7.95*

224 pages

640 Kristy and the Secret of Susan
Autism Society of North Carolina Bookstore
505 Oberlin Road
Suite 230
Raleigh, NC 27605-1345
919-743-0204
800-442-2762
Fax: 919-743-0208
www.www.autismsociety-nc.org

Tracey Sheriff, Chief Executive Officer
Paul Wendler, Chief Financial Officer
David Laxton, Director, Communications
Kay Walker, Director, Development

This book discusses Kristy and her new baby-sitting charge, Susan. Susan can't speak but sings beautifully. Susan is autistic. *$ 3.50*

641 Learning and Cognition in Autism
Kluwer Academic/Plenum Publishers
233 Spring Street
New York, NY 10013-1522
212-242-1490

Mads Soegaard, Editor-in-Chief

Collection of papers written by experts in the field of autism. Describes the cognitive and educational characteristics of people with autism and explains intervention techniques and strategies. Topics include motivating communication in children with autism and a chapter by a high-functioning woman with autism who discusses special learning problems and unique learning strengths that characterize their development and offers specific suggestions for working with people like herself. *$59.00*

368 pages ISBN 0-306448-71-8

642 Let Community Employment Be the Goal For Individuals with Autism
Autism Society of North Carolina Bookstore
505 Oberlin Road
Suite 230
Raleigh, NC 27605-1345
919-743-0204
800-442-2762
Fax: 919-743-0208
www.www.autismsociety-nc.org

Joanne Suomi, Author
Paul Wendler, Chief Financial Officer
David Laxton, Director, Communications
Kay Walker, Director, Development

A guide designed for people who are responsible for preparing individuals with autism to enter the work force. *$7.00*

60 pages

643 Let Me Hear Your Voice
Autism Society of North Carolina Bookstore
505 Oberlin Road
Suite 230
Raleigh, NC 27605-1345
919-743-0204
800-442-2762
Fax: 919-743-0208
www.www.autismsociety-nc.org

Catherine Maurice, Author
Paul Wendler, Chief Financial Officer
David Laxton, Director, Communications
Kay Walker, Director, Development

The Maruice family's second and third children were diagnosed with autism. This book recounts their experience with a home program using behavior therapy. *$13.95*

400 pages

644 Letting Go
Autism Society of North Carolina Bookstore
505 Oberlin Road
Suite 230
Raleigh, NC 27605-1345
919-743-0204
800-442-2762
Fax: 919-743-0208
www.www.autismsociety-nc.org

Philip Roth, Author
Paul Wendler, Chief Financial Officer
David Laxton, Director, Communications
Kay Walker, Director, Development

A book of poems about a journey, an emotional road of placing a child in a residential group home for children with autism. *$7.50*

640 pages

645 Management of Autistic Behavior
Pro-Ed Publications
8700 Shoal Creek Boulevard
Austin, TX 78757-6897
512-451-3246
800-897-3202
Fax: 512-451-8542
E-mail: info@proedinc.com

Donald D Hammill, Owner

Comprehensive and practical book that tells what works best with specific problems. *$41.00*

450 pages ISBN 0-890791-96-1

646 Mindblindness: An Essay on Autism and Theory of Mind
Autism Society of North Carolina Bookstore
505 Oberlin Road
Suite 230
Raleigh, NC 27605-1345
919-743-0204
800-442-2762
Fax: 919-743-0208
www.www.autismsociety-nc.org

Simon Baron-Cohen, Author
David Laxton, Director, Communications
Kay Walker, Director, Development

Interpretations and research into the theory of mindblindness in children with autism. *$19.95*

200 pages ISBN 0-262023-84-9

647 Mixed Blessings
Autism Society of North Carolina Bookstore
505 Oberlin Road
Suite 230
Raleigh, NC 27605-1345
919-743-0204
800-442-2762
Fax: 919-743-0208
www.autismsociety-nc.org

Danielle Steel, Author
Paul Wendler, Chief Financial Officer
David Laxton, Director, Communications
Kay Walker, Director, Development

A real-life family discusses the raising of their autistic son. *$19.95*

432 pages

648 More Laughing and Loving with Autism
Autism Society of North Carolina Bookstore
505 Oberlin Road
Suite 230
Raleigh, NC 27605-1345
919-743-0204
800-442-2762
Fax: 919-743-0208
www.autismsociety-nc.org

R Wayne Gilpin, Author
Paul Wendler, Chief Financial Officer
David Laxton, Director, Communications
Kay Walker, Director, Development

A collection of warm and humorous parent stories about raising a child with autism. *$9.95*

108 pages

649 Neurobiology of Autism
Johns Hopkins University Press
2715 N Charles Street
Baltimore, MD 21218-4319
410-516-6900
800-537-5487
Fax: 410-516-6998
www.www.press.jhu.edu

Kathleen Keane, Director
Stacey Armstead, Info Systems Manager
Kelly Rogers, Rights Manager
Jack Holmes, Director, Development

This 2nd edition discusses recent advances in scientific research that point to a neurobiological basis for autism and examines the clinical implications of this research. *$44.95*

272 pages Year Founded: 2005 ISBN 0-801856-80-9

650 News from the Border: a Mother's Memoir of Her Autistic Son
Houghton Mifflin Company
222 Berkeley Street
Boston, MA 02116-3760

617-351-5000
Fax: 617-351-1105
www.www.hmhco.com/

Barry O'Callaghan, CEO

A searingly honest account of the author's family experiences with autism. Raising an autistic child is the central, ongoing drama of her married life in this riveting account of acceptance and coping. *$22.95*

384 pages

651 Nobody Nowhere
Autism Society of North Carolina Bookstore
505 Oberlin Road
Suite 230
Raleigh, NC 27605-1345
919-743-0204
800-442-2762
Fax: 919-743-0208
www.www.autismsociety-nc.org

Donna Williams, Author
Paul Wendler, Chief Finacial Officer
David Laxton, Director, Communications
Kay Walker, Director, Development

An autobiography giving readers a tour of the author's life with autism. *$14.00*

219 pages

652 Parent Survival Manual
Autism Society of North Carolina Bookstore
505 Oberlin Road
Suite 230
Raleigh, NC 27605-1345
919-743-0204
800-442-2762
Fax: 919-743-0208
www.autismsociety-nc.org

Eric Schopler, Editor
Paul Wendler, Chief Financial Officer
David Laxton, Director, Communications
Kay Walker, Director, Development

Compiled from three hundred fifty anecdotes told by parents of autistic and developmentally disabled children. *$38.50*

224 pages

653 Parent's Guide to Autism
Autism Society of North Carolina Bookstore
505 Oberlin Road
Suite 230
Raleigh, NC 27605-1345
919-743-0204
800-442-2762
Fax: 919-743-0208
www.www.autismsociety-nc.org

Charles A Hart, Author
Paul Wendler, Chief Financial Officer
David Laxton, Director, Communications
Kay Walker, Director, Development

An essential handbook for anyone facing autism. *$14.00*

256 pages

654 Please Don't Say Hello
Human Sciences Press
233 Spring Street
New York, NY 10013-1522
212-620-8000
Fax: 212-807-1047
www.www.humansciencespress.com

Paul and his family moved into a new neighborhood. Paul's brother was autistic. The children thought that Eddie was retarded until they learned that there were skills that he could do better than they could. *$10.95*

47 pages ISBN 0-898851-99-8

655 Preschool Issues in Autism
Kluwer Academic/Plenum Publishers
233 Spring Street
New York, NY 10013-1522
212-242-1490
www.www.springer.com

Derk Haank, Chief Executive Officer
Martin Mos, Chief Operating Officer
Dr Ulrich Vest, Chief Financial Officer
Ralf Birkelbach, Executive Vice President

Combines some of the most important theory and data related to the early identifiction and intervention in autism and related disorders. Addresses clinical aspects, parental concerns and legal issues. Helps professionals understand and implement state-of-the-art services for young children and their families. *$54.00*

276 pages ISBN 0-306444-40-2

656 Psychoeducational Profile
Autism Society of North Carolina Bookstore
505 Oberlin Road
Suite 230
Raleigh, NC 27605-1345
919-743-0204
800-442-2762
Fax: 919-743-0208
www.www.autismsociety-nc.org

Tracey Sheriff, Chief Executive Officer
Paul Wendler, Chief Financial Officer
David Laxton, Director, Communications
Kay Walker, Director, Development

The PEP-R is a revision of the popular instrument that has been used for over twenty years to assess skills and behavior of autistic and communication-handicapped children who function between the ages of 6 months and 7 years. *$74.00*

657 Reaching the Autistic Child: a Parent Training Program
Brookline Books/Lumen Editions
8 Trumbell Road
Suite B-001
Northampton, MA 01060
413-584-0184
800-666-2665
Fax: 413-584-6184
www.brooklinebooks.com

Detailed case studies of social and behavioral change in autistic children and their families show parents how to implement the principles for improved socialization and behavior. Revised and updated 1998. *$15.95*

ISBN 1-571290-56-7

658 Record Books for Individuals with Autism
Indiana Institute on Disability and Community
Indiana University
2853 E Tenth Street
Bloomington, IN 47408-2601
812-855-9396
800-280-7010
Fax: 812-855-9630
TTY: 812-855-9396
E-mail: uap@indiana.edu
www.www.iidc.indiana.edu

Cathy Pratt, Center Director
Pamela Anderson, Outreach/Resource Specialist
Scott Bellini, PhD, Assistant Center Director
Donna Beasley, Adminstrative Program Secretary

This book was developed with parent information about an autistic child so that it is organized, easily accessible and can be copied as needed. *$5.00*

37 pages

659 Russell Is Extra Special
Autism Society of North Carolina Bookstore
505 Oberlin Road
Suite 230
Raleigh, NC 27605-1345
919-743-0204
800-442-2762
Fax: 919-743-0208
www.www.autismsociety-nc.org

Charles A Amenta, Author
Paul Wendler, Chief Financial Officer
David Laxton, Director, Communications
Kay Walker, Director, Development

A sensitive portrayal of an autistic boy written by his father. *$8.95*

32 pages

660 Schools for Students with Special Needs
Resources for Children with Special Needs
116 E 16th Street
Fifth Floor
New York City, NY 10003-2112
212-677-4650
Fax: 212-254-4070
E-mail: info@resourcesnyc.org
www.resourcesnyc.org

Rachel Howard, Executive Director
Vicky Garwood Burton, Executive Development Asst
Hilda Melendez, Family and Community Educator

The first complete book listing private day and residential schools for parents, caregivers and professionals seeking schools for students 5 and up with developmental, emotional, physical and learning disabilities in the NYC metro area. More than 400 schools and residential programs that serve children in the elementary through high school grades are listed with contact information, ages and populations served, class sizes and student-teacher ratios, special services and diplomas offered. Includes a 46-page section of Schools for Children with Autism Spectrum Disorders, as well as a guide with a list of websites on autism spectrum disorders. *$25.00*

342 pages

661 Sex Education: Issues for the Person with Autism
Indiana Institute on Disability and Community
Indiana University
2853 E Tenth Street
Bloomington, IN 47408-2601
812-855-9396
800-280-7010
Fax: 812-855-9630
TTY: 812-855-9396
E-mail: uap@indiana.edu

Michael McRobbie, President
Karen Adams, Chief of Staff
Kelly Kish, Deputy Chief of Staff

Discusses issues of sexuality and provides some methods of instruction for persons with autism. *$3.00*

18 pages

662 Siblings of Children with Autism: A Guide for Families
Autism Society of North Carolina Bookstore
505 Oberlin Road
Suite 230
Raleigh, NC 27605-1345
919-743-0204
800-442-2762
Fax: 919-743-0208
www.www.autismsociety-nc.org

Sandra L Harris, Author
Beth A Glasberg, Author
David Laxton, Director, Communications
Kay Walker, Director, Development

Offers information on the needs of a child with autism. *$16.95*

164 pages

663 Somebody Somewhere
Autism Society of North Carolina Bookstore
505 Oberlin Road
Suite 230
Raleigh, NC 27605-1345
919-743-0204
800-442-2762
Fax: 919-743-0208
www.autismsociety-nc.org

Donna Williams, Author
Paul Wendler, Chief Financial Officer
David Laxton, Director, Communications
Kay Walker, Director, Development

Offers a revealing account of the author's battle with autism. *$15.00*

256 pages

664 Soon Will Come the Light
Autism Society of North Carolina Bookstore
505 Oberlin Road
Suite 230
Raleigh, NC 27605-1345
919-743-0204
800-442-2762
Fax: 919-743-0208
www.autismsociety-nc.org

Thomas A McKean, Author
R Wayne Gilpin, Editor

David Laxton, Director, Communications
Kay Walker, Director, Development

Offers new perspectives on the perplexing disability of autism. *$19.95*

156 pages

665 Teaching Children with Autism: Strategies to Enhance Communication
Autism Society of North Carolina Bookstore
505 Oberlin Road
Suite 230
Raleigh, NC 27605-1345
919-743-0204
800-442-2762
Fax: 919-743-0208
www.autismsociety-nc.org

Kathleen Ann Quill, Editor
Paul Wendler, Chief Financial Officer
David Laxton, Director, Communications
Kay Walker, Director, Development

This valuable new book describes teaching strategies and instructional adaptations which promote communication and socialization in children with autism. *$34.95*

315 pages

666 Teaching and Mainstreaming Autistic Children
Love Publishing Company
9101 East Kenyon Avenue
Suite 2200
Denver, CO 80237-1854
303-221-7333
Fax: 303-221-7444
E-mail: lpc@lovepublishing.com
www.lovepublishing.com

Peter Knoblock, Author

Dr Knoblock advocates a highly organized, structured environment for autistic children, with teachers and parents working together. His premise is that the learning and social needs of autistic children must be analyzed and a daily program be designed with interventions that respond to this functional analysis of their behavior. *$39.95*

360 pages Year Founded: 1968 ISBN 0-891081-11-9

667 Ten Things Every Child with Autism Wishes You Knew
Future Horizons
721 West Abram Street
Arlington, TX 76013-6995
817-277-0727
800-489-0727
Fax: 817-277-2270
www.fhautism.com

Ellen Notbohm, Author
Jennifer Gilpin, Vice President
Kelly Gilpin, Editorial Director

Framed in both humor and compassion, the book defines the top ten characteristics that illuminate the minds and hearts of cildren with autism. Ellen's personal experiences.

200 pages

668 The Comprehensive Directory
Resources For Children with Special Needs
116 East 16th Street
5th Floor
New York, NY 10003-2164
212-677-4650
Fax: 212-254-4070
E-mail: info@resourcesnyc.org
www.resourcesnyc.org

Ellen Miller-Wachtel, Chair
Shon E Glusky, President
Rachel Howard, Executive Director
Stephen Stern, Director of Finance and Administ

The directory for everyone who needs to find services for children with disabilities and special needs. Designed for parents, caregivers and professionals, it includes more than 2, 500 agencies providing more than 4, 000 services and programs. *$30.00*

1096 pages Year Founded: 1983 ISBN 0-967836-51-4

669 The Hidden Child: Youth with Autism
Mason Crest Publishers
450 Parkway Drive
Suite D
Broomall, PA 19008-4017
610-543-6200
866-627-2665
Fax: 610-543-3878
E-mail: dtaylor@masoncrest.com
www.masoncrest.com

Sherry Bonice, Author
Dan Hilferty, President
Michelle Luke, Dir of Marketing, PR
Michael Toglia, Special Sales

Hope is the keyword for the autistic child's future. Through education, early intervention, and continued research, children with autism can live normal lives. Factual information about autism, the Autism Society of America, sibshops, and different educational treatments will expand the reader's knowledge of this condition. A fictional story told from a sibling's point of view helps the reader understand the effects autism has on individuals and family members.

128 pages ISBN 1-590847-38-9

670 Thinking In Pictures, Expanded Edition: My Life with Autism
Vintage
1745 Broadway
New York, NY 10019
212-782-9000
800-733-3000
Fax: 212-572-6043
E-mail: ecustomerservice@randomhouse.com
www.randomhouse.com

Temple Grandin, Author

304 pages ISBN 0-307275-65-5

671 Transition Matters from School to Independence
Resources for Children with Special Needs
116 East 16th Street
5th Floor
New York, NY 10003-2164
212-677-4650
Fax: 212-254-4070

E-mail: info@resourcesnyc.org
www.resourcesnyc.org

Ellen Miller-Wachtel, Chair
Shon E Glusky, President
Rachel Howard, Executive Director
Stephen Stern, Director of Finance and Administ

Youth with disabilities need special guidance when moving from school to adult life. Transition Matters covers every aspect of moving from high school to the world of postsecondary education, job training, employment and idependent living. This guide for parents, caregivers and educators presents a wealth of information about the transition process, and lists 1, 000 agencies and organizations that provide services for youth 14 and up. It explains entitlements and options and helps families navigate systems and procedures. *$15.00*

512 pages Year Founded: 1983 ISBN 0-967836-56-5

672 Ultimate Stranger: The Autistic Child
Autism Society of North Carolina Bookstore
505 Oberlin Road
Suite 230
Raleigh, NC 27605-1345
919-743-0204
800-442-2762
Fax: 919-743-0208
www.www.autismsociety-nc.org

Carl H Delacato, Author
Paul Wendler, Chief Financial Officer
David Laxton, Director, Communications
Kay Walker, Director, Development

Delacato's thesis is that autism is neuro-genic and not psycho-genic in origin. *$10.00*

240 pages

673 Understanding Autism
Fanlight Productions
32 Court Street
21st Floor
Brooklyn, NY 11201
718-488-8900
800-937-4113
Fax: 718-488-8642
E-mail: info@fanlight.com
www.fanlight.com

Suzanne Newman, Director

Parents of children with autism discuss the nature and symptoms of this lifelong disability, and outline a treatment program based on behavior modification principles. *$195.00*

ISBN 1-572951-00-1

674 Until Tomorrow: A Family Lives with Autism
Autism Society of North Carolina Bookstore
505 Oberlin Road
Suite 230
Raleigh, NC 27605-1345
919-743-0204
800-442-2762
Fax: 919-743-0208
www.autismsociety-nc.org

Dorothy Zeitz, Author
Paul Wendler, Chief Financial Officer
David Laxton, Director, Communications
Kay Walker, Director, Development

The central theme of this book is an effort to show what it is like to live with a child who cannot communicate. *$10.00*

675 When Snow Turns to Rain
Woodbine House
6510 Bells Mill Road
Bethesda, MD 20817-1636
301-897-3570
800-843-7323
Fax: 301-897-5838
E-mail: info@woodbinehouse.com
www.woodbinehouse.com

Craig B Schulze, Author

A gripping personal account of one family's experiences with autism. Chronicles a family's journey from parental bliss to devastation, as they learn that their son has autism. This book delves into diagnosis, treatments, and attitudes toward persons with autism. *$14.95*

216 pages Year Founded: 1985 ISBN 0-933149-63-8

676 Winter's Flower
Autism Society of North Carolina Bookstore
505 Oberlin Road
Suite 230
Raleigh, NC 27605-1345
919-743-0204
800-442-2762
Fax: 919-743-0208
www.autismsociety-nc.org

Ranae Johnson, Author
Paul Wendler, Chief Financial Officer
David Laxton, Director, Communications
Kay Walker, Director, Development

The story of Ranae Johnson's quest to rescue her son from a world of silence. A story of love, patience and dedication. *$12.95*

677 Without Reason
Autism Society of North Carolina Bookstore
505 Oberlin Road
Suite 230
Raleigh, NC 27605-1345
919-743-0204
800-442-2762
Fax: 919-743-0208
www.autismsociety-nc.org

Charles A Hart, Author
Paul Wendler, Chief Financial Officer
David Laxton, Director, Communications
Kay Walker, Director, Development

A story of a family coping with two generations of autism. *$19.95*

292 pages

Periodicals & Pamphlets

678 Autism Matters
Autism Society Ontario
1179 King Street West
Suite 004
Toronto, ON M6K 3-5
416-246-9592
800-472-7789
Fax: 416-246-9417

E-mail: mail@autismsociety.on.ca
www.autismsociety.on.ca

Covers society activities and contains information on autism. Recurring features include news of research, a calendar of events, reports of meetings, and book reviews. *$25.00*

10 pages 4 per year

679 Autism Research Review International
Autism Research Institute
4182 Adams Avenue
San Diego, CA 92116-2599
619-281-7165
Fax: 619-563-6840
www.autism.com

Stephen M Edelson, PhD, Executive Director
Jane Johnson, Managing Director
Valerie Paradiz , PhD, Director, ARI Autistic Global Ins
Rebecca McKenney, Office Manager

Discusses current research and provides information about the causes, diagnosis, and treatment of autism and related disorders. *$18.00*

8 pages 4 per year Year Founded: 1976 ISSN 0893-8474

680 Autism Society News
Utah Parent Center
230 West 200 South
Suite 1101
Salt Lake City, UT 84117-4428
801-272-1067
800-468-1160
Fax: 801-272-8907
www.utahparentcenter.org

Helen Post, Executive Director

Presents news, research information, and legislative updates regarding autism. Recurring features include a calendar of events and columns titled Parent Meetings, What's On in the News, Research News, Parent Corner, Legislative Summary, and A Big Thank You!

8 pages

681 Autism Spectrum Disorders in Children and Adolescents
Center for Mental Health Services: Knowledge Exchange Network
PO Box 42490
Washington, DC 20015
800-789-2647
Fax: 301-984-8796
TDD: 866-889-2647
E-mail: ken@mentalhealth.org
www.mentalhealth.org

Lee A Wilkinson, Author

This fact sheet defines autism, describes the signs and causes, discusses types of help available, and suggests what parents or other caregivers can do.

264 pages

682 Autism in Children and Adolescents
Center for Mental Health Services: Knowledge Exchange Network
PO Box 42557
Washington, DC 20015-557

800-789-2647
Fax: 301-984-8796
TDD: 866-889-2647
E-mail: ken@mentalhealth.org
www.mentalhealth.org.samhsa.gov

This fact sheet defines autism, describes the signs and causes, discusses types of help available, and suggests what parents or other caregivers can do.

2 pages Year Founded: 1997

683 Facts About Autism
Indiana Institute on Disability and Community
1 East 33rd Street
4th Floor
New York, NY 10016
212-252-8584
800-280-7010
Fax: 212-252-8676
TTY: 812-855-9396
E-mail: uap@indiana.edu
www.www.autismspeaks.org/

Liz Feld, President
Jennifer Bizub, Chief Human Resources Officer
Alec M Elbert, Chief Strategy and Development O
Jamitha Fields, Vice President - Community Affai

Provides concise information describing autism, diagnosis, needs of the person with autism from diagnosis through adulthood. Information on the Autism Society of America chapters in Indiana are listed in the back, along with a description of the Indiana Resource Center for Autism and suggested books to look for in the local library. Also available in Spanish. *$1.00*

684 Journal of Autism and Developmental Disorders
Springer Science & Business Media
Heidelberger Plate 3
14197 Berlin
Germany,
www.springer.com

Fred R. Volkmar, Editor-in-Chief

Features research and case studies involving the entire spectrum of interventions and advances in the diagnosis and classification of disorders.

6 per year Year Founded: 1842 ISSN 0162-3257

685 Sex Education: Issues for the Person with Autism
Autism Society of North Carolina Bookstore
955 Woodland Street
Nashville, TN 37206
615-385-2077
866-508-4987
Fax: 615-383-1176
E-mail: support@autismtn.org
www.www.autismtn.org

Nancy Dalrympale, Author
Susan Gray, Author
Lisa Ruble, Author
Kay Walker, Director, Development

Discusses issues of sexuality and provides methods of instruction for people with autism. *$4.00*

18 pages

686 The Source Newsletter
MAAP
PO Box 524
Crown Point, IN 46308-524
219-662-1311
Fax: 219-662-0638
E-mail: chart@netnitco.net

Story C Landis, Director
Wlater J Koroshetz, MD, Deputy Director
Caroline Lewis, Executive Officer

Newsletter from the Global Information and Support Network for More Advanced Persons with Austism and Asperger's Syndrome.

4 per year

687 Treatment of Children with Mental Disorders
National Institute of Mental Health
6001 Executive Boulevard
Room 8184, MSC 9663
Bethesda, MD 20892-9663
301-443-4513
866-615-6464
TTY: 301-443-8431
E-mail: nimhinfo@nih.gov
www.www.nimh.nih.gov/

Francis S Collins, MD, PhD, Director

A short booklet that contains questions and answers about therapy for children with mental disorders. Includes a chart of mental disorders and medications used.

Research Centers

688 Indiana Resource Center for Autism (IRCA)
1905 North Range Road
Bloomington, IN 47408-2601
812-855-6508
800-825-4733
Fax: 812-855-9630
TTY: 812-855-9396
E-mail: prattc@indiana.edu
www.www.iidc.indiana.edu/index.php?pageId=32

Cathy Pratt, PhD, BCBA-D, Center Director
David Mank, PhD, Director, Indiana Institute On Di
Doug Ryner, IT Director
Harriet L Figg, Business Manager/Fiscal Officer

Conducts outreach training and consultations, engage in research, develop and disseminate information on behalf of individuals across the autism spectrum, Aspergers syndrome, and other pervasive developmental disorders. Provides communities, organizations, agencies and families with the knowledge and skills to support children and adults in typical early intervention, school, community work and home.

689 TEACCH
CB# 6305
University of NC at Chapel Hill
Chapel Hill, NC 27599
919-966-2174
Fax: 919-966-4127
E-mail: teacch@unc.edu
www.teacch.com

Dr Laura Klinger, Director
Rebecca Mabe, Assistant Director of Business a

Walter Kelly, Business Officer
Mark Klinger, Director, Research

This organization is the division for the treatment and education of autistic and related communication handicapped children.

Video & Audio

690 Asperger's Unplugged, an Interview with Jerry Newport
Program Development Associates
32 Court St
21st Floor
Brooklyn, NY 11201
315-452-0643
800-876-1710
Fax: 718-488-8642
E-mail: info@disabilitytraining.com
www.disabilitytraining.com

Meet the man who answered a question in the film 'Rain Man' - How much is 4, 343 x 1, 234? - before the autistic savant character played by Dustin Hoffman answered it. Jerry Newport discovered Asperger's Syndrome while watching 'Rain Man' and has since become an engaging speaker and self-help organizer. This inspiring interview, available on VHS or DVD, supports teachers, staff developers and people with high functioning autism. 40 minutes. *$79.95*

691 Autism Spectrum Disorders and the SCERTS
Program Development Associates
32 Court St
21st Floor
Brooklyn, NY 11201
315-452-0643
800-876-1710
Fax: 718-488-8642
E-mail: info@disabilitytraining.com
www.disabilitytraining.com

Early intervention for children with Autism Spectrum Disorders. Shows a model in action with higher-functioning children who require less support. 105 minutes between three tapes. *$279.00*

Year Founded: 2004

692 Autism in the Classroom
Program Development Associates
32 Court St
21st Floor
Brooklyn, NY 11201
315-452-0643
800-876-1710
Fax: 718-488-8642
E-mail: info@disabilitytraining.com
www.disabilitytraining.com

Overviews symptoms, behaviors and treatments, and interviews children with autism, along with their parents and their teachers. 16 minutes. *$69.95*

Year Founded: 2004

693 Autism is a World
Program Development Associates
32 Court St
21st Floor
Brooklyn, NY 11201

315-452-0643
800-876-1710
Fax: 718-488-8642
E-mail: info@disabilitytraining.com
www.disabilitytraining.com

Takes a look inside the life of a woman who lives with the disorder. She explains how she feels, how she relates to others, her obsession and why her behavior can be so very different. Gives teachers and professionals striving to understand Autism Spectrum Disorder a glimpse from the inside out of this developmental disability. 40 minutes & can also be ordered as a DVD with special features. *$99.95*

Year Founded: 2004

694 Autism: A Strange, Silent World
Filmakers Library
3212 Duke Street
Alexandria, VA 22314
212-808-4980
E-mail: sales@alexanderstreet.com
www.filmakers.com

Sue Oscar, Manager

British educators and medical personnel offer insight into autism's characteristics and treatment approaches through the cameos of three children. 52 minutes. *$295.00*

695 Autism: A World Apart
Fanlight Productions
32 Court Street
21st Floor
Brooklyn, NY 11201
718-488-8900
800-876-1710
Fax: 718-488-8642
E-mail: fanlight@fanlight.com
www.fanlight.com

Karen Cunninghame, Author

In this documentary, three families show us what the textbooks and studies cannot; what it's like to live with autism day after day, raise and love children who may be withdrawn and violent and unable to make personal connections with their families. Video cassette. 29 minutes. *$199.00*

ISBN 1-572950-39-0

696 Autism: Being Friends
Indiana Institute on Disability and Community
Indiana University
2853 E Tenth Street
Bloomington, IN 47408-2601
812-855-9396
800-280-7010
Fax: 812-855-9630
TTY: 812-855-9396
E-mail: uap@indiana.edu

David Mank, Executive Director

This autism awareness videotape was produced specifically for use with young children. The program portrays the abilities of the child with autism and describes ways in which peers can help the child to be a part of the everyday world. *$10.00*

Year Founded: 1991

697 Avoiding The Turbulance: Guiding Families of Children Diagnosed with Autism
Program Development Associates
32 Court St
21st Floor
Brooklyn, NY 11201
315-452-0643
800-876-1710
Fax: 718-488-8642
E-mail: info@disabilitytraining.com
www.disabilitytraining.com

Focuses primarily on the best strategies of early intervention. Good resources for primary care medical providers and agency professionals involved in early intervention autism programs. 12 minutes. *$79.95*

Year Founded: 2005

698 Breakthroughs: How to Reach Students with Autism
ADD WareHouse
300 NW 70th Avenue
Suite 102
Plantation, FL 33317-2360
954-792-8100
800-233-9273
Fax: 954-792-8545
E-mail: websales@addwarehouse.com
www.addwarehouse.com

Karen Sewell, Author

This video is designed for instructors of children with autism, K-12. The program provides a fully-loaded teacher's manual with reproducible lesson plans that will take you through an entire school year as well as an award-winning video that demonstrates the instructional and behavioral techniques recommended in the manual. Covers math, reading, fine motor, self-help, vocational, social and life skills. Features a veteran instructor who was named 'Teacher of the Year' by the Autism Society of America. *$89.00*

243 pages Year Founded: 1990

699 Children and Autism: Time is Brain
Program Development Associates
PO Box 2038
Syracuse, NY 13220-2038
315-452-0643
800-543-2119
Fax: 315-452-0710
E-mail: info@disabilitytraining.com
www.disabilitytraining.com/autism

Video features Applied Behavior Analysis (ABA) as an autism treatment technique by focusing on two families raising a child with autism. Gives documentation on their interaction with therapists and behavior analysts. 28 minutes. *$99.95*

Year Founded: 2004

700 Dr. Tony Attwood: Asperger's Syndrome Volume 2 DVD
Program Development Associates
32 Court St
21st Floor
Brooklyn, NY 11201
315-452-0643
800-876-1710
Fax: 718-488-8642
E-mail: info@disabilitytraining.com
www.disabilitytraining.com

Following rave national reviews that autism expert Dr. Tony Attwood received for his Volume 1 introduction to Asperger's Syndrome, here's the new DVD of his latest conference presentations. Volume 2 leaps off the DVD screen with Dr. Attwood's interactive, in-depth, theory-of-mind approach to Asperger's. 180 minutes. *$109.95*

701 Going to School with Facilitated Communication
Syracuse University, Facilitated Communication Institute
370 Huntington Hall
Syracuse, NY 13244-1
315-443-9657
Fax: 315-443-2274
E-mail: fcstaff@sued.syr.edu
www.soeweb.syr.edu/thefci

Douglas Biklen, Author

A video in which students with autism and/or severe disabilities illustrate the use of facilitated communication focusing on basic principles fostering facilitated communication.

702 I'm Not Autistic on the Typewriter
Syracuse University, Facilitated Communication Institute
370 Huntington Hall
Syracuse, NY 13244-1
315-443-9657
Fax: 315-443-2274
E-mail: fcstaff@sued.syr.edu
www.soeweb.syr.edu/thefci

A video introducing facilitated communication, a method by which persons with autism express themselves.

11 pages

703 Interview with Dr. Pauline Filipek
Program Development Associates
PO Box 2038
Syracuse, NY 13220-2038
315-452-0643
800-543-2119
Fax: 315-452-0710
E-mail: info@disabilitytraining.com
www.disabilitytraining.com/autism

An interview that presents early stage developmental autism, with diagnosis and age-level comparisons, research, interventions and myths and false and future treatments. 14 minutes. *$79.95*

Year Founded: 2005

704 Matthew: Guidance for Parents with Autistic Children
Program Development Associates
PO Box 2038
Syracuse, NY 13220-2038
315-452-0643
800-543-2119
Fax: 315-452-0710
E-mail: info@disabilitytraining.com
www.disabilitytraining.com/autism

A resource video guide for parents of autistic children. Shows parents where they should go, who to consult and what did or did not work for Matthew and his parents. 28 minutes. *$79.95*

Year Founded: 2004

705 Rising Above a Diagnosis of Autism
Program Development Associates
32 Court St
21st Floor
Brooklyn, NY 11201
315-452-0643
800-876-1710
Fax: 718-488-8642
E-mail: info@disabilitytraining.com
www.disabilitytraining.com/autism

Focuses primarily on the period when a child receives a diagnosis of Autism. Meet with others who are involved somehow with autistic children, and hear recommendations from professionals and meet children that have Autism, PDD, Asperger's Syndrome or any other forms of Austism Spectrum Disorder. 30 minutes. *$99.95*

Year Founded: 2005

706 Rylee's Gift - Asperger Syndrome
Program Development Associates
PO Box 2038
Syracuse, NY 13220-2038
315-452-0643
Fax: 315-452-0710
E-mail: info@disabilitytraining.com
www.disabilitytraining.com

Martha Rylee, Author

This video or DVD spotlights Rylee - through his mother, grandparents, doctor, teacher - and adults with Asperger's Syndrome. Balances views of difficult transitions and meltdown behaviors, with sensory therapy, socialization and the amazing capabilities of people with this syndrome/gift. 56 minutes. *$89.95*

707 Straight Talk About Autism with Parents and Kids
ADD WareHouse
300 NW 70th Avenue
Suite 102
Plantation, FL 33317-2360
954-792-8100
800-233-9273
Fax: 954-792-8545
E-mail: websales@addwarehouse.com
www.addwarehouse.com

Jeff Schultz, Author

These revealing videos contain intimate interviews with parents of kids with autism and the young people themselves. Topics discussed include friends and social isolation, communication difficulties, hypersensitivities, teasing, splinter skills, parent support groups and more. One video focuses on childhood issues, while the second covers adolescent issues. Two 40 minute videos. *$99.00*

Year Founded: 1990

708 Struggling with Life: Asperger's Syndrome
Program Development Associates
PO Box 2038
Syracuse, NY 13220-2038

315-452-0643
Fax: 315-452-0710
E-mail: info@disabilitytraining.com
www.disabilitytraining.com

ABC News correspondent Jay Schadler's report on the neurological disorder called Asperger's focuses on the telling line between intense interests and obsessions. The latter may be an early symptom of the syndrome. This closed caption video is grounded on studies by Fred Voklmar at Yale that explore compulsive fixations and unreadable facial expressions, both of which are typical of Asperger's and inhibit normal peer interactions among children. VHS or DVD. 14 minutes. *$ 69.95*

Web Sites

709 www.aane.org
Asperger's Association of New England
Working advocacy group of Massachusetts parents of adults and teens with AS who have come together with the goal of getting state funding for residential supports for adults with AS. At the present time no state agency will provide these needed supports. Interested parents and AS adults are welcome to join this working group.

710 www.ani.ac
Autism Network International
This organization is run by and for the autistic people. The best advocates for autistic people are autistic people themselves. Provides a forum for autistic people to share information, peer support, tips for coping and problem solving, as well as providing a social outlet for autistic people to explore and participate in autistic social experiences. In addition to promoting self advocacy for high-functioning autistic adults, ANI also works to improve the lives of autistic people who, whether they are too young or because they do not have the communication skills, are not able to advocate for themselves. Helps autistic people by providing information and referrals for parenting and teachers. Also strives to educate the public about autism.

711 www.aspennj.org
Asperger Syndrome Education Network (ASPEN)
Regionally-based non-profit organization headquarted in New Jersey, with 11 local chapters, providing families and those individuals affected with Asperger Syndrome, PDD-NOS, High Function Autism, and related disorders. Provides education about the issues surrounding Asperger Syndrome and other related disorders. Support in knowing that they are not alone and in helping individuals with AS achieve their maximum potential. Advocacy in areas of appropriate educational programs and placement, medical research funding, and increased public awareness and understanding.

712 www.aspergerinfo.com
Aspergers Resource Links
AspergerInfo.com offers a safe place to ask questions, share experiences, and discuss treatments relating to Asperger Syndrome.

713 www.aspergers.com
Aspergers Resource Links
Asperger's Disorder Homepage

714 www.aspergersyndrome.org
Aspergers Resource Links

Barbara Kirby, Founder

A collection of web resources on Asperger's Syndrome and related topics. Hosted by the University of Delaware.

715 www.aspiesforfreedom.com
Aspies for Freedom

Aspies for Freedom (AFF) is a web site with chat rooms, forums and information relating to Austism and Asperger's Syndrome.

716 www.autism-society.org
Autism Society of America

Promotes lifelong access and opportunities for persons within the autism spectrum and their families, to be fully included, participating members of their communities through advocacy, public awareness, education and research related to autism.

717 www.autism.org
Center for the Study of Autism (CSA)

Located in the Salem/Portland, Oregon area. Provides information about autism to parents and professionals, and conducts research on the efficacy of various therapeutic interventions. Much of our research is in collaboration with the Autism Research Institute in San Diego, California.

718 www.autismresearchinstitute.org
Autism Research Institute

Devoted to conducting research on the causes of autism and on the methods of preventing, diagnosing and treating autism and other severe behavioral disorders of childhood.

719 www.autismservicescenter.org
Autism Services Center

Makes available technical assistance in designing programs. Provides supervised apartments, group homes, respite services, independent living programs and job-coached employment.

720 www.autismspeaks.org
National Alliance for Autism Research (NAAR)

National nonprofit, tax-exempt organization dedicated to finding the causes, preventions, effective treatments and, ultimately, a cure for the autism spectrum disorders. NAAR's mission is to fund, promote and support biomedical research into autism. Aims to have an aggressive and far-reaching research program. Seeks to encourage scientists outside the field of autism to apply their insights and experience to autism. Publishes a newsletter that focuses on developments in autism research. Supports brain banks and tissue consortium development.

721 www.autisticservices.com
Autistic Services

Dedicated to serving the unique lifelong needs of autistic individuals.

722 www.cfsny.org
Center for Family Support (CFS)

Devoted to the physical well-being and development of the retarded child and the sound mental health of the parents.

723 www.csaac.org
Community Services for Autistic Adults & Children

Enables individuals to achieve their highest potential and contribute as confident members in their community, instead of living in institutions.

724 www.cyberpsych.org
CyberPsych

Hosts the American Psychoanalyists Foundation, American Association of Suicideology, Society for the Exploration of Psychotherapy Intergration, and Anxiety Disorders Association of America. Also subcategories of the anxiety disorders, as well as general information, including panic disorder, phobias, obsessive compulsive disorder (OCD), social phobia, generalized anxiety disorder, post traumatic stress disorder, and phobias of childhood. Book reviews and links to web pages sharing the topics.

725 www.feat.org
Families for Early Autism Treatment

A nonprofit organization of parents and professionals, designed to help families with children who are diagnosised with autism or pervasive developmental disorder. It offers a network of support for families. FEAT has a Lending Library, with information on autism and also offers Support Meetings on the third Wednesday of each month.

726 www.iidc.indiana.edu
Indiana Resource Center for Autism (IRCA)

Conducts outreach training and consultations, engage in research and develop and disseminate info on behalf of individuals across the autism spectrum.

727 www.ladders.org
The Autism Research Foundation

A nonprofit, tax-exempt organization dedicated to researching the neurological underpinnings of autism and other related developmental brain disorders. Seeking to rapidly expand and accelerate research into the pervasive developmental disorders. To do this, time and efforts goes into investigating the neuropathology of autism in their laboratories, collecting and redistributing brain tissue to promising research groups for use by projects approved by the Tissue Resource Committee, studies frozen autistic brain tissue collected by TARF. They believe that only aggressive scientific and medical research will reveal the cure for this lifelong disorder.

728 www.maapservices.org
MAAP Services

Provides information and advice to people with Asperger Syndrome, Autism and Pervasive Developmental Disorders. Provides parents and professionals a chance to network with others to learn more within the autism spectrum.

729 www.mentalhealth.Samhsa.Gov
Center for Mental Health Services Knowledge Exchange Network

Information about resources, technical assistance, research, training, networks and other federal clearinghouses and fact sheets and materials.

730 www.mhselfhelp.org
National Mental Health Consumer's Self-Help Clearinghouse

Encourages the development and growth of consumer self-help groups.

731 www.nami.org
National Alliance on Mental Illness

From its inception in 1979, NAMI has been dedicated to improving the lives of individuals and families affected by mental illness.

732 www.necc.org
New England Center for Children

Serves students diagnosed with autism, learning disabilities, language delays, mental retardation, behavior disorders and related disabilities.

733 www.planetpsych.com
Planetpsych.com

Learn about disorders, their treatments and other topics in psychology. Articles are listed under the related topic areas. Ask a therapist a question for free, or view the directory of professionals in your area. If you are a therapist sign up for the directory. Current features, self-help, interactive, and newsletter archives.

734 www.resourcesnyc.org
Resources for Children with Special Needs

Gives a general introduction on autism, educational approaches, available resources, supplementary services, definitions and other related services are included.

735 www.son-rise.org
Son-Rise Autism Treatment Center of America

Training center for autism professionals and parents of autistic children. Programs focus on the design and implementation of home-based/child-centered alternatives.

736 www.thenadd.org
NADD-National Association for the Dually Diagnosed

Promotes the interest of professional and parent development with resources for individuals who have the coexistence of mental illness and mental retardation.

737 www.wrongplanet.net
Wrong Planet

WrongPlanet.net is a web community designed for individuals with Asperger's Syndrome and other PDDs. They provide a forum where members can communicate with each other, may read or submit essays or how-to guides about various subjects, and a chatroom for communication with other Aspies.

Conferences & Meetings

738 **Asperger Syndrome Education Network (ASPEN) Conference**
9 Aspen Circle
Edison, NJ 08820-2832
732-321-0880
E-mail: info@aspennj.org
www.www.aspennj.org

Lori Shery, President
Rich Meleo, Vice President
Elizabeth Yamashita, Vice President
Ann Hiller, Secretary

Annual conference.

Directories & Databases

739 **After School and More**
Resources for Children with Special Needs
116 E 16th Street
5th Floor
New York, NY 10003-2164
212-677-4650
Fax: 212-254-4070
E-mail: info@resourcenyc.org
www.resourcesnyc.org

Rachel Howard, Executive Director
Stephen Stern, Director , Finance and Administr
Todd Dorman, Director, Communications and Out
Helen Murphy, Director, Program and Fund Devel

The most complete directory of after school programs for children with disabilities and special needs in the metropolitan New York area focusing on weekend and holiday programs. *$15.00*

252 pages ISBN 0-967836-57-3

Cognitive Disorders

Introduction

Cognitive disorders are a group of conditions characterized by impairments in the ability to think, reason, plan and organize. There are three types of cognitive disorders; delirium, dementia (of which Alzheimer's Disease is the most common) and amnestic disorder.

Delirium is a relatively short-term condition in which the level of conciousness waxes and wanes. It is common in patients after surgery or during illness, as with high fever. It resolves when the underlying problem resolves. There are three categories of causes of delirium: a general medical condition; substance-induced; and multiple causes. An amnestic disorder, in contrast to delirium or dementia, is a condition in which only memory is impaired; for instance the person is unable to recall important facts or events, making it difficult to function normally. Dementia is a chronic impairment of multiple cognitive functions. Persons with dementia may have severe memory loss and also be unable to plan or prepare for events or to care for themselves.

Dementia, Alzheimer's type, is a progressive disorder that slowly kills nerve cells in the brain. While definitive treatments are lacking, there is a prodigious amount of research on the condition, some of which suggests that a vaccine may be developed to prevent the condition. Though such hopeful breakthroughs remain distant, there is much that families and patients can do when the condition is recognized and care and support are sought early in the disorder's progression. Since other, serious, treatable disorders can resemble Alzeimer's Disease, it is very important for individuals who are losing cognitive functions to be evaluated by a physician. Early detection of Alzheimer's Disease, with early treatment, may improve the chances for slowing the rate of decline.

Here we will describe only Alzheimer's dementia, the most prevalent Cognitive Disorder.

SYMPTOMS

- Langugage disorders;
- Impaired ability to carry out motor activities despite intact motor function;
- Failure to recognize or identify objects despite intact sensory perception;
- Disturbance in executive functioning (planning, organizing, sequencing, abstracting);
- The deficits cause impairment in social or occupational functioning and represent a decline from previous level of functioning;
- The course is gradual and continuous;
- The deficits are not due to central nervous system conditions such as Parkinson's Disease, other conditions known to cause dementia, and are not substance-induced;
- The deficits do not occur during the course of delirium and are not better accounted for by severe depression or schizophrenia.

ASSOCIATED FEATURES

Dementia, Alzheimer's type, generally begins gradually, not with deficits in cognition but with a marked change in personality. For instance, a person may suddenly become given to fits of anger for no apparent reason.

Soon, however, family and acquaintances may notice that the individual begins to mix up facts, or gets lost driving to a familiar place. In the early stages the afflicted individual may become aware of slipping cognitive functions, adding to confusion, fright and depression. After a period, lapses in memory grow more obvious; patients with Alzheimer's are apt to repeat themselves, and may forget the names of grandchildren or longtime friends. They may also be increasingly agitated and combative when family members or other caretakers try to correct them or help with accustomed tasks. The memory lapses in patients with Alzheimer's differ markedly from those in normal aging: a patient with Alzheimer's may often forget entire experiences and rarely remembers them later; the patient only grudgingly acknowledges lapses. In contrast, the individual with normal aging or depression is extremely concerned about, and may even exaggerate, the extent of memory loss. In Alzheimer's, skills deteriorate and a patient is increasingly unable to follow directions, or care for him/herself. Eventually the disease leads to death.

PREVALENCE

An estimated two percent to four percent of the population over age 65 has dementia, Alzheimer's type. Other types of dementia are believed to be much less common. Prevalance of the condition increases with age, particularly after age 75; in persons over 85, an estimated twenty percent have dementia, Alzheimer's type.

TREATMENT OPTIONS

There is no known cure or definitive treatment for dementia, Alzheimer's type. However, research has suggested avenues that involve drugs, such as THA, Donepezil, and Rivastigmine, for regulating acetylcholine, seratonin or norepinephrine in the brain. According to the American Psychiatric Association, some progress has been seen in slowing the death rate among nerve cells using a chemical known as Alcar (acetyl-l-carnitine). Psychiatrists treating patients with dementia, Alzheimer's type, may also be able to prescribe medications that can treat the depression and anxiety that accompanies the condition. And families are strongly encouraged to take advantage of adjunctive services including support groups, counseling and psychotherapy. There is a high incidence of depression among family members caring at home for persons with Alzheimer's Disease.

Associations & Agencies

741 Alzheimer's Association National Office
225 Noth Michigan Avenue
17th Floor
Chicago, IL 60601-7633
312-335-8700
800-272-3900
Fax: 866-699-1246
TDD: 312-335-5886
E-mail: info@alz.org
www.www.alz.org

Gerald Sampson, Chairman
Harry Johns, President and CEO
Richard Hovland, Chief Operations Officer
Angela Gieger, Chief Strategy Officer

Headquarters for the nation's leading organization for all those suffering with alzheimer's disease and their families and support network. Offers referrals, support groups, workshops, training seminars, publications.

Year Founded: 1980

742 Alzheimer's Disease Education and Referral Center
31 Center Drive, MSC 2292
Building 31, Room 5C27
Bethesda, MD 20892
301-495-3311
800-438-4380
Fax: 301-495-3334
TTY: 800-222-4225
E-mail: adear@nia.nih.gov
www.www.nia.nih.gov/alzheimers

Richard J Hodes MD, Director
Patrick Shirdon, Director of Management
Luigi Ferrucci, MD, PhD, Scietific Director
Marie A Bernard MD, Deputy Director

The ADEAR Center provides information about Alzheimer's Disease and related disorders to health professionals, patients and their families, and the public.

Year Founded: 1974

743 Brain Resources and Information Network (BRAIN)
NIH Neurological Institute
PO Box 5801
Bethesda, MD 20824-5801
301-496-5751
800-352-9424
Fax: 301-402-2186
TTY: 301-468-5981
E-mail: braininfo@ninds.nih.gov
www.ninds.nih.gov

Denise Dorsey, Chief Administrative Officer
Peter Soltys, Chief Information Officer
Story C Landis, PhD, Director
Marian Emr, Director, Office of Communication

Federal agency that supports research nationwide on disorders of the brain and nervous system. Website has updated neuroscience news and articles.

Year Founded: 1950

744 BrightFocus Foundation
22512 Gateway Center Drive
Clarksburg, MD 20871-2005
301-948-3244
800-437-2423
Fax: 301-258-9454
E-mail: info@brightfocus.org
www.www.brightfocus.org

Grace Frisone, Chairman
Stacy Pagos Haller, President and CEO
Michael H Barnett, Esq, Vice Chairman
Nicholas W Raymond, Treasurer

Provides information on treatment, symptoms risk factors and healthy exercises.

Year Founded: 1973

745 Caregiver Action Network
2000 M Street
Suite 400
Washington, DC 20036

202-772-5050
800-896-3650
E-mail: info@caregiveraction.org
www.www.caregiveraction.org

Jon Shanfield, Chair
John Schall, Chief Executive Officer
Lisa Winstel, Chief Operating Officer
Elizabeth Pearson, Treasurer and Secretary

Acts as a support and an advocate for family caregivers.

Year Founded: 1993

746 Center for Mental Health Services (CMHS)
1 Choke Cherry Road
Room 6-1057
Rockville, MD 20857
240-276-1310
877-726-4727
Fax: 240-276-1320
TDD: 800-487-4889
E-mail: info@mentalhealth.org
www.beta.samhsa.gov/about-us/who-we-are/offices-center

Michael E Etzinger, B.S.M.E, , M.B., SAMHSA Executive Officer, Director
Paolo Del Vecchio, M.S.W, Director, Center for Mental Healt
Deborah Baldwin, M.P.A, Acting Director, Consumer Affairs
Elizabeth Lopez, Ph.D, Acting Deputy Director

CMHS leads Federal efforts to treat mental illnesses by promoting mental health and by preventing the development or worsening of mental illness when possible. Congress created CMHS to bring new hope to adults who have serious mental illnesses and to children with serious emotional disorders. CMHS provides information about mental health via a toll-free the web site, and more than 600 publications. Developed for users of mental health services and their families, the general public, policy makers, providers, and the media.

Year Founded: 1992

747 Federation of Associations in Behavioral and Brain Sciences
750 First Street NorthEast
Suite 905
Washington, DC 20002
202-336-5920
Fax: 202-336-6183
E-mail: info@fabbs.org
www.www.fabbs.org

Susan T Fiske, PhD, President
Christine L Cameron, PhD, Executive Director
J Bruce Overmier, Treasurer
Victoria N Luine, PhD, Secretary

FABBS is a coalition to scietific societies that share an interest in advancing the sciences of mind, brain, and behavior. Understanding the human element of many of society's challenges in healthcare, conservation behavior, human conflicts, economic decision making and more is a key component to improving the welfare of individuals and our society.

Year Founded: 1980

748 National Association Councils on Developmental Disabilities
1825 K Street, North West
Suite 600
Washington, DC 20006
202-506-5813
800-950-6264
Fax: 703-524-9094
E-mail: info@nacdd.org
www.nacdd.org

Mathew McCollough, Treasurer and Chair, DC Council
Marshall Jones, Office Manager
Peggy Hathaway, Public Policy Manager
Sheryl Matney, Sr Manager, Counsel Services

A national membership organization representing the 55 State and Territorial Councils on Developmental Disabilities. An organization with the purpose of promoting and enhancing the outcomes of our member councils in developing and sustaining inclusive communities and self directed services and supports for individuals with developmental disabilities.

749 National Association for the Dually Diagnosed (NADD)
132 Fair Street
Kingston, NY 12401-4802
845-331-4336
800-331-5362
Fax: 845-331-4569
E-mail: info@thenadd.org
www.thenadd.org

Donna McNELIS, PhD, President
Robert J Fletcher DSW, Chief Executive Officer
Dan Baker, PhD, Vice President
Julia Pearce, Secretary

Nonprofit organization designed to promote interest of professional and parent development with resources for individuals who have the coexistence of mental illness and mental retardation. Provides conferences, educational services and training materials to professionals, parents, concerned citizens and service organizations.

Year Founded: 1983

750 National Mental Health Consumers' Self-Help Clearinghouse
1211 Chestnut Street
Suite 1100
Philadelphia, PA 19107-4103
215-751-1810
800-553-4539
Fax: 215-636-6312
E-mail: info@mhselfhelp.org
www.mhselfhelp.org

Joseph Rogers, Executive Director/ Founder
Susan Rogers, Director
Britani Nestel, Program Specialist
Christa Burkett, Technical Assistance Coordinator

A national consumer technical assistance center that has played a major role in the development of the mental health consumer movement.

Year Founded: 1986

751 National Niemann-Pick Disease Foundation
401 Madison Avenue
PO Box 49, Suite B
Fort Atkinson, WI 53538-49
920-563-0930
877-287-3672
Fax: 920-563-0931
E-mail: nnpdf@nnpdf.org
www.nnpdf.org

Leslie Hughes, NNPDF Board Chair
Lisa Chavez, Vice Chair
Nadine Hill, NNPDF Executive Director
Jill Flinton, Treasurer, Executive Committee

Offers support and funding for individuals with cognitive disorders and their support network.

Year Founded: 1992

752 SAMHSA's National Mental Health Information Center
1 Choke Cherry Road
Room 6-1057
Rockville, MD 20857
240-276-1310
800-789-2647
Fax: 240-221-4295
TDD: 866-889-2647
www.mentalhealth.smahsa.gov

Anna Marsh, PhD, Deputy Director

753 The Center for Family Support
2811 Zulette Avenue
Bronx, NY 10461
718-518-1500
Fax: 718-518-8200
www.cfsny.org

Steven Vernikoff, Executive Director
Virgil Seepersad, Director of Finance
Eileen Berg, Director of Quality Assurance
Barbara Greenwald, Associate Executive, Director

Service agency devoted to the physical well-being and development of the retarded child and the sound mental health of the parents. Helps families with retarded children with all aspects of home care including counseling, referrals, home aide service and consultation. Offers intervention for parents at the birth of a retarded child with in-home support, guidance and infant stimulation. Pioneered training of nonprofessional women as home aides to provide supportive services in homes.

Year Founded: 1954

Books

754 Agitation in Patients with Dementia: a Practical Guide to Diagnosis and Management
American Psychiatric Publishing, Inc.
1000 Wilson Boulevard
Suite 1825
Arlington, VA 22209-3901
703-907-7322
800-368-5777
Fax: 703-907-1091
E-mail: appi@psych.org
www.appi.org

George T Grossberg, M.D, Editor
Donald P Hay, M.D, Editor

Linda K Hay, R.N., Ph.D, Editor
John S Kennedy, M.D., F.R.C.P, Editor

Appealing to a wide audience of geriatric psychiatrists, primary care physicians and internists, general practitioners, nurses, social workers, psychologists, pharmacists and mental health care workers and practitioners in hospitals, nursing homes and clinics, this remarkable monograph offers practical direction on assessing and managing agitation in patients with dementia. *$57.00*

272 pages Year Founded: 2003 ISBN 0-880488-43-3

755 Alzheimer's Disease Sourcebook
Omnigraphics
155 West Congress
Suite 200
Detroit, MI 48226
313-961-1340
800-234-1340
Fax: 313-961-1383
E-mail: contact@omnigraphics.com
www.omnigraphics.com

Amy L. Sutton, Author

Omnigraphics is the publisher of the Health Reference Series, a growing consumer health information resource with more than 100 volumes in print. Each title in the series features an easy to understand format, nontechnical language, comprehensive indexing and resources for further information. Material in each book has been collected from a wide range of government agencies, professional associations, periodicals, and other sources. *$95.00*

637 pages Year Founded: 1985 ISBN 0-780811-50-8

756 Alzheimer's Disease: Activity-Focused Care, Second Edition
Therapeutic Resources
PO Box 16814
Cleveland, OH 44116-814
440-331-7114
888-331-7114
Fax: 440-331-7118
E-mail: contactus@therapeuticresources.com
www.therapeuticresources.com

Carly R. Hellen, OTR/L, Author

Provides practical and innovative strategies for care of people with Alzheimer's disease, emphasizing the activities that make up daily living - dressing, toileting, eating, exercising, and communication. The text is written from the viewpoint that activity-focused care promotes the resident's cognitive, physical, psychosocial, and spiritual well-being. *$559.95*

536 pages ISBN 0-750699-08-6

757 American Psychiatric Association Practice Guideline for the Treatment of Patients with Delirium
American Psychiatric Publishing, Inc.
1000 Wilson Boulevard
Suite 1825
Arlington, VA 22209-3901
703-907-7322
800-368-5777
Fax: 703-907-1091
E-mail: appi@psych.org
www.appi.org

Robert E Hales MD, Editor-in-Chief
Ron McMillen, Chief Executive Officer
John McDuffie, Editorial Director
Rebecca Rinehart, Publisher

Best practices examined from the group whose vision is a society that has available, accessible quality psychiatric diagnosis and treatment. *$47.95*

75 pages Year Founded: 1999 ISBN 0-890423-13-4

758 Behavioral Complications in Alzheimer's Disease
American Psychiatric Publishing, Inc.
1000 Wilson Boulevard
Suite 1825
Arlington, VA 22209-3901
703-907-7322
800-368-5777
Fax: 703-907-1091
E-mail: appi@psych.org
www.appi.org

Brian A. Lawlor, MD, Author

Practical management strategies for the identification, measurement and treatment of behavioral symptoms in patient with Alzheimer's disease. *$67.00*

303 pages Year Founded: 1995 ISBN 0-880484-77-0

759 Care That Works: A Relationship Approach to Persons with Dementia
Johns Hopkins University Press
2715 N Charles Street
Baltimore, MD 21218-4319
410-516-6900
800-537-5487
Fax: 410-516-6998

Jitka M. Zgola, Author

Provides caregivers the information with which they can develop their own approaches, evaluate their effectiveness, and continue to grow in skill and insight. Real life strategies for a challenging task. *$24.00*

272 pages Year Founded: 1999 ISBN 0-801860-25-6

760 Cognitive Therapy in Practice
WW Norton & Company
500 5th Avenue
New York, NY 10110-54
212-354-2907
800-233-4830
Fax: 212-869-0856
E-mail: npd@wwnorton.com

Jacqueline Persons, Author

Basic text for graduate studies in psychotherapy, psycholgy nursing social work and counseling. *$29.00*

256 pages Year Founded: 1989 ISBN 0-393700-77-0

761 Dementia: A Clinical Approach
Elsevier Health Sciences
11830 Westline Industrial Drive
St. Louis, MO 63146-3313
314-872-8370
800-568-5136
Fax: 314-432-1380
E-mail: orders@bhusa.com or custserv@bhusa.com
www.elsevier.com

Jeffrey L. Cummings, Author
Jeffrey L Cummings, Author

Third Edition, this is both a scholarly review of the dementias and a practical guide to their diagnosis and treatment. *$ 99.00*

432 pages Year Founded: 2003 ISBN 0-750674-70-9

762 Disorders of Brain and Mind: Volume 1
Cambridge University Press
32 Avenue of the Americas
New York, NY 10013-2473
212-337-5000
Fax: 212-691-3239
E-mail: newyork@cambrigde.org
www.www.cambridge.org

Maria A. Ron, Author
Anthony S. David, Author

Discusses various neuropsychiatry topics where the brain and mind come together. *$113.00*

388 pages Year Founded: 1534 ISBN 0-521778-51-0

763 Drug Therapy and Cognitive Disorders
Mason Crest Publishers
450 Parkway Drive
Suite D
Broomall, PA 19008-4017
610-543-6200
866-627-2665
Fax: 610-543-3878
E-mail: dtaylor@masoncrest.com
www.masoncrest.com

Sherry Bonice, Author
Carolyn Hoard, Author
Michelle Luke, Director, Marketing, PR
Michael Toglia, Special Sales

Alzheimer's disease is one of the most common cognitive disorder, one that affects millions of people. Patients, caregivers and loved ones all suffer as they experience the devastation of this often misunderstood disease. Researchers are working hard to find a cure for the symptoms of Alzheimer's and other cognitive disorders, and this book describes the most recent research. Coauthored by someone who has experienced the early stages of Alzheimer's firsthand, this volume will give readers a new understanding and appreciation of the treatment options for those who experience a cognitive disorder.

128 pages ISBN 1-590845-62-5

764 Progress in Alzheimer's Disease and Similar Conditions
American Psychiatric Publishing, Inc.
1000 Wilson Boulevard
Suite 1825
Arlington, VA 22209-3901
703-907-7322
800-368-5777
Fax: 703-907-1091
E-mail: appi@psych.org
www.appi.org

Leonard L Heston, M.D., Editor
Ron McMillen, Chief Executive Officer
John McDuffie, Editorial Director

Details advances in research on human genetics that is broadening our knowledge of Alzheimer's disease and other related afflictions. Describes disease mechanisms, in-

cluding prisons, that provide insight into the role environment plays in the development of disease. Includes stories about the pain inflicted by this disease on the patients and their family and friends as well as current efforts in management and treatment. *$77.00*

318 pages Year Founded: 1997 ISBN 0-880487-60-7

765 Treating Complex Cases: The Cognitive Behavioral Therapy Approach
John Wiley & Sons
111 River Street
Hoboken, NJ 07030-5774
201-748-6000
Fax: 201-748-6088
E-mail: info@wiley.com
www.wiley.com

Nicholas Tarrier, Author
Adrian Wells, Author
Gillian Haddock, Author

This book brings together some of the most experiences and expert cognitive behavioral therapists to share their specialist experience of formulation and treatment of complex problems such as co-morbidity, psychotic conditions, and chronic conditions. The experienced clinician will find: evidence-based approaches to assessment and formulation of complex cases; a wide range of problems not restricted to disorder categories, including anger, low self-esteem, abuse and shame; a concern with the realities of clinical practice which involves complex cases that do not fit into simple case conceptualisations or diagnostic categories. Copyright 2000. *$89.95*

458 pages Year Founded: 2000 ISBN 0-471978-39-8

766 Victims of Dementia: Service, Support, and Care
Haworth Press
10 Alice Street
Binghamton, NY 13904-1503
607-722-5857
800-429-6784
Fax: 607-721-0012
E-mail: getinfo@haworthpressinc.com
www.haworthpress.com

William Michael Clemmer, PhD, Editor

Provides an in depth look at the concept, construction and operation of Wesley Hall, a special living area at the Chelsea United Methodist retirement home in Michigan. *$27.95*

161 pages Year Founded: 1993 ISSN 978156024-265-9

Periodicals & Pamphlets

767 Alzheimer's Disease Research and the American Health Assistance Foundation
American Health Assistance Foundation
22512 Gateway Center Drive
Clarksburg, MD 20871-2005
301-948-3244
800-437-2423
Fax: 301-258-9454
E-mail: info@brightfocus.org
www.www.brightfocus.org

Grace Frisone, Chairman
Stacy Pagos Haller, President and CEO

Michael H Barnett, Esq, Vice Chairman
Nicholas W Raymond, Treasurer

Provides information on treatment, medication, medical referrals.

Video & Audio

768 A Change of Character
Fanlight Productions
32 Court Street
21st Floor
Brooklyn, NY 11201
718-488-8900
800-876-1710
Fax: 718-488-8642
E-mail: fanlight@fanlight.com
www.fanlight.com

Neal Goodman, Author

Truett Allen's personality changed drastically after a series of strokes resulted in damage to the frontal lobes of his brain. this captivating video features neuroscientist Dr. Elkhonon Goldberg, author of The Executive Brain, as well as neurologist and best-selling author Dr. Oliver Sacks.

769 Effective Learning Systems
5108 W 74th
St #390160
Minneapolis, MN 55439
239-948-1660
800-966-0443
Fax: 239-948-1664
E-mail: info@efflearn.com
www.effectivelearning.com

Robert E Griswold, President
Deirdre M Griswold, VP

Audio tapes for stress management, deep relaxation, anger control, peace of mind, insomnia, weight and smoking, self-image and self-esteem, positive thinking, health and healing. Since 1972, Effective Learning Systems has helped millions of people take charge of their lives and make positive changes. Over 75 titles available, each with a money-back guarantee. Price range $12-$14.

Year Founded: 1972

770 Understanding Mental Illness
Educational Video Network
1401 19th Street
Huntsville, TX 77340
936-295-5767
800-762-0060
Fax: 936-294-0233
E-mail: info at evn.org
www.www.evndirect.com

A video to learn and understand mental illness and how it affects you. *$79.95*

Year Founded: 2004 ISBN 1-589501-48-9

Web Sites

771 www.Nia.Nih.Gov/Alzheimers
Alzheimer's Disease Education and Referral
Fax: 301-495-3334

A division of the National Institute on Aging of the National Institute of Health. Solid information and a list of federally funded centers for evaluation, referral, treatment.

772 www.aan.com
American Academy of Neurology

Provides information for both professionals and the public on neurology subjects, covering Alzheimer's and Parkinson's diseases to stroke and migraine, includes comprehensive fact sheets.

773 www.agelessdesign.com
Ageless Design

Information on age related diseases such as Alzheimer's disease.

774 www.ahaf.org/alzdis/about/adabout.htm
American Health Assistance Foundation

Alzheimer's resource for patients and caregivers.

775 www.alz.co.uk
Alzheimer's Disease International

Umbrella organization of associations that support people with dementia.

776 www.alzforum.org
Alzheimer Research Forum

Information in layman's terms, plus many references and resources listed.

777 www.alzheimersbooks.com/
Alzheimer's Disease Bookstore

778 www.alzheimersupport.Com
AlzheimerSupport.com

Information and products for people dealing with Alzheimer's Disease.

779 www.biostat.wustl.edu
Washington University - Saint Louis

Page on Alzheimer's information, from basic care to friends and family networking experiences for support.

780 www.cyberpsych.org
CyberPsych

Hosts the American Psychoanalyists Foundation, American Association of Suicideology, Society for the Exploration of Psychotherapy Intergration, and Anxiety Disorders Association of America. Also subcategories of the anxiety disorders, as well as general information, including panic disorder, phobias, obsessive compulsive disorder (OCD), social phobia, generalized anxiety disorder, post traumatic stress disorder, and phobias of childhood. Book reviews and links to web pages sharing the topics.

781 www.mayohealth.org/mayo/common/htm/
MayoClinic.com

Information for dealing with Alzheimer's Disease.

782 www.mentalhealth.com
Internet Mental Health

On-line information and a virtual encyclopedia related to mental disorders, possible causes and treatments. News, articles, on-line diagnostic programs and related links. Designed to improve understanding, diagnosis and treatment of mental illness throughout the world. Awarded the Top Site Award and the NetPsych Cutting Edge Site Award.

783 www.mentalhealth.smahsa.gov
SMAHSA'S National Mental Health Information Center

US Department of Health and Human Services website with current Alzheimer's information.

784 www.mindstreet.com/training.html
Cognitive Therapy: A Multimedia Learning Program

The basics of cognitive therapy are presented.

785 www.ninds.nih.gov
National Institute of Neurological Disorders & Stroke

Neuroscience updates and articles.

786 www.noah-health.org/en/bns/disorders/ alzheimer.html
Ask NOAH About: Aging and Alzheimer's Disease

Links to brochures on medical problems of the elderly.

787 www.ohioalzcenter.org/facts.html
University Memory and Aging Center

Alzheimer's disease fact page.

788 www.planetpsych.com
Planetpsych.com

Learn about disorders, their treatments and other topics in psychology. Articles are listed under the related topic areas. Ask a therapist a question for free, or view the directory of professionals in your area. If you are a therapist sign up for the directory. Current features, self-help, interactive, and newsletter archives.

789 www.psych.org/clin_res/pg_dementia.cfm
American Psychiatric Association

Practice guidelines for the treatment of patients with Alzheimer's.

790 www.psychcentral.com
Psych Central

Personalized one-stop index for psychology, support, and mental health issues, resources, and people on the Internet.

791 www.rcpsych.ac.uk/info/help/memory
Royal College of Psychiatrists

Memory and Dementia

792 www.zarcrom.com/users/alzheimers
Alzheimer's Outreach

Detailed and practical information.

793 www.zarcrom.com/users/yeartorem
Year to Remember

A memorial site covering many aspects of Alzheimer's disease.

Conduct Disorder

Introduction

Conduct disorder is characterized by a repetitive and persistent pattern of behavior in which societal norms and the basic rights of others are violated. These behaviors can include physical harm to people or animals, damage to property, deceitfulness or theft, and extreme violations of rules. It is important to note that troublesome behavior can also result from adverse circumstances; the circumstances need to be fully investigated, and attempts to rectify adversity made, before Conduct Disorder is diagnosed. The diagnosis can be divided into two types, depending on the age of diagnosis: childhood-onset type and adolescent-onset type.

SYMPTOMS

• Aggression to people and animals, including bullying, picking fights, using weapons, physical cruelty to people and animals, stealing or forcing someone into sexual activity;
• Destruction of property;
• Deceitfulness or theft, including breaking into someone's house, lying to obtain goods or favors, or shoplifting;
• Violations of rules, including staying out past curfews, running away from home, and truancy from school.

ASSOCIATED FEATURES

Conduct disorder is often associated with early onset of sexual activity, drinking and smoking. The disorder leads to school disruption, problems with the police, sexually transmitted diseases, unplanned pregnancy, and injury from accidents and fights. Suicide and suicidal attempts are more common among adolescents with Conduct Disorder, probably both because they have a history of abuse and neglect and because their behavior results in adverse consequences. Individuals with Conduct Disorder appear to have little remorse for their acts, though they may learn that expressing guilt can diminish punishment; and they often show little or no empathy for the feelings, wishes, and well-being of others.

PREVALENCE

Prevalence of Conduct Disorder appears to have increased in recent years. For males under 18 years of age, rates range from six percent to sixteen percent; for females, rates range from two percent to nine percent.

TREATMENT OPTIONS

There is no agreement on the best way to treat conduct disorder, and approaves range from incarceration and 'tough love,' to individual and family psychotherapy. This condition is stressful for family members of the affected child or adolescent; it is crucial that they are supported and involved in the treatment.

Associations & Agencies

795 American Association of Children's Residential Centers
11700 West Lake Park Drive
Milwaukee, WI 53224
877-332-2272
E-mail: info@aacrc-dc.org
www.www.aacrc-dc.org

Christopher Bellonci, MD, President
Kari Sisson, National Director
Laurah Currey, Treasurer
Mary Hollie, Secretary

The American Association of Children's Residential Centers brings professionals together to advance the frontiers of knowledge pertaining to the spectrum of therapeutic living environments for children and adolescents with behavioral conduct disorders.

796 Association for Behavioral and Cognitive Therapies
305 Seventh Avenue
16th Floor
New York, NY 10001-6008
212-647-1890
Fax: 212-647-1865
E-mail: info@abct.org
www.www.abct.org/home

Dean McKay, PhD, President
Mary Jane Eimer, Executive Director
Karen Schmaling, PhD, Secretary-Treasurer
David Teisler, Director Of Communications

Membership listing of mental health professionals focusing in behavior therapy.

Year Founded: 1996

797 Career Assessment & Planning Services
Goodwill Industries
10596 Gandy Boulevard
St. Petersburg, FL 33702
727-523-1512
800-466-3945
Fax: 727-563-9300
E-mail: gw.marketing@goodwill-suncoast.com
www.goodwill-suncoast.org

Oscar J Horton, Chairman
R. Lee Waits, President and CEO Emeritus
Deborah A. Passerini, President, Board Officer
Martin W Gladysz, Senior Vice Chairman

Provides a comprehensive assessment, which can predict current and future employment and potential adjustment factors for physically, emotionally, or developmentally disabled persons who may be unemployed or underemployed. Assessments evaluate interests, aptitudes, academic achievements, and physical abilities (including dexterity and coordination) through coordinated testing, interviewing and behavioral observations.

Year Founded: 1954

798 Mental Health America
2000 North Beauregard Street
6th Floor
Alexandria, VA 22311
703-684-7722
800-969-6642
Fax: 703-684-5968
E-mail: info@mentalhealthamerica.net
www.mentalhealthamerica.net

Ann Boughtin, Chair
David Shern PhD, Interim President and CEO
Dianne Felton, Chief Operating Officer
Mike Turner, Vice President of Development

MHA. the leading advocacy organization addressing the full spectrum of mental conditions nationwide, works to inform, advocate, and enable access to quality behavioral health services fo all Americans. MHA's actions inform, support, and enable mental wellness and the recovery of conditions such as Conduct Disorders.

799 National Association for the Dually Diagnosed (NADD)
132 Fair Street
Kingston, NY 12401-4802
845-331-4336
800-331-5362
Fax: 845-331-4569
E-mail: info@thenadd.org
www.thenadd.org

Donna McNELIS, PhD, President
Robert J Fletcher DSW, Chief Executive Officer
Dan Baker, PhD, Vice President
Julia Pearce, Secretary

Nonprofit organization designed to promote interest of professional and parent development with resources for individuals who have the coexistence of mental illness and mental retardation. Provides conferences, educational services and training materials to professionals, parents, concerned citizens and service organizations.

Year Founded: 1983

800 National Dissemination Center
1825 Conneticut Ave NW
Suite 700
Washington, DC 20009
800-695-0285
TTY: 202-884-8200
E-mail: nichcy@fhi360.org
www.www.nichcy.org

NICHCY is the center that provides information to the nation on: disabilities in children and youth; programs for childeren and infants with disabilities; and research based information on effective practices for children with disabilities.

801 National Mental Health Consumers' Self-Help Clearinghouse
1211 Chestnut Street
Suite 1100
Philadelphia, PA 19107-4103
215-751-1810
800-553-4539
Fax: 215-636-6312
E-mail: info@mhselfhelp.org
www.mhselfhelp.org

Joseph Rogers, Executive Director/ Founder
Susan Rogers, Director
Britani Nestel, Program Specialist
Christa Burkett, Technical Assistance Coordinator

A national consumer technical assistance center that has played a major role in the development of the mental health consumer movement.

Year Founded: 1986

802 The Balanced Mind Foundation
730 N. Franklin Street
Suite 501
Chicago, IL 60654
312-642-0049
E-mail: info@thebalancedmind.org
www.www.thebalancedmind.org/

Paula Giovacchini, Director, Development
Nanci Schiman, Programs Manager
Shira Raider, Communications Manager
Lolli Ross, Family Response Team

The Balanced Mind guides families raising children with conduct disorders to answers, support, and stability they seek.

803 The Center for Family Support
2811 Zulette Avenue
Bronx, NY 10461
718-518-1500
Fax: 718-518-8200
www.cfsny.org

Steven Vernikoff, Executive Director
Virgil Seepersad, Director of Finance
Eileen Berg, Director of Quality Assurance
Barbara Greenwald, Associate Executive, Director

Service agency devoted to the physical well-being and development of the retarded child and the sound mental health of the parents. Helps families with retarded children with all aspects of home care including counseling, referrals, home aide service and consultation. Offers intervention for parents at the birth of a retarded child with in-home support, guidance and infant stimulation. Pioneered training of nonprofessional women as home aides to provide supportive services in homes.

Year Founded: 1954

Books

804 Antisocial Behavior by Young People
Cambridge University Press
32 Avenue of the Americas
New York, NY 10013-2473
212-337-5000
Fax: 212-691-3239
E-mail: newyork@cambrigde.org
www.www.cambridge.org

Michael Rutter, Author
Henri Giller, Author
Ann Hagell, Author

Written by a child psychiatrist, a criminologist and a social psychologist, this book is a major international review of research evidence on anti-social behavior. Covers all aspects of the field, including descriptions of different types of delinquency and time trends, the state of knowledge on the individuals, social-psychological and cultural factors involved and recent advances in prevention and intervention. *$53.00*

492 pages Year Founded: 1534 ISBN 0-521646-08-6

805 Bad Men Do What Good Men Dream: a Forensic Psychiatrist Illuminates the Darker Side of Human Behavior
American Psychiatric Publishing, Inc.
1000 Wilson Boulevard
Suite 1825
Arlington, VA 22209-3901
703-907-7322
800-368-5777
Fax: 703-907-1091
E-mail: appi@psych.org
www.appi.org

Robert I Simon, MD, Author

Provides insights into the minds of rapists, stalkers, serial killers, psychopaths, professional exploiters, and other individuals whose behavior both frightens and fascinates us. *$53.00*

339 pages Year Founded: 2008 ISBN 1-585622-94-8

806 Conduct Disorders in Childhood and Adolescence, Developmental Clinical Psychology and Psychiatry
Sage Publications
2455 Teller Road
Thousand Oaks, CA 91320-2234
805-499-0721
800-818-7243
Fax: 800-583-2665
E-mail: info@sagepub.com
www.sagepub.com

Alan E. Kazdin, Author

Conduct disorder is a clinical problem among children and adolescents that includes aggressive acts, theft, vandalism, firesetting, running away, truancy, defying authority and other antisocial behaviors. This book describes the nature of conduct disorder and what is currently known from research and clinical work. Topics include psychiatric diagnosis, parent psychopathology and child-rearing processes. Paperback also available. *$71.00*

191 pages Year Founded: 1995 ISBN 0-803971-81-8

807 Difficult Child
Bantam Doubleday Dell Publishing
1745 Broadway
New York, NY 10019-4343
212-782-9000
E-mail: ecustomerservice@randomhouse.com
www.randomhouse.com

Stanley Turecki, MD, Author
Leslie Tonner, Author

Help for parents dealing with behavioral problems. *$ 17.00*

320 pages Year Founded: 2000 ISBN 0-553380-36-2

808 Dysinhibition Syndrome How to Handle Anger and Rage in Your Child or Spouse
Hope Press
PO Box 188
Duarte, CA 91009-188
818-303-0644
800-321-4039
Fax: 626-358-3520
E-mail: dcomings@earthlink.net
www.hopepress.com

Rose Wood, Author

How to understand and handle rage and anger in your children or spouse. The book presents behavioral approaches that can be very effective and an understanding that can be family saving. *$18.96*

271 pages Year Founded: 1999 ISBN 1-878267-08-6

809 Helping Parents, Youth, and Teachers Understand Medications for Behavioral and Emotional Problems
American Psychiatric Publishing, Inc.
1000 Wilson Boulevard
Suite 1825
Arlington, VA 22209-3901
703-907-7322
800-368-5777
Fax: 703-907-1091
E-mail: appi@psych.org
www.appi.org

Mina K. Dulcan, MD, Editor

Resource Book of Medication Information Handouts, Second Edition. Valuable resource for anyone involved in evaluating psychiatric disturbances in children and adolescents. Provides a compilation of information sheets to help promote the dialogue between the patient's family, caregivers and the treating physician. *$101.00*

759 pages Year Founded: 2007 ISBN 1-585622-53-5

810 Preventing Antisocial Behavior Interventions from Birth through Adolescence
Guilford Press
72 Spring Street
New York, NY 10012-4068
212-431-9800
800-365-7006
Fax: 212-966-6708
E-mail: info@guilford.com

Bob Matloff, President
Seymour Weingarten, Editor-in-Chief

Establishes the crucial link between theory, measurement, and intervention. Brings together a collection of studies that utilize experimental approaches for evaluating intervention programs for preventing deviant behavior. Demonstrates both the feasibility and necessity of independent evaluation. Also shows how the information obtained in such studies can be used to test and refine prevailing theories about human behavior in general and behavior changes in particular. *$55.00*

391 pages Year Founded: 1992 ISBN 0-898628-82-2

811 Skills Training for Children with Behavior Disorders
Courage to Change
PO Box 486
Wilkes-Barre, PA 18703-486
800-440-4003
Fax: 800-772-6499
E-mail: customerservice@guidance-group.com
www.couragetochange.com

Michael L. Boomquist, Author

Written for both parents and therapists, this book provides backround, instructions, and many reproducible worksheets. Academic success, anger management, emotional well being and compliance/following rules are covered. *$36.00*

242 pages Year Founded: 1996 ISBN 1-572300-80-9

Periodicals & Pamphlets

812 Conduct Disorder in Children and Adolescents
PO Box 42557
Washington, DC 20015-557
800-789-2647
Fax: 240-747-5470
TDD: 866-889-2647
E-mail: ken@mentalhealth.org
www.mentalhealth.samhsa.gov

G Pirooz Shovelar, Editor
Edward B Searle, Deputy Director
414 pages

813 Mental, Emotional, and Behavior Disorders in Children and Adolescents
SAMHSA'S National Mental Health Information Center
PO Box 42557
Washington, DC 20015-557
800-789-2647
Fax: 240-747-5470
TDD: 866-889-2647
E-mail: ken@mentalhealth.org
www.mentalhealth.samhsa.gov

A Kathryn Power, MEd, Director
Edward B Searle, Deputy Director

This fact sheet describes mental, emotional, and behavioral problems that can occur during childhood and adolescence and discusses related treatment, support services, and research.

4 pages

814 Treatment of Children with Mental Disorders
National Institute of Mental Health
6001 Executive Boulevard
Room 8184, MSC 9663
Bethesda, MD 20892-9663
301-443-4513
866-615-6464
TTY: 301-443-8431
E-mail: nimhinfo@nih.gov
www.www.nimh.nih.gov/

Francis S Collins, MD, PhD

A short booklet that contains questions and answers about therapy for children with mental disorders. Includes a chart of mental disorders and medications used.

Year Founded: 2004

Research Centers

815 Child & Family Center
Menninger Clinic
21545 Centre Pointe Parkway
Santa Clarita, CA 91350
661-259-9439
800-351-9058
Fax: 661-255-6853
E-mail: webmaster@menninger.edu
www.www.childfamilycenter.org/

Steven Zimmer, Board Chair
Darrell Paulk, CEO
Bill Cooper, Vice Chair
Joan Aschoff, Executive Vice President of Prog

The Center's goals: to further develop emerging understanding of the impact of childhood maltreatment and abuse; to chart primary prevention strategies that will foster healthy patterns of caregiving and attachment and reduce the prevalence of maltreatment and abuse; to develop secondary prevention strategies that will promote early detection of attachment-related problems and effective interventions to avert the development of chronic and severe disorders; and to develop more effective treatment approaches for those individuals whose early attachment problems have eventuated in severe psychopathology.

Year Founded: 1976

Video & Audio

816 Active Parenting Now
Active Parenting Publishers
1220 Kennestone Circle
Suite 130
Marietta, GA 30066
770-429-0565
800-825-0060
Fax: 770-429-0334
E-mail: cservice@activeparenting.com

Michael Popkin, PhD, Author

A complete video-based parenting education program curriculum. Helps parents of children ages two to twelve raise responsible, courageous children. Emphasizes nonviolent discipline, conflict resolution and improved communication. With Leader's Guide, videotapes, Parent's Guide and more. Also available in Spanish. *$ 349.00*

Year Founded: 2002 ISBN 1-880283-89-1

817 Aggression Replacement Training Video: A Comprehensive Intervention for Aggressive Youth
Research Press
PO Box 7886
PO Box 9177
Champaign, IL 61826
217-352-3273
800-519-2707
Fax: 217-352-1221
E-mail: rp@researchpress.com
www.researchpress.com

Dr. Barry Glick, Author
Dr. John C. Gibbs, Author

This staff training video illustrates the training procedures in the Aggression Replacement Training (ART) book. It features scenes of adolescents participating in group sessions for each of ART's three interventions: Prosocial Skills, Anger Control, and Moral Reasoning. A free copy of the book accompanies the video program. *$35.95*

426 pages ISBN 0-878226-37-5

818 Understanding & Managing the Defiant Child
Courage to Change
1 Huntington Quadrangle
Suite: 1N03
Melville, NY 11747
800-962-1141
Fax: 800-262-1886
www.couragetochange.com

Russell A Barkley, PhD, Presenter

Understanding and Managing the Defiant Child provides a proven approach to behavior management. *$205.95*

819 Understanding Mental Illness
Educational Video Network
1401 19th Street
Huntsville, TX 77340
936-295-5767
800-762-0060
Fax: 936-294-0233
E-mail: info at evn.org
www.www.evndirect.com

A video to learn and understand mental illness and how it affects you. *$79.95*

Year Founded: 2004 ISBN 1-589501-48-9

820 **Understanding and Treating the Hereditary Psychiatric Spectrum Disorders**
Hope Press
PO Box 188
Duarte, CA 91009-188
818-303-0644
800-209-9182
Fax: 818-358-3520
E-mail: dcomings@earthlink.net
www.hopepress.com

David E Comings MD, Presenter

Learn with ten hours of audio tapes from a two day seminar given in May 1997 by David E Comings, MD. Tapes cover: ADHD, Tourette Syndrome, Obsessive-Compulsive Disorder, Conduct Disorder, Oppositional Defiant Disorder, Autism and other Hereditary Psychiatric Spectrum Disorders. Eight audio tapes. *$75.00*

Year Founded: 1997

Web Sites

821 **www.cyberpsych.org**
CyberPsych

Hosts the American Psychoanalyists Foundation, American Association of Suicideology, Society for the Exploration of Psychotherapy Intergration, and Anxiety Disorders Association of America. Also subcategories of the anxiety disorders, as well as general information, including panic disorder, phobias, obsessive compulsive disorder (OCD), social phobia, generalized anxiety disorder, post traumatic stress disorder, and phobias of childhood. Book reviews and links to web pages sharing the topics.

822 **www.planetpsych.com**
PlanetPsych.com

Learn about disorders, their treatments and other topics in psychology. Articles are listed under the related topic areas. Ask a therapist a question for free, or view the directory of professionals in your area. If you are a therapist sign up for the directory. Current features, self-help, interactive, and newsletter archives.

823 **www.psychcentral.com**
Psych Central

Personalized one-stop index for psychology, support, and mental health issues, resources, and people on the Internet.

Dissociative Disorders

Introduction

Dissociative Disorders are a cluster of mental disorders, characterized by a profound change in consciousness or a disruption in continuity of consciousness. People with a Dissociative Disorder may abruptly take on different personalities, or undergo long periods in which they do not remember anything that happened; in some cases, individuals may embark on lengthy international travels, returning home with no recollection of where they have been or why they had gone.

Dissociative Disorders are uncommon, mysterious and somewhat controversial; reports of Dissociative Disorders have grown more frequent in recent years and a degree of debate surrounds the validity of these reports. Some professionals say the disorders are far more rare than is reported, and that these individuals are highly vulnerable to the suggestions of others.

Dissociative Disorders are believed to be related in many cases to severe trauma, although the historical validity of these cases is difficult to determine. There are five types of Dissociative Disorders: Dissociative Amnesia; Dissociative Fugue; Dissociative Identity Disorder; Depersonalization Disorder; and Dissociative Disorder Not Otherwise Specified.

SYMPTOMS

Dissociative Amnesia
• One or more episodes of inability to recall important personal information, usually of a traumatic or stressful nature, that is too extensive to be explained by ordinary forgetfulness;
• The disturbance does not occur exclusively during the course of any other Dissociative Disorder and is not due to the direct physiological effects of a substance abuse or general medical condition;
• The symptoms cause clinically significant distress or impairment in social, occupational or other important areas of functioning.

Associative Fugue
• A sudden, unexpected travel away from home or work, with inability to recall one's past;
• Confusion about personal identity or assumption of a new identity;
• The disturbance does not occur exclusively during the course of any other Dissociative Disorder and is not due to the direct physiological effects of a substance or a general medical condition;
• The symptoms cause clinically significant distress or impairment in social, occupational, or other important areas of functioning.

Dissociative Identity Disorder
• The presence of two or more distinct identities or personality states that take control of the person's behavior;
• Inability to recall important personal information;
• The disturbance is not due to the direct physiological effects of a substance or a general medical condition.

Depersonalization Disorder
• Persistent or rec urrent experiences of feeling detached from one's body and mental processes;
• During the depersonalization experience, reality testing remains intact;
• The depersonalization causes clinically significant distress or impairment in social, occupational, or other important areas of functioning;
• The depersonalization does not occur during the course of another Dissociative Disorder or as a direct physiological effect of a substance or general medical condition;
• Akin to depersonalization (feeling one is not real) is derealization, which is feeling that one's environment and/or perceptions are not real.

ASSOCIATED FEATURES

Patients with any of the Dissociative Disorders may be depressed, and may experience depersonalization, or a feeling of not being in their own bodies. They often experience impairment in work or interpersonal relationships, and they may practice self-mutilation or have aggressive and suicidal impulses. They may also have symptoms typical of a Mood or Personality Disorder. Individuals with Dissociative Amnesia and Dissociative Identity Disorder (sometimes known as multiple personality disorder) often report severe physical and/or sexual abuse in childhood. Controversy surrounds the accuracy of these reports, in part because of the unreliability of some childhood memories. Individuals with Dissociative Identity Disorder may have symptoms typical of Post-Traumatic Stress Disorder, as well as Mood, Substance Abuse Related, Sexual, Eating or Sleep Disorders.

PREVALENCE

The prevalence of Dissociative Disorders is difficult to ascertain, and subject to controversy. The recent rise in the US in reports of Dissociative Amnesia and Dissociative Identity Disorder related to traumatic childhood abuse has been very controversial. Some say these disorders are overreported, the result of suggestibility in individuals and the unreliability of childhood memories. Others say the disorders are underreported, given the propensity for children and adults to dismiss or forget abusive memories and the tendency of perpetrators to deny or obscure their abusive actions. For Dissociative Fugue, a prevalence rate of 0.2 percent of the population has been reported. Dissociative Identity Disorder is diagnosed three to nine times more frequently in females than in males.

Associations & Agencies

825 Center for Mental Health Services (CMHS)
1 Choke Cherry Road
Room 6-1057
Rockville, MD 20857
240-276-1310
877-726-4727
Fax: 240-276-1320
TDD: 800-487-4889
E-mail: info@mentalhealth.org
www.beta.samhsa.gov/about-us/who-we-are/offices-center

Michael E Etzinger, B.S.M.E, , M.B., SAMHSA Executive Officer, Director
Paolo Del Vecchio, M.S.W, Director, Center for Mental Healt
Deborah Baldwin, M.P.A, Acting Director, Consumer Affairs
Elizabeth Lopez, Ph.D, Acting Deputy Director

CMHS leads Federal efforts to treat mental illnesses by promoting mental health and by preventing the development or worsening of mental illness when possible. Congress created CMHS to bring new hope to adults who have serious mental illnesses and to children with serious emotional disorders. CMHS provides information about mental health via a toll-free the web site, and more than 600 publications. Developed for users of mental health services and their families, the general public, policy makers, providers, and the media.

Year Founded: 1992

826   International Society for the Study of Trauma And Dissociation
8400 Westpark Drive
Second Floor
McLean, VA 22102
703-610-9037
Fax: 703-610-0234
E-mail: info@isst-d.org
www.www.isst-d.org

Philip J Kinsler, PhD, ABPP, President
Christine Forner, BA, BSW, MSW, Treasurer
Kevin J onnors, MS, MFT, Vice President
Martin Dorahy, PhD, Director

ISSTD seeks to advance clinical, scientific, and societel understanding about the prevalence and consequences of chronic trauma and dissociation.

827   National Association for the Dually Diagnosed (NADD)
132 Fair Street
Kingston, NY 12401-4802
845-331-4336
800-331-5362
Fax: 845-331-4569
E-mail: info@thenadd.org
www.thenadd.org

Donna McNELIS, PhD, President
Robert J Fletcher DSW, Chief Executive Officer
Dan Baker, PhD, Vice President
Julia Pearce, Secretary

Nonprofit organization designed to promote interest of professional and parent development with resources for individuals who have the coexistence of mental illness and mental retardation. Provides conferences, educational services and training materials to professionals, parents, concerned citizens and service organizations.

Year Founded: 1983

828   National Mental Health Consumers' Self-Help Clearinghouse
1211 Chestnut Street
Suite 1100
Philadelphia, PA 19107-4103
215-751-1810
800-553-4539
Fax: 215-636-6312
E-mail: info@mhselfhelp.org
www.mhselfhelp.org

Joseph Rogers, Executive Director/ Founder
Susan Rogers, Director
Britani Nestel, Program Specialist
Christa Burkett, Technical Assistance Coordinator

A national consumer technical assistance center that has played a major role in the development of the mental health consumer movement.

Year Founded: 1986

829   SAMHSA's National Mental Health Information Center
PO Box 42557
Washington, DC 20015-557
240-221-4021
800-789-2647
Fax: 240-221-4295
TDD: 866-889-2647
www.mentalhealth.samhsa.gov

A Kathryn Power, MEd, Director
Edward B Searle, Deputy Director

830   Sidran Institute
PO Box 436
Brooklandville, MD 21022-0436
410-825-8888
Fax: 410-560-0134
E-mail: info@sidran.org
www.www.sidran.org

Esther Giller, President, Director
Sheila Giller, Secretary/Treasurer
Tracy Howard, Book Sales/Office Manager
Ruta Mazelis, Editor, The Cutting Edge/Trainer

Sidran Institute provides useful, practical information for child and adult sufferers of Dissociative Disorders, for families and friends, and for the clinical and frontline service providers who assist in their recovery.

Year Founded: 1986

831   TARA Association for Personality Disorders
23 Greene Street
New York, NY 10013
212-966-6514
E-mail: info@tara4bpd.org
www.www.tara4bpd.org

Valerie Porr, MA, Founder, President
Michael Lionza, Vice President and Treasurer

Founded in 1994 in response to the realization that patients with personality disorders are stigmatized by the mental health community, as a group are: underdiagnosed, have little or no information on etiology, nosology, dissociationand treatment. TARA is the only national education and advocacy organization that provides information on Dissociative Disorders and BPD to families, consumers, and providers.

Year Founded: 1994

832   The Center for Family Support
2811 Zulette Avenue
Bronx, NY 10461
718-518-1500
Fax: 718-518-8200
www.cfsny.org

Steven Vernikoff, Executive Director
Virgil Seepersad, Director of Finance
Eileen Berg, Director of Quality Assurance
Barbara Greenwald, Associate Executive, Director

An agency that continues to develop new programs to serve families and individuals with their care needs. Currently offering services throughout the New York City region including: New Jersey, Long Island and the Lower Hudson Valley.

Year Founded: 1954

Books

833 Amongst Ourselves: A Self-Help Guide to Living with Dissociative Identity Disorder
NewHarbinger Publications
5674 Shattuck Avenue
Oakland, CA 94609-1662
510-652-0215
800-748-6273
Fax: 800-652-1613
E-mail: customerservice@newharbinger.com
www.newharbinger.com

Tracy Alderman, Author
Karen Marshall, Author

First person perspective of Dissociative Identity Disorder and practical suggestions to come to terms with and improve their lives. *$19.95*

240 pages Year Founded: 1973 ISBN 1-562241-22-5

834 Dialectical Behavior Therapy in Clinical Practice: Applications Across Disorders and Settings
Guilford Press
72 Spring Street
New York, NY 10012
800-365-7006
800-365-7006
Fax: 212-966-6708
E-mail: info@guilford.com
www.www.guilford.com

Linda A Dimeff, Editor
Kelly Koerner, Editor

This book presents applications for depression, substance dependence, eating disorders, psychosis, assaultive behaviors and other problems. *$42.50*

363 pages Year Founded: 1973 ISBN 1-572309-74-6

835 Dialectical Behavior Therapy with Suicidal Adolescents
Guilford Press
72 Spring Street
New York, NY 10012
800-365-7006
800-365-7006
Fax: 212-966-6708
E-mail: info@guilford.com
www.www.guilford.com

Alec L. Miller, Author
Jill H. Rathus, Author
Marsha M Linehan, Author

This book adapts the proven techniques of Dialectical Behavior Therapy among Dissociative Disorder sufferers to treatment. The authors take you step by step through understanding and assessing severe emotional dysregulation in teens and implementing individual family, family and group based interventions. *$42.50*

346 pages Year Founded: 1973 ISBN 1-593853-83-9

836 Dissociation Culture, Mind, and Body
American Psychiatric Publishing, Inc.
1000 Wilson Boulevard
Suite 1825
Arlington, VA 22209-3901
703-907-7322
800-368-5777
Fax: 703-907-1091
E-mail: appi@psych.org
www.appi.org

David Spiegel, MD, Editor

Combines cultural anthropology, congitive psychology, neurophysiology, and the study of psychosomatic illness to present the latest information on the dissociative process. Designed for professionals in cross cultural psychiatry and the influence of the mind on the body. *$83.00*

246 pages Year Founded: 1994 ISBN 0-880485-57-9

837 Dissociation and the Dissociative Disorders: DSM-V and Beyond
Routledge
270 Madison Avenue
New York, NY 10016-601
212-695-6599
www.routledgementalhealth.com

Paul F. Dell, Author
John A. O'Neil, Author

This book draws together and integrates the most recent scientific and conceptual foundations of dissociation and the dissociative disorders field. *$93.56*

898 pages Year Founded: 2009 ISBN 0-415957-85-4

838 Dissociative Child: Diagnosis, Treatment and Management
Sidran Institute
PO Box 436
Brooklandville, MD 21022-0436
410-825-8888
888-825-8249
Fax: 410-560-0134
E-mail: sidran@sidran.org
www.sidran.org

Joyanna L Silberg, PhD, Editor

This second groundbreaking edition addresses all aspects of caring for the dissociative child and adolescents. Contributors include experienced and eminent practitioners in the field of childhood DID. The section on diagnosis offers comprehensive coverage of various aspects of diagnosis, including diagnosis taxonomy, differential diagnosis, interviewing, testing and the special problems of male children and adolescents with DID. The section on treatment covers factors associated with positive theraputic outcome, therapeutic phases, the five-domain crisis model, promoting intergration in dissociative children, art therapy and group therapy. Includes ways school personnel can act to help the dissociative child, multiculturalism and other important information. *$37.00*

343 pages Year Founded: 1986

839 Drug Therapy and Dissociative Disorders
Mason Crest Publishers
450 Parkway Drive
Suite D
Broomall, PA 19008-4017

610-543-6200
866-627-2665
Fax: 610-543-3878
E-mail: dtaylor@masoncrest.com
www.masoncrest.com

Autumn Libal, Author
Dan Hilferty, President
Michelle Luke, Director, Marketing, PR
Michael Toglia, Special Sales

Dissociative disorders are some of the most controversial disorders in psychiatry today. Despite newfound recognition and numerous diagnosis the very existence of these disorders is still hotly debated in some academic circles. these disorders make us question our assumptions about memory, self, and personality, and shed unique light on the mysterious complexities of the human mind. From amnesia to multiple personalities, dissociative disorders present treatment challenges to psychotherapy and psychopharmacology alike. Through stories of individuals' struggles with dissociative disorders, this book provides both historical overview of treatment and reviews the most up-to-date treatments available today.

128 pages ISBN 1-590845-64-1

840 Got Parts? An Insider's Guide to Managing Life Successfully with Dissociative Identity Disorder
Loving Healing Press
5145 Pontiac Trail
Ann Arbor, MI 48105-9627
734-929-0881
888-761-6268
Fax: 734-663-6861
E-mail: info@lovinghealing.com
www.lovinghealing.com

A.T.W.

This book is directed towards people treating Dissociative Identity Disorder. It is a book for survivors written by a survivor. This book is filled with successful coping techniques and strategies to enhance the day to day functioning of a dult survivors of DID in relationships, work, and parenting.

132 pages Year Founded: 2003 ISBN 1-932690-03-4

841 Handbook for the Assessment of Dissociation: a Clinical Guide
American Psychiatric Publishing, Inc.
1000 Wilson Boulevard
Suite 1825
Arlington, VA 22209-3901
703-907-7322
800-368-5777
Fax: 703-907-1091
E-mail: appi@psych.org
www.appi.org

Marlene Steinberg, M.D., Author
Ron McMillen, Chief Executive Officer
John McDuffie, Editorial Director

Offers guidelines for the systematic assessment of dissociation and posttraumatic syndromes for clinicians and researchers. Provides a comprehensive overview of dissociative symptoms and disorders and an introduction to the use of the SCID-D, a diagnostic interview for the dissociative disorders. *$54.00*

450 pages Year Founded: 1995 ISBN 0-880486-82-1

842 Lost in the Mirror: An Inside Look at Borderline Personality Disorder
Sidran Institute
200 E Joppa Road
Suite 207
Baltimore, MD 21286-3107
410-825-8888
888-825-8249
Fax: 410-337-0747
E-mail: sidran@sidran.org
www.sidran.org

Richard A. Moskovitz, MD, Author
J G Goellner, Director Emertius
Stanley Platman, MD, Medical Advisor

Dr. Moskovitz considers BPD to be part of the dissociative continuum, as it has many causes, symptoms and behaviors in common with Dissociative Disorder. This book is intended for people diagnosed with BPD, their families and therapists. Outlines the features of BPD, including abuse histories, dissociation, mood swings, self harm, impulse control problems and many more. Includes an extensive resource section. *$13.95*

190 pages

843 New Hope for People with Borderline Personality Disorder
Three Rivers Press

Neil R. Bocklan, Author
Rob Viehman, Publisher
Amy England, Staff Writer

$18.95

Year Founded: 2004 ISBN 0-761527-18-4

844 Overcoming Borderline Personality Disorder: A Family Guide for Healing and Change
Oxford University Press

Valerie Porr, Author

a book for professional, families, and people suffering with Dissociative Disorders. *$24.95*

Year Founded: 2010 ISBN 0-195379-58-6

845 Rebuilding Shattered Lives: Responsible Treatment of Complex Post-Traumatic and Dissociative Disorders
John Wiley & Sons
111 River Street
Hoboken, NJ 07030-5774
201-748-6000
800-225-5945
Fax: 201-748-6088
E-mail: info@wiley.com
www.wiley.com

James A Chu, Author

Essential for anyone working in the field of trauma therapy. Part I discusses recent findings about child abuse, the changes in attitudes toward child abuse over the last two decades and the nature of traumatic memory. Part II is an overview of principles of trauma treatment, including symptom control, establishment of boundaries and therapist self-care. Part III covers special topics, such as dissociative identity disorder, controversies, hospitalization and acute care. *$ 73.95*

271 pages Year Founded: 1998 ISBN 0-471247-32-4

846 Skills Training Manual for Treating Borderline Personality Disorder
Guilford Press
72 Spring Street
New York, NY 10012
800-365-7006
800-365-7006
Fax: 212-966-6708
E-mail: info@guilford.com
www.www.guilford.com

Marsha M. Linehan, Author

This book is a step by step guide to teach clients four sets of skills: interpersonal effectiveness, emotion regulation, distress tolerance, and mindfulness. *$38.25*

180 pages Year Founded: 1973 ISBN 0-898620-34-4

847 The Abused Child Psychodynamic Understanding and Treatment
Guilford Press
72 Spring Street
New York, NY 10012
800-365-7006
800-365-7006
Fax: 212-966-6708
E-mail: info@guilford.com
www.www.guilford.com

Toni Vaughn Heineman, Author

The book traces the interplay of neurobiological and psychological facats of behavior to show how abuse derails normal development and how psychodynamic psychotherapy can reestablish emotional connections. *$34.00*

243 pages Year Founded: 1973 ISBN 1-572303-75-1

848 Traumatic Stress The Effects of Overwhelming Experience on Mind, Body, And Society
Guilford Press
72 Spring Street
New York, NY 10012
800-365-7006
800-365-7006
Fax: 212-966-6708
E-mail: info@guilford.com
www.www.guilford.com

Bessel A Van Der Kolk, Editor
Alexander C McFarlane, Editor
Lars Weisaeth, Editor

This best selling classic presents seminal theory and research on dissociation disorders. These leading editors and contributors comprehensively examine how trauma affects an individual's biology, conception of the world, and psychological functioning. *$42.50*

596 pages Year Founded: 1973 ISBN 1-572304-57-4

849 Treatment of Multiple Personality Disorder
American Psychiatric Publishing, Inc.
1000 Wilson Boulevard
Suite 1825
Arlington, VA 22209-3901
703-907-7322
800-368-5777
Fax: 703-907-1091
E-mail: appi@psych.org
www.appi.org

Bennett G Braun, M.D., Editor
Ron McMillen, Chief Executive Officer
John McDuffie, Editorial Director

Authorities in the Multiple Personality Disorder field merge clinical understanding and research into therapeutic approaches that can be employed in clinical practice. *$22.50*

228 pages Year Founded: 1986 ISBN 0-880480-96-3

850 Understanding Dissociative Disorders and Addiction
Sidran Institute
200 E Joppa Road
Suite 207
Townson, MD 21286-3107
410-825-8888
888-825-8249
Fax: 410-337-0747
E-mail: sidran@sidran.org
www.sidran.org

A Scott Winter, Author
J Gila Goellner, Director Emertius
Stanley Plantman, MD, Medical Advisor

This booklet discusses the origins and symptoms of dissociation, explains the links between dissociative disorder and chemical dependency. Addresses treatment options available to help in your recovery. The work book includes exercises and activities that help you acknowledge, accept and manage both your chemical dependency and your disociative disorder. *$7.20*

48 pages

851 Understanding Dissociative Disorders: A Guide for Family Physicians and Healthcare Workers
Crown House Publishing
6 Trowbridge Drive
Suite 5
Bethel, CT 06801-2882
203-778-1300

Marlene E. Hunter, Author

This volume outlines common presentations in the family physicians' practice, and offers realistic, practical answers to a multitude of questions. *$20.00*

Year Founded: 2009

Video & Audio

852 Different From You
Fanlight Publications
32 Court Street
21st Floor
Brooklyn, NY 11201
718-488-8900
800-876-1710
Fax: 718-488-8642
E-mail: fanlight@fanlight.com
www.fanlight.com

Milt L. Kogan, MD, MPH, Author
Demetrio Cuzzocrea, Author

As a result of the 'deinstituionalization' of mental patients, people with mental illnesses now make up a majority of the homeless in many areas. This video explores the problem through the work of a compassionate physician who cares for mentally ill people living on the streets and in inade-quate 'board and care' facilities in Los Angeles.

853 Understanding Mental Illness
Educational Video Network
1401 19th Street
Huntsville, TX 77340
936-295-5767
800-762-0060
Fax: 936-294-0233
E-mail: info at evn.org
www.www.evndirect.com

A video to learn and understand mental illness and how it affects you. *$79.95*

Year Founded: 2004 ISBN 1-589501-48-9

854 Understanding Personality Disorders DVD
Educational Video Network
1401 19th Street
Huntsville, TX 77340
936-295-5767
800-762-0060
Fax: 936-294-0233

Defines to adolescents what a personality disorder really is. *$89.95*

Year Founded: 2006

855 Understanding Self Destructive Behavior
Educational Video Network
1401 19th Street
Huntsville, TX 77340
936-295-5767
800-762-0060
Fax: 936-294-0233

helps adolescents learn how to deal with their destructive behavior due to their mental illness. *$129.95*

Year Founded: 2004

Web Sites

856 www.cyberpsych.org
CyberPsych

Hosts the American Psychoanalyists Foundation, American Association of Suicideology, Society for the Exploration of Psychotherapy Intergration, and Anxiety Disorders Association of America. Also subcategories of the anxiety disorders, as well as general information, including panic disorder, phobias, obsessive compulsive disorder (OCD), social phobia, generalized anxiety disorder, post traumatic stress disorder, and phobias of childhood. Book reviews and links to web pages sharing the topics.

857 www.fmsf.com
False Memory Syndrome Facts

Access to literature.

858 www.isst-D.Org
International Society for the Study of Dissociation

A nonprofit, professional society that promotes research and training in the identification and treatment of dissociative disorders, provides professional and public education about dissociative states, and serves as a catalyst for international communication and cooperation among clinicians and researchers working in this field.

859 www.planetpsych.com
Planetpsych.com

Learn about disorders, their treatments and other topics in psychology. Articles are listed under the related topic areas. Ask a therapist a question for free, or view the directory of professionals in your area. If you are a therapist sign up for the directory. Current features, self-help, interactive, and newsletter archives.

860 www.psychcentral.com
Psych Central

Personalized one-stop index for psychology, support, and mental health issues, resources, and people on the Internet.

861 www.sidran.org
Trauma Resource Area

Resources and Articles on Dissociative Experiences Scale and Dissociative Identity Disorder, PsychTrauma Glossary and Traumatic Memories.

Eating Disorders

Introduction

Eating is integral to human health, and for many people food is a pleasure that can be enjoyed without too much thought. But an increasing number of people (mostly, but not exclusively, women) have eating disorders, which cause them to use food and dieting in ways that are extremely unhealthy, even life-threatening. The two principal eating disorders are Anorexia Nervosa and Bulimia Nervosa; though different in the symptoms they manifest, the two disorders are quite similar in their underlying pathology: an obsessive concern with food, body image, and body weight.

The enormous increase in the incidence of obesity may lead to a formal classification of overating as a disorder. However, recent research reveals that the cause of obesity is not simply a lack of self-control, or too much self-indulgence, leading to the ingestion of too many calories. It appears that human beings are hard-wired, so to speak, to eat whenever food is available, and food is ever more available and more caloric. In addition, the eating patterns and weight of pregnany women seems to result is physiologic changes in their unborn babies, who are predisposed to become obese after birth regardless of diet.

Many people believe that eating disorders are, in part, culturally determined: in the Western world, and particularly the US, a pervasive cultural preference for slimness causes many people to spend extraordinary amounts of time, money and energy dieting and exercise to stay slim. At the same time, people are flooded with media; celebrations of anorexia, and suggested strategies for remaining thin, can be easily found on the Internet, on television, and in magazines. Cultural preference is likely to exert pressure on people, especially young women, who may be genetically or psychologically predisposed to the illness. It is important to be wary of media, including the Internet, which can expose young people to counterproductive influences. Overeating is another type of Eating Disorder, as it reflects the paradox that, as society values thinness more and more, more and more people are obese. Eating Disorders may do lasting physical damage; because of this, treatment must first restore a patient to a safe and healthy body weight. Treatment of the disorder is a long-term process, involving psychotherapy, family interventions and, for depressed or obsessional patients, antidepressant medication. Fortunately, most people who are appropriately treated can and do recover.

SYMPTOMS

Anorexia Nervosa:
• Refusal to maintain body weight at or above eighty-five percent of a minimally normal weight for age and height;
• Intense fear of gaining weight or becoming fat, even though underweight;
• Disturbance in the way one's body weight or shape is experienced, undue influence of body weight or shape on self-evaluation, or denial of the seriousness of the current low body weight;
• In menstruating females, the absence of at least three consecutive menstrual cycles;
• Physical damage often occurs, such as imbalances in body chemicals, which if severe can cause cardiac arrest; purging often erodes tooth enamel, in which case a dentist might make the diagnosis. Anorexia Nervosa is associated with

amenorrhea and infertility, which may lead patients to seek help from a gynecologist, who must then make the diagnosis.

Bulimia Nervosa:
• Recurrent episodes of binge eating characterized by eating more food than most people would eat during a similar period of time and under similar circumstances;
• A sense of loss of control over eating;
• Recurrent inappropriate behavior in order to prevent weight gain, such as self-induced vomiting or misuse of laxatives, and excessive fasting or exercise;
• The binge-eating and inappropriate behaviors both occur, on average, at least twice a week for three months;
• Self-evaluation is unduly influenced by body shape and weight;
• The disturbance does not occur exclusively during episodes of Anorexia Nervosa.

ASSOCIATED FEATURES

Patients with Anorexia Nervosa may be severely depressed, and may experience insomnia, irritability, and diminished interest in sex. These features may be exacerbated if the patient is severely underweight. People with Eating Disorders also share many of the features of Obsessive Compulsive Disorder. For instance, someone with an Eating Disorder may have an excessive interest in food; they may hoard food, or spend unusual amounts of time reading and researching about foods, recipes and nutrition. People with Anorexia Nervosa may also exhibit a strong need to control their environment, and may be socially and emotionally withdrawn.

Individuals with Bulimia Nervosa are often within the normal weight range, but prior to the development of the disorder they may be overweight. Depression and other Mood Disorders are common among people with bulimia, and patients often ascribe their bulimia to the Mood Disorders. In other cases, however, it appears that the Mood Disorders precede the Eating Disorders. Substance abuse occurs in about one-third of individuals with bulimia.

Anxiety Disorders are common, and fear of social situations can be a precipitating factor in binging episodes.

PREVALENCE

Prevalence studies in females have found rates of 0.5 to one percent for Anorexia Nervosa. There is only limited data for the prevalence of Anorexia Nervosa in males. The prevalence of Bulimia Nervosa among adolescent females is approximately one to three percent. The rate of the disorder among males is approximately one-tenth of that in females.

TREATMENT OPTIONS

Medications, especially the newest SSRIs (Selective Serotonin Reuptake Inhibitors, which were originally developed as antidepressants), have been found to be very effective in the treatment of Eating Disorders. They can help restore and build self-esteem, and thereby help the patient maintain a positive attitude as well as a safe and healthy body image and body weight.

Because of the physical damage that an Eating Disorder can do to a patient, nutritional counseling and monitoring is often vital to restore and maintain proper body weight.

It is critical to recognize that Eating Disorders are, in

addition to being life-threatening, extremely complex: simply restoring the patient to an acceptable body weight is not enough. Many patients have complex and conflicting psychological issues that trigger the compulsion to binge, or the morbid fear of gaining weight. These issues need to be addressed by psychotherapy. Forms of psychotherapy that may be useful in treating Eating Disorders include psychodynamic psychotherapy (in which longstanding and sometimes unconscious emotional issues related to the eating disorders are explored) and cognitive behavior therapy, which aims to identify the thought patterns that trigger the Eating Disorder and to establish healthy eating habits. Recent literature suggests that psychotherapeutic approaches are often more effective than medications in the treatment of Anorexia. Family involvement in treatment is critical, and peer pressure can be utilized to compel patients to maintain adequate nutrition. Eating Disorders are serious — untreated Anorexia can kill a patient — and treatment may be required over a course of many years.

Associations & Agencies

863   Alliance for Eating Disorders Awareness
1649 Forum Place
Suite 2
West Palm Beach, FL 33401
561-841-0900
866-662-1235
E-mail: info@allianceforeatingdisorders.com
www.www.allianceforeatingdisorders.com

Suzette Wexner, Board Chair
Johanna Kandel, Founder, CEO
Sharon Glynn, Director, Programming
Joann Hendelman, PhD, RN, FAED, Clinical Director

In October of 2000, The Alliance for Eating Disorders Awareness was created as a source of community outreach, education, awareness, and prevention of the various eating disorders currently plaguing the nation. Thier aim is to share the maeesage that recovery from these disorders is possible, and that individuals should not have to suffer or recover alone. They seek to educate individuals about the dangers of this epidemic and to reduce the rate and severity of eating disorders among people of all ages

Year Founded: 2000

864   Anorexia Nervosa and Related Eating Disorders
PO Box 5102
Eugene, OR 97405-102
541-344-1144
E-mail: jarinor@rio.com
www.anred.com

We are a nonprofit organization that provides information about anorexia nervosa, bulimia nervosa, binge eating diorder, and other less-well-known food and weight disorders.

865   Center for Mental Health Services (CMHS)
1 Choke Cherry Road
Room 6-1057
Rockville, MD 20857
240-276-1310
877-726-4727
Fax: 240-276-1320
TDD: 800-487-4889

E-mail: info@mentalhealth.org
www.beta.samhsa.gov/about-us/who-we-are/offices-center

Michael E Etzinger, B.S.M.E, , M.B., SAMHSA Executive Officer, Director
Paolo Del Vecchio, M.S.W, Director, Center for Mental Healt
Deborah Baldwin, M.P.A, Acting Director, Consumer Affairs
Elizabeth Lopez, Ph.D, Acting Deputy Director

CMHS leads Federal efforts to treat mental illnesses by promoting mental health and by preventing the development or worsening of mental illness when possible. Congress created CMHS to bring new hope to adults who have serious mental illnesses and to children with serious emotional disorders. CMHS provides information about mental health via a toll-free the web site, and more than 600 publications. Developed for users of mental health services and their families, the general public, policy makers, providers, and the media.

Year Founded: 1992

866   Change for Good Coaching and Counseling
3801 Connecticut Avenue NorthWest
Washington, DC 20008-4530
202-362-3009
Fax: 202-204-6100
E-mail: brockhansenlcsw@aol.com
www.change-for-good.org

Brock Hansen, LCSW, President

Coaching on learnable emotional skills to see goals clearly, harness resources and get moving toward a successful outcome.

867   Council on Size and Weight Discrimination (CSWD)
PO Box 305
Mount Marion, NY 12456-305
845-679-1209
Fax: 845-679-1206
E-mail: info@cswd.org
www.cswd.org

Miriam Berg, President
Lynn McAfee, Director of Medical Advocacy
William J. Fabrey, Media Project
Nancy Summer, Fund Raising

The Council on Size and Weight Discrimination is a not-for-profit group which works to change people's attitudes about weight. They act as consumer advocates for larger people, especially in the areas of medical treatment, job discrimination, and media images.

868   International Association of Eating Disorders Professionals Foundation
PO Box 1295
Pekin, IL 61555-1295
800-800-8126
800-800-8126
Fax: 800-800-8126
E-mail: iaedpmembers@earthlink.net
www.iaedp.com

James D Buck Runyan, MS, LMFT, CE, President
Bonnie Harken, Managing Director
Wendy Oliver-Pyatt, MD, FAED, C, Treasurer
Carolyn Costin, MA, Med, MFT, CEDS, Secretary

Offers professional counseling and assistance to the medical community, courts, law enforcement officials, and social welfare agencies.

Year Founded: 1985

869   Men Get Eating Disorders Too (MGEDT)
113 Queens Road
C/O Community Base
Brighton, BN1 3-G
845-634-1414
845-634-7650
E-mail: sam@mengetedstoo.co.uk
www.www.mengetedstoo.co.uk

Sam Thomas, Founder, Project Leader
Neil Holmes, Chairman
Hugh Smith, Trustee
Russell Delderfield, Trustee

Men Get Eating Disorders Too seeks awareness of eating disorders in men so men are able to recognize their symptoms and access support when they need it.

Year Founded: 2008

870   Multiservice Eating Disorders Association
288 Walnut Street
Suite 130
Newton, MA 02460
617-558-1881
866-343-MEDA
Fax: 617-558-1771
E-mail: info@medainc.org
www.www.medainc.org

Rebecca Manley, MS, Founder
Beth Mayer, LICSW, Executive Director
Lindsay Brady, Clinical Director
Susie Stockwell, Communications and Development D

MEDA is dedicated to the prevention and treatment of eating disorders and disordered eating. MEDA's mission is to prevent the continuing spread of eating disorders through educational awareness and early detection. MEDA serves as a support network and resource for clients, loved ones, clinicians, educators, and the general public.

Year Founded: 1994

871   National Alliance on Mental Illness
3803 North Fairfax Drive
Suite 100
Arlington, VA 22203
703-524-7600
800-950-6264
Fax: 703-524-9094
E-mail: helpline@nami.org
www.nami.org

Keris Jan Myrick, MBA, MS, PhD., President
Mary Giliberti, J.D, Executive Director
Jim Payne, J.D, First Vice President
David Levy, Chief Financial Officer

Nation's leading self-help organization for all those affected by severe brain disorders. Mission is to bring consumers and families with similar experiences together to share information about services, care providers, and ways to cope with the challenges of schizophrenia, manic depression, and other serious mental illnesses.

Year Founded: 1969

872   National Association for the Dually Diagnosed (NADD)
132 Fair Street
Kingston, NY 12401-4802
845-331-4336
800-331-5362
Fax: 845-331-4569
E-mail: info@thenadd.org
www.thenadd.org

Donna McNELIS, PhD, President
Robert J Fletcher DSW, Chief Executive Officer
Dan Baker, PhD, Vice President
Julia Pearce, Secretary

Nonprofit organization designed to promote interest of professional and parent development with resources for individuals who have the coexistence of mental illness and mental retardation. Provides conferences, educational services and training materials to professionals, parents, concerned citizens and service organizations.

Year Founded: 1983

873   National Association of Anorexia Nervosa and Associated Disorders (ANAD)
750 East Diehl Road
Suite 127
Naperville, IL 60563
630-577-1333
630-577-1330
Fax: 847-433-4632
E-mail: anadhelp@anad.org
www.anad.org

Laura Discipio, LCSW, Executive Director
Donna Rostamian, Community Organisational Manager
Melanie Zumm, Support Group Coordinator
Kyron Johnson-Brana, Administrative Assistant

Sponsors national and local programs to prevent eating disorders and assist people with eating disorders and their families. Provides a national clearinghouse of information and is a grassroots association for laypeople and professionals.

Year Founded: 1976

874   National Association to Advance Fat Acceptance (NAAFA)
PO Box 4662
Foster City, CA 94404-0662
916-558-6880
Fax: 415-373-0483
E-mail: naafa@naafa.org
www.www.naafaonline.com

Jason Docherty, Chairman
Lisa Tealer, Director of Programs and Treasur
Peggy Howell, Public Relations Director
Phyllis Warr, Member Services Director

Nonprofit organization dedicated to improving the quality of life for fat people. Opposes discrimination against fat people including discrimination in advertising, employment, fashion, medicine, insurance, social acceptance, the media, schooling and public accomodations. Monitors legislative activity and litigation affecting fat people. Publications: NAAFA Newsletter, bimonthly. Annual conference and symposium, always mid-August.

Year Founded: 1969

875 National Eating Disorders Association
165 West 46th Street
Suite 402
New York, NY 10036
212-575-6200
800-931-2237
Fax: 212-575-1650
E-mail: info@NationalEatingDisroders.org
www.nationaleatingdisorders.org

Ric Clark, Chairman
Lynn S Grefe, MA, President and Chief Executive Of
Russell Marx, MD, Treasurer and Chief Science Offi
Terry Marks, Chief Development Officer

Offers a national information phone line, an international treatment referral directory, and a support group directory. The organization sponsors an annual conference and offers a speakers' bureau with a wide range of eating disorder.

Year Founded: 2001

876 National Institute of Mental Health Eating Disorders Program
6001 Executive Boulevard
Room 6200, MSC 9663
Bethesda, MD 20892-9663
301-443-4513
866-615-6464
Fax: 301-443-4279
TTY: 301-443-8431
E-mail: nimhinfo@nih.gov
www.www.nimh.nih.gov

Tom Insel, MD, NIHM Director
William G Coleman, Scientific Director, NIMHD
Grace E O Ajao, Administrative Officer
Dionne D Draper, Administrative Officer

Mission is to reduce the burden of mental illness and behavior disorders through research on mind, brain and behavior. NIMH is committed to educating the public about mental disorders and has developed many booklets and fact sheets that provide the latest research-based information on these illnesses.

877 National Mental Health Consumers' Self-Help Clearinghouse
1211 Chestnut Street
Suite 1100
Philadelphia, PA 19107-4103
215-751-1810
800-553-4539
Fax: 215-636-6312
E-mail: info@mhselfhelp.org
www.mhselfhelp.org

Joseph Rogers, Executive Director/ Founder
Susan Rogers, Director
Britani Nestel, Program Specialist
Christa Burkett, Technical Assistance Coordinator

A national consumer technical assistance center that has played a major role in the development of the mental health consumer movement.

Year Founded: 1986

878 SAMHSA's National Mental Health Information Center
PO Box 42557
Washington, DC 20015-557

800-789-2647
Fax: 240-747-5470
TDD: 866-889-2647
E-mail: ken@mentalhealth.org
www.mentalhealth.samhsa.gov

A Kathryn Power, MEd, Director
Edward B Searle, Deputy Director

879 TOPS Take Off Pounds Sensibly
4575 South 5th Street
PO Box 070360
Milwaukee, WI 53207-360
414-482-4620
800-932-8677
Fax: 414-482-3955
E-mail: wondering@tops.org
www.www.tops.org

Beverly Staniak, Chairman
Barbara Cady, TOPS President
Nancy Maeasco, First Vice President
Sandra Seidlitz, Treasurer

TOPS is an international family of all ages, sizes, and shapes from all walk of life. Dedicated to helping each other Take Off and Keep Off Pounds Sensibly. We offer fellowship while you change to a healthier, new lifestyle andlearn to maintain it.

Year Founded: 1948

880 The Center for Family Support
2811 Zulette Avenue
Bronx, NY 10461
718-518-1500
Fax: 718-518-8200
www.cfsny.org

Steven Vernikoff, Executive Director
Virgil Seepersad, Director of Finance
Eileen Berg, Director of Quality Assurance
Barbara Greenwald, Associate Executive, Director

An agency that continues to develop new programs to serve families and individuals with their care needs. Currently offering services throughout the New York City region including: New Jersey, Long Island and the Lower Hudson Valley.

Year Founded: 1954

881 The National Association for Males with Eating Disorders, Inc
531 Mission Street
San Francisco, CA 94105
239-775-1145
877-780-0080
E-mail: chris@namedinc.org
www.www.namedinc.org

Christopher Clark, Executive Director

N.A.M.E.D.'s mission is to provide support to males with eating disorders, to educate the public on the issue, and to be a resource of information on the subject.

Year Founded: 2006

882 The National Coalition for a Healthy america
304 Tequesta Drive
Suite 200
Tequesta, FL 33469
877-843-2358
Fax: 561-746-4023

E-mail: info@forahealthyamerica.org
www.www.forahealthyamerica.org

Tara Weidenfeller, Executive Director
Rebecca Valenza, Program Manager

A non-profit coporation established in 2003 to combat the growing epidemics of obesity and related diseases across america. Their mission is to work in concert with state and local governments, non-profit organizations and institutions to develop and implement broad based walking and fitness initiatives that increase public awareness and participation in a healthy lifestyle program all socioeconomic strata .

Year Founded: 2003

Books

883 Anorexia Nervosa & Recovery: a Hunger for Meaning
Haworth Press
10 Alice Street
Binghamton, NY 13904-1503
607-722-5857
800-429-6784
Fax: 607-721-0012
E-mail: getinfo@haworthpress.com
www.haworthpress.com

Ellen Cole, Author
Karen Way, MA, Author
Esther D Rothblum, Author
Karly Way Schramm, Author

Presents the most objective, complete, and compassionate picture of what anorexia nervosa is about. *$19.95*

142 pages Year Founded: 1993 ISBN 0-918393-95-7

884 Beyond Anorexia
Cambridge University Press
32 Avenue of the Americas
New York, NY 10013-2473
212-337-5000
E-mail: newyork@cambrigde.org
www.www.cambridge.org

Catherine Garrett, Author

Beyond Anorexia is a sociological exploration of how people recover from what medicince lables 'eating disorders'. *$41.00*

260 pages Year Founded: 1534 ISBN 0-521629-83-6

885 Binge Eating: Nature, Assessment and Treatment
Guilford Press
72 Spring Street
New York, NY 10012-4068
212-431-9800
800-365-7006
Fax: 212-966-6708
E-mail: info@guilford.com

Bob Matloff, President

Informative and practical text brings together original and significant contributions from leading experts from a wide variety of fields. Detailed manual covers all those who binge eat, including those who are overweight. *$21.95*

419 pages ISBN 0-898628-58-X

886 Body Image Workbook: An 8 Step Program for Learning to Like Your Looks
NewHarbinger Publications
5674 Shattuck Avenue
Oakland, CA 94609-1662
510-652-0215
800-748-6273
Fax: 800-652-1613
E-mail: customerservice@newharbinger.com
www.newharbinger.com

Thomas Cash, PhD, Author

Workbook offering a program to help transform your relationship with your body. *$19.95*

240 pages Year Founded: 1973 ISBN 1-572240-62-8

887 Body Image, Eating Disorders, and Obesity in Youth
APA Books
750 First Street, NorthEast
Washington, DC 20002-4241
202-336-5500
800-374-2721
Fax: 202-336-5500
TDD: 202-336-6123
E-mail: order@apa.org
www.apa.org

Linda Smolak, PhD, Editor
J. Kevin Thompson, PhD, Editor

Provides for clinicians including research, assessment and treatment suggestions on body image disturbances and eating disorders in children and adolescents. *$49.95*

389 pages Year Founded: 1892 ISBN 1-433804-05-2

888 Brief Therapy and Eating Disorders
John Wiley & Sons
111 River Street
Hoboken, NJ 07030-5774
201-748-6000
Fax: 201-748-6088
www.wiley.com

Barbara McFarland, Author

Demonstrates how solution-focused brief therapy is one of the more efficient approaches in treating eating disorders. *$36.95*

284 pages ISBN 0-787900-53-2

889 Bulimia
Jossey-Bass Publishers
989 Martket Street
San Francisco, CA 94103-1708
415-433-1740
Fax: 415-433-0499
www.leadertoleader.org

Barbara G Baeur, PhD, Author
Wayne P Anderson, PhD, Author
Robert W Hyatt, MD, Author

A step-by-step guide to this complex disease. Filled with practical information and advice, this essential resource offers hope to millions of bulimics and their loved ones. *$17.95*

167 pages ISBN 0-787903-61-2

890 Bulimia Nervosa
University of Minnesota Press
111 Third Avenue South
Suite 290
Minneapolis, MN 55401-2520
612-627-1970
Fax: 612-627-1980
E-mail: ump@umn.edu
www.upress.umn.edu

James E. Mitchell, Author

A practical guide for health-care professionals to the diagnosis, treatment and management of bulimia by a leading expert in the field of eating disorders. Hardcover. *$27.95*

192 pages Year Founded: 1925 ISBN 0-816616-26-4

891 Bulimia Nervosa & Binge Eating: A Guide To Recovery
New York University Press
838 Broadway
3rd Floor
New York, NY 10003-4812
212-998-2575
Fax: 212-995-3833
www.nyupress.nyu.edu

Peter J Cooper, Author
Margie Guerra, Assistant Director
Monica McCormick, Program Officer

A self-help book designed to guide bilimics and binge-eaters to recovery. *$35.00*

170 pages ISBN 0-814715-22-2

892 Bulimia: a Guide to Recovery
Gurze Books
5145 B Avenida Encinas
Carlsbad, CA 92008
760-434-7533
800-756-7533
Fax: 760-434-5476
E-mail: info@gurze.net
www.www.gurzebooks.com

Lindsey Hall, Author
Leigh Cohn, M.A.T, Author

Guidebook offers a complete understanding of bulimia and a plan for recovery. Includes a two-week program to stop binging, things-to-do instead of binging, a two-week guide for support groups, specific advice for loved ones, and Eating Without Fear - Hall's story of self-cure which has inspired thousands of other bulimics. *$14.95*

280 pages Year Founded: 1980 ISBN 0-936077-31-X

893 Clinical Handbook of Eating Disorders: An Integrated Approach
Informa Healthcare
52 Vanderbilt Avenue
New York, NY 10017-3808
646-443-3976
Fax: 646-661-5054
E-mail: healthcare.enquiries@informa.com
www.informaworld.com

Timothy D Brewerton, Editor

Reviews the most current research on the assessment, epidemiology, etiology, risk factors, neurodevelopment, course of illness, and various empirically-based evaluation and treatment approaches relating to eating disorders-studying disordered eating in atypical patient populations, such as men, infants, and the elderly and highlighting gender, cultural, and age-related differences that have appeared in the study of these conditions.

740 pages

894 Controlling Eating Disorders with Facts, Advice and Resources
Oryx Press
88 Post Road W
Westport, CT 06880-4208
203-226-3571
Fax: 603-431-2214
E-mail: info@oryxpress.com
www.oryxpress.com

Raymond Lemberg, Editor

256 pages

895 Coping with Eating Disorders
Rosen Publishing Group
29 East 21st Street
New York, NY 10010-6209
212-777-3017
800-237-9932
Fax: 888-436-4643
E-mail: info@rosenpub.com
www.rosenpublishing.com

Barbara Moe, Author

Offers practical suggestions on coping with eating disorders. *$33.25*

149 pages Year Founded: 1950 ISBN 0-823921-33-6

896 Cult of Thinness
Oxford University Press
198 Madison Avenue
New York, NY 10016-4341
212-726-6400
800-445-9714
TTY: 800-445-9714
E-mail: custserv.us@oup.com
www.www.oup.com

Sharlene Nagy Hesse-Biber, Author

Discusses eating patterns and disorders and their relationship to emotional states and self-esteem. *$29.95*

288 pages Year Founded: 2006 ISBN 0-195178-78-4

897 Developmental Psychopathology of Eating Disorders: Implications for Research, Prevention and Treatment
Lawrence Erlbaum Associates
10 Industrial Avenue
Mahwah, NJ 07430-2253
201-825-3200
800-926-6577
Fax: 201-236-0072
E-mail: orders@erlbaum.com
www.erlbaum.com

Linda Smolak, Editor
Ruth H Striegel-Moore, Editor
Michael P Levine, Editor

This text provides backround material from developmental psychology and psychopathology - following the theory that eating problems and disorders are typically rooted in childhood. Applications are then outlined, including research, treatment, protective factors and primary prevention. *$79.95*

464 pages ISBN 0-805817-46-8

898   Disordered Eating Among Athletes
Human Kinetics Publishers
1607 North Market Street
PO Box 5076
Champaign, IL 61825-5076
800-747-4457
Fax: 217-351-1549
E-mail: orders@hkusa.com

Katherine Beals, Author

Gives readers the information they need to identify and address major eating disorders such as: anorexia, bulimia nervosa, and eating disorders not otherwise specified. *$50.00*

264 pages Year Founded: 2004 ISBN 0-736042-19-2

899   Eating Disorder Hope
5112 Golden Lane
Fort Worth, TX 76123
817-231-5184
800-986-4160
Fax: 817-887-4025
E-mail: info@eatingdisorderhope.com
www.www.eatingdisorderhope.com

Jaquelyn Ekern, MS, LPC, Founder and Director
Baxter Ekern, MBA, Vice President
Crystal Karges, MS, RDN, IBCLC, Special Projects
Manager

Eating Disorder Hope was founded in January 2005. Their mission is to offer hope, information, and resources to individual eating disorder sufferers, their family members, and treatment providers.

Year Founded: 2005

900   Eating Disorders & Obesity: a Comprehensive Handbook
Guilford Press
72 Spring Street
New York, NY 10012-4068
212-431-9800
800-365-7006
Fax: 212-966-6708
E-mail: info@guilford.com

Bob Matloff, President

Presents and integrates virtually all that is currently known about eating disorders and obesity in one authorative, accessible and eminently practical volume. *$57.95*

583 pages ISBN 0-898628-50-4

901   Eating Disorders Sourcebook
Omnigraphics
155 West Congress
Suite 200
Detroit, MI 48226
313-961-1340
800-234-1340
Fax: 313-961-1383
E-mail: contact@omnigraphics.com
www.omnigraphics.com

Sandra J Judd, Author/Editor

Omnigraphics is the publisher of the Health Reference Series, a growing consumer health information resource with more than 100 volumes in print. Each title in the series features an easy to understand format, nontechnical language, comprehensive indexing and resources for further information. Material in each book has been collected from a wide range of government agencies, professional associations, periodicals and other sources. *$78.00*

583 pages Year Founded: 1985 ISBN 0-780803-35-3

902   Eating Disorders and Obesity, Second Edition : A Comprehensive Handbook
The Guilford Press
72 Spring Street
New York, NY 10012-4019
212-431-9800
800-365-7006
Fax: 212-966-6708
E-mail: info@guilford.com

Bob Matloff, President

This unique handbook presents and integrates virtually all that is currently known about eating disorders and obesity in one authoritative, accessible, and eminently practical volume.

903   Eating Disorders: Reference Sourcebook
Oryx Press
88 Post Road W
Westport, CT 06880-4208
203-226-3571
Fax: 603-431-2214
E-mail: info@oryxpress.com
www.oryxpress.com

Raymond Lemberg, Author
Leigh Cohn, Author

Listings of 200 centers and groups for care and treatment of eating disorders, such as anorexia nervosa, bulimia nervosa, and compulsive overeating. *$49.95*

272 pages

904   Emotional Eating: A Practical Guide to Taking Control
Lexington Books
4501 Forbes Boulevard
Suite 200
Lanham, MD 20706-4346
301-459-3366
800-426-6420
Fax: 301-429-5748
www.lexingtonbook.com

Edward Abramson, Author

Using case histories he explores some of the causes of emotional eating (childhood programming, family life, sexual abuse) and the manifestos of emotional eating ('sneaky snaking', grazing, and binging). Of particular interest is the last chaper, which helps the reader determine whether or not it is a good or bad time to diet. While not a diet book or a 12-step primer, this is a tool for developing healthier ways of handling emotions and food. *$19.95*

208 pages ISBN 0-029002-15-X

905   Encyclopedia of Obesity and Eating Disorders
Facts on File
11 Penn Plaza
New York, NY 10001-2006

212-290-8090
800-322-8755
Fax: 212-678-3633

From abdominoplasty to Zung Rating Scale, this volume defines and explains these disorders, along with medical and other problems associated with them. *$50.00*

272 pages

906 Feminist Perspectives on Eating Disorders
Guilford Press
72 Spring Street
New York, NY 10012-4068
212-431-9800
800-365-7006
Fax: 212-966-6708
E-mail: info@guilford.com

Bob Matloff, President

Explores the relationship between the anguish of eating disorder sufferers and the problems of ordinary women. Examines the sociocultural pressure on women to conform to culturally ideal body types and how this affects individual self concept. Controversial topics include the relationship between sexual abuse and eating disorders, the use of medications and the role of hospitalization and 12-step programs. *$ 25.95*

465 pages ISBN 1-572301-82-1

907 Food for Recovery: The Next Step
Crown Publishing Group
201 E 50th Street
New York, NY 10022-7703
212-751-2600
www.randomhouse.com

Joseph D Beasley, Author
Susan Knightly, Author

A very practicle guide on every aspect needed by the patient and counselor to utilize nutrition as a therapeutic tool. *$ 14.00*

156 pages ISBN 0-517586-94-0

908 Golden Cage, The Enigma of Anorexia Nervosa
Random House
1745 Broadway 15-3
New York, NY 10019-4368
212-572-4985
Fax: 212-782-9052
www.randomhouse.com

Hilde Bruch, Author

One of the world's leading authorities offers a vivid and moving account of the causes, effects and treatment of this devastating disease. *$9.00*

174 pages ISBN 0-394726-88-X

909 Group Psychotherapy for Eating Disorders
American Psychiatric Publishing, Inc.
1000 Wilson Boulevard
Suite 1825
Arlington, VA 22209-3901
703-907-7322
800-368-5777
Fax: 703-907-1091
E-mail: appi@psych.org
www.appi.org

Heather Harper-Giuffre, Author
K. Roy MacKenzie, Author

The first book to fully explore the use of group therapy in the treatment of eating disorders. *$101.00*

374 pages Year Founded: 1992 ISBN 0-880484-19-0

910 Hunger So Wide and Deep
University of Minnesota Press
111 Third Avenue South
Suite 290
Minneapolis, MN 55401-2520
612-627-1970
Fax: 612-627-1980
E-mail: ump@umn.edu
www.upress.umn.edu

Becky W. Thompson, Author

$19.50

176 pages Year Founded: 1925 ISBN 0-816624-35-6

911 Hungry Self; Women, Eating and Identity
Harper Collins
10 East 53rd Street
New York, NY 10022-5299
212-207-7000
E-mail: feedback2@harpercollins.com
www.harpercollins.com

Kim Chernin, Author

Answers the need for help among the five million American women who suffer from eating disorders. Paperback. *$13.00*

240 pages Year Founded: 1817 ISBN 0-060925-04-3

912 Insights in the Dynamic Psychotherapy of Anorexia and Bulimia
Jason Aronson
506 Clemant Street
San Francisco, CA 94118-2324
415-387-2272
Fax: 415-387-2377
www.greenapplebooks.com

Joyce Kraus Aronson, Author

The clinical insights that guide the dynamic psychotheray of anorexic and bulimic patients. *$45.00*

288 pages ISBN 0-876685-68-8

913 Making Peace with Food
Harper Collins
10 East 53rd Street
New York, NY 10022-5299
212-207-7000
800-242-7737
E-mail: feedback2@harpercollins.com
www.www. harpercollins.com

Susan Kano, Author

For millions of diet-conscious Americans, the scientifically proven, step-by-step guide to overcoming repeated weight loss and gain, binge eating, guilt and anxieties about food and body image. *$15.00*

272 pages Year Founded: 1989 ISBN 0-060963-28-X

914 Obesity: Mechanisms & Clinical Management
Lippincott Williams &Wilkins
I 185 Avenue of the Americas
New York, NY 10013-1209
212-930-9500
800-638-3030
Fax: 212-869-3495
www.lww.com

Robert H. Eckel, MD, Author

A classic reference for clinicians dealing with obesity, this volume provides the most up-to-date research, preclinical and clinical information. *$139.00*

566 pages Year Founded: 2003 ISBN 0-781728-44-7

915 Overeaters Anonymous
Overeaters Anonymous
6075 Zenith Court NE
Rio Rancho, NM 87144-6424
505-891-2664
Fax: 505-891-4320
E-mail: NYOAMentroOffice@yahoo.com
www.www.oa.org/

Personal stories demonstrating the struggles overcome and accomplishments made. *$7.50*

204 pages Year Founded: 1958

916 Psychobiology and Treatment of Anorexia Nervosa and Bulimia Nervosa
American Psychiatric Publishing, Inc.
1000 Wilson Boulevard
Suite 1825
Arlington, VA 22209-3901
703-907-7322
800-368-5777
Fax: 703-907-1091
E-mail: appi@psych.org
www.appi.org

Katherine A. Halmi, MD, Editor

Combines clinical research concerning these distinct disorders and provides an overview of the psychobiology and treatment. *$101.00*

376 pages Year Founded: 1992 ISBN 0-880485-06-7

917 Psychosomatic Families: Anorexia Nervosa in Context
Harvard University Press
79 Garden Street
Cambridge, MA 02138-1400
617-495-2600
Fax: 617-495-5898
E-mail: contact_hup@harvard.edu
www.www.hup.harvard.edu

Salvador Minuchin, Author
Bernice L Rosman, Author
Lester Baker, Author

Hardcover. *$76.50*

351 pages Year Founded: 1913 ISBN 0-674722-20-0

918 Shame and Anger: The Criticism Connection
Change for Good Coaching and Counseling
3801 Connecticut Avenue NorthWest
Washington, DC 20008-4530
202-362-3009
Fax: 202-204-6100
E-mail: brockhansenlcsw@aol.com
www.change-for-good.org

Brock Hansen LCSW, Author

Coaching on learnable emotional skills to see goals clearly, harness resources and get moving toward a successful outcome. *$16.98*

226 pages ISBN 0-615135-81-6

919 Surviving an Eating Disorder: Perspectives and Strategies
Harper Collins
10 East 53rd Street
New York, NY 10022-5299
212-207-7000
E-mail: feedback2@harpercollins.com
www.www.harpercollins.com

Michele Siegel, Author
Judith Brisman, PhD, Author
Margot Weinshel, MSW, Author

Addresses the cutting-edge advances made in the field of eating disorders, discusses how the changes in health care have affected treatment and provides additional strategies for dealing with anorexia, bulimia and binge eating disorder. It also includes updated readings and a list of support organizations. A terrrific resource for those suffering from eating disorders, their families and professionals. Paperback. *$ 35.00*

288 pages Year Founded: 1817 ISBN 0-060952-33-4

920 Treating Eating Disorders
Jossey-Bass Publishers
10475 Crosspoint Boulevard
Indianapolis, IN 46256-3386
877-762-2974
Fax: 800-597-3299
E-mail: consumers@wiley.com
www.josseybass.com

Joellen Werne, Author

Details how some of the most eminent clinicians in the field combine and intergrate a wide variety of contemporary therapies — ranging from psychodynamic to systematic to cognitive behavioral—to successfully treat clients with anorexia nervosa, bulimia nervosa, and binge eating diorders. Filled with up to date information and important approaches to assessment and treatment, the book offers a hands-on approach that cogently illustrates both theory and technique. *$29.95*

377 pages ISBN 0-787903-30-2

921 When Food Is Love
Geneen Roth and Associates
PO Box 682
Aptos, CA 95001
703-401-0871
877-243-6336
Fax: 703-852-3956
E-mail: info@geneenroth.com
www.geneenroth.com

Geneen Roth, Author

Shows how dieting and compulsive eating often become a subsititue for intimacy. Drawing on painful personal experiece as well as the candid stories of those she has helped in her seminars, Roth claims the crucial issues that surrounds compulsive eating: need for control, dependency on melodrama, desire for what is forbidden, and the belief that the wrong move can mean catastrophe. She shows why many people overeat in an attempt to satisfy their emotional hunger, and why weight loss frequently just uncovers a new set of problems. This book will help readers break destructive, self-perpetuating patterns and learn to satisfy all the hungers - physical and emotional - that makes us human. *$13.98*

205 pages Year Founded: 1992

Periodicals & Pamphlets

922 Anorexia: Am I at Risk?
ETR Associates
4 Carbonero Way
Scotts Valley, CA 95066-4200
831-438-4060
800-321-4407
Fax: 831-438-3618
E-mail: customerservice@etr.org
www.etr.org

David Kitchen, MBA, Chief Operations Officer
Laurie Searson, Publisher
Sarah Stevens, Director, Product Development
Yvonne Collins, Sales Director

Offers a clear overview of anorexia; Lists symptoms; Explains helath problems.

923 Body Image
ETR Associates
4 Carbonero Way
Scotts Valley, CA 95066-4200
831-438-4060
800-321-4407
Fax: 831-438-3618
E-mail: support@etr.freshdesk.com
www.etr.org

David Kitchen, MBA, Chief Financial Officer
Talita Sanders, BS, Director, Human Resources
Coleen Cantwell, MPH, Director, Business Development Pl
Matt McDowell, BS, Director, Marketing

Discusses the difference between healthy and distorted body image; the link between poor body image and low self esteem; five point list to help people check out their own body image.

924 Bulimia
ETR Associates
4 Carbonero Way
Scotts Valley, CA 95066-4200
831-438-4060
800-321-4407
Fax: 831-438-3618
E-mail: customerservice@etr.org
www.etr.org

Bonnie Graves, Author
Laurie Searson, Publisher
Sarah Stevens, Director, Product Development
Yvonne Collins, Sales Director

Includes warning signs that someone's bulimic, health consequesnces of bulimia, and how to help a friend.

925 Eating Disorder Sourcebook
Gurze Books
PO Box 2238
Carlsbad, CA 92018-2238
760-434-7533
800-756-7533
Fax: 760-434-5476
E-mail: info@gurze.net
www.gurze.net

Carolyn Costin, Author
Lindsay Cohn, Co-Owner

Includes 125 books and tapes on eating disorders and related subjects for both lay and professional audiences, basic facts about eating disorders, a list of national organizations and treatment facilities. Also publishes a bimonthly newsletter for clinicians and are executive editors of Eating Disorders the Journal of Treatment and Prevention.

336 pages 1 per year

926 Eating Disorders
ETR Associates
4 Carbonero Way
Scotts Valley, CA 95066-4200
831-438-4060
800-321-4407
Fax: 831-438-3618
E-mail: support@etr.freshdesk.com
www.etr.org

David Kitchen, MBA, Chief Financial Officer
Talita Sanders, BS, Director, Human Resources
Coleen Cantwell, MPH, Director, Business Development Pl
Matt McDowell, BS, Director, Marketing

Includes anorexia and bulimia, eating patterns versus eating disorders, treatment and getting help.

927 Eating Disorders Factsheet
SAMHSA'S National Mental Health Information Center
PO Box 42557
Washington, DC 20015-557
800-789-2647
Fax: 240-747-5470
TDD: 866-889-2647
E-mail: ken@mentalhealth.org
www.mentalhealth.samhsa.gov

A Kathryn Power, MEd, Director
Edward B Searle, Deputy Director

This fact sheet provides basic information on the symptoms, medical complications, formal diagnosis, and treatment for anorexia nervousa and bulimia nervosa.

2 pages

928 Eating Disorders: Facts About Eating Disorders and the Search for Solutions
National Institute of Mental Health
6001 Executive Boulevard
Room 8184, MSC 9663
Bethesda, MD 20892-9663
301-443-4513
866-615-6464
TTY: 301-443-8431
E-mail: nimhinfo@nih.gov
www.www.nimh.nih.gov/

Francis S Collins PhD, Director

Eating is controlled by many factors, including appetite, food availability, family, peer, and cultural practices, and attempts at voluntary control. Dieting to a body weight leaner than needed for health is highly promoted by current fashion trends, sales campaigns for special foods, and in some activities and professions. Eating disorders involve serious disturbances in eating behavior, such as extreme and unhealthy reduction of food intake or severe overeating, as well as feelings of distress or extreme concern about body shape or weight. There is help, and there is every hope for recovery.

8 pages

929 Fats of Life
ETR Associates
4 Carbonero Way
Scotts Valley, CA 95066-4200
831-438-4060
800-321-4407
Fax: 831-438-3618
E-mail: customerservice@etr.org
www.etr.org

Caroline M Pond, Author
Laurei Searson, Publisher
Sarah Stevens, Director, Product Development
Yvonne Collins, Sales Director

Stresses that health, not body weight, is what's important; dispels myths about dieting; includes chart to help people determine their body mass index.

344 pages

930 Food and Feelings
ETR Associates
4 Carbonero Way
Scotts Valley, CA 95066-4200
831-438-4060
800-321-4407
Fax: 831-438-3618
E-mail: customerservice@etr.org
www.etr.org

David Kitchen, Chief Operations Officer
Laurie Searson, Publisher
Sarah Stevens, Director, Product Development
Yvonne Collins, Sales Director

Helps students recognize eating disorders; emphasizes the seriousness of eating disorders; encourages the sufferers to seek treatment.

931 Getting What You Want from Your Body Image
ETR Associates
4 Carbonero Way
Scotts Valley, CA 95066-4200
831-438-4060
800-321-4407
Fax: 831-438-3618
E-mail: support@etr.freshdesk.com
www.etr.org

Melinda M Mueller, Author
Laurie Searson, Publisher
Sarah Stevens, Director, Product Development
Yvonne Collins, Sales Director

Discusses topics such as the influence of the media, the truth about dieting, and body image survival tips.

8 pages

932 Restrictive Eating
ETR Associates
4 Carbonero Way
Scotts Valley, CA 95066-4200
831-438-4060
800-321-4407
Fax: 831-438-3618
E-mail: customerservice@etr.org
www.etr.org

David Kitchen, MBA, Chief Operations Officer
Laurie Searson, Publisher

Discusses the spectrum of eating patterns, signs of restrictive eating and why it is a problem, how to help a friend, and where to go for help.

933 Teen Image
ETR Associates
4 Carbonero Way
Scotts Valley, CA 95066-4200
831-438-4060
800-321-4407
Fax: 831-438-3618
E-mail: customerservice@etr.org
www.etr.org

Mary Nelson, President

Dispels unrealistic media images; offers ways to boost body image and self esteem; includes tips to maintain a good body image.

934 Working Together
National Association of Anorexia Nervosa and Associated Disorders
750 East Diehl Road
Suite 127
Naperville, IL 60563
630-577-1333
630-577-1330
Fax: 847-433-4632
E-mail: anadhelp@anad.org
www.anad.org

Laura Discipio, LCSW, Executive Director
Donna Rostamian, Community Organisational Manager
Melanie Zumm, Support Group Coordinator
Kyron Johnson-Brana, Administrative Assistant

Designed for individuals, families, group leaders and professionals concerned with eating disorders. Provides updates on treatments, resources, conferences, programs, articles by therapists, recovered victims, group members and leaders.

2 pages 4 per year Year Founded: 1976

Research Centers

935 Center for the Study of Anorexia and Bulimia
1841 Broadway 4th Floor
New York, NY 10023-7603
212-333-3444
Fax: 212-333-5444
E-mail: csab@icpnyc.orgg
www.www.icpnyc.org/csab/

Jill M Pollack, Director
Jill E Daino, Co-Director
Tracy McClair, CSAB Program Administrator

Established as a division of the Institute for Contemporary Psychotherapy in 1979 and is the oldest non-profit eating disorders clinic in New York City. Using an eclectic approach, the professional staff and affiliates are on the cutting edge of treatment in their field. The treatment staff includes social workers, psychologists, registered nurses and nutritionists, all with special training in the treatment of eating disorders.

Year Founded: 1979

936 Obesity Research Center
St. Luke's-Roosevelt Hospital
1111 Amsterdam Ave., Babcock 10
New York, NY 10025
212-523-4161
Fax: 212-523-4830
E-mail: katmarquez@chpnet.org
www.www.nyorc.org/

Lee C Bollinger, President
John H Coatsworth, Provost
Robert Kasdin, Sr Executive Vice President
Nicholas B Dirks, EVP, Arts ans Sciences

Helps reduce the the incidence of obesity and related diseases through leadership in basic research, clinical research, epidemiology and public health, patient care, and public education.

937 UAMS Psychiatric Research Institute
4224 Shuffield Drive
Little Rock, AR 72205
501-526-8100
Fax: 501-660-7542
E-mail: kramerteresal@uams.edu
www.www.psychiatry.uams.edu

Dan Rahn, MD, Chancellor

Combining research, education and clinical services into one facility, PRI offers inpatiend and outpatient services, with 40 psychiatric beds, therapy options, and specialized treatment for specific disorders, including: addictive eating, anxiety, deppressive and post-traumatic stress disorders. Research focuses on evidence-based care takes into consideration the education of future medical personnel while relying on research scientists to provide innovative forms of treatment. PRI includes the Center for Addiction Research as well as a methadone clinic.

938 University of Pennsylvania Weight and Eating Disorders Program
3535 Market Street
Suite 3108
Philadelphia, PA 19104-3313
215-898-7314
Fax: 215-898-2878
E-mail: cwilson@mail.med.upenn.edu
www.www.med.upenn.edu/weight/

Dwight L. Evans, MD, Chair

Conducts a wide variety of studies on the causes and treatment of weight-related disorders.

Support Groups & Hot Lines

939 Food Addicts Anonymous
529 N W Prima Vista Blvd.
#301 A
Port St. Lucie, FL 34983

772-878-9657
E-mail: faawso@bellsouth.net
www.foodaddictsanonymous.org

Linda Closy, Manager

The FAA program is based on the belief that food addiction is a bio-chemical disease. We share our experience, strength, and hope with others allows us to recover from this disease.

940 MEDA
92 Pearl Street
Newton, MA 02458-1529
617-558-1881
866-343-6332
E-mail: info@medainc.org
www.medainc.org

Rachel Benson, Clinical Programs Coordinator
Beth Mayer, LICSW, Executive Director
Lindsay Brady, LICSW, Clinical Director
Susie Stockwell, Communications and Development D

MEDA ia a nonprofit organization dedicated to the prevention and treatment of eating disorders and disordered eating. MEDA'S mission is to prevent the continuing spread of eating disorders through educational awareness and early detection. MEDA serves as a support network and resource for clients, loved ones, clinicians, educators and the general public.

941 National Center for Overcoming Overeating
PO Box 1257
Old Chelsea Station
New York, NY 10113-1257
212-875-0442
E-mail: webmaster@overcomingovereating.com
www.overcomingovereating.com

Is an educational and training organization working to end body hatred and dieting.

942 Overeaters Anonymous General Service Office
6075 Zenith Court, NorthEast
Rio Rancho, NM 87144-6424
505-891-2664
Fax: 505-891-4320
E-mail: info@oa.org
www.oa.org

OA offers a program of recovery from compulsive eating using the Twelve Steps and Twelve Traditions of OA. It addresses physical, emotional and spiritual well-being.

Year Founded: 1960

Video & Audio

943 Eating Disorder Video
Active Parenting Publishers
1955 Vaughn Road NW
Suite 108
Kennesaw, GA 30144-7808
770-429-0565
800-825-0060
Fax: 770-429-0334
E-mail: cservice@activeparenting.com

Features compelling interviews with several young people who have suffered from anorexia nervosa, bulimia and compulsive eating. Discusses the treatments, causes and techniques for prevention with field experts. *$39.95*

ISSN Q6456

Web Sites

944 **www.anred.com**
Anorexia Nervosa and Related Eating Disorders

The factual materials are detailed and organized.

945 **www.bulimia.us.com**
Bulimia: News & Discussion Forum

Eating disorders forum with news and information about bulimia, anorexia, male and teen eating disorders; treatment, help and resources information, events and inspirational stories.

946 **www.closetoyou.org/eatingdisorders**
Close to You

Information about eating disorders, anorexia, bulimia, binge eating disorder, and compulsive overeating.

947 **www.cyberpsych.org**
CyberPsych

Hosts the American Psychoanalyists Foundation, American Association of Suicideology, Society for the Exploration of Psychotherapy Intergration, and Anxiety Disorders Association of America. Also subcategories of the anxiety disorders, as well as general information, including panic disorder, phobias, obsessive compulsive disorder (OCD), social phobia, generalized anxiety disorder, post traumatic stress disorder, and phobias of childhood. Book reviews and links to web pages sharing the topics.

948 **www.edap.org**
Eating Disorders Awareness and Prevention

A source of educational brochures and curriculum materials.

949 **www.gurze.com**
Gurze Bookstore

Hundreds of books on eating disorders.

950 **www.healthyplace.com/Communities/**
Peace, Love, and Hope

Click on Body Views for information on body dysmorphic disorder.

951 **www.kidsource.com/nedo/**
National Eating Disorders Organization

Educational materials on dynamics, causative factors and evaluating treatment options.

952 **www.mentalhelp.net**
Anorexia Nervosa General Information

Introductory text on Anorexia Nervosa.

953 **www.mirror-mirror.org/eatdis.htm**
Mirror, Mirror

Relapse prevention for eating disorders.

954 **www.planetpsych.com**
Planetpsych.com

Learn about disorders, their treatments and other topics in psychology. Articles are listed under the related topic areas. Ask a therapist a question for free, or view the directory of professionals in your area. If you are a therapist sign up for the directory. Current features, self-help, interactive, and newsletter archives.

955 **www.psychcentral.com**
Psych Central

Personalized one-stop index for psychology, support, and mental health issues, resources, and people on the Internet.

956 **www.something-fishy.com**
Something Fishy Music and Publishing

Continuously educating the world on eating disorders to encourage every sufferer towards recovery.

Gender Identity Disorder

Introduction

With a wide scope of questions and confusion surrounding human sexuality and gender-explicit roles in the modern era, many children, adolescents and adults have been perplexed by the concepts of homosexuality and cross-gender identification. Homosexuality is a matter of sexual orientation: whether one is sexually attracted to men or women. The American Psychiatric Association ceased to classify homosexuality as an illness in 1973. Gender identity, in contrast, is a matter of what gender one feels oneself to be; people with Gender Identity Disorder feel that their psychological experience conflicts with the physical body with which they were born. Gender Identity Disorders can have serious social and occupational repercussions.

Diagnosis of Gender Identity Disorder requires two sets of criteria: (1) a heavy and persistent insistence that the individual is, or has a strong desire to be, of the opposite sex, and (2) a constant discomfort about his/her designated sex, a feeling of inappropriateness towards his/her biological designation. Typically, boys meeting critera for the disorder are predisposed to dressing as girls, drawing explicit pictures of females, playing with pre-designated feminine toys, fantasizing and role playing as females and interacting primarily with girls. Girls with the condition tend to participate in contact sports, have an aversion to wearing dresses, are often mistaken for boys due to attire and hair style, and may assert that they will develop in to men. For adolescents and adults, ostracism in school and the workplace is likely to occur, as is a profound inability to associate with others and poor relationships with family members and members of either sex.

There is a sharp divide among persons whose biological gender feels wrong; some insist that this is not a psychiatric disorder but rather a biological variant; others feel strongly that they have a psychiatric disorder. Some of this conviction is driven by the need to demonstrate 'medical necessity' in order for health insurance to cover hormonal or surgical interventions to make the individual look like the gender he or she feels they are.

SYMPTOMS

In boys
• A marked preoccupation with traditionally feminine activites;
• A preference for dressing as a girl;
• Attraction to stereotypical female games and toys;
• Portraying female characters in role playing;
• Assertion he is a girl;
• Insistence on sitting to urinate;
• Displaying disgust for his genitals, wishing to remove them.

In girls
• Aversion to traditional female attire;
• Shared interest in contact games;
• A preference for associating with boys;
• Refusing to urinate sitting down;
• Show little interest in playing with stereotypical female toys such as dolls;
• Assertion that she will grow a penis, not breasts;
• Identification with strong male figures.

In adolescents
• Ostracism in school and social situations;
• Social isolation, peer rejection and peer teasing;
• Significant cross-gender identification and mannerisms;
• Similar symptoms as children.

In adults
• Adoption of social roles, physical appearance, and mannerisms of opposite sex;
• Surgical and/or hormonal manipulation of biological state;
• Discomfort in being regarded by others, or functioning, as his/her designated sex;
• Cross-dressing;
• Transvestic Fetishism.

ASSOCIATED FEATURES

Those who have Gender Identity Disorder are at risk of mental and physical harm resulting, not from the condition itself, but from the reactions of other people to the condition. In children, a manifestation of Separation Anxiety Disorder, Generalized Anxiety Disorder and symptoms of Depression may result. For adolescents, depression and suicidal thoughts or ideas, as well as actual suicide attempts can result from prolonged feelings of ostracism by peers. Relationships with either one or both parents may weaken from resentment, lack of communication and misunderstanding; many with this disorder may drop out of or avoid school due to peer teasing. For many, lives are built around attempts to decrease gender distress. They are often preoccupied with appearance. In extreme cases, males with the disorder perform their own castration. Prostitution has been linked with the disorder because young people who are rejected by their families and ostracized by others may resort to prostitution as the only way to support themselves, a practice which increases the risk of acquiring sexually transmitted diseases. Some people with the disorder resort to substance abuse and other forms of abuse in an attempt to deal with the associated stress.

TREATMENT OPTIONS

Therapists who attempt to pathologize and 'cure' sexual orientation have been generally unsuccessful. So-called conversion therapy can cause more harm than good. In contrast, some people with Gender Identity Disorder decide to live as members of the opposite sex; some choose to undergo sex-change surgery. There is some controversy about the diagnosis; 'transsexual' groups protest that their condition, like homosexuality, should not be classified as a mental disease. Psychological assistance can help individuals to gain acceptance of themselves, and can teach methods of dealing with discrimination, prejudice and violence.

Associations & Agencies

958 Center for Mental Health Services (CMHS)
1 Choke Cherry Road
Room 6-1057
Rockville, MD 20857
240-276-1310
877-726-4727
Fax: 240-276-1320
TDD: 800-487-4889
E-mail: info@mentalhealth.org
www.beta.samhsa.gov/about-us/who-we-are/offices-center

Michael E Etzinger, B.S.M.E, , M.B., SAMHSA Executive Officer, Director
Paolo Del Vecchio, M.S.W, Director, Center for Mental Healt
Deborah Baldwin, M.P.A, Acting Director, Consumer Affairs
Elizabeth Lopez, Ph.D, Acting Deputy Director

CMHS leads Federal efforts to treat mental illnesses by promoting mental health and by preventing the development or worsening of mental illness when possible. Congress created CMHS to bring new hope to adults who have serious mental illnesses and to children with serious emotional disorders. CMHS provides information about mental health via a toll-free the web site, and more than 600 publications. Developed for users of mental health services and their families, the general public, policy makers, providers, and the media.

Year Founded: 1992

959 CenterLink
PO Box 24490
Ft Lauderdale, FL 33307
954-765-6024
954-765-6024
Fax: 954-206-0469
E-mail: centerlink@lgbtcenters.org
www.www.lgbtcenters.org

Terry Stone, CEO
Dr Scout , Director
Denise Spivak, Director of Member Relations and
Jake Tolan, Executive Assistant

CenterLink was founded in 1994 as a member based coalition to support the development of strong, sustainable LGBT communtiy centers. The organization has played an important role in supporting the growth of LGBT centers acroos the country addressing the challenges they face with gender orientation and sexual preference.

960 Gender Identity Disorder Reform Advocates
3895 Upham Street
Suite 40
Wheat Ridge, CO 80033
303-202-6466
888-462-8932
E-mail: kelley@gidreform.org
www.gidreform.org

Andrea Planelles, President
Olga C Baselga, Vice President
Riki Wilchins, Executive Director

Mental health and medical professional, clinicians, researchers, and scholars concerned about psychiatric nomenclature and diagnostic criteria for genedr variant, gender nonconforming, transgender, and transexual people to be specified in the Fifth Edition of the Diagnostic and Statistical Manual of Mental Disorders frothcoming from the American Psychiatric Association.

961 Human Rights Campaign
1640 Rhode Island Ave N.W.
Washington, DC 20036-3278
202-628-4160
800-777-4723
Fax: 202-347-5323
TTY: 202-216-1572
E-mail: info@hrc.org
www.www.hrc.org

Joe Solmonese, President
Susanne Salkind, Managing Director
Donna Payne, Director, Diversity
Cuc Vu, Chief Diversity Officer

Founded in 1980, HRC advocates on behalf of LGBT Americans, mobilizes grassroots actions in diverse communities, invests strategically to elect fair-minded individuals to office and educates the public about LGBT issues.

962 National Association for the Dually Diagnosed (NADD)
132 Fair Street
Kingston, NY 12401-4802
845-331-4336
800-331-5362
Fax: 845-331-4569
E-mail: info@thenadd.org
www.thenadd.org

Donna McNELIS, PhD, President
Robert J Fletcher DSW, Chief Executive Officer
Dan Baker, PhD, Vice President
Julia Pearce, Secretary

Nonprofit organization designed to promote interest of professional and parent development with resources for individuals who have the coexistence of mental illness and mental retardation. Provides conferences, educational services and training materials to professionals, parents, concerned citizens and service organizations.

Year Founded: 1983

963 National Coalition for LGBT Health
1325 Massachusetts Ave, NW
Suite 705
Washington, DC 20005
202-558-6828
Fax: 202-393-2241
E-mail: coalition@lgbthealth.net
www.lgbthealth.webolutionary.com/

Veronica Bayetti Flores, MPH, Board Co-Chair
JoAnne G Keatley, MSW, Board Co-Chair
Leslie Calman, PhD, Board Secretary
Terry Stone, Board Treasurer

The National Coalition for LGBT Health, a coalition of over 70 state and national organizational advocates and health services providers for lesbian, gay, bisexual, transgendered, and those with gender identity issues.

964 National Commission on Correctional Heath Care
1145 West Diversey Parkway
Chicago, IL 60614
773-880-1460
Fax: 773-880-2424
E-mail: info@ncchc.org
www.ncchc.org

Renee Kanan, MD, Chairman
Edward Harrison, CCHP, President
Thomas J Fagan, PhD, CCHP-MH, Treasurer
Jayne Russell, Med, CCHP-A, Secretary

The National Commission on Correctional Health Care is commited to improving the quality of healthcare for individuals with gender identity disorders.

Year Founded: 1983

965 National Gay and Lesbian Task Force
1325 Massachusetts Avenue NorthWest
Suite 600
Washington, DC 20005-4171
202-393-5177
Fax: 202-393-2241
E-mail: info@TheTaskForce.org
www.thetaskforce.org

Liebe Gadinsky, Co-Chair
Shilpen Patel, Co-Chair
Rea Carey, Executive Director
Brian Johnson, Chief Financial Officer

Offers community support for gay and lesbian individuals.

Year Founded: 1973

966 National Institute of Mental Health
6001 Executive Blvd
Room 6200, MSC 9663
Bethesda, MD 20892-9663
301-443-4513
866-615-6464
TTY: 301-443-8431
E-mail: nimhinfo@nih.gov
www.www.nimh.nih.go

Francis S Collins, PhD, Director

The mission of the National Institute of Mental Health is to reduce the burden of mental illness and behavioral disorders through research on mind, brain, and behavior.

967 National Mental Health Consumers' Self-Help Clearinghouse
1211 Chestnut Street
Suite 1100
Philadelphia, PA 19107-4103
215-751-1810
800-553-4539
Fax: 215-636-6312
E-mail: info@mhselfhelp.org
www.mhselfhelp.org

Joseph Rogers, Executive Director/ Founder
Susan Rogers, Director
Britani Nestel, Program Specialist
Christa Burkett, Technical Assistance Coordinator

A consumer-run national technical assistance center serving the mental health consumer movement. They connect individuals to self-help and advocacy resources, and offer expertise to self-help groups and other peer-run services for mental health consumers.

Year Founded: 1986

968 Parents and Friends of Lesbians and Gays
1828 L Street, NW
Suite 660
Washington, DC 20036
202-467-8180
Fax: 202-467-8194
E-mail: info@pflag.org
www.www.pflag.org

Rabbi David Horowitz, President
Jody M Huckaby, Executive Director
Elizabeth Kohm, Deputy Executive Director
Peggy Moore, Vice President

Organization of families and friends of lesbian and gay individuals, dedicated to offer support and understanding.

969 Parents, Families and Friends of Lesbians and Gays
1828 L Street, NW
Suite 660
Washington, DC 20036
202-467-8180
Fax: 202-467-8194
E-mail: info@pflag.org
www.www.pflag.org

Rabbi David Horowitz, President
Jody M Huckaby, Executive Director
Elizabeth Kohm, Deputy Executive Director
Peggy Moore, Vice President

A national non-profit organization with over 200, 000 members and supporters and over 500 affiliates in the United States.

970 SAMHSA's National Mental Health Information Center
PO Box 42557
Washington, DC 20015-557
240-221-4021
800-789-2647
Fax: 240-221-4295
TDD: 866-889-2647
www.mentalhealth.samhsa.gov

A Kathryn Power MEd, Director
Edward B Searle, Deputy Director

971 The Center for Family Support
2811 Zulette Avenue
Bronx, NY 10461
718-518-1500
Fax: 718-518-8200
www.cfsny.org

Steven Vernikoff, Executive Director
Virgil Seepersad, Director of Finance
Eileen Berg, Director of Quality Assurance
Barbara Greenwald, Associate Executive, Director

An agency that continues to develop new programs to serve families and individuals with their care needs. They currently offer services throughout the New York City region including: New Jersey, Long Island and the Lower Hudson Valley.

Year Founded: 1954

Books

972 Gender Identity Disorder: A Medical Dictionary, Bibliography, and Annotated Research Guide to Internet References
ICON Health Publications
7404 Trade Street
San Diego, CA 92121-3414
858-635-9414

Icon Group

This book was created for medical professionals, students, and members of the general public who want to conduct medical research using the most advanced tools available and spending the least amount of time doing so. *$28.95*

64 pages Year Founded: 2004 ISBN 0-497004-51-8

973 Handbook of Sexual and Gender Identity Disorder
John Wiley & Sons
111 River Street
Hoboken, NJ 07030-5774
201-748-6000
Fax: 201-748-6088
E-mail: info@wiley.com
www.wiley.com

David L. Rowland, Editor
Luca Incrocci, Editor

The Handbook of Sexual and Gender Identity Disorders provides mental health professionals a comprehensive yet practical guide to the understanding, diagnosis, and treatment of a variety of sexual problems. *$120.00*

696 pages Year Founded: 2008 ISBN 0-471767-38-1

974 Identity Without Selfhood
32 Avenue of the Americas
New York, NY 10013-2473
212-337-5000
E-mail: newyork@cambrigde.org
www.www.cambridge.org

Mariam Fraser, Author

226 pages Year Founded: 1534

975 Sexual Signatures: On Being a Man or a Woman
John Wiley & Sons
111 River Street
Hoboken, NJ 07030-5790
201-748-6000
Fax: 201-748-6088
E-mail: info@wiley.com
www.wiley.com

John Money, Author
Patricia Tucker, Author

Sexual differentiations begins before birth and extends through puberty, when the sexual hormones become active. Case histories of children born with sexual anomalies becoming satisfactorily 'masculine' or 'feminine.' This shows how strongly culture shapes gender-personalitites. *$19.95*

250 pages Year Founded: 1975 ISBN 0-471767-38-1

Periodicals & Pamphlets

976 Similarities and Differences Between Sexual Orientation and Gender Identity
PFLAG
PO Box 3313
San Luis Obispo, CA 93403
805-801-2186
E-mail: pflag.slo@gmail.com
www.pflagcentralcoastchapter.net

Moises Torreblanca, President
John Sullivan, Vice President
Val Barboza, Treasurer
Barabara Adams, Secretary

An explanation of the simialrities and differences of both a person sexual orientation and how they relate to gender.

977 The United Nations Speaks Out: Tackling Discrimination on Grounds of Sexual Orientation and Gender Identity
Unesco-Globe NY
E-mail: unescoglobe@gmail.com
www.www.unescoglobe.wordpress.com

Irina Bokova, UNESCO Director-General
Engida Getachew, Deputy Director-General, UNESCO
Year Founded: 2010

Support Groups & Hot Lines

978 Gender Trust
76 The Ridgeway
Astwood Bank, B96 6LX, WO
527-894-838
E-mail: info@gendertrust.org.uk
www.gendertrust.org.uk

Gender Trust is a listening ear, a caring support and an information centre for anyone with any question or problem concerning their gender identity, or whose loved one is struggling with gender identity issues.

979 TransYouth Family Allies
PO Box 1471
Holland, MI 49422-1471
888-462-8932
E-mail: info@imatyfa.org
www.imatyfa.org

Shannon Garcia, Founding Member, President
Lisa Gilinger, Vice President
Amy G., Founding Member, Treasurer
Kim Pearson, Founding Member, Training Direct

TYFA empowers children and families by partnering with educators, service providers and communities to develop supportive environments in which gender may be expressed and respected.

Year Founded: 2006

Web Sites

980 www.cyberpsych.org
CyberPsych

Presents information about psychoanalysis, psychotherapy and special topics such as anxiety disorders, the problematic use of alcohol, homophobia, and the traumatic effects of racism.

981 www.health.nih.gov
National Institutes of Health

Part of the U.S. Department of Health and Human Services that is the nation's medical research agency-making important medical discoveries that improve health and save lives.

982 www.healthfinder.gov
Healthfinder

Developed by the U.S. Department of Health and Human Services, a key resource for finding the best government and nonprofit health and human services information on the internet.

983 **www.intelihealth.com**
Aetna InteliHealth

Aetna InteliHealth's mission is to empower people with
trusted solutions for healthier lives.

984 **www.kidspeace.org**
KidsPeace

KidsPeace is a private charity dedicated to serving the behavioral and mental health needs of children,
preadolescents and teens.

985 **www.mayohealth.com**
Mayo Clinic Health Oasis

Their mission is to empower people to manage their health.
They accomplish this by providing useful and up-to-date
information and tools that reflect the expertise and standard
of excellence of Mayo Clinic.

986 **www.nlm.nih.gov**
National Library of Medicine

The National Library of Medicine (NLM), on the campus
of the National Institutes of Health in Bethesda, Maryland,
is the world's largest medical library. The Library collects
materials and provides information and research services in
all areas of biomedicine and health care

987 **www.planetpsych.com**
Planet Psych

The online resource for mental health information

988 **www.psychcentral.com**
Psych Central

The Internet's largest and oldest independent mental health
social network created and run by mental health professionals to guarantee reliable, trusted information and support
communities.

Conferences & Meetings

989 **Religion and Gender: Identity, Conflict, and**
Power Conference
Feminist Studies in Religion
Harvard Divinity School
45 Francis Avenue
Cambridge, MA 02138
617-384-8046
E-mail: fsr@fsrinc.org
www.www. fsrinc.org

Dr Pushpa Iyer, Conference Chair
Quinn Van Valler-Campbell, Conference Administrator
Judith Plaskow, Founding Editor
Elisabeth Sch☐ssler Fiorenza, Founding Editor

The conference will highlight the complex relationships between religion and gender in a global context. It seeks to
explore conflicts that arise at the nexus of gender and religion while simultaneously promoting spaces for empowerment that arise in these interactions.

Year Founded: 1983

Impulse Control Disorders

Introduction

Everyone has experienced a situation in which they are tempted to do something that is harmful to themselves or others. This kind of behavior only becomes a disorder when a person is repeatedly and persistently unable to resist a temptation which is always harmful to them or to others. Usually the person feels a rising tension before acting on the need, feels pleasure and relief when giving in to the impulse and, sometimes, feels remorse and guilt afterwards. Four different disorders are included in this category.

KLEPTOMANIA

Symptoms
• Recurrent failure to resist the impulse to steal objects; often they are objects the individual could have paid for or doesn't particularly want;
• Increased sense of tension immediately before the theft;
• Pleasure and relief during the stealing;
• The theft is not due to anger, delusions or hallucinations.
• Awareness that stealing is senseless and wrong;
• Feelings of depression and guilt after stealing.

Associated Features
Kleptomania should not be confused with thefts which are deliberate and for personal gain, or those that are sometimes done by adolescents on a dare or as a rite of passage. Kleptomania is strongly associated with Depression, Anxiety Disorders, and Eating Disorders.

Prevalence
Kleptomania appears to be very rare; fewer than five percent of shoplifters have the disorder. However, Kleptomania is usually kept secret by the person, so this estimate may be low. It is much more common among females than males and may continue in spite of convictions for shoplifting.

Treatment Options
Behavior therapy, which is psychotherapy focusing on changing the behavior, has had some success, as has anti-depressant medication. A combination of these is most likely to help the person curb the impulse to steal while treating some of the underlying problems.

PYROMANIA

Symptoms
• Purposefully setting fires more than once;
• Increased tension before the deed;
• Fascination with and curiosity about fire and its paraphernalia;
• Pleasure or relief when setting or watching fires;
• The fire is not set for financial gain, revenge, or political reasons.

Associated Features
Many with this disorder make complicated preparations for setting a fire, and seem not to care about the serious consequences. They may get pleasure from the destruction. Most juveniles who set fires also have symptoms of Attention-Deficit/Hyperactivity Disorder or Adjustment Disorder.

Prevalence

Over forty percent of people arrested for arson in the US are under 18, but among children, the disorder is rare. Fire setting occurs mostly among males, and is more common for males with alcohol problems, learning problems and poor social skills.

Treatment Options
There is no agreed-upon best treatment. Pyromania is difficult to treat because the person usually does not take responsibility for the fire setting, and is in denial. Psychotherapy focused on the individual and with the family have been helpful. There is some indication that antidepressants may be effective.

PATHOLOGICAL GAMBLING

Symptoms
• Recurrent gambling;
• Gambling distrupts family, personal and work activities;
• Preoccupation with gambling, thinking about past plays, planning future gambling and how to get money for more gambling;
• Seeks excitement more than money. Bets become bigger and risks greater to produce the needed excitement;
• Gambling continues despite repeated efforts to stop with accompanying restlessness and irritability;
• Person may gamble to escape depression, anxiety, guilt;
• Chasing losses may become a pattern;
• May lie to family, therapists, and others to conceal gambling;
• May turn to criminal behavior (forgery, fraud, theft) to get money for gambling;
• May lose job, relationships, career opportunities;
Bailout behavior, that is turning to family and others, when in desperate financial straits.

Associated Features
Compulsive gamblers are distorted in their thinking. They are superstitious, deny they have a problem, and may be overconfident. They believe that money is the cause of, and solution to, all their problems. They are often competitive and easily bored. They may be extravagantly generous and very concerned with other people's approval. Compulsive gamblers are prone to medical problems connected with stress, such as hypertension and migraine. They also have a higher rate of Attention-Deficit/Hyperactivity Disorder; up to seventy-five percent suffer from Major Depressive Disorder, one third from Bipolar Disorder, and more than fifty percent abuse alcohol. Twenty percent are reported to have attempted suicide.

Prevalence
Gambling takes different forms in different cultures, e.g. cock-fights, horse racing, the stock market. Although gambling opportunities have always been available, the proliferation and increasing accessibility of casinos and lotteries may be related to an increase in the prevalence of gambling problems. Both males and females can be compulsive gamblers. Men usually begin gambling in adolescence, women somewhat later.
Women are more likely to use gambling as an escape from Depression. The prevalence of pathological gambling is high and rising, now including between one percent and three percent of the adult US population.
It is estimated that half of pathological gamblers are women, though women only make up from two percent to four percent of Gamblers Anonymous. Women may not go to treatment programs because of greater stigma attached to

women gamblers.

Treatment Options

It is a difficult disorder to treat, but psychotherapy that concretely targets the behavior had limited success. Gamblers Anonymous, a 12-step program, may enable some to stop gambling. Treatment of the underlying disorders and involving family members may be helpful. It is important to note that, as specified in the American Psychiatric Association's Diagnostic and Statistical Manual of Mental Disorders, a psychiatric diagnosis, including this one, does not, and is not meant to, exonerate an individual from responsibility for criminal behavior.

TRICHOTILLOMANIA

Symptoms
• Repeated hair pulling so that hair loss is noticeable;
• Increasing tension just before the behavior or when trying to resist it;
• Pleasure or relief when pulling;
• Causes clear distress and problems in personal work, or social functioning.

Associated Features
Examining the hair root, pulling the hair between the teeth, or eating hairs (Trichophagia) may accompany Trichotillomania. Hair pulling is usually done in private or in the presence of close family members. Pain is not usually reported. The hair pulling is mostly denied and concealed by wigs, hairstyling and cosmetics. People with this disorder may also have Major Depressive Disorder, General Anxiety Disorder, Eating Disorder or Mental Retardation.

Prevalence
Among children, both males and females can have the disorder, but among adults, it is far more frequent in females. There are no recent prevalence figures for the general population, but in studies of college students, one percent to two percent have experienced Trichotillomania.

Treatment Options
There is no agreement about the cause of this disorder, making treatment more difficult. Professionals are often not consulted. Variable treatments that have been proposed include behavior therapy, hypnosis, and stress reduction. Medication has sometimes been helpful.

Associations & Agencies

991 Center for Mental Health Services (CMHS)
1 Choke Cherry Road
Room 6-1057
Rockville, MD 20857
240-276-1310
877-726-4727
Fax: 240-276-1320
TDD: 800-487-4889
E-mail: info@mentalhealth.org
www.beta.samhsa.gov/about-us/who-we-are/offices-center

Michael E Etzinger, B.S.M.E, , M.B., SAMHSA Executive Officer, Director
Paolo Del Vecchio, M.S.W, Director, Center for Mental Healt
Deborah Baldwin, M.P.A, Acting Director, Consumer Affairs
Elizabeth Lopez, Ph.D, Acting Deputy Director

CMHS leads Federal efforts to treat mental illnesses by promoting mental health and by preventing the development or worsening of mental illness when possible. Congress created CMHS to bring new hope to adults who have serious mental illnesses and to children with serious emotional disorders. CMHS pursues its mission by helping states improve and increase the quality and range of their treatment, rehabilitation, and support services for people with mental illness, their families and communities. It encourages a range of programs such as systems of care to respond to the increasing number of mental, emotional, and behavioral problems among America's children.

Year Founded: 1992

992 Mental Health Matters
Carron Consulting
19206 65th Pl NE
Kenmore, WA 98028
425-402-6934
E-mail: info@mental-health-matters.com
www.mental-health-matters.com

Provides a structured source of information about mental health issues. Offers detailed technical briefs on a variety of disorders, issues, symptoms, treatment modes, and medications.

993 National Association for the Dually Diagnosed (NADD)
132 Fair Street
Kingston, NY 12401-4802
845-331-4336
800-331-5362
Fax: 845-331-4569
E-mail: info@thenadd.org
www.thenadd.org

Donna McNELIS, PhD, President
Robert J Fletcher DSW, Chief Executive Officer
Dan Baker, PhD, Vice President
Julia Pearce, Secretary

The NADD's Mission is to advance mental wellness for persons with developmental disabilities through the promotion of excellence in mental health care. Providing educational services, training materials and conferences.

Year Founded: 1983

994 National Mental Health Consumers' Self-Help Clearinghouse
1211 Chestnut Street
Suite 1100
Philadelphia, PA 19107-4103
215-751-1810
800-553-4539
Fax: 215-636-6312
E-mail: info@mhselfhelp.org
www.mhselfhelp.org

Joseph Rogers, Executive Director/ Founder
Susan Rogers, Director
Britani Nestel, Program Specialist
Christa Burkett, Technical Assistance Coordinator

A national consumer technical assistance center that has played a major role in the development of the mental health consumer movement.

Year Founded: 1986

995 SAMHSA's National Mental Health Information Center
1 Choke Cherry Road
Rockville, MD 20857
877-786-4727
TDD: 866-889-2647
www.store.samhsa.gov/home

996 The Center for Family Support
2811 Zulette Avenue
Bronx, NY 10461
718-518-1500
Fax: 718-518-8200
E-mail: svernikoff@cfsny.org
www.cfsny.org

Steven Vernikoff, Executive Director
Virgil Seepersad, Director of Finance
Eileen Berg, Director of Quality Assurance
Barbara Greenwald, Associate Executive, Director

Committed to providing support and assistance to individuals with developmental and related disabilities, and to the family members who care for them.

Year Founded: 1954

997 The Shulman Center for Compulsive Theft, Spending & Hoarding
PO Box 250008
Franklin, MI 48025
248-358-8508
www.theshulmancenter.com

Terrence Daryl Shulman, JD, LMSW, , Founder/Director

Provides professional, confidential, comprehensive, and effective treatment for compulsive stealing, spending, and/or hoarding disorders. Serving individuals, couples, families, companies, and the community through education, assessment, & treatment. Vision is a world of emotional and financial health and balance, of honesty and deep self-esteem and self-worth for all.

Year Founded: 1992

998 Trichotillomania Learning Center
207 McPherson Street
Suite H
Santa Cruz, CA 95060-5863
831-457-1004
Fax: 831-427-5541
E-mail: info@trich.org
www.trich.org

Joanna Heitz, President
Jennifer Raikes, Executive Director
Deborah M. Kleinman, Treasurer
Brenda Cameron, Secretary

Works to improve the quality of life of children, adolescents and adults with trichotillomania and related body-focused repetitive disorders such as skin picking through information dissemination, education, outreach, alliance building, and support of research into the causes and treatment of these disorders.

Year Founded: 1991

Books

999 Angry All the Time: An Emergency Guide to Anger Control
NewHarbinger Publications
5674 Shattuck Avenue
Oakland, CA 94609-1662
510-652-0215
800-748-6273
Fax: 800-652-1613
E-mail: customerservices@newharbinger.com
www.newharbinger.com

Ronald T Potter-Efron MSW, PhD, Author

The book is organized to move readers along the shortest path to recovery. This edition includes tips for problem solving and directing anger in positive ways, new strategies for encouraging change, and a discussion of anger styles and the effects of jealousy on problem anger are just some of the engaging new concepts. *$16.95*

160 pages Year Founded: 1973 ISBN 1-572243-92-7

1000 Clinical Manual of Impulse-Control Disorders
American Psychiatric Publishing, Inc.
1000 Wilson Boulevard
Suite 1825
Arlington, VA 22209-3901
703-907-7322
800-368-5777
Fax: 703-907-1091
E-mail: appi@psych.org
www.appi.org

Eric Hollander, Author
Dan J. Stein, Author

Focuses on all of the different impulse-control disorders as a group.

368 pages Year Founded: 2006 ISBN 1-585621-36-1

1001 Drug Therapy and Impulse Control Disorders: Drugs & Psychology for the Mind & Body)
Mason Crest Publishers
450 Parkway Drive
Suite D
Broomall, PA 19008-4017
610-543-6200
866-627-2665
Fax: 610-543-3878
www.masoncrest.com

Autumn Libal, Author

The stories and information in this book will tell you more about impulse-control disorders, how they affect people's lives, and how they can be treated. *$24.95*

124 pages ISBN 1-590845-66-0

1002 Impulse Control Disorders: A Clinician's Guide to Understanding and Treating Behavioral Addictions
W.W. Norton & Company
500 Fifth Avenue
New York, NY 10110
212-354-5500
Fax: 212-869-0856
www.www.wwnorton.com

Jon E. Grant, Author

A comprehensive book on impulse control disorders topic for clinicians provides a screening instrument and a detailed method for assessing and treating them. *$26.95*

288 pages Year Founded: 2008

1003 Impulsivity and Compulsivity
American Psychiatric Publishing, Inc.
1000 Wilson Boulevard
Suite 1825
Arlington, VA 22209-3901
703-907-7322
800-368-5777
Fax: 703-907-1091
E-mail: appi@psych.org
www.appi.org

John M. Oldham, M.D., M.S., Editor
Eric Hollander, M.D., Editor
Andrew E. Skodol, M.D., Editor

Leading researchers and clinicians share their expertise on the phenomenological, biological, psychodynamic, and treatment aspects of these disorders. *$40.00*

312 pages Year Founded: 1996 ISBN 0-880486-76-7

1004 One Hundred Four Activities That Build
Sunburst Media
2 Skyline Drive
Suite 101
Hawthorne, NY 10532-2142
888-367-6368
Fax: 914-347-1805
E-mail: info@Childswork.com
www.Childswork.com

Full of interactive and fun games that can be used to encourage, modification of behavior, increase interaction with others, start discussions and build other life and social skills. *$23.95*

71 pages

1005 Out of Control: Gambling and Other Impulse Control Disorders
Chelsea House Publishers
132 West 31st Street
17th Floor
New York, NY 10001-3406
800-322-8755
Fax: 800-678-3633
E-mail: custserv@factsonfile.com
www.chelseahouse.infobasepublishing.com

Linda N. Bayer, Author

A ground-breaking series that provides up-to-date information on the history, causes and effects of, and treatment and therapies for problems affecting the human mind. *$35.00*

95 pages Year Founded: 2001 ISBN 0-791053-13-X

1006 Pyromania, Kleptomania, and Other Impulse Control Disorders
Enslow Publishers, Inc.
40 Industrial Road
Box 398, Department F61
Berkeley Heights, NJ 07922-0398
908-771-9400
800-398-2504
Fax: 908-771-0925
E-mail: customerservice@enslow.com
www.www.enslow.com

Julie Williams, Author

Describes the characterisitics of impulsive control disorders, from their early diagnoses and methods of treatment to today's available medications. *$26.60*

128 pages Year Founded: 1976 ISBN 0-766018-99-7

1007 Stop Me Because I Can't Stop Myself: Taking Control of Impulsive Behavior
McGraw-Hill Companies
PO Box 182604
Columbus, OH 43272
877-833-5524
Fax: 614-759-3749
E-mail: customer.service@mcgraw-hill.com
www.mcgraw-hill.com

S.W. Kim, Author
Jon E Grant, Author
Gregory Fricchione, Author

Offers the latest research and practical help for those who engage in all types of impulse-related behaviors.

224 pages Year Founded: 2004 ISBN 0-071433-68-6

1008 When Anger Hurts: Quieting The Storm Within
NewHarbinger Publications
5674 Shattuck Avenue
Oakland, CA 94609-1662
510-652-0215
800-748-6273
Fax: 800-652-1613
E-mail: customerservice@newharbinger.com
www.newharbinger.com

Matthew McKay, PhD, Author
Peter D Rogers, Author
Judith McKay, Author

Step-by-step guide to changing habitual, anger-generating thoughts while developing healthier, more effective ways of getting needs met. It is ideal for therapists who work with families or teach anger control and helpful for health professionals who treat the effects of Type A personality. *$16.95*

320 pages Year Founded: 1973 ISBN 1-572243-44-9

1009 Youth with Impulse-Control Disorders: On the Spur of the Moment
Mason Crest Publishers
450 Parkway Drive
Suite D
Broomall, PA 19008-4017
610-543-6200
866-621-2665
Fax: 610-543-3878
www.masoncrest.com

Kenneth McIntosh, Author
Phyllis Livingston, Author

128 pages Year Founded: 2008 ISBN 1-422204-47-2

Research Centers

1010 Impulse Control Disorders Clinic
University of Minnesota
231 Pillsbury Drive, South East.
240 Williamson Hall
Minneapolis, MN 55455-0213

612-625-2008
800-752-1000
Fax: 612-626-1693
TTY: 612-625-9051
www.impulsecontroldisorders.org

A group of doctors and trainees engaged in research in Impulse-Control Disorders (ICD) and Obsessive-Compulsive Disorder (OCD) and treating patients in a specialty clinic. Conducts research to elucidate pathophysiological links to the ICD and OCD and conducts clinical trials to come up with better and improved treatments for patients.

Support Groups & Hot Lines

1011 Gam-Anon Family Groups International Service Office, Inc.
PO Box 157
Whitestone, NY 11357-0157
718-352-1671
Fax: 718-746-2571
E-mail: gamanonoffice@gam-anon.org
www.gam-anon.org

A 12 Step self-help fellowship of men and women who have been affected by the gambling problems of a loved one.

1012 Gamblers Anonymous
PO Box 17173
Los Angeles, CA 90017
626-960-3500
Fax: 626-960-350
E-mail: isomain@gamblersanonymous.org
www.gamblersanonymous.org

Fellowship of men and women who share their experience, strength and hope with each other so that they may solve their common problem and help others recover from a gambling problem.

Year Founded: 1957

1013 Kleptomaniacs Anonymous
The Shulman Center for Compulsive Theft, Spending & Hoarding
PO Box 250008
Franklin, MI 48025
248-358-8508
www.kleptomaniacsanonymous.com

Terrence Shulman, JD, LMSW, Founder/Director

Kleptomaniacs And Shoplifters Anonymous (CASA) is a unique, independent and secular weekly self-help group.

Year Founded: 1992

1014 Trichotillomania Learning Center
207 McPherson Street
Suite H
Santa Cruz, CA 95060-5863
831-457-1004
Fax: 831-427-5541
E-mail: info@trich.org
www.trich.org

Joanna Heitz, President
Brenda Cameron, Secretary
Deborah M. Kleinman, Treasurer
Jennifer Raikes, Executive Director

Groups of individuals who get together and help one another understand about their disease. Also, they show each other different ways to prevent an attack from happening.

Year Founded: 1991

Video & Audio

1015 A Desperate Act
Trichotillomania Learning Center
207 McPherson Street
Suite H
Santa Cruz, CA 95060-5863
831-457-1004
Fax: 831-427-5541
E-mail: info@trich.org
www.trich.org

Joanna Heitz, President
Brenda Cameron, Secretary
Deborah M. Kleinman, Treasurer
Jennifer Raikes, Executive Director

A performance artist with TTM discusses her experiences in front of a live audience.

Year Founded: 1991

1016 Addictive Behavior: Drugs, Food and Relationships
Educational Video Network, Inc.
1401 19th Street
Huntsville, TX 77340
936-295-5767
800-762-0060
Fax: 936-294-0233
www.www.evndirect.com

Addiction is a serious and very real problem for many people. It can come in the forms of caffeine, heroin, food or love. Find out what makes one person more likely to develop an addiction than someone else, learn about the different types of addiction, the signs and the consequences.

1017 Anger Management-Enhanced Edition
Educational Video Network, Inc.
1401 19th Street
Huntsville, TX 77340
936-295-5767
800-762-0060
Fax: 936-294-0233
www.www.evndirect.com

Learn what causes anger and understand why our bodies react as they do when we're angry. Effective techniques for assuaging anger are discussed.

1018 Clinical Impressions: Identifying Mental Illness
Educational Training Videos
136 Granville St
Suite 200
Gahanna, OH 43230
Fax: 888-775-3919
www.educationaltrainingvideos.com

How long can mental illness stay hidden, especially from the eyes of trained experts? This program rejoins a group of ten adults- five of them healthy and five of them with histories of mental illness- as psychiatric specialists try to spot and correctly diagnose the latter. Administering a series of collaborative and one-on-one tests, including assessments of personality type, physical self-image, and rational thinking, the panel gradually makes decisions about who suffers from depression, bipolar disorder, bulimia, and social anxiety.

1019 Coping with Stress
Educational Video Network, Inc.
1401 19th Street
Huntsville, TX 77340
936-295-5767
800-762-0060
Fax: 936-294-0233
www.www.evndirect.com

Stress affects everyone, both emotionally and physically. For some, mismanaged stress can result in substance abuse, violence, or even suicide. This program answers the question, How can a person cope with stress?

1020 Dealing with ADHD: Attention Deficit/ Hyperactivity
Educational Video Network, Inc.
1401 19th Street
Huntsville, TX 77340
936-295-5767
800-762-0060
Fax: 936-294-0233
www.www.evndirect.com

Learn about attention deficit/hyperactivity disorder and learn what factors are thought to contribute to the development of this disorder. Other disorders that commonly co-exist with ADHD will be identified. The impulsivity and risk-taking behaviors of ADHD teens will be focused upon and tips that ADHD students can use to succeed academically will be provided. Laws that require schools to make special accommodations for ADHD students will be reviewed, and viewers will learn how to contact organizations that exist to help people who are dealing with ADHD.

1021 FRONTLINE: The Released
PBS
2100 Crystal Drive
Arlington, VA 22202
www.pbs.org

Will Lyman, Actor
Narrator
Miri Navasky, Director
Karen O'Connor, Director

The documentary states that of the 700, 000 inmates released from American prisons each year, half of them have mental disabilities. This work focused on those with severe problems who keep entering and exiting prison. Full of good information on the challenges they face with mental illnesses; housing, employment, stigmatization, and socialization.

Year Founded: 2009

1022 Mental Disorder
Educational Training Videos
136 Granville St
Suite 200
Gahanna, OH 43230
Fax: 888-775-3919
www.educationaltrainingvideos.com

What is abnormality? Using the case studies of two young women; one who has depression, one who has an anxiety disorder; as a springboard, this program presents three psychological perspective on mental disorder.

1023 No More Shame: Understanding Schizophrenia, Depression, and Addiction
Educational Training Videos
136 Granville St
Suite 200
Gahanna, OH 43230
Fax: 888-775-3919
www.educationaltrainingvideos.com

These programs examine research about the physiological, psychological, sociological, and cultural aspects of these disorders and their treatments. The goal of these programs is to explain what we do and do not know about each of these conditions, as well as to destigmatize the disorders by presenting them in the context of the same research process that is applied to all medical disorders.

1024 Obsessions: Understanding OCD
Educational Training Videos
136 Granville St
Suite 200
Gahanna, OH 43230
Fax: 888-775-3919
www.educationaltrainingvideos.com

Are compulsive hair-pulling, hand-washing, and even gambling learned behaviors or inherited diseases? Where do obsessions come from and how can they be managed so they do not dominate a person's life? This two-part series attempts to understand the roots of obsessive-compulsive disorder, or OCD, and looks at both standard and experimental treatment options.

1025 Our Personal Stories
Trichotillomania Learning Center
207 McPherson Street
Suite H
Santa Cruz, CA 95060-5863
831-457-1004
Fax: 831-427-5541
E-mail: info@trich.org
www.trich.org

Joanna Heitz, President
Brenda Cameron, Secretary
Deborah M. Kleinman, Treasurer
Jennifer Raikes, Executive Director

Documentary detailing 8 womens' personal experiences with TTM. *$28.00*

Year Founded: 1991

1026 Trichotillomania: Overview and Introduction to HRT
Trichotillomania Learning Center
207 McPherson Street
Suite H
Santa Cruz, CA 95060-5863
831-457-1004
Fax: 831-427-5541
E-mail: info@trich.org
www.trich.org

Joanna Heitz, President
Brenda Cameron, Secretary
Deborah M. Kleinman, Treasurer
Jennifer Raikes, Executive Director

A lecture on Behavior Therapy and Habit Reversal Training for TTM. *$30.00*

Year Founded: 1991

1027 Understanding Mental Illness
Educational Video Network, Inc.
1401 19th Street
Huntsville, TX 77340
936-295-5767
800-762-0060
Fax: 936-294-0233
www.www.evndirect.com

Contains information and classifications of mental illness. Mental illness can strike anyone, at any age. Learn about various organic and functional mental disorders as discussed and their causes and symptoms, and learn where to seek help for a variety of mental health concerns.

Web Sites

1028 www.apa.org/pubinfo/anger.html
Controlling Anger-Before It Controls You

From the American Psychological Association.

1029 www.cfsny.org
Center for Family Support

A not-for-profit human service agency that provides individualized support services and programs for individuals living with developmental and related disabilities, and for the families that care for them at home.

1030 www.cyberpsych.org
CyberPsych

Presents information about psychoanalysis, psychotherapy and special topics such as anxiety disorders, the problematic use of alcohol, homophobia, and the traumatic effects of racism.

1031 www.members.aol.com/AngriesOut
Get Your Angries Out

Guidelines for kids, teachers, and parents.

1032 www.mentalhelp.net/psyhelp/chap7
Anger and Aggression

Therapeutic approaches.

1033 www.mhselfhelp.org
National Mental Health Consumer's Self-Help Clearinghouse

A national consumer technical assistance center, has played a major role in the development of the mental health consumer movement.

1034 www.ncwd-youth.info/node/245
Center for Mental Health Services Knowledge Exchange Network

Information about resources, technical assistance, research, training, networks and other federal clearinghouses, fact sheets and materials.

1035 www.psychcentral.com
Psych Central

Internet's largest and oldest independent mental health social network created and run by mental health professionals to guarantee reliable, trusted information and support communities to you.

1036 www.stopbitingnails.com
Stop Biting Nails

Online organization created for those who bite their nails. Created a product which is used to prevent nailbiting.

1037 www.thenadd.org
National Association for the Dually Diagnosed

A not-for-profit membership association established for professionals, care providers and families to promote understanding of and services for individuals who have developmental disabilities and mental health needs.

Mood Disorders

Introduction

Mood disorders are psychiatric conditions in which the most prominent symptom is a consistent change in mood - either up, down, or both in alteration. They are common; they cause a large proportion of the disability world-wide, and they can be fatal. These are really whole-body diseases; many other symptoms go along with the mood change. There are changes in sleep, appetite, energy, and concentration, and many people have physical pain during episodes of depression. Some depressed people have irritability rather than sadness. Fortunately, there are effective treatments, both pharmacological and psychotherapeutic.

SYMPTOMS

Feelings of sadness are common to everyone, and quite natural in reaction to unfortunate circumstances. The death of a loved one, the end of a relationship, or other traumatic life experiences are bound to bring on the blues. But when feelings of sadness and despair persist beyond a reasonable period, arise for no particular reason, or begin to affect a person's ability to function, help is needed. Depression is a diagnosis made by a psychiatrist or other mental health professional to describe serious and prolonged symptoms of sadness or despair. While it is quite common, it is also a disease that no one should take lightly; depression can be deadly. Many people who are deeply depressed think about or actually try to commit suicide; some commit suicide. Even a relatively mild depresseion, if untreated, can disrupt marriages and relationships or impede careers. Such depressions cost the U.S. economy billions of dollars a year in lost productivity.

Symptoms

Depression is diagnosed when an individual experiences 1) persistent feelings of sadness or 2) loss of interest or pleasure in usual activities, in addition to five of the following symptoms for at least two weeks:
- Significant weight gain or loss unrelated to dieting;
- Inability to sleep or, conversely, sleeping too much;
- Restlessness and agitation;
- Fatigue or loss of energy;
- Feelings of worthlessness or guilt;
- Diminished ability to think or concentrate;
- Recurrentthoughts of death or suicide;
- Distress not caused by a medication or the symptoms of a medical illness.

Associated Features

Because depression can range from mild to severe, people who are depressed may exhibit a variety of behaviors. Often, people who are depressed are tearful, irritable, or brooding. Problems sleeping (either insomnia or sleeping too much) are common. People with Depression may worry unnecessarily about being sick or having a disease, or they may report physical symptoms such as headaches or other pains. Depression can seriously affect people's friendships and intimate relationships.

Depression can make people worry aout having a disease, but this is not a central symptom. Depression very frequently coexists with anxiety disorder. There is a genetic predisposition in some people.

Abuse of alcohol, presription drugs, or illegal drugs is also common among people who are depressed. The most serious risk associated with Depression is the risk of suicide: people who have tried to commit suicide are especially at risk. Individuals who have another mental disorder, such as Schizophrenia, in addition to Depression are also more likely to commit suicide.

Prevalence

Every year, more than 17 million Americans suffer some type of depressive illness. Depression does not discriminate; anyone can have it. Children, adults and the elderly are susceptible. Nevertheless, studies do indicate that women are twice as likely to have Depression as men. Depression has significant adverse effects on children's functioning and development; among adolescents, suicide id believed to be the fifth leading cause of death. Depression is also common among the elderly, and can be treated as an illness distinct from loneliness or sadness that may accompany old age.

Treatment Options

Depression is a medical disease and does not respond to the usual ways we have of cheering up ourselves or others. In fact, attempts to cheer depressed individuals may have the opposite and unfortunate consequence of making them feel worse, often because they are frustrated and feel guilty that others' well-meaning efforts do not help. If a person experiences the symptoms of Depression, he or she should seek treatment from a qualified professional. The vast majority of people with Depression get better when they are treated properly, and virtually everyone gets some relief from their symptoms.

A psychiatrist or other mental health professional should conduct a thorough evaluation, including and interview; a physical examination should be done by a primary care provider. On the basis of a complete evaluation, the appropriate treatment will be prescribed. Most likely, the treatment will be medication or psychotherapy, or both. Antidepressants usually take effect within three to six weeks after treatment has begun; it is important to give medications long enough to work, and to increase dosages or change or add medications ifdepression does not resolve completely.

The natural (untreated) course of a depressive episode is about nine months. Therefore treatment should be continued for at least that length of time even though the individual feels better. If treatment is discontinued prematurely, the depression is very likely to return. Depression is also a recurring disease; the risk of an episode after a first episode is 50%; after two episodes, 67%; and after three, over 90%. Therefore, some patients prefer to continue taking antidepressant medication indefinitely.

Dysthymic disorder is more low-level than chronic, with depressed mood consistently for at least two tears, than major depressive episodes, which last about nine months. Dysthymia can be treated with medication and psychotherapy as well.

Psychotherapy, or talk therapy, may be used to help the patient improve the way he or she thinks about things and deals with specific life problems. Individual, family, or couples therapy may be recommended, depending on the patient's life experiences. If the Depression is not severe, treatment can take a few weeks; if the Depression has been a longstanding problem, it may take much longer, but in many cases, a patient will experience improvement in 10-15 sessions.

ASSOCIATED FEATURES

Within days to a year after giving birth, women may experience a spectrum of psychological symptoms related to both the abrupt hormonal changes and the psychological and social demands of motherhood. The mildest of these symptoms, 'baby blues, ' is not a psychiatric condition. It consists of a few days of heightened emotionality starting within days after birth and resolving spontaneously. They may become concerned when the emotionality leads to tears, but women with 'baby blues, ' and their families, need only reassurance.

Postpartum depression is often a continuation of depression starting during or even before pregnancy. The symptoms, which are listed below, are much the same as those of depression occurring at any other time of life. The fact that the postpartum period is almost always associated with problems with sleep, appetite, libido, energy, and concentration makes those symptoms less useful for diagnosis at this time. Two cardinal questions are: 'Are you feeling sad most of the time?' and 'Are you unable to enjoy things that you usually enjoy?' Women with postpartum depression are preoccupied with concerns about their ability to be good mothers. Unlike an average, tired new mother, the depressed woman cannot enjoy her baby. She is often guilty and reluctant to tell her family about it because she knows she is supposed to appreciate her good fortune and be happy. Severe Postpartum Depression, or Postpartum Psychosis, that causes confusion, disorientation, delusions, and hallucinations, and can cause suicide or infanticide, is a serious medical condition demanding immediate professional attention. Fortunately, there is increasing awareness and understanding of postpartum depression among the general population.

Symptoms
In addition to the symptoms of Depression:
• Preoccupation with concerns of being a good mother;
• Inability to rest while the baby is sleeping;
• Inability to enjoy her baby accompanied with feelings of guilt.

Prevalence
Very mild depression after delivery, or 'baby blues, ' affects over half, perhaps up to 90% of postpartum women. Baby blues is actually not depression at all; rather it is a common condition characterized by sensitivity and emotionality, both happy and sad. Postpartum Depression affects approximately 10% of new mothers. Much postpartum depression is a continuation of depression that was already present during pregnancy.

Treatment Options
Treatment for Postpartum Depression is similar to treatment for depression in general. Possible risks of medications taken during pregnancy and breastfeeding have to be weighed against the risks of leaving the depression untreated. Women who discontinue antidepressant medication because they wish to become or have become pregnant are at a very high risk of relapse.

PREVALENCE

Bipolar Disorder (Manic Depression) is the name for a group of severe mental illnesses characterized by alterations between depression and manic euphoria or irritability.

The two states are not independent of each other, but part of the same illness. Individuals in the manic phase of Bipolar Disorder may feel exuberant, invincible, or even immortal. They may be awake for days at a time, and be able to work tirelessly; they may rush from one idea to the next carried by a nearly uncontrollable burst of energy that leaves others bewildered and unable to keep up. (Some extraordinarily creative people, Vincent Van Gogh, for example, have had Bipolar Disorder. Whether or not the disorder makes a positive contribution to creativity is a controversial question.)

In the depressed phase which follows a manic high, the patient may be suicidal. The depressed phase of the illness mirrors a major depressive episode. There are three forms of Bipolar Disorders: Bipolar I Disorder, Bipolar II Disorder, and Cyclothymic Disorder. Bipolar II Disorder consists of repeated depressive episodes interspersed with hypomaniac (not full blown mania) episodes. The individual with Cyclothymic Disorder has a history of at least two years of repeated episodes of elevated and depressed mood which don't meet all the criteria for mania or depression but which cause distress and/or decreased ability to function.

A number of researchers are closing in on genetic links to the illness. Like all mental disorders, however, the relationship between genetic physiologic, psychological, and environmental causes is complex. Lithium was the first medication found to be effective; several other medications are now available and effective. Many patients with Bipolar Disorders need a combination of medications to address both the manic and depressive aspects. While medication is quite effective, patients need psychotherapy as well, in order to address issues like compliance with medication, noting early signs of relapse, dealing with friends and family and environmental life stressors.

Symptoms
A **manic episode** consists of the following:

• A distinct period of abnormally and persistently elevated, expansive, or irritable mood, lasting at least one week;
• Inflated self-esteem or grandiosity;
• Decreased need for sleep;
• More talkative than usual;
• Flight of ideas (a succession of topics with little relationship to one another) or a subjective experience that thoughts are racing;
• Distractibility;
• Increase in goal-directed activity;
• Excessive involvement in activities that have a high potential for painful consequences;
• The mood disturbances are severe enough to cause impairment in social or occupational functioning;
• The symptoms are not due to the direct physiological effects of a substance.

The **depressive phase** of Bipolar Disorder consists of the following:

• Depressed mood most othe day, nearly every day, as indicated by either subjective report or observation;
• Markedly diminished interest or pleasure in almost all activities most of the day;

• Significant weight loss when not dieting, or weight gain, or decrease or increase in appetite nearly every day;
• Insomnia or hypersomnia nearly every night;
• Psychomotor agitation or retardation nearly every day;
• Fatigue or loss of evergy nearly every day;
• Feelings of worthlessness or excessive or inappropriate guilt nearly every day.

Associated Features
Bipolar Disorder is a severe mental illness that can cause extreme disruption to individual lives and careers, and to whole families. While manic, patients may spend all of a family's money, borrow great sums, engage in indiscriminate sexual activity, and behave in other ways that leave lasting negative effects. Suicide is a risk factor in the illness, and an estimated 10% to 15% of individuals with Bipolar I Disorder commit suicide. Abuse of children, spouses or other family members, or other types of violence, may occur during the manic phase of the illness. Untreated mania, during which the individual gets no sleep, little or no nutrition, and expends great quantities of energy, can result in death as well.

It is important for patients with depression to be carefully screened for any manic or hypomanic symptoms so that Bipolar Disorder can be diagnosed and the appropriate treatment prescribed. Most peo

TREATMENT OPTIONS

ple with Bipolar Disorder present, or are referred, for care while in the depressive state; it is essential that any individual diagnosed with depression be carefully evaluated to rule out bipolar disorder before antidepressany medication is prescribed. Antidepressany medication alone can precipitate a manic episode in an individual with Bipolar Disorder. The cycles of mood changes tend to become more frequent, shorter, and more intense as the patient gets older.

Disturbances in work, school or social functioning are common, resulting in frequent school truancy or failure, occupational failure, divorce, or episodic antisocial behavior. A variety of other mental disorders may accompany Bipolar Disorder; these include Anorexia Nervosa, Bulimia Nervosa, Attention Deficit/Hyperactivity Disorder, Panic Disorder, Social Phobia, and Substance-Abuse Related Disorder.

Prevalence
The prevalence of Bipolar I Disorder varies from 0.4% to 0.6% in the community. Community prevalence of Bipolar II Disorder is approximately 0.5%. The prevalence of Cyclothymic Disorder is estimated at 0.4% to 1%, and from 3% to 5% in clinics specializing in mood disorders.

Treatment Options
Lithium is the most commonly prescribed drug for Bipolar Disorder and is effective for stabilizing patients in the manic phase of the illness and preventing mood swings. However, compliance is a problem among patients both because of the nature of the condition (some patients may actually miss the high of their mood swings and other people often envy their enthusiasm, energy, and confidence) and because of the side effects associated with the drug. These include weight gain, excessive thirst, tremors and muscle weakness. Lithium is also very toxic in overdose. Blood levels of lithium must be measured daily or weekly to begin with, and in at least six-month intervals

thereafter. The disruptive nature of the condition also necessitates the use of psychotherapy and family therapy to help patients rebuild relationships, to maintain compliance with treatment and a positive attitude toward living with a chronic illness, and to restore confidence and self-esteem.

Anticonvulsants/mood stabilizers, such as Valproate, Carbamazepine, Lamotrigine, Gabapentin, and Topiramate have also become first-line treatments, as have several antipsychotic medications.

Education of the family is crucial for successful treatment, as is education of patients about the disorder and treatment.

Associations & Agencies

1039 Brain & Behavior Research Foundation
90 Park Avenue
16th Floor
New York, NY 10016
646-681-4888
800-829-8289
Fax: 516-487-6930
E-mail: info@bbrfoundation.org
www.bbrfoundation.org

Steve Lieber, Chairman of the Board
Jeffrey Borenstein, M.D, President and Chief Executive Of
Louis Innamorato, Vice president, Finance and Chief
Suzzane Golden, Vice President

The Brain and Behavior Research Foundation is committed to alleviating the suffering caused by mental illness by awarding grants that will lead to advances and break-throughs in scientific research.
Year Founded: 1981

1040 Center for Mental Health Services (CMHS)
1 Choke Cherry Road
Room 6-1057
Rockville, MD 20857
240-276-1310
877-726-4727
Fax: 240-276-1320
TDD: 800-487-4889
E-mail: info@mentalhealth.org
www.beta.samhsa.gov/about-us/who-we-are/offices-center

Michael E Etzinger, B.S.M.E, , M.B., SAMHSA Executive Officer, Director
Paolo Del Vecchio, M.S.W, Director, Center for Mental Healt
Deborah Baldwin, M.P.A, Acting Director, Consumer Affairs
Elizabeth Lopez, Ph.D, Acting Deputy Director

CMHS leads Federal efforts to treat mental illnesses by promoting mental health and by preventing the develop-ment or worsening of mental illness when possible. Con-gress created CMHS to bring new hope to adults who have serious mental illnesses and to children with serious emo-tional disorders. CMHS provides information about mental health via a toll-free the web site, and more than 600 publi-cations. Developed for users of mental health services and their families, the general public, policy makers, providers, and the media.
Year Founded: 1992

1041 Depression & Bi-Polar Support Alliance

730 North Franklin Street
Suite 501
Chicago, IL 60654-7225
312-642-0049
800-826-3632
Fax: 312-642-7243
E-mail: info@dbsalliance.org
www.dbsalliance.org

Cheryl T Magrini, MS.Ed, MTS, PhD, Chair
Allen Doederlein, President
Cindy Specht, ExecutiveVice president
Gregory E Ostfeld, Treasurer

Educates patients, families, professionals, and the public concerning the nature of depressive and manic-depressive illnesses as treatable medical diseases, fosters self-help for patients and families, works to eliminate discrimination and stigma, improves access to care, advocates for research toward the elimination of these illnesses.

1042 Depression & Related Affective Disorders Association (DRADA)

2330 West Joppa Road
Suite 100
Lutherville, MD 21093
410-583-2919
Fax: 410-614-3241
E-mail: drada@jhmi.edu
www.www.drada.org

Catherine Pollock, Executive Director
Elizabeth Boyce, Director Development

Non profit association whose mission is to alleviate the suffering arising from depression and manic depression by assisting self-help groups, providing education and information and lending support to research programs.

1043 Depression After Delivery

91 E Somerset Street
Raritan, NJ 08869-2129
908-575-9121
800-944-4773
Fax: 908-541-9713
E-mail: dadorg@earthlink.net
www.depressionafterdelivery.com

Joyce A Venis, RNC, President
Donna Cangialosi, Office Manager

24-hour information request line. Free information packet of referrals and volunteer contacts nationwide for women with postpartum disorders.

1044 Freedom From Fear

308 Seaview Avenue
Staten Island, NY 10305-2246
718-351-1717
Fax: 718-667-8893
E-mail: help@freedomfromfear.org
www.freedomfromfear.org

Irwin Freeman, President
Mary Guardino, Founder, Executive Director
Mark Sisti, PhD, 1st Vice President
Jonathan W Stewart, MD, Treasurer

A national non profit mental health advocacy association. The mission of FFF is to impact, in a positive way, the lives of all those affected by anxiety, depressive and related disorders through advocacy, education, research and community support.

Year Founded: 1984

1045 National Alliance on Mental Illness

3803 North Fairfax Drive
Suite 100
Arlington, VA 22203
703-524-7600
800-950-6264
Fax: 703-524-9094
E-mail: helpline@nami.org
www.nami.org

Keris Jan Myrick, MBA, MS, PhD., President
Mary Giliberti, J.D, Executive Director
Jim Payne, J.D, First Vice President
David Levy, Chief Financial Officer

The nation's largest grassroots mental health organization dedicated to building better lives for the millions of Americans affected by mental illness. NAMI advocates for access to services, treatment, supports and research and is steadfast in its commitment to raising awareness and building a community of hope for all those in need.

Year Founded: 1969

1046 National Association for the Dually Diagnosed (NADD)

132 Fair Street
Kingston, NY 12401-4802
845-331-4336
800-331-5362
Fax: 845-331-4569
E-mail: info@thenadd.org
www.thenadd.org

Donna McNELIS, PhD, President
Robert J Fletcher DSW, Chief Executive Officer
Dan Baker, PhD, Vice President
Julia Pearce, Secretary

Nonprofit organization designed to promote interest of professional and parent development with resources for individuals who have the coexistence of mental illness and mental retardation. Provides conferences, educational services and training materials to professionals, parents, concerned citizens and service organizations.

Year Founded: 1983

1047 National Institute of Mental Health

6001 Executive Boulevard
Room 6200, MSC 9663
Bethesda, MD 20892-9663
301-443-4513
866-615-6464
Fax: 301-443-4279
TTY: 301-443-8431
E-mail: nimhinfo@nih.gov
www.www.nimh.nih.gov

Tom Insel, MD, NIHM Director
William G Coleman, Scientific Director, NIMHD
Grace E O Ajao, Administrative Officer
Dionne D Draper, Administrative Officer

The mission of NIMH is to transform the understanding and treatment of mental illnesses through basic and clinical research, paving the way for prevention, recovery, and cure. For the Institute to continue fulfilling this vital public health mission, it must foster innovative thinking and ensure that a full array of novel scientific perspectives are used to further discovery in the evolving science of brain, behavior, and experience. In this way, breakthroughs in science can become breakthroughs for all people with mental illnesses.

1048 National Mental Health Consumers' Self-Help Clearinghouse

1211 Chestnut Street
Suite 1100
Philadelphia, PA 19107-4103
215-751-1810
800-553-4539
Fax: 215-636-6312
E-mail: info@mhselfhelp.org
www.mhselfhelp.org

Joseph Rogers, Executive Director/ Founder
Susan Rogers, Director
Britani Nestel, Program Specialist
Christa Burkett, Technical Assistance Coordinator

A national consumer technical assistance center that has played a major role in the development of the mental health consumer movement.

Year Founded: 1986

1049 Postpartum Support International

6706 SouthWest 54th Avenue
Portland, OR 97219
503-894-9453
800-944-4773
Fax: 503-894-9452
E-mail: support@postpartum.net
www.postpartum.net

Leslie Lowell Stoutenberg, RNC, President
Wendi N Davis, PhD, Executive Director
Sharon Gerdes, Public Relations and Marketing C
Robin Starkey Harpster, MA, Secretary

A non-profit organization whose mission is to promote awareness, prevention and treatment of mental health issues related to childbearing in every country worldwide.

Year Founded: 1987

1050 SAMHSA's National Mental Health Information Center

1 Choke Cherry Road
Rockville, MD 20857
877-786-4727
TDD: 866-889-2647
TTY: 301-443-9006
www.store.samhsa.gov

1051 The Balanced Mind Foundation

730 N. Franklin Street
Suite 501
Chicago, IL 60654
312-642-0049
E-mail: info@thebalancedmind.org
www.www.thebalancedmind.org

Susan Resko, M.M., Executive Director

The Balanced Mind Foundation guides families raising children with mood disorders to the answers, support and stability they seek.

1052 The Center for Family Support

2811 Zulette Avenue
Bronx, NY 10461
718-518-1500
Fax: 718-518-8200
E-mail: svernikoff@cfsny.org
www.cfsny.org

Steven Vernikoff, Executive Director
Virgil Seepersad, Director of Finance
Eileen Berg, Director of Quality Assurance
Barbara Greenwald, Associate Executive, Director

The Center for Family Support is committed to providing support and assistance to the individuals with developmental and related disabilities, and to the family members who care for them.

Year Founded: 1954

Books

1053 Against Depression
Viking Adult

375 Hudson Street
New York, NY 10014-3657
212-366-2372
Fax: 212-366-2933
E-mail: ecommerce@us.penguingroup.com
www.www.us.penguingroup.com

Peter D. Kramer, Author

A deeply felt, deeply moving book, grounded in time spent with the depressed. As his argument unfolds, Kramer becomes a crusader, the author of a compassionate polemic that is fiercely against depression and the devastation it causes. This book will offer hope to millions who suffer from depression, and radically alter the debate on its treatment.

368 pages Year Founded: 1936 ISBN 0-670034-05-3

1054 An Unquiet Mind: A Memoir of Moods and Madness
Random House

1745 Broadway
New York, NY 10019
212-782-9000
E-mail: ecustomerservice@randomhouse.com
www.randomhouse.com

Kay Redfield Jamison, Author

The author examines bipolar illness from the dual perspectives of the healer and the healed, revealing both its terrors and the cruel allure that at times prompted her to resist taking medication. An Unquiet Mind is a memoir of enormous candor, vividness, and wisdom- a deeply powerful book that has both transformed and saved lives. *$15.00*

224 pages ISBN 0-679763-30-9

1055 Anxiety and Depression in Adults and Children, Banff International Behavioral Science Series
Sage Publications, Inc.

2455 Teller Road
Thousand Oaks, CA 91320-2234
805-499-0721
800-818-7243
Fax: 800-583-2665
E-mail: info@sagepub.com
www.sagepub.com

Kenneth D. Craig, Author
Keith S. Dobson, Author

Collection of papers by well respected researchers in the field of anxiety and depression. Brings together desparate areas of research and integrates them in an informative and interesting way. Focuses on recent advances in treating anxiety and depression in adults and children. Topics include self-management therapy, assessing and treating sexually abused children and unipolar depression. Integrates empirical research with clinical applications. Paperback also available. *$46.95*

296 pages Year Founded: 1994 ISBN 0-803970-20-X

1056 Bipolar Disorder Survival Guide: What You and Your Family Need to Know
The Guilford Press
72 Spring Street
New York, NY 10012-4019
212-431-9800
800-365-7006
Fax: 212-966-6708
E-mail: info@guilford.com
www.www.guilford.com

David J. Miklowitz, PhD, Author

Gives ideas to the person diagnosed with the disorder how to come to terms with the diagnosis. Also shows who you should confide in and how to recognize mood swings. *$19.95*

342 pages Year Founded: 1973 ISBN 1-572305-25-8

1057 Bipolar Disorder for Dummies
John Wiley and Sons
111 River Street
Hoboken, NJ 07030-5774
201-748-6000
877-762-2974
Fax: 201-748-6088
E-mail: info@wiley.com
www.wiley.com

Candida Fink, MD, Author
Joe Kraynak, Author

Guide explains the brain chemistry behind the disease, and covers the latest medications and therapies. Sound advice and self-help techniques that everyone can use including children to ease and eliminate syptoms, function in a crisis, and plan ahead for manic or depressive episodes. *$19.99*

384 pages Year Founded: 2005 ISBN 0-764584-51-0

1058 Bipolar Disorders: A Guide to Helping Children & Adolescents
ADD WareHouse
300 NW 70th Avenue
Suite 102
Plantation, FL 33317-2360
954-792-8100
800-233-9273
Fax: 954-792-8545
E-mail: sales@addwarehouse.com
www.addwarehouse.com

Mitzi Waltz, Author

A million children and adolescents in the US may have childhood-onset bipolar disorder-including a significant number with ADHD. This new book helps parents and professionals recognize, treat and cope with bipolar disorders.

It covers diagnosis, family life, medications, talk therapies, school issues, and other interventions. *$24.95*

442 pages Year Founded: 2000 ISBN 1-565926-56-0

1059 Bipolar Disorders: Clinical Course and Outcome
American Psychiatric Publishing, Inc.
1000 Wilson Boulevard
Suite 1825
Arlington, VA 22209-3901
703-907-7322
800-368-5777
Fax: 703-907-1091
E-mail: appi@psych.org
www.appi.org

Joseph F. Goldberg, Editor
Martin Harrow, Editor

An important and much-needed resource, this book related empirical data on outcome with practical information on the prognosis, course, and potential complications of bipolar disorders in the modern era. Pulling together current knowledge from leading investigators in the field, it provides a concise, up-to-date summary of affective relapse, comorbid psychopathology, functional disability, and psychosocial outcome in contemporary bipolar disorders. *$49.95*

344 pages Year Founded: 1999 ISBN 0-880487-68-2

1060 Bipolar Puzzle Solution
Taylor and Francis
7625 Empire Drive
Florence, KY 41042-2919
800-634-7064
Fax: 800-248-4724
TDD: 703-516-7227
www.nami.org

Bryan L. Court, Author
Gerald E. Nelson, Author

An informative book on bipolar illness in a 187 question-and-answer format. *$18.50*

160 pages Year Founded: 1996

1061 Breaking the Patterns of Depression
Random House
1745 Broadway
New York, NY 10019-4343
212-782-9000
800-733-3000
Fax: 212-782-9052
E-mail: ecustomerservice@randomhouse.com
www.randomhouse.com

Michael D. Yapko, PhD, Author

Presents skills that enable readers to understand and ultimately avert depression's recurring cycles. Focusing on future prevention as well as initial treatment, the book includes over one hundred structured activities to help sufferers learn the skills necessary to become and remain depression-free. Translates the clinical literature on psychotherapy and antidepressant medication into understandable language. Defines what causes depression and clarifies what can be done about it. With this knowledge in hand, readers can control their depression, rather than having depression control them. *$13.95*

360 pages Year Founded: 1998 ISBN 0-385483-70-8

1062 Brilliant Madness: Living with Manic-Depressive Illness
Bantam Books
1745 Broadway
3rd Floor
New York, NY 10019-4368
212-782-9000
E-mail: bdpublicity@randomhouse.com

Patty Duke, Author
Gloria Hochman, Author

From what it's like to live with manic-depressive disorder to the latest findings on its most effective treatments, this compassionate and eloquent book provides profound insight into the challenge of mental illness. It offers hope for all those who suffer from mood disorders and for the family, friends, and physicians who love and care for them.

368 pages Year Founded: 1997 ISBN 0-553560-72-7

1063 Broken Connection: On Death and the Continuity of Life
American Psychiatric Publishing, Inc.
1000 Wilson Boulevard
Suite 1825
Arlington, VA 22209-3901
703-907-7322
800-368-5777
Fax: 703-907-1091
E-mail: appi@psych.org
www.appi.org

Robert Jay Lifton, Author

Exploration of the inescapable connections between death and life, the psychiatric disorders that arise from these connections, and the advent of the nuclear age which has jeopardized any attempts to ensure the perpetuation of the self beyond death. *$38.00*

512 pages Year Founded: 1996 ISBN 0-880488-74-3

1064 Carbamazepine and Manic Depression: A Guide
Madison Institute of Medicine
6515 Grand Teton Plaza
Suite 100
Madison, WI 53719
608-827-2470
Fax: 608-827-2444
E-mail: mim@miminc.org
www.www.miminc.org

James W. Jefferson, Author
Janet R. Medenwald, MD, Author
John H. Greist, Author

A concise guide to the use of carbamazepine for the treatment of manic depression with information about dosing, monitoring and side effects. *$5.95*

32 pages Year Founded: 1996 ISBN 1-890802-05-0

1065 Clinical Guide to Depression in Children and Adolescents
American Psychiatric Publishing, Inc.
1000 Wilson Boulevard
Suite 1825
Arlington, VA 22209-3901
703-907-7322
800-368-5777
Fax: 703-907-1091

E-mail: appi@psych.org
www.appi.org

Mohammad Shafii, Editor
Sharon Lee Shafii, Editor

The book begins with a discussion of depression's clinical manifestations, including epidemiology, neurobiology, and chronobiology of seasonal mood disorders. A section on diagnostic assessment and treatment addresses standardizes approaches to assessment and such treatment modalities as dynamic psychotherapy, group therapy, the latest advances in pharmacological treatment and inpatient treatment. A concluding section examines bipolar disorders clinical manifestations, natural history, genetics, and treatment. *$39.50*

320 pages Year Founded: 1991 ISBN 0-880483-56-3

1066 Consumer's Guide to Psychiatric Drugs
NewHarbinger Publications
5674 Shattuck Avenue
Oakland, CA 94609-1662
510-652-0215
800-748-6273
Fax: 800-652-1613
E-mail: customerservice@newharbinger.com
www.newharbinger.com

Mary C. Talaga, Author
John D. Preston, Author
John H. O'Neal, Author

Helps consumers understand what treatment options are available and what side effects to expect. Covers possible interactions with other drugs, medical conditions and other concerns. Explains how each drug works, and offers detailed information about treatments for depression, bipolar disorder, anxiety and sleep disorders, as well as other conditions. *$16.95*

340 pages Year Founded: 1973 ISBN 1-572241-11-X

1067 Depression Workbook: a Guide for Living with Depression
NewHarbinger Publications
5674 Shattuck Avenue
Oakland, CA 94609-1662
510-652-0215
800-748-6273
Fax: 800-652-1613
E-mail: customerservice@newharbinger.com
www.newharbinger.com

Mary Ellen Copeland, MS, MA, Author

Based on responses of participants sharing their insights, experiences, and strategies for living with extreme mood swings. *$ 19.95*

352 pages Year Founded: 1973 ISBN 1-572242-68-X

1068 Depression and Its Treatment
Grand Central Publishing

John H. Greist, MD, Author
James W. Jefferson, MD, Author

Depression is the most common psychological disorder, and at least ten percent of Americans will experience a major depression at some point in their lives. This clearly-written, straightforward guide explains depression and its causes and discusses treatments from drugs to psychotherapy. Developed by the American Psychiatric Press. *$19.95*

157 pages Year Founded: 1994

1069 Depression, the Mood Disease
Johns Hopkins University Press
2715 N Charles Street
Baltimore, MD 21218-4319
410-516-6900
800-537-5487
Fax: 410-516-6998

Francis Mark Mondimore, MD, Author

Explores the many faces of an illness that will affect as many as 36 million Americans at some point in their lives. Updated to reflect state-of-the-art treatment. *$12.76*

240 pages ISBN 0-801851-84-X

1070 Diagnosis and Treatment of Depression in Late Life: Results of the NIH Consensus Development Conference
American Psychiatric Publishing, Inc.
1000 Wilson Boulevard
Suite 1825
Arlington, VA 22209-3901
703-907-7322
800-368-5777
Fax: 703-907-1091
E-mail: appi@psych.org
www.appi.org

Lon S Schneider, M.D., Editor
Charles F Reynolds III, M.D, Editor
Barry D Lebowitz, Ph.D, Editor
Arnold Friedhoff, M.D, Editor

Provides comprehensive studies in early life depression versus late life depression, the prevalence of depression in the elderly and the risk factors involved. *$21.95*

550 pages Year Founded: 1993 ISBN 0-880485-56-6

1071 Divalproex and Bipolar Disorder: A Guide
Madison Institute of Medicine
6515 Grand Teton Plaza
Suite 100
Madison, WI 53719
608-827-2470
E-mail: mim@miminc.org
www.www.miminc.org

James W. Jefferson, MD, Author
John H. Greist, MD, Author

A concise, up-to-date booklet that provides the reader with an overview of bipolar disorder and its treatment with the medication, divalproex (sometimes referred to as valproate). Information an administration and dosage, patient monitoring, and possible side effects is included in the guide, as well as other information important to anyone taking divalproex for bipolar disorder. *$5.95*

32 pages

1072 Drug Therapy and Postpartum Disorders (Psychiatric Disorders: Drugs & Psychology for the Mind & Body)
Mason Crest Publishers
450 Parkway Drive
Suite D
Broomall, PA 19008-4017
610-543-6200
866-627-2665
Fax: 610-543-3878

E-mail: dtaylor@masoncrest.com
www.masoncrest.com

Autumn Libal, Author

Pregnancy, childbirth and early motherhood are supposed to be times filled with the joy and wonder of bringing a new life into the world. Unfortunately, many women find that the struggles of early motherhood are accompanied by multiple sorrows that clash with the sentimental ideal. New mothers may feel alone in their struggles, but depression after childbirth is far more common than most people realize. This book provides information about the psychiatric conditions that can accompany new motherhood and the treatments that can help.

128 pages ISBN 1-590846-70-6

1073 Emotions Anonymous Book
Emotions Anonymous International Service Center
PO Box 4245
Saint Paul, MN 55104-0245
651-647-9712
Fax: 651-647-1593
E-mail: info2gh99jsd@emotionsanonymous.org
www.EmotionsAnonymous.org

The Big Book of EA: A fellowship of men and women who share their experience, strength and hope with each other, that they may solve their common problem and help others recover from emotional illness. *$15.00*

261 pages ISBN 0-960735-65-5

1074 Encyclopedia of Depression (Facts on File Library of Health & Living)
Facts on File
132 W 31st Street
17th Floor
New York, NY 10001-3406
800-322-8755
Fax: 800-678-3633
E-mail: custserv@factsonfile.com
www.www.infobasepublishing.com

This volume defines and explains all terms and topics relating to depression. *$58.50*

170 pages

1075 Growing Up Sad: Childhood Depression and Its Treatment
WW Norton & Company
500 5th Avenue
New York, NY 10110-54
212-354-2907
800-233-4830
Fax: 212-869-0856
E-mail: npb@wwnorton.com

Leon Cytryn, Author
Donald H. McKnew Jr., Author

The authors have updated their classic study, Why Isn't Johnny Crying? that looks at the symptoms and treatment of childhood - onset depression. The authors give an authoritative summary of research, counsel prompt diagnosis, and assert that the disorder is treatable. *$25.00*

216 pages Year Founded: 1998 ISBN 0-393317-88-9

1076 Guildeline for Treatment of Patients with Bipolar Disorder
American Psychiatric Publishing, Inc.
1000 Wilson Boulevard
Suite 1825
Arlington, VA 22209-3901
703-907-7322
800-368-5777
Fax: 703-907-1091
E-mail: appi@psych.org
www.appi.org

Provides guidance to psychiatrists who treat patients with bipolar I disorder. Summarizes the pharmacologic, somatic, and psychotherapeutic treatments used for patients. *$22.50*

96 pages ISBN 0-890423-02-4

1077 Help Me, I'm Sad: Recognizing, Treating, and Preventing Childhood and Adolescent Depression
Penguin Publishers
375 Hudson Street
New York, NY 10014-3657
212-366-2372
800-847-5515
Fax: 212-366-2933
E-mail: ecommerce@us.penguingroup.com
www.www.us.penguingroup.com

David G. Fassler, Author
Lynne Dumas, Author

Discusses how to tell if your child is at risk; how to spot symptoms; depressions link with other problems and its impact on the family; teen suicide; finiding the right diagnosis, therapist, and treatment; and what you can do to help.

224 pages Year Founded: 1936 ISBN 0-140267-63-1

1078 Helping Someone with Mental Illness: A Compassionate Guide for Family, Friends, and Caregivers
Three Rivers Press
1745 Broadway
New York, NY 10019
212-782-9000
E-mail: ecustomerservice@randomhouse.com
www.randomhouse.com

Rosalynn Carter, Author
Susan Golant MA, Author

The authors address the latest breakthroughs in understanding, research, and treatment of schizophrenia, depression, manic depression, panic attacks, obsessive-compulsive disorder, and other mental disorders. *$19.00*

368 pages Year Founded: 1999 ISSN 9780812928983ISBN 0-812928-98-9

1079 Helping Your Depressed Teenager: a Guide for Parents and Caregivers
John Wiley & Sons
111 River Street
Hoboken, NJ 07030-5774
201-748-6000
800-225-5945
Fax: 201-748-6088
E-mail: info@wiley.com
www.wiley.com

Gerald D. Oster, Author
Sarah S. Montgomery, Author

A practical guide offering family solutions to a family problem. This book will sensitize you to the hidden struggles of adolescents and assist in understanding their multifaceted problems. The authors are experts in this field and have help countless youngsters confront and overcome their depressed mood. *$19.95*

208 pages Year Founded: 1994 ISBN 0-471621-84-6

1080 Lithium and Manic Depression: A Guide
Madison Institute of Medicine
6515 Grand Teton Plaza
Suite 100
Madison, WI 53719
608-827-2470
Fax: 608-827-2444
E-mail: mim@miminc.org
www.www.miminc.org

John Bohn, MD, Author
James W. Jefferson, MD, Author

A concise, up-to-date guide written by a leading expert on manic depression (bipolar disorder) and its treatment. This publication includes the most important information every patient taking lithium needs to know about lithium dosing, monitoring and side effects. *$5.95*

31 pages Year Founded: 1996 ISBN 1-890802-04-2

1081 Living Without Depression & Manic Depression: a Workbook for Maintaining Mood Stability
NewHarbinger Publications
5674 Shattuck Avenue
Oakland, CA 94609-1662
510-652-0215
800-748-6273
Fax: 800-652-1613
E-mail: customerservice@newharbinger.com
www.newharbinger.com

Mary Ellen Copeland, MS, MA, Author

Outlines a program that helps people achieve breakthroughs in coping and healing. Contents include: self advocacy, building a network of support, wellness lifestyle, symptom prevention strategies, self-esteem, mood stability, a career that works, trauma resolution, dealing with sleep problems, diet, vitamin and herbal therapies, dealing with stigma, medication side effects, psychotherapy, and counseling alternatives. *$18.95*

288 pages Year Founded: 1973 ISBN 1-879237-74-1

1082 Lonely, Sad, and Angry: a Parent's Guide to Depression in Children and Adolescents
ADD Warehouse
300 NorthWest 70th Avenue
Suite 102
Plantation, FL 33317-2360
954-792-8944
800-233-9273
Fax: 954-792-8545
E-mail: websales@addwarehouse.com
www.addwarehouse.com

Richard R. Morrissey, PhD, Author

Covers the symptoms of depression, its diagnosis, causes, treatment (including medication), suicide, and management strategies at home and at school. For parents and teenagers. $14.95

225 pages Year Founded: 1990

1083 Management of Bipolar Disorder: Pocketbook
American Psychiatric Publishing, Inc.
1000 Wilson Boulevard
Suite 1825
Arlington, VA 22209-3901
703-907-7322
800-368-5777
Fax: 703-907-1091
E-mail: appi@psych.org
www.appi.org

Robert E Hales MD, Editor-in-Chief
Ron McMillen, Chief Executive Officer
John McDuffie, Editorial Director

Contains the need for treatment, what defines bipolar disorders, spectrum of the disorder, getting the best out of treatment, treatment of mania and bipolar depression, preventing new episodes, special problems in treatment, mood stabilizers and case studies. $ 14.95

96 pages ISBN 1-853172-74-X

1084 Management of Depression
American Psychiatric Publishing, Inc.
1000 Wilson Boulevard
Suite 1825
Arlington, VA 22209-3901
703-907-7322
800-368-5777
Fax: 703-907-1091
E-mail: appi@psych.org
www.appi.org

Robert E Hales MD, Editor-in-Chief
Ron McMillen, Chief Executive Officer
John McDuffie, Editorial Director

Comprehensive text covers all the important issues in the management of depression. $39.95

136 pages ISBN 1-853175-47-1

1085 Mania: Clinical and Research Perspectives
American Psychiatric Publishing, Inc.
1000 Wilson Boulevard
Suite 1825
Arlington, VA 22209-3901
703-907-7322
800-368-5777
Fax: 703-907-1091
E-mail: appi@psych.org
www.appi.org

Paul J Goodnick, M.D., Editor
Ron McMillen, Chief Executive Officer
John McDuffie, Editorial Director

Diagnostic considerations, biological aspects, and treatment of mania. $59.95

440 pages Year Founded: 1998 ISBN 0-880487-28-3

1086 Manic-Depressive Illness: Bipolar Disorders and Recurrent Depression, 2nd Edition
Oxford University Press
198 Madison Avenue
New York, NY 10016

212-726-6000
E-mail: custserv.us@oup.com
www.www.oup.com/us/

Frederick K Goodwin, Author

The authors review the biological and genetic literature that has dominated the field in recent years and incorporate cutting-edge research conducted since publication of the first edition. They also update their surveys of psychological and epidemiological evidence, as well as that pertaining to diagnostice issues, course, and outcome, and they offer practical guidelines for differential diagnosis and clinical management.

1087 Mayo Clinic on Depression: Answers to Help You Understand, Recognize and Manage Depression
Mason Crest Publishers
370 Reed Road
Suite 302
Broomall, PA 19008-4017
866-627-2665
Fax: 610-543-3878
www.masoncrest.com

Keith G Kramlinger, MD, Author

Discusses factors that increase risk, indications of depression, what happens inside the brain, effective forms of psychotherapy, electroconvulsive therapy, new trends in treatment, self-care strategies for staying healthy, and more.

194 pages

1088 Mood Apart: The Thinker's Guide to Emotion and Its Disorders
William Morrow Paperbacks, Harper Collins Imprint
30 Bond Street
New York, NY 10012
212-253-1074
Fax: 212-253-1075
www.www.peterwhybrow.com/

Peter C. Whybrow, Author

An overview of depression and manic depression and the available treatments for them. $24.00

384 pages Year Founded: 1998 ISBN 0-060977-40-X

1089 Mood Apart: Thinker's Guide to Emotion & Its Disorders
Harper Collins
30 Bond Street
New York, NY 10012
212-253-1074
Fax: 212-253-1075
E-mail: sales@harpercollins.com
www.www.peterwhybrow.com/

Peter C. Whybrow, Author

Discussion of depression and mania includes symptoms, human costs, biological underpinnings, and therapies. Authoritatively written, it uses case histories, appendices, and historical references. $15.00

ISBN 0-060977-40-X

1090 Natural History of Mania, Depression and Schizophrenia
American Psychiatric Publishing, Inc.
1000 Wilson Boulevard
Suite 1825
Arlington, VA 22209-3901
703-907-7322
800-368-5777
Fax: 703-907-1091
E-mail: appi@psych.org
www.appi.org

George Winokur, M.D., Author
Ming T Tsuang, M.D., Ph.D., D, Author
John McDuffie, Editorial Director

An unusual look at the course of mental illness, based on data from the Iowa 500 Research Project. *$42.50*

384 pages Year Founded: 1996 ISBN 0-880487-26-7

1091 Overcoming Anxiety, Depression, and Other Mental Health Disorders in Children and Adults
Interdisciplinary Council on Development & Learning Disorders
4938 Hampden Lane
Suite 800
Bethesda, MD 20814
301-656-2667
E-mail: info@icdl.com
www.icdl.com

Dr Stanley I Greenspan, Author

Reveals strategies for family members as well as professionals from different disciplines to help both children and adults. The most common mental health disorders, including anxiety, depression, obsessive-compulsive patterns, ADD/ADHD, borderline states, and others, are discussed literally with a new set of eyeglasses.

168 pages ISBN 0-976775-88-3

1092 Overcoming Depression: The Definitive Resource for Patients and Families Who Live with Depression and Manic-Depression
Harper Collins
10 E 53rd Street
New York, NY 10022-5299
212-207-7000
www.harpercollins.com

Demitri Papolos, Author

Has become the book most often recommended by doctors to their depressed patients because it clearly and sympathetically presents state-of-the-art medical information and the solid, practical advice that patients and their families need to participate actively in diagnosis and treatment. Now featuring all-new data on the latest drugs, research, treatment, and medical insurance, it also includes a frank discussion of psychiatric therapy in the era of managed care. *$15.00*

432 pages Year Founded: 1997 ISBN 0-060927-82-8

1093 Pain Behind the Mask: Overcoming Masculine Depression
Haworth Press
711 Third Avenue
New York, NY 10017
212-216-7800
800-429-6784
Fax: 212-244-1563
E-mail: getinfo@haworthpress.com
www.haworthpress.com

John R Lynch, PhD, Author
Christopher Kilmartin, PhD, Author

Presents a model of masculinity based on the premise that men express depression through behaviors that distort the feelings and human conflicts they experience. *$22.95*

210 pages Year Founded: 1999 ISBN 0-789005-58-1

1094 Pastoral Care of Depression
Haworth Press
711 Third Avenue
New York, NY 10017
212-216-7800
800-429-6784
Fax: 212-244-1563
E-mail: getinfo@haworthpressinc.com
www.haworthpress.com

Binford W Gilbert, PhD, Author
Harold G Koenig, Author

Helps caregivers by overcoming the simplistic myths about depressive disorders and probing the real issues. *$17.95*

136 pages Year Founded: 1997 ISBN 0-789002-65-5

1095 Physician's Guide to Depression and Bipolar Disorders
McGraw-Hill Companies
PO Box 182604
Columbus, OH 43218-2604
877-833-5524
Fax: 614-759-3749
E-mail: customer.service@mcgraw-hill.com
www.mcgraw-hill.com

Dwight L Evans, MD, Author
Dennis S Charney, MD, Author
Lydia Lewis, Author

Offers a clear definitive instruction on drug treatments for bipolar disorders with the exact dosages needed. Crucial to a diagnosis and treatment is the ability to identify a patients symptoms. *$59.00*

400 pages Year Founded: 2005 ISBN 0-071441-75-1

1096 Post-Natal Depression: Psychology, Science and the Transition to Motherhood
Routledge
711 3rd Avenue
8th Floor
New York, NY 10017
212-216-7800
Fax: 212-563-2269
www.www.routledge.com

Paula Nicolson, Author

Challenges the expectation that it is normal to be a happy mother. It provides a radical critique of the traditional medical and social science explanations of post natal depression by supplying a systematic feminist psychological analysis of women's experiences following childbirth. This book makes an important contribution to the psychology of women and feminist research and will be of interest to psychologists, nurses, and doctors. *$23.95*

ISBN 0-415163-62-5

1097 Postpartum Mood Disorders
American Psychiatric Publishing, Inc.
1000 Wilson Boulevard
Suite 1825
Arlington, VA 22209-3901
703-907-7322
800-368-5777
Fax: 703-907-1091
E-mail: appi@psych.orgg
www.appi.org

Lee S Cohen, M.D., Editor
Ruta M Nonacs, M.D., Ph.D., Editor
John McDuffie, Editorial Director

Provides thorough coverage of a highly prevalent, but often misunderstood subject. *$38.50*

164 pages Year Founded: 2005 ISBN 0-880489-29-4

1098 Practice Guideline for Major Depressive Disorders in Adults
American Psychiatric Publishing, Inc.
1000 Wilson Boulevard
Suite 1825
Arlington, VA 22209-3901
703-907-7322
800-368-5777
Fax: 703-907-1091
E-mail: appi@psych.org
www.appi.org

Robert E Hales MD, Editor-in-Chief
Ron McMillen, Chief Executive Officer
John McDuffie, Editorial Director

Summarizes the specific forms of somatic, psychotherapeutic, psychosocial, and educational treatments developed to deal with major depressive order and its various subtypes. *$22.50*

1, 612 pages Year Founded: 2006 ISBN 0-890423-01-6

1099 Predictors of Treatment Response in Mood Disorders
American Psychiatric Publishing, Inc.
1000 Wilson Boulevard
Suite 1825
Arlington, VA 22209-3901
703-907-7322
800-368-5777
Fax: 703-907-1091
E-mail: appi@psych.org
www.appi.org

Paul J Goodnick, M.D., Editor
Ron McMillen, Chief Executive Officer
John McDuffie, Editorial Director

Helps clinicians and managed care administrators assign the correct somatic therapy. *$29.00*

260 pages Year Founded: 1995 ISBN 0-880484-94-2

1100 Prozac Nation: Young & Depressed in America, a Memoir
Houghton Mifflin Company
222 Berkeley Street
Boston, MA 02116-3760
617-351-5000
Fax: 617-351-1105

Elizabeth Wurtzel, Author

Struck with depression at 11, Wurtzel, now 27, chronicles her struggle with the illness. Witty, terrifying and sometimes funny, it tells the story of a young life almost destroyed by depression. *$19.95*

317 pages

1101 Questions & Answers About Depression & Its Treatment
Charles Press Publishers
230 North 21st Street
Suite 202
Philadelphia, PA 19103
215-561-2786
Fax: 215-600-1248
E-mail: mailbox@charlespresspub.com
www.charlespresspub.com

Ivan k Goldberg, MD, Author

All the questions you'd like to ask, with answers.

139 pages

1102 Seasonal Affective Disorder and Beyond: Light Treatment for SAD and Non-SAD Conditions
American Psychiatric Publishing, Inc.
1000 Wilson Boulevard
Suite 1825
Arlington, VA 22209-3901
703-907-7322
800-368-5777
Fax: 703-907-1091
E-mail: appi@psych.org
www.appi.org

Raymond W Lam, M.D., Editor
Ron McMillen, Chief Executive Officer
John McDuffie, Editorial Director

Summarizes issues around the therapeutic uses of light treatment. *$45.00*

344 pages Year Founded: 1998 ISBN 0-880488-67-0

1103 Talking to Depression: Simple Ways to Connect When Someone In Your Life Is Depressed
Penguin Group
375 Hudson Street
New York, NY 10014-3657
212-366-2372
800-847-5515
Fax: 212-366-2933
E-mail: ecommerce@us.penguingroup.com
www.www.us.penguingroup.com

Claudia J Strauss, Author
Martha Manning, Foreward

What to say and what not to say when a friend or family member is struggling with depression. *$14.00*

224 pages Year Founded: 1936 ISBN 0-451209-86-3

1104 Taming Bipolar Disorders
Alpha
677 Elm Street, Ste 112
PO Box 255
Royersford, PA 19468
800-992-9124
www.alphapub.com

Contains cutting-edge research and straightforward advice from the most respectable names on bipolar disorder, along with the most up-to-date information on mental health organizations, support and advocacy groups. *$17.95*

400 pages Year Founded: 2004 ISBN 1-592572-85-5

1105 The Cognitive Behavorial Workbook for Depression: A Step-by-Step Program
NewHarbinger Publications
5674 Shattuck Avenue
Oakland, CA 94609-1662
510-652-0215
800-748-6273
Fax: 800-652-1613
E-mail: customerservice@newharbinger.com
www.newharbinger.com

Dr William J Knaus, Ed.D., Author
Albert Ellis, Ph.D., Author

This type of cognitive behavioral therapy, called rational emotive behavior therapy (REBT) by Ellis, proved especially effective at relieving problems like anger, anxiety, and depression.

336 pages Year Founded: 1973

1106 Touched with Fire: Manic-Depressive Illness and the Artistic Temperament
Free Press
40 Main Street
Suite 301
Florence, MA 01062-3100
877-888-1533
Fax: 413-585-8904
www.freepress.net

Kay Redfield Jamison, Author

'We of the craft are all crazy.' -remarked Lord Byron about himself and his fellow poets.

325 pages Year Founded: 1996 ISBN 0-684831-83-X

1107 Treatment Plans and Interventions for Depression and Anxiety Disorders
Guilford Press
72 Spring Street
New York, NY 10012-4068
800-365-7006
Fax: 212-966-6708
E-mail: info@guilford.com
www.www.guilford.com

Robert L Leahy, Author
Stephen J.F Holland, Author
Lata K McGinn, Author

Provides information on treatments for seven frequently encountered disorders: major depression, generalized anxiety, panic, agoraphobia, PTSD, social phobia, specific phobia and OCD. Serving as ready to use treatment packages, chapters describe basic cognitive behavioral therapy techniques and how to tailor them to each disorder. Also featured are diagnostic decision trees, therapist forms for assessment and record keeping, client handouts and homework sheets. *$ 49.50*

490 pages Year Founded: 1973 ISBN 1-572305-14-2

1108 Treatment for Chronic Depression: Cognitive Behavioral Analysis System of Psychotherapy (CBASP)
Guilford Press
512 Glendale Drive
Richmond, VA 23229
804-740-7646
800-365-7006
Fax: 804-740-0305
E-mail: jmccull@vcu.edu
www.www.cbasp.org/

James P. McCullough Jr, PhD, Author

This book describes CBASP, a research based psychotherapeutic approach designed to motivate chronically depressed patients to change and help them develop needed problem solving and relationship skills. Filled with illustrative case material that brings challenging clinical situations to life, this book now puts the power of CBASP in the hands of the clinician. Readers are provided with two essential assets: an innovative framework for understanding the patient's psychopathology and a disciplined plan for helping the individual overthrow depression. *$35.00*

326 pages ISBN 1-572305-27-4

1109 When Nothing Matters Anymore: A Survival Guide for Depressed Teens
Free Spirit Publishing
217 Fifth Avenue North
Suite 200
Minneapolis, MN 55401-1299
612-338-2068
866-735-7323
Fax: 866-419-5199
E-mail: help4kids@freespirit.com
www.freespirit.com

Bev Cobain, R.N.C, Author

Written for teens with depression and those who feel despondent, dejected or alone. This powerful book offers help, hope, and potentially lifesaving facts and advice. *$13.95*

160 pages Year Founded: 1983 ISBN 1-575420-36-8

1110 Winter Blues: Seasonal Affective Disorder: What It Is and How to Overcome It
Guilford Press
72 Spring Street
New York, NY 10012-4068
212-431-9800
800-365-7006
Fax: 212-966-6708
E-mail: info@guilford.com

Norman Rosenthal, Author

Complete information about Seasonal Affective Disorder and its treatment. *$14.95*

355 pages Year Founded: 1998 ISBN 1-572303-95-6

1111 Yesterday's Tomorrow
Hazelden
PO Box 11
Center City, MN 55012-0176
651-213-4000
800-822-0080
www.www.hazelden.org

Barry Longyear, Author

At last, a meditation book that shows why and, more importantly, how recovery works written in no-nonsense language by a hard case who's been there, and been there, and been there. *$12.00*

384 pages ISBN 1-568381-60-3

1112 You Can Beat Depression: Guide to Prevention and Recovery
Impact Publishers
PO Box 6016
Atascadero, CA 93423-6016
805-466-5917
800-246-7228
Fax: 805-466-5919
E-mail: info@impactpublishers.com
www.impactpublishers.com

John Preston, Psy.D, Author

Includes material on prevention of depression, prevention of relapse after treatment, brief therapy interventions, exercise, other non medical approaches and the Prozac controversy. Helps readers recognize when and how to help themsevles, and when to turn to professional treatment. *$14.95*

176 pages Year Founded: 1970 ISBN 1-886230-40-4

Periodicals & Pamphlets

1113 Bipolar Disorder
National Institute of Mental Health
6001 Executive Boulevard
Room 6200, MSC 9663
Bethesda, MD 20892-9663
301-443-4513
866-615-6464
Fax: 301-443-4279
TTY: 301-443-8431
E-mail: nimhinfo@nih.gov
www.www.nimh.nih.gov

Tom Insel, MD, NIHM Director
William G Coleman, Scientific Director, NIMHD
Grace E O Ajao, Administrative Officer
Dionne D Draper, Administrative Officer

A detailed booklet that describes Bipolar Disorder symptons, causes, and treatments, with information on getting help and coping.

24 pages

1114 Coping With Unexpected Events: Depression & Trauma
Depression & BiPolar Support Alliance
730 North Franklin Street
Suite 501
Chicago, IL 60654-7225
312-642-0049
800-826-3632
Fax: 312-642-7243
E-mail: programs@dbsalliance.org
www.dbsalliance.org

Cheryl T Magrini, MS.Ed, MTS, PhD, Chair
Allen Doederlein, President
Cindy Specht, ExecutiveVice president
Gregory E Ostfeld, Treasurer

The mission of DBSA is to provide hope, help, and support to improve the lives of people living with mood disorders.

DBSA pursues and accomplishes this mission through peer-based, recovery-oriented, empowering services and resources when people want them, where they want them, and how they want to receive them.

1115 Coping with Mood Changes Later in Life
Depression & Bipolar Support Alliance
730 North Franklin Street
Suite 501
Chicago, IL 60654-7225
312-642-0049
800-826-3632
Fax: 312-642-7243
www.dbsalliance.org

Sue Bergeson, President

14 pages Year Founded: 2003

1116 DBSA Support Groups: An Important Step on the Road to Wellness
Depression and Bipolar Support Alliance
730 North Franklin Street
Suite 501
Chicago, IL 60654-7225
312-642-0049
800-826-3632
Fax: 312-642-7243
www.dbsalliance.org

Cheryl T Magrini, MS.Ed, MTS, PhD, Chair
Allen Doederlein, President
Cindy Specht, ExecutiveVice president
Gregory E Ostfeld, Treasurer

Support groups for people with depression or bipolar disorder to discuss the experiences, and helpful treatments.

10 pages Year Founded: 2003

1117 Depression
National Institute of Mental Health
6001 Executive Boulevard
Room 8184
Bethesda, MD 20892-1
301-443-4513
866-615-6464
TTY: 301-443-8431
E-mail: nimhinfo@nih.gov

This brochure gives descriptions of major depression, dysthymia and bipolar disorder (manic depression). It lists symptoms, gives possible causes, tells how depression is diagnosed and discusses available treatments. This brochure provides help and hope for the depressed person, family and friends.

23 pages

1118 Depression: Help On the Way
ETR Associates
4 Carbonero Way
Scotts Valley, CA 95066-4200
831-438-4060
800-321-4407
Fax: 831-438-3618
E-mail: support@etr.freshdesk.com
www.etr.org

David Kitchen, MBA, Chief Financial Officer
Talita Sanders, BS, Director, Human Resources
Coleen Cantwell, MPH, Director, Business Development Pl
Matt McDowell, BS, Director, Marketing

Includes symptoms of minor depression, major depression, and seasonal affective depression; treatment options and medication, and the importance of exercise and laughter. Sold in lots of 50.

1119 Depression: What Every Woman Should Know
National Institute of Mental Health
6001 Executive Boulevard
Room 8184, MSC 9663
Bethesda, MD 20892-9663
301-443-4513
866-615-6464
TTY: 301-443-8431
E-mail: nimhinfo@nih.gov
www.www.nimh.nih.gov/

This booklet discusses the symptoms of depression and some of the reasons that make women so vulnerable. It also discusses the types of therapy and where to go for help.

24 pages

1120 Finding Peace of Mind: Treatment Strategies for Depression and Bipolar Disorder
Depression and Bipolar Support Alliance
730 North Franklin Street
Suite 501
Chicago, IL 60654-7225
312-642-0049
800-826-3632
Fax: 312-642-7243
www.dbsalliance.org

Helps to build a good, cooperative relationship with your doctor by explaining some of the treatments for mood disorders and how they work. Also includes a guide for medication that has been frequently prescribed and new treatments that are being investigated.

20 pages Year Founded: 2003

1121 Getting Better Sleep: What You Need to Know
Depression and Bipolar Support Alliance
730 North Franklin Street
Suite 501
Chicago, IL 60654-7225
312-642-0049
800-826-3632
Fax: 312-642-7243
www.dbsalliance.org

Sue Bergeson, President

Describes some causes of sleep loss, and how sleep loss relates to bipolar disorder and depression. Also provides information on how to get better sleep.

1122 Introduction to Depression and Bipolar Disorder
Depression and Bipolar Support Alliance
730 North Franklin Street
Suite 501
Chicago, IL 60654-7225
312-642-0049
800-826-3632
Fax: 312-642-7243
www.dbsalliance.org

Sue Bergeson, President

Quick and easy-to-read brochure describing syptoms and treatments for mood disorders.

1123 Let's Talk About Depression
National Institute of Mental Health
6001 Executive Boulevard
Room 8184, MSC 9663
Bethesda, MD 20892-9663
301-443-4513
866-615-6464
TTY: 301-443-8431
E-mail: nimhinfo@nih.gov
www.www.nimh.nih.gov/

Facts about depression, and ways to get help. Target audience is teenaged youth.

1124 Major Depression in Children and Adolescents
PO Box 42557
Washington, DC 20015-557
800-789-2647
Fax: 240-747-5470
TDD: 866-889-2647
E-mail: ken@mentalhealth.org
www.mentalhealth.samhsa.gov

A Kathryn Power, MEd, Director
Edward B Searle, Deputy Director

2 pages

1125 McMan's Depression and Bipolar Weekly
McMan's Depression and Bipolar Web
PO Box 5093
Kendall Park, NJ 08824-5093
E-mail: mcman@mcmanweb.com
www.mcmanweb.com

John McManamy, Editor/Publisher

Online newsletter devoted to the issues of bipolar and depression disorders. There is no charge, just for you to understand different things about the disorders.

1126 Men and Depression
National Institute of Mental Health
6001 Executive Boulevard
Room 8184, MSC 9663
Bethesda, MD 20892-9663
301-443-4513
866-615-6464
TTY: 301-443-8431
E-mail: nimhinfo@nih.gov
www.www.nlmh.nih.gov/

Have you known a man who is grumpy, irritable, and has no sense of humor? Maybe he drinks too much or abuses drugs. Maybe he physically or verbally abuses his wife and his kids. Maybe he works all the time, or compulsively seeks thrills in high-risk behavior. Or maybe he seems isolated, withdrawn, and no longer interested in the people or activities he used to enjoy. Perhaps this man is you. Talk to a healthcare provider about how you are feeling, and ask for help.

36 pages

1127 Mood Disorders
Center for Mental Health Services: Knowledge Exchange Network
PO Box 42490
Washington, DC 20015
800-789-2647
Fax: 301-984-8796
TDD: 866-889-2647

E-mail: ken@mentalhealth.org
www.store.samhsa.gov

This fact sheet provides basic information on the symptoms, formal diagnosis, and treatment for bipolar disorder.

3 pages

1128 Myths and Facts about Depression and Bipolar Disorders
Depression and Bipolar Support Alliance
730 North Franklin Street
Suite 501
Chicago, IL 60654-7225
312-642-0049
800-826-3632
Fax: 312-642-7243
www.dbsalliance.org

Gives some myths about depression and bipolar disorder and the truths that combat them.

1129 New Message
Emotions Anonymous
PO Box 4245
Saint Paul, MN 55104-0245
651-647-9712
Fax: 651-647-1593
E-mail: info@EmotionsAnonymous.org
www.EmotionsAnonymous.org

Features stories and articles of recovery, plus the latest news from EA International. *$8.00*

4 per year

1130 Oxcarbazepine and Bipolar Disorder: A Guide
Madison Institute of Medicine
6515 Grand Teton Plaza
Suite 100
Madison, WI 53719
608-827-2470
Fax: 608-827-2444
E-mail: mim@miminc.org
www.factsforhealth.org

W Jefferson James, Author
John H Greist, Author
David J Katzelnick, MD, Author

This 31 page booklet provides patients with the information they need to know about the use of oxcarbazepine in the treatment of bipolar disorder, including information about proper dosing, medication management, and possible side effects. *$5.95*

31 pages

1131 Recovering Your Mental Health: a Self-Help Guide
SAMHSA'S National Mental Health Informantion Center
1 Choke Cherry Road
Rockville, MD 20857
877-726-4727
E-mail: ken@mentalhealth.org
www.mentalhealth.samhsa.gov

Mary Ellen Copeland, Author
Edward B Searle, Deputy Director

This booklet offers tips for understanding symptoms of depression and other conditions and getting help. Also details the advantages of counseling, medications available, op-

tions for professional help, relaxation techniques and paths to positive thinking.

32 pages

1132 Storm In My Brain
Depression & Bi-Polar Support Alliance
730 North Franklin Street
Suite 501
Chicago, IL 60654-7225
312-642-0049
800-826-3632
Fax: 312-642-7243
www.dbsalliance.org

Sue Bergeson, President
Ingrid Deetz, Program Director

Pamphlet free on the Internet or by mail. Discusses child or adolesent Bi-Polar symptoms.

1133 What to do When a Friend is Depressed: Guide for Students
National Institute of Mental Health
6001 Executive Boulevard
Room 8184
Bethesda, MD 20892-1
301-443-4513
866-615-6464
TTY: 301-443-8431
E-mail: nimhinfo@nih.gov
www.www.vamh.org

This brochure offers information on depression and its symptoms and suggests things a young person can do to guide a depressed friend in finding help. It is especially good for health fairs, health clinics, and school health units.

3 pages

1134 You've Just Been Diagnosed...What Now?
Depression and Bipolar Support Alliance
730 North Franklin Street
Suite 501
Chicago, IL 60654-7225
312-642-0049
800-826-3632
Fax: 312-642-7243
www.dbsalliance.org

Sue Bergeson, President

Pamphlet to help you understand about the disorder you have just been diagnosed with. Tells you basic facts about mood disorders and will help you work towards a diagnosis.

19 pages Year Founded: 2002

Research Centers

1135 Bipolar Clinic and Research Program
The Massachusetts General Hospital Bipolar Clinic & Research Program
50 Staniford Street
Suite 580
Boston, MA 02114-2540
617-726-5855
Fax: 617-726-6768
www.www.massgeneral.org

Michael Jellinek, MD, President
Laurie Ansorge Ball, Executive Director, MGH Departmen
Jerrold F Rosenbaum, MD, Chief of Psychiatry, MGH

Dedicated to providing quality clinical care, conducting clinically informative research, and educating our colleagues, patients, as well as the community.

1136 Bipolar Disorders Clinic
Standford School of Medicine
401 Quarry Road
Stanford, CA 94305-5723
650-723-3305
www.bipolar.stanford.edu

Terrence A Ketter, MD, Chief, Bipolar Disorders Clinic
Shelley Hill, MS, Clinical Research Coordinator

Offers an on-going clinical treatment, manage clinical trials and neuroimaging studies, lecture and teach seminar courses at Stanford University and train residents in the School of Medicine.

1137 Bipolar Research Program at University of Pennsylvania
3535 Market Street
6th Floor
Philadelphia, PA 19104-3413
215-898-4301
Fax: 215-898-0509
E-mail: balthrop@mail.med.upenn.edu
www.www.med.upenn.edu/psych/bipolar_research.html

Laszlo Gyulai, MD, Program Director
Chang-Gyu Hahn, MD, Ph.D., Clinical Team Member

Offers and conducts research on treatments for bipolar disorders. The program provides comprehensive care for persons with bipolar affective disorder (manic depressive illness), seasonal affective disorder, and rapid cycling bipolar disorder. Services offered for individuals who are in the ages of 18 or older include evaluations, consultations, and ongoing treatment options.

1138 Brain & Behavior Research Foundation
90 Park Avenue
16th Floor
New York, NY 10016
646-681-4888
800-829-8289
Fax: 516-487-6930
E-mail: info@bbrfoundation.org
www.bbrfoundation.org

Steve Lieber, Chairman of the Board
Jeffrey Borenstein, M.D, President and Chief Executive Of
Louis Innamorato, Vice president, Finance and Chief
Suzzane Golden, Vice President

Committed to alleviating the suffering caused by mental illness by awarding grants that will lead to advances and breakthroughs in scientific research. 100% of all donor contributions for research are invested in NARSAD Grants leading to discoveries in understanding causes and improving treatments of disorders in children and adults, such as depression, bipolar disorder, schizophrenia, autism, attention deficit hyperactivity disorder, and anxiety disorders like obsessive-compulsive and post-traumatic stress disorders.

Year Founded: 1981

1139 Epidemiology-Genetics Program in Psychiatry
John Hopkins University School of Medicine
PO Box 1997
Baltimore, MD 21203
888-289-4095
www.www.hopkinsmedicine.org

The research program is to help characterize the genetic (biochemical) developmental, and environmental components of bipolar disorder. The hope is that once scientists understand the biological causes of this disorder new medications and treatments can be developed.

1140 UAMS Psychiatric Research Institute
University of Arkansas for Medical Sciences
4224 Shuffield Drive
Little Rock, AR 72205
501-526-8100
Fax: 501-660-7542
E-mail: pri@umas.edu
www.psychiatry.uams.edu

Donald R Bobbitt, President
William Bowes, MS, Vice Chancellor, Finance And CFO
Roxane A Townsend, MD, Chief Executive Officer
Christina L Clark, BA, Chief of Staff

Combining research, education and clinical services into one facility, PRI offers inpatiend and outpatient services, with 40 psychiatric beds, therapy options, and specialized treatment for specific disorders, including: addictive eating, anxiety, deppressive and post-traumatic stress disorders. Research focuses on evidence-based care takes into consideration the education of future medical personnel while relying on research scientists to provide innovative forms of treatment. PRI includes the Center for Addiction Research as well as a methadone clinic.

1141 University of Texas: Mental Health Clinical Research Center
6363 Forest Park Road
7th Floor, Suite 749
Dallas, TX 75390-9121
214-648-3111
www.utsouthwestern.edu

Research activity of major and atypical depression.

1142 Yale Mood Disorders Research Program
Department of Psychiatry
300 George Street
Suite 901
New Haven, CT 06511-6624
203-785-2090
Fax: 203-785-2028
www.psychiatry.yale.edu

John H Krystal, Chair
Rajita Sinha, Chief, Psychology Section

MDRP is dedicated to understanding the science of mood disorders, including bipolar disorder and depression. The MDRP brings together a multi-disciplinary group of scientists from across the Yale campus in a highly collaborative research effort. Goals of the MDRP include the identification of biological markers for mood disorders and discovery of new treatment strategies.

Support Groups & Hot Lines

1143 Abraham Low Self-Help Systems
105 W. Adams Street
Suite 2940
Chicago, IL 60603
866-221-0302
Fax: 312-726-4446
E-mail: info@recoveryinternational.org
www.lowselfhelpsystems.org

Rudolph Pruden, Chair
John Rosenheim, 1st Vice Chair
Larry Kipperman, 2nd Vice Chair
Rudolph Pruden, Acting Treasurer

Mission is to use the cognitive-behavioral, peer-to-peer, self-help training system developed by Abraham Low, MD, to help individuals gain skills to lead more peaceful and productive lives.

1144 Depressed Anonymous
PO Box 17414
Louisville, KY 40217
502-569-1989
E-mail: info@depressedanon.com
www.depressedanon.com

Formed to provide therapeutic resources for depressed individuals of all ages. Works with the chronically depressed and those recently discharged from health facilities who were treated for depression.

1145 Emotions Anonymous International Service Center
PO Box 4245
Saint Paul, MN 55104-0245
651-647-9712
Fax: 651-647-1593
E-mail: info@EmotionsAnonymous.org
www.EmotionsAnonymous.org

Fellowship of men and women who share their experience, strength and hope with each other, that they may solve their common problem and help others recover from emotional illness.

Video & Audio

1146 A Madman's Journal
Educational Training Videos
136 Granville St
Suite 200
Gahanna, OH 43230
Fax: 888-775-3919
www.educationaltrainingvideos.com

For two years, the narrator of this program went through a nightmare, feeling a self-hatred and worthlessness beyond love and redemption that he described as the concentration camp of the mind. This video presents one man's attempt to convey the ordeal of severe depression by writing a memoir about the experience.

1147 Anger Management-Enhanced Edition
Educational Video Network, Inc.
1401 19th Street
Huntsville, TX 77340
936-295-5767
800-762-0060

Fax: 936-294-0233
www.www.evndirect.com

Learn what causes anger and understand why our bodies react as they do when we're angry. Effective techniques for assuaging anger are discussed.

1148 Beating Depression
Educational Training Videos
136 Granville St
Suite 200
Gahanna, OH 43230
Fax: 888-775-3919
www.educationaltrainingvideos.com

This program comes to grips with depression through the experiences of five patients whose backgrounds span the socioeconomic spectrum. Three cases of chronic depression, one of which is complicated by borderline personality disorder and another by alcohol abuse, and two cases of bipolar disorder, one of which is extreme, are presented.

1149 Bipolar Disorder: Shifting Mood Swings
Educational Training Videos
136 Granville St
Suite 200
Gahanna, OH 43230
Fax: 888-775-3919
www.educationaltrainingvideos.com

Different from the routine ups and downs of life, the symptoms of bipolar disorder are severe - even to the point of being life-threatening. In this insightful program, patients speak from their own experience about the complexities of diagnosis and the very real danger of suicide, while family members and close friends address the strain of the condition's cyclic behavior.

1150 Bundle of Blues
Fanlight Productions
32 Court Street
21st Floor
Brooklyn, NY 11201
718-488-8900
800-876-1710
Fax: 718-488-8642
E-mail: info@fanlight.com
www.fanlight.com

Serena Down, Author

The stories in this thoughtful documentary represent a range of experiences from minor postpartum depression through postpartum psychosis. It stresses that PDD can happen to any new mother, but that it can be managed. 13 minutes.

1151 Clinical Impressions: Identifying Mental Illness
Educational Training Videos
136 Granville St
Suite 200
Gahanna, OH 43230
Fax: 888-775-3919
www.educationaltrainingvideos.com

How long can mental illness stay hidden, especially from the eyes of trained experts? This program rejoins a group of ten adults- five of them healthy and five of them with histories of mental illness- as psychiatric specialists try to spot and correctly diagnose the latter. Administering a series of collaborative and one-on-one tests, including assessments of personality type, physical self-image, and rational thinking, the panel gradually makes decisions about who suffers from depression, bipolar disorder, bulimia, and social anxiety.

1152 Coping with Depression
NewHarbinger Publications
5674 Shattuck Avenue
Oakland, CA 94609-1662
510-652-0215
800-748-6273
Fax: 800-652-1613
E-mail: customerservice@newharbinger.com
www.newharbinger.com

Matthew McKay, Owner

60 minute videotape that offers a powerful message of hope for anyone struggling with depression. *$39.95*

Year Founded: 1973 ISBN 1-879237-62-8

1153 Coping with Stress
Educational Video Network, Inc.
1401 19th Street
Huntsville, TX 77340
936-295-5767
800-762-0060
Fax: 936-294-0233
www.www.evndirect.com

Stress affects everyone, both emotionally and physically. For some, mismanaged stress can result in substance abuse, violence, or even suicide. This program answers the question, How can a person cope with stress?

1154 Covert Modeling & Covert Reinforcement
NewHarbinger Publications
5674 Shattuck Avenue
Oakland, CA 94609-1662
510-652-0215
800-748-6273
Fax: 800-652-1613
E-mail: customerservice@newharbinger.com
www.newharbinger.com

Matthew McKay, Owner

Based on the essential book of cognitive behavioral techniques for effecting change in your life, Thoughts & Feelings. Learn step-by-step protocols for controlling destructive behaviors such as anxiety, obsessional thinking, uncontrolled anger, and depression. *$ 11.95*

Year Founded: 1973 ISBN 0-934986-29-0

1155 Dark Glasses and Kaleidoscopes: Living with Manic Depression
Depression and Bipolar Support Alliance
730 N Franklin Street
Suite 501
Chicago, IL 60654-7225
312-642-0049
800-826-3632
Fax: 312-642-7243
www.dbsalliance.org

Allen Doederlein, President
Cindy Specht, Executive Vice President
Lisa Goodale, Vice President, Peer Support Ser
Nancy Heffernan, Vice President, Finance and Admi

Dr. Kowatch speaks about the prevalence, diagnosis, comorbidity, medication treatment, and outcome of child/adolescent bipolar disorder. He addresses some of the unique traits of cild bipolar, as well as some factors that make it difficult to diagnose. He covers treatment options for both the manic and depressive phases in detail, using clinical studies as evidence. *$5.00*

1156 Day for Night: Recognizing Teenage Depression
DRADA-Depression and Related Affective Disorders Association
2330 W Joppa Road
Suite 100
Lutherville, MD 21093-4614
410-583-2919
Fax: 410-583-2964
E-mail: drada@jhmi.edu
www.drada.org

Catherine Pollock, Executive Director
Sallie Mink, Director Education
Vice Preside

In an effort to help teens gain a better understanding of depression, this video was created to build awareness of the illness and, in the process, save lives. Offering an in-depth look at the signs, symptoms and treatment of teenage depression, this video includes interviews with young people who are dealing with clinical depression and bipolar disorder. Featuring their families and friends, as well as interviews with health professionals, the video's goal is to provide education, support and hope to those suffering from this debilitating yet treatable disease. *$22.50*

1157 Dealing with Depression
Educational Video Network, Inc.
1401 19th Street
Huntsville, TX 77340
936-295-5767
800-762-0060
Fax: 936-294-0233
www.www.evndirect.com

As more and more young people are falling victim to depression, it is important to understand what causes it and to know how to get the help that can rid a person of this life-wrecking affliction.

1158 Dealing with Social Anxiety
Educational Video Network, Inc.
1401 19th Street
Huntsville, TX 77340
936-295-5767
800-762-0060
Fax: 936-294-0233
www.www.evndirect.com

Social anxiety is America's third-largest psychiatric disorder. It generally develops during the mid-teen years, and almost always before the age of 25. Understand what may trigger the development of anxiety and learn how it sometimes evolves into full-blown panic disorder, which is characterized by recurrent attacks of terror or fear. The consequences of social anxiety are examined and effective treatments are discussed.

1159 Depression & Anxiety Management
NewHarbinger Publications
5674 Shattuck Avenue
Oakland, CA 94609-1662
510-652-0215
800-748-6273
Fax: 800-652-1613

E-mail: customerservice@newharbinger.com
www.newharbinger.com

Matthew McKay, Owner

Offers step-by-step help for identifying the thoughts that make one anxious and depressed, confronting unrealistic and distorted thinking, and replacing negative mental patterns with healthy, realistic thinking. *$11.95*

Year Founded: 1973 ISBN 1-879237-46-6

1160 Depression: Fighting the Dragon
Fanlight Productions
32 Court Street
21st Floor
Brooklyn, NY 11201
718-488-8900
800-876-1710
Fax: 718-488-8642
E-mail: info@fanlight.com
www.fanlight.com

Sue Ridout, Author

Follows five people who have struggled for years to overcome this debilitating condition. Two of the five have family histories of the disease. Their moving personal stories are enriched by the perspectives of leading researchers, and by glimpses of the sophisticated brain-imaging technologies which now enable us to see what is happening in the human brain during depression and its treatment. *$149.00*

1161 FRONTLINE: The Released
PBS
2100 Crystal Drive
Arlington, VA 22202
www.pbs.org

Will Lyman, Actor
Narrator
Miri Navasky, Director
Karen O'Connor, Director

The documentary states that of the 700, 000 inmates released from American prisons each year, half of them have mental disabilities. This work focused on those with severe problems who keep entering and exiting prison. Full of good information on the challenges they face with mental illnesses; housing, employment, stigmatization, and socialization.

Year Founded: 2009

1162 Families Coping with Mental Illness
Mental Illness Education Project
25 West Street
Brookline Village, MA 01581
617-562-1111
800-343-5540
Fax: 617-779-0061
E-mail: info@miepvideos.org
www.miepvideos.org

Ten family members share their experiences of having a family member with schizophrenia or bipolar disorder. Designed to provide insights and support to other families, the tape also profoundly conveys to professionals the needs of families when mental illness strikes. In two versions: a 22-minute version ideal for short classes and workshops, and a richer 43-minute version with more examples and details. Discounted price for families/consumers. *$99.95*

1163 Kay Redfield Jamison: Surviving Bipolar Disorder
Educational Training Videos
136 Granville St
Suite 200
Gahanna, OH 43230
Fax: 888-775-3919
www.educationaltrainingvideos.com

Psychiatry professor and clinical psychologist Kay Redfield Jamison knows all about bipolar disorder- from the inside out. She talks frankly about her experiences with a mental illness that almost claimed her life.

1164 Living with Depression and Manic Depression
NewHarbinger Publications
5674 Shattuck Avenue
Oakland, CA 94609-1662
510-652-0215
800-748-6273
Fax: 800-652-1613
E-mail: customerservice@newharbinger.com
www.newharbinger.com

Matthew McKay, Owner

Describes a program based on years of research and hundreds of interviews with depressed persons. Warm, helpful, and engaging, this tape validates the feelings of people with depression while it encourages positive change. *$11.95*

Year Founded: 1973 ISBN 1-879237-63-6

1165 Mental Disorder
Educational Training Videos
136 Granville St
Suite 200
Gahanna, OH 43230
Fax: 888-775-3919
www.educationaltrainingvideos.com

What is abnormality? Using the case studies of two young women; one who has depression, one who has an anxiety disorder; as a springboard, this program presents three psychological perspective on mental disorder.

1166 No More Shame: Understanding Schizophrenia, Depression, and Addiction
Educational Training Videos
136 Granville St
Suite 200
Gahanna, OH 43230
Fax: 888-775-3919
www.educationaltrainingvideos.com

These programs examine research about the physiological, psychological, sociological, and cultural aspects of these disorders and their treatments. The goal of these programs is to explain what we do and do not know about each of these conditions, as well as to destigmatize the disorders by presenting them in the context of the same research process that is applied to all medical disorders.

1167 The Bonnie Tapes of Mental Illness
The Mental Illness Education Project
PO Box 470813
Brookline Village, MA 02447-813
617-562-1111
E-mail: info@miepvideos.org
www.miepvideos.org

Talks with a young woman with schizophrenia, how it has affected her and her family. Also talks with mental health professionals to see how she is handling everything. Talks about what happens when mental illness enters a family, and how the person with the illness feels, and what are steps to get better. Each video is $99.95

1168 Understanding Mental Illness
Educational Video Network, Inc.
1401 19th Street
Huntsville, TX 77340
936-295-5767
800-762-0060
Fax: 936-294-0233
www.www.evndirect.com

Contains information and classifications of mental illness. Mental illness can strike anyone, at any age. Learn about various organic and functional mental disorders as discussed and their causes and symptoms, and learn where to seek help for a variety of mental health concerns.

1169 Why Isn't My Child Happy? Video Guide
About Childhood Depression
ADD WareHouse
300 NW 70th Avenue
Suite 102
Plantation, FL 33317-2360
954-792-8100
800-233-9273
Fax: 954-792-8545
E-mail: websales@addwarehouse.com
www.addwarehouse.com

Sam Goldstein, PhD, Author

The first of its kind, this new video deals with childhood depression. Informative and frank about this common problem, this book offers helpful guidance for parents and professionals trying to better understand childhood depression. 110 minutes. *$55.00*

Year Founded: 1990

Web Sites

1170 www.befrienders.org
Samaritans International

Support, helplines, and advice.

1171 www.blarg.net/~charlatn/voices
Voices of Depression

Compilation of writings by people suffering from depression.

1172 www.bpso.org
BPSO-Bipolar Significant Others

Informational site intended to provide information and support to the spouses, families, friends and other loved ones of those who suffer from bi-polar.

1173 www.cfsny.org
Center for Family Services

Devoted to the physical well-being and development of the reatrded child and the sound mental health of the parents.

1174 www.cyberpsych.org
CyberPsych

Hosts the American Psychoanalysts Foundation, American Association of Suicideology, Society for the Exploration of Psychotherapy Intergration, and Anxiety Disorders Association of America. Also subcategories of the anxiety disorders, as well as general information, including panic disorder, phobias, obsessive compulsive disorder (OCD), social phobia, generalized anxiety disorder, post traumatic stress disorder, and phobias of childhood. Book reviews and links to web pages sharing the topics.

1175 www.dbsalliance.org
Depression & Bi-Polar Support Alliance

Mental health news updates and local support group information.

1176 www.emdr.com
EMDR Institute, Inc.

Discusses EMDR-Eye Movement Desensitization and Reprocessing-as an innovative clinical treatment for trauma, including sexual abuse, domestic violence, combat, crime, and those suffering from a number of other disorders including depressions, addictions, phobias and a variety of self-esteem issues.

1177 www.goodwill-suncoast.org
Suncoast Residential Training Center

Group home that serves individuals diagnosed as mentally retarded with a secondary diagnosis of psychiatric difficulties as evidenced by problem behavior.

1178 www.ifred.org
National Foundation for Depressive Illness

Support, helplines, and advice.

1179 www.klis.com/chandler/pamphlet/dep/
Jim Chandler MD

White paper on depression in children and adolesents.

1180 www.manicdepressive.org
The Massachusetts General Hospital Bipolar
Clinic/Research Program

Dedicated to providing quality clinical care, conducting clinically informative research, and educating colleagues, patients and the community.

1181 www.med.yale.edu
Yale University School of Medicine

Research center dedicated to understanding the science of mood disorders.

1182 www.mentalhealth.Samhsa.Gov
Center for Mental Health Services Knowledge
Exchange Network

Information about resources, technical assistance, research, training, networks, and other federal clearinghouses, fact sheets and materials.

1183 www.mhselfhelp.org
National Mental Health Consumer's Self-Help
Clearinghouse

Encourages the development and growth of consumer self-help groups.

1184 www.miminc.org
Bipolar Disorders Treatment Information Center

Provides information on mood stabilizers other than lithium for bipolar disorders.

1185 www.nami.org
National Alliance on Mental Illness

From its inception in 1979, NAMI has been dedicated to improving the lives of individuals and families affected by mental illness.

1186 www.nimh.nih.gov/publicat/depressionmenu.cfm
National Institute of Mental Health

National Institute of Mental Health offers brochures organized by topic. Depression discusses symptoms, diagnosis, and treatment options.

1187 www.nimh.nih.gov/publist/964033.htm
National Institute of Mental Health

Discusses depression in older years, symptoms, treatment, going for help.

1188 www.planetpsych.com
Planetpsych.com

Learn about disorders, their treatments and other topics in psychology. Articles are listed under the related topic areas. Ask a therapist a question for free, or view the directory of professionals in your area. If you are a therapist sign up for the directory. Current features, self-help, interactive, and newsletter archives.

1189 www.psychcentral.com
Psych Central

Personalized one-stop index for psychology, support, and mental health issues, resources, and people on the Internet.

1190 www.psychologyinfo.com/depression
Psychology Information On-line: Depression

Information on diagnosis, therapy, and medication.

1191 www.psycom.net/depression.central.html
Dr. Ivan's Depression Central

Medication-oriented site. Clearinghouse on all types of depressive disorders.

1192 www.queendom.com/selfhelp/depression/depression.html
Queendom

Articles, information on medication and support groups.

1193 www.shpm.com
Self Help Magazine

Articles and discussion forums, resource links.

1194 www.thebalancedmind.org/flipswitch
Flipswitch

Educational site dedicated to helping teens, parents and teachers understand symptoms of teenage depression. Provides resources for those ready to seek help.

1195 www.thenadd.org
NADD: National Association for the Dually Diagnosed

Promotes interest of professional and parent development with resources for individuals who have the coexistence of mental illness and mental retardation.

1196 www.utsouthwestern.edu
UT Southwestern Medical Center

Research to find the corticosteroid effects on the human brain, dual-diagnosed patients, and depression in asthma patients.

1197 www.wingofmadness.com
Wing of Madness: A Depression Guide

Accurate information, advice, support, and personal experiences.

Paraphilias (Perversions)

Introduction

Paraphilias are sexual disorders or perversions in which sexual intercourse is not the desired goal. Instead, the desire is to use non-human objects or non-sexual body parts for sexual activities sometimes involving the suffering of, or inflicting pain onto, non-consenting partners.

SYMPTOMS

• Recurrent, intense, sexually arousing fantasies, urges, or behavior involving the particular perversion for at least six months;
• The fantasies, urges, or behavior cause distress and/or disruption in the person's functioning in social, work, and interpersonal areas.

There are eight Paraphilias, described below, categorized as either victimless, or as victimizing someone who has not consented to the sexual activity, with relevant associated features.

Exhibitionism

The exposure of the genitals to a stranger or group of strangers. Sometimes the paraphiliac masturbates during exposure. The onset of this disorder usually occurs before age 18 and becomes less severe after age 40.

Fetishism

Using non-living objects, known as fetishes, for sexual gratification. Objects commonly used by men with the disorder include women's underwear, shoes, or other articles of women's clothing. The person often masturbates while holding, rubbing, or smelling the fetish object. This disorder usually begins in adolescence; it is chronic.

Frotteurism

Sexual arousal, and sometimes masturbation to orgasm, while rubbing against a non-consenting person. The behavior is usually planned to occur in a crowded place, such as on a bus, subway, or in a swimming pool, where detection is less likely. Frotteurism usually begins in adolescence, is most frequent between the ages of 15 and 25, then gradually declines.

Pedophilia

Sexual activity with a prepubertal child, generally 13 years or younger. The pedophiliac, him or herself, must be at least 16 and at least five years older than his victim when the behavior occurs. Pedophiliacs are usually attracted to children in one particular age range.
The frequency of the behavior may be associated with the degree of stress in the person's life. It usually begins in adolescence and is chronic. Pedophiles may be married, but have a higher than average incidence of marital discord.

Sexual Masochism

Acts of being bound, beaten, humiliated, or made to suffer in some other way in order to become sexually aroused. The behaviors can be self-inflicted or performed with a partner, and include physical bondage, blindfolding and humiliation. Masochistic sexual fantasies are likely to have been present since childhood. The activities themselves begin at different times but are common by early adulthood; they are usually chronic. The severity of the behaviors may increase over time.

Sexual Sadism

Acts in which the person becomes sexually excited through the physical or psychological suffering of someone else. Some Sexual Sadists may conjure up the sadistic fantasies during sexual activity without acting on them. Others act on their sadistic urges with a consenting partner (who may be a Sexual Masochist), or act on their urges with a non-consenting partner. The behavior may involve forcing the other person to crawl, be caged or tortured. Sadistic sexual fantasies are likely to have been present in childhood. The onset of the behavior varies but most commonly occurs by early adulthood. The disorder is usually chronic, and severity tends to increase over time. When the disorder is severe or coupled with Antisocial Personality Disorder, the person is likely to seriously injure or kill his victim.

Transvestic Fetishism

Consists of heterosexual males dressing in women's clothes and makeup then masturbating. When not cross dressed, the man looks like an ordinary masculine man. It is important to note that there is considerable controversy over this diagnosis; some people who cross dress seem to have little distress and function normally. This condition typically begins in childhood or adolescence. Often the cross dressing is not done publicly until adulthood.

Voyeurism

Peeping Tom disorder, involving the act of observing one or more unsuspecting persons (usually strangers) who are naked, in the process of undressing, or engaged in sexual activity, in order for the voyeur to become sexually excited. Sexual activity with the people being observed is not usually sought. The voyeur may masturbate during the observation or later. The onset of this disorder is usually before age 15. It tends to be chronic.

PREVALENCE

Paraphiliacs are almost exclusively male. Very few volunteer to disclose their activities or to seek treatment. It is estimated that most have deficits in interpersonal or sexual relationships. In one study, two thirds were diagnosed with Mood Disorders and fifty percent had alcohol or drug abuse problems.

Recent studies provide evidence that the great majority of Paraphiliacs are active in more than one form of sexually perverse behavior; less than ten percent have only one form; and thirty-eight percent engage in five or more different sexually deviant behaviors. In a survey of college students, it was found that young males often fantasize about forced sex, and almost half have engaged in some form of sexual misconduct or sexual behavior with someone younger than age 14.

At the same time, the incidence and prevalence of some sexual perversions are hard to estimate, or unknown, because they are rarely reported or the people involved do not come into contact with authorities.

TREATMENT OPTIONS

All the Paraphilias are difficult to treat. It is important for the professional making the diagnosis to take a very careful history, and to be sensitive to the presence of other, e.g., personality, disorders. Relapse is common.

Diagnostic techniques can be useful. Penile

plethysmography measures the degree of penile erection while the individual is exposed to visual sexual stimuli. Some people are treated in a formal Sex Offenders Program, developed for individuals arrested for and convicted of paraphilias that are crimes. Sometimes treatment occurs within the context of individual therapy where trust can be established. Others have been treated by means of conditioning techniques, e.g., where a fetish object is paired with an aversive stimulus such as mild electric shock. Medication is also used. Pedophilia is sometimes treated through so-called chemocastration which, through the use of female hormones or other medications, diminishes sexual appetite.

Treatment can be difficult because it is associated with the risk of reporting and punishment; many individuals do not have any real interest in being treated. They may deliberately deceive the professional, or deny the problem. Sex offenders are also more likely to exaggerate treatment gains, resist treatment, or end treatment prematurely. The fact that these conditions are classified as mental disorders does not relieve individuals who violate laws of criminal responsibility.

Associations & Agencies

1199 Center for Mental Health Services (CMHS)
1 Choke Cherry Road
Room 6-1057
Rockville, MD 20857
240-276-1310
877-726-4727
Fax: 240-276-1320
TDD: 800-487-4889
E-mail: info@mentalhealth.org
www.beta.samhsa.gov/about-us/who-we-are/offices-center

Michael E Etzinger, B.S.M.E, , M.B., SAMHSA Executive Officer, Director
Paolo Del Vecchio, M.S.W, Director, Center for Mental Healt
Deborah Baldwin, M.P.A, Acting Director, Consumer Affairs
Elizabeth Lopez, Ph.D, Acting Deputy Director

CMHS leads Federal efforts to treat mental illnesses by promoting mental health and by preventing the development or worsening of mental illness when possible. Congress created CMHS to bring new hope to adults who have serious mental illnesses and to children with serious emotional disorders. Helping states improve and increase the quality and range of their treatment, rehabilitation, and support services for people with mental illness, their families, and communities. Further, it encourages a range of programs such as systems of care to respond to the increasing number of mental, emotional, and behavioral problems among America's children.

Year Founded: 1992

1200 National Association for the Dually Diagnosed (NADD)
132 Fair Street
Kingston, NY 12401-4802
845-331-4336
800-331-5362
Fax: 845-331-4569
E-mail: info@thenadd.org
www.thenadd.org

Donna McNELIS, PhD, President
Robert J Fletcher DSW, Chief Executive Officer
Dan Baker, PhD, Vice President
Julia Pearce, Secretary

Nonprofit organization designed to promote interest of professional and parent development with resources for individuals who have the coexistence of mental illness and mental retardation. Provides conferences, educational services and training materials to professionals, parents, concerned citizens and service organizations.

Year Founded: 1983

1201 National Mental Health Consumers' Self-Help Clearinghouse
1211 Chestnut Street
Suite 1100
Philadelphia, PA 19107-4103
215-751-1810
800-553-4539
Fax: 215-636-6312
E-mail: info@mhselfhelp.org
www.mhselfhelp.org

Joseph Rogers, Executive Director/ Founder
Susan Rogers, Director
Britani Nestel, Program Specialist
Christa Burkett, Technical Assistance Coordinator

A national consumer technical assistance center that has played a major role in the development of the mental health consumer movement.

Year Founded: 1986

1202 SAMHSA's National Mental Health Information Center
1 Choke Cherry Road
Rockville, MD 20857
877-726-4727
www.mentalhealth.samhsa.gov

1203 The Center for Family Support
2811 Zulette Avenue
Bronx, NY 10461
718-518-1500
Fax: 718-518-8200
E-mail: svernikoff@cfsny.org
www.cfsny.org

Steven Vernikoff, Executive Director
Virgil Seepersad, Director of Finance
Eileen Berg, Director of Quality Assurance
Barbara Greenwald, Associate Executive, Director

The Center for Family Support is committed to providing support and assistance to individuals with developmental and related disabilities, and to the family members who care for them. Supporting individuals to live the lives they want, respecting diversity, individual choice and overall family needs, involving individuals in their communities, and delivering excellent, individualized support to all.

Year Founded: 1954

Books

1204 Emonics: A Systemic Analysis of Emotional Identity in the Etiology of Sexual Paraphilias
CreateSpace
7290 B. Investment Drive
Charleston, SC 29418

E-mail: Info@CreateSpace.com
www.createspace.com

Dr. Pierre F. Walter, Author

A daring new approach to grasping the reality of emosexual attraction, from not a sexological but a bioenergetic perspective. It is especially geared toward understanding the true nature and etiology of sexual paraphilias and pedoemotions.

232 pages Year Founded: 2012 ISBN 1-475031-24-6

1205 Gender Disorders and the Paraphilias
Intl Universities Pr Inc
59 Boston Post Rd.
Madison, CT 06443
203-245-4000
Fax: 203-245-0775
E-mail: info@iup.com
www.www.iup.com

William B. Arndt, Jr., Author

488 pages Year Founded: 1991 ISBN 0-823621-50-2

1206 Perversion (Ideas in Psychoanalysis)
National Book Network
4501 Forbes Boulevard
Suite 200
Lanham, MD 20706-4346
301-459-3366
800-462-6420
Fax: 301-429-5746
E-mail: customercare@nbnbooks.com
www.www.nbnbooks.com

Ivan Ward, Editor
Claire Pajaczkowska, Author

The concept of perversion is used to understand the unconscious dynamics of addiction, sexual abuse, delinquency, murder, sexual assault & even burglary. The concepts of narcissism, fetishism, voyeurism & sadomasochism are also useful as tools to analyze our culture, particularly in relation to film. *$7.24*

80 pages Year Founded: 1996 ISBN 1-840461-88-8

1207 Sex Crimes and Paraphilia
Prentice Hall Upper Saddle River, NJ
800-922-0579
www.pearsonhighered.com

Eric W. Hickey, Author

Offers a comprehensive examination of sex crimes, sex offenders, victims of sex crimes as well as intervention and treatment strategies. Examining a wide range of sex crimes ranging from non-violent offenses such as exhibitionism, voyeurism and obscene telephone calls to serial rapes and lust murders, this book looks to uncover the roots and causes of these behaviors to aid in the understanding of sex offenders and their crimes. *$60.98*

560 pages Year Founded: 2005 ISBN 0-131703-50-1

1208 Sexual Deviance, Second Edition: Theory, Assessment, and Treatment
The Guilford Press
72 Spring Street
New York, NY 10012
800-365-7006
Fax: 212-966-6708

E-mail: info@guilford.com
www.guilford.com

D. Richard Laws, PhD, Editor
William T. O'Donohue, PhD, Editor

This important work provides authoritative scientific and applied perspectives on the full range of paraphilias and other sexual behavior problems. For each major clinical syndrome, a chapter of psychopathology and theory is followed by a chapter on assessment and treatment. Challenges in working with sex offenders are considered in depth. New topics include an integrated etiological model, sexual deviance across the lifespan, Internet offenders, multiple paraphilias, neurobiological processes, the clinician as expert witness, and public health approaches.

642 pages Year Founded: 1973 ISBN 1-593856-05-9

1209 The Psychology of Lust Murder: Paraphilia, Sexual Killing, and Serial Homicide
Academic Press
1600 John F Kennedy Boulevard
Suite 1800
Philadelphia, PA 19103-2879
800-545-2522
Fax: 800-568-5136
E-mail: usbkinfo@elsevier.com
www.elsevier.com

Catherine Purcell, Author
Bruce Arrigo, Author

Systematically examines the phenomenon of paraphilia in relationship to the crime of lust murder. By synthesizing the relevant theories on sexual homicide and serial killing, the authors develop an original, timely, sensible model that accounts for the emergence and progression of paraphilias expressed through increasingly violent erotic fantasies. Going well beyond theoretical speculation, the authors apply their integrated model to the gruesome and chilling case of Jeffrey Dahmer. They convincingly demonstrate where and how their conceptual framework provides a more complete explanation of lust homicide than any other model available in the field today.

192 pages Year Founded: 1880 ISBN 0-123705-10-X

1210 The World of Perversion: Psychoanalysis and the Impossible Absolute of Desire
State University of New York Press
22 Corporate Woods Boulevard
3rd Floor
Albany, NY 12211-2504
518-472-5000
866-430-7869
Fax: 518-472-5038
E-mail: info@sunypress.edu
www.sunypress.edu

James Penney, Author

An original critique of queer theory, from a psychoanalysis perspective.

259 pages Year Founded: 1966 ISBN 0-791467-70-8

Video & Audio

1211 Clinical Impressions: Identifying Mental Illness
Educational Training Videos
136 Granville St
Suite 200
Gahanna, OH 43230
Fax: 888-775-3919
www.educationaltrainingvideos.com

How long can mental illness stay hidden, especially from the eyes of trained experts? This program rejoins a group of ten adults- five of them healthy and five of them with histories of mental illness- as psychiatric specialists try to spot and correctly diagnose the latter. Administering a series of collaborative and one-on-one tests, including assessments of personality type, physical self-image, and rational thinking, the panel gradually makes decisions about who suffers from depression, bipolar disorder, bulimia, and social anxiety.

1212 FRONTLINE: The Released
PBS
2100 Crystal Drive
Arlington, VA 22202
www.pbs.org

Will Lyman, Actor
Narrator
Miri Navasky, Director
Karen O'Connor, Director

The documentary states that of the 700, 000 inmates released from American prisons each year, half of them have mental disabilities. This work focused on those with severe problems who keep entering and exiting prison. Full of good information on the challenges they face with mental illnesses; housing, employment, stigmatization, and socialization.

Year Founded: 2009

1213 Understanding Mental Illness
Educational Video Network, Inc.
1401 19th Street
Huntsville, TX 77340
936-295-5767
800-762-0060
Fax: 936-294-0233
www.www.evndirect.com

Contains information and classifications of mental illness. Mental illness can strike anyone, at any age. Learn about various organic and functional mental disorders as discussed and their causes and symptoms, and learn where to seek help for a variety of mental health concerns.

Web Sites

1214 www.mentalhealth.com
Internet Mental Health

Website offers psychiatric diagnosis in the hope of reaching the two-thirds of individuals with mental illness who do not seek treatment.

1215 www.planetpsych.com
PlanetPsych

The online resource for mental health information.

1216 www.psychcentral.com
Psych Central

The Internet's largest and oldest independent mental health social network created and run by mental health professionals to guarantee reliable, trusted information and support communities to you.

Personality Disorders

Introduction

Personality is deeply rooted in our sense of ourselves and how others see us; it is formed from a complex interminling of genetic factors and life experience. Everyone has personality characteristics that are likable and unlikable, attractive and unattractive, to others. By adulthood, most of us have personality traits that are difficult to change. Sometimes, these deeply rooted personality traits can get in the way of our happiness, hinder relationships, and even cause harm to ourselves or others.

For example, a person may have a tendency to be deeply suspicious of other people with no good reason. Another person may assume a haughty, arrogant manner that is difficult to be around. Personality Disorders, by definition, do not cause symptoms, which are experiences that are troublesome to the individual. They consist of whole sets of distorted experiences of the outside world that pervade every or nearly every aspect of a person's life, causing traits and behaviors leading to interpersonal problems which only secondarily cause distress to the individual. The problem is blamed on other people. For example, people with dependent personality disorder feel that they need more care and protection than others, not that they are inordinately demanding of care and protection. People with narcissistic personality disorder feel that others do not respect them, not that they demand more attention and admiration than others; people with paranoid personality disorder feel that others are out to trick and cheat them, not that they are inordinately suspicious; people with obsessive personality disorder feel that others are sloppy, not that they are overly preoccupied with order and tidiness.

A diagnosis of a Personality Disorder should be distinguished from labeling someone as a bad or disagreeable person and not be used to stigmitize people who are simply unpopular, rebellious or otherwise unorthodox. A personality disorder is not simply a personality style, but a condition that interferes with successful living. A Personality Disorder refers to an enduring pattern or experience and behavior that is inflexible, long lasting (often beginning in adolescence or early childhood) and which leads to distress and impairment. Personality disorders frequently co-exist with depression and other mental disorders.

Ten distinct personality disorders have been identified:
• Paranoid Personality Disorder;
• Schiziod Personality Disorder;
• Schizotypal Personality Disorder;
• Antisocial Personality Disorder;
• Borderline Personality Disorder;
• Histrionic Personality Disorder;
• Narcissistic Personality Disorder;
• Avoidant Personality Disorder;
• Dependent Personality Disorder;
• Obsessive-Compulsive Personality Disorder.

SYMPTOMS

An enduring pattern of inner experience and behavior that deviates markedly from the expectations of the individual's culture:
• This pattern is manifested in two or more of the following areas: cognition, affectivity, interpersonal functioning, and impulse control;
• The enduring pattern is inflexible and pervasive across a broad range of personal and social situations;
• The enduring pattern leads to clinically significant distress or impairment in social, occupational, or other important areas of functioning;
• The pattern is stable and of long duration and its onset can be traced back at least to adolescence or early adulthood;
• The enduring pattern is not better accounted for as a manifestation or consequence of another mental disorder;
• The enduring pattern is not due to the direct physiological effects of a substance or a general medical condition.

TREATMENT OPTIONS

Most people who suffer from a Personality Disorder do not see themselves as having psychological problems, and therefore do not seek treatment. For those who do, the most effective treatment is long-term (at least one year) psychotherapy. People with Personality Disorders generally seek treatment only because they are distressed about the behavior of those around them. It is important for a patient to find a mental health professional with expert knowledge and experience in treating personality disorders. Some therapists specialize in treating Borderline Personality Disorder. Antisocial Personality disorder is notably difficult to treat, especially in extreme cases, when the affected individual lacks all concern for others.

Psychotherapy encourages patients to talk about their suspicions, doubts and other personality traits that have a negative impact on their lives, and therefore helps to improve social interactions.

Psychotherapeutic treatment should include attention to family members, stressing the importance of emotional support, reassurance, explanation of the disorder, and advice on how to manage and respond to the patient. Group therapy is helpful in many situations.

Antipsychotic medication can be useful in patients with certain Personality Disorders, specifically Schizotypal and Borderline Disorders.

Associations & Agencies

1218 Career Assessment & Planning Services
Goodwill Industries-Suncoast, Inc.
10596 Gandy Boulevard
St. Petersburg, FL 33702-1427
727-523-1512
888-279-1988
TDD: 727-579-1068
E-mail: gw.marketing@goodwill-suncoast.com
www.goodwill-suncoast.org

Oscar J Horton, Chairman
R. Lee Waits, President and CEO Emeritus
Deborah A. Passerini, President, Board Officer
Martin W Gladysz, Senior Vice Chairman

Provide a comprehensive assessment to help physically, emotionally or developmentally disabled persons develop a plan for employment. In addition to making employment and training recommendations, Goodwill identifies community resources that could improve the quality of life for those who are unprepared for immediate placement in employment.
Year Founded: 1954

1219 Center for Mental Health Services (CMHS)
1 Choke Cherry Road
Room 6-1057
Rockville, MD 20857
240-276-1310
877-726-4727
Fax: 240-276-1320
TDD: 800-487-4889
E-mail: info@mentalhealth.org
www.beta.samhsa.gov/about-us/who-we-are/offices-center

*Michael E Etzinger, B.S.M.E, , M.B., SAMHSA Executive
Officer, Director*
*Paolo Del Vecchio, M.S.W, Director, Center for Mental
Healt*
*Deborah Baldwin, M.P.A, Acting Director, Consumer
Affairs*
Elizabeth Lopez, Ph.D, Acting Deputy Director

CMHS leads Federal efforts to treat mental illnesses by
promoting mental health and by preventing the development or worsening of mental illness when possible. Congress created CMHS to bring new hope to adults who have
serious mental illnesses and to children with serious emotional disorders. CMHS provides information about mental
health via a toll-free the web site, and more than 600 publications. Developed for users of mental health services and
their families, the general public, policy makers, providers,
and the media.

Year Founded: 1992

1220 National Alliance on Mental Illness
3803 North Fairfax Drive
Suite 100
Arlington, VA 22203
703-524-7600
800-950-6264
Fax: 703-524-9094
E-mail: helpline@nami.org
www.nami.org

Keris Jan Myrick, MBA, MS, PhD., President
Mary Giliberti, J.D, Executive Director
Jim Payne, J.D, First Vice President
David Levy, Chief Financial Officer

The nation's largest grassroots mental health organization
dedicated to building better lives for the millions of Americans affected by mental illness. NAMI advocates for access
to services, treatment, supports research and is steadfast in
its commitment to raising awareness and building a community of hope for all of those in need.

Year Founded: 1969

**1221 National Association for the Dually Diagnosed
(NADD)**
132 Fair Street
Kingston, NY 12401-4802
845-331-4336
800-331-5362
Fax: 845-331-4569
E-mail: info@thenadd.org
www.thenadd.org

Donna McNELIS, PhD, President
Robert J Fletcher DSW, Chief Executive Officer
Dan Baker, PhD, Vice President
Julia Pearce, Secretary

Nonprofit organization designed to promote interest of professional and parent development with resources for individuals who have the coexistence of mental illness and
mental retardation. Provides conference, educational services and training materials to professionals, parents, concerned citizens and service organizations.

Year Founded: 1983

**1222 National Mental Health Consumers' Self-Help
Clearinghouse**
1211 Chestnut Street
Suite 1100
Philadelphia, PA 19107-4103
215-751-1810
800-553-4539
Fax: 215-636-6312
E-mail: info@mhselfhelp.org
www.mhselfhelp.org

Joseph Rogers, Executive Director/ Founder
Susan Rogers, Director
Britani Nestel, Program Specialist
Christa Burkett, Technical Assistance Coordinator

A national consumer technical assistance center that has
played a major role in the development of the mental health
consumer movement.

Year Founded: 1986

**1223 SAMHSA's National Mental Health
Information Center**
1 Choke Cherry Road
Rockville, MD 20857
877-726-4727
TDD: 866-889-2647
www.mentalhealth.samhsa.gov

1224 The Center for Family Support
2811 Zulette Avenue
Bronx, NY 10461
718-518-1500
Fax: 718-518-8200
E-mail: svernikoff@cfsny.org
www.cfsny.org

Steven Vernikoff, Executive Director
Virgil Seepersad, Director of Finance
Eileen Berg, Director of Quality Assurance
Barbara Greenwald, Associate Executive, Director

The Center for Family Support is committed to providing
support and assistance to individuals with developmental
and related disabilities, and to the family members who
care for them.

Year Founded: 1954

Books

**1225 Biology of Personality Disorders, Review of
Psychiatry**
American Psychiatric Publishing, Inc.
1000 Wilson Boulevard
Suite 1825
Arlington, VA 22209-3901
703-907-7322
800-368-5777
Fax: 703-907-1091
E-mail: appi@psych.org
www.appi.org

Kenneth R. Silk, Editor

An all-inclusive guide for the study of the etiology and the treatment of personality disorders. For the many patients who suffer from personality disorders and the physicians who have the challenge of successfully treating them, this book is a welcome reference. *$25.00*

176 pages Year Founded: 1998 ISBN 0-880488-35-2

1226 Borderline Personality Disorder
American Psychiatric Publishing, Inc.
1000 Wilson Boulevard
Suite 1825
Arlington, VA 22209-3901
703-907-7322
800-368-5777
Fax: 703-907-1091
E-mail: appi@psych.org
www.appi.org

John G. Gunderson, M.D., Author
Paul S Links, M.D., F.R.C.P.C, Author
John McDuffie, Editorial Director

Guide to the diagnosis and treatment of borderline personality disorder. *$34.00*

366 pages Year Founded: 2008 ISBN 0-880486-89-9

1227 Borderline Personality Disorder:
Multidimensional Approach
American Psychiatric Publishing, Inc.
1000 Wilson Boulevard
Suite 1825
Arlington, VA 22209-3901
703-907-7322
800-368-5777
Fax: 703-907-1091
E-mail: appi@psych.org
www.appi.org

Joel Paris, M.D., Author
Ron McMillen, Chief Executive Officer
John McDuffie, Editorial Director

Practical approach to the management of patients with BPD. *$33.00*

232 pages Year Founded: 1994 ISBN 0-880486-55-4

1228 Borderline Personality Disorder: A Patient's
Guide to Taking Control
W.W. Norton & Company, Inc.
500 Fifth Avenue
New York, NY 10110
212-354-2907
800-233-4830
Fax: 212-869-0856
E-mail: npb@wwnorton.com
www.books.wwnorton.com/books/

The Patient's Guide is your clients' means to begin to take command of their lives by following the therapeutic course described in these books. Provides a step-by-step cognitive program wich in worksheets and exercises to facilitate your clients' personal process of self-examination and problem solving.

ISBN 0-393703-53-3

1229 Borderline Personality Disorder: Etilogy and
Treatment
American Psychiatric Publishing, Inc.
1000 Wilson Boulevard
Suite 1825
Arlington, VA 22209-3901
703-907-7322
800-368-5777
Fax: 703-907-1091
E-mail: appi@psych.org
www.appi.org

Robert E Hales MD, Editor-in-Chief
Ron McMillen, Chief Executive Officer
John McDuffie, Editorial Director

Provides empirical data as the basis for progress in understanding and treating the borderline patient. *$50.00*

420 pages ISBN 0-880484-08-X

1230 Borderline Personality Disorder: Tailoring the
Psychotherapy to the Patient
American Psychiatric Publishing, Inc.
1000 Wilson Boulevard
Suite 1825
Arlington, VA 22209-3901
703-907-7322
800-368-5777
Fax: 703-907-1091
E-mail: appi@psych.org
www.appi.org

Leonard Horwitz, Ph.D, Author
Glen O Gabbard, M.D, Author
Jon G Allen, Ph.D, Author
Donald B Colson, Ph.D, Author

Emphasizes how the clinician should decide between the use of supportive as opposed to expressive techniques, depending upon the characteristics of the patient. *$34.00*

272 pages Year Founded: 1996 ISBN 0-880486-89-9

1231 Borderline Personality Disorder: The Latest
Assessment and Treatment Strategies
Jones & Bartlett Learning
5 Wall Street
Burlington, MA 01803-4211
978-443-5000
800-832-0034
Fax: 978-443-8000
E-mail: info@jblearning.com
www.jblearning.com

Melanie Dean, PhD, Author

7 typical characteristics of those with BPD, differential diagnostic concerns, treatment strategies for interpersonal, cognitive, dialectical behavior, and group therapy, 13 predisposing factors for suicide, 4 psychometric assessment tools, new self-report and interview instruments, treatment dialogue examples for vaious theoretical approaches, comparison table of 6 classes of medications used to treat BPD and 6 key relapse prevention treatment strategies.

88 pages Year Founded: 1983

1232 Challenging Behaviour, Third Edition
Cambridge University Press
32 Avenue of the Americas
New York, NY 10013-2473

212-337-5000
E-mail: newyork@cambridge.org
www.www.cambridge.org

Eric Emerson, Author
Stewart L Einfield, Author

This edition contains significantly expanded sections on the emergence and development of challenging behaviour and strategies for prevention, at the level of both individuals and service systems. Essential reading for students undertaking professional training in health and related aspects of intellectual disabilities, including psychologists, psychiatrists, nurses, teachers and social workers. This book is a key text for professional staff delivering health, educational and social care services to people with intellectual disabilities.

224 pages Year Founded: 1534 ISBN 0-521728-93-5

1233 Clinical Assessment and Management of Severe Personality Disorders
American Psychiatric Publishing, Inc.
1000 Wilson Boulevard
Suite 1825
Arlington, VA 22209-3901
703-907-7322
800-368-5777
Fax: 703-907-1091
E-mail: appi@psych.org
www.appi.org

Paul S Links, M.D., F.R.C.P.C, Editor
Ron McMillen, Chief Executive Officer
John McDuffie, Editorial Director

Focuses on issues relevant to the clinician in private practice, including the diagnosis of a wide range of personality disorders and alternative management approaches. *$33.00*

250 pages Year Founded: 1995 ISBN 0-880484-88-8

1234 Cognitive Analytic Therapy & Borderline Personality Disorder: Model and the Method
John Wiley & Sons
111 River Street
Hoboken, NJ 07030-5774
201-748-6000
877-762-2974
Fax: 201-748-6088
E-mail: info@wiley.com
www.wiley.com

Anthony Ryle, Author

This book documents CAT's recent theoretical and practical developments is a must for anyone interested in CAT itself and in integrative approaches, for those interested in brief, psychodynamically informed therapy, or indeed for those interested in developments in psychology generally. *$70.00*

206 pages Year Founded: 1997 ISBN 0-471976-18-0

1235 Cognitive Therapy of Personality Disorders, Second Edition
The Guilford Press
72 Spring Street
New York, NY 10012
212-431-9800
800-365-7006
Fax: 212-966-6708
E-mail: info@guilford.com
www.guilford.com

Aaron T. Beck, M.D., Author
Arthur Freeman, Author
Denise D. Davis Ph.D., Author

This landmark work was the first to present a cognitive framework for understanding and treating personality disorders.

412 pages Year Founded: 1973 ISBN 1-572308-56-7

1236 Developmental Model of Borderline Personality Disorder: Understanding Variations in Course and Outcome
American Psychiatric Publishing, Inc.
1000 Wilson Boulevard
Suite 1825
Arlington, VA 22209-3901
703-907-7322
800-368-5777
Fax: 703-907-1091
E-mail: appi@psych.org
www.appi.org

Patricia Hoffman Judd, Ph.D, Author
Thomas H McGlashan, M.D., Author
John McDuffie, Editorial Director

Landmark work on this difficult condition. Emphasizes a developmental approach to BPD based on treatment of inpatients at Chestnut Lodge in Rockville, Maryland, during the years through 1975. Using information gleaned from the original clinical notes and follow-up studies, the authors present four intriguing case studies to chart the etiology, long-term course, and clinical manifestations of BPD. *$34.95*

248 pages Year Founded: 2003 ISBN 0-880485-15-9

1237 Disordered Personalities
Rapid Psychler Press
2014 Holland Avenue
Suite 374
Port Huron, MI 48060-1994
519-667-2335
888-779-2453
Fax: 888-779-2457
E-mail: rapid@psychler.com
www.psychler.com

David J. Robinson, MD, Author

Provides a comprehensive, practical and entertaining overview of the DSM-IV personality disorders. The diagnostic, theoretical and therapeutic principles relevant to understanding character pathology are detailed in the introductory chapters. *$39.95*

430 pages Year Founded: 2005 ISBN 1-894328-09-4

1238 Disorders of Narcissism: Diagnostic, Clinical, and Empirical Implications
American Psychiatric Publishing, Inc.
1000 Wilson Boulevard
Suite 1825
Arlington, VA 22209-3901
703-907-7322
800-368-5777
Fax: 703-907-1091
E-mail: appi@psych.org
www.appi.org

Elsa Ronningstam, Ph.D., Editor
Ron McMillen, Chief Executive Officer
John McDuffie, Editorial Director

Addresses important subjects at the forefront of the study of narcissism, including cognitive treatment, normal narcissism, pathological narcissism and suicide, and the connection between pathological narcissism, trauma, and alexithymia. *$42.50*

512 pages Year Founded: 1998 ISBN 0-880487-01-1

1239 Drug Therapy and Personality Disorders
Mason Crest Publishers
450 Parkway Drive
Suite D
Broomall, PA 19008-4017
610-543-6200
866-627-2665
Fax: 610-543-3878
E-mail: dtaylor@masoncrest.com
www.masoncrest.com

Shirley Brinkerhoff, Author

What is a personality disorder? Can it be treated? If so, how? What can people do about their troublsome symptoms? These are just a few of the questions Drug Therapy and Personality Disorders answers. Learn about these common forms of mental illness and the treatments that bring new hope to those who suffer with them.

128 pages Year Founded: 2004 ISBN 1-590845-71-4

1240 Fatal Flaws: Navigating Destructive Relationships with People with Disorders of Personality and Character
American Psychiatric Publishing, Inc.
1000 Wilson Boulevard
Suite 1825
Arlington, VA 22209-3901
703-907-7322
800-368-5777
Fax: 703-907-1091
E-mail: appi@psych.org
www.appi.org

Stuart C. Yudofsky, Author

Featuring case vignettes from nearly 30 years of Dr. Yudofsky's clinical practice and incorporating the knowledge of gifted clinicians, educators, and research scientists with whom he has collaborated throughout that time.

512 pages Year Founded: 2005

1241 Field Guide to Personality Disorders: A Companion to Disordered Personalities
Rapid Psychler Press
2014 Holland Avenue
Suite 374
Port Huron, MI 48060-1994
519-667-2335
888-779-2453
Fax: 888-779-2457
E-mail: rapid@psychler.com
www.psychler.com

David J. Robinson, MD, Author

Practical introduction to the DSM-IV personality disorders. Covers diagnosis, theoretical and therapeutic principles. Each chapter covers a different personality Synopsis of the text Disordered Personalities. *$19.95*

212 pages Year Founded: 2005 ISBN 1-894328-10-8

1242 Get Me Out of Here: My Recovery from Borderline Personality Disorder
Hazelden
PO Box 11
Center City, MN 55012-0011
651-213-4200
800-257-7810
Fax: 651-213-4793
E-mail: info@hazelden.org
www.hazelden.org

Rachel Reiland, Author

With astonishing honesty, Reiland's memoir reveals what mental illness feels like and looks like from the inside, and how healing from such a devastating disease is possible through intensive therapy and the support of loved ones.

464 pages Year Founded: 1949 ISBN 1-592850-99-5

1243 I Hate You, Don't Leave Me: Understanding the Borderline Personality
Avon, Imprint of Harper Collins Publishers
10 East 53rd Street
11th Floor
New York, NY 20706-1002
212-207-7528
800-242-7737
E-mail: orders@harpercollins.com
www.harpercollins.com

Jerold J. Kreisman MD, Author
Hal Strauss, Author

For years BPD was difficult to describe, diagnose, and treat. But now, for the first time, Dr. Jerold J. Kreisman and health writer Hal Straus offer much-needed professional advice, helping victims and their families to understand and cope with this troubling, shockingly widespread affliction.

288 pages Year Founded: 1991 ISBN 0-380713-05-5

1244 Lost in the Mirror: An Inside Look at Borderline Personality Disorder
Sidran Institute
200 E Joppa Road
Suite 207
Baltimore, MD 21286-3107
410-825-8888
888-825-8249
Fax: 410-337-0747
E-mail: sidran@sidran.org
www.sidran.org

Richard A. Moskovitz, MD, Author

Dr. Moskovitz considers BPD to be part of the dissociative continuum, as it has many causes, symptoms and behaviors in common with Dissociative Disorder. This book is intended for people diagnosed with BPD, their families and therapists. Outlines the features of BPD, including abuse histories, dissociation, mood swings, self harm, impulse control problems and many more. Includes an extensive resource section. *$13.95*

190 pages

1245 Management of Countertransference with Borderline Patients
American Psychiatric Publishing, Inc.
1000 Wilson Boulevard
Suite 1825
Arlington, VA 22209-3901

703-907-7322
800-368-5777
Fax: 703-907-1091
E-mail: appi@psych.org
www.appi.org

Glen O Gabbard, M.D, Author
Sallye M. Wilkinson, Ph.D., Author
John McDuffie, Editorial Director

Open and detailed discussion of the emotional reactions that clinicians experience when treating borderline patients. *$34.50*

272 pages Year Founded: 1994 ISBN 0-880785-63-9

1246 Personality Disorders in Modern Life
John Wiley & Sons
111 River Street
Hoboken, NJ 07030-5774
201-748-6000
877-762-2974
Fax: 201-748-6088
E-mail: info@wiley.com
www.wiley.com

Carrie M. Millon, Author
Sarah Meagher, Author
Seth Grossman, Author
Rowena Ramnath, Author

Exploring the continuum from normal personality tests to the diagnosis amd treatment of severe cases of personality disorders.

624 pages Year Founded: 2004 ISBN 0-471237-34-5

1247 Personality and Psychopathology
American Psychiatric Publishing, Inc.
1000 Wilson Boulevard
Suite 1825
Arlington, VA 22209-3901
703-907-7322
800-368-5777
Fax: 703-907-1091
E-mail: appi@psych.org
www.appi.org

C. Robert Cloninger, Editor

Compiles the most recent findings from more than 30 internationally recognized experts. Analyzes the association between personality and psychopathology from several interlocking perspective, descriptive, developmental, etiological, and therapeutic. *$58.50*

544 pages Year Founded: 1999 ISBN 0-880489-23-5

1248 Role of Sexual Abuse in Etiology of Borderline Personality Disorder
American Psychiatric Publishing, Inc.
1000 Wilson Boulevard
Suite 1825
Arlington, VA 22209-3901
703-907-7322
800-368-5777
Fax: 703-907-1091
E-mail: appi@psych.org
www.appi.org

Mary C. Zanarini, Editor

Presenting the latest generation of research findings about the impact of traumatic abuse on the development of BPD. This book focuses on the theoretical basis of BPD, includ-

ing topics such as childhood factors associated with the development, the relationship of child sexual abuse to dissociation and self-mutilation, severity of childhood abuse, borderline symptoms and family environment. Twenty six contributors cover every aspect of BPD as it relates to childhood sexual abuse. *$65.00*

264 pages Year Founded: 1996 ISBN 0-880484-96-9

1249 Stop Walking on Eggshells: Taking Your Life Back When Someone You Care About Has Borderline Personality Disorder
NewHarbinger Publications
5674 Shattuck Avenue
Oakland, CA 94609-1662
510-652-0215
800-748-6273
Fax: 800-652-1613
E-mail: customerservice@newharbinger.com
www.newharbinger.com

Paul T. Mason, MS, Author
Randi Kreger, Author

Stop Walking on Eggshells has helped nearly half a million people with friends and family members suffering from BPD understand this destructive disorder, set boundaries, and help their loved ones stop relying on dangerous BPD behaviors. This fully revised edition has been updated with the very latest BPD research and includes coping and communication skills you can use to stabilize your relationship with the BPD sufferer in your life. *$15.95*

288 pages Year Founded: 1973 ISBN 1-572241-08-X

1250 Structured Interview for DSM-IV Personality (SIDP-IV)
American Psychiatric Publishing, Inc.
1000 Wilson Boulevard
Suite 1825
Arlington, VA 22209-3901
703-907-7322
800-368-5777
Fax: 703-907-1091
E-mail: appi@psych.org
www.appi.org

Bruce Pfohl, M.D, Author
Nancee Blum, M.S.W, Author
Mark Zimmerman, M.D, Author

Semistructured interview uses nonperorative questions to examine behavior and personality traits from the patient's perspective. *$21.95*

48 pages Year Founded: 1997 ISBN 0-880489-37-5

1251 The Angry Heart: Overcoming Borderline and Addictive Disorders: An Interactive Self-Help Guide
NewHarbinger Publications
5674 Shattuck Avenue
Oakland, CA 94609-1662
510-652-0215
800-748-6273
Fax: 800-652-1613
E-mail: customerservice@newharbinger.com
www.newharbinger.com

Joseph Santoro, Author
Ronald Jay Cohen, Author

The emotional turmoil and impulsive behavior that characterize borderline personality disorder are so often accompanied by alcoholism or drug abuse that some estimates suggest that as many as half of the millions of people with substance abuse prolems may have a masked borderline personality disorder. This self-help guide offers a range of exercises and step-by-step techniques to help you come to terms with the destructive aspects of your lifestyle *$15.95*

272 pages Year Founded: 1973 ISBN 1-572240-80-6

1252 The Borderline Personality Disorder Survival Guide: Everything You Need to Know About Living with BPD
NewHarbinger Publications
5674 Shattuck Avenue
Oakland, CA 94609-1662
510-652-0215
800-748-6273
Fax: 800-652-1613
E-mail: customerservice@newharbinger.com
www.newharbinger.com

Alex L Chapman, Author
Kim L Gratz, Author

This book provides answers to many questions one might have about BPD: what is it, how long does it last, what other problems co-occur with BPD?

256 pages Year Founded: 1973 ISBN 1-572245-07-7

1253 Understanding the Borderline Mother: Helping Her Children Transcend the Intense, Unpredictable, and Volatile Relationship
Jason Aronson
4501 Forbes Blvd
Suite 200
Lanham, MD 20706
301-459-3366
Fax: 301-429-5748
www.www.rowmanlittlefield.com

Christine Ann Lawson, Author

Vividly describes how mothers who suffer from borderline personality disorder produce children who may flounder in life even as adults, futilely struggling to reach the safety of a parental harbor, unable to recognize that their borderline parent lacks a pier, or even a discernible shore. Four character profiles describe different symptom clusters that include the waif mother, the hermit mother, the queen mother, and the witch. Addressing the adult children of borderlines and the therapists who work with them, Dr. Lawson shows how to care for the waif without rescuing her, to attend to the hermit without feeding her fear, to love the queen without becoming her subject, and to live with the witch without becoming her victim. *$37.50*

352 pages Year Founded: 2002

Support Groups & Hot Lines

1254 Out of the FOG
www.www.outofthefog.net

Providing information and support to the family members and loved-ones of individuals who suffer from a personality disorder. A supportive, close-knit community encouraging one another through the many challenges that come with having a family member or significant other who has a personality disorder. FOG stands for Fear, Obligation, and Guilt, feelings which often result from being in a relationship with a person who suffers from a Personality Disorder.

Year Founded: 2007

1255 Paranoid Personality Disorder Forum
Mental Health Matters
www.www.psychforums.com/paranoid-personality/

A helpful user to user forum for support and information about Paranoid Personality Disorders.

1256 S.A.F.E. Alternatives
7115 W North Avenue
PMB 319
Oak Park, IL 60302-1002
708-366-9066
800-366-8288
Fax: 708-366-9065
E-mail: info@selfinjury.com
www.selfinjury.com

Karen Conterio, CEO & Founder
Wendy Lader, PhD, M.Ed, Clinical Director
Michelle Seliner MSW, LCSW, Chief Operating Officer
Joni Nowicki, BA, Admissions Coordinator

A world-renowned treatment program that in it's more than twenty years of operation has helped thousands of people successfully end self-injurious behavior. A treatment team of experts uses therapy, education, and support to empower clients to identify healthier ways to cope with emotional distress. The S.A.F.E. Alternatives philosophy and model of treatment focus on shifting control to the client, empowering them to make healthy choices, including the choice to not self-injure.

Year Founded: 1986

Video & Audio

1257 Anger Management-Enhanced Edition
Educational Video Network, Inc.
1401 19th Street
Huntsville, TX 77340
936-295-5767
800-762-0060
Fax: 936-294-0233
www.www.evndirect.com

Learn what causes anger and understand why our bodies react as they do when we're angry. Effective techniques for assuaging anger are discussed.

1258 Beating Depression
Educational Training Videos
136 Granville St
Suite 200
Gahanna, OH 43230
Fax: 888-775-3919
www.educationaltrainingvideos.com

This program comes to grips with depression through the experiences of five patients whose backgrounds span the socioeconomic spectrum. Three cases of chronic depression, one of which is complicated by borderline personality disorder and another by alcohol abuse, and two cases of bipolar disorder, one of which is extreme, are presented.

1259 Clinical Impressions: Identifying Mental Illness
Educational Training Videos
136 Granville St
Suite 200
Gahanna, OH 43230

Fax: 888-775-3919

www.educationaltrainingvideos.com

How long can mental illness stay hidden, especially from the eyes of trained experts? This program rejoins a group of ten adults- five of them healthy and five of them with histories of mental illness- as psychiatric specialists try to spot and correctly diagnose the latter. Administering a series of collaborative and one-on-one tests, including assessments of personality type, physical self-image, and rational thinking, the panel gradually makes decisions about who suffers from depression, bipolar disorder, bulimia, and social anxiety.

1260 Dealing with Social Anxiety
Educational Video Network, Inc.
1401 19th Street
Huntsville, TX 77340
936-295-5767
800-762-0060
Fax: 936-294-0233
www.www.evndirect.com

Social anxiety is America's third-largest psychiatric disorder. It generally develops during the mid-teen years, and almost always before the age of 25. Understand what may trigger the development of anxiety and learn how it sometimes evolves into full-blown panic disorder, which is characterized by recurrent attacks of terror or fear. The consequences of social anxiety are examined and effective treatments are discussed.

1261 FRONTLINE: The Released
PBS
2100 Crystal Drive
Arlington, VA 22202
www.pbs.org

Will Lyman, Actor
Narrator
Miri Navasky, Director
Karen O'Connor, Director

The documentary states that of the 700, 000 inmates released from American prisons each year, half of them have mental disabilities. This work focused on those with severe problems who keep entering and exiting prison. Full of good information on the challenges they face with mental illnesses; housing, employment, stigmatization, and socialization.

Year Founded: 2009

1262 Lost in the Mirror: Women with Multiple Personalities
Educational Training Videos
136 Granville St
Suite 200
Gahanna, OH 43230
Fax: 888-775-3919
www.educationaltrainingvideos.com

In this program, ABC News anchors Diane Sawyer and Sam Donaldson study the causes and key signs of dissociative identity disorder and the fragmented lives of two people dealing with its effects.

1263 Mental Disorder
Educational Training Videos
136 Granville St
Suite 200
Gahanna, OH 43230

Fax: 888-775-3919

www.educationaltrainingvideos.com

What is abnormality? Using the case studies of two young women; one who has depression, one who has an anxiety disorder; as a springboard, this program presents three psychological perspective on mental disorder.

1264 Multiple Personality Disorder: In the Shadows
Educational Training Videos
136 Granville St
Suite 200
Gahanna, OH 43230
Fax: 888-775-3919
www.educationaltrainingvideos.com

This program shows how therapy can integrate the multiple personalities and make a patient whole again. Following two MPD patients and health care professionals, the program traces the struggles and triumphs in treating this disorder.

1265 Understanding Mental Illness
Educational Video Network, Inc.
1401 19th Street
Huntsville, TX 77340
936-295-5767
800-762-0060
Fax: 936-294-0233
www.www.evndirect.com

Contains information and classifications of mental illness. Mental illness can strike anyone, at any age. Learn about various organic and functional mental disorders as discussed and their causes and symptoms, and learn where to seek help for a variety of mental health concerns.

1266 Understanding Personality Disorders
Educational Video Network, Inc.
1401 19th Street
Huntsville, TX 77340
936-295-5767
800-762-0060
Fax: 936-294-0233
www.www.evndirect.com

For many people, the onset of a psychological disorder goes undiagnosed and untreated, and, as a result, they face a constant, if not impossible, struggle to maintain good mental health. This can be especially true when individuals suffer from a personality disorder. However, with identification and understanding, crippling personality disorders can be brought out of the shadows of ignorance and into the light of treatment.

Web Sites

1267 www.cyberpsych.org
CyberPsych
Presents information about psychoanalysis, psychotherapy and special topics such as anxiety disorders, the problematic use of alcohol, homophobia, and the traumatic effects of racism

1268 www.mentalhealth.com
Internet Mental Health
Offers online psychiatric diagnosis in the hope of reaching the two-thirds of individuals with mental illness who do not seek treatment.

1269 **www.mhsanctuary.com/borderline**
Borderline Personality Disorder Sanctuary

Borderline personality disorder education, communities,
support, books, and resources.

1270 **www.nimh.nih.gov/publicat/ocdmenu.cfm**
Obsessive-Compulsive Disorder

Introductory handout with treatment recommendations.

1271 **www.ocdhope.com/ocd-families.php**
OCD Resource Center of Florida

1272 **www.outofthefog.net**
Out of the FOG

Information and support for those with a family member or
loved one who suffers from a personality disorder.

1273 **www.planetpsych.com**
Planetpsych.com

The online resource for mental health information.

1274 **www.psychcentral.com**
Psych Central

The Internet's largest and oldest independent mental health
social network created and run by mental health professionals to guarantee reliable, trusted information and support
communities to you.

Post Traumatic Stress Disorder

Introduction

Post-traumatic stress disorder, or PTSD, is one of the Anxiety Disorders receiving particular attention because it affects a significant number of individuals returning from war zones, as well as those affected by terrorism and natural disasters. Post-traumatic stress disorder has been recognized for over a hundred years at least. During and after World War I, traumatized soldiers' symptoms of hypersensitivity, avoidance, and other characteristics of what we now call PTSD were called 'shell shock' in the past. PTSD continues to be identified with military service, but it is not limited to members of the military. It can affect adults and children exposed to terrifying and dangerous events in any circumstances: natural disasters, physical and/or sexual attack, acts of terrorism, and accidents, for example. By definition, the precipitating event must be outside the bounds of everyday human experience and the individual must feel helpless to protect him or herself from the event. Women appear to be somewhat more vulnerable to PTSD than men.

SYMPTOMS

PTSD symptoms occur in three categories: re-experiencing, heightened emotional arousal, and numbing.
Re-experiencing is the group of symptoms we hear most about. These include:
• Intense anxiety when the individual is exposed to a situation reminiscent of the event;
• Recurrent distressing flashbacks, nightmares and/or dreams of the event;
• Acting or feeling as if the traumatic event were taking place immediately in the present. At these times, physiologic changes, such as a fast heartbeat, breathlessness, or gastrointestinal symptoms occur along with the anxiety.
Heightened emotional arousal includes:
• Jumpiness, where the individual responds to ordinary touch or noises as though they were a signal of mortal danger;
• Extreme avoidance of stimuli associated with the trauma;
• Bouts of anger out of proportion to a situation.
Numbing refers to:
• Diminished general responsiveness;
• Desensitization of emotional response whether the events affect them or those close to them.

Duration of the disturbance is more than one month, and the disturbance causes clinically significant distress or impairment. It is easy to see how any or all of these symptoms not only cause terrible distress for the individual, but are incomprehensible and disturbing to members of the family.

ASSOCIATED FEATURES

The recognition of PTSD as a disorder has been a great relief to those current and past members of the military who had had no explanation for symptoms that are extremely painful to them and disruptive to their families when they return from active duty. Instead of being grateful to have survived, and able to relax and enjoy the safety and affection at home, they are irritable and jumpy. Now that their symptoms have a name, they can seek treatment. Increasing knowledge about PTSD has also benefited other individuals with previously unexplained symptoms, including those who had been diagnosed as having a personality disorder, specifically borderline personality disorder.
For example, women who developed symptoms as a result

of domestic violence had been labeled 'borderline', which made it seem that they, rather than their abusers, were responsible for their symptoms. Under these circumstances, a loving and capable, but symptomatic, mother might have lost custody of her children to the abusive partner who was the cause of her symptoms.

PREVALENCE

Most people exposed to a particular traumatic event do not develop PTSD. Some of the vulnerability is genetic. Because we might assume that people repeatedly exposed to trauma, for example those living in war zones or other dangerous areas, would develop resistance to the resulting anxiety, it is especially important to note that the opposite is true; people who have been traumatized in the past are more likely to develop PTSD after a future traumatic event.

TREATMENT OPTIONS

There is some controversy over the best way to treat PTSD. After 9/11, volunteer counselors of all sorts offered to work with survivors and those traumatized in the course of trying to rescue people or retrieve human remains. However, it seems that encouraging people to talk about a trauma right after it happens is generally not helpful. Many people exposed to trauma would rather go to a safe, and, if possible, familiar, place; take care of any immediate needs like food, clothing, or shelter, and do comforting things like take a bath and spend time with friends and loved ones.

Medications, including paroxetine and sertraline, can help with symptoms but are not a cure for PTSD. Non-pharmacologic treatments have been more successful. The underlying concept is the elimination of traumatic memories by gradual and controlled exposure of the patient to memories or reminders of the traumatic event or events, in a safe environment. One method is called Eye Movement Desensitization and Reprocessing, or EMDR. Therapists have a patient make specific eye movements or, more recently, listen to beep tones, while bringing traumatic memories to mind. There is considerable controversy over the need for the eye movements or beep tones. Patients have achieved better resolution of symptoms by recounting the memories and their feelings (not immediately after the event) to a therapist. Therapists may also help patients who are avoiding places or situations to gradually tolerate exposure to them.

Currently, psychiatrists are in active discussions with military leaders to address the following problem. While it is a relief to know that one's symptoms are part of a recognized illness that affects many others, and while access to treatment can require medical diagnosis, there is also stigma against having a mental illness. Only recently did the President of the United States agree to give veterans afflicted with PTSD the same recognition of battle-related injuries, with medals of honor for example, that are given to those with more obvious bodily injuries. Members of the military continue to be concerned, sometimes with good reason, that having a psychiatric diagnosis will adversely affect their military careers. The ongoing discussions may enable us to develop a special descriptive term, other than 'disorder' for PTSD resulting from the trauma of war.

Associations & Agencies

1276 Association of Traumatic Stress Specialists
500 Old Buncombe Road
500 Old Buncombe Road
Greenville, SC 29617
864-294-4337
Fax: 864-294-4384
E-mail: admin@atss.info
www.atss.info

Chrys Harris, PhD., CTS, President
Bill Mc Dermott, C.Psych, CTS, Vice President
Linda Hood, B.A., CTSS, Secretary
Diane Travers, LCSW, CTS, Chair of Certification Board

Helps the traumatized through international service, education and professional development

1277 Career Assessment & Planning Services
Goodwill Industries-Suncoast, Inc.
10596 Gandy Boulevard
St. Petersburg, FL 33702-1427
727-523-1512
888-279-1988
TDD: 727-579-1068
E-mail: gw.marketing@goodwill-suncoast.com
www.goodwill-suncoast.org

Oscar J Horton, Chairman
R. Lee Waits, President and CEO Emeritus
Deborah A. Passerini, President, Board Officer
Martin W Gladysz, Senior Vice Chairman

Provide a comprehensive assessment to help physically, emotionally or developmentally disabled persons develop a plan for employment. In addition to making employment and training recommendations, Goodwill identifies community resources that could improve the quality of life for those who are unprepared for immediate placement in employment.

Year Founded: 1954

1278 Center for Mental Health Services (CMHS)
1 Choke Cherry Road
Room 6-1057
Rockville, MD 20857
240-276-1310
877-726-4727
Fax: 240-276-1320
TDD: 800-487-4889
E-mail: info@mentalhealth.org
www.beta.samhsa.gov/about-us/who-we-are/offices-center

Michael E Etzinger, B.S.M.E, , M.B., SAMHSA Executive Officer, Director
Paolo Del Vecchio, M.S.W, Director, Center for Mental Healt
Deborah Baldwin, M.P.A, Acting Director, Consumer Affairs
Elizabeth Lopez, Ph.D, Acting Deputy Director

CMHS leads Federal efforts to treat mental illnesses by promoting mental health and by preventing the development or worsening of mental illness when possible. Congress created CMHS to bring new hope to adults who have serious mental illnesses and to children with serious emotional disorders. CMHS provides information about mental health via a toll-free the web site, and more than 600 publications. Developed for users of mental health services and their families, the general public, policy makers, providers, and the media.

Year Founded: 1992

1279 International Society for Traumatic Stress Studies
111 Deer Lake Road
Suite 100
Deerfield, IL 60015-1591
847-480-9028
Fax: 847-480-9282
E-mail: istss@istss.org
www.www.istss.org/Home.htm

Nancy Kassam-Adams, PhD, President
Meaghan O'Donnell, PhD, Vice President
Rick Koepke, Executive Director
Grete A Dyb, MD, PhD, Treasurer

Provides a forum for sharing research, clinical strategies, public policy concerns and theoretical formulation on trauma in the US and worldwide. Dedicated to discovery and dissemination of knowledge and to the stimulation of policy, program and services.

Year Founded: 1985

1280 Mental Health America
2000 North Beauregard Street
6th Floor
Alexandria, VA 22311
703-684-7722
800-969-6642
Fax: 703-684-5968
E-mail: info@mentalhealthamerica.net
www.www.mentalhealthamerica.net

Ann Boughtin, Chair
David L Shern, Ph.D., Interim President and CEO
Dianne Felton, Chief Operating Officer
Mike Turner, VP of Development

MHA is the leading advocacy agency addressing the full spectrum of mental and substance use conditions and their effects nationwide. MHA's actions inform, support, and enable mental wellness and recovery from mental illness including anxiety and post traumatic stress disorder.

1281 National Alliance on Mental Illness
3803 North Fairfax Drive
Suite 100
Arlington, VA 22203
703-524-7600
800-950-6264
Fax: 703-524-9094
E-mail: helpline@nami.org
www.nami.org

Keris Jan Myrick, MBA, MS, PhD., President
Mary Giliberti, J.D, Executive Director
Jim Payne, J.D, First Vice President
David Levy, Chief Financial Officer

Nation's leading self-help organization for all those affected by severe brain disorders. Mission is to bring consumers and families with similar experiences together to share information about services, care providers, and ways to cope with the challenges of schizophrenia, manic depression, and other serious mental illnesses.

Year Founded: 1969

1282 National Association for the Dually Diagnosed (NADD)
132 Fair Street
Kingston, NY 12401-4802
845-331-4336
800-331-5362
Fax: 845-331-4569
E-mail: info@thenadd.org
www.thenadd.org

Donna McNELIS, PhD, President
Robert J Fletcher DSW, Chief Executive Officer
Dan Baker, PhD, Vice President
Julia Pearce, Secretary

Nonprofit organization designed to promote interest of professional and parent development with resources for individuals who have the coexistence of mental illness and mental retardation. Provides conferences, educational services and training materials to professionals, parents, concerned citizens and service organizations.

Year Founded: 1983

1283 SAMHSA's National Mental Health Information Center
1 Choke Cherry Rd.
Rockville, MD 20857
240-221-4021
877-786-4727
Fax: 240-221-4295
TDD: 866-889-2647
www.store.samhsa.gov

1284 The Center for Family Support
2811 Zulette Avenue
Bronx, NY 10461
718-518-1500
Fax: 718-518-8200
E-mail: svernikoff@cfsny.org
www.cfsny.org

Steven Vernikoff, Executive Director
Virgil Seepersad, Director of Finance
Eileen Berg, Director of Quality Assurance
Barbara Greenwald, Associate Executive, Director

The Center for Family Support is committed to providing support and assistance to individuals with developmental and related disabilities, and to the family members who care for them.

Year Founded: 1954

Books

1285 After the Crash: Assessment and Treatment of Motor Vehicle Accident Survivors
American Psychological Publishing
750 First Street, NorthEast
Washington, DC 20002-4242
202-336-5500
800-374-2721
Fax: 202-336-5518
TDD: 202-336-6123
TTY: 202-336-6123
www.apa.org

Edward B Blanchard, PhD, ABPP, Author
Edward J Hickling, PsyD, Author
Suzanne Bennett-Johnson, PhD, President

In this timely second edition, written in a clear and lucid style and illustrated by a wealth of charts, guides, case studies, and clinical advice, the authors report on new, international research and provide updates on their own long-standing research protocols within the groundbreaking Alabny MVA Project. *$29.95*

475 pages   Year Founded: 1892 ISBN 1-591470-70-6

1286 Aging and Post Traumatic Stress Disorder
American Psychiatric Publishing, Inc.
1000 Wilson Boulevard
Suite 1825
Arlington, VA 22209-3901
703-907-7322
800-368-5777
Fax: 703-907-1091
E-mail: appi@psych.org
www.appi.org

Robert E Hales MD, Editor-in-Chief
Rebecca D Rinehart, Publisher
John McDuffie, Editorial Director

Provides both literature reviews and data about animal and clinical studies and training for important current concepts of aging, the stress response and the interaction between them. *$85.00*

280 pages   ISBN 0-880485-13-5

1287 Children and Trauma: A Guide for Parents and Professionals
Courage to Change
303 Crossways Park Drive
Woodbury, NY 11797
800-440-4003
Fax: 800-772-6499
www.couragetochange.com

Cynthia Monahon, Author

Teaches parents and professionals about the effects of such ordeals on children and offers a blueprint for restoring a child's sense of safety and balance. Offers hope and reassurance for parents. The author suggests straightforward ways to help kids through tough times, and also describes in detail the warning signs that indicate a child needs professional help. Monahon helps adults understand psychological trauma from a child's point of view and explores the ways both parents and professionals can help children heal. *$19.95*

240 pages   Year Founded: 1997 ISBN 0-787910-71-6

1288 Coping with Post-Traumatic Stress Disorder
Rosen Publishing Group
29 East 21st Street
New York, NY 10010-6209
212-777-3017
800-237-9932
Fax: 888-436-4643
E-mail: info@rosenpub.com
www.rosenpublishing.com

Carolyn Simpson, Author
Dwain Simpson, Author

$33.25

176 pages   Year Founded: 1950 ISBN 0-823934-56-X

1289 Coping with Trauma: A Guide to Self Understanding

8730 Georgia Avenue
Suite 600
Silver Spring, MD 20910-3643
240-485-1001
E-mail: AnxDis@adaa.org
www.adaa.org

Jon G Allen, Author
Michelle Alonso, Communications/Membership

1290 Coping with Trauma: A Guide to Self Understanding

1000 Wilson Boulevard
Suite 1825
Arlington, VA 22209-3901
703-907-7322
800-368-5777
Fax: 703-907-1091
E-mail: appi@psych.org
www.appi.org

Robert E Hales MD, Editor-in-Chief
Ron McMillen, Chief Executive Officer
John McDuffie, Editorial Director
Jon G Allen, Author

385 pages

1291 Effecive Treatments for PTSD: Practice Guidelines from the International Society for Traumatic Stress Studies
The Guilford Press
72 Spring Street
New York, NY 10012-4019
212-431-9800
800-365-7006
Fax: 212-966-6708
E-mail: info@guilford.com

Bob Matloff, President
Edna Foa, Author
Terence Keane, Author
Matthew Friedman, Author

The treatment guidelines presented in this book were developed under the auspices of the PTSD Treatment Guidelines Task Force established by the Board of Directors. *$38.25*

658 pages Year Founded: 2010 ISBN 1-609181-49-9

1292 Effective Treatments for PTSD
Guilford Press
72 Spring Street
New York, NY 10012-4068
212-431-9800
800-365-7006
Fax: 212-966-6708
E-mail: info@guilford.com

Bob Matloff, President

Represents the collaborative work of experts across a range of theoretical orientations and professional backgrounds. Addresses general treatment considerations and methodological issues, reviews and evaluates the salient literature on treatment approaches for children, adolescents and adults. *$44.00*

379 pages ISBN 1-572305-84-3

1293 Handbook of PTSD: Science and Practice
The Guilford Press
72 Spring Street
New York, NY 10012-4019
212-431-9800
800-365-7006
Fax: 212-966-6708
E-mail: info@guilford.com

Bob Matloff, President
Seymour Weingarten, Editor-in-Chief
Matthew Friedman, Author

Unparalleled in its breadth and depth, this state-of-the-art handbook reviews the latest scientific advances in understanding trauma and PTSD. *$42.50*

592 pages Year Founded: 2010 ISBN 1-609181-74-1

1294 Haunted by Combat: Understanding PTSD in War Veterans
Rowman & Littlefield Publishers
4501 Forbes Boulevard
Suite 200
Lanham, MD 20706
301-459-3366
301-459-5748
Fax: 301-429-5748
www.rowman.com

Daryl S Paulson, Author
Stanley Krippner, Author
Jeff Harris, Vice President of Credit
Mike Cornell, Vice President of Operations

Across history, the condition has been called soldier's heart, shell shock, or combat fatigue. *$18.99*

226 pages Year Founded: 2010 ISBN 1-442203-91-4

1295 I Can't Get Over It: Handbook for Trauma Survivors
NewHarbinger Publications
5674 Shattuck Avenue
Oakland, CA 94609
510-652-0215
800-748-6273
Fax: 800-652-1613
E-mail: customerservice@newharbinger.com
www.newharbinger.com

Aphrodite T Matsakis, PhD, Author

Guides readers through the healing process of recovering from Post Traumatic Stress Disorder. From the emotional experience to the process of healing, this book is written for survivors of all types of trauma including war, sexual abuse, crime, family violence, rape and natural catastrophes. *$16.95*

416 pages Year Founded: 1973 ISBN 1-572240-58-X

1296 Managing Traumatic Stress Risk: A Proactive Approach
Charles C Thomas Publisher Ltd.
2600 South First Street
Springfield, IL 62794-9265
217-789-8980
800-258-8980
Fax: 217-789-9130
www.ccthomas.com

This volume represents the first systematic review of critical incident and disaster hazards, the contextual factors that influence risk, and their implications for traumatic stress risk management. It provides the hazard assessment and risk analysis information which, combined with information on resilience, facilitates the systematic analysis of traumatic stress risk and proactive and methodical development of mitigation and risk reduction strategies. This book is also available in paperback for $41.95. *$61.95*

258 pages Year Founded: 2004 ISBN 0-398075-17-4

1297 Post-Traumatic Stress Disorder: Assessment, Differential Diagnosis, and Forensic Evaluation
Professional Resource Press
PO Box 3197
Sarasota, FL 34230-3197
941-343-9601
800-443-3364
Fax: 941-343-9201
E-mail: orders@prpress.com
www.prpress.com

Carroll L Meek, Author, Editor

A concise yet thorough examination of PTSD. An excellent resource for psychologists, psychiatrists, and lawyers involved in litigation concerning PTSD. *$26.95*

264 pages Year Founded: 1990 ISBN 0-943158-35-4

1298 Posttraumatic Stress Disorder in Litigation: Guidelines for Forensic Assessment
American Psychiatric Publishing, Inc.
1000 Wilson Boulevard
Suite 1825
Arlington, VA 22209-3901
703-907-7322
800-368-5777
Fax: 703-907-1091
E-mail: appi@psych.org
www.appi.org

Robert I Simon, M.D., Editor
Ron McMillen, Chief Executive Officer
John McDuffie, Editorial Director

This essential collection by 13 leading US experts sheds important new light on forensic guidelines for effective assessment and diagnosis and determination of disability, serving both plaintiffs and defendants in litigation involving PTSD claims. Mental health and legal professionals, third-party payers, and interested laypersons will welcome this balanced approach to a complex and difficult field. *$44.95*

272 pages Year Founded: 2003 ISBN 1-585620-66-1

1299 Posttraumatic Stress Disorder: A Guide
6515 Grand Teton Plaza
Suite 100
Madison, WI 53719
608-827-2470
Fax: 608-827-2444
E-mail: mim@miminc.org
www.www.miminc.cor

John H. Greist, MD, Author
James W. Jefferson, MD, Author
David J. Katzelnick, MD, Author

68 pages Year Founded: 2007

1300 Rebuilding Shattered Lives: Responsible Treatment of Complex Post-Traumatic and Dissociative Disorders
John Wiley & Sons
111 River Street
Hoboken, NJ 07030-5774
201-748-6000
800-225-5945
Fax: 201-748-6088
E-mail: info@wiley.com
www.wiley.com

James A Chu, Author

Essential for anyone working in the field of trauma therapy. Part I discusses recent findings about child abuse, the changes in attitudes toward child abuse over the last two decades and the nature of traumatic memory. Part II is an overview of principles of trauma treatment, including symptom control, establishment of boundaries and therapist self-care. Part III covers special topics, such as dissociative identity disorder, controversies, hospitalization and acute care. *$ 73.95*

271 pages Year Founded: 1998 ISBN 0-471247-32-4

1301 Risk Factors for Posttraumatic Stress Disorder
1000 Wilson Boulevard
Suite 1825
Arlington, VA 22209-3901
703-907-7322
800-368-5777
Fax: 703-907-1091
E-mail: appi@psych.org
www.appi.org

Robert E Hales MD, Editor-in-Chief
Ron McMillen, Chief Executive Officer
John McDuffie, Editorial Director

320 pages

1302 Take Charge: Handling a Crisis and Moving Forward
American Institute for Preventive Medicine
30445 Northwestern Highway
Suite 350
Farmington Hills, MI 48334-3107
248-539-1800
800-345-2476
Fax: 248-539-1808
E-mail: aipm@healthy.net
www.HealthyLife.com

Don R Powell, PhD, President/CEO
Elaine Frank, M.Ed, R.D, Vice President
Jeanette Karwan, Director, Product Development

Take Charge helps people effectively live their lives after September 11th. This full color booklet provides just the right amount of information to effectively address the many concerns people have today. It will help people to be prepared for any kind of disaster, be it a terrorist attack, fire or flood. *$4.25*

32 pages Year Founded: 1983

1303 Traumatic Stress: Effects of Overwhelming Experience on Mind, Body and Society
Guilford Press
72 Spring Street
New York, NY 10012-4068

212-431-9800
800-365-7006
Fax: 212-966-6708
E-mail: info@guilford.com
Besell van der Kolk, Author
Alexander McFarlane, Author

The current state of research and clinical knowledge on traumatic stress and its treatment. Contributions from leading authorities summarize knowledge emerging. Addresses the uncertainties and controversies that confront the field of traumatic stress, including the complexity of posttraumatic adaptations and the unproven effectiveness of some approaches to prevention and treatment. *$42.50*

596 pages Year Founded: 2006 ISBN 1-572300-88-4

1304 Trust After Trauma: A Guide to Relationships for Survivors and Those Who Love Them
NewHarbinger Publications
5674 Shattuck Avenue
Oakland, CA 94609-1662
510-652-0215
800-748-6273
Fax: 800-652-1613
E-mail: customerservice@newharbinger.com
www.newharbinger.com

Aphrodite T Matsakis, PhD, Author

Survivors guided through process of strengthening existing bonds, building new ones, and ending cycles of withdrawal and isolation. *$24.95*

352 pages Year Founded: 1973 ISBN 1-572241-01-2

1305 Understanding Post Traumatic Stress Disorder and Addiction
Sidran Institute
200 E Joppa Road
Suite 207
Baltimore, MD 21286-3107
410-825-8888
888-825-8249
Fax: 410-337-0747
E-mail: sidran@sidran.org
www.sidran.org

Katie Evans, Author

This booklet discusses PTSD, how to recognize it and how to begin a dual recovery program from chemical dependency and PTSD. The workbook includes information to enhance your understanding of PTSD, activities to help identify the symptoms of dual disorders, a self evaulation of your recovery process and ways to handle situations that may trigger PTSD. *$7.20*

48 pages

1306 Who Gets PTSD? Issues of Posttraumatic Stress Vulnerability
Charles C Thomas Publisher Ltd.
2600 South First Street
Springfield, IL 62704
217-789-8980
800-258-8980
Fax: 217-789-9130
E-mail: books@ccthomas.com
www.ccthomas.com

John M. Violanti, Author, Editor
Douglas Paton, Editor

Major topics in the text include: assessing psychological distress and physiological vulnerability in police officers, personal, organizational, and contextual influences in stress vulnerability; differences in vulnerability to posttraumatic deprivation: gender differences in police work , stress and trauma, trauma types, etc. *$ 46.95*

216 pages Year Founded: 1927 ISBN 3-980761-89-

Periodicals & Pamphlets

1307 Helping Children and Adolescents Cope with Violence and Disasters
National Institute of Mental Health
6001 Executive Boulevard
Room 8184, MSC 9663
Bethesda, MD 20892-9663
301-443-4513
866-615-6464
TTY: 301-443-8431
E-mail: nimhinfo@nih.gov
www.www.nimh.nih.gov/

A booklet that describes what parents can do to help children and adolescents cope with violence and disasters.

1308 Let's Talk Facts About Post-Traumatic Stress Disorder
American Psychiatric Publishing, Inc.
1000 Wilson Boulevard
Suite 1825
Arlington, VA 22209-3901
703-907-7322
800-368-5777
Fax: 703-907-1091
E-mail: appi@psych.org
www.appi.org

Robert E Hales MD, Editor-in-Chief
Ron McMillen, Chief Executive Officer
John McDuffie, Editorial Director

$12.50

8 pages Year Founded: 2005 ISBN 0-890423-63-6

Video & Audio

1309 Anxiety Disorders
American Counseling Association
5999 Stevenson Avenue
Alexandria, VA 22304-3304
703-823-9800
800-347-6647
Fax: 703-823-0252
TDD: 703-823-6862
E-mail: webmaster@counseling.org
www.counseling.org

Cirecie A. West-Olatunji, President
Richard Yep, Executive Director
Thelma Daley, Treasurer

Increase your awareness of anxiety disorders, their symptoms, and effective treatments. Learn the effect these disorders can have on life and how treatment can change the quality of life for people presently suffering from these disorders. Includes 6 audiotapes and a study guide. *$140.00*

Year Founded: 1952

1310 Treating Trauma Disorders Effectively
Colin A Ross Institute for Psychological Trauma
1701 Gateway
Suite 349
Richardson, TX 75080-3546
972-918-9588
Fax: 972-918-9069
E-mail: rossinst@rossinst.com
www.rossinst.com

Dr Colin A Ross, MD, Founder, President
Melissa Caldwell, Manager

A training video that gives a comprehensive overview of clinical interventions with trauma patients. The video teaches advanced techniques for treating Dissociative Identity Disorder, Post Traumatic Stress Disorder, & trauma related Depression, Anxiety, Addictions, and Borderline Personality Disorder. The video's teaching modalities consist of case examples, with dramatic reenactments, and narrator discussion by Colin Ross, M.D. The teaching methods used clearly demonstrate effective therapeutic techniques that are backed by years of experience and research.
$85.00

Year Founded: 1995

Web Sites

1311 www.apa.org/practice/traumaticstress.html
American Psychological Association

Provides tips for recovering from disasters and other traumatic events.

1312 www.bcm.tmc.edu/civitas/caregivers.htm
Caregivers Series

Sophisticated articles describing the effects of childhood trauma on brain development and relationships.

1313 www.cyberpsych.org
CyberPsych

CyberPsych presents information about psychoanalysis, psychotherapy and topics like anxiety disorders, substance abuse, homophobia, and traumas. It hosts mental health organizations and individuals with content of interest to the public and professional communities. There is also a free therapist finder service.

1314 www.icisf.org
International Critical Incident Stress Foundation

A nonprofit, open membership foundation dedicated to the prevention and mitigation of disabling stress by education, training and support services for all emergency service professionals. Continuing education and training in emergency mental health services for psychologists, psychiatrists, social workers and licensed professional counselors.

1315 www.mentalhealth.com
Internet Mental Health

On-line information and a virtual encyclopedia related to mental disorders, possible causes and treatments. News, articles, on-line diagnostic programs and related links. Designed to improve understanding, diagnosis and treatment of mental illness throughout the world. Awarded the Top Site Award and the NetPsych Cutting Edge Site Award.

1316 www.ncptsd.org
National Center for PTSD

Aims to advance the clinical care and social welfare of U.S. Veterans through research, education and training on PTSD and stress-related disorders

1317 www.planetpsych.com
PlanetPsych

Learn about disorders, their treatments and other topics in psychology. Articles are listed under the related topic areas. Ask a therapist a question for free, or view the directory of professionals in your area. If you are a therapist sign up for the directory. Current features, self-help, interactive, and newsletter archives.

1318 www.psychcentral.com
Psych Central

Personalized one-stop index for psychology, support, and mental health issues, resources, and people on the Internet.

1319 www.ptsdalliance.org
Post Traumatic Stress Disorder Alliance

Website of the Post Traumatic Stress Disorder Alliance.

1320 www.sidran.org
Sidran Institute, Traumatic Stress Education & Advocacy

Helps people understand, recover from, and treat traumatic stress (including PTSD), dissociative disorders, and co-occuring issues, such as addictions, self injury, and suicidality.

1321 www.sidran.org/trauma.html
Trauma Resource Area

Resources and Articles on Dissociative Experiences Scale and Dissociative Identity Disorder, PsychTrauma Glossary and Traumatic Memories.

1322 www.trauma-pages.com
David Baldwin's Trauma Information Pages

Focus primarily on emotional trauma and traumatic stress, including PTSD (Post-traumatic Stress Disorder) and dissociation, whether following individual traumatic experience(s) or a large-scale disaster.

Psychosomatic (Somatizing) Disorders

Introduction

Officially known as Somatizing Disorders, the disorders in this category are characterized by multiple physical symptoms or the conviction that one is ill despite negative medical examinations and laboratory tests. Those who have a Somatizing Disorder persist in believing they are ill, or experience physical symptoms over long periods, and their beliefs negatively affect all areas of their functioning. Two main types of Somatizing Disorders are Hypochondriasis, which consists of being convinced that one is ill despite evidence to the contrary, and Somatization Disorder, consisting of experiencing physical symptoms without a discernible basis.

Facititious disorder and malingering are also conditions in which physical symptoms are not caused by an identifiable general medical condition, but in these conditions, the symptoms are deliberately and consiously produced. A malingerer deliberately complains or mimics symptoms to achieve a specific goal, such as winning a medical mapractice suit or obtaining disability insurance.

Individuals with Factitious Disorder deliberately cause significant medical conditions in themselves, for example by introducing fecal contamination intravenously, or taking insulin to the point of severe hypoglycemia. The motivations for this behavior are unclear. Once the diagnosis is suspected, and the suspicion is conveyed to the patient, these individuals nearly always flee the medical care venue and are unwilling to undergo more definitive diagnostic examinations.

SYMPTOMS

HYPOCHONDRIASIS

• Pre occupation with fears of having a serious illness based on a misinterpretation of bodily symptoms or sensations;
• The preoccupation persists in spite of medical reassurance;
• The preoccupation is a source of distress and difficulty in social, work, and other areas;
• The duration of the preoccupation is at least six months.

SOMATIZATION DISORDER

• A history beginning before age 30 and continuing over years, resulting in a search for treatment or clear difficulties in social, work or interpersonal areas;
• Four pain symptoms related to at least four anatomical areas or functions;
• Two gastrointestinal problems other than pain, e.g. nausea, diarrhea;
• One sexual sympton other than pain, e.g. irregular menstruation, sexual disinterest, erectile dysfunction;
• One pseudoneurological symptom other than pain, e.g., weakness, double vision;
• Symptoms cannot be explained by a medical condition;
• When a medical condition exists, physical complaints and social difficulties are greater than normal.

ASSOCIATED FEATURES

The person with either of these Somatizing Disorders visits many doctors, but physical examinations and negative lab results neither reassure them nor resolve their symptoms. They often believe they are not getting proper respect or attention, and, indeed, they may be viewed in medical settings as troublesome, because their problems are 'all in their heads.' Persons with these disorders often suffer from anxiety and depression as well. Physical symptoms appearing after the somatization diagnosis is made, however, should not be dismissed completely out of hand. Sufferers can have general medical disorders at the same time as Somatizing Disorders.

The person may be treated by several doctors at once, which can lead to unwitting and possibly dangerous combinations of treatments. There may be suicide threats and attempts, and deteriorating personal relationships. Individuals with these disorders often have associated Personality Disorders, such as Histrionic, Borderline, or Antisocial Personality Disorder.

PREVALENCE

Hypochondriasis is equally common in both sexes. Its prevalence in the general population is not known. In general medical practice, four percent to nine percent of patients have the disorder. It is usually chronic.

Somatization Disorder was once thought to be mainly a disease of women, but occurs in both sexes. It is slightly less common among men in the general population of the US than in other countries, but not uncommon in general medical practice. It is more common among Puerto Rican and Greek men, which suggests that cultural factors influence the sex ratios.

TREATMENT OPTIONS

These disorders are chronic by definition, and are difficult to manage. Repeated reassurance is not successful. The aim is to limit the extent to which the physical concerns and symptoms preoccupy an individual's thoughts and activities, and drain family emotional and financial resources. Individuals suffering from these disorders often resist mental health referral because they interpret it, sometimes correctly, as an indication that their symptoms are not being taken seriously. Treatment, whether by the primary care or mental health professional or both, should focus on maintaining function despite the symptoms. It is important that the psychological management and treatment is coordinated with medical treatment if possible by one physician only; one person should oversee all the medical treatment, including the psychological, so that care does not become fragmented and/or repetitive as the patient sees many different clinicians. Some individuals with Hypochondriasis respond to treatment which combines medication with intensive behavioral and cognitive techniques to manage anxiety and modify beliefs about the origin and course of physical symptoms.

People with hypochondriasis and somatization disorders do not deliberatley produce or falsely complain of physical symptoms; their beliefs and behaviors are engendered by psychological conflict, and often by modeling on someone who was important to them when they were growing up.

Associations & Agencies

1324 Academy of Psychosomatic Medicine
5272 River Road
Suite 630
Bethesda, MD 20816-1453
301-718-6520
Fax: 301-656-0989
E-mail: apm@apm.org
www.www.apm.org

Philips R Muskin, MD, Chair, Foundation of APM
Linda L.M Workley, MD, President
James Vrac, Executive Director
Steven A Epstein, MD, Vice President

Represents psychiatrists dedicated to the advancement of medical science, education, and healthcare for persons with comorbid psychiatric and general medical conditions and provides national and international leadership in the furtherance of those goals. Promotes a global agenda of excellence in clinical care for patients with comorbid psychiatric and general medical conditions by actively influencing the direction and process of research and public policy and promoting interdisciplinary education. Also created the Foundation of the Academy of Psychosomatic Medicine, a scientific foundation supporting education and research programs.

1325 Career Assessment & Planning Services
Goodwill Industries-Suncoast
10596 Gandy Boulevard
St. Petersburg, FL 33702
727-523-1512
Fax: 727-563-9300
E-mail: gw.marketing@goodwill-suncoast.com
www.goodwill-suncoast.org

Oscar J Horton, Chairman
R. Lee Waits, President and CEO Emeritus
Deborah A. Passerini, President, Board Officer
Martin W Gladysz, Senior Vice Chairman

Provide a comprehensive assessment to help physically, emotionally or developmentally disabled persons develop a plan for employment. In addition to making employment and training recommendations, Goodwill identifies community resources that could improve the quality of life for those who are unprepared for immediate placement in employment.

Year Founded: 1954

1326 Center for Mental Health Services (CMHS)
1 Choke Cherry Road
Room 6-1057
Rockville, MD 20857
240-276-1310
877-726-4727
Fax: 240-276-1320
TDD: 800-487-4889
E-mail: info@mentalhealth.org
www.beta.samhsa.gov/about-us/who-we-are/offices-center

Michael E Etzinger, B.S.M.E, , M.B., SAMHSA Executive Officer, Director
Paolo Del Vecchio, M.S.W, Director, Center for Mental Healt
Deborah Baldwin, M.P.A, Acting Director, Consumer Affairs
Elizabeth Lopez, Ph.D, Acting Deputy Director

CMHS leads Federal efforts to treat mental illnesses by promoting mental health and by preventing the development or worsening of mental illness when possible. Congress created CMHS to bring new hope to adults who have serious mental illnesses and to children with serious emotional disorders. CMHS provides information about mental health via a toll-free the web site, and more than 600 publications. Developed for users of mental health services and their families, the general public, policy makers, providers, and the media.

Year Founded: 1992

1327 Institute for Contemporary Psychotherapy
1841 Broadway, 60th Street
4th Floor
New York, NY 10023-7608
212-333-3444
Fax: 212-333-5444
www.icpnyc.org

Ron Taffel, PhD, Chairman
Sue Warshal, Ph.D., MBA, Executive Director
Fred Lipschitz, PhD, Treasurer, Co-Founder
Mary Labiento, Associate Director of Operations

The Institute is composed of a group of 150 professionally trained, licensed psychotherapists who offer a full ranger of psychotherapeutic services, including individual and group psychotherapy, and psychoanalysis in addition to more specialized treatment services.

Year Founded: 1971

1328 National Association for the Dually Diagnosed (NADD)
132 Fair Street
Kingston, NY 12401-4802
845-331-4336
800-331-5362
Fax: 845-331-4569
E-mail: info@thenadd.org
www.thenadd.org

Donna McNELIS, PhD, President
Robert J Fletcher DSW, Chief Executive Officer
Dan Baker, PhD, Vice President
Julia Pearce, Secretary

Nonprofit organization designed to promote interest of professional and parent development with resources for individuals who have the coexistence of mental illness and mental retardation. Provides conference, educational services and training materials to professionals, parents, concerned citizens and service organizations.

Year Founded: 1983

1329 National Mental Health Consumers' Self-Help Clearinghouse
1211 Chestnut Street
Suite 1100
Philadelphia, PA 19107-4103
215-751-1810
800-553-4539
Fax: 215-636-6312
E-mail: info@mhselfhelp.org
www.mhselfhelp.org

Joseph Rogers, Executive Director/ Founder
Susan Rogers, Director
Britani Nestel, Program Specialist
Christa Burkett, Technical Assistance Coordinator

A national consumer technical assistance center that has played a major role in the development of the mental health consumer movement.

Year Founded: 1986

1330 SAMHSA'S National Mental Health Information Center
PO Box 42557
Washington, DC 20015-557
800-789-2647
Fax: 240-747-5470
TDD: 866-889-2647
E-mail: ken@mentalhealth.org
www.mentalhealth.samhsa.gov

A Kathryn Power, MEd, Director
Edward B Searle, Deputy Director

1331 The Center for Family Support
2811 Zulette Avenue
Bronx, NY 10461
718-518-1500
Fax: 718-518-8200
www.cfsny.org

Steven Vernikoff, Executive Director
Virgil Seepersad, Director of Finance
Eileen Berg, Director of Quality Assurance
Barbara Greenwald, Associate Executive, Director

An agency that continues to develop new programs to serve families and individuals with their care needs. They currently offer services throughout the New York City region including: New Jersey, Long Island and the Lower Hudson Valley.

Year Founded: 1954

Books

1332 Concise Guide to Psychopharmacology
American Psychiatric Publishing, Inc.
1000 Wilson Boulevard
Suite 1825
Arlington, VA 22209-3901
703-907-7322
800-368-5777
Fax: 703-907-1091
E-mail: appi@psych.org
www.appi.org

Lauren B Marangell, M.D, Author
James M Martinez, M.D, Author
John McDuffie, Editorial Director
Lauren B Marangell MD, Author

The definitive pocket reference for convenient everyday use. This invaluable clinical companion begins with an overview of the general principles relevant to the safe and effective use of psychotropic medications. Subsequent chapters focus on the major classes of psychotropic medications and the disorders for which they are prescribed.
$47.95

260 pages Year Founded: 2006 ISSN 9781585622559ISBN 1-585622-55-9

1333 Disorders of Simulation: Malingering, Factitious Disorders, and Compensation Neurosis
Psychosocial Press
59 Boston Post Road
Madison, CT 06443-2130
203-245-4000
Fax: 203-245-0775

Grant L. Hutchinson, Author

The book suggests that patients who suffer from disorders of simulation should be considered to have a bona fide problem, one deserving of mental health attention, understanding, analysis, and treatment.

1334 Do No Harm? Munchhausen Syndrome by Proxy
Independent Publishers Group
814 North Franklin Street
Chicago, IL 60610-3813
312-337-0747
800-888-4741
Fax: 312-337-5985
E-mail: frontdesk@ipgbook.com
www.ipgbook.com

Craig McGill, Author

The syndrome that causes parents and care workers to harm their children to get attention is separating many families. But has the fertile imagination of social workers and the publicc turned MSBP into the trendy disorder of our time? McGill traces the 25-year history of the disorder and examines high profile cases from six countries. He produces compelling stories from parents and care workers and asks what can be done to protect parents from being wrongly accused. *$16.95*

240 pages Year Founded: 1971 ISBN 1-901250-48-2

1335 Drug Therapy and Psychosomatic Disorders
Mason Crest Publishers
450 Parkway Drive
Suite D
Broomall, PA 19008-4017
610-543-6200
866-627-2665
Fax: 610-543-3878
E-mail: dtaylor@masoncrest.com
www.masoncrest.com

Autumn Libal, Author

How can doctors treat pain and illness in the body that are caused by the mind? In this book, learn more about Kevin's story, what psychosomatic disorders are, and how these phantom disorders can be treated.

128 pages Year Founded: 2004 ISBN 1-590845-73-0

1336 Essentials of Psychosomatic Medicine
American Psychiatric Publishing, Inc.
1000 Wilson Boulevard
Suite 1825
Arlington, VA 22209-3901
703-907-7322
800-368-5777
Fax: 703-907-1091
E-mail: appi@psych.org
www.appi.org

James L. Levenson, Author

This condensed version of The American Psychiatric Publishing Textbook of Psychosomatic Medicine focuses on psychiatric care for medically ill patients. Presents that portion of the larger work devoted to specific disorders, enabling the practitioner to assist patients with comorbid psychiatric and general medical illnesses complicating each other's management.

604 pages Year Founded: 2007

1337 Hypochondria: Woeful Imaginings
University of California Press
2120 Berkeley Way
Berkeley, CA 94704-5804
510-642-4247
Fax: 510-643-7127
E-mail: askucp@ucpress.edu
www.ucpress.edu

Susan Baur, Author

Susan Baur illuminates the process by which hypochondriacs come to adopt and maintain illness as a way of life. $25.00

260 pages Year Founded: 1989 ISBN 0-520067-51-7

1338 Mind-Body Problems: Psychotherapy with Psychosomatic Disorders
Jason Aronson
230 Livingston Street
Northvale, NJ 07647-1726
570-342-1320
800-782-0015
Fax: 201-767-1576
www.aronson.com

Janet Schumacher Finell, Author

Animated case reports on specific disorders- anorexia, arthritis, irritable bowel syndrome, even (speculatively) miscarriage- balance consideration of developmental questions and treatment issues (transference/countertransference) and techniques. $70.00

376 pages Year Founded: 1977 ISBN 1-568216-54-8

1339 Munchausen by Proxy: Identification, Intervention, and Case Management
Routledge
270 Madison Avenue
New York, NY 10016-601
770-385-9799
E-mail: louisalasher@mindspring.com
www.www.mbpexpert.com/

Louisa J. Lasher, Author
Louisa Lasher, Author

This step-by-step guide will help you identify and manage cases of this unique form of child maltreatment. This skills-base, practical book contains a thorough, up-to-date overview of MBP and includes suggestions for identifying and reporting to child protection agencies, investigating and gathering evidence, and legal and court procedures. Its easy readability and immediate applicability make this text a valuable tool in identifying and preventing this form of child abuse.

384 pages Year Founded: 2004 ISBN 0-789012-17-0

1340 Munchausen's Syndrome by Proxy
World Scientific Publishing Company
27 Warren Street
Suite 401-402
Hackensack, NJ 07601-5477
201-487-9655
800-227-7562
Fax: 201-487-9656
E-mail: wspc@wspc.com
www.worldscibooks.com

Gwen Adshead, Editor
Deborah Brooke, Editor

This book reviews the current state of knowledge of Munchausen's Syndrome by Proxy, a type of child abuse which causes wide concern. Two main areas are covered: new directions in research, and treatment of the perpetrator in and outside the family. Unlike other books, this volume provides a multidisciplinary perspective, with input from social workers, pediatricians, child-psychiatrists and lawyers, among others. It also offers an international perspective, with contributors from the USA, Canada and Australia. $53.00

252 pages Year Founded: 1981 ISBN 1-860941-34-6

1341 Phantom Illness: Recognizing, Understanding, and Overcoming Hypochondria
Houghton Mifflin Company
222 Berkeley Street
Boston, MA 02116-3760
617-351-5000
Fax: 617-351-1105
E-mail: inquiries@hmco.com
www.houghtonmifflinbooks.com

Carla Cantor, Author

Offers hope to those who suffer from the debilitating disorder of hypochondria. Carla Cantor's long, dark road to hypochondria began when she crashed a car, killing a friend of hers. She couldn't forgive herself, and a few years later began imagining that she was suffering from Lupus. Many years and two hospitalizations later, she wrote this book not only about her experiences, but about hypochondria in general, now more politely referred to as a somatoform disorder. $15.00

351 pages ISBN 0-395859-92-1

1342 Playing Sick?: ntangling the Web of Munchausen Syndrome, Munchausen by Proxy, Malingering, and Factitious Disorde
Routledge Publishing
270 Madison Avenue
New York, NY 10016-601
212-695-6599

Marc D. Feldman, Author

Taken from bizarre cases of real patients, the first book to chronicle the devastating impact of phony illnesses-factitious disorders and Munchausen syndrome-on patients and caregivers alike. Based on years of research and clinical practics, this book provides the clues that can help practitioners and family members recognize these disorders, avoid invasive procedures, and sort out the motives that drive people to hurt themselves and deceive others. With insight and years of hands-on experience, Feldman shows how to get these emotionally ill patients the psychiatric help they need. $27.50

328 pages ISBN 0-415949-34-7

1343 Playing Sick?: Untangling the Web of Munchausen Syndrome, Munchausen by Proxy, Malingering, and Factitious Disorder
Routledge
7625 Empire Drive
Florence, KY 41042-2919
800-634-7064
Fax: 800-248-4724
E-mail: orders@taylorandfrancis.com
www.www.routledge.com

Maura May, Publisher

Based on years of research and clinical practice, this book provides the clues that can help practitioners and family members recognize these disorders, avoid invasive procedures, and sort out the motives that drive people to hurt themselves and deceive others.

1344 Somatoform and Factitious Disorders (Review of Psychiatry)
American Psychiatric Publishing, Inc.
1000 Wilson Boulevard
Suite 1825
Arlington, VA 22209-3901
703-907-7322
800-368-5777
Fax: 703-907-1091
E-mail: appi@psych.org
www.appi.org

Katherine A Phillips, M.D., Editor
Ron McMillen, Chief Executive Officer
John McDuffie, Editorial Director

Offers clinicians a broad synthesis of the current knowledge about somatoform and factitious disorders.

216 pages Year Founded: 2001

1345 The Divided Mind: The Epidemic of Mindbody Disorders
HarperCollins Publishers
10 East 53rd Street
New York, NY 10022-5299
212-207-7000
Fax: 212-207-6964
E-mail: feedback2@harpercollins.com
www.harpercollins.com

John E. Sarno, Author

Traces the history of psychosomatic medicine, including Freud's crucial role as well as his failures. Most important, it describes the psychology of the human condition that is responsible for the broad range of psychosomatic illness. Dr. Sarno believes that the failure of medicine's practitioners to recognize and appropriately treat mindbody disorders had produced public health and economic problems of major proportions in the United States.

400 pages Year Founded: 1817 ISBN 0-060851-78-3

1346 What Your Patients Need to Know about Psychiatric Medications
American Psychiatric Publishing, Inc.
1000 Wilson Boulevard
Suite 1825
Arlington, VA 22209-3901
703-907-7322
800-368-5777
Fax: 703-907-1091

E-mail: appi@psych.org
www.appi.org

Robert E Hales MD, Author
Robert H. Chew, Ph.D., Author
Stuart C. Yudofsky, MD, Author

This book includes all major classes of medications, along with detailed information on specific agents - information that's more in-depth and easier to understand than what can be obtained from pharmacies or found on the Internet.
$87.00

441 pages Year Founded: 2009 ISSN 9781585623563

Periodicals & Pamphlets

1347 Asher Meadow Newsletter
18209 Smoke House Court
Germantown, MD 20874-2425
www.www.abysse.info

Asher Meadow is a wholly-owned non-profit subsidiary of American Marvels, an Internet development company that provides a newsletter for survivors of MSBP.

Video & Audio

1348 Clinical Impressions: Identifying Mental Illness
Educational Training Videos
136 Granville St
Suite 200
Gahanna, OH 43230
Fax: 888-775-3919
www.educationaltrainingvideos.com

How long can mental illness stay hidden, especially from the eyes of trained experts? This program rejoins a group of ten adults- five of them healthy and five of them with histories of mental illness- as psychiatric specialists try to spot and correctly diagnose the latter. Administering a series of collaborative and one-on-one tests, including assessments of personality type, physical self-image, and rational thinking, the panel gradually makes decisions about who suffers from depression, bipolar disorder, bulimia, and social anxiety.

1349 Coping with Stress
Educational Video Network, Inc.
1401 19th Street
Huntsville, TX 77340
936-295-5767
800-762-0060
Fax: 936-294-0233
www.www.evndirect.com

Stress affects everyone, both emotionally and physically. For some, mismanaged stress can result in substance abuse, violence, or even suicide. This program answers the question, How can a person cope with stress?

1350 Dealing with Depression
Educational Video Network, Inc.
1401 19th Street
Huntsville, TX 77340
936-295-5767
800-762-0060
Fax: 936-294-0233
www.www.evndirect.com

As more and more young people are falling victim to depression, it is important to understand what causes it and to know how to get the help that can rid a person of this life-wrecking affliction.

1351 Dealing with Social Anxiety
Educational Video Network, Inc.
1401 19th Street
Huntsville, TX 77340
936-295-5767
800-762-0060
Fax: 936-294-0233
www.www.evndirect.com

Social anxiety is America's third-largest psychiatric disorder. It generally develops during the mid-teen years, and almost always before the age of 25. Understand what may trigger the development of anxiety and learn how it sometimes evolves into full-blown panic disorder, which is characterized by recurrent attacks of terror or fear. The consequences of social anxiety are examined and effective treatments are discussed.

1352 FRONTLINE: The Released
PBS
2100 Crystal Drive
Arlington, VA 22202
www.pbs.org

Will Lyman, Actor
Narrator
Miri Navasky, Director
Karen O'Connor, Director

The documentary states that of the 700, 000 inmates released from American prisons each year, half of them have mental disabilities. This work focused on those with severe problems who keep entering and exiting prison. Full of good information on the challenges they face with mental illnesses; housing, employment, stigmatization, and socialization.

Year Founded: 2009

1353 Mental Disorder
Educational Training Videos
136 Granville St
Suite 200
Gahanna, OH 43230
Fax: 888-775-3919
www.educationaltrainingvideos.com

What is abnormality? Using the case studies of two young women; one who has depression, one who has an anxiety disorder; as a springboard, this program presents three psychological perspective on mental disorder.

1354 Mind-Body Problems: Psychotherapy with Psychosomatic Disorders
Jason Aronson, Inc.- Rowman Littlefield Imprint
4501 Forbes Blvd.
Suite 200
Lanham, MD 20706
301-459-3366
Fax: 301-429-5748
www.rowmanlittlefield.com

Janet Schumacher Finell, Author

The opening paper profitably links psychosomatic disorders to alexithymia, the absence or deadening of feeling, the inability to identify or express emotion.

376 pages Year Founded: 1977 ISBN 1-568216-54-8

1355 Neurotic, Stress-Related, and Somatoform Disorders
Educational Training Videos
136 Granville St
Suite 200
Gahanna, OH 43230
Fax: 888-775-3919
www.educationaltrainingvideos.com

This program, filmed in the UK, discusses the following disorders and their differential diagnoses; phobic anxiety; anxiety; obsessive-compulsive disorder, from minor to acute; stress reaction and adjustment; and dissociative disorders. Sub-disorders discussed include Korsakov's syndrome; agoraphobia and social phobia; generalized anxiety and mixed-anxiety-and-depressive disorder; panic disorder; and post-traumatic stress syndrome. Patients suffering from each disorder exhibit the various symptoms in interviews conducted by psychiatrists.

1356 Somatoform Disorders: A Medicolegal Guide
Cambridge University Press
32 Ave of the Americas
New York, NY 10013-2473
212-337-5000
E-mail: newyork@cambridge.org
www.cambridge.org

Michael Trimble, Author

This book is an in-depth, clinically oriented review of the somatoform disorders and related clinical manifestations (such as chronic fatigue syndrome) and how they appear in a medico-legal setting. The volume is aimed at clinicians and lawyers who deal with injury claims where these disorders impact much more frequently than generally recognized.

268 pages Year Founded: 2011 ISBN 0-521169-25-9

1357 Understanding Mental Illness
Educational Video Network, Inc.
1401 19th Street
Huntsville, TX 77340
936-295-5767
800-762-0060
Fax: 936-294-0233
www.www.evndirect.com

Contains information and classifications of mental illness. Mental illness can strike anyone, at any age. Learn about various organic and functional mental disorders as discussed and their causes and symptoms, and learn where to seek help for a variety of mental health concerns.

Web Sites

1358 www.mbpexpert.com
MBP Expert Services

Expert services from Louisa J Lasher, MA, provides Munchausen by Proxy maltreatment training, case consultation, technical assistance, and expert witness services in an objective manner and in the best interest of the child or children involved.

1359 www.mentalhealth.com
Internet Mental Health

Offers online psychiatric diagnosis in the hope of reaching the two-thirds of individuals with mental illness who do not seek treatment.

1360 **www.msbp.com**
Mothers Against Munchausen Syndrome by Proxy Allegations

Begun in response to the fast growing number of false allegations of Munchausen Syndrome by Proxy.

1361 **www.munchausen.com**
Munchause Syndrome

Dr. Marc Feldman's Munchausen Syndrome, Malingering, Factitious Disorder, & Munchausen by Proxy page. Includes articles, related book list, personal stories and links.

1362 **www.planetpsych.com**
Planetpsych.com

Online resource for mental health information

1363 **www.psychcentral.com**
Psych Central

The Internet's largest and oldest independent mental health social network created and run by mental health professionals to guarantee reliable, trusted information and support communities to you.

Schizophrenia

Introduction

Schizophrenia is an old term meaning, approximately, 'split personality.' While the name of the diagnosis survives, the concept of split personality is outdated. This is a misuse of the term.

Schizophrenia is a devastating disease of the brain that severely impairs an individual's ability to think, feel and function normally. Though not a common disorder, it is one of the most destructive, disrupting the lives of sufferers, as well as of family members and loved ones. Long misunderstood, people with Schizophrenia and their families have also borne a burden of stigma in addition to the burden of their illness.

Although family and other environmental stressors can play a role in precipitating or exacerbating episodes of illness, theories that the disease is caused by poor parenting have been discredited. Much has been learned about the disease in recent years and treatments have improved markedly.

Schizophrenia is a largely genetically determined disorder of the brain. One theory is that it is a disorder of information processing resulting from a defect in the prefrontal cortex of the brain. Because this system is defective, an individual with Schizophrenia is easily overwhelmed by the amount of information and stimuli coming from the environment. Schizophrenia causes hallucinations, which are sensory experiences in the absence of actual stimuli (hearing voices when no one is speaking), and delusions, which are bizarre beliefs (tThat the individual is God, that the television is conveying messages specifically aimed at the individual, that some power is removing the individual's thoughts from his or her mind). Speech may be tangential or confused. These are called 'positive symptoms.' The individual also loses some normal behaviors and experiences, engaging in little behavior or social interaction. These are called 'negative symptoms.' Schizophrenia is a chronic disease and, once diagnosed, a person often needs treatment the rest of his or her life. However, great strides have been made in treating the disease and many individuals with schizophrenia can hold jobs, marry, parent children, and have gratifying and productive lives.

SYMPTOMS

So-called 'Positive' symptoms (experiences not shared by people in society):
• Delusions or false and bizarre beliefs;
• Hallucinations;

Negative symptoms (the loss of normal behaviors):
• Withdrawing from social contact;
• Speaking less;
• Losing interest in things and the ability to enjoy them;
• Disorganized speech;
• Grossly disorganized or catatonic behavior (extremely agitated or zombie-like);
• The symptoms cause social and occupational dysfunction;
• Signs of the disturbance persist for at least six months;
• The symptoms must not be related to mood or depressive disorders, substance abuse or general medical conditions.

ASSOCIATED FEATURES

People with Schizophrenia, because their disease causes difficulty in perceiving their environment and responding to it normally, often act strange, and have odd beliefs. They sometimes react to stimuli (voices or images originating inside their brains) as though they were originating in their environment; hallucinations and delusions can make a person's behavior appear bizarre to others. Anhedonia, the inability to enjoy pleasurable activities, is common in Schizophrenia, as are sleep disturbances and abnormalities of psychomotor activity. The latter may take the form of pacing, rocking, or immobility. Negative symptoms can be more disabling than positive ones. Family members often become annoyed because they think the individual is just lazy. Schizophrenia takes many forms, and there are a number of subtypes of the illness, including paranoid schizophrenia.

Individuals with untreated Schizophrenia, under the influence of hallucinations and delusions, have a slightly greater propensity for violence than the general population, but only when there is co-existing alcohol or substance abuse, which is quite common. Schizophrenia is known as a heterogenous disease, meaning that the illness takes many forms, depending on a variety of individual characteristics and circumstances. Patients who receive appropriate treatment are not more violent than the general population.

The life expectancy of people with Schizophrenia is shorter than the general population for a varietyof reasons: suicide is common among people with the disease and people with Schizophrenia often have both poor medical care and poor health.

PREVALENCE

The first episode of Schizophrenia usually occurs in teenage years, although some cases may occur in the late thirties or forties. Onset prior to puberty is rare, though cases as early as five year olds have been reported. Women have a later average of onset and a better prognosis. Estimates of the prevalence of Schizophrenia vary widely around the world, but probably about one percent of the world population has the disease.

TREATMENT OPTIONS

Medications can diminish or eliminate many of the positive symptoms of Schizophrenia. Older medications, such as Haldol, are effective and inexpensive, but cause more side effects than newer medications, such as Zyprexa and Geodon. Clozapine was the first and is still one of the most effective treatments, but it causes a low incidence of a life-threatening blood disorder; therefore people who take it must have blood tests at regular intervals. The newer medications are more effective in treating the negative, as well as the positive, symptoms.

Often, patients report that antipsychotic medications make them feel foggy, or lethargic. Antipsychotic medications can have serious side effects, including Tardive Dyskinesia, which consists of involuntary muscular movements. The newer antipsychotic medications are less sedating and have a decreased risk of causing Tardive Dyskinesia, but are associated with significant weight gain and increased risk of diabetes. There is considerable public controversy as to whether the weight gain, and risk of diabetes associated with the newer medications, along with their cost, outweigh their advantages.

Having Schizophrenia interferes with taking care of oneself and getting proper medical care in several ways; Schizophrenia often depletes financial resources so that patients cannot afford medication, nutrition, and medical care. Untreated Schizophrenia can also interfere with an individual's ability to understand signs and symptoms of medical disorders. Compliance with medication is often a problem, and failure to continue taking medication is a major cause of relapse. For this reason, treatment should include supportive therapy, in which a psychiatrist or other mental health professional provides counseling aimed at helping the patient maintain a positive and optimistic attitude focused on staying healthy. Other forms of therapy, such as social skills training, have also found some success and may be useful in helping a person with schizophrenia learn appropriate social and interpersonal behavior. It is important to note that psychotic illness does not necessarily affect all aspects of an individual's thinking. People with schizophrenia may have bizarre beliefs or behaviour in one sphere of life but be perfectly able to make decisions and function in other areas. In addition, it is crucial not to destroy an individual or family's hopes of a normal life by communicating the message that schizophrenia is hopeless.

Paranoid schizophrenia is especially difficult to treat. Paranoia, the irrational conviction that other people, institutions (the FBI), or alien beings are attempting to harm the individual, prevents the individual from forming trusting relationships with care providers and adhering to effective treatment regimens. The individual with paranoid schizophrenia can appear convincingly lucid in order to obtain release from care, while continuing to hold psychotic beliefs.

Associations & Agencies

1365 Brain & Behavior Research Foundation

90 Park Avenue
16th Floor
New York, NY 10016
646-681-4888
800-829-8289
Fax: 516-487-6930
E-mail: info@bbrfoundation.org
www.bbrfoundation.org

Steve Lieber, Chairman of the Board
Jeffrey Borenstein, M.D, President and Chief Executive Of
Louis Innamorato, Vice president, Finance and Chief
Suzzane Golden, Vice President

The Brain and Behavior Research Foundation is committed to alleviating the suffering caused by mental illness by awarding grants that will lead to advances and break-throughs in scientific researhc. 100% of all donor contributions for research are invested in NARSAD Grants leading to discoveries in understanding causes and improving treatments of disorders in children and adults, such as depression, bipolar disorder, schizophrenia, autism, attention deficit hyperactivity disorder, and anxiety disorders like obsessive-compulsive and post-traumatic stress disorders.

Year Founded: 1981

1366 Career Assessment & Planning Services

Goodwill Industries-Suncoast
10596 Gandy Boulevard
St. Petersburg, FL 33702-1427

727-523-1512
Fax: 727-563-9300
E-mail: gw.marketing@goodwill-suncoast.com
www.goodwill-suncoast.org

Oscar J Horton, Chairman
R. Lee Waits, President and CEO Emeritus
Deborah A. Passerini, President, Board Officer
Martin W Gladysz, Senior Vice Chairman

Provides a comprehensive assessment, which can predict current and future employment and potential adjustment factors for physically, emotionally, or developmentally disabled persons who may be unemployed or underemployed. Assessments evaluate interests, aptitudes, academic achievements, and physical abilities (including dexterity and coordination) through coordinated testing, interviewing and behavioral observations.

Year Founded: 1954

1367 Center for Mental Health Services (CMHS)

1 Choke Cherry Road
Room 6-1057
Rockville, MD 20857
240-276-1310
877-726-4727
Fax: 240-276-1320
TDD: 800-487-4889
E-mail: info@mentalhealth.org
www.beta.samhsa.gov/about-us/who-we-are/offices-center

Michael E Etzinger, B.S.M.E, , M.B., SAMHSA Executive
Officer, Director
Paolo Del Vecchio, M.S.W, Director, Center for Mental
Healt
Deborah Baldwin, M.P.A, Acting Director, Consumer
Affairs
Elizabeth Lopez, Ph.D, Acting Deputy Director

CMHS leads Federal efforts to treat mental illnesses by promoting mental health and by preventing the development or worsening of mental illness when possible. Congress created CMHS to bring new hope to adults who have serious mental illnesses and to children with serious emotional disorders. CMHS provides information about mental health via a toll-free the web site, and more than 600 publications. Developed for users of mental health services and their families, the general public, policy makers, providers, and the media.

Year Founded: 1992

1368 Mental Health America

2000 N. Beauregard Street
6th Floor
Alexandria, VA 22311-1739
703-684-7722
800-969-6642
Fax: 703-684-5968
E-mail: infoctr@nmha.org
www.mentalhealthamerica.net

Ann Boughtin, Chair
David Shern PhD, Interim President and CEO
Dianne Felton, Chief Operating Officer
Mike Turner, Vice President of Development

Formerly known as the National Mental Health Association, Mental Health America is the country's leading non-profit dedicated to helping ALL people live mentally healthier lives. Good mental health is fundamental to the health and well-being of every person and of the nation as a whole.

1369 National Alliance on Mental Illness
3803 North Fairfax Drive
Suite 100
Arlington, VA 22203
703-524-7600
800-950-6264
Fax: 703-524-9094
E-mail: helpline@nami.org
www.nami.org

Keris Jan Myrick, MBA, MS, PhD., President
Mary Giliberti, J.D, Executive Director
Jim Payne, J.D, First Vice President
David Levy, Chief Financial Officer

Nation's leading self-help organization for all those affected by severe brain disorders. Mission is to bring consumers and families with similar experiences together to
share information about services, care providers, and ways
to cope with the challenges of schizophrenia, manic depression, and other serious mental illnesses.

Year Founded: 1969

**1370 National Association for the Dually Diagnosed
(NADD)**
132 Fair Street
Kingston, NY 12401-4802
845-331-4336
800-331-5362
Fax: 845-331-4569
E-mail: info@thenadd.org
www.thenadd.org

Donna McNELIS, PhD, President
Robert J Fletcher DSW, Chief Executive Officer
Dan Baker, PhD, Vice President
Julia Pearce, Secretary

Nonprofit organization designed to promote interest of professional and parent development with resources for individuals who have the coexistence of mental illness and
mental retardation. Provides conference, educational services and training materials to professionals, parents, concerned citizens and service organizations.

Year Founded: 1983

**1371 National Mental Health Consumers' Self-Help
Clearinghouse**
1211 Chestnut Street
Suite 1100
Philadelphia, PA 19107-4103
215-751-1810
800-553-4539
Fax: 215-636-6312
E-mail: info@mhselfhelp.org
www.mhselfhelp.org

Joseph Rogers, Executive Director/ Founder
Susan Rogers, Director
Britani Nestel, Program Specialist
Christa Burkett, Technical Assistance Coordinator

A national consumer technical assistance center that has
played a major role in the development of the mental health
consumer movement.

Year Founded: 1986

**1372 SAMHSA'S National Mental Health
Information Center**
1 Choke Cherry Road
Rockville, MD 20857

800-789-2647
Fax: 240-747-5470
TDD: 866-889-2647
E-mail: ken@mentalhealth.org
www.mentalhealth.samhsa.gov

A Kathryn Power, MEd, Director
Edward B Searle, Deputy Director

1373 The Center for Family Support
2811 Zulette Avenue
Bronx, NY 10461
718-518-1500
Fax: 718-518-8200
www.cfsny.org

Steven Vernikoff, Executive Director
Virgil Seepersad, Director of Finance
Eileen Berg, Director of Quality Assurance
Barbara Greenwald, Associate Executive, Director

The Center for Family Support is committed to providing
support and assistance to individuals with developmental
and related disabilities, and to the family members who
care for them.

Year Founded: 1954

Books

1374 Biology of Schizophrenia and Affective Disease
American Psychiatric Publishing, Inc.
1000 Wilson Boulevard
Suite 1825
Arlington, VA 22209-3901
703-907-7322
800-368-5777
Fax: 703-907-1091
E-mail: appi@psych.org
www.appi.org

Stanley J. Watson, MD, PhD, Editor

Provides a state-of-the-art look at the biological basis of
several mental illness from the perspective of the researchers making these discoveries. This outstanding reference
tool explores the explosive progress in the fields of biochemistry, molecular genetics, neuroscience, and brain circuit anatomy and the resultant advances in nearly every
aspect of the biology of the brain and mental illness. The
book also discusses treatment issues, including the mechanisms of action of antidepressants and atypical
antipsychotic drugs. *$58.50*

560 pages Year Founded: 1995 ISBN 0-880487-46-7

**1375 Breakthroughs in Antipsychotic Medications: A
Guide for Consumers, Families, and Clinicians**
National Alliance on Mental Illness
2107 Wilson Boulevard
Suite 300
Arlington, VA 22201-3080
703-524-7600
800-950-6264
Fax: 703-524-9094
TDD: 703-516-7227
E-mail: generalinquiry@center4si.com
www.homeless.samhsa.gov

Ronald J. Diamond, Author
Ruth Ross, Author
Patricia L. Scheifler, Author
Peter J. Weiden, Author

Helps consumers and their families weigh the pros and cons of switching from older antipsychotics to newer ones. Answers frequently asked questions about antipsychotics and guides readers through the process of switching. Includes fact sheets on the new medications and their side effects. *$22.95*

208 pages Year Founded: 1999 ISBN 0-393703-03-7

1376 Concept of Schizophrenia: Historical Perspectives
American Psychiatric Publishing, Inc.
1000 Wilson Boulevard
Suite 1825
Arlington, VA 22209-3901
703-907-7322
800-368-5777
Fax: 703-907-1091
E-mail: appi@psych.org
www.appi.org

John G. Howells, Editor

The authors question whether there is a psychodynamics of schizophrenia and discuss the insights that spring from this field of inquiry. Presenting material on the concept of schizophrenia this work shows how historical research can be of value to contemporary clinical practice. *$65.00*

211 pages Year Founded: 1991 ISBN 0-880481-08-0

1377 Contemporary Issues in the Treatment of Schizophrenia
American Psychiatric Publishing, Inc.
1000 Wilson Boulevard
Suite 1825
Arlington, VA 22209-3901
703-907-7322
800-368-5777
Fax: 703-907-1091
E-mail: appi@psych.org
www.appi.org

Christian L. Shriqui, MD, Editor
Henry A. Nasrallah, MD, Editor

Covers the spectrum of therapeutic approaches to the disorder- biological, pharmacologica, and psychosocial- as well as presenting a wealth of new research on the course and outcome of schizophrenia. This volume should be a welcome addition to the libraries of psychiatrists, psychiatric residents, psychologists, and other health professionals working with schizophrenia. *$99.95*

889 pages Year Founded: 1995 ISBN 0-880486-81-3

1378 Drug Therapy and Schizophrenia
Mason Crest Publishers
450 Parkway Drive
Suite D
Broomall, PA 19008-4017
610-543-6200
866-627-2665
Fax: 610-543-3878
E-mail: gbaffa@nationalhighlights.com
www.masoncrest.com

Shirley Brinkerhoff, Author

This volume provides a concise description of this disease, which is considered the most severe of the mental disorders. The book also includes a brief account of the disease in history, as well as explanations of how the brain operates and how psychiatric drugs work within the brain. Many

case studies are presented to help readers better understand the nature of this difficult and potentially devastating mental disorder.

128 pages ISBN 1-590845-74-9

1379 Encyclopedia of Schizophrenia and Other Psychotic Disorders
Facts on File
132 W 31st Street
17th Floor
New York, NY 10001-3406
212-613-2800
800-322-8755
E-mail: custserv@factsonfile.com

Richard Noll, Author

Details recent theories and research findings on schizophrenia and psychotic disorders, together with a complete overview of the field's history. *$65.00*

368 pages Year Founded: 2000 ISBN 0-816040-70-2

1380 Family Care of Schizophrenia: a Problem-solving Approach to the Treatment of Mental Illness
Guilford Press
72 Spring Street
New York, NY 10012-4068
212-431-9800
800-365-7006
Fax: 212-966-6708
E-mail: info@guilford.com
www.www.guilford.com

Jeffrey L. Boyd, Author
Ian R.H. Falloon, Author
Christine W McGill, Author

Falloon and his colleagues have developed a model for the broad-based community treatment of schizophrenia and other severe forms of mental illness that taps this underutilized potential. The goal of their program is not merely the reduction of stress that can trigger florid episodes, but also the restoration of the patient to a level of social functioning that permits employment and socialization with people outside the family. As the author demonstrates, families can, with proper guidance, be taught to modulate intrafamilial stress, whether it derives from family tensions or external life events. *$27.95*

451 pages Year Founded: 1973 ISBN 0-898629-23-3

1381 Family Work for Schizophrenia: a Practical Guide
American Psychiatric Publishing, Inc.
1000 Wilson Boulevard
Suite 1825
Arlington, VA 22209-3901
703-907-7322
800-368-5777
Fax: 703-907-1091
E-mail: appi@psych.org
www.appi.org

Liz Kuipers, Author
J.P. Leff, Author
Dominic Lam, Author

The techniques and strategies included in the guide are clearly described for use by clinical practitioners and are illustrated by case examples. The guide has been further enriched with the authors' experience of working with families over the ten years since the first edition was published.

1382 First Episode Psychosis
American Psychiatric Publishing, Inc.
1000 Wilson Boulevard
Suite 1825
Arlington, VA 22209-3901
703-907-7322
800-368-5777
Fax: 703-907-1091
E-mail: appi@psych.org
www.appi.org

Robert E Hales MD, Editor-in-Chief
Ron McMillen, Chief Executive Officer
John McDuffie, Editorial Director

Professional discussion of early Psychosis presentation. *$39.95*

160 pages ISBN 1-853174-35-1

1383 Group Therapy for Schizophrenic Patients
American Psychiatric Publishing, Inc.
1000 Wilson Boulevard
Suite 1825
Arlington, VA 22209-3901
703-907-7322
800-368-5777
Fax: 703-907-1091
E-mail: appi@psych.org
www.appi.org

Nick Kanas, M.D., Author
Ron McMillen, Chief Executive Officer
John McDuffie, Editorial Director

Acquaints mental health practitioners with this cost-effective method of treatment. *$29.00*

184 pages Year Founded: 1996 ISBN 0-880481-72-2

1384 Guidelines for the Treatment of Patients with Schizophrenia
American Psychiatric Publishing, Inc.
1000 Wilson Boulevard
Suite 1825
Arlington, VA 22209-3901
703-907-7322
800-368-5777
Fax: 703-907-1091
E-mail: appi@psych.org
www.appi.org

Robert E Hales MD, Editor-in-Chief
Ron McMillen, Chief Executive Officer
John McDuffie, Editorial Director

Provides therapists with a set of patient care strategies that will aid their clinical decison making. Describes the best and most appropriate treatments available to patients. *$22.50*

160 pages ISBN 0-890423-09-1

1385 How to Cope with Mental Illness In Your Family: A Guide for Siblings and Offspring
Health Source
1404 K Street, NW
Washington, DC 20005-2401
202-789-7303
800-713-7122
Fax: 202-789-7899

E-mail: healthsourcebooks@psych.org
www.healthsourcebooks.org

Diane T Marsh, Author
Rex M Dickens, Author

This book explores the nature of illnesses such as schizophrenia, major depression, while providing the tools to overcome the devasting effects of growing up or living in a family where they exist. Readers are led through the essential stages of recovery, from revisiting their childhood to revising their family legacy, and ultimately, to reclaiming their life. *$14.00*

206 pages ISBN 0-874779-23-5

1386 Innovative Approaches for Difficult to Treat Populations
American Psychiatric Publishing, Inc.
1000 Wilson Boulevard
Suite 1825
Arlington, VA 22209-3901
703-907-7322
800-368-5777
Fax: 703-907-1091
E-mail: appi@psych.org
www.appi.org

Scott W Henggeler, Ph.D, Editor
Alberto W Santos, M.D., Editor
John McDuffie, Editorial Director

Firsthand look at the future direction of clinical services. Focuses on services for individuals who use the highest proportion of mental health resources and for whom traditional services have not been effective. *$65.00*

552 pages Year Founded: 1997 ISBN 0-880486-80-5

1387 Me, Myself, and Them: A Firsthand Account of One Young Person's Experience with Schizophrenia
Oxford University Press
198 Madison Avenue
New York, NY 10016-4341
800-445-9714
Fax: 919-677-1303
E-mail: custserv.us@oup.com
www.oup.com/us

Kurt Snyder, Author
Raquel E Gur, MD, Author
Linda Wasmer Andrews, Author

Offers hope to young people who are struggling with schizophrenia, helping them to understand and manage the challenges of this illness and go on to lead healthy lives.

192 pages Year Founded: 1896 ISBN 0-195311-22-1

1388 Natural History of Mania, Depression and Schizophrenia
American Psychiatric Publishing, Inc.
1000 Wilson Boulevard
Suite 1825
Arlington, VA 22209-3901
703-907-7322
800-368-5777
Fax: 703-907-1091
E-mail: appi@psych.org
www.appi.org

George Winokur, M.D, Author
Ming T Tsuang, M.D., Ph.D, Author
John McDuffie, Editorial Director

An unusual look at the course of mental illness, based on data from the Iowa 500 Research Project. *$42.50*

384 pages Year Founded: 1996 ISBN 0-880487-26-7

1389 New Pharmacotherapy of Schizophrenia
American Psychiatric Publishing, Inc.
1000 Wilson Boulevard
Suite 1825
Arlington, VA 22209-3901
703-907-7322
800-368-5777
Fax: 703-907-1091
E-mail: appi@psych.org
www.appi.org

Alan F Breier, M.D, Editor
Ron McMillen, Chief Executive Officer
John McDuffie, Editorial Director

Discusses the new class of antipsychotic agents that promise superior efficacy and more favorable side-effects; offers an improved understanding of how to employ existing pharmachotherapeutic agents. *$32.50*

264 pages Year Founded: 1996 ISBN 0-880484-91-8

1390 Office Treatment of Schizophrenia
American Psychiatric Publishing, Inc.
1000 Wilson Boulevard
Suite 1825
Arlington, VA 22209-3901
703-907-7322
800-368-5777
Fax: 703-907-1091
E-mail: appi@psych.org
www.appi.org

Robert E Hales MD, Editor-in-Chief
Ron McMillen, Chief Executive Officer
John McDuffie, Editorial Director

Examines options in outpatient treatment of schizophrenic patients. *$31.00*

208 pages

1391 Practicing Psychiatry in the Community: a Manual
American Psychiatric Publishing, Inc.
1000 Wilson Boulevard
Suite 1825
Arlington, VA 22209-3901
703-907-7322
800-368-5777
Fax: 703-907-1091
E-mail: appi@psych.org
www.appi.org

Jerome V Vaccaro, M.D, Editor
Gordon H Clark, Jr., M.D., M.Di, Editor
John McDuffie, Editorial Director

Addressess the major issues currently facing community psychiatrists. *$67.50*

534 pages Year Founded: 1996 ISBN 0-880486-63-5

1392 Prenatal Exposures in Schizophrenia
American Psychiatric Publishing, Inc.
1000 Wilson Boulevard
Suite 1825
Arlington, VA 22209-3901
703-907-7322
800-368-5777
Fax: 703-907-1091
E-mail: appi@psych.org
www.appi.org

Ezra S Susser, M.D., Dr.P.H, Editor
Alan S Brown, M.D, Editor
Jack M Gorman, M.D, Editor

Considers a range of epigenetic elements thought to interact with abnormal genes to produce the onset of illness. Attention to the evidence implicating obstetric complications, prenatal infection, autoimmunity and prenatal malnutrition in brain disorders. *$36.50*

296 pages Year Founded: 1999 ISBN 0-880484-99-3

1393 Psychiatric Rehabilitation of Chronic Mental Patients
American Psychiatric Publishing, Inc.
1000 Wilson Boulevard
Suite 1825
Arlington, VA 22209-3901
703-907-7322
800-368-5777
Fax: 703-907-1091
E-mail: appi@psych.org
www.appi.org

Robert P Liberman, M.D., Editor
Ron McMillen, Chief Executive Officer
John McDuffie, Editorial Director

Provides highly detailed prescriptions for assessment and treatment techniques with case examples and learning exercises. *$28.00*

319 pages Year Founded: 1987 ISBN 0-880482-01-X

1394 Psychoses and Pervasive Development Disorders in Childhood and Adolescence
American Psychiatric Publishing, Inc.
1000 Wilson Boulevard
Suite 1825
Arlington, VA 22209-3901
703-907-7322
800-368-5777
Fax: 703-907-1091
E-mail: appi@psych.org
www.appi.org

Robert E Hales MD, Editor-in-Chief
Ron McMillen, Chief Executive Officer
John McDuffie, Editorial Director

Provides a concise summary of currently knowledge of psychoses and pervasive developmental disorders of childhood and adolescence. Discusses recent changes in aspects of diagnosis and definition of these disorders, advances in knowledge, and aspects of treatment. *$46.50*

368 pages ISBN 1-882103-01-7

1395 Return From Madness
Jason Aronson
200 Livingston Street
Northvale, NJ 07647

201-767-4093
800-782-1005
Fax: 201-767-1576
www.aronson.com

Kathleen Degen, Author
Ellen Nasper, Author

The authors describe group therapy that helps patients identify and cope with unexpected, intense feelings such as sadness or painful memories of childhood trauma, increase their interpersonal skills, and advance their sense of self beyond that of their label as mental patients. Degen and Nasper show how to build on the phenomenal changes that the new medications provide. *$50.00*

256 pages ISBN 1-568216-25-4

1396 Schizophrenia

1000 Wilson Boulevard
Suite 1825
Arlington, VA 22209-3901
703-907-7322
800-368-5777
Fax: 703-907-1091
E-mail: appi@psych.org
www.appi.org

Robert E Hales MD, Editor-in-Chief
Ron McMillen, Chief Executive Officer
John McDuffie, Editorial Director

760 pages

1397 Schizophrenia Revealed: From Neurons to Social Interactions
W.W. Norton & Company
500 Fifth Avenue
New York, NY 10110
212-354-2907
Fax: 212-869-0856
www.books.wwnorton.com/books/

Drake McFeely, CEO

In this much-needed book, and expert in the neurocognition of schizophrenia, presents an integrated overview of schizophrenia covering a wide range of topics in lively, understandable proze. He outlines a neurodevelopmental model of schizophrenia, discusses neurocognitive indicators of genetic vulnerability, the introduction of a new generation of medications, recent findings from brain imaging, cognitive remediation, and the determinants of functional outcome. He presents a modern view of schizophrenia based on neuroscience that goes far beyond the symptoms of the illness.

224 pages Year Founded: 2003

1398 Schizophrenia and Genetic Risks
National Alliance on Mental Illness
2107 Wilson Boulevard
Suite 300
Arlington, VA 22201-3080
703-524-7600
800-950-6264
Fax: 703-524-9094
TDD: 703-516-7227
E-mail: info@nami.org
www.nami.org

Irving I. Gottesman, Author
Steven O. Moldin, Author

Provides basic facts about schizophrenia and its familial distribution so consumers and mental health workers can become informed enough to initiate appropriate actions. Includes suggested resources.

17 pages Year Founded: 1999 ISBN 9-997725-94-8

1399 Schizophrenia and Manic Depressive Disorder
National Alliance for the Mentally Ill
2107 Wilson Boulevard
Suite 300
Arlington, VA 22201-3080
703-525-0686
800-950-6264
TDD: 703-516-7227
E-mail: info@nami.org
www.nami.org

E Fuller Torrey, Author

Explores the biological roots of mental illness with a primary focus on schizophrenia. *$27.00*

312 pages ISBN 0-465072-85-2

1400 Schizophrenia and Primitive Mental States
Jason Aronson Publishing
276 Livingston Street
Northvale, NJ 07647
570-342-1320
800-782-0015
Fax: 201-767-1576
www.aronson.com

Peter L. Giovacchini, Author

In this volume, renowned therapist Peter Giovacchini shows readers how to do more for psychotic patients than rely on medication to reduce their florid symptoms. Instead, he demonstrates how schizophrenic patients can be offered true cure and the possibility of living a full and related life through intensive psychotherapeutic treatment. *$50.00*

288 pages ISBN 0-765700-27-1

1401 Schizophrenia in a Molecular Age
American Psychiatric Publishing, Inc.
1000 Wilson Boulevard
Suite 1825
Arlington, VA 22209-3901
703-907-7322
800-368-5777
Fax: 703-907-1091
E-mail: appi@psych.org
www.appi.org

Carol A Tamminga, M.D, Editor
Ron McMillen, Chief Executive Officer
John McDuffie, Editorial Director

Explores the multidimensional phenotype of schizophrenia, and use of molecular biology and anti-psychotic medications. Reviews the implications of early sensory procesing and subcortical involvement of cognitive dysfuntion in schizophrenia. Functional neuroimaging applied to the syndrome of schizophrenia. *$26.50*

204 pages Year Founded: 1999 ISBN 0-880489-61-8

1402 Schizophrenia: From Mind to Molecule
American Psychiatric Publishing, Inc.
1000 Wilson Boulevard
Suite 1825
Arlington, VA 22209-3901

703-907-7322
800-368-5777
Fax: 703-907-1091
E-mail: appi@psych.org
www.appi.org

Nancy C Andreasen, M.D., Ph.D, Editor
Ron McMillen, Chief Executive Officer
John McDuffie, Editorial Director

Provides a thorough look at schizophrenia that includes neurobehavioral studies, traditional and emerging technologies, psychosocial and medical treatments, and future research opportunities. *$34.00*

294 pages Year Founded: 1994 ISBN 0-800489-50-2

1403 Schizophrenia: Straight Talk for Family and Friends
William Morrow & Company
10 East 53rd Street
New York, NY 10022-5244
212-872-1133
Fax: 212-872-1199
www.signal-capital.com

Maryellen Walsh, Author

This compassionate survival manual explains the malady and its effects, treatments, and prospects, as well as widespread myths and actual experiences. *$17.95*

Year Founded: 1985

1404 Stigma and Mental Illness
American Psychiatric Publishing, Inc.
1000 Wilson Boulevard
Suite 1825
Arlington, VA 22209-3901
703-907-7322
800-368-5777
Fax: 703-907-1091
E-mail: appi@psych.org
www.appi.org

Paul J Fink, M.D, Editor
Allan Tasman, M.D., Editor
John McDuffie, Editorial Director

Collection of firsthand accounts on how society has stigmatized mentally ill individuals, their families and their caregivers. *$36.00*

256 pages Year Founded: 1992 ISBN 0-880484-05-5

1405 Surviving Schizophrenia: A Manual for Families, Consumers and Providers
Harper Collins
10 E 53rd Street
New York, NY 10022-5299
212-207-7000
800-242-7737

Since its first publication nearly twenty years ago, this has become the standard reference book on this disease, helping thousands of patients, families and mental health professionals to better deal with the condition. Dr. Fuller Torrey explains the nature causes, symptoms, and treatment of this often misunderstood illness. This fully revised 4th edition of Surviving Schizophrenia is a must-have for the multitude of people affected both directly and indirectly by this serious, yet treatable, disorder. *$15.00*

544 pages ISBN 0-060959-19-3

1406 The Complete Family Guide to Schizophrenia: Helping Your Loved One Get the Most Out of Life
The Guilford Press
72 Spring Street
New York, NY 10012-4019
212-431-9800
800-365-7006
Fax: 212-966-6708
E-mail: info@guilford.com

Bob Matloff, President
Kim T Mueser, Author
Susan Gingerich, Author

This book walks readers through a range of treatment and support options that can lead to a better life for the entire family. Individual chapters hightlight special issues for parents, siblings, and partners, while other sections provide tips for dealing with problems including cognitive difficulties, substance abuse, and psychosis.

1407 Treating Schizophrenia
Jossey-Bass / John Wiley & Sons
111 River Street
Hokoken, NJ 07030-5790
201-748-6000
Fax: 201-748-6088
E-mail: custserv@wiley.com
www.wiley.com

Sophia Vinogradov, Author

Using case studies from their own practices, the contributors describe how to conduct a successful assessment of schizophrenia. They then explore in detail the major treatment methods, including inpatient treatment, individual therapy, family therapy, group therapy, and the crucial role of medication. Th authors also address the timely issue of treating schizophrenia in the era of managed care. *$ 121.60*

372 pages Year Founded: 1995

1408 Understanding Schizophrenia: Guide to the New Research on Causes & Treatment
Free Press
40 Main St.
Suite 301
Florence, MA 01062
877-888-1533
Fax: 413-585-8904
E-mail: consumer.customerservice@simonandschuster.com
www.simonsays.com

Richard Keefe, Author
Philip D Harvey, Author

Two noted researchers provide an accessible, timely guide to schizophrenia, discussing the nature of the disease, recent advances in understanding brain structure and function, and the latest psychological and drug treatments. *$25.95*

283 pages Year Founded: 1994 ISBN 0-029172-47-0

1409 Water Balance in Schizophrenia
American Psychiatric Publishing, Inc.
1000 Wilson Boulevard
Suite 1825
Arlington, VA 22209-3901
703-907-7322
800-368-5777
Fax: 703-907-1091

E-mail: appi@psych.org
www.appi.org

David B. Schnur, Editor
Darrell G. Kirch, Editor

Represents the first attempt to provide clinicians with a consolidated guide to polydipsia-hyponatremia, associated with schizophrenia. Here, some of the foremost experts in the field address a variety of issues pertinent to both researchers and clinicians. All clinicians who treat schizophrenic patients will find this book an indispensable reference. Whenever possible, the editors provide details regarding methodolody and explicit management guidelines. They even include a detailed description of an inpatient polydipsia unit, as well as a comprehensive review of drug treatment. *$54.95*

360 pages Year Founded: 1996 ISBN 0-880484-85-3

Periodicals & Pamphlets

1410 Schizophrenia
National Institute of Mental Health
6001 Executive Boulevard
Room 8184
Bethesda, MD 20892-1
301-443-4513
866-615-6464
TTY: 301-443-8431
E-mail: nimhinfo@nih.gov

This booklet answers many common questions about schizophrenia, one of the most chronic, severe and disabling mental disorders. Current research-based information is provided for people with schizophrenia, their family members, friends and the general public about the symptoms and diagnosis of schizophrenia, possible causes, treatments and treatment resources.

28 pages Year Founded: 1999

1411 Schizophrenia Fact Sheet
SAMHSA'S National Mental Health Information Center
PO Box 42557
Washington, DC 20015-557
800-789-2647
Fax: 240-747-5470
TDD: 866-889-2647
E-mail: ken@mentalhealth.org
www.mentalhealth.samhsa.gov

This fact sheet provides information on the symptoms, diagnosis, and treatment for schizophrenia.

2 pages

1412 Schizophrenia Research
1600 John F Kennedy Boulevard
Suite 1800
Philadelphia, PA 19103-2879
212-633-3730
800-545-2522
Fax: 800-535-9935
E-mail: usbkinfo@elsevier.com
www.elsevier.com

H.A Nasrallah, Editor-in-Chief
L.E DeLisi, Editor-in-Chief

The journal of choice for international researchers and clinicians to share their work with the global schizophrenia research community. Publishes novel papers that really contribute to understanding the biology and treatment of schizophrenic disorders; Schizophrenia Research brings together biological, clinical and psychological research in order to stimulate the synthesis of findings from all disciplines involved in improving patient outcomes in schizophrenia.

Year Founded: 1880 ISSN 0920-9964

Research Centers

1413 Brain & Behavior Research Foundation
90 Park Avenue
16th Floor
New York, NY 10016
646-681-4888
800-829-8289
Fax: 516-487-6930
E-mail: info@bbrfoundation.org
www.bbrfoundation.org

Steve Lieber, Chairman of the Board
Jeffrey Borenstein, M.D, President and Chief Executive Of
Louis Innamorato, Vice president, Finance and Chief
Suzzane Golden, Vice President

Committed to alleviating the suffering caused by mental illness by awarding grants that will lead to advances and breakthroughs in scientific research. 100% of all donor contributions for research are invested in NARSAD Grants leading to discoveries in understanding causes and improving treatments of disorders in children and adults, such as depression, bipolar disorder, schizophrenia, autism, attention deficit hyperactivity disorder, and anxiety disorders like obsessive-compulsive and post-traumatic stress disorders.

Year Founded: 1981

1414 Schizophrenia Research Branch: Division of Clinical and Treatment Research
6001 Executive Boulevard
Room 7122, MSC 9625
Bethesda, MD 20892-1
301-443-9233
866-615-6464
Fax: 301-443-5158
TTY: 301-443-8431
E-mail: sarah.morris@nih.gov
www.www.nimh.nih.gov

Sarah E Morris, PhD, Program Chief

Plans, supports, and conducts programs of research, research training, and resource development of schizophrenia and related disorders. Reviews and evaluates research developments in the field and recommends new program directors. Collaborates with organizations in and outside of the National Institute of Mental Health (NIMH) to stimulate work in the field through conferences and workshops.

Support Groups & Hot Lines

1415 Common Ground Sanctuary
1410 S. Telegraph
Bloomfield Hills, MI 48302
248-456-8150
800-231-1127
Fax: 248-456-8147
E-mail: contactus@commongroundsanctuary.org
www.www.commongroundsanctuary.org

Tony Rothschild, President & CEO
Steve Mitchell, Board Chair
Gary Dembs, Secretary
Charles Schmidt, Treasurer

A 24-hour nonprofit agency dedicated to helping youths, adults and families in crisis. Through its crisis line and in person through various programs, Common Ground Sanctuary provides professional and compassionate service to more than 40, 000 people a year, with most services provided free of charge. Mission is to provide a lifeline for individuals and families in crisis, victims of crime, persons with mental illness, people trying to cope with critical situations and runaway and homeless youth.

Year Founded: 1998

1416 Family-to-Family: National Alliance on Mental Illness

3803 N. Fairfax Drive
Suite 100
Arlington, VA 22203
703-524-7600
888-999-6264
Fax: 703-524-9094
E-mail: info@nami.org
www.nami.org

The NAMI Family-to-Family Education Program is a free, 12-week course for family caregivers of individuals with severe mental illnesses. The course is taught by trained family members, all instruction and course materials are free to class participants, and over 300, 000 family members have graduated from this national program.

Video & Audio

1417 Bonnie Tapes
Mental Illness Education Project, Inc.
25 West Street
Westborough, MA 01581
617-562-1111
E-mail: info@miepvideos.org
www.miepvideos.org

Bonnie's account of coping with schizophrenia will be a revelation to people whose view of mental illness has been shaped by the popular media. She and her family provide an intimate view of a frequently feared, often misrepresented, and much stigmatized illness-and the human side of learning to live with a psychiatric disability.

Year Founded: 1997

1418 Clinical Impressions: Identifying Mental Illness
Educational Training Videos
136 Granville St
Suite 200
Gahanna, OH 43230
Fax: 888-775-3919
www.educationaltrainingvideos.com

How long can mental illness stay hidden, especially from the eyes of trained experts? This program rejoins a group of ten adults- five of them healthy and five of them with histories of mental illness- as psychiatric specialists try to spot and correctly diagnose the latter. Administering a series of collaborative and one-on-one tests, including assessments of personality type, physical self-image, and rational thinking, the panel gradually makes decisions about who suffers from depression, bipolar disorder, bulimia, and social anxiety.

1419 Dark Voices: Schizophrenia
Educational Training Videos
136 Granville St
Suite 200
Gahanna, OH 43230
Fax: 888-775-3919
www.educationaltrainingvideos.com

This program seeks to understand how schizophrenia touches the lives of patients and their family members while examining the disease's etiology and pathology. A Discovery Channel Production.

1420 FRONTLINE: The Released
PBS
2100 Crystal Drive
Arlington, VA 22202
www.pbs.org

Will Lyman, Actor
Narrator
Miri Navasky, Director
Karen O'Connor, Director

The documentary states that of the 700, 000 inmates released from American prisons each year, half of them have mental disabilities. This work focused on those with severe problems who keep entering and exiting prison. Full of good information on the challenges they face with mental illnesses; housing, employment, stigmatization, and socialization.

Year Founded: 2009

1421 Families Coping with Mental Illness
Mental Illness Education Project
PO Box 470813
Brookline Village, MA 02447-813
617-562-1111
800-343-5540
Fax: 617-779-0061
E-mail: info@miepvideos.org
www.miepvideos.org

Christine Ledoux, Executive Director

Designed to provide insights and support to other families, the tape also has profound messages for professionals about the needs of families when mental illness strikes. *$68.95*

Year Founded: 1997

1422 Mental Disorder
Educational Training Videos
136 Granville St
Suite 200
Gahanna, OH 43230
Fax: 888-775-3919
www.educationaltrainingvideos.com

What is abnormality? Using the case studies of two young women; one who has depression, one who has an anxiety disorder; as a springboard, this program presents three psychological perspective on mental disorder.

1423 My Name is Walter James Cross: The Reality of Schizophrenia
Educational Training Videos
136 Granville St
Suite 200
Gahanna, OH 43230
Fax: 888-775-3919
www.educationaltrainingvideos.com

Walter James Cross tried to kill himself and failed, so he decided to tell his story instead. Created by a psychiatrist who has worked for many years with schizophrenic patients, this compelling dramatic monologue presents an acurate depiction of a devastating, costly, much maligned, and misunderstood illness.

1424 No More Shame: Understanding Schizophrenia, Depression, and Addiction
Educational Training Videos
136 Granville St
Suite 200
Gahanna, OH 43230
Fax: 888-775-3919
www.educationaltrainingvideos.com

These programs examine research about the physiological, psychological, sociological, and cultural aspects of these disorders and their treatments. The goal of these programs is to explain what we do and do not know about each of these conditions, as well as to destigmatize the disorders by presenting them in the context of the same research process that is applied to all medical disorders.

1425 To See What I See - The Stigma of Mental Illness
Northern Lakes Community Mental Health

People served by Northern Lakes Community Mental Health have come together as Stigma Busters - creating artwork, photographs, recovery stories, media campaigns, personal testimonies, buttons, and other projects for the purpose of eliminating the stigma associated with mental illness and spreading the word that recovery is possible. This is their story.

1426 Understanding Mental Illness
Educational Video Network, Inc.
1401 19th Street
Huntsville, TX 77340
936-295-5767
800-762-0060
Fax: 936-294-0233
www.www.evndirect.com

Contains information and classifications of mental illness. Mental illness can strike anyone, at any age. Learn about various organic and functional mental disorders as discussed and their causes and symptoms, and learn where to seek help for a variety of mental health concerns.

Web Sites

1427 www.cyberpsych.org
CyberPsych

Presents information about psychoanalysis, psychotherapy and special topics such as anxiety disorders, the problematic use of alcohol, homophobia, and the traumatic effects of racism.

1428 www.hopkinsmedicine.org/epigen
Epidemology-Genetics Program in Psychiatry

Research program to help characterize the genetic, developmental and environmental componenets of bipolar disorder and schizophrenia.

1429 www.mentalhealth.com
Internet Mental Health

Offers online psychiatric diagnosis in the hope of reaching the two-thirds of individuals with mental illness who do not seek treatment.

1430 www.naminys.org
National Alliance on Mental Illness

From its inception in 1979, NAMI has been dedicated to improving the lives of individuals and families affected by mental illness.

1431 www.planetpsych.com
Planetpsych.com

The online resource for mental health information.

1432 www.psychcentral.com
Psych Central

The Internet's largest and oldest independent mental health social network created and run by mental health professionals to guarantee reliable, trusted information and support communities to you.

1433 www.schizophrenia.com
Schizophrenia

A non-profit community providing in-depth information, support and education related to schizophrenia, a disorder of the brain and mind.

1434 www.schizophrenia.com/discuss/
Schizophrenia

On-line support for patients and families.

1435 www.schizophrenia.com/newsletter/buckets/ success.html
Schizophrenia

Success stories including biographical accounts, links to stories of famous people who have schizophrenia, and personal web pages.

Sexual Disorders

Introduction

It is not possible to know what degree of sexual interest, desire, or activity is 'normal'; at best, we have averages, not indications of the optimal state. A Sexual Disorder is diagnosed when lack of desire or activity is repeated, persists over time and causes distress or interferes with the person's functioning in other important areas of life. Sexual Disorders are divided into four groups: Disorders of Sexual Desire; Disorders of Sexual Arousal; Orgasmic Disorders; and Disorders involving Sexual Pain. It is essential to know whether the problem is lifelong or was precipitated by a recent event, and whether it occurs only with a particular partner or in a particular situation. It is also essential not to make assumptions about sexual activity based on age, socioeconomic status, or sexual orientation. The only way to know about an individual's sexual life is to ask.

SEXUAL DESIRE DISORDERS SYMPTOMS

Hypoactive Sexual Desire Disorder (HSDD)
• Persistent or repeated lack of sexual fantasies and desire for sexual activities;
• The lack of sexual fantasies and desire cause marked distress or interpersonal problems.

Sexual Aversion Disorder (SAD)
• Persistent or repeated extreme aversion to, and avoidance of, all or almost all genital sexual contact with a sexual partner;
• The aversion causes marked distress or interpersonal problems.

Associated Features
The person with a Sexual Desire Disorder commonly has a poor body image and avoids nudity. In HSDD, a person does not initiate sexual activity, or respond to the partner's initiation attempts. The disorder is often associated with the inability to achieve orgasm in women, and the inability to achieve an erection in men. It can also be associated with other psychiatric and medical problems, including a history of sexual trauma and abuse.

Prevalence
HADD is common in both men and women but twice as many women as men report it. It is estimated at twenty percent overall, and as high as sixty-five-percent among those seeking treatment for sexual disorders. The prevalence of SAD is unknown.

SEXUAL AROUSAL DISORDER SYMPTOMS

Female Sexual Arousal Disorder (FSAD)
• Persistent or repeated inability to attain or maintain adequate lubrication-swelling (sexual excitement) response throughout sexual activity;
• The disorder causes clear distress or interpersonal problems.

Male Erectile Disorder (MED)
• Persistent or repeated inability to maintain an adequate erection throughout sexual activity;
• The disorder causes clear distress or interpersonal problems.

Associated Features

While both these disorders are common, men tend to be more upset by it than women. Contributing issues include performance anxiety (especially in men), fear of failure, inadequate stimulation, and relationship conflicts. Other problems are also associated with FSAD and MED, such as childhood sexual trauma, sexual identity concerns, religious orthodoxy, depression, lack of intimacy or trust, and power conflicts. MED is frequently associated with diabetes, peripheral nerve disorders, and hypertension, and is a side effect of a variety of medications; men with MED must be evaluated for these conditions. In addition, the medications used to treat MED are contraindicated in some medical conditions, such as heart conditions.

Prevalence
Prevalence information varies for FSAD. In one study, 13.6 percent of women overall reported a lack of lubrication during most or all sexual activity; twenty-three percent had such problems occasionally; and 4, 4.2 percent of post-menopausal women reported having lubrication problems. In a study of happily married couples, about one third of women complained of difficulty in achieving or maintaining sexual excitement.

Erectile difficulties in men are estimated to be very common, affecting 20-30 million men in the US. The frequency of erectile problems increases steeply with age. In one survey, fifty-two percent of men aged 40-70 reported erectile problems, with three times as many older men reporting difficulties. The disorder is common among married, single, heterosexual and homosexual men.

Treatment Options
In FSAD, a cognitive-behavioral psychotherapy is often recommended, including practical help such as the use of water-soluble lubricating products. Hormone treatment, such as testosterone-estrogen compounds, is sometimes helpful.

An array of treatments is available for Male Erectile Dysfunction, including prosthetic devices for physiological penile problems. In cases of hormonal problems, testosterone treatments have had some results. (However, the use of testosterone to treat sexual disorders in menopausal women is controversial and can have serious side effects.) Viagra is producing success for male erectile dysfunction, as are two newer medications for MED, vardenafil (Levitra) and tadalafil (Cialis).

When sexual problems are limited to a particular partner or situation, psychotherapy (individual or couple) is necessary to resolve the difficulty.

ORGASMIC DISORDER SYMPTOMS

Female and Male Orgasmic Disorders
• Persistent or repeated delay in, or absence of, orgasm despite a normal sexual excitement phase;
• The disorder causes clear distress or interpersonal problems.

Premature Ejaculation
• Persistent or recurring ejaculation with minimal sexual stimulation before, upon, or shortly after penetration and earlier than desired;
• The disorder causes clear distress or interpersonal problems.

Associated Features

When FOD or MOD occur only in certain situations, difficulty with desire and arousal are often also present.

All of these disorders are associated with poor body image, self-esteem or relationship problems. In FOD or MOD, medical or surgical conditions can also play a role, such as multiple sclerosis, spinal cord injury, surgical prostatectomy (males), and some medications. PE is likely to be very distruptive. Some males may have had the disorder all their lives, for others it may be situational. Few illnesses or drugs are associated with PE.

Prevalence

FOD is probably the most frequent sexual disorder among females. Among those who have sought sex therapy twenty-four percent to thirty-seven percent report the problem. In general population samples, 15.4 percent of premenopausal women report the disorder, and 34.7 percent of postmenopausal women do so. More single than married women report that they have never had an orgasm. There is no association between FOD and race, socioeconomic status, education, or religion. MOD is relatively rare; only three percent to eight percent of men seeking treatment report having the disorder, though there is a higher prevalence among homosexual males (ten percent to fifteen percent).

PE is very common: twenty-five percent to forty percent of adult males report having, or having had, this problem.

Treatment Options

Psychotherapeutic treatments are similar to those for Sexual Desire and Sexual Arousal Disorders. In both males and females with Orgasmic Disorders there may be a lack of desire, performance anxiety, and fear of impregnation or disease. Therapy should take into account contextual and historical information concerning the onset and course of the problem. Cognitive-behavioral methods to help change the assumptions and thinking of the person have sometimes been helpful.

SEXUAL PAIN DISORDER SYMPTOMS

Dyspareunia

• Recurring or persistent pain with sexual intercourse in a male or female;
• The disorder causes clear distress or interpersonal problems.

Vaginismus

• Persistent or recurrent involunatry spasm of the vagina that interferes with sexual intercourse;
• The disorder causes clear distress or interpersonal problems.

Associated Features

Both Dyspareunia and Vaginismus may be associated with lack of desire or arousal. Women with Vaginismus tend to avoid gynecological exams, and the disorder is most often associated with psychological and interpersonal issues. Various physical factors are associated with Dyspareunia, such as pelvic inflammatory disease, hymenal or childbirth-related scarring, and vulvar vestibulitis. Dyspareunia is not a clear symptom of any physical condition. In women it is often combined with Depression and interpersonal conflicts. Other associated psychosocial factors include religious orthodoxy, low self-esteem, poor body image, poor couple communication, and history of sexual trauma.

Prevalence

Dyspareunia is frequent in females but occurs infrequently in males. Vaginismus is seen quite often in sex therapy clinics - in fifteen percent to seventeen percent of women coming for treatment.

Treatment Options

Probably the most successful treatment for women with these disorders is the reinsertion of a graduated sequence of dilators in the vagina. The woman's sexual partner should be present, and a participant in this treatment. This treatment should be done in conjunction with relaxation training, sensate focusing exercises, (which help people focus on the pleasures of sex rather than the performance) and sex therapy.

General Treatment Options

The professional making the diagnosis of a Sexual Disorder should be trained and experienced in Sexual Disorders and sex therapy. It is important to know whether or not a medical or medication issue is present. However, many with these disorders do not seek treatment. Their lack of desire for sex is often combined with a lack of desire for sex therapy. Even with therapy, relapse is commonly reported. Treatments that have had some success are ones that challenge the cognitive assumptions and distortions of client(s), e.g., that sex should be perfect, that without intercourse and without both partners having an orgasm it isn't real sex. Therapy often also includes sensate focusing in which the person is encouraged and trained to give up the role of agitated spectator to love-making in favor of participating in it. A sexual history should be part of every mental health evaluation, and patients receiving psychotropic medications should be asked about sexual side effects. Having information about sexual function before medication is prescribed will prevent pre-existing sexual problems from being confused with any that may result from medication.

Associations & Agencies

1437 National Association for the Dually Diagnosed (NADD)
132 Fair Street
Kingston, NY 12401-4802
845-331-4336
800-331-5362
Fax: 845-331-4569
E-mail: info@thenadd.org
www.thenadd.org

Donna McNELIS, PhD, President
Robert J Fletcher DSW, Chief Executive Officer
Dan Baker, PhD, Vice President
Julia Pearce, Secretary

A non profit membership association established for professionals, care providers and families to promote understanding of and services for individuals who have developmental disabilites and mental health needs. The mission of NADD is to advance mental wellness for persons with developmental disabilities through the promotion of excellence in mental health care.

Year Founded: 1983

1438 National Mental Health Consumers' Self-Help Clearinghouse
1211 Chestnut Street
Suite 1100
Philadelphia, PA 19107-4103
215-751-1810
800-553-4539
Fax: 215-636-6312
E-mail: info@mhselfhelp.org
www.mhselfhelp.org

Joseph A Rogers, Executive Director/ Founder
Susan Rogers, Director
Britani Nestel, Program Specialist
Christa Burkett, Technical Assistance Coordinator

A national consumer technical assistance center that has played a major role in the development of the mental health consumer movement.

Year Founded: 1986

1439 SAMHSA'S National Mental Health Information Center
1 Choke Cherry Road
Rockville, MD 20857
800-789-2647
Fax: 240-747-5470
TDD: 866-889-2647
E-mail: ken@mentalhealth.org
www.mentalhealth.samhsa.gov

A Kathryn Power, Director
Edward B Searle, Deputy Director

1440 The Center for Family Support
2811 Zulette Avenue
Bronx, NY 10461
718-518-1500
Fax: 718-518-8200
E-mail: svernikoff@cfsny.org
www.cfsny.org

Steven Vernikoff, Executive Director
Virgil Seepersad, Director of Finance
Eileen Berg, Director of Quality Assurance
Barbara Greenwald, Associate Executive, Director

The Center for Family Support is committed to providing support and assistance to individuals with developmental and related disabilities, and to the family members who care for them.

Year Founded: 1954

Books

1441 Back on Track: Boys Dealing with Sexual Abuse
Sidran Institute
PO Box 436
Brooklandville, MD 21022-0436
410-825-8888
888-825-8249
Fax: 410-560-0134
E-mail: sidran@sidran.org
www.sidran.org

Leslie Bailey Wright, Author
Mindy B Loiselle, Author

Written for boys age ten and up, this wookbook addresses adolescent boys directly, answering commonly asked ques-

tions, offering concrete suggestions for getting help and dealing with unspoken concerns such as homosexuality. Contains descriptions of what therapy may be like and brief explanations of social services and courts, as well as sections on family and friends. Exercises and interesting graphics break up the text. The book's important message is TELL: Just keep telling until someone listens who STOPS the abuse. *$14.00*

126 pages Year Founded: 1986 ISBN 1-884444-43-1

1442 Dangerous Sex Offenders: a Task Force Report of the American Psychiatric Association
American Psychiatric Publishing, Inc.
1000 Wilson Boulevard
Suite 1825
Arlington, VA 22209-3901
703-907-7322
800-368-5777
Fax: 703-907-1091
E-mail: appi@psych.org
www.appi.org

Robert E Hales MD, Editor-in-Chief
Ron McMillen, Chief Executive Officer
John McDuffie, Editorial Director

Topics in this volume on sexually dangerous offenders include: epidemiology of sex offenders; sexual predator commitment laws; juvenile sex offenders; and pharmacological treatment of sexual offenders. *$40.95*

210 pages Year Founded: 1999 ISBN 0-890422-80-X

1443 Handbook of Sexual and Gender Identity Disorders
John Wiley & Sons
111 River Street
Hoboken, NJ 07030-5774
201-748-6000
877-762-2974
Fax: 201-748-6088
E-mail: info@wiley.com
www.wiley.com

David L. Rowland, Editor
Luca Incrocci, Editor

The Handbook of Sexual and Gender Identity Disorders provides mental health professionals a comprehensive yet practical guide to the understanding, diagnosis, and treatment of a variety of sexual problems. *$95.00*

696 pages Year Founded: 2008 ISBN 0-471767-38-7

1444 Interviewing the Sexually Abused Child
American Psychiatric Publishing, Inc.
1000 Wilson Boulevard
Suite 1825
Arlington, VA 22209-3901
703-907-7322
800-368-5777
Fax: 703-907-1091
E-mail: appi@psych.org
www.appi.org

Robert E Hales MD, Editor-in-Chief
Ron McMillen, Chief Executive Officer
John McDuffie, Editorial Director

Guide for mental health professionals who need to know if a child has been sexually abused. Presents guidelines on the structure of the interview and covers the use of free play, toys, and play materials by focusing on the investigate interview of the suspected victim. *$27.95*

80 pages ISBN 0-880486-12-0

1445 Masculinity and Sexuality: Selected Topics
American Psychiatric Publishing, Inc.
1000 Wilson Boulevard
Suite 1825
Arlington, VA 22209-3901
703-907-7322
800-368-5777
Fax: 703-907-1091
E-mail: appi@psych.org
www.appi.org

Jennifer Downey, Author/Editor
Richard C. Friedman, Editor

Sheds light on clinical issues important in the treatment of all male patients. Sexual experiences and related attitudes of patients and therapists influence symptoms, treatment, and outcome across diverse diagnostic categories. Chapters cover clinical issues related sexual thoughts, impulses, and desires and the way they are organized into erotic fantasies including the differences that exist in the way ment and women experience sexual fantasy. *$37.50*

172 pages Year Founded: 1999 ISBN 0-880489-62-6

1446 Principles and Practice of Sex Therapy
The Guilford Press
72 Spring Street
New York, NY 10012-4019
212-431-9800
800-365-7006
Fax: 212-966-6708
E-mail: info@guilford.com

Sandra R. Leiblum, Ph.D., Editor/Author

Provides a comprehensive guide to assessment and treatment of all of the major female and male sexual dysfunctions. Leading authorities demonstrate effective ways to integrate psychological, interpersonal, and medical interventions. Every chapter includes detailed clinical examples illustrating the process of therapy and the factors that influence treatment outcomes. *$95.00*

Year Founded: 2006 ISBN 1-593853-49-1

1447 Quickies: The Handbook of Brief Sex Therapy
W.W. Norton & Company
500 Fifth Avenue
New York, NY 10110
212-354-2907
Fax: 212-869-0856
www.wwnorton.com

Shelley K. Green, Author
Douglas Flemons, Author

The authors gather a wonderful array of approaches to brief sex therapy, each presented by a well known therapist in the field. Pleasure and humor are highlighted, the office and the bed, as readers are reminded that the point of sex therapy is a sexual change.

ISBN 0-393705-27-7

1448 Sexual Aggression
American Psychiatric Publishing, Inc.
1000 Wilson Boulevard
Suite 1825
Arlington, VA 22209-3901

703-907-7322
800-368-5777
Fax: 703-907-1091
E-mail: appi@psych.org
www.appi.org

Jon A Shaw, M.D., Editor

Appropriate diagnosis and treatment options are presented. *$64.00*

360 pages Year Founded: 1999 ISBN 0-880487-57-7

1449 Therapy for Adults Molested as Children: Beyond Survival
Springer Publishing Company
11 West 42nd Street
15th Floor
New York, NY 10036-8002
212-431-4370
877-687-7476
Fax: 212-941-7842
E-mail: cs@springerpub.com
www.springerpub.com

John Briere, PhD, Author

Substantially expanded and updated, this classic volume provides therapists with detailed information on how to treat sexual abuse survivors more effectively. Dr. Briere offers an integrated theory of postabuse symptom development and suggests certain core phenomena that account for many of the psychosocial difficulties associated with childhood sexual abuse. *$39.95*

270 pages Year Founded: 1950 ISBN 0-826156-41-X

1450 Treating Intellectually Disabled Sex Offenders: A Model Residential Program
Safer Society Foundation
PO Box 340
Brandon, VT 05733-0340
802-247-3132
Fax: 802-247-4233
E-mail: gina@safersociety.org
www.safersociety.org

James Haaven, Author
Roger Little, Author
Dan Petre-Miller, Author

Describes how the intensive residential specialized Social Skills Program at Oregon State Hospital combines the principles of respect, self-help, and experiential learning with traditional sex-offender treatment methods. *$24.00*

152 pages ISBN 1-884444-30-X

Video & Audio

1451 Clinical Impressions: Identifying Mental Illness
Educational Training Videos
136 Granville St
Suite 200
Gahanna, OH 43230
Fax: 888-775-3919
www.educationaltrainingvideos.com

How long can mental illness stay hidden, especially from the eyes of trained experts? This program rejoins a group of ten adults- five of them healthy and five of them with histories of mental illness- as psychiatric specialists try to spot and correctly diagnose the latter. Administering a series of collaborative and one-on-one tests, including assessments of personality type, physical self-image, and rational thinking, the panel gradually makes decisions about who suffers from depression, bipolar disorder, bulimia, and social anxiety.

1452 FRONTLINE: The Released
PBS
2100 Crystal Drive
Arlington, VA 22202
www.pbs.org

Will Lyman, Actor
Narrator
Miri Navasky, Director
Karen O'Connor, Director

The documentary states that of the 700, 000 inmates released from American prisons each year, half of them have mental disabilities. This work focused on those with severe problems who keep entering and exiting prison. Full of good information on the challenges they face with mental illnesses; housing, employment, stigmatization, and socialization.

Year Founded: 2009

Web Sites

1453 www.emdr.com
EMDR Institute

Eye Movement Desensitization and Reprocessing (EMDR) integrates elements of many effective psychotherapies in structured protocols that are designed to maximize treatment effects. These include psychodynamic, cognitive behavioral, interpersonal, experiential, and body-centered therapies.

1454 www.mentalhealth.com
Internet Mental Health

Offers online psychiatric diagnosis in the hope of reaching the two-thirds of individuals with mental illness who do not seek treatment.

1455 www.planetpsych.com
Planetpsych.com

Online resource for mental health information.

1456 www.priory.com/sex.htm
Sexual Disorders

Diagnoses and treatments.

1457 www.psychcentral.com
Psych Central

The Internet's largest and oldest independent mental health social network created and run by mental health professionals to guarantee reliable, trusted information and support communities to you.

1458 www.shrinktank.com
Shrinktank

Psychology-related programs, shareware and freeware.

1459 www.xs4all.nl/~rosalind/cha-assr.html
Support and Information on Sex Reassignement

The purpose of this newsgroup is to provide a supportive and informative environment for people who are undergo-

ing or who have undergone sex reassignment surgery (SRS) and for their relatives and significant others.

Sleep Disorders

Introduction

Sleep Disorders are a group of disorders characterized by extreme distruptions in normal sleeping patterns. These include Primary Insomnia, Primary Hypersomnia, Narcolepsy, Breathing-related Sleep Disorder, Circadian Rhythm Sleep Disorder, Substance Abuse Induced Sleep Disorder, Nightmare Disorder and Sleep Terror Disorder. Primary Insomnia consists of the inability to sleep, with excessive daytime sleepiness, for at least one month, as evidenced by either prolonged sleep episodes or daytime sleep episodes that occur almost daily. Narcolepsy is characterized by chronic, involuntary and irresistible sleep attacks; a person with the disorder can suddenly fall asleep at any time of the day and during nearly any activity, including driving a car.

Breathing-related Sleep Disorder is diagnosed when sleep is distrupted by an obstruction of the breathing apparatus. Circadian Rhythm Sleep Disorder is a disruption of normal sleep patterns leading to a mismatch between the schedule required by a person's environment and his or her sleeping patterns; i.e., the individual is irresistibly sleepy when he or she is required to be awake, and awake at those times that he or she should be sleeping. Nightmare Disorder is diagnosed when there is a repeated occurrence of frightening dreams that lead to waking. Sleep Terror Disorder is the repeated occurrence of sleep terrors, or abrupt awakenings from sleeping with a shriek or a cry.

SYMPTOMS

This discussion addresses the disorder with the greatest prevalence: Primary Insomnia. A diagnosis of Primary Insomnia is made if the following criteria are met:

• Difficulty initiating or maintaining sleep or nonrestorative sleep for at least one month;
• The impairment causes clinically significant distress or impairment in social, occupational or other important areas of functioning;
• The disturbance does not occur exclusively during the course of other sleep-related disorders;
• The disturbance is not due to another general medical or psychiatric disorder, or the direct physiological effects of a substance.

ASSOCIATED FEATURES

Individuals with primary insomnia have a history of light sleeping. Interpersonal or work-related problems typically arise because of lack of sleep. Accidents and injuries may result from lack of attentiveness during waking hours, and sleep inducing, tranquillizer, or other medications are liable to be misused or abused. Once general medical problems are ruled out, a careful sleep history will often reveal that the individual has poor sleep habits or is reacting to an adverse life situation. These problems can then be addressed with advice or psychotherapy.

PREVALENCE

Surveys indicate a one-year prevalence of insomnia complaints in thirty percent to forty percent of adults, though the percentage of those who would have a diagnosis of Primary Insomnia is unknown. In clinics specializing in Sleep Disorders, about fifteen percent to twenty-five percent of individuals with chronic insomnia are diagnosed with Primary Insomnia.

TREATMENT OPTIONS

Treatment for Sleep Disorders includes an examination by a primary care physician to determine physical condition and sleeping habits, and a discussion with a somnologist, a professional trained in Sleep Disorders, or other mental health professional, to determine the individual's emotional state.

Referrals may be made to sleep clinics, which can be situated in hospitals, or sleep disorder centers in hospitals, universities or psychiatric institutions. To determine the cause of sleep disturbances, an individual in a sleep clinic or sleep disorder center may undergo interviews, psychological tests and laboratory observation — sleeping in the sleep laboratory while various functions are monitored. Medications that may be part of treatment for Sleep Disorders include drugs known as Hypnotics, or sleeping pills, including temazepam, Ambien, Sonata, and Lunesta. Some medications are more helpful with falling, and others with staying, asleep; a new formulation of Ambien has been developed in an attempt to address both. Sleep medications can lose effectiveness if taken over extended periods; use should always be supervised by a physician. Many cases will resolve with improved sleep hygiene, and treatment of pain and other remediable causes. There is also a new drug, Provigil, which helps people with Narcoleopsy to stay awake.

Associations & Agencies

1461 American Academy of Dental Sleep Medicine
2510 North Frontage Road
Darien, IL 60561
630-737-9761
Fax: 630-737-9790
E-mail: info@aadsm.org
www.www.aadsm.org

B. Gail Demko, DMD, President
Michael Simmons, DMD, Director
Todd Morgan, DMD, Director
Leslie C Dort, DDS, Secretary/Treasurer

Promotes research on the use of oral appliances and dental surgery for the treatment of sleep disordered breathing and provides training and resources for those who work directly with patients. The organization builds bridges and forms relationships with the medical community, especially in sleep centers, and other professional groups who play an integral part of the sleep disorders treatment and research team. The AADSM also reaches out to the community at large, working toward the creation of a positive public awareness of sleep disorders and the role of the dentist in recognition and treatment of sleep breathing disorders.
Year Founded: 1991

1462 American Academy of Sleep Medicine
2510 North Frontage Road
Darien, IL 60561
630-737-9700
Fax: 630-737-9790
E-mail: inquiries@aasmnet.org
www.aasmnet.org

M Safwan Badr, MD, President
Jerome A Barrett, Executive Director

Ronald D Chervin, MD, MS, Secretary/Treasurer
Timothy I Morgenthaler, MD, President-Elect

The only professionaly society dedicated exclusively tothe medical subspecialty of sleep medicine. As the leading voice in the field of sleep medicin, the AASM sets standards and promotes excellence in health care, education and research. Members specialize in studying, diagnosing and treating disorders of sleep and daytime alertness such as insomnia, narcolepsy and obstructive sleep apnea. The leader in setting standards and promoting excellence in sleep medicine health care, education and research.

Year Founded: 1975

1463 Narcolepsy Network

129 Waterwheel Lane
North Kingstown, RI 02852
401-667-2523
888-292-6522
Fax: 401-633-6567
E-mail: NarNet@narcolepsynetwork.org
www.narcolepsynetwork.org

Sara Kowalczyk, MA, MPH, President
Eveline Honig, MD, MPH, Executive Director
Matt Patterson, MD, PhD, Vice President
Louise O'Connell, Treasurer

A non profit organization dedicated to individuals with narcolepsy and related sleep disorders. Mission is to provide services to educate, advocate, support and improve awareness of this neurological sleep disorder.

Year Founded: 1986

1464 National Alliance on Mental Illness

3803 North Fairfax Drive
Suite 300
Arlington, VA 22203
703-524-7600
800-950-6264
Fax: 703-524-9094
E-mail: helpline@nami.org
www.nami.org

Keris Jan Myrick, MBA, MS, PhD., President
Mary Giliberti, J.D, Executive Director
Jim Payne, J.D, First Vice President
David Levy, Chief Financial Officer

Nation's leading self-help organization for all those affected by severe brain disorders. Mission is to bring consumers and families with similar experiences together to share information about services, care providers, and ways to cope with the challenges of schizophrenia, manic depression, and other serious mental illnesses.

Year Founded: 1969

1465 National Association for the Dually Diagnosed (NADD)

132 Fair Street
Kingston, NY 12401-4802
845-331-4336
800-331-5362
Fax: 845-331-4569
E-mail: info@thenadd.org
www.thenadd.org

Donna McNELIS, PhD, President
Robert J Fletcher DSW, Chief Executive Officer
Dan Baker, PhD, Vice President
Julia Pearce, Secretary

Nonprofit organization designed to promote interest of professional and parent development with resources for individuals who have the coexistence of mental illness and mental retardation. Provides conference, educational services and training materials to professionals, parents, concerned citizens and service organizations.

Year Founded: 1983

1466 National Mental Health Consumers' Self-Help Clearinghouse

1211 Chestnut Street
Suite 1100
Philadelphia, PA 19107-4103
215-751-1810
800-553-4539
Fax: 215-636-6312
E-mail: info@mhselfhelp.org
www.mhselfhelp.org

Joseph A Rogers, Executive Director/ Founder
Susan Rogers, Director
Britani Nestel, Program Specialist
Christa Burkett, Technical Assistance Coordinator

A national consumer technical assistance center that has played a major role in the development of the mental health consumer movement.

Year Founded: 1986

1467 National Sleep Foundation

1010 North Glebe Road
Suite 310
Arlington, VA 22201
703-243-1697
E-mail: nsf@sleepfoundation.org
www.sleepfoundation.org

Christopher Drake, PhD, Chairman
Charles A Czeisler, PhD, MD, Vice Chairman
David M. Cloud, MBA, Chief Executive Officer
Daniel B Brown, Treasurer

Alerting the public, healthcare providers and policymakers to the live-and-death importance of adequate sleep is central to the mission of NSF. NSF is dedicated to improving the quality of life for Americans who suffer from sleep problems and disorders. This means helping the public better understand the importance of sleep and the benefits of good sleep habits, and recognizing the signs of sleep problems so that they can be properly diagnosed and treated.

1468 SAMHSA'S National Mental Health Information Center

1 Choke Cherry Blvd
Rockville, MD 20857
877-726-4727
TDD: 866-889-2647
E-mail: ken@mentalhealth.org
www.mentalhealth.samhsa.gov

A Kathryn Power, MEd, Director
Edward B Searle, Deputy Director

1469 The Center for Family Support

2811 Zulette Avenue
Bronx, NY 10461
718-518-1500
Fax: 718-518-8200
E-mail: svernikoff@cfsny.org
www.cfsny.org

Steven Vernikoff, Executive Director
Virgil Seepersad, Director of Finance
Eileen Berg, Director of Quality Assurance
Barbara Greenwald, Associate Executive, Director

An agency that continues to develop new programs to serve families and individuals with their care needs. They currently offer services throughout the New York City region including: New Jersey, Long Island and the Lower Hudson Valley.

Year Founded: 1954

Books

1470 100 Q&A About Sleep and Sleep Disorders, Second Edition
Jones and Bartlett Publishers, Inc.
5 Wall Street
Burlington, MA 01803
978-443-5000
800-832-0034
Fax: 978-443-8000
E-mail: info@jblearning.com
www.jblearning.com

Sudhansu Chokroverty, MD, FRCP, FA, Author

The only text available to provide both the doctor's and patient's views, giving you authoritative, practical answers to the common questions about sleep and sleep disorders. Written by an expert on the subject, with insider commentary from actual patients, this book is an invaluable resource for anyone struggling with the medical, psychological, or emotional turmoil of these conditions.

188 pages Year Founded: 1983 ISBN 0-763741-20-5

1471 A Woman's Guide to Sleep Disorders
McGraw-Hill
1221 Avenue of the Americas
New York, NY 10020-1095
212-904-2000
www.mcgraw-hill.com

Meir H. Kryger, MD, Author

The first comprehensive book written about sleep disorders in women by a leading medical expert in the field. Dr. Kryger provides a thorough overview of sleep disorders among women. He shows how to determine whether a sleep problem is a disorder, help pinpoint causes, and what can be done to help. A resource guide, sleep questionnaire, and worksheet are included to assist the reader, and her doctor, in evaluating her condition.

337 pages Year Founded: 2004 ISBN 0-071425-27-6

1472 Concise Guide to Evaluation and Management of Sleep Disorders
American Psychiatric Publishing, Inc.
1000 Wilson Boulevard
Suite 1825
Arlington, VA 22209-3901
703-907-7322
800-368-5777
Fax: 703-907-1091
E-mail: appi@psych.org
www.appi.org

Martin Reite, Author
Michael Weissberg, M.D, Author
John Ruddy, Author

Overview of sleep disorders medicine, sleep physiology and pathology, insomnia complaints, excessive sleepiness disorders, parasomnias, medical and psychiatric disorders and sleep, medications with sedative-hypnotic properties, special problems and populations. *$29.95*

395 pages Year Founded: 2009 ISBN 0-880489-06-5

1473 Drug Therapy and Sleep Disorders
Mason Crest Publishers
450 Parkway Drive
Suite D
Broomall, PA 19008-4017
610-543-6200
866-627-2665
Fax: 610-543-3878
E-mail: dtaylor@masoncrest.com
www.masoncrest.com

Joan Esherick, Author

What are sleep disorders? Which drugs do doctors prescribe to treat them? What risks and benefits are involved? This book answers these and other questions by examining various sleep disorders, their symptoms and causes, common treatments, the drugs used to treat them, and how sleep drugs affect the brain.

128 pages ISBN 1-590845-76-5

1474 Getting a Good Night's Sleep A Cleveland Clinic Guide
Cleveland Clinic Press
9500 Euclid Avenue
Cleveland, OH 44195
216-444-2200
800-223-2273
TTY: 216-444-0261
www.cchealth.clevelandclinic.org/publications

Nancy Foldvary-Schaefer, Author

This book gives the sleepless what they need; real, substantive information from a source that is trusted by people all over the world. It provides a straightforward and clear examination of sleep problems and serves as a complete home reference for anyone.

228 pages Year Founded: 2006 ISBN 1-596240-14-8

1475 Parasomnias, An Issue of Sleep Medicine Clinics
Saunders: Elsevier, Health Sciences Division
1600 John F. Kennedy Blvd
Suite 1800
Philadelphia, PA 19103-2899
215-239-3900
800-523-1649
Fax: 215-239-3990
www.www.us.elsevierhealth.com

Mark Pressman, PhD, D.ABSM, Author

Articles examine disorders such as sleepwalking, sleep sex, sleep violence, sleep eating, and diagnostic methods of these. The issue also delves into forensic concerns, especially with regard to sleep violence. Other types of parasomnias discussed include sleep talking and sleep enuresis.

Year Founded: 2011 ISBN 1-455779-92-X

1476 Principles and Practice of Sleep Medicine
Elsevier, Inc.
1600 John F. Kennedy Boulevard.
Suite 1800
Philadelphia, PA 19103-2822
215-239-3900
800-523-1649
Fax: 215-239-3990
www.www.us.elsevierhealth.com

Meir H. Kryger, MD, Author/ Editor
Thomas Roth, PhD, Author/ Editor
William C. Dement, MD, PhD, Author/ Editor

Delivers the comprehensive, dependable guidance you
need to effectively diagnose and manage even the most
challenging sleep disorders. Updates to genetics and circadian rhythms, occupational health, sleep in older people,
memory and sleep, physical examination of the patient,
comorbid insomnias, and much more keep physicians current on the newest areas of the field. A greater emphasis on
evidence-based approaches helps you make the most
well-informed clinical decisions. *$329.00*

1766 pages Year Founded: 2011 ISBN 1-437707-31-1

1477 Say Good Night to Insomnia: The Six-Week,
Drug-Free Program Developed at Harvard
Medical School
Henry Holt and Company
175 Fifth Avenue
New York, NY 10010
646-307-5151
Fax: 212-633-0748
E-mail: customerservice@mpsvirginia.com
www.us.macmillan.com

Gregg D. Jacobs, PhD, Author
Dr. Herbert Benson, Introduction

The first clinician to offer proof that insomnia can be overcome without drugs, Dr. Jacob's program provides techniques for: eliminating sleeping pills, establishing
sleep-promoting habits and lifestyle practices, changing
negative stressful thoughts about sleep, implementing relaxation and stress-reduction techniques, enhancing peace
of mind and reducing negative emotions.

256 pages Year Founded: 1999 ISBN 0-805055-48-7

1478 Sleep Apnea: Pathogenesis, Diagnosis, and
Treatment
Informa Healthcare
52 Vanderbilt Ave.
New York, NY 10017
212-520-2777
866-861-0135
E-mail: books@informa.com
www.informahealthcare.com

Allan I. Pack, MBChB PhD, Author, Editor

Considers the relationship between obstructive sleep apnea
(OSA) and cardiovascular disease, right and left ventricular
dysfunction, and hypertension. A must-have, in-depth
guide for pulmonologists; physiologists; chest, pulmonary,
thoracic, and cardiovascular physicians and surgeons; car-
diologists; respiratory therapists; clinical neurologists;
sleep disorder specialists; and medical school students.

570 pages Year Founded: 2002 ISBN 0-824703-12-X

1479 Sleep Disorders Sourcebook
Omnigraphics
155 West Congress
Suite 200
Detroit, MI 48226
313-961-1340
800-234-1340
Fax: 313-961-1383
E-mail: contact@omnigraphics.com
www.omnigraphics.com

Sandra J Judd, Author/Editor

Gathering information from government and relevant
agency sources, this consumer reference addresses the biology of sleep, changing sleep needs throughout life, how to
improve sleep quality and quantity, the diagnosis and treatment of specific sleep disorders in adults and children, and
conditions that affect sleep. The volume includes a glossary, directory of resources, and suggested further reading.
$ 78.00

561 pages Year Founded: 1985 ISBN 1-780807-43-X

1480 Sleep Medicine Essentials
Wiley-Blackwell
111 River Street
Hoboken, NJ 07030-5774
201-748-6000
Fax: 201-748-6088
E-mail: info@wiley.com
www.wiley.com

Teofilo L. Lee-Chiong, Author

This is a concise, convenient, practical, and affordable
handbook on sleep medicine. It consists of forty topic-fo-
cused chapters written by a panel of international experts
covering a range of topics including insomnia, sleep apnea,
narcolepsy, parasomnias, circadian sleep disorders, sleep in
the elderly, sleep in children, sleep among women, and
sleep in the medical, psychiatric, and neurological
disorders.

280 pages Year Founded: 2009 ISBN 0-470195-66-5

1481 Sleep and Pain
Intl Association for the Study of Pain
1510 H Street, NorthWest
Suite 600
Washington, DC 20005-1020
202-524-5300
Fax: 202-524-5301
E-mail: IASPdest@iasp-pain.org
www.iasp-pain.org

Gilles Lavigne, Editor
Barry J. Sessle, Editor
Manon Choiniere, Editor
Peter J. Soja, Editor

Many in the research and clinical communities are becoming increasingly aware of the interactions between sleep
disorders and chronic pain syndromes. There are a number
of obstacles on the path to better patient care, and there is
considerable room for improvement in the way knowledge
is shared between professionals in the sleep and pain communities. This book serves as the first step toward enhancing communication between the sleep and pain
communities with the intent of improving patient care.

474 pages Year Founded: 1974 ISBN 0-931092-80-0

1482 The Dana Guide to Brain Health: A Practical Family Reference from Medical Experts
The Dana Foundation
505 Fifth Avenue
6th Floor
New York, NY 10017
212-223-4040
Fax: 212-317-8721
E-mail: danainfo@dana.org
www.dana.org

Floyd E Bloom, MD, Editor
M. Flint Beal, MD, Editor
David J. Kupfer, MD, Editor

A milestone in health publishing, the first major home medical reference on the brain, the Dana Guide is based on the contributions of more than 100 of America's most distinguished scientists and clinicians. The most authoritative, comprehensive, and clearly written guide to the bodily organ that is the key to our everyday health. No home should be without it.

Year Founded: 2007

1483 The Parasomnias and Other Sleep-Related Movement Disorders
Cambridge University Press
32 Avenue of the Americas
New York, NY 10013-2473
212-337-5000
E-mail: newyork@cambrigde.org
www.www.cambridge.org

Michael J. Thorpy, MD, Editor
Giuseppe Plazzi, MD, Editor

The first authoritative review on the parasomnias - disorders that cause abnormal behavior during sleep - this book contains many topics never before covered in detail. Appropriate behavioral and pharmacological treatments are addressed in detail. Sleep specialists, neurologists, psychiatrists, psychologists, and other healthcare professionals with an interest in sleep disorders will find this book essential reading.

356 pages Year Founded: 1534 ISBN 0-521111-57-9

Periodicals & Pamphlets

1484 Narcolepsy In the Classroom
Narcolepsy Network
129 Waterwheel Lane
North Kingstown, RI 02852
401-667-2523
888-292-6522
Fax: 401-633-6567
E-mail: NarNet@narcolepsynetwork.org
www.narcolepsynetwork.org

Sara Kowalczyk, MA, MPH, President
Eveline Honig, MD, MPH, Executive Director
Mark Patterson, MD, PhD, Vice President
Louise O'Connell, Treasurer

Concerned about a sleepy student? Essential information for school nurses, administrators, special education teams, parents, teachers, and students.

Year Founded: 1986

1485 Narcolepsy Q&A
Narcolepsy Network
129 Waterwheel Lane
North Kingstown, RI 02852
401-667-2523
888-292-6522
Fax: 401-633-6567
E-mail: NarNet@narcolepsynetwork.org
www.narcolepsynetwork.org

Sara Kowalczyk, MA, MPH, President
Eveline Honig, MD, MPH, Executive Director
Mark Patterson, MD, PhD, Vice President
Louise O'Connell, Treasurer

Common questions about narcolepsy for doctors' offices, public service buildings as well as psychiatrist offices and sleep study programs.

Year Founded: 1986

1486 Narcolepsy and You
Narcolepsy Network
129 Waterwheel Lane
North Kingstown, RI 02852
401-667-2523
888-292-6522
Fax: 401-633-6567
E-mail: NarNet@narcolepsynetwork.org
www.narcolepsynetwork.org

Sara Kowalczyk, MA, MPH, President
Eveline Honig, MD, MPH, Executive Director
Mark Patterson, MD, PhD, Vice President
Louise O'Connell, Treasurer

This booklet provides information about narcolepsy and tips on how to live a healthy life with this often misunderstood condition.

16 pages Year Founded: 1986

1487 Sleep and Breathing
American Academy of Dental Sleep Medicine
2510 North Frontage Road
Darien, IL 60561
630-737-9761
Fax: 630-737-9790
E-mail: info@aadsm.org
www.www.aadsm.org

B. Gail Demko, DMD, President
Michael Simmons, DMD, Director
Todd Morgan, DMD, Director
Leslie C Dort, DDS, Secretary/Treasurer

The official peer-reviewed journal of the AADSM, features the most recent original research in dental sleep medicine. Timely and original studies on the management of the upper airway during sleep in addition to common sleep disorders and disruptions, including sleep apnea, insomnia and shiftwork. Coverage includes patient studies and studies that emphasize the principles of physiology and pathophysiology or illustrate novel approaches to diagnosis and treatment.

4x per year Year Founded: 1991

Research Centers

1488 Sleep Studies
eRiver Neurology of New York, LLC
21 Fox Street
Suite 102
Poughkeepsie, NY 12601-4723
845-452-9750
Fax: 845-452-9751
E-mail: JM@eRiverNeurology.com
www.eriverneurology.com/Sleep%20Disorders%20Lab.ht
m

The all-night sleep study is frequently used by sleep physicians to evaluate adult patients when they are sleeping. This laboratory tet is extremely valuable for diagnosing and treating many sleep disorders, including neurologic disorders, movement disorders and breathing disorders at night. Sleep studies are generally easy to tolerate, comfortable for patients, and give sleep physicians the information they need to accurately diagnose and treat the sleep disorder.

Support Groups & Hot Lines

1489 ASAA A.W.A.K.E. Network
American Sleep Apnea Association (ASAA)
6856 Eastern Avenue NW
Suite 203
Washington, DC 20012
202-293-3650
Fax: 202-293-3656
www.stanford.edu/~dement/sleeplinks.html#so

Plays a crucial role in the ASAA's educational and avocacy efforts. A.W.A.K.E. is an acronym for Alert, Well, And Keeping Energetic. A mutual-help support group for persons affected by sleep apnea, composed of more than 200 groups in 45 states. Meetings are held regularly and guest speakers are often invited to address the group. Topics may include advice on complying with CPAP therapy, legal issues affecting those with sleep apnea, weight loss, treatment options such as oral appliances, and new research findings. Baltimore, New York, California, Oakland California, and Western Pennsylvania are just a few of the many locations of A.W.A.K.E. groups.

1490 Night Terrors Forum
Night Terrors Resource Center
www.www.nightterrors.org/forum.htm

David W. Richards, Site Administrator

Helping people understand that there are medical solutions and reasons for Night Terrors. Information on causes, medications, personal stories, sleep stages, and frequently asked questions about night terrors.

Year Founded: 1996

1491 eHealthForum Sleep Disorder Support Forum
www.ehealthforum.com/health/sleep_disorders.html#b

A health community featuring member and doctor discussions ranging from a specific symptom to related conditions, treatment options, medication, side effects, diet, and emotional issues surrounding medical sleep conditions.

Video & Audio

1492 Clinical Impressions: Identifying Mental Illness
Educational Training Videos
136 Granville St
Suite 200
Gahanna, OH 43230
Fax: 888-775-3919
www.educationaltrainingvideos.com

How long can mental illness stay hidden, especially from the eyes of trained experts? This program rejoins a group of ten adults- five of them healthy and five of them with histories of mental illness- as psychiatric specialists try to spot and correctly diagnose the latter. Administering a series of collaborative and one-on-one tests, including assessments of personality type, physical self-image, and rational thinking, the panel gradually makes decisions about who suffers from depression, bipolar disorder, bulimia, and social anxiety.

1493 Coping with Stress
Educational Video Network, Inc.
1401 19th Street
Huntsville, TX 77340
936-295-5767
800-762-0060
Fax: 936-294-0233
www.www.evndirect.com

Stress affects everyone, both emotionally and physically. For some, mismanaged stress can result in substance abuse, violence, or even suicide. This program answers the question, How can a person cope with stress?

1494 Effective Learning Systems
5108 W 74th
St #390160
Minneapolis, MN 55439
952-943-1660
800-966-0443
www.effectivelearning.com

Audio tapes for stress management, deep relaxation, anger control, peace of mind, insomnia, weight and smoking, self-image and self-esteem, positive thinking, health and healing. Since 1972, Effective Learning Systems has helped millions of people take charge of their lives and make positive changes. Over 75 titles available.

Year Founded: 1972

1495 Insomnia
Educational Training Videos
136 Granville St
Suite 200
Gahanna, OH 43230
Fax: 888-775-3919
www.educationaltrainingvideos.com

An inability to sleep is far more than a nuisance- it's a genuine health problem. This program examines insomnia from a medical perspective, exploring the physical, emotional, and psychological aspects of the disorder. Interview with doctors who specialize in treating sleep difficulties provide historical background on the affliction, the personal and professional hazards it can present, and dietary and behavioral adjustments that can improve the quality of sleep.

1496 Mental Disorder
Educational Training Videos
136 Granville St
Suite 200
Gahanna, OH 43230
Fax: 888-775-3919
www.educationaltrainingvideos.com

What is abnormality? Using the case studies of two young women; one who has depression, one who has an anxiety disorder; as a springboard, this program presents three psychological perspective on mental disorder.

1497 Understanding Mental Illness
Educational Video Network, Inc.
1401 19th Street
Huntsville, TX 77340
936-295-5767
800-762-0060
Fax: 936-294-0233
www.www.evndirect.com

Contains information and classifications of mental illness. Mental illness can strike anyone, at any age. Learn about various organic and functional mental disorders as discussed and their causes and symptoms, and learn where to seek help for a variety of mental health concerns.

Web Sites

1498 ehealthforum.com/health/sleep_disorders.
html#b
eHealthForum Sleep Disorder Support Forum

A health community featuring member and doctor discussions ranging from a specific symptom to related conditions, treatment options, medication, side effects, diet, and emotional issues surrounding medical sleep conditions.

1499 www.aadsm.org
American Academy of Dental Sleep Medicine

Promotes research on the use of oral appliances and dental surgery for the treatment of sleep disordered breathing and provides training and resources for those who work directly with patients. The organization builds bridges and forms relationships with the medical community, especially in sleep centers, and other professional groups who play an integral part of the sleep disorders treatment and research team. The AADSM also reaches out to the community at large, working toward the creation of a positive public awareness of sleep disorders and the role of the dentist in recognition and treatment of sleep breathing disorders.

1500 www.aasmnet.org
American Academy of Sleep Medicine

A professional society that is dedicated exclusively to the medical subspecialty of sleep medicine.

1501 www.cyberpsych.org
CyberPsych

Presents information about psychoanalysis, psychotherapy and special topics such as anxiety disorders, the problematic use of alcohol, homophobia, and the traumatic effects of racism.

1502 www.mentalhealth.com
Internet Mental Health

Offers on-line psychiatric diagnosis in the hope of reaching the two-thirds of individuals with mental illness who do not seek treatment.

1503 www.narcolepsynetwork.org
Narcolepsy Network
www.narcolepsynetwork.org

A non profit organization dedicated to individuals with narcolepsy and related sleep disorders. Mission is to provide services to educate, advocate, support and improve awareness of this neurological sleep disorder.

1504 www.nhlbi.nih.gov/about/ncsdr
National Institute of Health National Center on Sleep Disorders

The Center seeks to fulfill its goal of improving the health of Americans by serving four key functions: research, training, technology transfer, and coordination.

1505 www.nightterrors.org/forum.htm
Night Terrors Resource Center, Night Terrors Forum

Helping people understand that there are medical solutions and reasons for Night Terrors. Information on causes, medications, personal stories, sleep stages, and frequently asked questions about night terrors.

1506 www.nlm.nih.gov/medlineplus/sleepdisorders.
html
MEDLINEplus on Sleep Disorders

Compilation of links directs you to information on sleep disorders.

1507 www.planetpsych.com
Planetpsych.com

Online resource for mental health information.

1508 www.psychcentral.com
Psych Central

The Internet's largest and oldest independent mental health social network created and run by mental health professionals to guarantee reliable, trusted information and support communities to you.

1509 www.reggiewhitefoundation.org
Reggie White Sleep Disorders Research & Education Foundation, Inc.

Helping provide CPAP treatment equipment to those people who might otherwise be unable to secure the needed equipment. CPAP equipment is provided to patients who qualify for the foundation's assistance and who have a current prescription for it. Co-founded by Reggie White's wife, Sara, who recognized the role of her husbands sleep disorder in cutting his life short. Started the Foundation to help people of all economic backgrounds to understand the symptoms and risks of sleep disorders.

1510 www.sdrfoundation.org
Sleep Disorder Relief Foundation
www.sdrfoundation.org

A public non profit organization founded to: assist the underpriveleged suffering from sleep disorders by creating a network of relief, further the field of sleep medicine through organizing and funding sleep disorder researcch, and spread domestic and international awareness about the importance of sleep and the prevalence of sleep disorders.

1511 www.sleepfoundation.org
National Sleep Foundation

Alerting the public, healthcare providers and policymakers to the live-and-death importance of adequate sleep is central to the mission of NSF. NSF is dedicated to improving the quality of life for Americans who suffer from sleep problems and disorders. This means helping the public better understand the importance of sleep and the benefits of good sleep habits, and recognizing the signs of sleep problems so that they can be properly diagnosed and treated.

1512 www.stanford.edu/~dement/sleeplinks.html#so
ASAA A.W.A.K.E. Network

Plays a crucial role in the ASAA's educational and avocacy efforts. A.W.A.K.E. is an acronym for Alert, Well, And Keeping Energetic. A mutual-help support group for persons affected by sleep apnea, composed of more than 200 groups in 45 states. Meetings are held regularly and guest speakers are often invited to address the group. Topics may include advice on complying with CPAP therapy, legal issues affecting those with sleep apnea, weight loss, treatment options such as oral appliances, and new research findings. Baltimore, New York, California, Oakland California, and Western Pennsylvania are just a few of the many locations of A.W.A.K.E. groups.

1513 www.uic.edu/nursing/CNSHR/index.html
Center for Narcolepsy, Sleep & Health Research

Primary goal is to conduct important basic, clinical and bio-behavioral research for improving, preserving or promoting health through good sleep. The Center also aims to continue as an important source of sleep science and health expertise for colleagues, aspiring sleep researchers, clinicians, patients and families. Researching sleep and sleep-related disorders; educating young scientists for productive careers in sleep research; and transferring technologies and knowledge developed through research into practice or into the private sector.

Tic Disorders

Introduction

A tic is described as an involuntary, sudden, rapid, recurrent, non-rhythmic motor movement or vocalization. Four disorders are associated with tics: Chronic Motor or Vocal Tic Disorder, Transient Tic Disorder, Tic Disorder Not Otherwise Specified, and Tourette's Syndrome. Tourette's Syndrome is the most extreme case, consisting of multiple motor tics and one or more vocal tics, and will be the focus of this chapter. The vocalizations of Tourette's Syndrome can consist of grunts, obscenities, or other words the individual otherwise would not make. They are disruptive and profoundly embarrassing.

SYMPTOMS

• Multiple motor, as well as one or more vocal tics have been present during the illness, not necessarily at the same time;
• The tics occur many times during a day (often in bouts) nearly every day or intermittently throughout for more than one year, and during this period there was never a tic-free period of more three consecutive months;
• The disturbance causes clear distress or difficulties in social, work, or other areas;
• The onset is before age 18;
• The involuntary movements or vocalizations are not due to the direct effects of a substance (e.g., stimulants) or a general medication condition.

ASSOCIATED FEATURES

Between ten percent and forty percent of people with Tourette's Syndrome also have echolalia (automatically repeating words spoken by others) or echopraxia (imitating someone else's movements). Fewer than ten percent have coprolalia (the involuntary uterance of obscenities).

There seems to be a clear association between tic disorders, such as Tourette's Syndrome, and Obsessive Compulsive Disorder (OCD). As many as twenty percent to thirty percent of people with OCD report having or having had tics, and between five percent and seven percent of those with OCD also have Tourette's Syndrome. In studies of patients with Tourette's Syndrome it was found that thirty-six percent to fifty-two percent also meet the criteria for OCD. This is evidence that Tourette's Syndrome and Obsessive Compulsive Disorder share a genetic basis or some underlying pathological/physiological disturbance. The genetic evidence is further strengthened by the concordance rate in twins (i.e., the likelihood that if one member of the pair has the disorder, the other will also develop it): in identical twins, who have the same genes, the concordance is fifty-three percent, whereas in fraternal twins, who are no more closely related than other siblings, it is eight percent.

Other conditions commonly associated with Tourette's Syndrome are hyperactivity, distractibility, impulsivity, difficulty in learning, emotional disturbances, and social problems. The disorder causes social uneasiness, shame, self-consciousness, and depression. The person may be rejected by others and may develop anxiety about the tics, negatively affecting social, school, and work functioning. In severe cases, the disorder may interfere with everyday activities like reading and writing.

PREVALENCE

Tourette's Syndrome is reported in a variety of ethnic and cultural groups. It is one and one-half to three times more common in males than females and about 10 times more prevalent in children and adolescents than in adults. Overall prevalence is estimated at between four and five people in 10, 000.

While the age of onset can be as early as two years, it commonly begins during childhood or early adolescence. The median age for the development of tics is seven years. The disorder usually lasts for the life of the person, but there may be periods of remission of weeks, months, or years. The severity, frequency, and variability of the tics often diminish during adolescence and adulthood. In some cases, tics can disappear entirely by early adulthood.

TREATMENT OPTIONS

Many treatments have been tried. Haloperidol, an antipsychotic drug, is the most effective; it acts directly on the brain source of the tic, counteracting the overactivity, and can have a calming effect, but also can have unfortunate side effects. In very severe, disabling cases of OCD, brain surgery is an option. SSRIs (Selective Serotonin Reuptake Inhibitors) have also been effective in some cases of Tic Disorders. Symptoms of the disorder usually diminish with increasing age, and many people learn to live with them.

Associations & Agencies

1515 Centers for Disease Control and Prevention
Division of Human Development and Disability
1600 Clifton Road
MS E-88
Atlanta, GA 30333
800-232-4636
TTY: 888-232-6348
E-mail: cdcinfo@cdc.gov
www.cdc.gov/ncbddd/tourette/index.html

Offers information and links to other helpful sites. Facts, concerns & conditions, data & statistics, research, education & training, free materials, information for families and health professionals all about tic disorders and tourette syndrome.

1516 National Alliance on Mental Illness
3803 North Fairfax Drive
Suite 100
Arlington, VA 22203
703-524-7600
800-950-6264
Fax: 703-524-9094
E-mail: helpline@nami.org
www.nami.org

Keris Jan Myrick, MBA, MS, PhD., President
Mary Giliberti, J.D, Executive Director
Jim Payne, J.D, First Vice President
David Levy, Chief Financial Officer

Nation's leading self-help organization for all those affected by severe brain disorders. Mission is to bring consumers and families with similar experiences together to share information about services, care providers, and ways to cope with the challenges of schizophrenia, manic depression, and other serious mental illnesses.

Year Founded: 1969

1517 National Association for the Dually Diagnosed (NADD)
132 Fair Street
Kingston, NY 12401-4802
845-331-4336
800-331-5362
Fax: 845-331-4569
E-mail: info@thenadd.org
www.thenadd.org

Donna McNELIS, PhD, President
Robert J Fletcher DSW, Chief Executive Officer
Dan Baker, PhD, Vice President
Julia Pearce, Secretary

Nonprofit organization designed to promote interest of professional and parent development with resources for individuals who have the coexistence of mental illness and mental retardation. Provides conference, educational services and training materials to professionals, parents, concerned citizens and service organizations.

Year Founded: 1983

1518 National Mental Health Consumers' Self-Help Clearinghouse
1211 Chestnut Street
Suite 1100
Philadelphia, PA 19107-4103
215-751-1810
800-553-4539
Fax: 215-636-6312
E-mail: info@mhselfhelp.org
www.mhselfhelp.org

Joseph Rogers, Executive Director/ Founder
Susan Rogers, Director
Britani Nestel, Program Specialist
Christa Burkett, Technical Assistance Coordinator

A national consumer technical assistance center that has played a major role in the development of the mental health consumer movement. The consumer movement strives for dignity, respect, and opportunity for those with mental illnesses. Consumers- those who receive or have received mental health services- continue to reject the label of those who cannot help themselves.

Year Founded: 1986

1519 National Tourette Syndrome Association
42-40 Bell Boulevard
Bayside, NY 11361-2874
718-224-2999
888-486-8738
Fax: 718-279-9596
E-mail: ts@tsa-usa.org
www.tsa-usa.org

Michael Wolff, Chairman
Annetta Hewko, President
Julie Noulas, Vice President, Finance
J Mark Levine, Vice President, Development

Raising public awareness and counter media stereotypes about TS. Program development, education and medical programs, government outreach, adherence to TSA's mission, maximizing efforts, minimizing expenses, TeamTSA events, awareness month, publications, chapter relations, research grants, scientific and medical conferences, are on-going efforts of TSA's full-time professional staff. Volun-

teers of extraordinary dedication and professional merit serve on TSA's Board of Directors, Medical Advisory Board (MAB), and Scientific Advisory Board (SAB).

Year Founded: 1972

1520 SAMHSA'S National Mental Health Information Center
1 Choke Cherry Road
Rockville, MD 20857
877-726-4727
E-mail: ken@mentalhealth.org
www.mentalhealth.samhsa.gov

1521 The Center for Family Support
2811 Zulette Avenue
Bronx, NY 10461
718-518-1500
Fax: 718-518-8200
E-mail: svernikoff@cfsny.org
www.cfsny.org

Steven Vernikoff, Executive Director
Virgil Seepersad, Director of Finance
Eileen Berg, Director of Quality Assurance
Barbara Greenwald, Associate Executive, Director

The Center for Family Support is committed to providing support and assistance to individuals with developmental and related disabilities, and to the family members who care for them.

Year Founded: 1954

Books

1522 A Mind of Its Own: Tourette's Syndrome: a Story and a Guide
Oxford University Press
198 Madison Avenue
New York, NY 10016-4341
212-726-6000
800-445-9714
Fax: 919-677-1303
E-mail: custserv.us@oup.com
www.www.oup.com/us/

Ruth Dowling Bruun, Author
Bertel Bruun, Author

In spite of the attention paid to Tourette's syndrome in recnt years, there was still no book which explains the condition to patients and their families in an informative, comprehensive, and accessible manner. This book fills that need. It presents factual information on all important aspects of TS along with a composite case history. The story of Michael Lockman, who typifies the average child with TS, is woven into the factual text which contains information on symptomology, diagnosis, natural history, biochemistry, genetics, associated disorders, treatment and related topiccs.

174 pages Year Founded: 1994 ISBN 0-195065-87-5

1523 Adam and the Magic Marble
Hope Press
PO Box 188
Duarte, CA 91009-188
800-321-4039
Fax: 626-358-3520
E-mail: dcomings@earthlink.net
www.hopepress.com

Adam Buehrens, Author
Carol Buehrens, Author

Exciting reading for all ages, and a must for those who have been diagnosed with Tourette syndrome or other disabilities. An up-beat story of three heros, two with Tourette syndrome, one with cerebal palsy. Constantly taunted by bullies, the boys find a marble full of magic power, they aim a spell at the bullies and the adventure begins. *$6.95*

108 pages

1524 Children with Tourette Syndrome: A Parent's Guide (Special Needs Collection)
ADD WareHouse
300 NorthWest 70th Avenue
Suite 102
Plantation, FL 33317-2360
954-792-8944
800-233-9273
Fax: 954-792-8545
E-mail: websales@addwarehouse.com
www.addwarehouse.com

Tracy Haerle, Editor
Jim Eisenreich, Foreword

This handbook for parents of children and teenagers with Tourette Syndrome offers up-to-date informaion and compassionate advice for dealing with what is perhaps one of the most misunderstood and misdiagnosed neurological disorders. Written by a team of professionals and parents, this book covers medical, educational, legal, family life, daily care and emotional issues. *$17.00*

361 pages Year Founded: 1990 ISBN 0-933149-44-1

1525 Don't Think About Monkeys: Extraordinary Stories Written by People with Tourette Syndrome
Hope Press
Fax: 626-358-3520
E-mail: dcomings@earthlink.net
www.hopepress.com

Adam Ward Seligman, Editor
John S Hilkevich, Editor

A remarkable collection of stories written by fourteen people who live with Tourette syndrome. Ranging from three teenagers learning to come to grips with treatment to adults encountering discrimination, the collection represents the incredible diversity of a disorder as diverse as life itself. The drama of living with a disability and the comedy of a Tourette syndrome conference show the range of a book that Oliver Sacks called, A fascinatingly varied book! *$12.95*

200 pages Year Founded: 1992 ISBN 1-878267-33-7

1526 Echolalia: an Adult's Story of Tourette Syndrome
Hope Press
Fax: 626-358-3520
E-mail: dcomings@earthlink.net
www.hopepress.com

Adam Ward Seligman, Author

Echolalia is the story of best selling writer Jackson Evans, who is diagnosed as having Tourette syndrome, a complex genetic disorder characterized by tics and vocal noises (including obscenities), and obsessive-compulsive behavior. At first, he is grateful for the answers it brings him, but

Jackson soon realizes that the real problems are just beginning. The story is told in a style that captures the rhythms that soothe the Tourette. It ends with the ultimate truth- the answer isn't in being diagnosed, the answer is in living with the diagnosis. *$11.95*

165 pages Year Founded: 1991 ISBN 1-878267-31-0

1527 Hi, I'm Adam: a Child's Book About Tourette Syndrome
Hope Press
Fax: 626-358-3520
E-mail: dcomings@earthlink.net
www.hopepress.com

Adam Buehrens, Author

A child's story of how it feels to have Tourette syndrome and hyperactivity (attention deficit hyperactivity disorder). *$4.95*

35 pages Year Founded: 1990 ISBN 1-878267-29-9

1528 I Can't Stop!: A Story About Tourette Syndrome
Albert Whitman & Company
250 South Northwest Highway
Suite 320
Park Ridge, IL 60068-4272
847-581-2800
800-255-7675
Fax: 847-581-0039
E-mail: mail@awhitmanco.com
www.albertwhitman.com

Holly L. Niner, Author
Meryl Treatner, Illustrator

Kindergarten-Grade 4 level, An introduction for parents and teachers gives more information about it an notes that tics are common among children. The plot and primarily one-dimensional characters are devices to educate readers about TS. There is a lot of dialogue, and the students in Nathan's class represent diverse cultures. Very few books are available for young audiences on this medical concern; what's out there tends to be nonfiction for older readers. Thus, this title does fill a void.

32 pages Year Founded: 1919 ISBN 0-807536-20-2

1529 Neurodevelopmental Disabilities: Clinical Care for Children and Young Adults
Springer
11 West 42nd Street
15th Floor
New York, NY 10036
212-431-4370
877-687-7476
Fax: 212-941-7842
E-mail: cs@springerpub.com
www.springerpub.com

Dilip R. Patel, Editor
Donald E. Greydanus, Editor
Hatim A. Omar, Editor
Joav Merrick, Editor

Increasingly more and more children with developmental disabilities survive into adulthood. Pediatricians and other clinicians are called upon to care for an increasing number of children with developmental disabilities in their practice and thus there is a need for a practical guide specifically written for pediatricians and primary care clinicians that addresses major concepts of neurodevelopmental pediatrics.

350 pages Year Founded: 1950 ISBN 9-400706-26-X

1530 RYAN: A Mother's Story of Her Hyperactive/ Tourette Syndrome Child
Hope Press
Fax: 626-358-3520
E-mail: dcomings@earthlink.net
www.hopepress.com

Susan Hughes, Author

A moving and informative story of how a mother struggled with the many behavioral problems presented by her son with Tourette syndrome, ADHD and oppositional defiant disorder. *$9.95*

153 pages Year Founded: 1990 ISBN 1-878267-25-6

1531 Raising Joshua: One Mother's Story of the Challenges of Parenting a Child With Tourette Syndrome
Hope Press
Fax: 626-358-3520
E-mail: dcomings@earthlink.net
www.hopepress.com

Sheryl Johnson Hamer, RN, Author

The harrowing and heartwarming story of Josh, a boy caught in Tourette Syndrome, and Attention Deficit Hyperactivity Disorder, as told by his mother. The true story of two souls caught in a modern jungle of medical ignorance, powerful drugs, and the ravaging behavior of a mysterious condition. Their indomitable spirits of love and courage help them walk hand in hand through their special world. *$14.95*

150 pages Year Founded: 1997 ISBN 0-965750-16-7

1532 Tics and Tourette Syndrome: A Handbook for Parents and Professionals
Jessica Kingsley Publishers
400 Market Street
Suite 400
Philadelphia, PA 19106
215-922-1161
866-416-1078
Fax: 215-922-1474
E-mail: hello.usa@jkp.com
www.jkp.com

Uttom Chowdhury, Author
Isobel Heyman, Foreword

This essential guide to tic disorders and Tourette Syndrome tackles problems faced both at home and at school, such as adjusting to the diagnosis, the effect on siblings and classroom difficulties. Dr. Chowdhury offers advice on how to manage symptoms, describing psychological techniques such as habit reversal and massed practice and reviewing available medical treatments. In clear, accessible language, this book explains the clinical signs and symptoms of Tourette and related conditions, and their possible causes. Presenting practical strategies for dealing with associated difficulties, including low self-esteem, anger management and bullying, this book will be invaluable to parents, teachers, social workers and other professionals.

160 pages Year Founded: 1987 ISBN 1-843102-03-X

1533 Tourette Syndrome and Human Behavior
Hope Press
110 Mill Run
Monrovia, CA 91016-1658
Fax: 626-358-3520
E-mail: dcomings@earthlink.net
www.hopepress.com

David E. Comings, Author

The story of how Tourette syndrome provides insights into the cause and treatment of a wide range of human behavioral problems. It covers diagnosis, associated behaviors including ADHD, learning disorders, dyslexia, conduct disorder, OCD, alcoholism, drug abuse, obesity, depression, panic attacks, phobias, night terrors, bed wetting, sleep disturbances, lying, stealing, inappropriate sexual behavior, and others: brain structure and chemistry, treatment and implications for society, over 2, 500 references, 30-page Tourette Syndrom-Human Behavior Questionnaire, and Extensive index. *$39.95*

850 pages Year Founded: 1990 ISBN 1-878267-28-0

1534 Tourette's Syndrome- Tics, Obsession, Compulsions: Developmental Psychopathology & Clinical Care
John Wiley & Sons
605 3rd Avenue
New York, NY 10158-180
212-850-6301
E-mail: info@wiley.com

James F. Leckman, Author
Donald J. Cohen, Author

Edited by two of the leading international authorities on Tourette's Syndrome and tic-related, obsessive-compulsive disorders, this book is the most up-to-date edited reference covering this neuropsychiatric disorder and related disorders from a variety of perspectives. Featuring contributors from the world-renowned Yale Child Study Center, this volume introduces a groundbreaking developmental framework for understanding Tourette's-defined by persistent motor and vocal tics and frequently associated with obsessions, compulsions, and attentional difficulties- and maps out the diagnosis, genetics, manifestations, and treatment. This comprehensive resource describes the major categories of disorders. *$189.00*

584 pages Year Founded: 2001 ISBN 0-471160-37-7

1535 Tourette's Syndrome: The Facts, Second Edition
Oxford University Press
198 Madison Avenue
New York, NY 10016-4341
212-726-6400
800-451-7556

Mary Robertson, Editor
Andrea Cavanna, Editor

This text explains the causes of the syndrome, how it is diagnosed, and how to cope if you have been recently diagnosed. It provides information on the treatment and therapies that are available, and advice on how individuals can manage their symptoms. It clearly explains the different presentations that can affect individuals, covering a spectrum from very mild to more uncommon severe forms of TS, and also discusses disorders that can be mistaken for TS. This edition contains new chapters focusing on education, employment and empowerment, and famous and successful people who acheived their goals despite their diagnosis. *$ 19.95*

110 pages Year Founded: 2008 ISBN 0-198523-98-X

1536 Treating Tourette Syndrome and Tic Disorders: A Guide for Practitioners
The Guilford Press
72 Spring Street
New York, NY 10012
800-365-7006
Fax: 212-966-6708
E-mail: info@guilford.com
www.guilford.com

Douglas W. Woods, PhD, Editor
John C. Piacentini, PhD, Editor
John T. Walkup, MD, Editor
Peter Hollenbeck, PhD, Foreword

Grounded in a comprehensive model of Tourette syndrome (TS) and related disorders, this state-of-the-art volume provides a multidisciplinary framework for assessment and treatment. Leading authorities present the latest knowledge on the neurobehavioral underpinnings of TS, its clinical presentation, and how to distinguish it from frequently encountered co-occurring disorders, such as obsessive-compulsive disorder and attention-deficit/hyperactivity disorder. Strategies for managing symptoms and providing effective support to children and families are thoroughly detailed, with an emphasis on integrating medication and psychosocial therapies. Several chapters also address clinical work with adults with TS.

287 pages Year Founded: 1973 ISBN 1-593854-80-3

1537 What Makes Ryan Tick: A Family's Triumph over Tourette Syndrome and Attention Deficiency Hyperactivity Disorder
Hope Press
Fax: 626-358-3520
E-mail: dcomings@earthlink.net
www.hopepress.com

Susan Hughes, Author

A follow-up to Susan Hughes best selling book RYAN - A Mother's Story of her Hyperactivity Tourette Syndrome Child, covering his particularly difficult teenage years.

303 pages Year Founded: 1996 ISBN 1-878267-35-3

Research Centers

1538 Child Neurology and Developmental Center
1510 Jericho Turnpike
New Hyde Park, NY 11040
516-352-2500
Fax: 516-352-2573
www.childbrain.com

Rami Grossmann, M.D.

Pediatric neurology practice of Rami Grossmann, M.D. in New York. Neurologists are highly trained to treat disorders of the nervous system. This includes diseases of the brain, spinal cord, nerves, and muscles. Common problems that Dr. Grossmann diagnoses and treats include the following: AD/HD, Autism, a form of PDD, Developmental delays, Epilepsy, Headaches, Learning difficulties, and Tic Disorders.

1539 KidsHealth
The Nemours Foundation
10140 Centurion Parkway
Jacksonville, FL 32256
904-697-4100
Fax: 904-697-4220
E-mail: comments@KidsHealth.org
www.kidshealth.org

Alfred I. duPont, Nemour's Foundation Creator
Neil Izenberg, MD, Editor-in-Chief & Founder

KidsHealth is more than just the facts about health. As part of The Nemours Foundation's Center for Children's Health Media, KidsHealth also provides families with perspective, advice, and comfort about a wide range of physical, emotional, and behavioral issues that affect children and teens. The Nemours Center for Children's Health Media is a part of The Nemours Foundation, a nonprofit organization created by philanthropist Alfred I. duPont in 1936 and devoted to improving the health of children.

Year Founded: 1936

Support Groups & Hot Lines

1540 DailyStrength: Tourette Syndrome Support Forum
3280 Peachtree Rd
Suite 600
Atlanta, GA 30305
www.dailystrength.org

DailyStrength is a subsidiary of Sharecare, Inc., the first truly interactive healthcare ecosystem giving consumers the ability to ask, learn, and act on the questions of health. DailyStrength was created and operated by some very passionate and dedicated people that get great satisfaction knowing that this site can be a positive force for everyone who faces challenges in their lives.

Video & Audio

1541 After the Diagnosis...The Next Steps
Tourette Syndrome Association
42-40 Bell Boulevard
Suite 205
Bayside, NY 11361-2874
718-224-2999
888-486-8738
Fax: 718-279-9596
E-mail: ts@tsa-usa.org
www.tsa-usa.org

Judit Ungar, President
Gary Frank, EVP
Mark Levine, VP Development
Richard Dreyfuss, Narrator

When the diagnosis is Tourette Syndrome, what do you do first? How do you sort out the complexities of the disorder? Whose advice do you follow? What steps do you take to lead a normal life? Six people with TS—as different as any six people can be—relate the sometimes difficult, but finally triumphant path each took to lead the rich, fulfilling life they now enjoy. Narrated by Academy Award-winning actor, Richard Dreyfuss, the stories are refreshing blends of poignancy, fact, and inspiration illustrating that a diagnosis of TS can be approached with confidence and hope. Includes comments by family and friends, teachers, counselors and leading medical authorities on Tourette Syndrome.

A must-see for the newly diagnosed child, teen or adult. *$35.00*

Year Founded: 1972

1542 Clinical Counseling: Toward a Better Understanding of TS
Tourette Syndrome Association
42-40 Bell Boulevard
Suite 205
Bayside, NY 11361-2874
718-224-2999
888-486-8738
Fax: 718-279-9596
E-mail: ts@tsa-usa.org
www.tsa-usa.org

Judit Ungar, President
Gary Frank, EVP
Mark Levine, VP Development
Dylan McDermott, Narrator

Certain key issues often surface during the counseling sessions of people wwith TS and their families. These important areas of concern are explored for counselors, social workers, educators, psychologists and other allied professionals. Expert clinical practitioners offer invaluable insights for those working with people affected by Tourette Syndrome. *$30.00*

Year Founded: 1972

1543 Clinical Impressions: Identifying Mental Illness
Educational Training Videos
136 Granville St
Suite 200
Gahanna, OH 43230
Fax: 888-775-3919
www.educationaltrainingvideos.com

How long can mental illness stay hidden, especially from the eyes of trained experts? This program rejoins a group of ten adults- five of them healthy and five of them with histories of mental illness- as psychiatric specialists try to spot and correctly diagnose the latter. Administering a series of collaborative and one-on-one tests, including assessments of personality type, physical self-image, and rational thinking, the panel gradually makes decisions about who suffers from depression, bipolar disorder, bulimia, and social anxiety.

1544 Complexities of TS Treatment: Physician's Roundtable
Tourette Syndrome Association
42-40 Bell Boulevard
Suite 205
Bayside, NY 11361-2874
718-224-2999
888-486-8738
Fax: 718-279-9596
E-mail: ts@tsa-usa.org
www.tsa-usa.org

Judit Ungar, President
Gary Frank, EVP
Mark Levine, VP Development

Three of the most highly regarded experts in the diagnosis and treatment of Tourette Syndrome offer insight, advice and treatment strategies to fellow physicians and other healthcare professionals. *$ 30.00*

Year Founded: 1972

1545 Family Life with Tourette Syndrome... Personal Stories
Tourette Syndrome Association
42-40 Bell Boulevard
Suite 205
Bayside, NY 11361-2874
718-224-2999
888-486-8738
Fax: 718-279-9596
E-mail: ts@tsa-usa.org
www.tsa-usa.org

Judit Ungar, President
Gary Frank, EVP
Mark Levine, VP Development

In extended, in-depth interviews, all the people engagingly profiled in After the Diagnosis. The Next Steps, reveal the individual ways they developed to deal with TS. Each shows us that the key to leading a successful life in spite of having TS, is having a loving, supportive network of family and friends. Available in its entirety or as separate vignettes. *$50.00*

Year Founded: 1972

1546 Understanding and Treating the Hereditary Psychiatric Spectrum Disorders
Hope Press
PO Box 188
Duarte, CA 91009-188
818-303-0644
800-209-9182
Fax: 818-358-3520
E-mail: dcomings@earthlink.net
www.hopepress.com

David E Comings MD, Presenter

Learn with ten hours of audio tapes from a two day seminar given in May 1997 by David E Comings, MD. Tapes cover: ADHD, Tourette Syndrome, Obsessive-Compulsive Disorder, Conduct Disorder, Oppositional Defiant Disorder, Autism and other Hereditary Psychiatric Spectrum Disorders. Eight Audio tapes. *$75.00*

Year Founded: 1997

Web Sites

1547 www.mentalhealth.com
Internet Mental Health

Offers online psychiatric diagnosis in the hope of reaching the two-thirds of individuals with mental illness who do not seek treatment.

1548 www.planetpsych.com
Planetpsych.com

Online resource for mental health information.

1549 www.psychcentral.com
Psych Central

The Internet's largest and oldest independent mental health social network created and run by mental health professionals to guarantee reliable, trusted information and support communities to you.

1550 www.tourette-syndrome.com
Tourette Syndrome

Online community devoted to children and adults with
Tourette Syndrome disorder and their families, friends,
teachers, and medical professionals. Provides an interactive
meeting place for those interested in Tourette Syndrome or
people wanting to help others who have TS.

1551 www.tourettesyndrome.net
Tourette Syndrome Plus

Parent and teacher friendly site on Tourette Syndrome, Attention Deficit Disorder, Executive Dysfunction, Obessive
Compulsive Disorder, and related conditions.

1552 www.tsa-usa.org
Tourette Syndrome Association

Web site of the association dedicated to identifying the
cause, finding the cure and controlling the effects of TS.

Information Services

1553 Tourette Syndrome Plus
Leslie E. Packer, PhD
940 Lincoln Place
North Bellmore, NY 11710-1016
516-785-2653
E-mail: admin@tourettesyndrome.net
www.www.tourettesyndrome.net

Leslie E. Packer, PhD

Information on Tourette Syndrome PLUS the Associated
Disorders.

Pediatric & Adolescent Issues

Introduction

The media is full of reports about supposed epidemics of psychiatric medications in children, and, tragically, from time to time, stories of children who commit suicide or murder. Parents, other relatives, guardians, and teachers are understandably concerned about not missing the signs of a treatable disorder while, at the same time, not subjecting the child to unnecessary and potentially stigmatizing diagnosis and treatment. No one can say for sure whether there are more cases of bipolar disorder in children now than ten or twenty years ago. Whenever there is publicity about any medical disorder, the number of diagnoses goes up. Some of those accurately diagnosed would have been overlooked in the past. Others are diagnosed and treated without a full evaluation. As noted in the chapter on autism spectrum disorders, while awareness of the diagnosis has brought more children to diagnosis and treatment, it seems that the actual incidence of the condition has increased in recent years; the reasons are still unknown. The American Academy of Child and Adolescent Psychiatry (http://www.aacap.org/) provides accurate and useful information to help those responsible for children decide: whether a child's behavior is normal for his or her age; if a child is being adversely influenced by circumstances; what is a warning sign for mental disorder; and what constitutes a mental disorder.

In general, a child or adolescent is evaluated not only on the basis of particular behaviors that cause concern, but also with respect to meeting the milestones expected at his or her age. A child should be increasingly able to relate to other people, both children and adults, and to learn. An untreated mental disorder can deprive a child of essential years of social and educational growth. Anyone concerned about a child should start with the child's pediatrician. A child should not be given a diagnosis or prescribed medication without a complete physical health evaluation, specialized observation, and interviews with parents, teachers, and others familiar with the him or her. There is a shortage of fully qualified experts in child and adolescent mental health; it may require considerable persistence to assure that a child receives the attention necessary, but it will be worthwhile. There should be no hesitation to obtain a second opinion. Heatlh professionals should be able to explain why a child was or wasn't given a specific diagnosis, and the pros and cons of the treatment choices.

Note: Vaccinations do not cause autism, and going un-vaccinated exposes both a child to diseases that can be serious, even fatal, and all those the child comes in contact with, before the signs of the disease are evident.

Associations & Agencies

1555 AHRC New York City
83 Maiden Lane
New York, NY 10038-4812
212-780-2500
Fax: 212-777-5893
TTY: 800-662-1220
E-mail: webmaster@ahrcnyc.org
www.ahrcnyc.org

Laura J Kennedy, President
Amy West, Chief Financial Officer

Michael Decker, Chief Operating Officer
Gary Lind, Executive Director

Developmentally disabled children and adults, their families, and interested individuals. Provides support services, training programs, clinics, schools and residential facilities to the developmentally disabled. Formerly known as the Association for the Help of Retarded Children.

1556 American Academy of Child and Adolescent Psychiatry
3615 Wisconsin Avenue NW
Washington, DC 20016-3007
202-966-7300
800-333-7636
Fax: 202-966-2891
www.www.aacap.org

Virginia Anthony, Executive Director
Earl Magee, Administrator
William Bernet, Treasurer

Professional medical organization comprised of child and adolescent psychiatrist trained to promote healthy development and to evaluate, diagnose, and treat children and adolescents and their families who are affected by disorders of feeling, thinking, learning and behavior. Child and adolescent psychiatrists are physicians who are uniquely qualified to integrate knowledge about human behavior, social, and cultural perspectives with scientific, humanistic, and collaborative approaches to diagnosis, treatment and the promotion of mental health.

1557 American Academy of Pediatrics
141 Northwest Point Boulevard
Elk Grove Village, IL 60007-1098
847-434-4000
800-433-9016
Fax: 847-434-8000
E-mail: cme@aap.org
www.aap.org

James M Perrin, MD, FAAP, President
Errol R. Alden, MD, FAAP, Executive Director/CEO
Sandra Hassink, MD, FAAP, President-Elect

An organization of 60, 000 pediatricians committed to the optimal physical, mental, and social health and well-being for all infants, children, adolescents, and young adults.

Year Founded: 1929

1558 American Pediatrics Society
3400 Research Forest Drive
Suite B7
The Woodlands, TX 77381-4259
281-419-0052
Fax: 281-419-0082
E-mail: info@aps-spr.org
www.aps-spr.org

Alan L Schwartz, M.D, PhD, President
Donna M Ferriero, M.D, M.S, Vice President
Debbie Anagnostelis, Executive Director
Judy L Aschner, M.D, Secretary/Treasurer

Society of professionals working with pediatric health care issues; offers seminars and a variety of publications.

1559 Association for Children's Mental Health
6017 West Steet Joseph Highway
Suite 200
Lansing, MI 48917

517-372-4016
888-226-4543
Fax: 517-372-4032
E-mail: acmhmalisa@aol.com
www.acmh-mi.org

Gail Lanphear, President
Rosemary Allen, Vice President
Jane Shank, Executive Director
Dalis Smith, Secretary

Provides information, support, resources, referral and advocacy for children and youth with mental, emotional, or behavioral disorders and their families

Year Founded: 1989

1560 Federation for Children with Special Needs (FCSN)

529 Main Street
Suite 1M3
Boston, MA 02129
617-236-7210
800-331-0688
Fax: 617-241-0330
E-mail: fcsninfo@fcsn.org
www.fcsn.org

James F. Whalen, President
Rich Robinson, Executive Director
William Henderson, Ed.D, Director Emeritus
Michael Weiner, Treasurer

Provides information, support, and assistance to parents of children with disabilities, their professional partners, and their communities. Committed to listening to and learning from families, and encouraging full participation in community life by all people, especially those with disabilities.

1561 Lifespire

1 Whitehall Street
9th Floor
New York, NY 10004
212-741-0100
Fax: 212-463-9814
E-mail: info@lifespire.org
www.lifespire.org

Jeffrey Goodman, Chairman
Mark Van Voorst, CEO/ President
Keith Lee, Chief Financial Officer
Tom Lydon, Chief Operating Officer

Committed to the principle that all individuals with a developmental disability are able to become contributing members to their family and community. It is Lifespire's aim to provide these individuals with the assistance and support necessary so that they can attain the skills needed to maintain themselves in their community in the most integrated and independent manner possible.

Year Founded: 1951

1562 Mentally Ill Kids in Distress (MIKID)

2642 East Thomas Road
Phoenix, AZ 85016
602-253-1240
800-356-4543
Fax: 602-253-1250
E-mail: familyresource@MIKID.org
www.mikid.org

Iiene Dode, President
Sue Gilbertson, Vice President

Faron Jack, Chief Executive Officer
Sue Knabe, MAPC, LPC, LISAC, Clinical Director, Interim COO

Mission is to provide support and assistance to families in Arizona with behaviorally challenged children, youth, and young adults. Offers information centers, assistance by phone email or in person, support groups, educational meetings, referral to excellent resources, and direct support services.

Year Founded: 1987

1563 National Dissemination Center for Children with Disabilities

1825 Connecticut Ave NW
Suite 700
Washington, DC 20009
800-695-0285
Fax: 202-884-8441
TTY: 202-884-8200
E-mail: nichcy@aed.org
www.nichcy.org/

NICHCY is the center that provides information to the nation on: disabilities in children and youth; programs and services for infants, children, and youth with disabilities; IDEA, the nation's special education law; and research-based information on effective practices for children with disabilities.

1564 National Federation of Families for Children's Mental Health

9605 Medical Center Drive
Suite 280
Rockville, MD 20850-6390
240-403-1901
Fax: 240-403-1909
E-mail: ffcmh@ffcmh.org
www.ffcmh.org

Sandra Spencer, Executive Director
Lynda Gargan, Senior Managing Director
Lizette Albright, Finance Director

Through a family and youth-driven approach, children and youth emotional, behavioral, and mental health challenges and their families obtain needed supports and services so that children grow up healthy and able to maximize their potential.

Year Founded: 1989

1565 National Technical Assistance Center for Children's Mental Health

Box 571485
Washington, DC 20057-1485
202-687-5000
Fax: 202-687-1954
TTY: 202-687-5503
E-mail: childrensmh@georgetown.edu
www.gucchd.georgetown.edu/67211.html

Year Founded: 1986

1566 Parents Helping Parents

Sobrato Center for Nonprofits
1400 Parkmoor Avenue
Suite 100
San Jose, CA 95126
408-727-5775
855-727-5775

Fax: 408-286-1116
www.php.com

Susan Cistulli, Board Chair
Mary Ellen Peterson, MA, Executive Director/CEO
Paul Schutz, Chief Financial Officer
Christopher Baker, Board Treasurer

A nonprofit agency that meets the needs of children with any special need and their families. This includes children of all ages and all backgrounds who have a need for special services due to any special need, including but not limited to illness, cancer, accidents, birth defects, neurological conditions, premature birth, learning or physical disabilities, mental health issues, and attention deficit (hyperactivity) disorder, to name a few.

Year Founded: 1976

1567 Pilot Parents: PP
Ollie Webb Center
1941 South 42nd Street
Suite 122
Omaha, NE 68105-2942
402-346-5220
Fax: 402-342-4857
www.olliewebbinc.org/arc/pilot.shtml

Laurie Ackermann, Executive Director
Annie Anderson, Family Services Director
Janet Miler, Program Director
Lisa Dougherty, Human Resource Manager

Parents, professionals and others concerned with providing emotional and peer support to new parents of children with special needs. Sponsors a parent-matching program which allows parents who have had sufficient experience and training.

1568 Research and Training Center for Children's Mental Health
University of South Florida
13301 Bruce B Downs Blvd.
Tampa, FL 33612-3807
813-974-4661
Fax: 813-974-6257
www.http://rtckids.fmhi.usf.edu/

Robert M Friedman, Ph.D., Center Director
Albert Duchnowski, PhD, Deputy Director
Krista Kutash, Ph.D., Deputy Director

Initiated to address the need of improved services and outcomes for children with serious emotional/behavioral disabilities and their families. Conducting research, synthesizing and sharing existing knowledge, provided training and consultation, and serving as a resource for other researchers, policy makers, administrators in the public system, and organizations representing parents, consumers, advocates, professional societies, and practitioners.

Year Founded: 1984

1569 Research and Training Center on Family Support and Children's Mental Health
Portland State University/Regional Research Institute
PO Box 751
Portland State University
Portland, OR 97207-751
503-725-4040
Fax: 503-725-4180

E-mail: rtcpubs@pdx.edu
www.rtc.pdx.edu

Nicole Ave, Public Information/Outreach
Janet Walker, Director of Research

Dedicated to promoting effective community based, culturally competent, family centered services for families and their children who are or may be affected by mental, emotional or behavioral disorders. This goal is accomplished through collaborative research partnerships with family members, service providers, policy makers, and other concerned persons. Major efforts in dissemination and training include: An annual conference, an award winning web site to share information about child and family mental services and policy issues which includes Focal Point, a national bulletin regarding family support and children's mental health.

1570 Resources for Children with Special Needs
116 East 16th Street
5th Floor
New York, NY 10003-2164
212-677-4650
Fax: 212-254-4070
E-mail: info@resourcesnyc.org
www.resourcesnyc.org

Ellen Miller-Wachtel, Chair
Shon E Glusky, President
Rachel Howard, Executive Director
Stephen Stern, Director of Finance and Administ

New York City's only independent nonprofit organization that works for families and children with all special needs, across all boroughs, to understand, navigate, and access the services needed to ensure that all children have the opportunity to develop their full potential. RCSN serves families of children and young adults with all special needs- social, cognitive, physical, and behavioral- with a focus on the city's highest-needs families and communities, and the organizations that serve them.

Year Founded: 1983

1571 The Center for Family Support
2811 Zulette Avenue
Bronx, NY 10461
718-518-1500
Fax: 718-518-8200
E-mail: svernikoff@cfsny.org
www.cfsny.org

Steven Vernikoff, Executive Director
Virgil Seepersad, Director of Finance
Eileen Berg, Director of Quality Assurance
Barbara Greenwald, Associate Executive, Director

A not for profit human service agency that provides individualized support services and programs for individuals living with developmental disabilities, and for the families that care for them.

Year Founded: 1954

1572 Young Adult Institute and Workshop (YAI)
460 W 34th Street
New York, NY 10001-2382
212-273-6100
www.yai.org

Matthew Sturiale, L.C.S.W., Chief Executive Officer
Marco Damiani, M.A., Executive Vice President, Innova

Sanjay Dutt, Chief Financial Officer
Roberta G Koenigsberg, J.D., Chief Compliance Officer

Serves more than 15, 000 people of all ages and levels of mental retardation, developmental and learning disabilities. Provides a full range of early intervention, preschool, family supports, employment training and placement, clinical and residential service.

Year Founded: 1957

1573 Youth Services International
6000 Cattleridge Drive
Suite 200
Sarasota, FL 34232-6064
941-953-9199
Fax: 941-953-9198
E-mail: YSIWEB@youthservices.com
www.ysii.com

Premier provider in the Youth Care Industry of educational and developmental services that change, dramatically, the thinking and behavior of troubled youth. Offering the most comprehensive programs and services available to government agencies serving at-risk youth. YSI has been recognized for its dynamic approach to rehabilitating juveniles through integrated programs, staff mentoring and environments to promote learning and change.

1574 ZERO TO THREE: National Center for Infants, Toddlers, and Families
1255 23rd Street, NorthWest
Suite 350
Washington, DC 20037
202-638-1144
800-899-4301
Fax: 202-638-0851
E-mail: oto3@presswarehouse.com
www.zerotothree.org

Ann Pleshette Murphy, President
Matthew E. Melmet, JD, Executive Director
Ross Thompson, PhD, Vice President
Laura Shiflett, Chief Financial and Administrati

A national, nonprofit organization that informs, trains, and supports professionals, policymakers, and parents in their efforts to improve the lives of infants and toddlers. Mission is to promote the health and development of infants and toddlers.

Books

1575 After School and More
Resources for Children with Special Needs
116 East 16th Street
5th Floor
New York, NY 10003-2164
212-677-4650
Fax: 212-254-4070
E-mail: info@resourcenyc.org
www.resourcesnyc.org

Ellen Miller-Wachtel, Chair
Shon E Glusky, President
Rachel Howard, Executive Director
Stephen Stern, Director of Finance and Administ

The most complete directory of after school programs for children with disabilities and special needs in the metropolitan New York area focusing on weekend and holiday programs. *$15.00*

252 pages Year Founded: 1983 ISBN 0-967836-57-3

1576 Aggression Replacement Training: A Comprehensive Intervention for Aggressive Youth
Research Press
PO Box-7886
Champaign, IL 61826
217-352-3273
800-519-2707
Fax: 217-352-1221
E-mail: rp@researchpress.com
www.researchpress.com

Dr Barry Glick, Author
Dr John C Gibbs, Author

Aggression Replacement Training (ART) offers a comprehensive intervention program designed to teach adolescents to understand and replace aggression and antisocial behavior with positive alternatives. The book is designed to be user-friendly and teacher-oriented. It contains summaries of ART's outcome evaluations and it discusses recent applications in schools and other settings. *$24.95*

426 pages Year Founded: 1968 ISBN 0-878223-79-7

1577 Bibliotherapy Starter Set
The Guidance Group
303 Crossways Park Dr
Woodbury, NY 11797-2099
800-962-1141
Fax: 800-262-1886
E-mail: info@Childswork.com
www.Childswork.com

Beth Ann Marcozzi, Author

Eight popular books for helping children ages four - twelve. Titles include Self Esteem, Divorce, ADHD, Feelings, and Anger. *$105.00*

1578 Book of Psychotherapeutic Homework
Childs Work/Childs Play
303 Crossways Park Dr
Woodbury, NY 11797-2099
800-962-1141
Fax: 800-262-1886
E-mail: info@Childswork.com
www.Childswork.com

Lawrence E Shapiro, Author

More than 80 home activities to guarantee your therapy won't lose momentum. Appropriate for ages five - ten. *$20.95*

Year Founded: 2001 ISBN 1-882732-55-3

1579 Breaking the Silence: Teaching the Next Generation About Mental Illness
NAMI Queens/Nassau
1981 Marcus Avenue
Suite C-117
Lake Success, NY 11042
516-326-0797
Fax: 516-437-5785
E-mail: btslessonplans@aol.com
www.www.btslessonplans.org/

Janet Susin, Author
Lorraine Kaplan, Author
Louise Slater, Author

Breaking the Silence (BTS) is an innovative teaching package which includes lesson plans, games and posters on serious mental illness for three grade levels: upper elementary, middle and high school. It is designed to fight stigma by putting a human face on mental illness, replacing fear and ridicule with compassion. BTS meets national health standards.

1580 CARE Child and Adolescent Risk Evaluation: A Measure of the Risk for Violent Behavior
Research Press
Dept 24 W
PO Box 9177
Champaign, IL 61826-9177
217-352-3273
800-519-2707
Fax: 217-352-1221
E-mail: rp@researchpress.com
www.researchpress.com

Dr Kathryn Siefert, Author

The CARE was developed as a prevention tool to identify youth, as early as possible, who are at risk for committing acts of violence. Unlike other evaluation programs, CARE includes a case management planning form that provides the information needed to develop a risk management intervention plan. The CARE Kit includes 25 assessment forms, 25 case management planning forms and manual. *$75.00*

50 pages

1581 Camps 2009-2010
Resources for Children with Special Needs
116 E 16th Street
5th Floor
New York, NY 10003-2164
212-677-4650
Fax: 212-254-4070
E-mail: info@resourcenyc.org
www.resourcesnyc.org

Rachel Howard, Executive Director

The guide includes a dozen new camps and updates on more than 300 camps and programs that provide a wide range of summer activities for children with emotional, developmental, learning and physical disabilities, health issues and other special needs. Day camps in the New York metro area are included as well as sleepaway camps in the Northeast. *$25.00*

133 pages Year Founded: 2009 ISBN 0-967836-57-3

1582 Children and Trauma: A Guide for Parents and Professionals
Courage to Change
303 Crossways Park Drive
Woodbury, NY 11797
800-440-4003
Fax: 800-772-6499
www.couragetochange.com

Cynthia Monahon, Author

Teaches parents and professionals about the effects of such ordeals on children and offers a blueprint for restoring a child's sense of safety and balance. Offers hope and reassurance for parents. The author suggests straightforward ways to help kids through tough times, and also describes in detail the warning signs that indicate a child needs professional help. Monahon helps adults understand psychological trauma from a child's point of view and explores the

ways both parents and professionals can help children heal. *$19.95*

240 pages Year Founded: 1997 ISBN 0-787910-71-6

1583 Children in Therapy: Using the Family as a Resource
WW Norton & Company
500 5th Avenue
New York, NY 10110-54
212-354-2907
800-233-4830
Fax: 212-869-0856
E-mail: npb@wwnorton.com
www.wwnorton.com

Drake McFeely, CEO

This anthology presents theoretical perspectives of five different competency-based approaches: solution-oriented brief therapy, narrative therapy, collaborative language systems therapy, internal family systems therapy, and emotionally focused family therapy.

ISBN 0-393704-85-8

1584 Childs Work/Childs Play
303 Crossways Park Dr
Woodbury, NY 11797-2099
800-962-1141
Fax: 800-262-1886
E-mail: info@Childswork.com
www.Childswork.com

Catalog of books, games, toys and workbooks relating to child development issues such as recognizing emotions, handling uncertainty, bullies, ADD, shyness, conflicts and other things that children may need some help navigating.

1585 Creative Therapy with Children & Adolescents
Impact Publishers
PO Box 6016
Atascadero, CA 93423-6016
805-466-5917
800-246-7228
Fax: 805-466-5919
E-mail: info@impactpublishers.com
www.impactpublishers.com

Angela Hobday, M.Sc, Author
Kate Ollier, M.Psych, Author

Over 100 activities that can be used in working with children, adolescents, and families. Encourages creativity in therapy and assists therapists in talking with children to facilitate change. From simple ideas to fresh innovations, the activities are designed to be used as tools to supplement a variety of therapeutic approaches, and can be tailored to each child's needs. Therapists will find practical help in gaining rapport with clients who find it difficult to talk about feelings and experiences. Each activity is categorized according to the child's needs or the purpose of the activity, and cross-referenced by problem, activity, and by the features of each game/exercise. *$21.95*

192 pages Year Founded: 1970 ISBN 1-886230-19-6

1586 Don't Feed the Monster on Tuesdays!: The Children's Self-Esteem Book
ADD WareHouse
300 NorthWest 70th Avenue
Suite 102
Plantation, FL 33317-2360

954-792-8944
800-233-9273
Fax: 954-792-8545
E-mail: websales@addwarehouse.com
www.addwarehouse.com

Adolph J. Moser, Author
Nancy R. Thatch, Editor
David Melton, Illustrator

Strikes right at the heart of the basic elements of self-esteem. It presents valuable information to children that will help them understand the importance of their self worth. A friendly book that children ages 4 to 10 will love. *$18.95*

55 pages Year Founded: 1990 ISBN 0-933849-38-9

1587 Don't Pop Your Cork on Mondays: The Children's Anti-Stress Book
ADD WareHouse
300 NorthWest 70th Avenue
Suite 102
Plantation, FL 33317-2360
954-792-8944
800-233-9273
Fax: 954-792-8545
E-mail: websales@addwarehouse.com
www.addwarehouse.com

Adolph J. Moser, Author
Dav Pilkey, Illustrator

In this very informative and highly entertaining handbook for children, Dr. Adolph Moser offers practical approaches and effective techniques to help young people deal with stress. *$18.95*

48 pages Year Founded: 1990 ISBN 0-933849-18-4

1588 Don't Rant and Rave on Wednesdays: The Children's Anger-Control Book
ADD WareHouse
300 NorthWest 70th Avenue
Suite 102
Plantation, FL 33317-2360
954-792-8944
800-233-9273
Fax: 954-792-8545
E-mail: websales@addwarehouse.com
www.addwarehouse.com

Adolph Moser, Author
Nancy R. Thatch, Editor
David Melton, Illustrator

This book will delight both children and adults. It's informative and it's fun because Dr. Moser examines the complex feelings of human anger with the proper blend of sensitivity and humor. And David Melton's colorful illustrations are bright and witty. *$18.95*

61 pages Year Founded: 1990 ISBN 0-933849-54-0

1589 Essentials of Lewis's Child and Adolescent Psychiatry
Lippincott Williams & Wilkins
333 Seventh Avenue
19th & 20th Floors
New York, NY 10001
301-223-2300
800-933-6525
www.lww.com

Fred R. Volkmar, Author
Andres Martin, MD MPH, Author

Companion guide to: Lewis's child and adolescent psychiatry.

432 pages Year Founded: 1998 ISBN 0-781775-02-7

1590 Forms for Behavior Analysis with Children
Research Press
Dept 12W
PO Box 9177
Champaign, IL 61826-9177
217-352-3273
800-519-2707
Fax: 217-352-1221
E-mail: rp@researchpress.com
www.researchpress.com

Joseph R. Cautela, Author
Julie Cautela, Author
Sharon Esonis, Author

A unique collection of 42 reproducible assessment forms designed to aid counselors and therapists in making proper diagnoses and in developing treatment plans for children and adolescents. Different assessment formats are included, ranging from direct observations and interviews to informant ratings and self-reports. Certain forms are to be filled out by children and adolescents, while others are to be completed by parents, school personnel, significant others or the therapist. *$ 39.95*

208 pages ISBN 0-878222-67-7

1591 Forms-5 Book Set
Childs Work/Childs Play
303 Crossways Park Dr
Woodbury, NY 11797-2099
800-962-1141
Fax: 800-262-1886
E-mail: info@Childswork.com
www.Childswork.com

Five-book pack with reproducible forms titled: Oppositional Child, Children with OCD, Counseling Children, ADHD Child and Socially Fearful Child. *$125.00*

1592 Handbook of Infant Mental Health 3rd Edition
The Guilford Press
72 Spring Street
New York, NY 10012
800-365-7006
Fax: 212-966-6708
E-mail: info@guilford.com
www.guilford.com

Charles H. Zeanah Jr., MD, Editor

Widely regarded as the standard reference in the field, this state-of-the-art handbook offers a comprehensive analysis of developmental, clinical, and social aspects of mental health from birth to the preschool years. Leading authorities explore models of development; biological, family, and sociocultural risk and protective factors; and frequently encountered disorders and disabilities. Evidence-based approaches to assessment and treatment are presented, with an emphasis on ways to support strong parent-child relationships. The volume reviews the well-documented benefits of early intervention and prevention and describes applications in mental health, primary care, childcare, and child welfare settings.

622 pages Year Founded: 1973 ISBN 1-606233-15-7

1593 I Wish Daddy Didn't Drink So Much
Childs Work/Childs Play
303 Crossways Park Dr
Woodbury, NY 11797-2099
800-962-1141
Fax: 800-262-1886
E-mail: info@Childswork.com
www.Childswork.com

Judith Vigna, Author

A young girl shares her feelings and frustrations about her alcoholic father's behavior. *$6.95*

32 pages ISBN 0-807535-26-5

1594 I'm Somebody, Too!
ADD WareHouse
300 NW 70th Avenue
Suite 102
Plantation, FL 33317-2360
954-792-8944
800-233-9273
Fax: 954-792-8545
E-mail: sales@addwarehouse.com
www.addwarehouse.com

Harvey C Parker, Owner

When her brother responds to therapy for ADD, Emily no longer knows what her family role should be. *$13.00*

159 pages

1595 Kid Power Tactics for Dealing with Depression
Childswork/Childsplay
303 Crossways Park Drive
Woodbury, NY 11797
800-962-1141

Nicholas Dubuque, Author
Susan Dubuque, Author

Written by an 11 year-old boy with depression and his mother, inclues 15 strategies to deal with depression. *$12.95*

47 pages Year Founded: 1996 ISBN 1-882732-48-0

1596 Lewis's Child and Adolescent Psychiatry: A Comprehensive Textbook, 4th Edition
Lippincott Williams & Wilkins
333 Seventh Avenue
19th & 20th Floors
New York, NY 10001
301-223-2300
800-933-6525
www.lww.com

Fred R. Volkmar, Editor
Andres Martin, Editor

Established for fifteen years as the standard work in the field, this classic text emphasizes the relationship between basic science and clinical research and integrates scientific principles with the realities of drug interactions. Companion website provides instant access to the complete, fully searchable text.

1088 pages Year Founded: 1998 ISBN 0-781762-14-6

1597 My Body is Mine, My Feelings are Mine
Childs Work/Childs Play
303 Crossways Park Dr
Woodbury, NY 11797-2099

800-962-1141
Fax: 800-262-1886
E-mail: info@Childswork.com
www.Childswork.com

Susan Hoke, LCSW, ACSW, Author
Bruce Van Patter, Illustrator
Charles Brenna, Designer

For ages 3 - 8. First part to be read to children, the second part teaches adults how to educate children about body safety. Sexual victimization can be prevented through explanation of how to identify inappropriate touching and what to do about it. *$20.95*

78 pages Year Founded: 1995 ISBN 1-882732-24-3

1598 My Listening Friend: A Story About the Benefits of Counseling
Childs Work/Childs Play
303 Crossways Park Dr
Woodbury, NY 11797-2099
800-962-1141
Fax: 800-262-1886
E-mail: info@Childswork.com
www.Childswork.com

P J Michaels, Author
Anna Dewdney, Illustrator

For ages five - twelve, explores the feelings a child has the first time they see a counselor. Written from the point of view of the child. *$14.50*

57 pages Year Founded: 2001 ISBN 1-588150-43-7

1599 Neurodevelopmental Disabilities: Clinical Care for Children and Young Adults
Springer
11 West 42nd Street
15th Floor
New York, NY 10036
212-431-4370
877-687-7476
Fax: 212-941-7842
E-mail: cs@springerpub.com
www.springerpub.com

Dilip R. Patel, Editor
Donald E. Greydanus, Editor
Hatim A. Omar, Editor
Joav Merrick, Editor

Increasingly more and more children with developmental disabilities survive into adulthood. Pediatricians and other clinicians are called upon to care for an increasing number of children with developmental disabilities in their practice and thus there is a need for a practical guide specifically written for pediatricians and primary care clinicians that addresses major concepts of neurodevelopmental pediatrics.

350 pages Year Founded: 1950 ISBN 9-400706-26-X

1600 Preventing Maladjustment from Infancy Through Adolescence
Sage Publications
2455 Teller Road
Thousand Oaks, CA 91320-2234
805-499-0721
800-818-7243
Fax: 800-583-2665
E-mail: info@sagepub.com
www.sagepub.com

Annette U Rickel, Author
Larue Allen, Author

Authoritative and thoroughly researched, this book examines the theoretical and historical issues of prevention with children and youth, and delineates those factors which place the individual at risk. It will serve as an excellent text for advanced level undergraduate and graduate courses courses dealing with preventive interventions for infants, children, and adolescents.

160 pages Year Founded: 1987 ISBN 0-803928-68-8

1601 Psychotherapy with Infants and Young Children: Repairing the Effects of Stress and Trauma on Early Attachement
The Guilford Press
72 Spring Street
New York, NY 10012
800-365-7006
Fax: 212-966-6708
E-mail: info@guilford.com
www.guilford.com

Alicia F. Lieberman, PhD, Author
Patricia Van Horn, PhD, Author

This eloquent book presents an empirically supported treatment that engages parents as the most powerful agents of their young children's healthy development. The book provides a comprehensive theoretical framework together with practical strategies for combining play, developmental guidance, trauma-focused interventions, and concrete assistance with problems of living. It is grounded in extensive clinical experience and important research on early development, attachment, neurobiology, and trauma.

366 pages Year Founded: 1973 ISBN 1-609182-40-5

1602 Saddest Time
Childs Work/Childs Play
303 Crossways Park Dr
Woodbury, NY 11797-2099
800-962-1141
Fax: 800-262-1886
E-mail: info@Childswork.com
www.Childswork.com

Norma Simon, Author

Helps children ages 6 - 12 understand that death is sad and sometimes tragic, but it is also part of life. *$13.95*

Year Founded: 1999 ISBN 0-613141-80-6

1603 Schools for Students with Special Needs
Resources for Children with Special Needs
116 E 16th Street
Fifth Floor
New York City, NY 10003-2112
212-677-4650
Fax: 212-254-4070
E-mail: info@resourcesnyc.org
www.resourcesnyc.org

Rachel Howard, Executive Director

The first complete book listing private day and residential schools for parents, caregivers and professionals seeking schools for students 5 and up with developmental, emotional, physical and learning disabilities in the NYC metro area. More than 400 schools and residential programs that serve children in the elementary through high school grades are listed with contact information, ages and populations served, class sizes and student-teacher ratios, special ser-

vices and diplomas offered. Includes a 46-page section of Schools for Children with Autism Spectrum Disorders, as well as a guide with a list of websites on autism spectrum disorders. *$25.00*

342 pages

1604 Teen Relationship Workbook
Childs Work/Childs Play
303 Crossways Park Dr
Woodbury, NY 11797-2099
516-349-5520
800-962-1141
Fax: 800-262-1886
E-mail: info@childswork.com
www.childswork.com

Kerry Moles, Author
Amy L Leutenberg-Brodsky, Illustrator

A reproducible workbook, this hands-on tool helps teens develop healthy relationships and prevent dating abuse and domestic violence. *$44.95*

135 pages

1605 Thirteen Steps to Help Families Stop Fighting Solve Problems Peacefully
Childs Work/Childs Play
303 Crossways Park Dr
Woodbury, NY 11797-2099
800-962-1141
Fax: 800-262-1886
E-mail: info@Childswork.com
www.Childswork.com

Sharon Hernes Silverman, Author

Candid views on why families fight, and solutions to conflict. *$15.95*

Year Founded: 2001 ISBN 1-882732-77-4

1606 What Works When with Children and Adolescents: A Handbook of Individual Counseling Techniques
Research Press
PO Box-7886
Champaign, IL 61826
217-352-3273
800-519-2707
Fax: 217-352-1221
E-mail: rp@researchpress.com
www.researchpress.com

Dr Ann Vernon, Author

This practical handbook is designed for counselors, social workers and psychologists in schools and mental health settings. It offers over 100 creative activities and effective interventions for individual counseling with children and adolescents (ages 6-18). Dr. Vernon provides strategies for establishing a therapeutic relationship with students who are sometimes apprehensive or opposed to counseling. Several case studies are included to help illustrate the counseling techniques and interventions. The book also includes a chapter on working with parents and teachers. *$39.95*

384 pages Year Founded: 1968 ISBN 0-878224-38-6

Periodicals & Pamphlets

1607 Helping Hand
Performance Resource Press
1270 Rankin Drive
Suite F
Troy, MI 48083-2843
248-588-7733
800-453-7733
Fax: 248-588-6633
www.store.amplifiedlifenetwork.com

Lyle Labardee, MS, LPC, NCC, President

A newsletter on child and adult behavioral health.

4 pages 9 per year

1608 Treatment of Children with Mental Disorders
National Institute of Mental Health
6001 Executive Boulevard
Room 8184, MSC 9663
Bethesda, MD 20892-9663
301-443-4513
866-615-6464
TTY: 301-443-8431
E-mail: nimhinfo@nih.gov
www.www.nimh.nih.gov/

Ruth Dubois, Assistant Chief

A booklet with answers to frequently asked questions about the treatment of mental disorders in children, includes a medications chart.

Research Centers

1609 Child Neurology and Developmental Center
1510 Jericho Turnpike
New Hyde Park, NY 11040
516-352-2500
Fax: 516-352-2573
www.childbrain.com

Rami Grossmann, M.D.

Pediatric neurology practice of Rami Grossmann, M.D. in New York. Neurologists are highly trained to treat disorders of the nervous system. This includes diseases of the brain, spinal cord, nerves, and muscles. Common problems that Dr. Grossmann diagnoses and treats include the following: AD/HD, Autism, a form of PDD, Developmental delays, Epilepsy, Headaches, Learning difficulties, and Tic Disorders.

1610 KidsHealth
The Nemours Foundation
10140 Centurion Parkway
Jacksonville, FL 32256
904-697-4100
Fax: 904-697-4220
E-mail: comments@KidsHealth.org
www.kidshealth.org

Alfred I. duPont, Nemour's Foundation Creator
Neil Izenberg, MD, Editor-in-Chief & Founder

KidsHealth is more than just the facts about health. As part of The Nemours Foundation's Center for Children's Health Media, KidsHealth also provides families with perspective, advice, and comfort about a wide range of physical, emotional, and behavioral issues that affect children and teens. The Nemours Center for Children's Health Media is a part of The Nemours Foundation, a nonprofit organization cre-

ated by philanthropist Alfred I. duPont in 1936 and devoted to improving the health of children.

Year Founded: 1936

Support Groups & Hot Lines

1611 Alateen and Al-Anon Family Groups
1600 Corporate Landing Parkway
Virginia Beach, VA 23454-5617
757-563-1600
888-425-2666
Fax: 757-563-1655
E-mail: wso@al-anon.org
www.al-anon.alateen.org

Mary Ann Keller, Director Members Services

Strength and hope for friends and families of problem drinkers.

1612 Girls and Boys Town of New York
281 Park Avenue South
5th Floor
New York, NY 10010
212-725-4260
800-448-3000
Fax: 212-725-4385
www.www.boystown.org

Guy Cleveland, Chairman
John C. Scott, Ph.D., Board Secretary
Jennifer Armstrong, Senior Vice President of New Pro
Crystal Denunzio, Vice President of Business Devel

Crisis intervention and referrals.

Year Founded: 1990

1613 Kidspeace National Centers
4085 Independence Drive
Schnecksville, PA 18078
800-257-3223
Fax: 610-391-8280
E-mail: kpinfo@kidspeace.org.
www.kidspeace.org

Mary Jane Willis, Chairman
William R Isemann, President & CEO
James Horan, Executive VP, CFO, Treasurer
Michael Slack, EVP, Business Development

Mission is to give hope, help and healing to children, families and communities. Helping people in need overcome challenges and transform their lives by providing emotional and physical healthcare and educational services in an atmosphere of teamwork, compassion and creativity.

1614 National Youth Crisis Hotline
5331 Mount Alifan Drive
San Diego, CA 92111-2622
800-448-4663
www.1800hithome.com/

Information and referral for runaways, and for youth and parents with problems.

1615 One Place for Special Needs
One Place for Special Needs, Ltd.
PO Box 9701
Naperville, IL 60567
E-mail: info@oneplaceforspecialneeds.com
www.oneplaceforspecialneeds.com

Dawn Villarreal, Founder

An information network and social community that allows the disability community to share resources and make connections in their own neighborhood. And a place where those who actively work with those who have disabilities can let families learn about their products, program and services.

Year Founded: 2002

1616 Rainbows

1360 Hamilton Parkway
Itasca, IL 60143
847-952-1770
800-266-3206
Fax: 847-952-1774
E-mail: info@rainbows.org
www.rainbows.org

Anthony Taglia, Chair
Bob Thomas, Executive Director and CEO
Burt Heatherly, CFO

The largest international children's charity dedicated solely to helping youth successfully navigate the very difficult grief process. Every day, children are touched by emotional suffering caused by a death, divorce, deployment of a family member, incarceration of a loved one, or any of a multitude of significant event traumas including natural or manmade disasters.

Year Founded: 1983

1617 SADD: Students Against Destructive Decisions

255 Main Street
Marlborough, MA 01752-5505
508-481-3568
877-723-3462
Fax: 508-481-5759
E-mail: info@sadd.org
www.sadd.org

Danna Mauch, PhD, Chairman
Penny Wells, President and CEO
Susan Scarola, Treasurer
James E Champagne, Secretary/Clerk

Providing students with the best prevention tools possible to deal with the issues of underage drinking, other drug use, risky and impaired driving, and other destructive decisions.

Year Founded: 1981

Video & Audio

1618 Aggression Replacement Training Video: A Comprehensive Intervention for Aggressive Youth
Research Press
PO Box 7886
PO Box 9177
Champaign, IL 61826
217-352-3273
800-519-2707
Fax: 217-352-1221
E-mail: rp@researchpress.com
www.researchpress.com

This staff training DVD features scenes of adolescents participating in group sessions for each of ART's three interventions. Viewers will see a prosocial skills training group, an anger management session, and a moral reasoning group. *$125.00*

ISBN 0-878225-91-0

1619 Anger Management-Enhanced Edition
Educational Video Network, Inc.
1401 19th Street
Huntsville, TX 77340
936-295-5767
800-762-0060
Fax: 936-294-0233
www.www.evndirect.com

Learn what causes anger and understand why our bodies react as they do when we're angry. Effective techniques for assuaging anger are discussed.

1620 Are the Kids Alright?
Fanlight Productions
32 Court Street
21st Floor
Brooklyn, NY 11201
718-488-8900
800-876-1710
Fax: 718-488-8642
E-mail: orders@fanlight.com
www.fanlight.com

Karen Bernstein, Author
Ellen Spiro, Author

Filmed in courtrooms, correctional institutions, treatment centers, and family homes, this searing documentary documents the results of the tragic decline in mental health services for children and adolescents at risk.

1621 Bipolar Disorder: Shifting Mood Swings
Educational Training Videos
136 Granville St
Suite 200
Gahanna, OH 43230
Fax: 888-775-3919
www.educationaltrainingvideos.com

Different from the routine ups and downs of life, the symptoms of bipolar disorder are severe - even to the point of being life-threatening. In this insightful program, patients speak from their own experience about the complexities of diagnosis and the very real danger of suicide, while family members and close friends address the strain of the condition's cyclic behavior.

1622 Bipolar Focus, Bipolar Disorder Audio and Video Files: Bipolar and Children/Adolescents
Bipolar Focus
www.pendulum.org/video/videospecial.htm

Website with list of playable video and audio files on topics including: children and mental health, antipsychotics in special populations: pediatrics and adolescents, mental health in childre, parts I and II, mental health and illness in teenagers, adult minds- mental health in early adulthood, college students and mental health, and pregnancy and the mind.

1623 Case Studies in Childhood Obsessive-Compulsive Disorder
Educational Training Videos
136 Granville St
Suite 200
Gahanna, OH 43230
Fax: 888-775-3919
www.educationaltrainingvideos.com

This edition of Primetime tracks the treatment of Bridget, Rocco, and Michelle as they attempt to reclaim their lives and overcome the stigma associated with the disorder. Original ABC News broadcast title: Kids Battle Obsessive-Compulsive Disorder.

1624 Children: Experts on Divorce
Courage to Change
1 Huntington Quadrangle
Suite: 1N03
Melville, NY 11747
800-962-1141
Fax: 800-262-1886
www.couragetochange.com/

Dede L Pitts, CEO

This DVD should be played for divorcing parents in your waiting room or client library. Children, ages 5-17, speak of what they need from their parents, what helps and what hurts. Judges, mediators, therapists and Karl Malone also appear on camera. DVD makes parents more ready to collaborate and make agreements that will benefit their children. Have a box of tissues handy. *$34.95*

1625 Chill: Straight Talk About Stress
Childs Work/Childs Play
303 Crossways Park Dr
Woodbury, NY 11797-2099
800-962-1141
Fax: 800-262-1886
E-mail: info@Childswork.com
www.Childswork.com

Encourages youth to recognize, analyze and handle the stresses in their lives. 22 minutes. *$96.95*

1626 Clinical Impressions: Identifying Mental Illness
Educational Training Videos
136 Granville St
Suite 200
Gahanna, OH 43230
Fax: 888-775-3919
www.educationaltrainingvideos.com

How long can mental illness stay hidden, especially from the eyes of trained experts? This program rejoins a group of ten adults- five of them healthy and five of them with histories of mental illness- as psychiatric specialists try to spot and correctly diagnose the latter. Administering a series of collaborative and one-on-one tests, including assessments of personality type, physical self-image, and rational thinking, the panel gradually makes decisions about who suffers from depression, bipolar disorder, bulimia, and social anxiety.

1627 Coping with Emotions
Educational Video Network, Inc.
1401 19th Street
Huntsville, TX 77340
936-295-5767
800-762-0060
Fax: 936-294-0233
www.evndirect.com

Anger, indifference, sadness, confusion and ecstatic happiness are emotions that manifest themselves frequently during the teen years. The hormones that change the body physically also have a great effect on a teenager's emotions. Discover the gamut of emotions that rule a teenager's life and what can be done to control them.

1628 Coping with Stress
Educational Video Network, Inc.
1401 19th Street
Huntsville, TX 77340
936-295-5767
800-762-0060
Fax: 936-294-0233
www.www.evndirect.com

Stress affects everyone, both emotionally and physically. For some, mismanaged stress can result in substance abuse, violence, or even suicide. This program answers the question, How can a person cope with stress?

1629 Dark Voices: Schizophrenia
Educational Training Videos
136 Granville St
Suite 200
Gahanna, OH 43230
Fax: 888-775-3919
www.educationaltrainingvideos.com

This program seeks to understand how schizophrenia touches the lives of patients and their family members while examining the disease's etiology and pathology. A Discovery Channel Production.

1630 Dealing with ADHD: Attention Deficit/ Hyperactivity
Educational Video Network, Inc.
1401 19th Street
Huntsville, TX 77340
936-295-5767
800-762-0060
Fax: 936-294-0233
www.www.evndirect.com

Learn about attention deficit/hyperactivity disorder and learn what factors are thought to contribute to the development of this disorder. Other disorders that commonly co-exist with ADHD will be identified. The impulsivity and risk-taking behaviors of ADHD teens will be focused upon and tips that ADHD students can use to succeed academically will be provided. Laws that require schools to make special accommodations for ADHD students will be reviewed, and viewers will learn how to contact organizations that exist to help people who are dealing with ADHD.

1631 Dealing with Depression
Educational Video Network, Inc.
1401 19th Street
Huntsville, TX 77340
936-295-5767
800-762-0060
Fax: 936-294-0233
www.www.evndirect.com

As more and more young people are falling victim to depression, it is important to understand what causes it and to know how to get the help that can rid a person of this life-wrecking affliction.

1632 Dealing with Grief
Educational Video Network, Inc.
1401 19th Street
Huntsville, TX 77340
936-295-5767
800-762-0060
Fax: 936-294-0233
www.www.evndirect.com

Grief allows us to acknowledge and mourn our losses so we can reconcile our feelings and move forward in life. Learn how to deal with your grief and become a better person for having gone through it.

1633 Dealing with Social Anxiety
Educational Video Network, Inc.
1401 19th Street
Huntsville, TX 77340
936-295-5767
800-762-0060
Fax: 936-294-0233
www.www.evndirect.com

Social anxiety is America's third-largest psychiatric disorder. It generally develops during the mid-teen years, and almost always before the age of 25. Understand what may trigger the development of anxiety and learn how it sometimes evolves into full-blown panic disorder, which is characterized by recurrent attacks of terror or fear. The consequences of social anxiety are examined and effective treatments are discussed.

1634 Don't Kill Yourself: One Survivor's Message
Educational Training Videos
136 Granville St
Suite 200
Gahanna, OH 43230
Fax: 888-775-3919
www.educationaltrainingvideos.com

This is the story of a young man, David, who at 16 years of age survived a suicide attempt. Now 22, he shares the events of his life leading up to the attempt, including how low self-esteem led to drug addiction, and how the addiction encouraged the sense that life was no longer worth living.

1635 Fetal Alcohol Syndrome and Effect DVD
Hazelden
15251 Pleasant Valley Road
PO Box 11
Center City, MN 55012-0011
651-213-4200
800-328-9000
Fax: 651-213-4793
E-mail: info@hazelden.org
www.hazelden.org

Mark Mishek, President and CEO
James A. Blaha, Vice President Finance and Admin
Ann Bray, General Counsel and Vice Preside
Sharon Birnbaum, Corporate Director of Human Reso

Excellent for women in treatment, addiction professionals, and community education programs, the video is centered on the work being done with children affected by fetal alcohol and their families. It provides a factual definition of Fetal Alcohol Syndrome and Effect, explains how children are diagnosed and, most importantly, vividly illustrates the positive prognosis possible for fetal alcohol children. Medical and educational professionals, biological and adoptive parents and siblings, and the children themselves speak in this video about FAS. *$225.00*

Year Founded: 1949

1636 Legacy of Childhood Trauma: Not Always Who They Seem
Research Press
Dept 24 W
PO Box 9177
Champaign, IL 61826-9177
217-352-3273
800-519-2707
Fax: 217-352-1221
E-mail: rp@researchpress.com
www.researchpress.com

Russell Pense, VP Marketing

Focuses on the connection between so-called delinquent youth and the experience of childhood trauma such as emotional, sexual, or physical abuse. The video features the unique stories of four young adults who are survivors of childhood trauma. They candidly discuss their troubled childhood and teenage years and reveal how, with the help of caring adults, they were able to salvage their lives. The caregivers, who helped these young adults through their teenage years, are joined by other helping professionals who provide thorough discussions of diagnosis and treatment issues. They offer valuable guidelines and insights on working with adolescents who have experienced childhood trauma. *$195.00*

1637 Mental Disorder
Educational Training Videos
136 Granville St
Suite 200
Gahanna, OH 43230
Fax: 888-775-3919
www.educationaltrainingvideos.com

What is abnormality? Using the case studies of two young women; one who has depression, one who has an anxiety disorder; as a springboard, this program presents three psychological perspective on mental disorder.

1638 Overcoming Obstacles and Self-Doubt
Educational Video Network, Inc.
1401 19th Street
Huntsville, TX 77340
936-295-5767
800-762-0060
Fax: 936-294-0233
www.www.evndirect.com

When feelings of self-doubt are combined with the sudden appearance of an overwhelming obstacle, the situation can be emotionally crippling.

1639 Suicide among Teens
Educational Video Network, Inc.
1401 19th Street
Huntsville, TX 77340
936-295-5767
800-762-0060
Fax: 936-294-0233
www.www.evndirect.com

Suicide devastates surviving loved ones. Find out why it should never be considered as a solution and learn how to recognize warning signs in a suicidal person.

1640 Teenage Anxiety, Depression, and Suicide
Educational Video Network, Inc.
1401 19th Street
Huntsville, TX 77340

936-295-5767
800-762-0060
Fax: 936-294-0233
www.www.evndirect.com

This program can provide helpful insight to those in need of assistance.

1641 Understanding Mental Illness
Educational Video Network, Inc.
1401 19th Street
Huntsville, TX 77340
936-295-5767
800-762-0060
Fax: 936-294-0233
www.www.evndirect.com

Contains information and classifications of mental illness. Mental illness can strike anyone, at any age. Learn about various organic and functional mental disorders as discussed and their causes and symptoms, and learn where to seek help for a variety of mental health concerns.

1642 Understanding Personality Disorders
Educational Video Network, Inc.
1401 19th Street
Huntsville, TX 77340
936-295-5767
800-762-0060
Fax: 936-294-0233
www.www.evndirect.com

For many people, the onset of a psychological disorder goes undiagnosed and untreated, and, as a result, they face a constant, if not impossible, struggle to maintain good mental health. This can be especially true when individuals suffer from a personality disorder. However, with identification and understanding, crippling personality disorders can be brought out of the shadows of ignorance and into the light of treatment.

1643 Why Isn't My Child Happy? Video Guide About Childhood Depression
ADD WareHouse
300 NW 70th Avenue
Suite 102
Plantation, FL 33317-2360
954-792-8100
800-233-9273
Fax: 954-792-8545
E-mail: sales@addwarehouse.com
www.addwarehouse.com

Sam Goldstein, PhD, Author

The first of its kind, this new video deals with childhood depression. Informative and frank about this common problem, this book offers helpful guidance for parents and professionals trying to better understand childhood depression. 110 minutes. *$55.00*

Year Founded: 1990

Web Sites

1644 www.Al-Anon-Alateen.org
Al-Anon and Alateen

AA literature may serve as an introduction.

1645 www.CHADD.org
CHADD: Children/Adults with Attention Deficit/Hyperactivity Disorder

Offers support for individuals, parents, teachers, professionals, and others.

1646 www.aacap.org
American Academy of Child and Adolescent Psychiatry

Represents over 6, 000 child and adolescent psychiatrists, brochures availible online which provide concise and up-to-date material on issues ranging from children who suffer from depression and teen suicide to stepfamily problems and child sexual abuse.

1647 www.adhdnews.com/Advocate.htm
Advocating for Your Child

1648 www.adhdnews.com/sped.htm
Special Education Rights and Responsibilities

Writing IEP's and TIEPS. Pursuing special education services.

1649 www.couns.uiuc.edu
Self-Help Brochures

Address issues teens deal with.

1650 www.freedomvillageusa.com
Freedom Village USA

Faith-based home for troubled teens.

1651 www.kidshealth.org/kid/feeling/index.html
Dealing with Feelings

Ten readings. Examples are: Why Am I So Sad; Are You Shy; Am I Too Fat or Too Thin; and A Kid's Guide to Divorce.

1652 www.naturalchild.com/home
Natural Child Project

Articles by experts.

1653 www.nichcy.org
National Dissemination Center for Children with Disabilities

Excellent information in English and Spanish.

1654 www.nospank.net
Project NoSpank

Site for those against paddling in schools.

1655 www.oneplaceforspecialneeds.com
One Place for Special Needs, Ltd.

1656 www.parenthood.com
Parenthood.Com

A leading online destination for moms, mothers-to-be, and families.

1657 www.wholefamily.com
About Teens Now

Addresses important issues in teens lives.

1658 www2.mc.duke.edu/pcaad
Duke University's Program in Child and Anxiety
Disorders

Suicide

Introduction

Suicide is an event, not a mental disorder, but it is the lethal consequence of some mental disorders. Suicide involves a complex interaction of psychological, neurological, medical, social, and family factors.

Most professionals distinguish at least two suicide groups: those who actually kill themselves, i.e. completed suicides; and those who attempt it, usually harming themselves, but survive. Those who succeed in killing themselves are nearly always suffering from one or more psychiatric disorders, most commonly depression, often along with alcohol or substance abuse. Some individuals plan suicide very carefully, taking steps to insure that they will not be discovered and rescued, and they use lethal means (shooting themselves, or jumping from high places). Some act impulsively, reacting to a life disappointment by jumping off a nearby bridge. Some suicide attempts or gestures use means that make discovery and rescue probable, and are not likely to be lethal (e.g. taking insufficient pills). Some people make repeated suicide attempts. Unfortunately, recurrent suicidal gestures cannot be dismissed; each unsuccesful attempt increases the likelihood of a completed suicide.

ASSOCIATED FEATURES

Nine of ten suicides are associated with some form of mental disorder, especially Depression, Schizophrenia, Alcohol/Substance Abuse, Bipolar Disorder, and Anxiety Disorders. In addition, Personality Disorders have been diagnosed in one-third to one-half of people who kill themselves. These suicides often occur in younger people who live in an environment where drug and alcohol abuse, as well as violence, are common. The most common personality disorders associated with suicide are Borderline Personality Disorder, Antisocial Personality Disorder, and Narcissistic Personality Disorder. Among people with schizophrenia, especially those suffering from Paranoid Schizophrenia, suicide is the main reason for premature death.

Drug and alcohol abuse is risk factor for suicide. In a recent study among 113 young people who killed themselves in California, fifty-five percent had some kind of substance abuse problems, usually long-standing and including several different drugs.

Some suicides result from insufficiently treated, severe, debilitating, or terminal physical illness. The pain, restricted function, and dread of dependence can all contribute to suicidal behavior, especially in illnesses such as Huntington's Disease, cancer, MS, spinal cord injuries and AIDS. Some or many of these risk factors are present in most completed suicides. Depression and suicide are not inevitable for people with severe general medical diagnoses. The recognition and treatment of depression, when it does occur, can prevent many suicides.

PREVALENCE

Suicide is the ninth leading cause of death in the United States and the third leading cause among 15-24 year-olds. It is estimated that over five million people have suicidal thoughts, though there are only 30, 000 deaths from it each year. This may be a serious underestimate, however, since suicide is still stigmatized and often goes unreported. In the general population there are 11.2 suicides reported for every 100, 000 people. The incidence among 5-14 year-olds is 0.7 percent per 100, 000; even very young children can commit suicide. The rate among 15-19 year-olds, 13.2 percent per 100, 000, has recently increased sharply. Boys are more likely to complete suicide than girls, largely because they use more lethal means, such as firearms. Compared to other countries, guns are particularly common in the U.S. as a means of suicide. Children who kill themselves often have a history of antisocial behavior, and depression and suicide is more common in their families than in families in general.

More males than females commit suicide, both among adults and adolescents. Among adults, the most likely suicides are among men who are widowed, divorced, or single, who lack social support, who are unemployed, who have a diagnosed mental disorder (especially Depression), who have a physical illness, a family history of suicide, who are in psychological turmoil, who have made previous attempts, who use or abuse alcohol, and/or who have easy access to firearms. Among adolescents, the most likely suicides are married males (or unwed and pregnant females), who have suffered from parental abuse or absence, who have academic problems, affect disorders (especially Bipolar Disorder), who are substance abusers, suffer from AD/HD or epilepsy, who have Conduct Disorder, problems with impulse control, a family history of suicide, and/or access to firearms. Keeping guns in the home is a suicide risk for both males and females.

Elderly people (those over age 65) are more likely than any other age group to commit suicide. While only twelve percent of the population is elderly, twenty percent of all those who kill themselve are elderly. As in other population groups, elderly men are more likely to kill themselves than elderly woman but the difference between the sexes is much bigger in this age group than in other age groups. Among all ages, the rate of suicide for men is about 20 per 100, 000 and for women five per 100, 000. Among the elderly, the rate for men is about 42 per 100, 000 and for women about six and one-half per 100, 000. Thus the great overall gender differences become even bigger among the elderly and more so as the elderly get older. The highest rate of suicide is among elderly white men, probably because their economic and social status drops severely with age, and because they may lack good social support systems and be reluctant to ask for help.

Although all the factors discussed here are risk factors, it should be kept in mind that 99.9 percent of those at risk do not commit suicide.

TREATMENT OPTIONS

Considering the risk factors, a professional must first make a careful assessment, taking all the risk factors into account, including the availabilty of weapons, pill and other lethal means, as well as whether or not the person has conveyed the intention to commit suicide, and whether the method the patient plans to use is available (one can only jump off a bridge if there is a bridge, or drive into a wall if one has access to a vehicle). Every individual who feels that life is not worth living, or who is contemplating suicide, should be asked about guns in the home and should be encouraged to remove them. The same is true for medications that are dangerous in overdose.

Someone who has no thought of death or has thoughts of death that are not connected with suicide is at a lower risk than someone who is thinking about suicide. Among those who are thinking of it, those who have not worked out the means of committing suicide are at a lower risk than those who have thought of a specific method of carrying it out. Treatment is partly based on the level of intervention that is believed to be required. If the person is seriously depressed and is also anxious, tense and angry, and in overwhelming psychological anguish, the risk is more acute. The first priority is to ensure the safety of the client. To that end, hospitalization may be necessary.

After safety is assured, treatment is aimed at the underlying disorder. It may include psychological support, medication, and other therapies: group, art, dance/movement, music. Professional treatment should involve working with the family when possible, and other medical staff, e.g. a physician, and should include regular reassessments.

In cases of Personality Disorders, there may be anger and aggression, and the suicidal thoughts and ideas may be chronic or repetitive. This is a particular strain on professionals, patients, and family. They all must work together to understand the chronocity of the condition, and the fact that suicide cannot always be prevented. It is essential to develop a working alliance between the therapist and client, based on trust, mutual respect, and on the client's belief that the therapist genuinely cares about him/her. At the same time, the therapist must set limits on patient demands to prevent 'burn out'.

Reassessments include getting information from other professionals involved in treating the patient, including medication with the prescribing physician, and from family members or others significant in the life of the client who should participate in planning and following up. Assessment must also include assessment of the client's ability to understand and participate in the treatment, information about his/her psychological state (hopeless, despairing, depressed) and cognitive competence.

Associations & Agencies

1660 American Association of Suicidology
5221 Wisconsin Avenue NorthWest
Washington, DC 20015
202-237-2280
Fax: 202-237-2282
www.suicidology.org

William Bill Schmitz Jr, PsyD, President
Alan L Berman, PhD, ABPP, Executive Director
Karen Kanefield, Director, Training and Accreditat
Amy Boland, CPA, Treasurer

AAS is a membership organization for all those involved in suicide prevention and intervention, or touched by suicide. AAS is a leader in the advancement of scientific and programmatic efforts in suicide prevention through research, education and training, the development of standards and resources, and survivor support services.

Year Founded: 1968

1661 Break the Silence
821 Landis Street
Scranton, PA 18504

800-784-2433
E-mail: BTSSaveALife@aol.com
www.break-the-silence.org

Denise Burne Fein, President/Founder

A non profit organization whose basis and foundation came from first-hand knowledge and experience that inpatient safety is not always provided to those in need of protection, causing a desperate need for a watch-dog organization like Break the Silence.

Year Founded: 2007

1662 Byron Peter Foundation for Hope
31 Hartfort Pike
No. Scituate, RI 02857
401-647-9295
www.byronpeterfoundation.org

Marilynn Hammond, President and Founder
Seth W Harrington, Vice President
Phoebe M Harrington, Secretary/Treasurer

A non profit foundation formed to honor the life of Byron Peter Harrington II, a young man who tragically took his own life. The Foundation's mission is to inspire troubled young people with hope for a strong future. Striving to provide opportunities of hope for at-risk youth, including those at risk due to depression, illegal drug use, or possible suicide.

1663 Grief Guidance Inc.
PO Box 32789
Palm Beach Gardents, FL 33420-2789
561-625-6751
Fax: 561-625-6751
E-mail: info@griefguidance.com
www.griefguidance.com

Doreen Cammarata, Founder

A company created by Doreen Cammarata to promote intervention services for suicide survivors.

1664 National Alliance on Mental Illness
3803 North Fairfax Drive
Suite 100
Arlington, VA 22203
703-524-7600
800-950-6264
Fax: 703-524-9094
E-mail: helpline@nami.org
www.nami.org

Keris Jan Myrick, MBA, MS, PhD., President
Mary Giliberti, J.D, Executive Director
Jim Payne, J.D, First Vice President
David Levy, Chief Financial Officer

Nation's leading self-help organization for all those affected by severe brain disorders. Mission is to bring consumers and families with similar experiences together to share information about services, care providers, and ways to cope with the challenges of schizophrenia, manic depression, and other serious mental illnesses.

Year Founded: 1969

1665 National Center for the Prevention of Youth Suicide
American Association of Suicidology
5221 Wisconsin Avenue NorthWest
Washington, DC 20015

202-237-2280
Fax: 202-237-2282
E-mail: ajkulp@suicidology.org
www.suicidology.org/ncpys

William Bill Schmitz Jr, PsyD, President
Alan L Berman, PhD, ABPP, Executive Director
Amy Kulp, MS, Director, National Center for Pre
Karen Kanefield, Director, Training and Accreditat

Many youth give warning signs if they are considering taking their lives, and intervening can save their lives. Strong communities, safe schools, and supportive families all help the development of healthy youth. For youth struggling with mental illness and or substance abuse, effective services make a difference. The National Center disseminates the warning signs of suicide through web outreak, partners with other organizations to increase development of best practices in suicide prevention, and developing strategies to move prevention efforts upstream.

Year Founded: 1968

1666 National Organization for People of Color Against Suicide
PO Box 75571
Washington, DC 20001
202-549-6039
800-273-8255
Fax: 866-899-5317
E-mail: info@nopcas.org
www.nopcas.com

Donna Barnes, PhD, CoFounder/President/Executive Di
Doris Smith, CoFounder/Vice President/Treasur
Les Franklin, CoFounder

NOPCAS serves as the only national organization of its kind addressing the issue of suicide prevention and intervention, specifically in communities of color. Primary focus and mission is to increase suicide education and awareness. Offering unique opportunities for outreach partnerships and community education efforts directed at communities of color across the nation.

1667 National P.O.L.I.C.E. Suicide Foundation
7015 Clarke Road
Seaford, DE 19973
302-536-1214
866-276-4615
E-mail: redoug2001@aol.com
www.psf.org

Robert E. Douglas, Jr., Founder and Executive Director
Carolyn Douglas, Administrative Assistant

This foundation provides educational training seminars for emergency responders, primarily associated with law enforcement on the issue of police suicide. Providing police suicide awareness and prevention training programs and support services that will meet the psychological, emotional, and spiritual needs of law enforcement, on every level, and their families.

Year Founded: 1997

1668 SAMHSA'S National Mental Health Information Center
1 Choke Cherry Road
Rockville, MD 20857
877-726-4727
E-mail: ken@mentalhealth.org
www.mentalhealth.samhsa.gov

A Kathryn Power, MEd, Director
Edward B Searle, Deputy Director

1669 Screening for Mental Health, Inc. (SMH)
One Washington Street
Suite 304
Wellesley Hills, MA 02481
781-239-0071
800-273-8255
Fax: 781-431-7447
E-mail: smhinfo@mentalhealthscreening.org
www.mentalhealthscreening.org

Douglas George Jacobs, MD, President & Medical Director
Wilfred Labiosa, Chief Executive Officer
Candice Porter.LICSW, Chief Development Officer
John Della Vecchia, Chief Technology Officer

Dedicated to promoting the improvement of mental health by providing the public with education, screening, and treatment resources. SMH pioneered the concept of large-scale mental health screening and education programs with its flagship program, National Depression Screening Day (NDSD). SMH programs - provided both in person and online - educate, raise awareness, and screen individuals for depression, bipolar disorder, generalized anxiety disorder, post traumatic stress disorder, eating disorders, alcohol use disorders, and suicide.

Year Founded: 1991

1670 Suicide Awareness Voices of Education (SAVE)
8120 Penn Avenue South
Suite 470
Bloomington, MN 55431
952-946-7998
www.save.org

Joseph W. Stackhouse, President
Daniel J Reidenberg, PSY.D, FAPA, Executive Director
Patrick M. Klinger, Vice President
Kevin Rohe, Treasurer

One of the nation's first organizations dedicated to the prevention of suicide and was a co-founding member of the National Council for Suicide Prevention. Leading national non profit organization with staff dedicated to prevent suicide. Based on the foundation and belief that suicide should no longer be considered a hidden or taboo topic and that through raising awareness and educating the public, we can SAVE lives.

Year Founded: 1990

1671 Survivors of Loved Ones' Suicides (SOLOS)
8310 Ewing Halsell Drive
San Antonio, TX 78229
210-885-7069
E-mail: solossanantonio@gmail.com
www.www.solossa.org

Tony Mata, SOLOS Facilitator
Angie Navarette, SOLOS Facilitator

Organization to help provide support for the families and friends who have suffered the suicide loss of a loved one.

Year Founded: 1987

1672 The Jason Foundation, Inc.
18 Volunteer Drive
Hendersonville, TN 37075

615-264-2323
888-881-2323
Fax: 615-264-0188
E-mail: contact@jasonfoundation.com
www.jasonfoundation.com

Clark Flatt, President
Michele Ray, Sr. Vice President/CEO
Deanne Ray, Vice President/COO/Treasurer
Brett Marciel, Director of Publlic Relations an

An educational organization dedicated to the awareness and prevention of youth suicide. JFI believes that awareness and education are the first steps to prevention.

1673 Yellow Ribbon Suicide Prevention Program
Light for Life Foundation International
3790 West 75th Avenue
PO Box 644
Westminster, CO 80036-0644
303-429-3530
Fax: 303-426-4496
E-mail: ask4help@yellowribbon.org
www.yellowribbon.org

Dale Emme, Executive Director
Dar Emme, Deputy Director

Dedicated to preventing suicide and attempts by making suicide prevention accessible to everyone and removing barriers to help by empowering individuals and communities through leadership, awareness and education, and by collaborating and partnering with support networks to reduce stigma and help save lives.

Year Founded: 1994

Books

1674 Adolescent Suicide
American Psychiatric Publishing, Inc.
1000 Wilson Boulevard
Suite 1825
Arlington, VA 22209-3901
703-907-7322
800-368-5777
Fax: 703-907-1091
E-mail: appi@psych.org
www.appi.org

Presents techniques that allow psychiatrists and other professionals to respond to signs of distress with timely therapeutic intervention. It also suggests measures of anticipatory prevention. Adolescent Suicide presents an overview of adolescent suicidal behavior. It explores risk factors, the identification and evaluation of the suicidal adolescent, and approaches to therapy. *$38.95*

210 pages Year Founded: 1996 ISBN 0-873182-08-9

1675 Adolescent Suicide: A School-Based Approach to Assessment and Intervention
Research Press
Dept 12 W
PO Box 9177
Champaign, IL 61826-9177
217-352-3273
800-519-2707
Fax: 217-352-1221
E-mail: rp@researchpress.com
www.researchpress.com

Dr William G Kirk, Author

Presents the information required to accurately identify potentially suicidal adolescents and provides the skills necessary for effective intervention. The book includes many case examples derived from information provided by parents, mental health professionals and educators, as well as adolescents who have considered suicide or survived suicide attempts. An essential resource for school counseling staff, psychologists, teachers and administrators. *$16.95*

175 pages Year Founded: 1993 ISBN 0-878223-36-3

1676 After a Suicide: An Activity Book for Grieving Kids
The Dougy Center
PO Box 86852
Portland, OR 97286
503-775-5683
866-775-5683
E-mail: help@dougy.org
www.dougy.org

In this hands-on, interactive workbook, children who have been exposed to a suicide can learn from other grieving kids. The workbook includes drawing activities, puzzles, stories, advice from other kids and helpful suggestions for how to navigate the grief process after a suicide death.

48 pages Year Founded: 2001 ISBN 1-890534-06-4

1677 Anatomy of Suicide: Silence of the Heart
Charles C Thomas Publisher Ltd.
2600 S First Street
Springfield, IL 62704-4730
217-789-8980
800-258-8980
Fax: 217-789-9130
E-mail: books@ccthomas.com
www.ccthomas.com

Louis Everstine, Author

The author explores the scope of this problem which involves clinical and ethical issues; the myth of depression; the path to suicide; unfinished business; staying alive; early warnings; first interventions; the self-contract; cases in point; and the future of suicide. Written for psychologists, counselors, and mental health professionals, this book is an excellent resource that will further our understanding of suicide and seek new ways for prevention. *$42.95*

153 pages Year Founded: 1998 ISSN 0-398-06803-8ISBN 0-398068-02-X

1678 Exuberance: The Passion for Life
Knopf Publishing Group
1745 Broadway
New York, NY 10019-4343
212-782-9000
Fax: 212-940-7390
E-mail: knopfpublicity@randomhouse.com
www.knopfdoubleday.com

Kay Redfield Jamison, Author

An exploration of exuberance and how it fuels our most important creative and scientific achievements. In a fascinating and intimate coda to the rest of the book, renowned scientists, writers, and politicians share their thoughts on the forms and role of exuberance in their own lives. Original, inspiring, authoritative, Exuberance brims with the very energy and passion that it celebrates.

416 pages Year Founded: 2004 ISBN 0-375401-44-X

1679 Harvard Medical School Guide to Suicide Assessment and Intervention
Jossey-Bass / Wiley & Sons
111 River Street
Hoboken, NJ 07030-5774
201-748-6000
Fax: 201-748-6088
E-mail: info@wiley.com
www.wiley.com

Douglas G. Jacobs, Editor

This vital resource is the definitive guide for helping mental health professionals determine the risk for suicide and appropriate interventions for suicidal or at-risk patients. Created primarily for mental health clinicians, the book is a hands-on guide for those who are often the first line of defense for assessing if a patient or client is suicidal. *$59.95*

736 pages Year Founded: 1998 ISBN 0-787943-03-7

1680 In the Wake of Suicide: Stories of the People Left Behind
Jossey-Bass / Wiley & Sons
10475 Crosspoint Blvd.
Indianapolis, IN 46256
877-762-2974
Fax: 800-597-3299
E-mail: consumers@wiley.com
www.wiley.com

Victoria Alexander, Author

Offers survivors the understanding, compassion, and hope they need to guide them on their own path in the wake of this most painful loss. Breathtaking stories of incredible power for anyone struggling to find the meaning in the suicidal death of a loved one and for all readers seeking writing that moves and inspires. *$27.00*

256 pages Year Founded: 1998 ISBN 0-787940-52-6

1681 Left Alive: After a Suicide Death in the Family
Charles C Thomas Publisher Ltd.
2600 S 1st Street
Springfield, IL 62704-4730
217-789-8980
800-258-8980
Fax: 217-789-9130
E-mail: books@ccthomas.com
www.ccthomas.com

Linda Rosenfeld, Author
Marilynne Prupas, Author

$21.95

100 pages Year Founded: 1984 ISBN 0-398066-50-7

1682 My Son...My Son: A Guide to Healing After Death, Loss, or Suicide
Bolton Press Atlanta
1090 Crest Brook Lane
Roswell, GA 30075-3403
770-645-1886
Fax: 770-649-0999
E-mail: contactus@boltonpress.com
www.boltonpress.com

Iris Bolton, Author
Curtis Mitchell, Collaborator

A moving story of love, loss and recovery that will grab your heart, nourish your soul and open your eyes. A must read for anyone who has experienced a great loss and is

trying to find some path out of the darkness of their despair or to understand those that are.

120 pages Year Founded: 1983 ISBN 0-961632-60-7

1683 Night Falls Fast: Understanding Suicide
Vintage Books A Division Of Random House
1745 Broadway
20th Floor
New York, NY 10019
212-782-9000
800-733-3000
Fax: 212-302-7985
E-mail: ecustomerservice@randomhouse.com
www.randomhouse.com

Kay Redfield Jamison, Author

Tragically timely: suicide has become one of the most common killers of Americans between the ages of fifteen and forty-five. Weaving together a historical and scientific exploration of the subject with personal essays on individual suicides, the author not only brings her remarkable conpassion and literary skill but also all of her knowledge and research to bear on this devastating problem. This is a book that helps us to understand the suicidal mind, to recognize and come to the aid of those at risk, and to comprehend the profound effects on those left behind. It is critical reading for parents, educators, and anyone wanting to understand this tragic epidemic.

448 pages ISBN 0-375701-47-8

1684 No Time to Say Goodbye: Surviving the Suicide of a Loved One
Three Rivers Press
1745 Broadway
New York, NY 10019
212-782-9000
E-mail: ecustomerservice@randomhouse.com
www.randomhouse.com

Carla Fine, Author

With No Time to Say Goodbye, the author brings suicide survival from the darkness into light, speaking frankly about the overwhelming feelings of confusion, guilt, shame, anger, and loneliness that are shared by all survivors. Fine draws on her own experience and on conversations with many other survivors- as well as on the knowledge of counselors and mental health professionals.

272 pages Year Founded: 1999 ISBN 0-385485-51-4

1685 Someone I Love Died by Suicide: A Story for Child Survivors and Those Who Care for Them
Grief Guidance Inc.
PO Box 32789
Palm Beach Gardents, FL 33420-2789
561-625-6751
Fax: 561-625-6751
E-mail: info@griefguidance.com
www.griefguidance.com

Doreen Cammarata, Author

This book is designed for adult caregivers to read to surviving youngsters following a suicidal death. Although the language used in the book is simplistic enough to be read along with children ultimately stimulating family discussion, it can be beneficial to all who have been tragically devastated by suicide. It is recommended for this book to be utilized in conjunction with therapy.

40 pages Year Founded: 2001 ISBN 0-970933-29-0

1686 Suicidal Patient: Principles of Assessment, Treatment, and Case Management
American Psychiatric Publishing, Inc.
1000 Wilson Boulevard
Suite 1825
Arlington, VA 22209-3901
703-907-7322
800-368-5777
Fax: 703-907-1091
E-mail: appi@psych.org
www.appi.org

John A. Chiles, Author
Kirk D. Strosahl, Author

Presents a clinical approach and valuable assessment strategies and techniques. Demonstrates an easy to use innovative clinical model with specific stages of treatment and associated interventions outlined for inpatient and outpatient settings. *$45.50*

282 pages Year Founded: 1995 ISBN 0-800485-54-X

1687 Suicide Over the Life Cycle
American Psychiatric Publishing, Inc.
1000 Wilson Boulevard
Suite 1825
Arlington, VA 22209-3901
703-907-7322
800-368-5777
Fax: 703-907-1091
E-mail: appi@psych.org
www.appi.org

Susan J. Blumenthal, Editor
David J. Kupfer, Editor

This book attempts to solve the mystery of suicide by filling in the gaps in our understanding about risk factors and treatment of suicidal patients, and by integrating and translating current knowledge about suicidal behavior into practical treatment considerations. This book brings together the research studies and clinical experience of more than 40 internationally recognized contributors who paint an insightful and thought-provoking portrait of the suicidal patient at various stages of the life span. A comprehensive guide, this superb text is a practical and encyclopedic compendium of assessment and intervention strategies that the clinician can use in day-to-day treatment of suicidal patients.

828 pages Year Founded: 1990 ISBN 0-880483-07-5

1688 Understanding and Preventing Suicide: New Perspectives
Charles C Thomas Publisher Ltd.
PO Box 19265
Springfield, IL 62794-9265
217-789-8980
800-258-8980
Fax: 217-789-9130
E-mail: books@ccthomas.com
www.ccthomas.com

David Lester, Author

Seven perspectives for understanding and preventing suicidal behavior, illustrating their implications for prevention. This book discusses suicide from a crimnological perspective, and whether the theories in it have any applicability to suicidal behavior, both in furthering our understanding of suicide and in seeing new ways to prevent suicide. Armed with this information, we may move far toward understand-

ing and preventing suicide in the twenty-first century. *$35.95*

121 pages Year Founded: 1990 ISSN 0-398-06235-8ISBN 0-398057-09-5

1689 Why Suicide? Answers to 200 of the Most Frequently Asked Questions about Suicide, Attempted Suicide, and Assisted Suicide
HarperOne
10 East 53rd Street
New York, NY 10022
212-207-7000
www.harpercollins.com

Eric Marcus, Author

$14.95

256 pages Year Founded: 1996 ISBN 0-062511-66-9

Periodicals & Pamphlets

1690 Suicide Talk: What To Do If You Hear It
ETR Associates
4 Carbonero Way
Scotts Valley, CA 95066-4200
831-438-4060
800-321-4407
Fax: 831-438-3618
E-mail: support@etr.freshdesk.com
www.etr.org

David Kitchen, MBA, Chief Financial Officer
Talita Sanders, BS, Director, Human Resources
Coleen Cantwell, MPH, Director, Business Development Pl
Matt McDowell, BS, Director, Marketing

Includes suicide warning signs, how to help a friend, and ways to relieve stress. *$16.00*

1691 Suicide: Fast Fact 3
SAMHSA'S National Mental Health Information Center
PO Box 42557
Washington, DC 20015-557
800-789-2647
Fax: 240-747-5470
TDD: 866-889-2647
E-mail: ken@mentalhealth.org
www.mentalhealth.samhsa.gov

A Kathryn Power MEd, Director
Edward B Searle, Deputy Director

This fact card provides statistics and a list of resources on suicide.

Year Founded: 2000

1692 Suicide: Who Is at Risk?
ETR Associates
4 Carbonero Way
Scotts Valley, CA 95066-4200
831-438-4060
800-321-4407
Fax: 831-438-3618
E-mail: customerservice@etr.org
www.etr.org

Infinite Mind, Author

Includes warning signs, symptoms, and what to do. *$ 16.00*

Research Centers

1693 American Foundation for Suicide Prevention
120 Wall Street
29th Floor
New York, NY 10005
212-363-3500
888-333-2377
Fax: 212-363-6237
E-mail: info@afsp.org
www.afsp.org

Nancy Farrell, M.P.A, Chairman
Yeates Conwell, M.D, President
Maria Oquendo, M.D, Vice President
Robert Gebbia, Chief Executive Officer

AFSP has been at the forefront of a wide range of suicide prevention initiatives, each designed to reduce loss of life from suicide. AFSP is investing in groundbreaking research, new educational campaigns, innovative demonstration projects and critical policy work. Also expanding assistance to people whose lives have been affected by suicide, reaching out to offer support and offering opportunities to become involved in prevention.

Year Founded: 1987

Support Groups & Hot Lines

1694 Covenant House Nineline
461 Eighth Avenue
New York, NY 10001
212-613-0300
800-388-3888
Fax: 212-629-3756
www.nineline.org

Andrew P. Bustillo, Board Chair
Kevin Ryan, President and CEO

Nationwide crisis/suicide hotline.

Year Founded: 1972

Video & Audio

1695 A Madman's Journal
Educational Training Videos
136 Granville St
Suite 200
Gahanna, OH 43230
Fax: 888-775-3919
www.educationaltrainingvideos.com

For two years, the narrator of this program went through a nightmare, feeling a self-hatred and worthlessness beyond love and redemption that he described as the concentration camp of the mind. This video presents one man's attempt to convey the ordeal of severe depression by writing a memoir about the experience.

1696 Bipolar Disorder: Shifting Mood Swings
Educational Training Videos
136 Granville St
Suite 200
Gahanna, OH 43230
Fax: 888-775-3919
www.educationaltrainingvideos.com

Different from the routine ups and downs of life, the symptoms of bipolar disorder are severe - even to the point of being life-threatening. In this insightful program, patients speak from their own experience about the complexities of diagnosis and the very real danger of suicide, while family members and close friends address the strain of the condition's cyclic behavior.

1697 Clinical Impressions: Identifying Mental Illness
Educational Training Videos
136 Granville St
Suite 200
Gahanna, OH 43230
Fax: 888-775-3919
www.educationaltrainingvideos.com

How long can mental illness stay hidden, especially from the eyes of trained experts? This program rejoins a group of ten adults- five of them healthy and five of them with histories of mental illness- as psychiatric specialists try to spot and correctly diagnose the latter. Administering a series of collaborative and one-on-one tests, including assessments of personality type, physical self-image, and rational thinking, the panel gradually makes decisions about who suffers from depression, bipolar disorder, bulimia, and social anxiety.

1698 Coping with Stress
Educational Video Network, Inc.
1401 19th Street
Huntsville, TX 77340
936-295-5767
800-762-0060
Fax: 936-294-0233
www.www.evndirect.com

Stress affects everyone, both emotionally and physically. For some, mismanaged stress can result in substance abuse, violence, or even suicide. This program answers the question, How can a person cope with stress?

1699 Dealing with Depression
Educational Video Network, Inc.
1401 19th Street
Huntsville, TX 77340
936-295-5767
800-762-0060
Fax: 936-294-0233
www.www.evndirect.com

As more and more young people are falling victim to depression, it is important to understand what causes it and to know how to get the help that can rid a person of this life-wrecking affliction.

1700 Dealing with Grief
Educational Video Network, Inc.
1401 19th Street
Huntsville, TX 77340
936-295-5767
800-762-0060
Fax: 936-294-0233
www.www.evndirect.com

Grief allows us to acknowledge and mourn our losses so we can reconcile our feelings and move forward in life. Learn how to deal with your grief and become a better person for having gone through it.

1701 Don't Kill Yourself: One Survivor's Message
Educational Training Videos
136 Granville St
Suite 200
Gahanna, OH 43230
Fax: 888-775-3919
www.educationaltrainingvideos.com

This is the story of a young man, David, who at 16 years of age survived a suicide attempt. Now 22, he shares the events of his life leading up to the attempt, including how low self-esteem led to drug addiction, and how the addiction encouraged the sense that life was no longer worth living.

1702 FRONTLINE: The Released
PBS
2100 Crystal Drive
Arlington, VA 22202
www.pbs.org

Will Lyman, Actor
Narrator
Miri Navasky, Director
Karen O'Connor, Director

The documentary states that of the 700,000 inmates released from American prisons each year, half of them have mental disabilities. This work focused on those with severe problems who keep entering and exiting prison. Full of good information on the challenges they face with mental illnesses; housing, employment, stigmatization, and socialization.

Year Founded: 2009

1703 Suicide among Teens
Educational Video Network, Inc.
1401 19th Street
Huntsville, TX 77340
936-295-5767
800-762-0060
Fax: 936-294-0233
www.www.evndirect.com

Suicide devastates surviving loved ones. Find out why it should never be considered as a solution and learn how to recognize warning signs in a suicidal person.

1704 Teenage Anxiety, Depression, and Suicide
Educational Video Network, Inc.
1401 19th Street
Huntsville, TX 77340
936-295-5767
800-762-0060
Fax: 936-294-0233
www.www.evndirect.com

This program can provide helpful insight to those in need of assistance.

Web Sites

1705 www.afsp.org
American Foundation for Suicide Prevention
AFSP has been at the forefront of a wide range of suicide prevention initiatives, each designed to reduce loss of life from suicide. AFSP is investing in groundbreaking research, new educational campaigns, innovative demonstration projects and critical policy work. Also expanding assistance to people whose lives have been affected by suicide, reaching out to offer support and offering opportunities to become involved in prevention.

1706 www.break-the-silence.org
Break the Silence
www.break-the-silence.org

A non profit organization whose basis and foundation came from first-hand knowledge and experience that inpatient safety is not always provided to those in need of protection, causing a desperate need for a watch-dog organization like Break the Silence.

1707 www.friendsforsurvival.org
Friends for Survival
Assisting anyone who has suffered the loss of a loved one through suicide death.

1708 www.griefguidance.com
Grief Guidance Inc.
A company created by Doreen Cammarata to promote intervention services for suicide survivors.

1709 www.jasonfoundation.com
The Jason Foundation, Inc.
An educational organization dedicated to the awareness and prevention of youth suicide. JFI believes that awareness and education are the first steps to prevention.

1710 www.mentalhealth.samhsa.gov
Substance Abuse & Mental Health Services Administration
Information about resources, technical assistance, research, training, networks, and other federal clearing houses, and fact sheets and materials. Information specialists refer callers to mental health resources in their communities as well as state, federal and nonprofit contacts.

1711 www.nami.org
National Alliance on Mental Illness
Nation's leading self-help organization for all those affected by severe brain disorders. Mission is to bring consumers and families with similar experiences together to share information about services, care providers, and ways to cope with the challenges of schizophrenia, manic depression, and other serious mental illnesses.

1712 www.nineline.org
Covenant House Nineline
Nationwide crisis/suicide hotline.

1713 www.nopcas.com
National Organization for People of Color Against Suicide
NOPCAS serves as the only national organization of its kind addressing the issue of suicide prevention and intervention, specifically in communities of color. Primary focus and mission is to increase suicide education and awareness. Offering unique opportunities for outreach partnerships and community education efforts directed at communities of color across the nation.

1714 www.psf.org
National P.O.L.I.C.E. Suicide Foundation
This foundation provides educational training seminars for emergency responders, primarily associated with law en-

forcement on the issue of police suicide. Providing police suicide awareness and prevention training programs and support services that will meet the psychological, emotional, and spiritual needs of law enforcement, on every level, and their families.

1715 www.save.org
Suicide Awareness Voices of Education (SAVE)

One of the nation's first organizations dedicated to the prevention of suicide and was a co-founding member of the National Council for Suicide Prevention. Leading national non profit organization with staff dedicated to prevent suicide. Based on the foundation and belief that suicide should no longer be considered a hidden or taboo topic and that through raising awareness and educating the public, we can SAVE lives.

1716 www.solossa.org
Survivors of Loved Ones' Suicides (SOLOS)

Organization to help provide support for the families and friends who have suffered the suicide loss of a loved one.

1717 www.suicide.supportgroups.com
SupportGroups

An online support group community bringing people together around life's challenges by providing concise, up-to-date information and a meeting place for individuals, their friends and families, and professionals who offer pathways to help.

1718 www.suicidology.org
American Association of Suicidology

AAS is a membership organization for all those involved in suicide prevention and intervention, or touched by suicide. AAS is a leader in the advancement of scientific and programmatic efforts in suicide prevention through research, education and training, the development of standards and resources, and survivor support services.

1719 www.yellowribbon.org
Yellow Ribbon Suicide Prevention Program

Dedicated to preventing suicide and attempts by making suicide prevention accessible to everyone and removing barriers to help by empowering individuals and communities through leadership, awareness and education, and by collaborating and partnering with support networks to reduce stigma and help save lives.

Associations & Organizations

National

1720 Abraham Low Self-Help Systems
105 W. Adams Street
Suite 2940
Chicago, IL 60603
866-221-0302
Fax: 312-726-4446
E-mail: inquiries@recovery-inc.com
www.lowselfhelpsystems.org

Rudolph Pruden, Chair
John Rosenheim, 1st Vice Chair
Larry Kipperman, 2nd Vice Chair
Rudolph Pruden, Acting Treasurer

The mission of Abraham Low Self-Help Systems is to use the cognitive-behavioral, peer-to-peer, self-help training system developed by Abraham Low, MD, to help individuals gain skills to lead more peaceful and productive lives. The organization meets this mission by providing mental health self-help groups, telephone and online meetings, The Power to Change for Schools and The Power to Change for Corrections.

Year Founded: 1989

1721 Advocates for Human Potential (AHP)
490-B Boston Post Road
Sudbury, MA 01776-3022
978-443-0055
Fax: 978-443-4722
E-mail: cgalland@ahpnet.com
www.ahpnet.com

Alexandra Gasper, Director of New Business and Pro
Charlie Galland, Chief Operating Officer
Charles R. Galland, JD, MBA, COO

Excels in research and evaluation; technical assistance and training; system and program development, including strategic planning and information management; and resource development and dissemination. Staff is expert in content areas critical to addressing the behavioral health needs of vulnerable populations: mental health policy and services, substance abuse treatment and prevention, co-occurring disorders, workforce development, electronic medical records, homelessness, housing, employment program development, trauma, domestic violence, and criminal justice.

Year Founded: 1980

1722 American Academy of Child and Adolescent Psychiatry
3615 Wisconsin Avenue NW
Washington, DC 20016-3007
202-966-7300
Fax: 202-966-2891
E-mail: communications@aacap.org
www.aacap.org

Paramjit T. Joshi, M.D, President
Aradhana Sood, M.D., Secretary
David G. Fassler, M.D, Treasurer
Paramjit T. Joshi, MD, President-Elect

The AACAP is the leading national professional medical association dedicated to treating and improving the quality of life for children, adolescents, and families affected by these disorders. Members actively research, evaluate, diag-nose, and treat psychiatric disorders and pride themselves on giving direction to and responding quickly to new developments in addressing the health care needs of children and their families. Widely distributes information in an effort to promote an understanding of mental illnesses and remove the stigma associated iwth them; advance efforts in prevention of mental illnesses, and assure proper treatment and access to services for children and adolescents.

Year Founded: 1953

1723 American Academy of Pediatrics
141 NW Point Boulevard
Elk Grove Village, IL 60007-1098
847-434-4000
800-433-9016
Fax: 847-434-8000
E-mail: cme@aap.org
www.aap.org

James M. Perrin, MD, FAAP, President
Errol R. Alden, MD, FAAP, Executive Director/CEO
Errol R. Alden, MD, FAAP, Executive Director/CEO

Mission of the AAP is to attain optimal physical, mental, and social health and well-being for all infants, children, adolescents and young adults. A professional membership organization of 60, 000 primary care pediatricians, pediatric medical sub-specialists and pediatric surgical specialists.

Year Founded: 1930

1724 American Association for Geriatric Psychiatry
7910 Woodmont Avenue
Suite 1050
Bethesda, MD 20814-3004
301-654-7850
Fax: 301-654-4137
E-mail: main@aagponline.org
www.aagponline.org

David C. Steffens, MD, MHS, President
Christine deVries, Chief Executive Officer/Executiv
Denise Disque, Office Manager/Executive Assista
Kate McDuffie, Director, Communications & Marke

The only national association that has products, activities and publications which focus exlusively on the challenges of geriatric psychiatry. Practitioners, researchers, educations, students, the public - anyone interested in improving the mental health of the elderly - have relied on AAGP as the key driver for progress for elderly mental health care.

Year Founded: 1978

1725 American Association on Intellectual and Developmental Disabilities (AAIDD)
501 3rd Street NW
Suite 200
Washington, DC 20001
202-387-1968
800-424-3688
Fax: 202-387-2193
E-mail: anam@aaidd.org
www.aaidd.org

James R. Thompson, PhD, President
Margaret Nygren, EdD, Executive Director and CEO
Paul D. Aitken, CPA, Director, Finance & Administrati
Ajith Mathew, Contracts Manager

Providing worldwide leadership in the field of intellectual and developmental disabilities. The oldest and largest interdisciplinary organization of professionals and citizens concerned about intellectual and developmental disabilities. Tireless promoters of progressive policies, sound research, effective practices and universal human rights for people with intellectual and developmental disabilities.

Year Founded: 1876

1726 American Holistic Health Association

PO Box 17400
Anaheim, CA 92817-7400
714-779-6152
E-mail: mail@ahha.org
www.ahha.org

Suzan V. Walter, MBA, President
Gena E. Kadar, DC, CNS, Secretary
Susan J. Negus, HHD, Treasurer

The leading national resource connecting people with vital solutions for reaching a higher level of wellness. Dedicated to promoting holistic principles: honoring the whole person (mind, body, spirit) and encouraging people to actively participate in their own health and healthcare.

Year Founded: 1989

1727 American Network of Community Options and Resources (ANCOR)

1101 King Street
Suite 380
Alexandria, VA 22314-2962
703-532-7850
Fax: 703-535-7860
E-mail: ancor@ancor.org
www.ancor.org

Dave Toeniskoetter, President
Renee L. Pietrangelo, PhD, Chief Executive Officer
Cindy Allen de Ramos, Finance Manager
Debra Langseth, Education and Foundation Directo

A national trade association representing private providers of community living and employment supports and services to individuals with disabilities. As a nonprofit organization, ANCOR successfully addresses the needs and interests of private providers before Congress and federal agencies, continually advocating for the crucial role private providers play in enhancing and supporting the lives of people with disabilities and their families.

1728 American Pediatrics Society

3400 Research Forest Drive
Suite B-7
The Woodlands, TX 77381-4259
281-419-0052
Fax: 281-419-0082
E-mail: info@aps-spr.org
www.aps-spr.org

Debbie Anagnostelis, Executive Director
Kate Culliton, Accounting Manager
Belinda Thomas, PAS, Education Program Director
Barbara Anagnostelis, Student Research Coordinator

Advancing academic pediatrics and fostering the research and career development of investigators engaged in the health and well-being of children and youth.

1729 American Psychiatric Association

1000 Wilson Boulevard
Suite 1825
Arlington, VA 22209-3901
703-907-7300
888-357-7924
E-mail: apa@psych.org
www.psych.org

John M. Oldham, MD, President
Dilip V. Jeste, MD, President-Elect
Roger Peele, MD, Secretary
David Fassler, MD, Treasurer

The world's largest psychiatric organization. It is a medical specialty society representing more than 36, 000 psychiatric physicians from the United States and around the world. Its member physicians work together to ensure humane care and effective treatment for all persons with mental disorders, including intellectual developmental disorders and substance use disorders. APA is the voice and conscience of modern psychiatry. Members are primarily medical specialists who are psychiatrists or in the process of becoming psychiatrists.

Year Founded: 1844

1730 American Psychological Association

750 First Street NE
Washington, DC 20002-4242
202-336-5500
800-374-2721
TDD: 202-336-6123
TTY: 202-336-6123
www.apa.org

Nadine J. Kaslow, PhD, President
Norman B. Anderson, Chief Executive Officer and Exec
L. Michael Honaker, PhD, Deputy Chief Executive Officer
Ellen G. Garrison, PhD, Senior Policy Advisor

Seeks to advance psychology as a science, a profession, and as a means of promoting health, education and human welfare.

1731 American Speech-Language-Hearing Association

2200 Research Blvd
Rockville, MD 20850-3289
301-269-5700
800-638-8255
Fax: 301-296-8580
TTY: 301-296-5650
E-mail: actioncenter@asha.org
www.asha.org

Elizabeth S. McCrea, President
Barbara K. Cone, Vice President for Academic Affa
Howard Goldstein, Vice President for Science and R
Edie R. Hapner, Vice President for Planning

The professional, scientific, and credentialing association for members and affiliates who are audiologists, speech-language pathologists, and speech, languard, and hearing scientists in the United States and internationally. Support personnel in audiology and speech-language pathology alson affiliate with ASHA.

Year Founded: 1925

1732 Association for Behavioral Health and Wellness

1325 G Street, NW
Suite 500
Washington, DC 20005
202-449-7660
Fax: 202-449-7659

E-mail: info@abhw.org
www.www.abhw.org

Kyle Raffaniello, Chair
Pamela Greenberg, MPP, President and CEO
Rebecca Murow Klein, Associate Director, Government A
Michael Golinkoff, Ph.D., MBA, Treasurer

An association of the nation's leading behavioral health and wellness companies. These companies provide an array of services related to mental health, substance use, employee assistance, disease management, and other health and wellness programs to over 110 million people in both the public and private sectors.

Year Founded: 1994

1733 Association of Mental Health Librarians (AMHL)

140 Old Orangeburg Rd.
Orangeburg, NY 10962
845-398-6576
Fax: 845-398-5551
E-mail: moss@nki.rfmh.org
www.mhlib.org

Stuart Moss, President

A professional organization of individuals working in the field of mental health information delivery. Members come from a variety of settings: inpatient hospitals, academic and research institutions, and psychiatric and psychological agencies. AMHL provides opportunities for its members to enhance their professional skills, encourages research activities in mental health librarianship, and strengthens the role of the librarian within the mental health community.

1734 Attitudinal Healing International

One Gate Six Road
Suite E
Sausalito, CA 94965-3100
877-244-3392
E-mail: info@ahinternational.org
www.ahinternational.org

Gerald G. Jampolsky, MD, Founder
Diane V. Cirincione, PhD, Executive Director
Paige Peterson, Chief Consult/Growth & Devel.
Lynne Law, International Liaison

Attitudinal Healing is based on the principle that it is not other people or situations that cause us distress. Rather, it is our own thoughts and attitudes that are responsible. AHInternational's mission is to create, develop, and support the official home portal for Attitudinal Healing and to help facilitate the organic creation and growth of independent centers, groups, and individuals worldwide. Hundreds of locations worldwide.

Year Founded: 1975

1735 Bazelon Center for Mental Health Law

1101 15th Street NW
Suite 1212
Washington, DC 20005-5002
202-467-5730
Fax: 202-223-0409
TDD: 202-467-4232
E-mail: communications@bazelon.org
www.bazelon.org

Robert Bernstein, President & CEO
Ira Burnim, Director

Jennifer Mathis, Deputy Director
Lewis Bossing, Senior Staff Attorney

National legal advocate for people with mental disabilities. Through precedent-setting litigation and in the public policy arena, the Bazelon Center works to advance and preserve the rights of people with mental illnesses and development disabilities.

Year Founded: 1972

1736 Bellefaire Jewish Children's Bureau

1 Pollock Circle
22001 Fairmont Blvd.
Cleveland, OH 44118
216-932-2800
800-879-2522
E-mail: info@bellfairejcb.org
www.bellefairejcb.org

Provides a variety of behavioral health, education, and prevention services for children, adolescents and their families. Serves children, families and young adults throughout the United States through its residential and autism treatment programs. Bellefaire JCB also meets the needs of children, internationally, through its Hague-accredited international adoption program.

Year Founded: 1868

1737 Best Buddies International (BBI)

100 SE 2nd Street
Suite 2200
Miami, FL 33131-2100
305-374-2233
800-892-8339
Fax: 305-374-5305
www.bestbuddies.org

David M. Quilleon, Senior Vice President, Major Gif
Alina M. Shriver, Vice President, Art & Merchandis
JR Fry, Vice President, Best Buddies Cha
Jen Miller, Vice President, Finance

An international organization that has grown from one original chapter to almost 1, 500 middle school, high school, and college chapters worldwide. Best Buddies programs engage participants in each of the 50 United States, and in 50 countries around the world.

Year Founded: 1989

1738 Bethesda Lutheran Communities

600 Hoffmann Drive
Watertown, WI 53094-6204
920-261-3050
800-369-4636
Fax: 920-261-8441
E-mail: john.bauer@mailblc.org
www.bethesdalutherancommunities.org

Dr. John E. Bauer, President & CEO
John Twardos, Vice President of Operations
Jack Tobias, Vice President of Finance
Michael Hoffman, Vice President of Human Resource

Mission is to enhance the lives of people with intellectual and developmental disabilities through services that share the good news of Jesus Christ.

1739 Black Mental Health Alliance (BMHA)

200 E Lexington St
Suite 10
Baltimore, MD 21202

410-338-2642
Fax: 410-338-1771
E-mail: bhealthall@blackmentalhealth.com
www.blackmentalhealth.com

Jan A. Desper, Executive Director
Cherly Maxwell, Program Manager

BMHA promotes appropriate mental health care, service delivery and theoretical understanding of all the mental health programs. An organization that provides training, education, consultation, public information, support groups, and resource referrals regarding mental health and related issues. Primary mission of BMHA is to provide a forum and promote a holistic, culturally relevant approach to the development and maintenance of optimal mental health programs and services for African Americans and other people of color.

Year Founded: 1984

1740 Canadian Art Therapy Association

26 Earl Grey Road
Toronto ON, ZZ
416-461-9420
www.catainfo.ca

Olena Darewych, President
Lucille Proulx, Vice President
Heather Stump, Secretary
Gilda Raimondi, Treasurer

A non profit organization promoting Art Therapy in Canada. Objectives are; to encourage professional growth of Art Therapy through the exchange and collaboration of Art Therapists; to maintain national standards of training, practice and professional registration; to foster research and publications in Art Therapy; to increase awareness of Art Therapy as an important mental health discipline within the community Services.

Year Founded: 1977

1741 Canadian Federation of Mental Health Nurses

1 Concorde Gate; Suite 109
Toronto ON M3z 3n6,
416-867-7443
Fax: 416-867-3739
E-mail: yvonne.currie@cdha.nshealth.ca
www.cfmhn.org

Lisa Crawley Beames, President
Joanne Jones, President Elect
Elly Spencer, Finance Director
Sherette Currie, Membership Director

The CFMHN is a national voice for psychiatric and mental health (PMH) nursing in Canada. It is an associate group of the Canadian Nurses' Association (CNA), for which it provides expertise for the specialty in matters relating to mental health nursing. Primary objectives are to assure national leadership in the development and applications of nursing standards that inform and affect psychiatric and mental health nursing practice; examine and influence government policy, and address national issues related to mental health and mental illness; communicate and collaborate with national and international groups that share professional interests; and, facilitate excellence in psychiatric and mental health nursing by providing members with educational opportunities.

Year Founded: 1988

1742 Canadian Mental Health Association
Canadian Mental Health Association

1110-151 Slater Street
595 Montreal Road, Suite 303
Ottawa, ON K1P 5H3,
613-745-5522
Fax: 613-745-5522
E-mail: info@cmha.ca
www.cmha.ca

David Copus, Chair
Irene Merie, Vice-Chair
Cal Crocker, Treasurer
Susan Grohn, Secretary

As a nation-wide, voluntary organization, the Canadian Mental Health Association promotes the mental health of all and supports the resilience and recovery of people experiencing mental illness. The CMHA accomplishes this mission through advocacy, education, research and services. Research and information services, sponsored research projects, workshops, seminars, pamphlets, newsletters and resource centres. Programs assist with employment, housing, early intervention for youth, peer support, recreation services for people with mental illness, stress reduction workshops and public education campaigns for the community. Also acts as a social advocate to encourage public action and commitment to strengthening community mental health services and legislation.

Year Founded: 1918

1743 Center for Mental Health Services (CMHS)

1 Choke Cherry Road
Rockville, MD 20857
240-276-1310
Fax: 240-276-1320
TDD: 866-889-2647
www.samhsa.gov/about/cmhs.aspx

Paolo Del Vecchio, Acting Director
Anna Marsh, Ph.D., Deputy Director

CMHS leads Federal efforts to treat mental illness by promoting mental health and by preventing the development or worsening of mental illness when possible. Congress created CMHS to bring new hope to adults who have serious mental illnesses and to children with serious emotional disorders. Helping states improve and increase the quality and range of their treatment, rehabilitation, and support services for people with mental illness, their families, and communities. Further, it encourages a range of programs; such as systems of care; to respond to the increasing number of mental, emotional, and behavioral problems among America's children. Supports outreach and case management programs for thousands of mentally ill homeless.

Year Founded: 1992

1744 Center for the Study of Issues in Public Mental Health
Nathan S Kline Institute for Psychiatric Research

140 Old Orangeburg Road
Orangeburg, NY 10962-1157
845-398-6594
Fax: 845-398-6592
E-mail: ashendenpc@aol.com
www.csipmh.rfmh.org

Carole Siegel, PhD, Director
Mary Jane Alexander, PhD, Director for Research/CSIPMH
Peter C. Ashenden, Executive Director

The Center is committed to developing and conducting research within the contents of a rigorous research program that is strongly influenced by the requirements of a public mental health system and, in turn, influences the development of policy and practice in this arena.

1745 Centre for Addiction and Mental Health

1001 Queen Street West
30-60 White Squirrel Way
Toronto ON M6J 1H4, ZZ
416-535-8501
800-463-6273
E-mail: info@camh.net
www.camh.net

Catherine Zahn, President & CEO of CAMH
Darrell Gregersen, President/CEO CAMH Foundation
Lori Spadorcia, Executive Director

CAMH is Canada's leading addiction and mental health organization, integrating specialized clinical care with innovative research, education, health promotion and policy development. Fully affiliated with the University of Toronto, and is a Pan American Health Organization/World Health Organization Collaborating Centre. CAMH combines clinical care, research, education, policy and health promotion to transform the lives of people affected by mental health and addiction issues.

Year Founded: 1998

1746 Child & Parent Resource Institute (CPRI)

600 Sanatorium Road
London ON N6H 3W7,
519-858-2774
877-494-2774
Fax: 519-858-3913
E-mail: Gillian.Kriter@ontario.ca
www.cpri.ca

Dr. Shannon L. Stewart, Research/Education Prog. Mgr.

A tertiary centre that provides highly specialized voluntary services to children and youth with multi complex, severe behavioural disturbances and/or developmental challenges that impacts the child/youth in all areas i.e. home, school, and/or community. 100% funded by the Ontario Ministry of Children and Youth Services and services are offered at no charge.

1747 Community Access

2 Washington Street
9th Floor
New York, NY 10004
212-780-1400
Fax: 212-780-1412
www.communityaccess.org

Stephen H. Chase, President
Jessica Catlow, Secretary
Cal Hedigan, Deputy CEO
Steve Coe, CEO

Community Access assists people with psychiatric disabilities in making the transition from shelters and institutions to independent living. Providing safe, affordable housing and support services, and advocating for the rights of people to live without fear or stigma. Provides a range of housing, job skills, employment placement and professional support services to help break the cycle of homelessness, institutionalization and/or incarceration that often complicates the lives of people who have a history of mental ill-

ness. Creating pathways to meaningful and successful community life.

Year Founded: 1974

1748 Council for Learning Disabilities

11184 Antioch Road
Box 405
Overland Park, KS 66210
913-491-1011
Fax: 913-491-1012
E-mail: CLDinfo@cldinternational.org
www.www-council-for-learning-disabilities.org

Silvana Watson, President
Diane Bryant, Vice President
Rebecca Shankland, Secretary
Dave Majsterek, Treasurer

An international organization that promotes evidence-based teaching, collaboration, research, leadership, and advocacy. CLD is comprised of professionals who represent diverse disciplines and are committed to enhancing the education and quality of life for individuals with learning disabilities and others who experience challenges in learning.

1749 Council on Quality and Leadership (CQL)

100 West Road
Suite 300
Towson, MD 21204
410-583-0060
Fax: 410-832-7226
E-mail: info@thecouncil.org
www.thecouncil.org

CQL offers consultation, accreditation, training and certification services to organizations and systems that share the vision of dignity, opportunity and community for all people. Providing leadership to improve the quality of life for people with disabilities, people with mental illness, and older adults.

Year Founded: 1969

1750 Emotions Anonymous International Service Center

PO Box 4245
St. Paul, MN 55104-0245
651-647-9712
Fax: 651-647-1593
E-mail: info@EmotionsAnonymous.org
www.EmotionsAnonymous.org

Fellowship of men and women who share their experience, strength and hope with each other, that they may solve their common problem and help others recover from emotional illness.

1751 Eye Movement Desensitization and Reprocessing International Association (EMDRIA)

5806 Mesa Drive
Suite 360
Austin, TX 78731
512-451-5200
866-451-5200
Fax: 512-451-5256
E-mail: info@emdria.org
www.emdria.org

Mark Nickerson, LICSW, President
Mark G. Doherty, CAE, Executive Director

Gayla Turner, CAE, Deputy Executive Director
Nicole Evans, Communications Specialist

A professional association where EMDR practitioners and EMDR researchers seek the highest standards for the clinical use of EMDR. EMDR is an accepted psychotherapy by leading mental health organizations throughout the world for the treatment of a variety of symptoms and conditions.

Year Founded: 1995

1752 Families Anonymous, Inc.
701 Lee St.
Suite 670
Des Plaines, IL 60016
847-294-5877
800-736-9805
Fax: 847-294-5837
E-mail: famanon@familiesanonymous.org
www.familiesanonymous.org

A 12 Step fellowship for the families and friends who have known a feeling of desperation concerning the destructive behavior of someone very near to them, whether caused by drugs, alcohol, or related behavioral problems. Any concerned person is encouraged to attend meetings, even if there is only a suspicion of a problem.

1753 Federation for Children with Special Needs (FCSN)
The Schrafft Center
529 Main Street
Suite 1M3
Boston, MA 02129
617-236-7210
800-331-0688
Fax: 617-241-0330
E-mail: fcsninfo@fcsn.org
www.fcsn.org

James F. Whalen, President
Rich Robison, Executive Director
Sara Miranda, Associate Executive Director - P
John Sullivan, Associate Executive Director - T

The federation provides information, support, and assistance to parents of children with disabilities, their professional partners and their communities. Promotes the active and informed participation of parents of children with disabilities in shaping, implementing, and evaluating public policy that affects them.

Year Founded: 1974

1754 Federation of Families for Children's Mental Health
9605 Medical Center Drive
Ste. 280
Rockville, MD 20850-6390
240-403-1901
Fax: 240-403-1909
E-mail: ffcmh@ffcmh.org
www.ffcmh.org

Sandra Spencer, Executive Director
Lizzette Albright, Finance Director
Lynda Gargan, Senior Managing Director
Nicole Marshall, Projects & Logistics Manager

A national family-run organization linking chapters and state organizations focused on the issues of children and youth with emotional, behavioral, or mental health needs and their families. Works to develop and implement policies, legislation, funding mechanisms, and service systems that utilize the strengths of families. Its emphasis on advocacy offers families a voice in the formation of national policy, services and supports for children with mental health needs and their families. Through a family and youth-driven approach, children emotional, behavioral, and mental health challenges and their families obtain needed supports and services so that children grow up healthy and able to maximize their potential.

Year Founded: 1989

1755 Gam-Anon Family Groups International Service Office
PO Box 157
Whitestone, NY 11357-0157
718-352-1671
Fax: 718-746-2571
E-mail: gamanonoffice@gam-anon.org
www.gam-anon.org

The self-help organization of Gam-Anon is a life saving instrument for the spouse, family or close friends of compulsive gamblers.

1756 Genetic Alliance
4301 Connecticut Avenue NW
Suite 404
Washington, DC 20008-2369
202-966-5557
Fax: 202-966-8553
E-mail: info@geneticalliance.org
www.geneticalliance.org; www.diseaseinfosearch.org

Sharon Terry, CEO
Natasha Bonhomme, Vice President of Strategic Deve
Rachel Koren, Program Assistant
Tetyana Murza, MES, Managing Director

Genetic Alliance is the world's leading nonprofit health advocacy organization committed to transforming health through genetics and promoting an environment of openness centered on the health of individuals, families, and communities.

Year Founded: 1986

1757 Healing for Survivors
PO Box 8405
Fresno, CA 93747-8405
559-442-3600
Fax: 559-442-3600
E-mail: jankister@email.com
www.healingforsurvivors.org

Jan Kister, Director/Founder

A community based non profit organization dedicated to provideing education, counseling, resources, and a safe place for individuals and families impacted by physical, emotional and/or sexual abuse to pursue wholeness and healing.

1758 Hincks-Dellcrest Centre
440 Jarvis Street
Toronto ON, ZZ
416-924-1164
Fax: 416-924-8208
E-mail: info@hincksdellcrest.org
www.hincksdellcrest.org

Donna Duncan, President & CEO
Valerie Campbell, Interim President & CEO

Dr. Marshall Korenblum, Psychiatrist-in-Chief
Annabelle Rocha, Vice-President, Corporate Servic

A leading edge, non profit children's mental health centre offering a comprehensive range of innovative mental health services to infants, children, youth, and their families. Dedicated to promoting optimal social, emotional, and behavioral well-being in infants, children, youth, and their families, and to contributing to the achievement of healthy communities. Each year, more than 8, 000 children and families are helped through a variety of prevention, early intervention, outpatient, and residential treatment programs.

Year Founded: 1998

1759 Hong Fook Mental Health Association

3320 Midland Avenue, 2/F
Unit 201
Scarborough, ON
416-493-4242
Fax: 416-493-2214
E-mail: info@hongfook.ca
www.hongfook.ca

Katherine Wong, President
Lin Fang, Vice President
Jessica Luey, Vice President
Terence Chan, Treasurer

Hong Fook Mental Health Association aims to facilitate access to mental health services by people with linguistic and cultural barriers. We operate with 'Holistic Health, ' 'Empowerment' and 'Capacity Building' guiding principles. Our 'Continuum of Services' ranges from Health Promotion, Intake and Referrals, Consulatation/Liason, Intensive Case Management, Supportive Housing with Case Management, Self Help Initiatives, to Family Initiatives.

1760 Human Services Research Institute

7690 SW Mohawk St.
Bldg K.
Tualatin, OR 97062
503-924-3783
Fax: 503-924-3789
www.hsri.org

Valerie Bradley, President
Faythe Aiken, Research Assistant
Julie Bershadsky, Research Associate
Teresita Camacho-Gonsalves, Senior Research Specialist

Assists state and federal government to enhance services and support people with mental illness and people with mental retardation.

Year Founded: 1976

1761 Institute of Living- Anxiety Disorders Center; Center for Cognitive Behavioral Therapy
The Institute of Living/Hartford Hospital

80 Seymour Street
Hartford, CT 06102
860-545-5000
800-673-2411
Fax: 840-545-7156
www.harthosp.org/instituteofliving/

David Tolin, Director

Provide state-of-the-art treatments with proven effectiveness, conducting meaningful research on the nature and treatment of anxiety, and educating mental health professionals in research and treatment.

1762 Institute on Violence, Abuse and Trauma at Alliant International University

10065 Old Grove Road
San Diego, CA 92131
858-527-1860
Fax: 858-527-1743
E-mail: ivat@alliant.edu
www.www.fvsai.org

Robert Geffner, PhD, President
Sandi Capuano Morrison, MA, Executive Director
Malou Indon, Administrative Manager/Marketing
Diana Agostini, Special Projects & Development C

Strives to be a comprehensive resource, training and research center dealing with all aspects of violence, abuse and trauma. IVAT interfaces with Alliant International University's academic schools and centers, which provide resource support and educational training. Through a focus on collaborations with various partering organizations, IVAT desires to bridge gaps and help improve current systems of care on a local, national, and global level.

Year Founded: 2005

1763 International Society of Psychiatric-Mental Health Nurses

2424 American Lane
Madison, WI 53704-3102
608-443-2463
866-330-7227
Fax: 608-443-2474
E-mail: info@ispn-psych.org
www.ispn-psych.org

Evelyn Parrish, PhD, APRN, President
Edilma L Yearwood, PhD, BC, FAAN, ACAPN Division Director
Susan Benson, DNP, MSN, AGPN Division Director
Margaret Plunkett, APRN, MSN, Treasurer

The mission of ISPN is to unite and strengthen the presence and the voice of specialty psychiatric-mental health nursing while influencing health care policy to promote equitable, evidence-based and effective treatment and care for individuals, families and communities. Purpose is to: unite and strengthen the presence and voice of specialty psychiatric-mental health (PMH) nurses, promote equitable quality care for individuals and families with mental health problems, enhance the ability of PMH nurses to work collaboratively on issue facing the profession, provide expanded opportunities for networking and leadership development, and impact healthcare policy to facilitate effective use of human and financial resources.

Year Founded: 1999

1764 Judge Baker Children's Center

53 Parker Hill Avenue
Boston, MA 02120-3225
617-232-8390
Fax: 617-232-8399
E-mail: info@jbcc.harvard.edu
www.jbcc.harvard.edu

Stephen Schaffer, Interim President and COO
Elizabeth Fitzsimons, Director of Development
Alan L Kaye, CPA, MBA, Director of Finance
Nina Rodriguez, Director of Facilities

A nonprofit organization dedicated to improving the lives of children whose emotional and behavioral problems threaten to limit their potential. Integrating education, service, research, and training, the Center is the oldest child mental health organization in New England and a national leader in the field of children's mental health. Promoting the best possible mental health of children through the integration of research, intervention, training and advocacy.

Year Founded: 1917

1765 Learning Disabilities Association of America

4156 Library Road
Pittsburgh, PA 15234-1349
412-341-1515
Fax: 412-344-0224
E-mail: info@ldaamerica.org
www.LDAAmerica.org

Patricia H. Latham, President
Mary-Clare Reynolds, Executive Director
Heather Nicklow, Accounting Manager
Andrea Turkheimer, Director of Program Committee Su

LDA's mission is to create opportunities for success for all individuals affected by learning disabilities and to reduce the incidence of learning disabilities in future generations.

Year Founded: 1963

1766 Life Development Institute

18001 N 79th Avenue
Building E-71
Glendale, AZ 85308-8396
623-773-2774
866-736-7811
Fax: 623-773-2788
E-mail: info@life-development-inst.org
www.lifedevelopmentinstitute.org

LDI is a special education school dedicated to motivating and inspiring its students to seek and experience success. Learning disability program staff and administrators are devoted to actively working with and supporting parents to help their child succeed and be independent for life.

1767 Lifespire

1 Whitehall Street
9th Floor
New York, NY 10004
212-741-0100
Fax: 212-463-9814
E-mail: info@lifespire.org
www.lifespire.org

Jeffrey Goodman, Chair
Mark van Voorst, Chief Executive Officer / Presid
Keith Lee, Chief Financial Officer
Tom Lydon, COO

Lifespire is committed to the principle that all individuals with a developmental disability are able to become contributing members to their family and community. It is Lifespire's aim to provide these individuals with the assistance and support necessary so that they can attain the skills needed to maintain themselves in their community in the most integrated and independent manner possible.

Year Founded: 1951

1768 Menninger Clinic

12301 Main Street
Houston, TX 77035
713-275-5000
800-351-9058
Fax: 713-275-5107
www.www.menningerclinic.com

Ian Aitken, President & CEO
Kenny J. Klein, CPA, Sr VP & CFO
John Oldham, MD, MS, Sr VP & Chief of Staff
Pam Greene, PhD, RN, Sr VP & Chief Nursing Officer

Menninger is a leading psychiatric hospital dedicated to treating individuals with mood, personality, anxiety and addictive disorders, teaching mental health professionals and advancing mental healthcare through research.

1769 Mental Health and Aging Network (MHAN) of the American Society on Aging (ASA)

American Society on Aging
575 Market St.
Suite 2100
San Francisco, CA 94105-2869
415-974-9600
800-537-9728
Fax: 415-974-0300
E-mail: info@asaging.org
www.asaging.org

Louis Colbert, Chairperson
Robert Stein, President & CEO
Robert R. Lowe, Chief Operating Officer
Carole Anderson, Vice President of Education

Dedicated to improving the supportive interventions for older adults with mental health problems and their caregivers by: Creating a cadre of professionals with expertise in geriatric mental health, Assuring that service professionals are multi capable, Improving the systems of care, Providing a voice for the underserved and Advocating for the services that advance quality of life for our clients.

Year Founded: 1954

1770 Mental Illness Education Project, Inc.

25 West Street
Westborough, MA 01581
617-562-1111
800-343-5540
Fax: 617-779-0061
E-mail: info@miepvideos.org
www.miepvideos.org

Christine Ledoux, Executive Director

Engaged in the production of video-based educational and support materials for the following specific populations: people with psychiatric disabilities; families, mental health professionals, special audiences, and the general public. The Project's videos are designed to be used in hospital, clinical and educational settings, and at home by individuals and families.

1771 NYSARC, Inc.

393 Delaware Avenue
Delmar, NY 12054
518-439-8311
Fax: 518-439-1893
E-mail: info@nysarc.org
www.nysarc.org

John A. Schuppenhauer, President
Joseph M Bognanno, Vice President, Western Region
Lori Martindale, Treasurer
Maryann Bruner, Secretary

Improving the quality of life for people with intellectual and other developmental disabilities by providing support, information, direction, and services for people with intellectual and other developmental disabilities; having one of the best servicce delivery systems in the nation, including family members, self-advocates, and professionals in all matters; and continually building training and educational opportunities into all aspects of NYSARC, Inc.

Year Founded: 1949

1772 Nathan S Kline Institute for Psychiatric Research
140 Old Orangeburg Road
Orangeburg, NY 10962-1157
845-398-5500
Fax: 845-398-5510
E-mail: webmaster@nki.rfmh.org
www.www.rfmh.org/nki

Donald C. Goff, MD, Director
Antonio Convit, M.D., Deputy Director
Thomas O. O'Hara, MBA, Deputy Director Administration

A facility of the New York State Office of Mental Health that has earned a national and international reputation for its pioneering contributions in psychiatric research, especially in the areas of psychopharmacological treatments for schizophrenia and major mood disorders, and in the application of computer technology to mental health services. A broad range of studies are conducted at NKI, including basic, clinical, and services research. All work is intended to improve care for people suffering from these complex, psychobiologically-based, severely disabling mental disorders.

1773 National Alliance on Mental Illness
3803 N. Fairfax Dr.
Suite 100
Arlington, VA 22203
703-524-7600
888-999-6264
Fax: 703-524-9094
E-mail: helpline@nami.org
www.nami.org

Kevin B. Sullivan, President
Michael J. Fitzpatrick, Executive Director
Peggy Stedman, CFO
Lynn Borton, COO

The nation's largest grassroots mental health organization dedicated to building better lives for the millions of Americans affected by mental illness. NAMI advocates for access to services, treatment, supports and research and is steadfast in its commitment to raising awareness and building a community of hope for all of those in need. Improving the lives of individuals and families affected by mental illnesses. Financial contributions allow NAMI to offer an array of programs, initiatives and activities in support of the NAMI mission.

Year Founded: 1979

1774 National Association for Rural Mental Health
25 Massachusetts Ave NW
Ste 500
Washington, DC 20001
202-942-4276
Fax: 320-202-1833
E-mail: info@narmh.org
www.narmh.org

Jerry Parker, President
Lori Irvine, Membership Chair, Secretary
David Weden, Treasurer

Provides a forum for rural mental health professionals and advocates to: identify and solve challenges; work cooperatively toward improving the delivery of rural mental health services; promote the unique needs and concerns of rural mental health policy and practice issues. Sponsors an annual conference where rural mental health professionals benefit from the sharing of knowledge and resources.

Year Founded: 1977

1775 National Association for the Dually Diagnosed (NADD)
132 Fair Street
Kingston, NY 12401-4802
845-331-4336
800-331-5362
Fax: 845-331-4569
E-mail: info@thenadd.org
www.thenadd.org

Donna McNelis, PhD, President
Dr Robert Fletcher, Executive Director, Founder, CEO
Dan Baker, PhD, Vice President
L Jarrett Barnhill, MD, Treasurer

Nonprofit organization designed to promote interest of professional and parent development with resources for individuals who have the coexistence of mental illness and mental retardation. Provides conference, educational services and training materials to professionals, parents, concerned citizens and service organizations.

Year Founded: 1983

1776 National Association of State Mental Health Program Directors
66 Canal Center Plaza
Suite 302
Alexandria, VA 22314-1568
703-739-9333
Fax: 703-548-9517
E-mail: roy.praschil@nasmhpd.org
www.nasmhpd.org

Robert W. Glover, PhD, Executive Director
Jay Meek, CPA, MBA, CFO
Joan Gillece, PhD, Project Manager
Justin Harding, JD, Senior Policy Associate

The only national association to represent state mental health commissioners/directors and their agencies. A private non profit membership organization, NASMHPD helps set the agenda and determine the direction of state mental health agency interests across the country, including state mental health planning, service delivery, and evaluation. The association provides members with the opportunity to exchange diverse views and experiences, learning from one another in areas vital to effective public policy development and implementation. Provides a broad array of services designed to identify and respond to critical policy issues, cutting-edge consultation, training, and technical assistance.

Year Founded: 1959

1777 National Center for Learning Disabilities
381 Park Avenue South
Suite 1401
New York, NY 10016-8829
212-545-7510
888-575-7373
Fax: 212-545-9665
www.ncld.org

Frederic M. Poses, Chairman
James H. Wendorf, Executive Director
Alan Bendich, Director, Finance and Operations
Kevin Hager, Chief Communications and Engagem

The NCLD's mission is to ensure success for all individual with learning disabilities in school, at work and in life. They connect parents with resources, guidance and support to advocate effectively for their children, deliver evidence-based tools, resources and professional development to educators to improve student outcomes, develop policies and engage advocates to strengthen educational rights and opportunities.

Year Founded: 1977

1778 National Center on Addiction and Substance Abuse (CASA) at Columbia University

633 3rd Avenue
19th Floor
New York, NY 10017-6706
212-841-5200
Fax: 212-956-8020
E-mail: contact@casacolumbia.org
www.casacolumbia.org

Jeffery B. Lane, Chairman
Joseph A. Califano, Founder and Chairman Emeritus
Samuel A. Ball, President and Chief Executive Of
Susan P. Brown, Vice President and Director of F

The National Center on Addiction and Substance Abuse (CASA) at Columbia University is a science-based, multidisciplinary organization focused on transforming society's understanding of and responses to substance use and the disease of addiction. Founded in 1992 by Former U.S. Secretary of Health, Education, and Welfare Joseph A. Califano, Jr., CASA remains the only national organization that assembles under one roof all of the professional skill needed to research and develop proven, effective ways to prevent and treat substance abuse and addiction to all substances - alcohol, nicotine as well as illegal, prescription and performance enhancing drugs - in all sectors of society.

Year Founded: 1992

1779 National Council for Behavioral Health

1701 K Street NW
Suite 400
Washington, DC 20006
202-684-7457
Fax: 202-386-9391
E-mail: communications@thenationalcouncil.org
www.TheNationalCouncil.org

Jeffery Walter, Chairman
Linda Rosenburg, President
Mohini Venkatesh, VP, Practice Improvement
Jeannie Campbell, Executive Vice President And COO

The unifying voice of America's behavioral health organizations. Committed to providing comprehensive, quality care that affords every opportunity for recovery and inclusion in all aspects of community life. The National Council advocates for public policies in mental and behavioral health that ensure that people who are ill can access comprehensive healthcare services, and also offer state-of-the-science education and practice improvement resources so that service are efficient and effective.

1780 National Disability Rights Network, Inc.

900 2nd Street NE
Suite 211
Washington, DC 20002-3560
202-408-9514
Fax: 202-408-9520
TDD: 202-408-9521
E-mail: info@ndrn.org
www.ndrn.org

Rocky Nichols, President
Kim Moody, Vice President
Curtis L. Decker, JD, Executive Director
Monica Ball, Program Support Specialist

NDRN was established under the Protection and Advocacy for Individuals with Mental Illness (PAIMI) Act. PAIMI programs protect and advocate for the legal rights of persons with mental illness. The programs investigate reports of abuse or neglect and provide technical assistance, information, and legal counseling. Publishes a free, quarterly newsletter, P&A News.

Year Founded: 1982

1781 National Empowerment Center

599 Canal Street
Lawrence, MA 01840-1244
978-685-1494
800-769-3728
Fax: 978-681-6426
www.power2u.org

Daniel B Fisher, MD, PhD, Executive Director
Oryx Cohen, MPA, Technical Assitance Center Direc
Judene Shelley, MPH, Director, Special Projects
Leah Harris, MA, Communication Development Direct

Mission is to carry a message of recovery, empowerment, hope and healing to people with lived experience with mental health issues, trauma, and/or extreme states.

1782 National Federation of Families for Children's Mental Health

9605 Medical Center Drive
Suite 280
Rockville, MD 20850
240-403-1901
Fax: 240-403-1909
E-mail: ffcmh@ffcmh.org
www.www.ffcmh.org

Sandra Spencer, Executive Director
Lizzette Albright, Finance Director
Corey Brown, Webmaster/Social Marketing TA Pr
Lynda Gargan, Senior Managing Director

FFCMH provides families and youth with knowledge on current policy issues. They view family and youth involvement in the research agenda about children's mental health to be essential, and offer high quality curricula which have been developed through thorough and inclusive processes with continuous quality improvement feedback loops at every step. Trainings are comprehensive, outcome-focused, and are tailored to the community's requests. Attention has been paid to all current details and requirements, as well as to cultural competence.

1783 National Institute of Drug Abuse (NIDA)
Office of Science Policy & Communications, Public Information Branch
6001 Executive Boulevard
Room 5213
Bethesda, MD 20892-9561
301-443-6245
Fax: 301-443-7397
E-mail: information@nida.nih.gov
www.drugabuse.gov

Glenda Conroy, Director, Management
David Daubert, Deputy Director, Management
Mark Swieter, Ph.D., Acting Director

NIDA has made a concerted effort to better understand and address the need for research on drug abuse and addiction among health disparity populations, particularly racial/ethnic minority populations who experience disproportionate consequences of drug use and involvement.

1784 National Institute of Mental Health Information Resources and Inquiries Branch
6001 Executive Boulevard
Room 8184, MSC 9663
Bethesda, MD 20892-1
301-443-4513
866-615-6464
TTY: 301-443-8431
E-mail: nimhinfo@nih.gov
www.www.nimh.nih.gov/

One of 27 components of the National Institutes of Health, the Federal government's principal biomedical and behavioral research agency.

1785 National Mental Health Association
2000 N Beauregard Street
6th Floor
Alexandria, VA 22311-1748
703-684-7722
800-969-6642
Fax: 703-684-5968
TTY: 800-433-5959
www.mentalhealthamerica.net

Ann Boughtin, Chair of the Board
David L. Shern, Ph.D., Interim President and CEO
Dianne Felton, Chief Operating Officer
Mike Turner, Vice President of Development

Dedicated to improving treatments, understanding and services for adults and children with mental health needs. Working to win political support for funding for school mental health programs. Provides information about a wide range of disorders, such as panic disorder, obsessive-compulsive disorder, post traumatic stress, generalized anxiety disorder and phobias. Also advocates for programs to diagnose and treat children in juvenille justice systems.

1786 National Mental Health Consumers' Self-Help Clearinghouse
1211 Chestnut Street
Suite 1207
Philadelphia, PA 19107-4103
215-751-1810
800-553-4539
Fax: 215-636-6312
E-mail: info@mhselfhelp.org
www.mhselfhelp.org

Joseph Rogers, Executive Director
Susan Rogers, Director
Christa Burkett, Technical Assistance Coordinator
Britani Nestel, Program Specialist

A national consumer technical assistance center that has played a major role in the development of the mental health consumer movement.

Year Founded: 1986

1787 National Network for Mental Health
3575 Quakerbridge Rd.
St. Catharine ON, ZZ
905-682-2423
888-406-4663
Fax: 905-682-7469
E-mail: info@nnmh.ca
www.nnmh.ca

Constance McKnight, Executive Director

The purpose of the NNMH is to advocate, educate and provide expertise and resources that benefit the Canadian consumer/survivor community. The focus of the organization is to network with Candian consumer/survivors and family and friends of consumer/survivors to provide opportunities for resource sharing, information distribution and education on issues impacting persons living with mental health issues/illness/disability.

1788 National Organization on Disability
77 Water Street
Suite 204
New York, NY 10005
646-505-1191
Fax: 646-606-1184
E-mail: info@nod.org
www.nod.org

Thomas J Ridge, Chairman
Carol Glazer, President
Charles F Day, Vice Chairman
Cory Olicker Henkel, Chief Operating Officer

NOD is demonstrating new employment practices and models of service delivery, evaluating results, and sharing successful approaches for widespread replication. Conducting research on disability employment issues, including the field's most widely used polls on meployment trends and the quality of life for people with disabilities. Working in partnership with employers, schools, the military, service providers, researchers, and disability advocates. Current employment progrmas are benefiting high school students with disabilities, seriously injured service members returning from Iraq and Afghanistan, employers seeking to become more disability friendly, and state governments engaged in policy reform.

Year Founded: 1982

1789 National Rehabilitation Association
PO Box 150235
Alexandria, VA 22315
703-836-0850
888-258-4295
Fax: 703-836-0848
TDD: 703-836-0849
E-mail: info@nationalrehab.org
www.www.nationalrehab.org

David Beach, PhD, CRC, CPM, President
Patricia Leahy, Interim Executive Director

Patricia Leahy, Governmental Affairs Director
Veronica Hamilton, Office Manager

Founded in 1925. Concerned with the rights of people with disabilities, our mission is to provide advocacy, awareness and career advancement for professionals in the fields of rehabilitation. Our members include rehab counselors, physical, speech and occupational therapists, job trainers, consultants, independent living instructors and other professionals involved in the advocacy of programs and services for people with disabilities.

Year Founded: 1927

1790 New Hope Foundation

PO Box 201
Kensington, MD 20895-201
301-946-6395
800-705-4673
Fax: 301-946-1402
www.newhopefoundation.org

Tony Comerford, PhD, President & CEO
David Roden, LCSW, LCADC, Vice President & COO

A nonprofit corporation serving those in need of treatment for alcoholism, drug addiction and compulsive gambling. Over the years, New Hope has expanded its capacity and capabilities to include specialized programming for adolescents, woment and those with co-occuring disorders. Today, New Hope ranks among the nation's leading organizations of this type, constantly striving to advance the quality of addiction treatment through ongoing professional education and participation in select research projects.

1791 Parents Helping Parents
Sobrato Center for Nonprofits

1400 Parkmoor Avenue
Suite 100
San Jose, CA 95126
408-727-5775
855-727-5775
Fax: 408-286-1116
www.php.com

Suzanne Cistulli, Board Chair
Mary Ellen Peterson, MA, Executive Director/CEO
Paul Schutz, Chief Financial Officer
Christopher Baker, Board Treasurer

PHP's mission is to help children and adults with special needs receive the support and services they need to reach their full potential by providing information, training and resources to build strong families and improve systems of care.

Year Founded: 1976

1792 Partnership for Workplace Mental Health
c/o American Psychiatric Foundation

1000 Wilson Blvd
Suite 1825
Arlington, VA 22209-3901
703-907-8561
Fax: 703-907-7851
E-mail: mleftwich@psych.org
www.workplacementalhealth.org

Clare Miller, Director
Mary Claire Kraft, Promgram Manager
Kate Burke, Associate Director
Nancy Spangler, PhD, Consultant

The Partnership works with businesses to ensure that employees and their families living with mental illness, including substance use disorders, receive effective care. It does so in recognition that employers purchase healthcare for millions of American workers and their families.

1793 Sidran Traumatic Stress Institute

PO Box 436
Brooklandville, MD 21022-0436
410-825-8888
Fax: 410-560-0134
E-mail: sidran@sidran.org
www.sidran.org

Esther Giller, President and Director
Tracy Howard, Book Sales/Office Manager
Ruta Mazelis, Editor, The Cutting Edge/Trainer
Mary Lou Kenney, Consultant

Sidran Institute provides useful, practical information for child and adult survivors of any type of trauma, for families/friends, and for the clinical and frontline service providers who assist in their recovery. Sidran's philosophy of education through collaboration brings together great minds (providers, survivors, and loved ones) to develop comprehensive programs to address the practical, emotional, spiritual and medical needs of trauma survivors.

Year Founded: 1986

1794 The Center for Family Support

333 Seventh Avenue
9th Floor
New York, NY 10001
212-629-7939
Fax: 212-239-2211
E-mail: eberg@cfsny.org
www.cfsny.org

Steven Vernikoff, Executive Director
Barbara Greenwald, Associate Executive Director
Eileen Berg, Director of Quality Assurance
Virgil Seepersad, Director of Finance

Committed to providing support and assistance to individuals with developmental and related disabilities, and to the family members who care for them. Supporting individuals to live the lives they want; respecting diversity, individual choice, and overall family needs; providing families with the support they need at all stages of life; involving individuals in the communities; and delivering excellent, individualized support to all.

Year Founded: 1954

1795 Thresholds

4101 N Ravenswood Avenue
Chicago, IL 60613
773-572-5500
E-mail: thresholds@thresholds.org
www.thresholds.org

Jana Barbe, President
Mark Ishaug, M.A., Chief Executive Officer
Debbie Pavick, L.C.S.W., Chief Clinical Officer
Gavin Farry, M.B.A., C.P.A., Chief Administrative and Financi

Thresholds has created innovative, award-winning programs that honor and respect people with mental illnesses and helps give them the tools to create a meaningful life. Strong leadership, and enduring vision, and a solid belief in the resilience and value of all individuals has made Thresholds one of the nation's most successful and respected provider of services for people with severe mental illness. Developing innovative programs that have served as nationwide models for others around the world. Organization that serves people with severe and persistent mental illness with a range of programs designed with the individual's recovery as a goal.

1796 VOR

836 S. Arlington Heights Rd.
#351
Elk Grove Village, IL 60007
877-399-4867
Fax: 847-253-0675
E-mail: info@vor.net
www.vor.net

Ann Knighton, President
Julie Huso, Executive Director
Tamie Hopp, Director of Government Relations
Geoffrey Dubrowsky, Treasurer

Through national programs, VOR achieves its mission to unite advocates, educate and assist families, organizations, public officials, and individuals concerned with the quality of life and choice for persons with intellectual disabilities within a full array of residential options, including community and facility-based care. The only national organization to advocate for a full range of quality residential options and services, including own home, family home, community-based service options. VOR advocates that the final determination of what is appropriate depends on the unique abilities and needs of the individual and desires of the family and guardians.

Year Founded: 1983

1797 Warren Grant Magnuson Clinical Center

9000 Rockville Pike
Building 10, Room 1C255
Bethesda, MD 20892-1
301-496-2563
Fax: 301-402-2984
E-mail: occc@cc.nih.gov
www.cc.nih.gov

Maureen E. Gormley, MPH, MA, RN, Chief Operating Officer
Maria D. Joyce, MBA, CPA, Chief Financial Officer
Clare Hastings, PhD, RN, FAA, Chief Nurse Officer
John I. Gallin, MD, Clinical Center Director

Established as the research hospital of the National Institutes of Health. Designed with patient care facilities close to research laboratories so new findings of basic and clinical scientists can be quickly applied to the treatment of patients. Upon referral by physicians, patients are admitted to NIH clinical studies.

Year Founded: 1953

1798 Willowglen Academy; Wisconsin, Inc.

5151 West Silver Spring Drive
Milwaukee, WI 53218
414-225-4460
866-225-4459
Fax: 414-225-4475
E-mail: john.yopps@phoenixcaresystems.com
www.phoenixcaresystems.com/wi/

Nathan Neiger, MS, Executive Director
La Kelvin B Hill, Associate Executive Director
Dawn Reese, Admissions Coordinator

As a wholly owned subsidiary of Phoenix Care Systems, Inc, Willowglen Academy provides therapeutic residential treatment and educational services to children, adolescents and young adults with mental health, emotional, cognitive and developmental disabilities. Our accrediting bodies include COA, CARF and JCAHO.

1799 World Federation for Mental Health Secretariat

PO BOX 807
Suite 101
Occoquan, VA 22125
703-490-6926
Fax: 703-494-6518
E-mail: info@wfmh.com
www.wfmh.org

George Christodoulou, President
Ellen R Mercer, Vice President, Program Developm
Larry Cimino, Corporate Secretary
Helen Millar, Treasurer

An international organization to advance the prevention of mental and emotional disorders, the proper treatment and care of those with such disorders, and the promotion of mental health. The Federation has responded to international mental health crises through its role as the only worldwide grassroots advocacy and public education organization in the mental health field. The organization's broad and diverse membership makes possible collaboration among governments and non-governmental organizations to advance the cause of mental health services, research, and policy advocacy worldwide.

Year Founded: 1948

1800 Young Adult Institute and Workshop (YAI)

460 West 34th Street
New York, NY 10001-2382
212-273-6100
www.yai.org

Matthew Sturiale, L.C.S.W., CEO
Sanjay Dutt, Chief Financial Officer
Roberta G. Koenigsberg, J.D., Chief Compliance Officer
Karen Wegmann, M.B.A., Chief Business Officer

Serves more than 15, 000 people of all ages and levels of mental retardation, developmental and learning disabilities. Provides a full range of early intervention, preschool, family supports, employment training and placement, clinical and residential services, as well as recreation and camping services. YAI/National Intitute for People with Disabilities is also a professional organization, nationally renowned for its publications, conferences, training seminars, video training tapes and innovative television programs.

Year Founded: 1957

1801 Youth Services International

6000 Cattleridge Drive
Suite 200
Sarasota, FL 34232
941-953-9199
Fax: 941-953-9198
E-mail: YSIWEB@youthservices.com
www.youthservices.com

Premier provider in the youth care industry of educational and developmental services that change, dramatically, the thinking and behavior of troubled youth.

1802 ZERO TO THREE: National Center for Infants, Toddlers, and Families
1255 23rd Street, NW
Suite 350
Washington, DC 20037
202-638-1144
800-899-4301
Fax: 202-638-0851
E-mail: oto3@presswarehouse.com
www.zerotothree.org

Ann Pleshette Murphy, President
Matthew E Melmed JD, Executive Director

Publishes book, pamphlets, and curricula with a focus on the social and emotional development of infants, toddlers, and their families. Publications include the Diagnostic Classification of Mental Health and Developmental Disorders of Infancy and Early Childhood, Revised, Early Development and the Brain, Caring for Infants and Toddlers in Groups, Learning Happens (DVD), and the Magic of Everyday Moments. Publishes the Zero to Three journal (six yearly issues), a theme-based professional publication, sponsors the National Training Institute, an annual professional training conference in December, provides resources for parents and offers a fellows program.

State

Alabama

1803 Horizons School
15th Avenue South
Birmingham, AL 35205
205-322-6606
800-822-6242
Fax: 205-322-6605
www.horizonsschool.org

Don Lutomski, President
Jade K. Carter, Executive Director
Brian Geiger, Assistant Director
Anita Bosley, Public Relations and Development

College based, non degree program for students with specific learning disabilities and other mild learning problems. This specially-designed, two-year program prepares individuals for successful transitions to the community. Classes teach life skills, social skills and career training.

Year Founded: 1991

1804 Mental Health Board of North Central Alabama
1316 Somerville Road SE
Suite 1
Decatur, AL 35601
256-355-5904
800-365-6008
Fax: 256-355-6092
E-mail: mentalhealth@mhcnca.org
www.mhcnca.org

David Fuller, President
William Hudson, Vice-President
Doris Todd, Secretary
Carolyn Stair, Treasurer
Year Founded: 1967

1805 Mental Health Center of North Central Alabama
1316 Somerville Road SE
Suite 1
Decatur, AL 35601
256-355-5904
800-365-6008
E-mail: mentalhealth@mhcna.org
www.mhcnca.org

David Fuller, President
William Hudson, Vice-President
Doris Todd, Secretary
Carolyn Stair, Treasurer

Provides treatment, education and assitance to people affected by mental health problems.

Year Founded: 1967

1806 NAMI Alabama (National Alliance on Mental Illness)
1401 I-85
Suite A
Montgomery, AL 36106-2861
334-396-4797
800-626-4199
Fax: 334-396-4794
E-mail: wlaird@namialabama.org
www.namialabama.org

Sue Guffey, President
Ricky Hatcher, 1st Vice President
James Walsh, 2nd Vice President
Joel Willis, Treasurer

An organization comprised of local support and advocacy groups throughout the state dedicated to improving the quality of life for persons with a mental illness in Alabama.

Year Founded: 1979

Alaska

1807 Mental Health Association in Alaska
4045 Lake Otis Parkway
Suite 209
Anchorage, AK 99508-5227
907-563-0880
Fax: 907-563-0881
www.alaska.net/~mhaa/

Virginia L. Hostman, M.S., Chairman
Janet McGillivary, M.Ed., President & CEO
William F. Hostman, B.A., Assistant to the CEO

1808 National Alliance on Mental Illness: Alaska
PO Box 201753
Anchorage, AK 99520-1753
907-277-1300
800-478-4462
Fax: 907-277-8456
E-mail: alaskanami@gmail.com
www.nami.org/sites/alaska

Shirley Holloway, President
Scott Owens, Vice-President
Dick Farris, Treasurer
Kay Smith, Secretary

A nonprofit, support, education and advocacy organization of consumers, families and friends of people with severe brain disorders such as schizophrenia, schizoaffective disorder, bipolar disorder, major depressive disorder, obsessive-compulsive disorder, panic and anxiety disorders and attention deficit/hyperactivity disorder.

Arizona

1809 Community Partnership of Southern Arizona
4575 E Broadway
Tucson, AZ 85711-3509
520-325-4268
800-959-1063
Fax: 520-325-1441
E-mail: nogra@cpsa-rhba.org
www.www.cpsaarizona.org

Neal J. Cash, President & Chief Executive Offi
Charles Andrade, BS, Chief Financial Officer
Bethanne Enoki, MA, SPHR, Chief Human Resources Officer
Edward M. Gentile, DO, MBA, FAPA, Chief Medical Officer

Administrative organization responsible for the coordination of behavioral health treatment and preventitive services in southern and southeastern Arizona. We are a local community based nonprofit organization that is dedicated to ensuring the provision of accessible high quality and cost effective behavioral health services for adults and children.

1810 Devereux Arizona Treatment Network
444 Devereux Drive
PO Box 638
Villanova, PA 19085
480-998-2920
800-345-1292
Fax: 480-443-5587
www.devereux.org

Robert Q. Kreider, President and CEO
Margaret McGill, Senior Vice President & Chief Op
Robert C. Dunne, Senior Vice President & Chief Fi
Marilyn B. Benoit, M.D., Senior Vice President & Chief Cl

National non-profit treatment centers for emotional disorders.

Year Founded: 1983

1811 Mental Health Association of Arizona
501 N. 44th St.
Suite 300
Phoenix, AZ 85008
480-982-5305
800-642-4407
Fax: 480-994-4744
E-mail: info@mhaarizona.org
www.mhaarizona.org

Charles Japson, Executive Director
Julie Clark, Community Education

Allfiliate of the National Mental Health Association, we support all people with mental disorders to achieve respect and dignity, to reach their full potential and to be free from stigma and prejudice.

Year Founded: 1954

1812 Mentally Ill Kids in Distress (MIKID)
2642 E. Thomas Road
Phoenix, AZ 85016
602-253-1240
800-356-4543
Fax: 602-840-3409
E-mail: Phoenix@mikid.org
www.mikid.org

Steve Carter, President, Board of Directors
Vicki L Johnson, Executive Director
Sue Gilbertson, Founder

Mission is to provide support and assistance to families in Arizona with behaviorally challenged children, youth, and young adults.

Year Founded: 1984

1813 National Alliance on Mental Illness: Arizona
5025 E. Washington Street
Suite # 112
Phoenix, AZ 85034
602-244-8166
800-626-5022
Fax: 602-252-1349
E-mail: namiaz@namiaz.org
www.namiaz.org

Cheryl Fanning, President

The mission of NAMI Arizona shall be to serve as an alliance of local Arizona Affiliates of NAMI and their members and associate members who are dedicated to the eradication of mental illnesses and to the improvement of the quality of life of persons whose lives are affected by these diseases.

Arkansas

1814 Arkansas Alliance for the Mentally Ill
1012 Autumn Road
Suite 1
Little Rock, AR 72211-3704
501-661-1548
800-844-0381
Fax: 501-312-7540
E-mail: nami-ar@namiarkansas.org
www.www.namiarkansas.org

Rick Owen, President
Kim Arnold, Executive Director

Dedicated to improving the lives of individuals and families affected by mental illness.

1815 National Alliance on Mental Illness: Arkansas
1012 Autumn Road
Suite 1
Little Rock, AR 72211-3704
501-661-1548
800-844-0381
Fax: 501-312-7540
E-mail: nami-ar@namiarkansas.org
www.www.namiarkansas.org

Rick Owen, President
Kim Arnold, Executive Director

A non-profit, grassroots organization dedicated to improving the lives of persons with severe mental illness, their families, and their communities. Formerly known as Arkansas Alliance for the Mentally Ill (AAMI), NAMI Arkansas operates a statewide organization and coordinates a network of affiliates, support groups and field services throughout the state.

California

1816 Assistance League of Southern California
1360 North Street
Andrews Plaza
Hollywood, CA 90028-8529
323-469-1973
Fax: 323-469-5896
E-mail: email@assistanceleague.net
www.www.assistanceleaguela.org

Floran Fowkes, President
Susan Thalken, Vice President
Andy Goodman, Treasurer
Patricia Mulville, Secretary

Provides mental health services to children over 5 years of age, individuals and families. Parent education and domestic violence classes are available. Services in English, Spanish and Armenian.

Year Founded: 1919

1817 California Alliance for the Mentally Ill
National Alliance for the Mentally Ill
1851 Heritage Lane
Suite 150
Sacramento, CA 95815
916-567-0163
Fax: 916-567-1757
E-mail: nami.california@namicalifornia.org
www.namicalifornia.org

Dorothy Hendrickson, President
Jessica Cruz, Executive Director
Steven Kite, Deputy Director
Carla Coale, Accounting Manager

Nation's leading self-help organization for all those affected by severe brain disorders. Mission is to bring consumers and families with similar experiences together to share information about services, care providers, and ways to cope with the challenges of schizophrenia, manic depression, and other serious mental illnesses. The California office answers questions from hundreds of individuals and groups outside NAMI who turn to us for accurate information about mental illness, NAMI affiliates near them, and where to turn for help.

Year Founded: 1977

1818 California Association of Marriage and Family Therapists

7901 Raytheon Road
San Diego, CA 92111-1606
858-292-2638
Fax: 858-292-2666
E-mail: jepstein@camft.org
www.camft.org

Guillermo Alvarez, LMFT, President
Victoria Campbell, LMFT, Chief Financial Officer
Jill Epstein, J.D., Executive Director
Cathy Atkins, J.D., Deputy Executive Director

Independent professional organization representing the interests of licensed marriage and family therapists. Dedicated to advancing the profession as an art and a science, to maintaining high standards of professional ethics, to upholding the qualifications for the profession and to expanding the recognition and awareness of the profession.

88 pages 6 per year Year Founded: per ISSN 1540-2770

1819 California Association of Social Rehabilitation Agencies

815 Marina Vista, Suite D
PO Box 388
Martinez, CA 94553-38
925-229-2300
Fax: 925-229-9088
E-mail: casra@casra.org
www.casra.org

Betty Dahlquist, Executive Director
David Holden, Deputy Director
Marianne Baptista, Director of Training and Educati
Sheryle Stafford, Public Policy

Dedicated to improving services and social conditions for people with psychiatric disabilities by promoting their recovery, rehabilitation and rights. A diagnosis is not a destiny.

Year Founded: 1989

1820 California Health Information Association

1915 N Fine Avenue
Suite 104
Fresno, CA 93727-1565
559-251-5038
Fax: 559-251-5836
E-mail: info@californiaihia.org
www.californiaihia.org

Lavonne La Moureaux, Executive Director
Marilyn R Taylor, Operations Manager

LaVonne LaMoureaux, RHIA, CAE, Executive Director
Marilyn R. Taylor, RHIT, Operations Manager

Nonprofit association that provides leadership, education, resources and advocacy for California's health information management professionals. Contributes to the delivery of quality patient care through excellence in health information management practice.

1821 California Institute for Mental Health

2125 19th Street
2nd Floor
Sacramento, CA 95818
916-556-3480
Fax: 916-556-3483
E-mail: sgoodwin@cimh.org
www.cimh.org

Mark Refowitz, Chairman
Sandra Naylor Goodwin, PhD, M, President and CEO
Doretha Williams-Flournoy, MS, Deputy Director, Chief Operating
Michelle Elder, Chief Financial Officer

Promoting excellence in mental health services through training, technical assistances, research and policy development.

1822 California Psychiatric Association (CPA)

1029 K Street
Suite 28
Sacramento, CA 95814
916-442-5196
Fax: 916-442-6515
E-mail: calpsych@worldnet.att.net
www.calpsych.org

Barbara Gard, Executive Director
Randall Hagar, Government Affairs Director
Lila Schmall, CPA Associate Executive Director

Represents psychiatrists and the interests of their patients as those interests are affected by state government. CPA is area six of the American Psychiatric Association, and is composed of members of APA's five district branches in California.

1823 California Psychological Association

1231 I Street
Suite 204
Sacramento, CA 95814-2933
916-286-7979
Fax: 916-286-7971
E-mail: cpa@cpapsych.org
www.cpapsych.org

Robert deMayo, President
Patricia VanWoerkom, Director Administration & Direct
Jo Linder-Crow, Chief Executive Officer
Pat Jaspin, Director, Accounting

A non-profit professional association for licensed psychologists and others affiliated with the delivery of psychological services.

Year Founded: 1948

1824 Calnet

3625 East Thousand Oaks Blvd
Suite 178
Westlake Village, CA 91362
805-778-0055
Fax: 805-778-0054
www.calnetcare.com

Craig Lambdin, Chairman
Cary Quashen, Vice Chairman of the Board
Steven Wright, Secretary-Treasurer
Bill Redder, Director

A not-for-profit network founded to connect accredited mental health and chemical dependency treatment providers with insurers and managed care organizations

Year Founded: 1983

1825 Community Resource Council
PO Box 443
Hackensack, NJ 07601
201-343-4900
www.www.crchelpline.org/

Barry Leedy, Executive Director

Agency provides groups and classes to all ages. Sliding fee scale.

1826 Filipino American Service Group
135 N Park View Street
Los Angeles, CA 90026-5215
213-487-9804
Fax: 213-487-9806
E-mail: fasgi@fasgi.org
www.fasgi.org

Steve D. Popkin, Chairman
Rich Cabael, Vice-Chairman
Ralph Bernardino, Secretary
Emelyn Gamboa, Treasurer

FASGI focuses on promoting the physical health and mental well-being of underserved, low-income seniors. It aims to improve the quality of life of all members of the community in Historic Filipinotown and the Greater Los Angeles Area.

Year Founded: 1981

1827 Five Acres: Boys and Girls Aid Society of Los Angeles County
760 W Mountain View Street
Altadena, CA 91001-4925
626-798-6793
TTY: 626-204-1375
E-mail: for5acres@earthlink.com
www.5acres.org

John Reithl, Chairman
Don Bishop, Vice Chair Finance
Rustin Mork, Vice Chair Business Affairs
Chanel Boutakidis, Chief Executive Officer

Works to: prevent child abuse and neglect, care for, treat and educate emotionally disturbed, abused and neglected children and their families in residential and outreach programs, advance the welfare of children and families by research, advocacy and collaboration, strive for the highest standards of excellence by professionals and volunteers, and provide research and educational resources to families, the community and professionals for the prevention and treatment of child abuse and neglect.

Year Founded: 1888

1828 Gold Coast Alliance for the Mentally Ill
520 N Main Street, Room 203
PO Box 1088
Angels Camp, CA 95222-1088
209-736-4264
Fax: 209-736-4264

E-mail: gcami@goldrush.com
www.nami.org

Laurie Flynn, Executive Director

Local chapter of the national self-help organization (NAMI) for all those affected by severe brain disorders. Mission is to bring consumers and families with similar experiences together to share information about services, care providers, and ways to cope with the challenges of schizophrenia, manic depression, and other serious mental illnesses.

1829 Health Services Agency: Mental Health
1080 Emeline Avenue
Santa Cruz, CA 95060-1966
831-454-4000
Fax: 831-454-4770
TDD: 831-454-2123
E-mail: info@santacruzhealth.org
www.santacruzhealth.org

Rama Khalsa PhD, Health Services Administrator
David McNutt MD, County Health Officer

Exists to protect and improve the health of the people in Santa Cruz County. Provides programs in environmental health, public health, medical care, substance abuse prevention and treatment, and mental health. Clients are entitled to information on the costs of care and their options for getting health insurance coverage through a variety of programs.

1830 National Alliance on Mental Illness: California
1851 Heritage Lane
Suite 150
Sacramento, CA 95815
916-567-0163
Fax: 916-567-1757
E-mail: nami.california@namicalifornia.org
www.namicalifornia.org

Dorothy Hendrickson, President
Jessica Cruz, Executive Director
Steven Kite, Deputy Director
Carla Coale, Accounting Manager

An organization of families and individuals whose lives have been affected by serious mental illness. We advocate for lives of quality and respect, without discrimination and stigma, for all our constituents. We provide leadership in advocacy, legislation, policy development, education and support throughout California.

1831 National Association of Mental Illness: California
1851 Heritage Lane
Suite 150
Sacramento, CA 95815
916-567-0163
Fax: 916-567-1757
E-mail: nami.california@namicalifornia.org
www.namicalifornia.org

Dorothy Hendrickson, President
Jessica Cruz, Executive Director
Steven Kite, Deputy Director
Carla Coale, Accounting Manager

Provides support, information and education for families of seriously mentally ill individuals. NAMI California's efforts focus on support, referral, advocacy, research and education. Available are the Journal Magazine, videos, educational classes, and support groups.

1832 National Health Foundation
Hospital Association of Southern California
1000 Town Center Drive
Suite 300
Oxnard, CA 93036
805-351-3727
Fax: 805-650-6456
E-mail: mclark@hasc.org
www.hasc.org

John Calderone, Ph.D., Chair
Jim Barber, President
Mark Gamble, Senior Vice President/Chief Oper
Marty Gallegos, Senior Vice President, Health Po

Charitable affiliate whose mission is to improve and enhance the health of the underserved by developing and supporting inovative programs that can become independently viable, systemic solutions to gaps in healthcare access and delivery and have potential to be replicated nationally.

1833 Orange County Psychiatric Society
17322 Murphy Avenue
Irvine, CA 92614
949-250-3157
Fax: 949-398-8120
www.ocps.org

Holly Appelbaum, Manager

Works to improve public awareness of mental illness and increase financial support.

1834 UCLA Department of Psychiatry &
Biobehavioral Sciences
C8-871 Neuropsychiatry Institute
Box 951759
Los Angeles, CA 90095-1759
310-825-0511
www.psychiatry.ucla.edu

Programs for clinical research treatment for adults and children suffering from psychiatric illness.

1835 United Advocates for Children of California
2035 Hurley Way
Suite 290
Sacramento, CA 95825
916-643-1530
Fax: 916-643-1592
TTY: 916-643-1532
E-mail: information@uacc4families.org
www.www.uacf4hope.org

Carmen Diaz, President
Mary Jane Gross, Treasurer
Errol Campbell, Secretary

A nonprofit organization that works on behalf of children and youth with serious emotional disturbances and their families.

Year Founded: 1933

Colorado

1836 Adolescent and Family Institute of Colorado
10001 W 32nd Avenue
Wheat Ridge, CO 80033-5601

303-238-1231
Fax: 303-238-0500
www.aficonline.com

Mary Panio, Administrator

A licensed and accredited adolescent psychiatric and substance abuse 24 hour facility.

Year Founded: 1982

1837 CAFCA
1120 Lincoln Street
Suite 701
Denver, CO 80203-2137
720-570-8402
Fax: 720-570-8408
E-mail: info@cafca.net
www.cafca.net

Bentley Smith, President
Skip Barber, Executive Director
Monica Mendoza, Executive Assistant Director

The services provided by member agencies include: adoption, alcohol and drug treatment, day treatment, education, family support and preservation, foster care, group homes, independent living, kinship care, mental health treatment and counseling, pregnancy counseling, residential care at all levels, services for homeless and runaway youth, services for sexually reactive youth, sexual abuse services and transitional living.

1838 CHINS UP Youth and Family Services
10 North Farragut Avenue
Colorado Springs, CO 80909
719-636-2122
Fax: 719-634-0482
E-mail: info@griffithcenters.org
www.chinsup.org

Beth Millern, CEO
Lee Patke, COO of Residential Services
Ken Lingle, Community Programs Director
Laura Patke, Chief Clinical Director

A division of The Griffith Centers for Children, Chins Up is a nonprofit multi-service agency serving children and families in the child welfare and juvenile justice systems. Chins Up strives to heal the broken lives of children and families.

Year Founded: 1974

1839 Colorado Health Networks-Value Options
7150 Campus Drive
Suite 300
Colorado Springs, CO 80920-6553
719-538-1430
800-804-5040
Fax: 719-538-1433
www.valueoptions.com

Heyward R. Donigan, President and Chief Executive Of
Douglas Thompson, M.S., M.B.A., Executive Vice President and Chi
Kyle A. Raffaniello, Executive Vice President and Chi
Dan Risku, J.D., Executive Vice President and Gen

CHN is comprised of partnerships between ValueOptions and seven community mental health centers.

Year Founded: 1983

1840 Federation of Families for Children's Mental Health: Colorado Chapter
7475 West Fifth Avenue
Suite 307
Lakewood, CO 80226
303-893-7984
877-792-8886
Fax: 303-433-1605
E-mail: tdillingham@coloradofederation.org
www.coloradofederation.org

Randy Garfield, President/Chair
Sarah Davidon, Vice President
Tom Dillingham, Executive Director
Lacey Berumen, Deputy Director

To promote mental health for all children, youth and families.

1841 Mental Health Association of Colorado
1385 S. Colorado Blvd.
Ste. 610
Denver, CO 80222
303-377-3040
800-456-3249
Fax: 303-377-4920
www.mhacolorado.org

Donald J. Mares, President and CEO
Laura Cordes, Vice President of External Affai
Moe Keller, Vice President of Public Policy
Jamie Gulick, Vice President of Programs & Com

A nonprofit association providing leadership to address the full range of mental health issues in Colorado. The association is a catalyst for improving diagnosis, care and treatment for people of all ages with mental health problems.

Year Founded: 1953

1842 National Alliance on Mental Illness: Colorado
2280 S. Albion Street
Suite 201
Denver, CO 80222
303-321-3104
888-566-6264
Fax: 303-321-0912
E-mail: admin@namicolorado.org
www.namicolorado.org

Greg C. Coleman, President
Scott Glaser, Executive Director
Cheri Bishop, Director of Education Programs
Catherine Benavidez Clayton, Director of Multicultural Progra

A statewide nonprofit organization whose mission is to give strength and hope to individuals with mental illness and their families.

Connecticut

1843 Connecticut National Alliance on Mental Illness
576 Farmington Avenue
5th Floor
Hartford, CT 06105
860-882-0236
800-215-3021
E-mail: namicted@namict.org
www.nami.org

Marisa Walls, President
Kate Mattias MPH JD, Executive Director

Supports families and consumers whose lives are impacted by serious mental illness; educate families, people with mental illnesses and the general public about brain disorders such as schizophrenia, bipolar disorder, obsessive compulsive disorder, and severe depression among other and advocate for improved treatment and services for all individuals with mental illnesses, including increased research that will lead to more effective treatment.

1844 National Alliance on Mental Illness: Connecticut
576 Farmington Avenue
5th Floor
Hartford, CT 06105
860-882-0236
800-215-3021
Fax: 860-882-0240
E-mail: namicted@namict.org
www.namict.org

Marisa Walls, President
Kate Mattias, Executive Director
Shelly Blackman, Administrative Coordinator
Daniela Giordano, MSW, Public Policy Director

NAMI-CT is the only Connecticut organization affiliated with NAMI, the nation's leading grassroots family and consumer organization dedicated to improving the lives of people with serious mental illnesses and their families.

1845 Thames Valley Programs
189 Storrs Rd.
Mansfield Center, CT 06250-1683
860-456-1311
800-426-7792
www.natchaug.org

Corey Gartner, Manager

The Thames Valley Programs offer a continuum of care services with the goal of stabilization for children and adolescents who suffer from a broad range of behavioral and emotional problems. Programs utilize a positive, goal oriented approach to treatment that emphasizes patients' strength and success in the effort to maintain recovery and desired outcomes. Individualized, highly structured treatment programs offered at Thames Valley include: Partial Hospital Program, Intensive Outpatient Program, and Extended Day Program.

Year Founded: 1954

1846 Women's Support Services
158 Gay Street
PO Box 341
Sharon, CT 06069
860-364-1900
Fax: 860-364-5767
E-mail: info@wssdv.org
www.www.wssdv.org/

Lori A. Rivenburgh, Executive Director

Support and advocacy for those affected by domestic violence and abuse as well as women in transition in the towns of Cannan, Cornwall, Kent, North Cannan, Salisbury, and Sharon, CT and nearby NY and MA.

Delaware

1847 Delaware Alliance for the Mentally Ill
2400 W 4th Street
Wilmington, DE 19805-3306

302-427-0787
888-427-2643
Fax: 302-427-2075
E-mail: namide@namide.org
www.namide.org

Mary Berger, President
Edward M. McNally, Esq., Secretary
Julius Meisel, Ph.D., Treasurer

A statewide organization of families, mental health consumers, friends and professionals dedicated to improving
the quality of life for those affected by life changing brain
diseases such as schizophrenia, bipolar disorder and major
depression.

1848 Mental Health Association of Delaware

100 W 10th Street
Suite 600
Wilmington, DE 19801-6604
302-654-6833
800-287-6423
www.www.mhainde.org/wp/

Janet M Brown, President
James Lafferty, Executive Director
Sandra M Rodriguez, Vice President
Lawrence G Boyer, Treasurer

To deliver mental health education, advocacy and support,
and to collaborate to provide mental health leadership in
Delaware

Year Founded: 1932

1849 National Alliance on Mental Illness: Delaware

2400 W 4th Street
Wilmington, DE 19805-3306
302-427-0787
888-427-2643
Fax: 302-427-2075
E-mail: namide@namide.org
www.namide.org

Mary Berger, President
Edward M. McNally, Esq., Secretary
Julius Meisel, Ph.D., Treasurer

A statewide organization of families, mental health consumers, friends, and professionals dedicated to improving
the quality of life for those affected by life-changing brain
diseases such as schizophrenia, bipolar disorder, and major
depression.

1850 National Association of Social Workers: Delaware Chapter

100 W. 10th Street
Suite 608
Wilmington, DE 19801
302-288-0931
E-mail: naswae@aol.com
www.naswde.org

Eleanor Mary Kiesel, President
Debra A.H. O'Neal, Vice President
Norwood James Coleman, Jr., Treasurer
Stefanie Streets, Secretary

Works to enhance the professional growth and development
of its members, to create and maintain professional standards, and to advance sound social policies.

District of Columbia

1851 Department of Health and Human Services/OAS

200 Independence Avenue SW
Washington, DC 20201-4
202-619-0257
877-696-6775
www.www.hhs.gov

Andrea Palm, Chief of Staff (COS)
Daniel R. Levinson, Inspector General
William B. Schultz, General Counsel
Kathleen Sebelius, HHS Secretary

The DHHS is the United States government's principal
agency for protecting the health of all Americans and providing essential human services, especially for those who
are least able to help themselves.

Florida

1852 Family Network on Disabilities

2196 Main St
Suite K
Dunedin, FL 34698-5694
727-523-1130
800-825-5736
Fax: 727-523-8687
E-mail: fnd@fndusa.org
www.fndusa.org

Jennifer Morgan-Byrd, President
Tracy Stewart, Vice President/Treasurer/Parliam
Richard La Belle, Executive Director
Christine Goulbourne, Director of Programs

Family Network on Disabilities is a national network of individuals of all ages who may be at-risk, have disabilities,
or have special needs, and their families, professionals and
concerned citizens. The mission of Family Network on
Disabilities is to ensure through collaboration that individuals have full access to family-driven support, education, information, resources and advocacy, and to serve families of
children with disabilities ages birth through 26, who have a
full range of disabilities as described in section 602.3 of
IDEA.

Year Founded: 1985

1853 Florida Alcohol and Drug Abuse Association

2868 Mahan Drive
Suite 1
Tallahassee, FL 32308
850-878-2196, Fax: 850-878-6584
E-mail: fadaa@fadaa.org
www.fadaa.org

Doug Leonardo, President
Mark Fontaine, MSW, CAP, Executive Director
Frank Rabbito, Vice President
Angie Durbin, Director, Finance and Human Resou

Statewide membership organization that represents more
than 100 community-based substance abuse treatment and
prevention agencies throughout Florida. FADAA has provided advocacy for substance abuse programs and the clients they serve for the past 30 years, as well as quality
training programs for substance abuse professionals and
up-to-date information on substance abuse to the general
public.

Year Founded: 1981

1854 Florida Federation of Families for Children's Mental Health
734 Shadeville Highway
Crawfordville, FL 32327-2405
850-926-3514
877-926-3514
Fax: 413-480-2947
E-mail: ejwells@sprynet.com
www.fifionline.org

Conni Wells

A nationally affiliated parent-run organization focused on the needs of children and youth with emotional, behavioral or mental disorders and their families.

1855 Florida Health Care Association
307 W Park Avenue
PO Box 1459
Tallahassee, FL 32301-1457
850-224-3907
Fax: 850-681-2075
www.fhca.org

Scott J. Allen, President
J. Emmett Reed, CAE, Executive Director
Kristen Knapp, APR, CAE, Director of Communications
Tony Marshall, Senior Director of Reimbursement

FHCA is dedicated to providing the highest quality care for elderly, chronically ill, and disabled individuals.

Year Founded: 1954

1856 Florida Health Information Management Association
7510 Ehrlich Road
Tampa, FL 33625-1462
813-358-8598
Fax: 813-792-9442
E-mail: fhima@infionline.net
www.fhima.org

Alice Noblin, PhD, RHIA, CCS, President
Erin Head, RHIA, Chief Delegate
Carolyn Glavan, MS RHIA, Executive Director
Kaley Schnitker, Student Liaison

Fosters professional development for its members, promotes privacy and quality of health information through education, communication and advocacy.

1857 Florida National Alliance for the Mentally Ill
PO Box 961
Tallahassee, FL 32302
850-671-4445
877-626-4352
Fax: 850-671-5272
E-mail: Info@namiflorida.org
www.www.namiflorida.org

Dr. Rajiv Tandon, President
Paula Kegelman, Second Vice President
Carol Weber, Program Director
Ken DeCerchio, Treasurer

Nation's leading self-help organization for all those affected by severe brain disorders. Mission is to bring consumers and families with similar experiences together to share information about services, care providers, and ways to cope with the challenges of schizophrenia, manic depression, and other serious mental illnesses.

1858 Mental Health Association of West Florida
840 W Lakeview Avenue
Pensacola, FL 32501-1967
850-438-9879
Fax: 850-438-5901
www.www.mhawfl.org/

Offers special information and referrals for families of mental health.

Year Founded: 1957

1859 National Alliance on Mental Illness: Florida
PO Box 961
Suite 6
Tallahassee, FL 32302
850-671-4445
877-626-4352
Fax: 850-671-5272
E-mail: Info@namiflorida.org
www.www. namiflorida.org

Dr. Rajiv Tandon, President
Paula Kegelman, Second Vice President
Carol Weber, Program Director
Ken DeCerchio, Treasurer

Contains thirty-four affiliates in communities throughout Florida that provide education, advocacy, and support groups for people with mental illness and their loved ones.

1860 National Association of Social Workers Florida Chapter
1931 Dellwood Drive
Tallahassee, FL 32303-4815
850-224-2400
800-352-6279
Fax: 850-561-6279
E-mail: naswfl@naswfl.org
www.naswfl.org

Mitch Rosenwald, President
Cori Bauserman, LCSW, Vice President
Rikki A. Vidak, LCSW, Secretary
Mark A. Lazarus, LCSW, Treasurer

NASW is a membership organization for professional social workers in Florida. NASWFL provides: continuing education, information center, advocacy for employment and legislation.

Georgia

1861 Georgia Association of Homes and Services for Children
50 Hurt Plaza
Suite 1555
Atlanta, GA 30303
404-572-6170
Fax: 404-572-6171
E-mail: norman@gahsc.org
www.gahsc.org

Normer Adams, Executive Director

GAHSC is an association that is dedicated to supporting those who care for children who are at risk of abuse and neglect. Member agencies of GAHSC include family foster care, community group homes, education programs and others.

1862 Georgia Parent Support Network

1381 Metropolitan Parkway
Atlanta, GA 30310-4455
404-758-4500
800-832-8645
Fax: 404-758-6833
E-mail: slsmith2@ix.netcom.com
www.gpsn.org

Kathy Dennis, President
Sue L. Smith, Ed.D., Chief Executive Officer
Brett Barton, LPC, Chief Operating Officer
Linda Seay, Treasurer

The Georgia Parent Support Network is dedicated to providing support, education and advocacy for children and
youth with mental illness, emotional disturbances and behavioral difference and their families.

1863 Grady Health Systems: Central Fulton CMHC

80 Jesse Hill Jr Drive S.E.
Atlanta, GA 30303-3031
404-616-4307
www.gradyhealthsystem.org

Michael Young, CEO
Clayton Sheptherd, Treasurer

Grady Health System improves the health of the community by providing quality, comprehensive health care in a
compassionate, culturally competent, ethical and fiscally
responsible manner. Grady maintains its commitment to the
underserved of Fulton and DeKalb counties, while also providing care for residents of metro Atlanta and Georgia.
Grady leads through its clinical exellence, innovative research and progressive medical education and training.

Year Founded: 1982

1864 National Alliance on Mental Illness: Georgia

3180 Presidential Dr
Suite A
Atlanta, GA 30340-3916
770-234-0855
800-728-1052
Fax: 770-234-0237
E-mail: namigeorgia@namiga.org
www.namiga.org

Martee Horne, President
Eric Spencer, Executive Director
Jean Dervan, Program Director
Pat Strode, CIT Administrator

The purpose of NAMI Georgia, Inc. is to relieve the suffering and improve the quality of life for mentally ill Geor-
gians and their families.

Hawaii

1865 Hawaii Families As Allies

99-209 Moanalua Road
Suite 305
Aiea, HI 96701
808-487-8785
866-361-8825
Fax: 808-487-0514
E-mail: hfaa@hfaa.net
www.www.hfaa.net

Linda Machado, Executive Director
Charlene Daraban, Family Resource Specialist
Leinaala Launiu, Youth Specialist Coordinator
Shanelle Lum, Public Policy/Information Specia

Parent Advocacy group for those with children who have
mental disorders.

1866 National Alliance on Mental Illness: Hawaii

770 Kapiolani Boulevard
Suite 613
Honolulu, HI 96813-5212
808-591-1297
Fax: 808-591-2058
E-mail: info@namihawaii.org
www.namihawaii.org

Carol Kozlovich, President
Carol Denis, First Vice President
Robert Collesano, Second Vice President
Dana Anderson, Secretary

Nation's leading self-help organization for people living
with mental illness and their families. Provides education,
support and advocacy for consumers, families and care givers on the challanges of living with schizophrenia, bipolar,
and other serious mental illnesses.

Idaho

1867 Idaho Alliance for the Mentally Ill

PO Box 95
Hailey, ID 83333
208-242-7430
800-572-9940
Fax: 208-673-6685
E-mail: namiidaho@yahoo.com
www.www.nami.org/sites/namiidaho

Kathleen Mercer, Chairman
Tom Hanson, President
Kim Jardine-Dickerson, Vice President
Michael Sandvig, BS, Treasurer

NAMI Idaho is a non-profit, tax exempt family organization for people with brain disorders.

Year Founded: 1991

1868 National Alliance on Mental Illness: Idaho

PO Box 95
Hailey, ID 83333
208-242-7430
E-mail: namiidaho@yahoo.com
www.nami.org/sites/namiidaho

Tom Hanson, President
Kim Jardine-Dickerson, Vice President
Michael Sandvig, BS, Treasurer
Kathleen Mercer, Secretary

A nationwide organization dedicated to support, education
and advocacy on behalf of people with a mental illness and
their families.

Year Founded: 1991

Illinois

1869 Allendale Association

PO Box 1088
Lake Villa, IL 60046-1088
847-356-2351
888-255-3631
Fax: 847-356-0289
www.allendale4kids.org

Connie Borucki, Senior Vice President of Human R
Vanessa L. Genger, Vice President of Development &

Dr. Sandra E.J. Clavelli, Director of Clinical Training
Judy Griffeth, Placement Director

The Allendale Association is a private, non-profit organization dedicated to the excellence and innovation in the care, education, treatment and advocacy for troubled children, youth and their families.

Year Founded: 1897

1870 Baby Fold

108 E Wilow Street
Normal, IL 61761
309-452-1170
Fax: 309-452-0115
E-mail: info@thebabyfold.org
www.www.thebabyfold.org/

The Baby Fold is a multi-service agency that provides Residential, Special Education, Child Welfare, and Family Support Services to children and families in central Illinois.

Year Founded: 1902

1871 Chaddock

205 S 24th Street
Quincy, IL 62301-4492
217-222-0034
888-242-3625
Fax: 217-222-3865
E-mail: kehmen@chaddock.org
www.chaddock.org

Debbie Reed, President/CEO
Linda Harcharick, Director of Finance
Amy Hyer, Director of Human Resources
Matt Obert, Director of Quality Assurance

A faith-based, not-for-profit organization dedicated to providing hope and healing to children and families. Chaddock specializes in developmental trauma and attachment and provides a wide-range of services including child and adolescent residential treatment, independent living program, group home, special education school serving children 6 to 21, three levles of foster care and adoption

Year Founded: 1853

1872 Chicago Child Care Society

5467 S University Avenue
Chicago, IL 60615-5193
773-643-0452
Fax: 773-643-0620
www.cccsociety.org

Dorri McWhorter, President
Robert Lindstrom, Vice President
Deborah Hagman-Shannon, Ph.D., Executive Director
Curt Holderfield, LCSW, Associate Director

Chicago Child Care Society exists to protect vulnerable children and strengthen their families. We strive to be among the premier providers of high quality and effective child welfare services. We believe the quality of life for future generations depends upon the quality of care provided for children today. We believe children should be provided with services and opportunities that will enable them to reach their optimism physical, mental and social development. We believe all the children are entitled to the protection and nurturing care of adults, preferably within their birth families. However, if family can't fulfill these basic functions, we believe society, by either public or private means should provide the best alternative care.

Year Founded: 1949

1873 Children's Home Association of Illinois

2130 N Knoxville Avenue
Peoria, IL 61603-2497
309-685-1047
Fax: 309-687-7299
www.chail.org

Clete Winkelmann, President & CEO
Melissa Riddle, Vice President, Chief Financial
Danial Haligas, Executive Vice President
Lou Tenarvitz, Vice President, Development

Nonprofit, non-sectarian multiple program and social service organization. Giving children a childhood and future by protecting them, teaching them, healing them and by building strong communities and loving families.

1874 Coalition of Illinois Counselors Organization

PO Box 1086
Northbrook, IL 60065-1086
815-787-0515
E-mail: imhca@imhca.org
www.cico-il.org

Daniel Stasi, Executive Director

The Coalition has as its purpose representation of and advocacy for all Illinois counselros and master's level psychologists, their organization and their clients, in relations to government in all its branches and agencies; relevant segments of the private sector, such as insurance, managed care, business and industry, and other mental health providers, health and human services organization and professions

1875 Family Service Association of Greater Elgin Area

1140 N. McLean Blvd.
Suite I
Elgin, IL 60123
847-695-3680
E-mail: JZahm@fsaelgin.org
www.fsaelgin.org

Lisa La Forge, Executive Director
Dr. Sandra Angelo, Dir. Consumer Credit Counseling
Jon A Zahm, Developmental/Community Rel.

A non-profit agancy, Family Service Association has served the Greater Elgin Area since 1931. Supported both publicly and privately, most of the funding is received from such local sources as United Ways, corporate and individual contributions and client fees.

1876 Human Resources Development Institute

222 S Jefferson Street
Chicago, IL 60661-5603
312-441-9009
Fax: 312-441-9019
E-mail: Info@hardi.org
www.hrdi.org

Joel K. Johnson, President and CEO
Miller Anderson, COO

Community based behavioral health and human services organization. This nonprofit agency on the south side of Chicago, is concerned with mental health and substance abuse solutuions. Offering more than 40 programs at 20 sites.

Year Founded: 1974

1877 Illinois Alcoholism and Drug Dependency Association
937 South Second Street
Springfield, IL 62704-2701
217-528-7335
Fax: 217-528-7340
www.iadda.org

Bruce Suardini, Chairman
Sara Moscato Howe, Chief Executive Officer
Eric Foster, Chief Operating Officer
Jerry Scogmo, Treasurer

IADDA is a statewide organization established in 1967 respresenting more than 100 prevention and treatment agencies, as well as individuals who are interested in the substance abuse field. The Association advocates for sound public policy that will create healthier families and safer communites. IADDA members educate government officials in Springfield and Washington, and work to increase the public understanding of substance abuse and addiction.

Year Founded: 1967

1878 Larkin Center
1212 Larkin Avenue
Elgin, IL 60123-6098
847-695-5656
Fax: 847-695-0897
www.larkincenter.org

Dennis L Graf MS, Executive Director
Richard Peterson MSW, Executive Director
Martine Lyle, Admissions And QA Director
Michelle Potter MS LCPC, Clinical Director

Our mission is achieved through the efforts of Larkins Center's team of skilled professionals in creative cooperation with the community.

Year Founded: 1896

1879 Little City Foundation (LCF)
1760 W Algonquin Road
Palatine, IL 60067-4799
847-358-5510
Fax: 847-358-3291
E-mail: people@littlecity.org
www.littlecity.org

Matthew B. Schubert, President
Douglas A. Wilson, Vice President
Shawn E. Jeffers, Executive Director
Ed Hockfield, Chief Development Officer

The mission of Little City Foundation is to provide state of the art services to help children and adults with mental retardation or other developmental emotional and behavioral challenges to lead meaningful, productive, and dignified lives.

1880 Metropolitan Family Services
One North Dearborn
Suite 1000
Chicago, IL 60602
312-986-4000
Fax: 312-986-4289
E-mail: contactus@metrofamily.org
www.metrofamily.org

Tony W. Hunter, Chair
Ricardo Estrada, President & CEO
Colleen M. Jones, Executive Vice President & Chief
Denis Hurley, Chief Financial Officer

Our mission is to help Chicago - area families become strong, stable and self-sufficient.

Year Founded: 1857

1881 National Alliance on Mental Illness: Illinois
218 West Lawrence
Springfield, IL 62704-2612
217-522-1403
800-346-4572
Fax: 217-522-3598
E-mail: namiil@sbcglobal.net
www.il.nami.org

Hugh Brady, President
Lora Thomas, Executive Director
Brian Allen, Vice President
Mike Bach, Director

A state-wide organization comprised of local Illinois Affiliates dedicated to the task of eradicating mental illness and improving the lives of persons with mental illness and their families.

Indiana

1882 Indiana Resource Center for Autism (IRCA)
1905 North Range Road
Bloomington, IN 47408-2601
812-855-6508
800-825-4733
Fax: 812-855-9630
TTY: 812-855-9396
E-mail: prattc@indiana.edu
www.iidc.indiana.edu/irca

Cathy Pratt PhD, BCBA-D, Center Director
Donna Beasley, Administrative Program Secretary
Pamela Anderson, Outreach/Resource Specialist
Melissa Dubie, MS, Research Associate

Conducts outreach training and consultations, engage in research, develop and disseminate information on behalf of individuals across the autism spectrum, Aspergers syndrome, and other pervasive developmental disorders. Provides communities, organizations, agencies and families with the knowledge and skills to support children and adults in typical early intervention, school, community work and home.

1883 National Alliance on Mental Illness: Indiana
PO Box 22697
Indianapolis, IN 46222-697
317-925-9399
800-677-6442
Fax: 317-925-9398
E-mail: nfo@namiindiana.org
www.namiindiana.org

Joshua G. Sprunger, M.A., Executive Director
Joanne Abbott, Program Director
Marianne Halbert, J.D., Criminal Justice Program Directo
Linda Williams, Program Coordinator

Dedicated to improving the quality of life for those persons who are affected by mental illness.

Iowa

1884 Iowa Federation of Families for Children's Mental Health
106 South Booth
PO Box 362
Anamosa, IA 52205
319-462-2187
888-400-6302
Fax: 319-462-6789
E-mail: help@iffcmh.org
www.www.iffcmh.org

Lori Reynolds, Executive Director
Heidi Reynolds, Program Director

Our mission is to link families to community, county and state partners for needed support and services; and to promote system change that will enable families to live in a safe, stable and respectful environment.

1885 National Alliance of Mental Illness Iowa
5911 Meredith Drive
Suite E
Des Moines, IA 50322-1903
515-254-0417
800-417-0417
Fax: 515-254-1103
E-mail: info@namiiowa.com
www.www.namiiowa.com/

Diane Banasiak, President
Nancy Hale, Executive Director
Jeff Grell, 1st Vice President
Shelly Kramer, 2nd Vice President

NAMI is dedicated to the education of mental illnesses and to the improvement of the quality of life of all whose lives are affected by these diseases.

1886 National Alliance on Mental Illness: Iowa
5911 Meredith Drive
Suite E
Des Moines, IA 50322-1903
515-254-0417
800-417-0417
Fax: 515-254-1103
E-mail: info@namiiowa.com
www.namiiowa.com

Diane Banasiak, President
Nancy Hale, Executive Director
Marijke Hodgson, Education Coordinator and Walk M
John Rowley, Administrative Assistant

Mission is to raise public awareness and concern about mental illness, to foster research, to improve treatment and to upgrade the system of care for the people of Iowa.

Year Founded: 1979

Kansas

1887 Keys for Networking: Kansas Parent Information & Resource Center
900 South Kansas Avenue
Suite 301
Topeka, KS 66612
785-233-8732
800-499-8732
Fax: 785-235-6659

E-mail: jadams@keys.org
www.keys.org

Mary Ellen Conlee, President
Greg Whittaker, Treasurer
Juan Perez, Secretary
Cheryl Renolds-Buckley, Secretary

A non-profit organization providing information, support, and training to families in Kansas whose children who have educational, emotional, and/or behavioral problems.

1888 National Alliance on Mental Illness: Kansas
610 SW 10th Ave
#203
Topeka, KS 66612-1674
785-233-0755
800-539-2660
Fax: 785-233-4804
E-mail: info@namiKansas.org
www.www.namikansas.org

Rick Cagan, Executive Director

Nation's leading self-help membership organization for all those affected by severe brain disorders. Mission is to provide peer support, education, advocacy and research on behalf of persons affected by serious mental illness and their family members.

Kentucky

1889 Children's Alliance
718 6th Avenue South
Seattle, WA 98104
206-324-0340
800-854-KIDS
Fax: 206-325-6291
E-mail: seattle@childrensalliance.org
www.www.childrensalliance.org/

Tom Rembiesa, Chair
Paola Maranan, Executive Director
Nancy Norman, Finance and Operations Director
Jon Gould, Deputy Director

Our mission is to shape public policy, inform constituencies and provide leadership in advocacy for Kentucky's children and families.

Year Founded: 1983

1890 KY-SPIN
10301-B Deering Road
Louisville, KY 40272-4000
502-937-6894
800-525-7746
Fax: 502-937-6464
E-mail: spininc@kyspin.com
www.kyspin.com

Non-profit organization dedicated to promoting programs which will enable persons with disabilities and their families to enhance their quality of life.

Year Founded: 1988

1891 Kentucky Alliance for the Mentally Ill
808 Monticello Street
Building 103
Somerset, KY 42501
606-451-6935
800-257-5081
Fax: 606-677-4052

E-mail: namiky@bellsouth.net
www.namikyadvocacy.com/

Wendy Morris, Chairman
Bertha Diaz-Story, 1st Vice Chair
Dr. Sean Reilley, 2nd Vice Chair
Cathy Epperson, Executive Director

Nation's leading self-help organization for all those affected by severe brain disorders. Mission is to bring consumers and families with similar experiences together to share information about services, care providers, and ways to cope with the challenges of schizophrenia, manic depression, and other serious mental illnesses.

1892 Kentucky Partnership for Families and Children

207 Homes Street
1st Floor
Frankfort, KY 40621
502-875-1320
800-369-0855
Fax: 502-875-1399
E-mail: kpfc@kypartneship.org
www.kypartnership.org

Carol W Cecil, Executive Director
Kate Tilton, Program Coordinator
Carmilla Ratliff, Youth Empowerment Specialist
Barbara Greene, Project Coordinator

Non-profit organization focused on the need of children and youth with emotional, behavioral or mental disorders and their families. Kentucky state chapter of the Federation of Families for Children's Mental Health.

1893 Kentucky Psychiatric Association

649 Charity Court
Suite #13
Frankfort, KY 40601
502-695-4843
877-597-7924
Fax: 502-695-4441
E-mail: kpma@timewarnercable.com
www.kyppsych.org

Mark S. Wright, MD, President
Theresa Walton, Executive Director

A non-profit association of medical doctors who have completed a psychiatry residency.

1894 National Alliance on Mental Illness: Kentucky

808 Monticello Street
Building 103
Somerset, KY 42501
606-451-6935
800-257-5081
Fax: 606-677-4052
E-mail: namiky@bellsouth.net
www.ky.nami.org

Wendy Morris, Chair
Bertha Diaz-Story, 1st Vice Chair
Dr. Sean Reilley, 2nd Vice Chair
Charlotte Stogsdill, Secretary

NAMI Kentucky is a self-help organization that is part of a nation-wide network devoted to improving the lives of the seriously mentally ill and decreasing the prevailing stigma associated with mental illness.

1895 National Association of Social Workers: Kentucky Chapter

304 West Liberty Street
Suite 201
Louisville, KY 40202-3035
800-526-8098
Fax: 502-589-3602
E-mail: naswky@aol.com
www.www.nasw-ky.affiniscape.com

Professional membership organization, for state social workers.

1896 ValueOptions

240 Corporate Boulevard
Norfolk, VA 23502-4847
757-459-5100
www.valueoptions.com

Heyward R. Donigan, President and Chief Executive Of
Douglas Thompson, M.S., M.B.A., Executive Vice President and Chi
Kyle A. Raffaniello, Executive Vice President and Chi
Dan Risku, J.D., Executive Vice President and Gen

Supports the unique needs of client organizations with traditional managed care products, integrated behavioral health care services, as well as wellness and prevention initiatives and work/life programs.

Louisiana

1897 Louisiana Federation of Families for Children's Mental Health

5627 Superior Drive
Suite A-2
Baton Rouge, LA 70816-6085
225-293-3508
800-224-4010
Fax: 225-293-3510
E-mail: info@laffcmh.org
www.laffcmh.org

Anthony D. Beasley, President
Shana Sears, Vice President
Cynthia Cobb, Secretary

A parent-run organization focused on the needs of children and youth with emmotional, behavioral or mental disorders and their families.

Year Founded: 1991

1898 National Alliance on Mental Illness: Louisiana

5534 Galeria Dr.
Suite A
Baton Rouge, LA 70816
225-924-3900
800-437-0303
Fax: 225-291-6244
E-mail: info@namilouisiana.org
www.namilouisiana.org

Ms. Stephani Boyd, President
Mitch Bergeron, Vice President
Greg Mullowney, Treasurer
Juliana Fort, Secretary

Dedicated to the eradication of mental illnesses and to the improvement of the quality of life for persons of all ages who are affected by mental illnesses

Year Founded: 1984

Maine

1899 National Alliance on Mental Illness: Maine
1 Bangor Street
Augusta, ME 04330-4701
207-622-5767
800-464-5767
Fax: 207-621-8430
E-mail: info@namimaine.org
www.namimaine.org

Jenna Mehnert, MSW, Executive Director
Christine Canty Brooks, Director of Peer and Family Prog
Sophie M Gabrion, MS, Mental Health Outreach Coordinat
Gilles Soucy, Criminal Justice Coordinator

Dedicated to improving the lives of all people affected by
mental illness NAMI Maine provides services across the
entire state of Maine. Available on Twitter and FaceBook.

Year Founded: 1977

Maryland

1900 Community Behavioral Health Association of Maryland: CBH
18 Egges Lane
Cantonsville, MD 21228-4511
410-788-1865
Fax: 410-788-1768
E-mail: mdcbh@aol.com
www.www.mdcbh.org/

Herbert Cromwell, Executive Director

Professional association for Maryland's network of community behavioral health programs operating in the public
and private sectors.

1901 Maryland Psychiatric Research Center
655 West Baltimore Street
Baltimore, MD 21201-1559
410-402-7666
Fax: 410-402-7198
www.www.mprc.umaryland.edu

Dr. William Carpenter Jr, Director

To study the manifestations, causes, and innovative treatment of zchizophrenia.

Year Founded: 1807

1902 Mental Health Association of Maryland
1301 York Road
Suite 505
Lutherville, MD 21093
443-901-1550
800-572-6426
Fax: 443-901-0038
E-mail: info@mhamd.org
www.mhamd.org

Stuart B. Silver, MD, President
Linda J. Raines, Chief Executive Officer
Lea Ann Browning McNee, Deputy Director
Adrienne Ellis, Director of the Maryland Parity

The Mental Health Association of Maryland is dedicated to
promoting mental health, preventing mental disorders and
achieving victory over mental illness through advocacy, education, research and service.

1903 National Alliance on Mental Illness: Maryland
10630 Little Patuxent Pkwy
Suite 475
Columbia, MD 21044-3264
410-884-8691
877-878-2371
Fax: 410-884-8695
E-mail: info@namimd.org
www.namimd.org

Chris Griffin, President
Kate Farinholt, Executive Director
Jessica Honke, Policy and Advocacy Director
Kristin Knott, Program, Training, and Events Co

A grassroots organization dedicated to education, support
and advocacy for persons with mental illnesses, their families and the wider community.

1904 National Association of Social Workers: Maryland Chapter
5750 Executive Drive
Suite 208
Baltimore, MD 21228-1767
410-788-1066
800-867-6776
Fax: 410-747-0635
E-mail: nasw.md@verizon.net
www.nasw-md.org

Cherie Cannon, President
Anna Williams, Vice President
Daphne McClellan, Ph.D., Executive Director
John Costa, Deputy Director

The mission of the NASW-MD chapter is to support, promote and advocate for the social work profession and its
clients, promote just and equitable social policies and for
the health and welfare of the people of Maryland.

1905 National Federation of Families for Children's Mental Health
Attn: Marion Mealing, Admin Asst
9605 Medical Center Drive
Rockville, MD 20850
240-403-1901
Fax: 240-403-1909
E-mail: ffcmh@ffcmh.org
www.ffcmh.org/

Sandra Spencer, Executive Director
Lizzette Albright, Finance Director
Lynda Gargan, Senior Managing Director
Nicole Marshall, Projects & Logistics Manager

A national family-run organization serves to: provide advocacy at the national level for the rights of children and
youth with emotional, behavioral and mental health challenges and their families; provide leadership and technical
assistance to a nation-wide network of family run organizations; and collaborate with family run and other child serving organization to transform mental health care in
America. The vision of the Federation is, through a family
driven approach, to obtain the needed support and services
for children and youth with these challenges in order for
these children to grow up healthy and be able to maximize
their potential.

1906 Sheppard Pratt Health System
6501 N Charles Street
Baltimore, MD 21204-6893

410-938-3800
888-938-4207
E-mail: info@sheppardpratt.org
www.www.sheppardpratt.org

Steven S Sharfstein, CEO
Dr Robert Roca, VP & Medical Director

1907 Survey & Analysis Branch
5600 Fishers Lane
Rockwall II Suite 15C
Rockville, MD 20857-1
301-443-3343
Fax: 301-443-7926
www.samhsa.gov

Dr. Ronald Manderscheid, Branch Chief

Federally funded agency studying mental health issues.

Massachusetts

1908 Bridgewell
471 Broadway
Lynn, MA 01904-2649
781-593-1088
Fax: 781-593-5731
E-mail: info@bridgewell.org
www.bridgewell.org

Robert Stearns, President and Chief Executive Of

Private, non-profit corporation that provides residential, clinical, recreation, day and employment, work training, affordable housing, and multi-cultural and community education services for people with disabilities, their families, and advocates in Northeastern Massachusetts.

1909 CASCAP
231 Somerville Avenue
Floor 10
Somerville, MA 02143
617-492-5559
Fax: 617-492-6928
TTY: 617-234-2992
E-mail: info@cascap.org
www.cascap.org

Mr. Shawn Luther, Chair
Michael Haran, Chief Executive Officer
Mr. Tony Loftis, Clerk
Mr. Thomas M Sadtler, MSW, MBA, Treasurer

Committed to improving the quality of life for members of the community who may be disadvantaged by poverty, disability, or age. Our purpose is to help thos we serve achieve optimal levels of personal autonomy and community integration.

Year Founded: 1973

1910 Concord Family and Youth Services A Division of Justice Resource Institute
160 Gould Street
Suite 300
Needham, MA 02494-2300
781-559-4900
Fax: 978-263-3088
www.jri.org

Arden O'Connor, Chairperson
Andy Pond, MSW, MAT, President
Gregory Canfield, MSW, Executive Vice President
Deborah Reuman, MBA, Chief Financial Officer

Concord Family and Youth Services, a division of the non-profit Justice Resource Institute, Inc., has been providing help to adolescents, young adults and families since 1814. Programs include a group home for boys, a therapeutic high school in Acton, two residential schools for girls, as well as, parenting and adoption support services through First Connections.

1911 Depression and Bipolar Support Alliance of Boston
115 Mill Street
PO Box 102
Belmont, MA 02478
617-855-2795
Fax: 617-855-3666
E-mail: info@dbsaboston.org
www.dbsaboston.org

Michele O'Shea, President
John Parente, Vice President
Dennis Hagler, Treasurer

DBSA-BOSTON is a resource for people with affective disorders and their families and friends.

1912 Jewish Family and Children's Services
1430 Main Street
Waltham, MA 02451
781-647-5327
E-mail: info@jfcsboston.org
www.jfcsboston.org

Robin Neiterman, President
Alan Jacobson, Senior VP Programs
Rimma Zefland, Chief Executive Officer
Keene Metzger, Chief Financial Officer

Cares for individuals and families by providing exceptional human service and health care programs, guided by Jewish traditions of social responsibility, compassion, and respect for all members of the community. Available on FaceBook.

1913 Massachusetts Behavioral Health Partnership
1000 Washington Street
Suite 310
Boston, MA 02118-5002
617-790-4000
800-495-0086
Fax: 617-790-4128
www.masspartnership.com

Elizabeth O'Brien, Manager

The Massachusetts Behavioral Health Partnership manages the mental health and substance abuse services for MassHealth Members who select the Division's Primary Care Clinician Plan.

Year Founded: 1996

1914 Massachusetts National Alliance on Mental Illness
529 Main Street
Suite 1M17
Boston, MA 02129
617-580-8541
800-370-9085
Fax: 617-580-8673
E-mail: namimass@aol.com
www.namimass.org

Steve Rosenfeld, President
Laurie Martinelli, Executive Director

Marilyn DeSantis, Bookkeeper/Donor Relations
Karen Gromis, Events and Walk Manager

Nation's leading self-help organization for all those affected by severe brain disorders. Mission is to bring consumers and families with similar experiences together to share information about services, care providers, and ways to cope with the challenges of schizophrenia, manic depression, and other serious mental illnesses.

1915 Mental Health and Substance Abuse Corporations of Massachusetts
251 W Central Street
Suite 21
Natick, MA 01760-3758
508-647-8385
Fax: 508-647-8311
E-mail: vdigravio@ABHmass.org
www.www.mhsacm.org/

Vic DiGravio, President/CEO
Sara Hartman, Vice President, Mental Health
Constance Peters, Vice President for Addiction Ser
Amanda Gilman, Director of Public Policy and Re

To promote community-based mental health and substance abuse services as the most appropriate, clinically effective, and cost-sensitive method for providing care to individuals in need.

1916 Parent Professional Advocacy League
45 Bromfield Street
10th Floor
Boston, MA 02108
617-542-7860
866-815-8122
Fax: 617-542-7832
E-mail: info@ppal.net
www.ppal.net

Earl N. Stuck, Chair
Lisa Lambert, Executive Director
Deborah A. Fauntleroy, MSW, Associate Director
Meri Viano, Senior Regional Manager

Provides support, education, and advocacy around issues related to children's mental health

Michigan

1917 Borgess Behavioral Medicine Services
1521 Gull Road
Kalamazoo, MI 49048-1640
269-226-7000
Fax: 269-226-7396
www.borgess.com

James Devlin, Chair
William M. Harrison, Secretary
Susan Pozo, PhD, Treasurer

Offers patients and families a wide array of services to address their mental health concerns.

1918 Boysville of Michigan
8759 Clinton Macon Road
Clinton, MI 49236-9569
517-423-7455
Fax: 517-423-5442
E-mail: info@hccsnet.org
www.boysville.org

Tim Patton, Chairperson
Francis Boylan, Executive Director
Sharon Berkobien, Program Operations Director
John Meszaros, Admissions Director

Boysville of Michigan works with one thousand plus boys and girls and their families on a daily basis in both residential and community based programs throughout Michigan and northwestern Ohio.

Year Founded: 1948

1919 Macomb County Community Mental Health
22550 Hall Road
5th Floor
Clinton Twp., MI 48036
586-469-5258
Fax: 586-307-3898
www.macombcountymi.gov

Ricco Bono, Manager

Provides a wide variety of mental health treatment and support services to adults and children with mental illness, developmental disabilities, and substance abuse treatment needs.

1920 Michigan Alliance for the Mentally Ill
921 N Washington Avenue
Lansing, MI 48906-5137
517-485-4049
800-331-4264
Fax: 517-485-2333
E-mail: namimichigan@acd.net
www.www.namimi.org

Hubert Huebl, President

Nation's leading self-help organization for all those affected by severe brain disorders. Mission is to bring consumers and families with similar experiences together to share information about services, care providers, and ways to cope with the challenges of schizophrenia, manic depression, and other serious mental illnesses.

Year Founded: 1979

1921 Michigan Association for Children with Emotional Disorders: MACED
230233 Southfield Road
Suite 219
Southfield, MI 48076
248-433-2200
Fax: 248-433-2299
E-mail: info@michkids.org
www.michkids.org

Samuel L Davis, Clinical Director

Ensures that children with serious emotional disorders receive appropriate mental health and educational services so that they reach their full potential. To provide support to families and to encourage community understanding of the need for specialized programs for their children.

1922 Michigan Association for Children's Mental Health
6017 W St Joseph Highway
Suite 200
Lansing, MI 48823-3104
517-372-4016
888-226-4543
Fax: 517-372-4032
www.acmh-mi.org

Gail Lanphear, President
Jane Shank, Executive Director
Mary Porter, Business Manager
Lois DeMott, Administrative Assistant

Provides information, support, resources, referral and advocacy for children and youth with mental, emotional, or behavioral disorders and their families

1923 National Alliance on Mental Illness: Michigan

921 N Washington Avenue
Lansing, MI 48906-5137
517-485-4049
800-331-4264
Fax: 517-485-2333
E-mail: namimichigan@acd.net
www.www.namimi.org

Hubert Huebl, President

To assist affiliates, provide support, promote education, pursue advocacy and encourage research on mental illness.
Year Founded: 1979

1924 Southwest Counseling & Development Services

1700 Waterman Street
Detroit, MI 48209-2022
313-841-8900
Fax: 313-841-3756
www.swsol.org

Seth Lloyd, Chair
John Vancamp, President
Lenora Hardy-Foster, Executive Director
Joseph Tardella, Executive Director, Southwest Co

A mental health agency working to promote community well being. The mission is to enhance the well being of individuals, families and the community by providing effective leadership and innovative, quality mental health services.

1925 Woodlands Behavioral Healthcare Network

960 M-60 East
Cassopolis, MI 49031-9339
269-445-3043
www.woodlandsbhn.org

Kathy Boes, CEO

Provides community mental health services.

Minnesota

1926 NASW Minnesota Chapter

Iris Park Place, Suite 340
1885 University Avenue W
Saint Paul, MN 55104-3458
651-293-1935
Fax: 651-293-0952
E-mail: email@naswmn.org
www.nasw-heartland.org

Alan Ingram, Executive Director

To promote the profession of Social Work by establishing and maintaining professional standards and by advancing the authority and credibility of Social Work; to provide services to its members by supplying opportunities for professional development and leadership and by enhancing communication among its members; to advocate for clients by promoting political action and community education.

1927 National Alliance on Mental Illness: Minnesota

800 Transfer Road
Suite 7A
Saint Paul, MN 55114-1414
651-645-2948
888-473-0237
Fax: 651-645-7379
E-mail: namihelps@namimn.org
www.www.namihelps.org

Barb Lindberg, President
Sue Abderholden, Executive Director
Morgan Caldwell, Peer Programming Assistant
Donna Fox, Program Director

A non-profit organization dedicated to improving the lives of adults and children with mental illness and their families. NAMI-MN offers programs of education, support and advocacy, and supports research efforts.
Year Founded: 1976

1928 North American Training Institute: Division of the Minnesota Council on Compulsive Gambling

314 W Superior Street
Suite 508
Duluth, MN 55802-1868
218-722-1503
888-989-9234
Fax: 218-722-0346
E-mail: info@nati.org
www.nati.org

Elizabeth George, Executive Director

The NATI conducts web based clinical courses to provide specific knowledge and advanced training leading to national certification for professionals in the prevention, treatment, and rehabilitation of patholgical gamblers.
Year Founded: 1988

1929 Pacer Center

8161 Normandale Boulevard
Minneapolis, MN 55437-1044
952-838-9000
888-248-0822
Fax: 952-838-0199
TTY: 952-838-0190
E-mail: pacer@pacer.org
www.pacer.org

Paul Luehr, Board President
Alison Bakken, Board Vice-President
Paula Goldberg, Executive Director
Dan Levinson, Board Secretary

To expand opportunities and anhance the quality of life of children and young adults with disabilities and their families, based on the concept of parents helping parents.
Year Founded: 1977

Mississippi

1930 Mississippi Alliance for the Mentally Ill

411 Briarwood Drive
Suite 401
Jackson, MI 39206-3058
601-899-9058
800-357-0388
Fax: 601-956-6380

E-mail: namimiss1@aol.com
www.nami.org

Debbie Waller, President
Melissa Difatta, Interim-Executive Director
Ricky Quinn, Program Director
Christy Bradshaw, Administrative Assistant

Nation's leading self-help organization for all those affected by severe brain disorders. Mission is to bring consumers and families with similar experiences together to share information about services, care providers, and ways to cope with the challenges of schizophrenia, manic depression, and other serious mental illnesses.

Year Founded: 1981

1931 National Alliance on Mental Illness: Mississippi

2618 Southerland Street
Suite 401
Jackson, MS 39216
601-899-9058
803-357-0388
Fax: 601-899-9058
E-mail: stateoffice@namims.org
www.nami.org/sites/namimississippi

Anette Giessner, President
Shirley Montgomery, Executive Director

Year Founded: 1989

Missouri

1932 Depressive and Bipolar Support Alliance (DBSA)

730 N Franklin Street
Suite 501
Chicago, IL 60654-7225
800-826-3632
Fax: 312-642-7243
E-mail: info@dbsalliance.org
www.dbsalliance.org

Cheryl T. Magrini, MS.Ed, MTS, P, Chair
Allen Doederlein, President
Cindy Specht, Executive Vice President
Lisa Goodale, Vice President, Peer Support Ser

The Depression and Bipolar Support Alliance is the leading patient-directed national organization focusing on the most prevalent mental illnesses. The organization fosters an environment of understanding about the impact and management of these life threatening illnesses by providing up-to-date, scientifically based tools and information written in language the general public can understand.

Year Founded: 1985

1933 Missouri Alliance for the Mentally Ill

1001 SW Boulevard
Suite E
Jefferson City, MO 65109-2501
573-634-7727
800-374-2138
Fax: 573-761-5636
E-mail: mocami@aol.com
www.www.nami.org/MST

Steven R Wilhelm, President
Cindi Keele, Executive Director

The Missouri Coalition of Alliance for the Mentally Ill is a family organization for persons with brain disorders. It has 15 active chapters throughout Missouri.

1934 Missouri Institute of Mental Health

5400 Arsenal Street
Saint Louis, MO 63139
314-516-8400
Fax: 314-877-6405
www.www.mimh.edu

Dedicated to providing research, evaluation, policy and training expertise to the Missouri Department of Mental Health, other state agencies, service provider agencies, and other organizations and individuals seeking information related to mental health and other related policy areas.

1935 National Alliance on Mental Illness: Missouri

1001 Southwest Boulevard
Suite E
Jefferson City, MO 65109-2501
573-634-7727
800-374-2138
Fax: 573-761-5636
E-mail: sonyabaumgartner@yahoo.com
www.www.nami.org/MST

Tim Harlan, President
Cindi Keele, Executive Director

Montana

1936 Mental Health Association of Montana

205 Haggerty Lane Suite 170
PO Box 88
Bozeman, MT 59771
406-587-7774
E-mail: info@montanamentalhealth.org
www.montanamentalhealth.org

Dan Aune, LCSW, Executive Director
Michelle Aune, Housing, Community Development
Julio Brionez, MS, Warmline/Prevention/Outreach

A statewide education and advocacy organization. Mission is to work for good mental health for all; and for social justice as well as quality services for persons with mental illnesses.

1937 National Alliance on Mental Illness: Montana

616 Helena Avenue
Suite 218
Helena, MT 59601-3654
406-443-7871
Fax: 406-862-6357
E-mail: info@namimt.org
www.namimt.org

Gary Popiel, President
Matthew Kuntz, Executive Director

Supports, educates and advocates for Montanans with severe mental illnesses and their families.

Nebraska

1938 Department of Health and Human Services Division of Public Health

Licensure Unit
Lincoln, NE 68508-4986
402-471-2115
E-mail: marie.mcclatchey@nebraska.gov
www.dhhs.ne.gov

Joseph M. Acierno, MD, JD, Director
Helen Meeks, Administrator of Licensure Unit

The Licensure Unit's mission is to assure the public that health-related practices provided by individuals, facilities and programs are safe, of acceptable quality, and that the cost of expanded services is justified by the need.

1939 Mutual of Omaha's Health and Wellness Programs

Mutual of Omaha Plaza
Omaha, NE 68175-1
402-342-7600
800-238-9354
Fax: 402-351-2775
E-mail: grouphealth@mutualofomaha.com.
www.mutualofomaha.com

Daniel P Neary, CEO

Mutual of Omaha's Health and Wellness Programs provide assistance and professional support in a variety of areas including family concerns; depression/anxiety; gambling and other addictions; parenting issues; drug/alcohol abuse; grief issues and life changes.

1940 National Alliance on Mental Illness: Nebraska

415 South 25th Avenue
Omaha, NE 68131
402-345-8101
877-463-6264
Fax: 402-346-4070
E-mail: nami.nebraska@nami.org
www.naminebraska.org

Nancy Kelley, PhD., President
Steve Spelic, Vice President
Mary Thunker, Secretary

The office of NAMI Nebraska, a non-profit organization dedicated to providing support, education and advocacy to and for anyone whose life has been touched by a mental illness

1941 National Association of Social Workers: Nebraska Chapter

650 'J' St.
Ste. #208
Lincoln, NE 68508
402-477-7344
877-816-6279
Fax: 402-477-0374
E-mail: naswne@naswne.org
www.naswne.org

Andrea M. Phillips, President
Susan M. Kloch, Vice President
Terry Martin Werner, Executive Director
Amy West, Secretary

Nebraska chapter is an affiliate of the National Association of Social Workers with a membership of six hundred plus.

1942 Nebraska Family Support Network

3568 Dodge Street
Suite 2
Omaha, NE 68131-3851
402-345-0791
800-245-6081
Fax: 402-444-7722
E-mail: info@nefamilysupport.org
www.nefamilysupportnetwork.org

Chinedu Igbokwe, Board President
Tim Flott, Vice President

Dan Jackson, Executive Director
Steven Bauer, Program Director

1943 Pilot Parents: PP
Ollie Webb Center

1941 S 42nd Street
Suite 122
Omaha, NE 68105-2942
402-346-5220
Fax: 402-346-5253
E-mail: info@olliewebb.org
www.olliewebbinc.org

Laurie Ackermann, Executive Director

Parents, professionals and others concerned with providing emotional and peer support to new parents of children with special needs. Sponsors a parent-matching program which allows parents who have had sufficient experience and training in the care of their own children to share their knowledge and expertise with parents of children recently diagnosed as disabled. Publications: The Gazette, newsletter, published 6 times a year. Also has chapters in Arizona and limited other states.

Nevada

1944 National Alliance on Mental Illness: Carson City, NV Carson City, NV 89701-6122

775-246-7364
E-mail: ruthpax@yahoo.com
www.nami.org

Ruth Paxton, Contact

Part of the nation's leading self-help organization for all those affected by severe brain disorders. Mission is to bring consumers and families with similar experiences together to share information about services, care providers, and ways to cope with the challenges of schizophrenia, manic depression, and other serious mental illnesses.

1945 Nevada Principals' Executive Program

2101 South Jones Boulevard
Suite 120
Las Vegas, NV 89146-3106
702-388-8899
800-216-5188
Fax: 702-388-2966
E-mail: pepinfo@nvpep.org
www.nvpep.org

Karen Taycher, Executive Director
Natalie Filipic, Director of Operations
Stephanie Vrsnik, Community Development Director
Robin Kincaid, Educational Services Director

To strengthen and renew the knowledge, skills, and beliefs of public school leaders so that they might help improve the conditions for teaching and learning in schools and school districts.

New Hampshire

1946 Monadnock Family Services

64 Main Street
Suite 301
Keene, NH 03431-3701
603-357-4400
Fax: 603-355-3833
E-mail: rboyd@mfs.org
www.mfs.org

John Santos, Chair
Nancy Vincent, Vice Chair
Jill Batty, Treasurer
Jane Larmon, Secretary

A nonprofit community mental health center serving the mental health needs of families, buisness and other public and private organizations with comprehensive continuum of education, prevention and treatment services.

1947 National Alliance on Mental Illness: New Hampshire

85 North State Street
Concord, NH 03301
603-225-5359
800-242-6264
Fax: 603-228-8848
E-mail: info@naminh.org
www.naminh.org

Elizabeth Merry, President
Michael Cohen, Executive Director

A statewide education, support and advocacy organization working for a quality, comprehensive mental health service system.

1948 New Hampshire Alliance for the Mentally Ill

85 North State Street
Concord, NH 03301
603-225-5359
800-242-6264
Fax: 603-228-8848
E-mail: info@naminh.org
www.naminh.org

Michael Cohen, Executive Director
Sam Adams, President

Nation's leading self-help organization for all those affected by severe brain disorders. Mission is to bring consumers and families with similar experiences together to share information about services, care providers, and ways to cope with the challenges of schizophrenia, manic depression, and other serious mental illnesses.

New Jersey

1949 Association for Children of New Jersey

35 Halsey Street
2nd Floor
Newark, NJ 07102-3000
973-643-3876
Fax: 973-643-9153
E-mail: advocates@acnj.org
www.acnj.org

Cecilia Zalkind, Executive Director
Mary Coogan, Assistant Director
Carla Ross, Operations Manager
Diane Dellanno, Policy Analyst

Association for Children of New Jersey is a statewide non-profit child advocacy organization. They work on behalf of children and families by conducting research, developing and supporting legislation, and maintaining oversight of the policies and programs of New Jersey administrative agencies. An advocate on a broad range of issues affecting New Jersey's children and families, special areas of interest include: budget advocacy; public policy; early education; child health; community advocacy and outreach. ACNJ operates a Children's Legal Resource Center to meet the demand for information on the status of the law and

children's rights. Other ACNJ web sites are: www.kidlaw.org and www.makekidscountnj.org
Year Founded: 1847

1950 Disability Rights New Jersey

210 S Broad Street
3rd Floor
Trenton, NJ 08608-2404
609-292-9742
800-922-7233
Fax: 609-777-0187
TTY: 609-633-7106
E-mail: advocate@drnj.org
www.drnj.org

Joseph B Young, Executive Director
Maritza Williams, Intake Coordinator
Lillie Lowe-Reid, CAP, Coordinator/PABSS Project Direct
Rachel Parsio, Senior Staff Advocate

Legal and non legal advocacy, information and referral, technical assistance and training, outreach and education in support of the human, civil, and legal rights of people with disabilities in New Jersey.
Year Founded: 1994

1951 Jewish Family Service of Atlantic and Cape May Counties

607 North Jerome Avenue
Margate, NJ 08402-1527
609-822-1108
Fax: 609-882-1106
www.jfsatlantic.org

Mitchell Gurwicz, President
Andea Steinberg, LCSW, Executive Director
Beverly Rubin, Vice President
Richard Wise, MD, Vice President

Multi-service familty counseling agency dedicated to promoting, strengthening and preserving individual, family, and community weel-being in a manner consistent with Jewish philosophy and values.
Year Founded: 1930

1952 Mental Health Association of New Jersey

1562 US Highway 130
North Brunswick, NJ 08902-3090
732-940-0991
Fax: 732-940-0355
E-mail: naminj@optonline.net
www.naminj.org

Mark Perrin, President
Sylvia Axelrod, Executive Director
Phil Lubitz, Associate Director
Aruna Rao, Associate Director

Nation's leading self-help organization for all those affected by severe brain disorders. Mission is to bring consumers and families with similar experiences together to share information about services, care providers, and ways to cope with the challenges of schizophrenia, manic depression, and other serious mental illnesses.

1953 National Alliance on Mental Illness: New Jersey

1562 US Highway 130
North Brunswick, NJ 08902-3090
732-940-0991
Fax: 732-940-0355

E-mail: info@naminj.org
www.naminj.org

Mark Perrin, President
Sylvia Axelrod, Executive Director
Phil Lubitz, Associate Director
Aruna Rao, Associate Director

A statewide non profit organization dedicated to improving the lives of individuals and families who are affected by mental illness. Also provides education, support and systems advocacy to empower families and persons with mental illness.

Year Founded: 1985

1954 New Jersey Association of Mental Health Agencies

The Neuman Building
3575 Quakerbridge Road, Suite 102
Mercerville, NJ 08619-1205
609-838-5488
Fax: 609-838-5489
E-mail: njamha@njamha.org
www.njamha.org

Ann DeMuzio, Human Resources Specialist
Ron Gordon, Associate Director, IT Project
Tom Leach, Director, Public Affairs
Shauna Moses, Associate Executive Director

To champion opportunities that advance its members' ability to deliver accessible, quality, efficient and effective integrated behavioral health care services to mental health consumers and their families.

Year Founded: 1951

1955 New Jersey Psychiatric Association

PO Box 428
Bedminster, NJ 07921
908-719-2222
Fax: 908-719-4747
E-mail: info@njpsychiatry.org
www.www.psychnj.org/index.htm

Theresa M Miskimen MD, President
Carla A Ross, Executive Director

A professional organization of about 100 physicians qualified by training and experience in the treatment of mental illness.

Year Founded: 1935

New Mexico

1956 National Alliance on Mental Illness: New Mexico

6001 Marble NE, Suite 8
PO Box 3086
Alburquerque, NM 87190-3086
505-260-0154
Fax: 505-260-0342
E-mail: naminm@aol.com
www.nm.nami.org

Becky Beckett, President
Kim Ahlbom, Additional Contact

New York

1957 Compeer

259 Monroe Avenue
Suite B1
Rochester, NY 14607-3632
585-546-8280
800-836-0475
Fax: 585-325-2558
E-mail: compeerp@rochester.rr.com
www.compeer.org

J. Theodore Smith, Chair
Johanna Ambrose, CEO and President
Barb Mestler, Affiliate Program Specialist
Nancy Dhurjaty, Project Specialist

National nonprofit organization which matches community volunteers in supportive friendship relationships with children and adults recieving mental health treatment.

Year Founded: 1973

1958 Families Together in New York State

737 Madison Avenue
Albany, NY 12208
518-432-0333
888-326-8644
Fax: 518-434-6478
E-mail: info@ftnys.org
www.ftnys.org

Vicki McCarthy, President
CEO and Pres Pierce, Executive Director
Anne Kuppinger, Director of Training & Credentia
Tracie Killar, Communications Director

Non-profit, parent-run organization that strives to establish a unified voice for children with emotional, behavioral, and social challenges.

1959 Finger Lakes Parent Network, Inc.

25 W Steuben Street
Bath, NY 14810
607-776-2164
800-934-4244
Fax: 607-776-4327
E-mail: flpninc25@flpn.org
www.flpn.org

Pamela Maglier, President
Sue M arosek, Vice President
Patti DiNardo, Executive Director
Jeannine Struble, Assistant Director

A parent-governed organization, focused on the needs of children and youth with emotional, behavioral, and /or mental disorders and their families. Supports and empowers families so that they can improve the quality of their lives and help their child to achieve his/her full potential within the community.

Year Founded: 1990

1960 Healthcare Association of New York State

1 Empire Drive
Rensselaer, NY 12144-5729
518-431-7600
Fax: 518-431-7915
E-mail: info@hanys.org
www.hanys.org

Dennis P. Whalen, President
Valerie Grey, Executive Vice President, Policy
Richard Cook, Chief Operating Officer

Serves as the primary advocate for more than 550 non-profit and public hospitals, health systems, long-term care, home care, hospice, and other health care organizations throughout New York State.

1961 Mental Health Association in Dutchess County

253 Mansion Street
Poughkeepsie, NY 12601
845-473-2500
Fax: 845-473-4870
E-mail: mhadc@hvc.rr.com
www.www.mhadc.com/

The Mental Health Association in Dutchess County is a voluntary, not-for-profit dedicated to the promotion of mental health, the prevention of mental illness and the improved care and treatment of persons with mental illnesses.

1962 Mental Health Association in Orange County Inc

73 James P Kelly Way
Middletown, NY 10940
845-342-2400
800-832-1200
Fax: 845-343-9665
E-mail: mha@mhaorangeny.com
www.mhaorangeny.com

David Goggins, President of the Board
Nadia Allen, Executive Director

Seeks to promote the positive mental health and emotional well-being of Orange County residents, working towards reducing the stigma of mental illness, developmental disabilities, and providing support to victims of sexual assault and other crimes.

1963 National Association of Social Workers New York State Chapter

188 Washington Avenue
Albany, NY 12210-2394
518-463-4741
800-724-6279
Fax: 518-463-6446
E-mail: info@naswnys.com
www.naswnys.org

Debra Fromm-Faria, President
Lenora Colaruotolo, LMSW, Vice President
Reinaldo Cardona, MSSW, LCSW, Executive Director
Karin Carreau, MSW, Director of Policy

The National Association of Social Workers is the largest membership organization of professional social workers in the world, with more than 155, 000 members. NASW works to enhance the professional growth and development of its members, to create and maintain professional standards, and to advance sound social policies.

Year Founded: 1955

1964 New York Association of Psychiatric Rehabilitation Services

194 Washington Avenue
Suite 400
Albany, NY 12210
518-436-0008
Fax: 518-436-0044

E-mail: nyaprs@aol.com
www.nyaprs.org

Maura Kelly, Co-President
Steven Coe, Co-President
Harvey Rosenthal, Executive Director
Michelle Jensen, Vice President

New York Association of Psychiatric Services (NYAPRS) is a statewide coalition of New Yorkers, who are in recovery from mental illness and the professionals who work alongside them in rehabilitation and peer support services located throughout New York State. NYAPRS' mission is to promote the partnership of consumers, providers and families seeking to increase opportunities for community integration and independence for persons who have experienced a mental illness.

Year Founded: 1981

1965 New York Business Group on Health

386 Park Avenue S
Suite 703
New York, NY 10016-8832
212-252-7440
E-mail: nybgh@nybgh.org

Laurel Pickering, Executive Director
Janaera J Gaston MPA, Programs Director

NYBGH is a not-for-profit coalition of 150 businesses and is the only organization in the New York Metropolitan area exclusively devoted to employer health benefit issues. The mission is to provide leadership and knowledge to employers to promote a value-based, market-driven healthcare system.

1966 State University of New York at Stony Brook
Department of Psychiatry and Behavioral Science

101 Nicolls Road
Stony Brook, NY 11794
631-632-6000
E-mail: registrar_office@stonybrook.edu
www.www.stonybrook.edu/

Evelyn Petralia, Manager
Gabrielle Carlson, MD, Director of Child Psychiatry
Regina T Cline, JD, Administrator

1967 Westchester Alliance for the Mentally Ill

101 Executive Boulevard
Suite 2
Elmsford, NY 10523-1316
914-592-5458
Fax: 914-592-5458
E-mail: info@namiwestchester.org
www.www.namiwestchester.org

Stamatia Pappas, President

Provides support and education for families who are feeling alone and in pain with a member of their family suffering from mental illness; no meeting fee.

North Carolina

1968 Autism Society of North Carolina

505 Oberlin Road
Suite 230
Raleigh, NC 27605-1345
919-743-0204
800-442-2762
Fax: 919-743-0208

E-mail: info@autismsociety-nc.org
www.www.autismsociety-nc.org

Beverly Moore, Chair
Tracey Sheriff, Chief Executive Officer
Paul Wendler, Chief Financial Officer
Sharon Jeffries-Jones, Vice Chair

Committed to providing support and promoting opportunities which enhance the lives of individuals within the autism spectrum and their families

1969 National Alliance on Mental Illness: North Carolina

309 W Millbrook Road
Suite 121
Raleigh, NC 27609-4394
919-788-0801
800-451-9682
Fax: 919-788-0906
E-mail: mail@naminc.org
www.naminc.org

Mike Mayer, President
Debra Dihoff, Executive Director
Megan Fazekas-King, Communications Specialist
Robin Kellogg, Development Director

The mission of NAMI North Carolina is to improve the quality of life for individuals and their families living with the debilitating effects of severe and persistent mental illness. We work to protect the dignity of people living with brain disorders through advocacy, education, and support.

1970 National Association of Social Workers: North Carolina Chapter

412 Morson Street
PO Box 27582
Raleigh, NC 27611-7582
919-828-9650
800-280-6207
Fax: 919-828-1341
E-mail: naswnc@naswnc.org
www.naswnc.org

Katherine Boyd, Executive Director
Valerie Arendt, MSW, MPP, Associate Executive Director
Kay Castillo, BSW, Director of Advocacy, Policy & L
Hope Venetta, Director of Professional Develop

NASW is a membership organization that promotes, develops, and protects the practice of social work and social workers. NASW also seeks to enhance the effective functioning and well-being of individuals, families, and communities through its work and through advocacy.

1971 North Carolina Alliance for the Mentally Ill

309 W. Millbrook Road
Ste. 121
Raleigh, NC 27609-4394
919-788-0801
800-451-9682
Fax: 919-788-0906
E-mail: mail@naminc.org
www.naminc.org

Debra G. Dihoff, MA, Executive Director
Megan Fazekas-King, Communications Specialist
Jai Harris, Data Entry/Membership Specialist
Gloria Harrison, Helpline Manager

Nation's leading self-help organization for all those affected by severe brain disorders. Mission is to bring con-

sumers and families with similar experiences together to share information about services, care providers, and ways to cope with the challenges of schizophrenia, manic depression, and other serious mental illnesses.

1972 North Carolina Mental Health Consumers Organization

PO Box 27042
Raleigh, NC 27611-7042
919-832-2285
800-326-3842
Fax: 919-828-6999
E-mail: info@ncmhco.org
www.www.ncmhco.org/

NC MHCO is a private non-profit organization not affilated with NAMI NC. This organization has been providing advocacy and support to adults with mental illness since 1989.

North Dakota

1973 National Association of Social Workers: North Dakota Chapter

1120 College Dr, Suite 100
PO Box 1775
Bismarck, ND 58503
701-223-4161
Fax: 701-223-4161
E-mail: info@naswnd.org
www.www.nasw-heartland.org/displaycommon.cfm?an=1&suba

Tom Tupa, Executive Director

NASW Dakotas, serves the critical and diverse needs of the entire social work profession.

1974 North Dakota Federation of Families for Children's Mental Health

PO Box 3061
Bismarck, ND 58502-3061
701-222-3310
E-mail: carlottamccleary@bis.midco.net
www.ndffcmh.org

Carlotta McCleary, Executive Director

To provide support and informatin to families of children and adolescents with serious emotional, behavioral, or mental disorders.

Year Founded: 1994

Ohio

1975 National Alliance on Mental Illness: Ohio

1225 Dublin Rd.
Suite 125
Columbus, OH 43215
614-224-2700
800-686-2646
Fax: 614-224-5400
E-mail: amiohio@amiohio.org
www.namiohio.org

Bob Spada, President
Stacey Smith, Director of Operations
Terry Russell, Executive Director
Peg Morrison, Director of Programs

Nation's leading selp-help organization for all those affected by severe brain disorders. Mission is to bring consumers and families with similar experiences together to share information about services, care providers and ways to cope with the challenges of schizophrenia, manic depression, and other serious mental illnesses. Available on FaceBook.

1976 National Association of Social Workers: Ohio Chapter

33 N Third Street
Suite 530
Columbus, OH 43215-3514
614-461-4484
Fax: 614-461-9793
E-mail: info@naswoh.org
www.naswoh.org

Danielle Smith, MSW, MA, LSW, Executive Director
Dorothy Martindale, BSSW, LSW, Membership Associate

The mission of NASW is to strengthen, support, and unify the social work profession, to promote the development of social work standards and practice, and to advocate for social policies that advance social justice and diversity.

1977 Ohio Association of Child Caring Agencies

1151 Bethel Road
Suite 104B
Columbus, OH 43220
614-461-0014
Fax: 614-228-7004
E-mail: PWyman@oacca.org
www.oacca.org

Dr Jeffrey Greene, President
Mark M Mecum, Executive Director
Debra Rex, Treasurer
Chris Wolf, Secretary

The Ohio Association of Child Caring Agencies is to promote and strengthen a fully-integrated, private/public network of high-quality services for Ohio's children and their families through advocacy, education, and support of member agencies.

Year Founded: 1973

1978 Ohio Council of Behavioral Healthcare Providers

35 E Gay Street
Suite 401
Columbus, OH 43215-3138
614-228-0747
Fax: 614-228-0740
E-mail: staff@ohiocouncil-bhp.org
www.ohiocouncil-bhp.org

Hubert Wirtz, CEO
Brenda Cornett, Associate Director for Membershi
Peg Burns, Associate Director
Teresa Lampl, Associate Director

A trade association representing provider organizations throughout Ohio which provide behavioral healthcare services to their communities.

1979 Ohio Department of Mental Health

30 E Broad Street
36th Floor
Columbus, OH 43215-3430
614-466-2596
877-275-6364
TDD: 614-752-9696
TTY: 614-752-9696

E-mail: questions@mha.ohio.gov
www.mha.ohio.gov/

Cheri L Walter, Chief Executive Officer

State agency responsible for oversight and funding of public mental health programs and services.

1980 Planned Lifetime Assistance Network of Northeast Ohio

5010 Mayfield Road
Lyndhurst, OH 44124
216-504-6483
Fax: 216-321-0021
E-mail: info@planNEohio.org
www.www.jfsa-cleveland.org

Philip Cohen, Board Chair
Susan Bichsel, PhD, President and CEO
David Hlavac, MBA, Vice President and CFO
Ethan Cohen, Treasurer

Provides individualized home-based social services and advocacy to assist families who have a neurobiologically disabled family member to function at their maximum. LISW staff provides therapy and works with existing service providers to ensure quality of care. Offers a wide range of community-based, social, and recreational activities for its participants.

Year Founded: 1989

1981 Positive Education Program

3100 Euclid Avenue
Cleveland, OH 44115-2508
216-361-4400
Fax: 216-361-8600
E-mail: pepgen@pepcleve.org
www.www.pepcleve.org/

Frank A Fecser Ph D, Executive Director
Tom Valore Ph D, Program Director

The Positive Education Program (PEP) is to help troubled and troubling children and their families build skills to grow and learn successfully.

Year Founded: 1971

1982 Six County

2845 Bell Street
Zanesville, OH 43701-1794
740-454-9766
Fax: 740-588-6452
E-mail: info@sixcounty.org
www.sixcounty.org

Helping community mental health needs in Coshocton, Guernsey, Morgan, Muskingum, Noble and Perry counties. In addition to the traditional treatment services, specialized services have been developed to reach people with ever changing needs. Employee assistance, sheltered employment, intensive outpatient, and residential services.

Oklahoma

1983 National Alliance on Mental Illness: Oklahoma

4200 Perimeter Center Dr
Suite 150
Oklahoma City, OK 73107-3925
405-230-1900
800-583-1264
Fax: 405-230-1903

E-mail: nami-ok@swbell.net
www.ok.nami.org

Paula Walker, President
Traci Cook, Executive Director
Andrea Michaels, Operations & Communications Dire
Lisa Buck, Development Director

1984 Oklahoma Alliance for the Mentally Ill
4200 Perimeter Center Dr
Suite 150
Oklamhoma City, OK 73107-3925
405-230-1900
800-583-1264
Fax: 405-230-1903
E-mail: nami-OK@swbell.net
www.ok.nami.org

Paula Walker, President
Traci Cook, Executive Director
Andrea Michaels, Operations & Communications Dire
Lisa Buck, Development Director

Nation's leading self-help organization for all those affected by severe brain disorders. Mission is to bring consumers and families with similar experiences together to
share information about services, care providers, and ways
to cope with the challenges of schizophrenia, manic depression, and other serious mental illnesses.

1985 Oklahoma Mental Health Consumer Council
3200 NW 48th
Suite 102
Oklahoma City, OK 73112-5911
405-604-6975
888-424-1305
www.omhcc.org

Becky Tallent, Executive Director

Oregon

1986 National Alliance for Mental Illness: Oregon
4701 SE 24th Ave.
Suite E
Portland, OR 97202-1552
503-230-8009
800-343-6264
Fax: 503-230-2751
E-mail: namioregon@namior.org
www.nami.org/sites/namioregon

Kim Schneiderman, President
Christopher Bouneff, Executive Director
Michelle Madison, Events and Outreach Manager
Peter Link, Education Programs Manager

Dedicated to improving the quality of life for individuals
with mental illness and their families.

1987 National Alliance on Mental Illness: Oregon
4701 SE 24th Ave.
Suite E
Portland, OR 97202-1552
503-230-8099
800-343-6264
Fax: 503-230-2751
E-mail: namioregon@namior.org
www.nami.org/sites/namioregon

Kim Schneiderman, President
Christopher Bouneff, Executive Director

Michelle Madison, Events and Outreach Manager
Peter Link, Education Programs Manager

A statewide grassroots organization dedicated to improving
the quality of life for individuals with mental illness and
their families through support, education, and advocacy.

1988 Oregon Family Support Network
1300 Broadway St. NE
Suite #403
Salem, OR 97301
503-363-8068
800-323-8521
Fax: 503-390-3161
E-mail: ofsn@ofsn.org
www.ofsn.org

David de Fiebre, President
Sandy Bumpus, Executive Director
Leah Skipworth, Operations Manager
Janelle Rasmussen, Bookkeeper

Oregon families supporting Oregon families with children
and adolescents with emotional, behavioral, mental and/or
physical challenges and special needs.

1989 Oregon Psychiatric Association
PO Box 21571
Keizer, OR 97307
503-406-2526
800-533-7031
Fax: 503-406-2526
E-mail: info@oregonpsychiatric.org
www.www.orpsych.org/

John McCulley, Executive Secretary

To ensure human care and effective treatment for all persons with mental disorder, including mental retardation and
substance-related disorders.

Pennsylvania

**1990 American Anorexia/Bulimia Association of
Philidelphia**
PO Box 1287
Langhorne, PA 19047-6287
215-221-1864
Fax: 215-702-8944
E-mail: mail.aabaphila@yahoo.com
www.aabaphila.org

The American Anorexia/Bulimia Association of
Philidelphia is non-profit, providing services and programs
for anyone interested in or affected by, Anorexia, Bulimia
and/or related disorders. Its purpose is to aid in the education and prevention of these life threatening disorders. Referral programs and support groups assist in the treatment
and recovery process.

1991 Health Federation of Philadelphia
1211 Chestnut Street
Suite 801
Philadelphia, PA 19107-4120
215-567-8001
Fax: 215-567-7743
E-mail: healthfederation@healthfederation.org
www.healthfederation.org

Patricia Deitch, Board Chair
Phyllis Cater, Board Secretary/ Treasurer
Natalie Levkovich, Executive Director

A private, non-profit membership organization which provides shared services to a consortium of community and federally qualified health centers in Philadelphia.

Year Founded: 1983

1992 Mental Health Association of Southeastern Pennsylvania (MHASP)

1211 Chestnut Street
Suite 1100
Philadelphia, PA 19107-4103
215-751-1800
800-688-4226
Fax: 215-636-6300
E-mail: mha@mhasp.org
www.mhasp.org

Carol Boylan, Chairman
Michael Brody, Chief Executive Officer
Joseph Rogers, Chief Advocacy Officer
Jacob Bowling, Director

The Mental Health Association of Southeastern Pennsylvania (MHASP) is a nonprofit citizen's organization that develops, supports and promotes innovative education and advocacy programs. MHASP serves adults, children and family members through our programs and advocacy efforts. It is the mission of the Mental Health Association of Southeastern Pennsylvania to develop, maintain, and promote innovative education and advocacy programs and mental health services in the five counties we represent in a culturally competent manner, serving as a role model and technical assistance resource for state and national organizations and constituencies.

Year Founded: 1951

1993 National Alliance on Mental Illness: Pennsylvania

2149 North 2nd Street
Harrisburg, PA 17110-1005
717-238-1514
800-223-0500
Fax: 717-238-4390
E-mail: nami-pa@nami.org
www.nami-pa.org

Richard H. Rugen, President
Gwen DeYoung, Vice President
Tim Grumbacher, Secretary
Bill Kennedy, Treasurer

A statewide non-profit organization dedicated to helping mental health consumers and their families rebuild their lives and conquer the challenges posed by severe and persistent mental illness.

1994 Pennsylvania Alliance for the Mentally Ill

2149 N 2nd Street
Harrisburg, PA 17110-1005
717-238-1514
800-223-0500
Fax: 717-238-4390
E-mail: nami-pa@nami.org
www.nami-pa.org

Richard H. Rugen, President
Gwen DeYoung, Vice President
Tim Grumbacher, Secretary
Bill Kennedy, Treasurer

The largest statewide non-profit organization dedicated to helping mental health consumers and their families rebuild

their lives and conquer the challenges posed by severe and persistent mental illness.

1995 Pennsylvania Psychiatric Society

777 East Park Drive
PO Box 8820
Harrisburg, PA 17105-8820
717-558-7750
800-422-2900
Fax: 717-558-7841
E-mail: papsych@pamedsoc.org
www.papsych.org

A disctrict branch of the American Psychiatric Association, the PPS has 1, 800 member physicians practicing in the field of psychiatry. The mission of the Society is to fully represent Pennsylvania Psychiatrists in advocating for their profession and their patients, and to assure access to psychiatric services of high quality, through activities in education, shaping of legislation and upholding ethical standards.

1996 University of Pittsburgh Medical Center

200 Lothrop Street
Pittsburgh, PA 15213-2582
412-647-2345
800-533-8762
Fax: 412-647-4801
E-mail: upmcweb@upmc.edu
www.upmc.com

Jeffrey A Romoff, President

The University of Pittsburgh Medical Center is the leading health care system in western Pennsylvania and one of the largest nonprofit integrated health care systems in the United States.

Rhode Island

1997 National Alliance on Mental Illness: Rhode Island

154 Waterman Street
Unit 5B Lower Level
Providence, RI 02906-3116
401-331-3060
800-749-3197
Fax: 401-274-3020
E-mail: chaznami@cox.net
www.namirhodeisland.org

Marcia Boyd, Esq., President
Chaz J. Gross, Executive Director
David Bainer, Vice President
Kathy Carland, Secretary

The mission of NAMI Rhode Island is to educate the public about mental illness; to offer resources and support to all whose lives are touched by mental illness; to advocate at every level to ensure the rights and dignity of those with mental illness; and to promote research in the science and treatment of mental illness.

1998 Parent Support Network of Rhode Island

1395 Atwood Avenue
Suite 114
Johnston, RI 02919
401-467-6855
800-483-8844
Fax: 401-467-6903

E-mail: c.ciano@psnri.org
www.mentalhealth.samhsa.gov/

Linda Winfield, Board President
George McDonough, Vice President
Cathy Ciano, Executive Director
Brenda Alejo, Peer Mentor Program Director

Organization of families supporting families with children and youth who are at risk for or have serious behavioral, emotional, and/or mental health challenges, having consideration for their backround and values. The goals of PSN are to: strengthen and preserve families; enable families in advocacy; extend social networks, reduce family isolation and develop social policy systems of care. Parent Support Network accomplishes these goals through providing advocacy, education and training, promoting outreach and public awareness, facilitating social events for families, participating on committees responsible for developing, implementing and evaluating policies and systems of care.

South Carolina

1999 Federation of Families of South Carolina
810 Dutch Square Blvd
Ste 205
Columbia, SC 29210
803-772-5210
866-779-0402
Fax: 803-772-5212
www.fedfamsc.org

Kathleen Scharer, President
Roxann McKinnon, Vice President
Diane Revels Flashnick, Executive Director
Donna Shaw, Staff Support Specialist

Nonprofit organization established to serve the families of children with any degree of emotional, behavioral or psychiatric disorder. The services and programs by the Federation are designed to meet the individual needs of families around the state. Through support networks, educational materials, publications, conferences, workshops and other activities, the Federation provides many avenues of support for families of children with emotional, behavioral or psychiatric disorders.

2000 National Alliance on Mental Illness: South Carolina
PO Box 1267
Columbia, SC 29202-1267
803-733-9592
800-788-5131
Fax: 803-733-9593
E-mail: namisc@namisc.org
www.namisc.org

Jim Hayes, MD, President
Bill Lindsey, Executive Director
Corinne Matthews, Office Manager
Betsey O'Brien, Director of Education and Family

Year Founded: 1986

2001 South Carolina Alliance for the Mentally Ill
PO Box 1267
5000 Thurmond Mall Boulevard, Suite 338
Columbia, SC 29201-2390
803-733-9592
800-788-5131
Fax: 803-733-9593

E-mail: namisc@namisc.org
www.namisc.org

Jim Hayes, MD, President
Bill Lindsey, Executive Director
Corinne Matthews, Office Manager
Betsey O'Brien, Director of Education and Family

Non-profit with 17 local groups throughout the state. Provide support, education and advocacy for families and friends of people with serious mental illness.

Year Founded: 1986

2002 South Carolina Alliance for the Mentally Ill
PO Box 2538
Columbia, SC 29202-2538
803-779-7849
800-788-5131
Fax: 803-733-9593
www.nami.org

Bill Lindsey, Executive Director

Nation's leading self-help organization for all those affected by severe brain disorders. Mission is to bring consumers and families with similar experiences together to share information about services, care providers, and ways to cope with the challenges of schizophrenia, manic depression, and other serious mental illnesses.

South Dakota

2003 Brookings Alliance for the Mentally Ill
PO Box 88808
PO Box 221
Brookings, SD 57109
605-271-1871
800-551-2531
E-mail: namisd@midconetwork.com
www.nami.org/sites/NAMISouthDakota

Wendy Giebink, Executive Director

Nation's leading self-help organization for all those affected by severe brain disorders. Mission is to bring consumers and families with similar experiences together to share information about services, care providers, and ways to cope with the challenges of schizophrenia, manic depression, and other serious mental illnesses.

2004 National Alliance on Mental Illness: South Dakota
PO Box 88808
Sioux Falls, SD 57109-8808
605-271-1871
800-551-2531
Fax: 605-271-1871
E-mail: namisd@midconetwork.com
www.nami.org/sites/namisouthdakota

Wendy Giebink, Executive Director
Phyllis Arends, Executive Director

Provides education and support for individuals and families impacted by brain-based disorders (mental illnesses), advocate for the development of a comprehensive system of services and lessen the stigma in the general public.

Tennessee

2005 Memphis Business Group on Health

5050 Poplar Avenue
Suite 509
Memphis, TN 38157-509
901-767-9585
Fax: 901-767-6592
E-mail: information@memphisbusinessgroup.org
www.memphisbusinessgroup.org

Christie Upshaw Travis, Chief Executive Officer
Janis M Slivinski, Administrative Assistant
Tara Hill, Project Coordinator

To facilitate the purchase of efficient and effective health care services for the Memphis community.

Year Founded: 1985

2006 National Alliance on Mental Illness: Tennessee

1101 Kermit Drive
Suite 605
Nashville, TN 37217-5110
615-361-6608
800-467-3589
Fax: 615-361-6698
E-mail: jfladen@namitn.org
www.namitn.org

Dick Baxter, President
Jeff Fladen, Executive Director
Roger Stewart, Deputy Director
Susan Ezzell, Finance Coordinator

NAMI Tennessee is a grassroots, non-profit made up of families, consumers and professionals. We are dedicated to improving quality of life for people with mental illness and their families.

2007 Tennessee Alliance for the Mentally Ill

1101 Kermit Drive
Suite 605
Nashville, TN 37217
615-361-6608
800-771-5491
Fax: 615-361-6698
E-mail: jfladen@namitn.org
www.namitn.org/

Dick Baxter, President
Jeff Fladen, Executive Director
Roger Stewart, Deputy Director
Susan Ezzell, Finance Coordinator

Nation's leading self-help organization for all those affected by severe brain disorders. Mission is to bring consumers and families with similar experiences together to share information about services, care providers, and ways to cope with the challenges of schizophrenia, manic depression, and other serious mental illnesses.

2008 Tennessee Association of Mental Health Organization

42 Rutledge Street
Nashville, TN 37210-2043
615-244-2220
800-568-2642
Fax: 615-254-8331
E-mail: tamho@tamho.org
www.tamho.org

Ellyn Wilbur, Executive Director
Alysia Williams, Director of Policy and Advocacy
Teresa Fuqua, Director of Member Services
Laura Jean, Office Manager

State wide trade association representing primarily community mental health centers, community-owned corporations that have historically served the needs of the mentally ill and chemically dependent citizens of Tennessee regardless of their ability to pay.

2009 Tennessee Mental Health Consumers' Association

3931 Gallatin Pike
Nashville, TN 37216
615-250-1176
888-539-0393
Fax: 615-383-1176
E-mail: info@tmhca-tn.org
www.tmhca-tn.org

Anthony Fox, President/Chief Executive Office
Stacey Murphy, Vice President of Administrative
Carolina George, Vice President of Clinical Servi
Lori Abbot Rash, Vice President of Support Servic

A not for profit organization whose members are mental health consumers and other individuals and groups who support our mission. TMHCA recognizes our members as individuals whose life experiences and dreams for the future are invaluable in the structuring of ourplans and policies.

Year Founded: 1988

2010 Tennessee Voices for Children

701 Bradford Avenue
Nashville, TN 37204
615-269-7751
800-670-9882
Fax: 615-269-8914
E-mail: TVC@tnvoices.org
www.tnvoices.org

Dick Blackburn, President
Paula Sandidge, M.D., Board Secretary
Chad Poff, Board Treasurer

Speaks out as active advocates for the emotional and behavioral well-being of children and their families. A non-profit organization of families, professionals, business and community leaders, and government representatives committed to improving and expanding services related to the emotional and behavioral well-being of children. Available on FaceBook and LinkedIn.

Year Founded: 1990

2011 Vanderbilt University: John F Kennedy Center for Research on Human Development

110 Magnolia Circle
Peabody College
Nashville, TN 37203
615-322-8240
Fax: 615-322-8236
TDD: 615-343-2958
E-mail: kc@vanderbilt.edu
www.kc.vanderbilt.edu

Pat Leavitt PhD, Center Acting Director
Jan Rosemergy PhD, Director Communications

Research and research training related to disorders of thinking, learning, perception, communication, mood and emotion caused by disruption of typical development. Available services include behavior analysis clinic, referrals, lectures and conferences, and a free quarterly newsletter.

Year Founded: 1963

Texas

2012 Children's Mental Health Partnership
1210 San Antonio Street
Suite 200
Austin, TX 78701
512-454-3706
Fax: 512-454-3725
E-mail: mhainfo@mhatexas.org
www.mhatexas.org

A coalition of human services providers, parents, educators and juvenile court professionals who care about the special mental health needs of Austin area youth and families.

Year Founded: 1935

2013 Depression and Bipolar Support Alliance Greater Houston
3800 Buffalo Speedway
Suite 300
Houston, TX 77098
713-600-1131
Fax: 713-600-1137
E-mail: dbsahouston@dbsahouston.org
www.www.dbsahouston.org

Mary Collins, President & CEO
Jennifer Strich, LPC-S, NCC, Vice President of Programs

Depression and Bipolar Support Alliance Greater Houston provides free and confidential peer support groups for individuals living with, and family and friends affected by, depression and bipolar disorders.

2014 Jewish Family Service of Dallas
5402 Arapaho Road
Dallas, TX 75248-6905
972-437-9950
Fax: 972-437-1988
E-mail: info@jfsdallas.org
www.jfsdallas.org

Michael Fleisher, Chief Executive Officer
Cathy Barker, Chief Operating Officer
Beth Donahue, Director, Marketing Communicatio
Allison Harding, Director, Career and Employment

2015 Jewish Family Service of San Antonio
12500 NW Military Hwy
#250
San Antonio, TX 78231-1871
210-302-6808
Fax: 210-349-6952
E-mail: johnsonb@jfs-sa.org
www.www.jfs-sa.org/

Ilene Kramer, President
M.H. Levine, Executive Director
Susan Gordon, Secretary
David Scotch, Treasurer

2016 Mental Health America of Southeast Texas
505 Orleans
Suite 301
Beaumont, TX 77701

409-833-9657
Fax: 409-833-3522
www.mhatexas.org

Jayne Bordelon, Executive Director

Non-profit agency offering free information, referral services, educational programs, and advocay to all of Jefferson, Orange, and Hardin Counties

2017 Mental Health Association
1210 San Antonio Street
Suite 200
Austin, TX 78701
512-454-3706
Fax: 512-454-3725
E-mail: mhainfo@mhatexas.org
www.mhatexas.org

Jayne Bordelon, Executive Director

Year Founded: 1935

2018 National Alliance on Mental Illness: Texas
Fountain Park Plaza III
2800 South IH35, Suite 140
Austin, TX 78704-5700
512-693-2000
800-633-3760
Fax: 512-693-8000
E-mail: rpeyson@namitexas.org
www.namitexas.org

Andrea Hazlitt, President
Chris Scroggin, Executive Director
Kelly Jeschke, Membership Coordinator/Office Ma
Patti Haynes, Education Director

The mission of NAMI Texas is to improve the lives of all persons affected by serious mental illness by providing support, education and advocacy through a grassroots network.

2019 Texas Counseling Association (TCA)
1204 San Antonio
Suite 201
Austin, TX 78701-1870
512-472-3403
800-580-8144
Fax: 512-472-3756
E-mail: jan@txca.org
www.txca.org

Jan Friese, Executive Director

The Texas Counseling Association is dedicated to providing leadership, advocacy and education to promote the growth and development of the counseling profession and those that are served.

2020 Texas Psychological Association
1464 E. Whitestone Blvd
Suite 410
Cedar Park, TX 78613
512-528-8400
888-872-3435
Fax: 888-511-1305
E-mail: admin@texaspsyc.org
www.texaspsyc.org/

David White, Executive Director
Sherry Reisman, Assistant Executive Director
Brian Stagner, PhD, Director of Professional Affairs
Amanda McCoy, Office Manager/Communications Co

2021 Texas Society of Psychiatric Physicians
401 W 15th Street
Suite 675
Austin, TX 78701-1665
512-370-1533
E-mail: TxPsychiatry@aol.com
www.tsge.org

Michael Guirl, MD, FACG, President
Ira Flax, Secretary
Stephen Utts, Treasurer

2022 University of Texas Southwestern Medical Center
5323 Harry Hines Boulevard
Dallas, TX 75390-7200
214-648-3111
www.www.utsouthwestern.edu/

Daniel K Podolsky, M.D., President
J. Gregory Fitz, M.D., Executive Vice President for Aca
Willis C Maddrey, M.D., Assistant to the President
Amanda Billings, Interim Vice President for Devel

Year Founded: 1943

Utah

2023 Healthwise of Utah
3110 State Office Building
Suite 30270
Salt Lake City, UT 84114
801-538-3800
800-439-3805
www.insurance.utah.gov

Todd E. Kiser, Insurance Commissioner

2024 National Alliance on Mental Illness: Utah
1600 W. 2200 S.
Suite 202
West Valley City, UT 84119
801-323-9900
877-230-6264
Fax: 801-323-9799
E-mail: education@maniut.org
www.namiut.org

Brian Miller, President
Rebecca Glathar, Executive Director
Tracy Bunner, Accounts Specialist
Mary Burchett, Outreach Specialist

NAMI Utah's mission is to ensure the dignity and improve the lives of those who live with mental illness and their families through support, education and advocacy.

2025 Utah Parent Center
230 West 200 South
Suite 1101
Salt Lake City, UT 84117-4428
801-272-1051
800-468-1160
Fax: 801-272-8907
E-mail: info@utahparentcenter.org
www.utahparentcenter.org

Helen Post, Executive Director
Jennie Gibson, Associate Director

The Utah Parent Center is a statewide nonprofit organization founded in 1984 to provide training, information, referral and assistance to parents of children and youth with all disabilities: physical, mental, learning and emotional. Staff at the center are primarily parents of children and youth with disabilities who carry out the philosophy of Parents Helping Parents.

2026 Utah Psychiatric Association
310 E 4500 Sth
Suite 500
Salt Lake City, UT 84107
801-747-3500
Fax: 801-747-3501
E-mail: paige@utahmed.org
www.www.utahpsychiatricassociation.org

Paige De Mille, Executive Director
Year Founded: 1951

Vermont

2027 Fletcher Allen Health Care
111 Colchester Avenue
Burlington, VT 05401-1416
802-847-0000
800-358-1144
www.www.fletcherallen.org

Melinda L Estes, MD, President/CEO
Richarad Magnuson, CFO
Angeline Marano, COO
Theresa Alberghini Dipalma, VP/Government External Affairs

2028 National Alliance on Mental Illness: Vermont
132 South Main Street
Waterbury, VT 05676-1519
802-244-1396
800-639-6480
Fax: 802-244-1405
E-mail: info@namivt.org
www.namivt.org

Ann Cummins, Chairman
Wendy Beinner, President/CEO
Wendy Beinner, Director
Chelsea Smiley, Office Manager

NAMI-Vermont is a statewide volunteer organization comprised of family members, friends, and individuals affected by mental illness. We have experienced the struggles and have joined together in membership to help ourselves and others by providing support, information, education and advocacy.

Year Founded: 1983

2029 Retreat Healthcare
Anna Marsh Lane
PO Box 803
Brattleboro, VT 05302-803
802-257-7755
800-738-7328
Fax: 802-258-3791
TDD: 802-258-8770
www.retreathealthcare.org/

Richard T Palmisano, President/CEO
Gregory A Miller, VP Medical Affairs
Robert Soucy, COO
John E Blaha, VP/CFO

2030 Vermont Alliance for the Mentally Ill
132 South Main Street
Waterbury, VT 05676-1585
802-244-1396
800-639-6480
Fax: 802-244-1405
E-mail: info@namivt.org
www.namivt.org

Ann Cummins, Chairman
Wendy Beinner, President/CEO
Wendy Beinner, Director
Chelsea Smiley, Office Manager

Nation's leading self-help organization for all those affected by severe brain disorders. Mission is to bring consumers and families with similar experiences together to share information about services, care providers, and ways to cope with the challenges of schizophrenia, manic depression, and other serious mental illnesses.

Year Founded: 1983

2031 Vermont Federation of Families for Children's Mental Health
600 Blair Park Road
PO Box 1577
Williston, VT 05495
802-244-1955
800-639-6071
Fax: 802-828-2135
E-mail: vffcmh@vffcmh.org
www.vffcmh.org

Ted Tighe, President
Sherry Schoenberg, Vice President
Kathy Holsopple, Executive Director
Matt Wolf, Young Adult Coordinator

Supports families and children where a child or youth, age 0-22, is experiencing or at risk to experience emotional, behavioral, or mental health challenges.

Virginia

2032 Garnett Day Treatment Center
University of Virginia Health System/UVHS
1 Garnet Center Drive
Charlottesville, VA 22911-8572
434-977-3425
Fax: 434-977-8529
www.healthsystem.virginia.edu/internet/homehealth/

Byrd S Leavell Jr, MD, President UVHS

2033 NAMI
3803 N. Fairfax Drive
Suite 100
Arlington, VA 22203
703-524-7600
888-999-6264
Fax: 703-524-9094
www.nami.org

Michael Fitzpatrick, Executive Director
Lynn Borton, COO

Dedicated to the eradication of mental illnesses and to the improvement of the quality of life of all whose lives are affected by these diseases.

2034 National Alliance on Mental Illness: Virginia
PO Box 8260
Richmond, VA 23226-260
804-285-8264
888-486-8264
Fax: 804-285-8464
E-mail: namiva@verizon.net
www.namivirginia.org

Barbara Collins, President
Kristin Yavorsky, MSW, 2nd Vice President
Mira Signer, Executive Director
Danny Aldred, Administrative Assistant

Created in 1985 to provide support, education, and advocacy for consumers and families in Virginia affected by mental illness. It is our mission to improve the lives of all those who are affected by serious brain disorders and to fight the stigma that surrounds mental illness.

2035 Parent Resource Center
Division of Special Education And Student Services
Virginia Department of Education
P O Box 2120
Richmond, VA 23218-2120
804-371-7421
800-422-2083
Fax: 804-559-6835
E-mail: judy.hudgins@doe.virginia.gov
www.doe.virginia.gov/VDOE/sess

Patricia I. Wright, Superintendent of Public Instruc

Washington

2036 A Common Voice
Hope Center, Lakewood Boys/Girls Club
10402 Kline Street SW
Lakewood, WA 98499
253-537-2145
E-mail: acvsherry@msn.com
www.acommonvoice.org

Marge Critchlow, Director
Sharon Lyons, Assistant Director

A parent driven, nonprofit organization funded by Washington State Mental Health. Their goal is to provide support, technical assistance, and to bring Pierce County parents together who have experience raising children with complex needs, facilitaing partnership between communities, systems, familes, and schools.

Year Founded: 1995

2037 Children's Alliance
718 6th Avenue South
Seattle, WA 98104
206-324-0340
Fax: 206-325-6291
E-mail: seattle@childrensalliance.org
www.childrensalliance.org

Tom Rembiesa, Chairman
Paola Maranan, Executive Director
Nancy Norman, Finance and Operations Director
Jon Gould, Deputy Director

Washington's statewide child advocacy organization. We champion public policies and practices that deliver the essentials that kids need to thrive — confidence, stability, health and safety.

Year Founded: 1983

2038 Mental Health & Spirituality Support Group
Nami Eastside-Family Resource Center
16315 NE 87th Street
Suite B-3
Redmond, WA 98052-3537
425-489-4084
E-mail: info@nami-eastside.org
www.nami-eastside.org/

Paul Beatty, Co - President
Manka Dhingra, Co - President
Shari Shovlin, Vice President
Michael C.Maloney, Secretary

Nation's leading self-help organization for all those affected by severe brain disorders. Mission is to bring consumers and families with similar experiences together to share information about services, care providers, and ways to cope with the challenges of schizophrenia, manic depression, and other serious mental illnesses.

2039 National Alliance on Mental Illnes: Whidbey Island Oak Harbor, WA 98277-8802
360-675-7358
Fax: 360-675-7358
E-mail: info@namiwi.org
www.namiwi.org

Margaret Houlihan

Nation's leading self-help organization for all those affected by severe brain disorders. Mission is to bring consumers and families with similar experiences together to share information about services, care providers, and ways to cope with the challenges of schizophrenia, manic depression, and other serious mental illnesses.

2040 National Alliance on Mental Illness: Washington
7500 Greenwood Avenue North
Seattle, WA 98103
206-783-4288
800-782-9264
E-mail: office@namiwa.org
www.www.namiwa.org/

Gordon Bopp, President
Year Founded: 1979

2041 North Sound Regional Support Network
North Sound Mental Health Administration
117 North First Street
Suite 8
Mount Vernon, WA 98273-2858
360-416-7013
800-684-3555
Fax: 360-419-7017
TTY: 360-419-9008
E-mail: nsmha@nsmha.org
www.nsmha.org

Kurt Aemmer, Quality Specialist
Annette Calder, Executive Assistant
Julie de Losada, Quality Specialist Coordinator
Shari Downing, Accounting Specialist

It is the purpose of the North Sound Regional Support Network (NSRSN) to ensure the provision of quality and integrated mental health services for the five counties (San Juan, Skagit, Snohomish, Island, and Whatcom) served by the NSRSN Prepaid Health Plan (PHP). We join together to enhance our community's mental health and support recovery for people with mental illness served in the North Sound region, through high quality culturally competent services.

2042 Nueva Esperanza Counseling Center
720 W Court Street
Suite 8
Pasco, WA 99301-4178
509-545-6506

Maria A Morcuende

2043 Pierce County Alliance for the Mentally Ill
PO Box 111923
Tacoma, WA 98411-1923
253-677-6629
E-mail: info@namipierce.org
www.nami.org

Bob Winslow, President
LaDonna Barnwell, Vice President
Virginia C. Peterson, Programs Contact
Karen I. Davis, Programs Contact

Nation's leading self-help organization for all those affected by severe brain disorders. Mission is to bring consumers and families with similar experiences together to share information about services, care providers, and ways to cope with the challenges of schizophrenia, manic depression, and other serious mental illnesses.

2044 Sharing & Caring for Consumers, Families Alliance for the Mentally Ill
NAMI-Eastside Family Resource Center
16315 NE 87th Street
Suite B-11
Redmond, WA 98052-3537
425-885-6264
E-mail: info@nami-eastside.org
www.nami-eastside.org/

Paul Beatty, Co - President
Manka Dhingra, Co - President
Shari Shovlin, Vice President
Michael C.Maloney, Secretary

Nation's leading self-help organization for all those affected by severe brain disorders. Mission is to bring consumers and families with similar experiences together to share information about services, care providers, and ways to cope with the challenges of schizophrenia, manic depression, and other serious mental illnesses.

2045 South King County Alliance for the Mentally Ill
515 West Harrison Street
Suite 215
Kent, WA 98032-4403
253-854-6264
E-mail: NAMIskc@qwestoffice.net
www.nami.org/sites/NAMISouthKingCounty

John Corr, President
Sandy Klungness

Nation's leading self-help organization for all those affected by severe brain disorders. Mission is to bring consumers and families with similar experiences together to share information about services, care providers, and ways to cope with the challenges of schizophrenia, manic depression, and other serious mental illnesses.

2046 Spanish Support Group Alliance for the Mentally Ill
NAMI-Eastside
2601 Elliott Avenue
Suite 4143
Seattle, WA 98121-1399
425-747-7892
E-mail: remmedicalraulmunoz@comcast.net
www.nami-eastside.org/

Paul Beatty, Co - President
Manka Dhingra, Co - President
Shari Shovlin, Vice President
Michael C.Maloney, Secretary

Nation's leading self-help organization for all those affected by severe brain disorders. Mission is to bring consumers and families with similar experiences together to share information about services, care providers, and ways to cope with the challenges of schizophrenia, manic depression, and other serious mental illnesses.

2047 Spokane Mental Health
107 South Division Street
Spokane, WA 99202-1510
509-838-4651
Fax: 509-458-7456
www.fbhwa.org

David Panken, CEO
Jennifer Allen, UC Coordinator

Since 1970, Spokane Mental Health, a not-for-profit organization, has served children, families, adults and elders throughout Spokane County. Our professional staff provides quality treatment and rehabilitation for those with mental illness and co-occurring disorders. These services include crisis response services; individual, family and group therapy; case management and support; vocational rehabilitation; psychiatric and psychological services; medication management and consumer education. We tailor services to the unique needs and strengths of each person seeking care.

2048 Washington Advocates for the Mentally Ill
NAMI Eastside Family Resource Center
16315 NE 87th Street
Suite B-11
Redmond, WA 98052-3537
425-885-6264
800-782-9264
E-mail: info@nami-eastside.org
www.nami-eastside.org/

Paul Beatty, Co - President
Manka Dhingra, Co - President
Shari Shovlin, Vice President
Michael C.Maloney, Secretary

Nation's leading self-help organization for all those affected by severe brain disorders. Mission is to bring consumers and families with similar experiences together to share information about services, care providers, and ways to cope with the challenges of schizophrenia, manic depression, and other serious mental illnesses.

2049 Washington Institute for Mental Illness Research and Training
Washington State University, Spokane
PO Box 1495
Spokane, WA 99210-1495

509-358-7514
Fax: 509-358-7619
www.spokane.wsu.edu/research&service/

Michael Hendrix, Director
Sandie Kruse, Training Coordinator

Governmental organization focusing on mental illness research.

2050 Washington State Psychological Association
PO Box 95168
Seattle, WA 98145-2168
206-547-4220
Fax: 206-547-6366
E-mail: wspa@wapsych.org
www.wapsych.org

Kathleen Hosfeld, Interim Executive Director
Lucy Homans, EdD, Director of Professional Affairs
Kevand Topping, Member Services Coordinator

To support, promote and advance the science, education and practice of psychology in the public interest.
Year Founded: 1947

West Virginia

2051 CAMC Family Medicine Center of Charleston
PO Box 1547
Suite 108
Charleston, WV 25326
304-347-4600
Fax: 304-347-4621
www.www.camc.org

Robert M D'Alessandri, MD, Vice President Health Sciences

2052 Mountain State Parent Child and Adolescent Contacts
1201 Garfield Street
McMechen, WV 26003-9062
304-233-5399
800-244-5385
Fax: 304-233-3847
www.mspcan.org

Joyce Floyd, President
Hope Coleman, Vice President
Jackie Hensley, Secretary
Donna Moss, Treasurer

A private non-profit, family-run organization that improves outcomes for children with serious emotional disorders and their families.

Wisconsin

2053 National Alliance on Mental Illness: Wisconsin
4233 West Beltline Highway
Madison, WI 53711-3814
608-268-6000
800-236-2988
Fax: 608-268-6004
E-mail: nami@namiwisconsin.org
www.namiwisconsin.org

Jim Connors, President
Thomas Christensen, Vice President
Kathy Rohr, Secretary
Julianne Carbin, MSW, Executive Director

The mission of NAMI Wisconsin is to improve the quality of life of people affected by mental illnesses and to promote recovery.

Year Founded: 1977

2054 Wisconsin Alliance for the Mentally Ill
NAMI-Wisconsin
4233 West Beltline Highway
Madison, WI 53711-3814
608-268-6000
800-236-2988
E-mail: nami@namiwisconsin.org
www.namiwisconsin.org

Jim Connors, President
Thomas Christensen, Vice President
Kathy Rohr, Secretary
Julianne Carbin, MSW, Executive Director

Self-help organization for all those affected by severe brain disorders. Mission is to bring consumers and families with similar experiences together to share information about services, care providers, and ways to cope with the challangs of schizophrenia, manic depression, and other serious mental illnesses.

Year Founded: 1977

2055 Wisconsin Association of Family and Child Agency
131 W Wilson Street
Suite 901
Madison, WI 53703-3259
608-257-5939
Fax: 608-257-6067
www.wafca.org

Linda A Hall, Executive Director
Kathy Markeland, Associate Director
Carla Shedivy, Projects Manager

2056 Wisconsin Family Ties
16 N Carroll Street
Suite 230
Madison, WI 53703-2783
608-267-6888
800-422-7145
Fax: 608-267-6801
E-mail: info@wifamilyties.org
www.wifamilyties.org

Hugh Davis, Executive Director
Joan Maynard, Information Referral Coordinator

Wyoming

2057 Central Wyoming Behavioral Health at Lander Valley
1320 Bishop Randall Drive
Lander, WY 82520-3939
307-332-4420
800-788-9446
Fax: 307-332-3548
www.landerhospital.com/patientservices.htm

Rebecca K Smith

2058 National Alliance on Mental Illness: Wyoming
137 W 6th St
Casper, WY 82601
307-265-2573
888-882-4968

Fax: 307-265-0968
E-mail: info@namiwyoming.org
www.www.namiwyoming.org

Marty Coe, President
Gerard Baumstarck, Vice President
Tammy Noel, Executive Director
Becky Spahn, Office Manager/Marketing Coordin

To improve the quality of life for those who suffer from depression, bipolar disorder, schizophrenia, obsessive compulsive disorder, panic disorder, autism, borderline personality disorder and other severe and persistent mental illnesses that affect the brain

2059 Uplift
4007 Greenway Street
Suite 201
Cheyenne, WY 82001-4434
307-778-8686
888-875-4383
Fax: 307-778-8681
E-mail: uplift@wyoming.com
www.upliftwy.org/

Brenden McKinney, President
Peggy Nikkel, Executive Director
Sandy Reoff-Elledge, Vice President

Wyoming Chapter of the Federation of Families for Children's Mental Health. Providing support, education, advocacy, information and referral for parents and professionals focusing on emotional, behavioral and learning needs of children and youth.

2060 Wyoming Alliance for the Mentally Ill
NAMI Wyoming
PO Box 1883
Casper, WY 82602
307-265-2573
888-882-4968
Fax: 307-265-0968
E-mail: namiwyominginfo@gmail.com
www.nami.org

Tammy Noel, Executive Director

Nation's leading self-help organization for all those affected by severe brain disorders. Mission is to bring consumers and families with similar experiences together to share information about services, care providers, and ways to cope with the challenges of schizophrenia, manic depression, and other serious mental illnesses.

Government Agencies

Federal

2061 Administration for Children and Families
370 L'Enfant Promenade SW
Washington, DC 20447
202-401-4802
Fax: 202-401-5706
www.acf.hhs.gov/index.html

Jeannie Chaffin, Director of the Office of Commun
Yolanda J. Butler, Deputy Director of the Office
Lauren Christopher, Chief Energy Program Operations
Seth Hassett, Director of the Division of Stat

Responsible for federal programs that promotes the economic and social well-being of families, children, individuals, and communities.

2062 Administration for Children, Youth and Families
US Department of Health & Human Services
370 L'Enfant Promenade SW
Washington, DC 20447
202-401-4802
Fax: 202-401-5706
www.www.acf.hhs.gov

Jeannie Chaffin, Director of the Office of Commun
Yolanda J. Butler, Deputy Director of the Office
Lauren Christopher, Chief Energy Program Operations
Seth Hassett, Director of the Division of Stat

Advises Health and Human Services department on plans and programs related to early childhood development; operates the Head Start day care and other related child service programs; provides leadership, advice, and services that affect the general well-being of children and youths.

2063 Administration on Aging
1 Massachusetts Avenue
Suites 4100 & 5100
Washington, DC 20201-1
202-619-0724
Fax: 202-357-3555
E-mail: aclinfo@acl.hhs.gov
www.aoa.gov

Kathy Greenlee, Secretary for Aging
Vacant , Principal Deputy Asst Secretary
Edwin Walker, Dept Asst Secretary Operations
Dan Berger, Director, Management Budget

One of the nation's largest providers of home and community-based care for older persons and their caregivers. The mission is to promote the dignity and independence of older people, and help society prepare for an aging population.

2064 Administration on Developmental Disabilities
US Department of Health & Human Services
370 L'Enfant Promenade SW
Washington, DC 20447
202-401-4802
Fax: 202-690-6904
www.www.acf.hhs.gov

Jeannie Chaffin, Director of the Office of Commun
Yolanda J. Butler, Deputy Director of the Office
Lauren Christopher, Chief Energy Program Operations
Seth Hassett, Director of the Division of Stat

Develops and administers programs protecting rights and promoting independence, productivity and inclusion; funds state grants, protection and advocacy programs, University Affiliated Programs and other national projects.

2065 Agency for Healthcare Research and Quality: Office of Communications and Knowledge Transfer
540 Gaither Road
Suite 2000
Rockville, MD 20850-6649
301-427-1104
E-mail: info@ahrq.org
www.ahrq.org

Richard Kronick, Ph.D., Director
Boyce Ginieczki, Ph.D., Acting Deputy Director
Paul N Casale, MD, F.A.C.E, Director, Quality
Helen Darling, MA, President

Provides policymakers and other health care leaders with information needed to make critical health care decisions.

2066 Association of Maternal and Child Health Programs (AMCHP)
2030 M Street NW
Suite 350
Washington, DC 20036-2435
202-775-0436
Fax: 202-775-0061
E-mail: lramo@amchp.org
www.amchp.org

Millie Jones, PA, , President
Barbara Laur, MS, Interim Chief Executive Office
Lacy Fehrenbach, MPH, CPH, Director; Region III Liaison; Pr
Matt Algee, Senior Accountant; Organizationa

National non-profit organization representing state public health workers. Provides leadership to assure the health and well-being of women of reproductive age, children, youth, including those with special health care needs and their families.

2067 Center for Mental Health Services Homeless Programs Branch
Substance Abuse and Mental Health Services Administration
1 Choke Cherry Road
Rockville, MD 20857-1
240-276-1310
Fax: 240-276-1320
www.samhsa.gov

Paolo del Vecchio, M.S.W., Director
Elizabeth Lopez, Ph.D., Acting Deputy Director
Deborah Baldwin, M.P.A., Consumer Affairs, Acting Directo
Mark Weber, Director, Communications

Federal agency concerned with the prevention and treatment of mental illness and the promotion of mental health. Homeless Programs Branch administers a variety of programs and activities. Provides professional leadership for collaborative intergovernmental initiatives designed to assist persons with mental illnesses who are homeless. Also supports a contract for the National Resource Center on Homelessness and Mental Illness.

2068 Center for Substance Abuse Treatment
Substance Abuse Mental Health Services
Administration
1 Choke Cherry Road
Rockville, MD 20857-1
240-276-1660
Fax: 240-276-1670
www.samhsa.gov

Anna Marsh, Deputy Director, Mental Health
Frences M Harding, Director, Sub Abuse Prevention
H Westley Clark, Director, Sub Abuse Treatment
Peter Delany, Director, Behavioral Health

CSAT promotes the quality and availability of community based substance abuse treatment services for individuals and families who need them. CSATÆworks with Sates and community based groups to improve and expand existing subsance abouse treatment services under the Substance Abuse Prevention and Treatment Block Grant Program.

2069 Centers for Disease Control & Prevention
1600 Clifton Road
Atlanta, GA 30333
404-639-3311
800-311-3435
E-mail: cdcinfo@cdc.gov
www.cdc.gov

Robert Delaney, Plant Manager

Protecting the health and safety of people — at home and abroad, providing credible information to enhance health decisions, and promoting health through strong partnership. Serves as the national focus for developing and applying disease prevention and control, environmental health, and health promotion in education activities designed to improve the health of the people of the United States.

2070 DC Department of Mental Health
Government of the District of Columbia
64 New York Avenue, NE
4th Floor
Washington, DC 20002-3329
202-673-7440
888-793-4357
Fax: 202-673-3433
TDD: 202-673-7500
E-mail: dbh@dc.gov
www.dmh.dc.gov

Stephen J Baron, Director
Vincent C Gray, DC Mayor

The goal of the Department of Mental Health is to develop, support, and oversee a comprehensive, community-based, consumer-driven, culturally competent, quality mental health system. This system should be responsive and accessible to children, youths, adults, and their families. It should leverage continuous positive change through its ability to learn and to partner. It should also ensure that mental health providers are accountable to consumers and offer services that promote recovery from mental illness.

2071 Equal Employment Opportunity Commission
131 M Street, NE
Washington, DC 20507-1
202-663-4900
800-669-4000
TTY: 800-663-4494
E-mail: info@eeoc.gov
www.www.eeoc.gov

Milton A. Mayo Jr., Inspector General
Stuart J Ishimaru, Commissioner
Constance S Barker, Commissioner
Chai Feldblum, Commissioner

To eradicate employment discrimination at workplace.

Year Founded: 1965

2072 Health Care For All(HCFA)
30 Winter Street
10th Floor
Boston, MA 02108-4720
617-350-7279
Fax: 617-451-5838
TTY: 617-350-0974
E-mail: mcdonough@hcfama.org
www.www.hcfama.org

Amy Whitcomb Slemmer, Executive Director
Amilton Baptista, Community Education Coordinator
Kathryn Bicego, Consumer Assistance Program Mana
Rosemarie Boardman, Director of Finance and Operatio

2073 Health Systems and Financing Group
Health Resources and Services Administration
1818 H Street, NW
5600 Fishers Lane
Washington, DC 20433
202-473-1000
www.www.worldbank.org

Jim Yong Kim, President
Sri Mulyani Indrawati, Managing Director and Chief Oper
Bertrand Badr,, Managing Director and World Bank
Kaushik Basu, Chief Economist and Senior Vice

The World Bank will help develop low and middle income countries to improve peoples health and to guard against the poverty that can result from sudeen illness. POor families often tap into savings or sell they own to cover the costs of medical care. As a result, all to often people end up falling below the poverty line.

Year Founded: 1944

2074 Health and Human Services Office of Assistant
Secretary for Planning & Evaluation
200 Independence Avenue SW
Washington, DC 20201-4
202-619-0257
877-696-6775
www.aspe.hhs.gov

Ruth Katz, Acting Deputy Assistant Secretar
Rima Cohen, Acting Assistant Secretary for P
Kirsten Beronio, Director, Division of Behavioral
William Marton, Director, Division of Disability

ASPE is the principal advisor to the Secretary of the U.S. Department of Health and Human Services on policy development, and is responsible for major activities in policy coordination, legislation development, strategic planning, policy research, evaluation, and economic analysis.

Year Founded: 1972

2075 Information Resources and Inquiries Branch
National Institute of Mental Health
6001 Executive Boulevard
Room 8184
Bethesda, MD 20892-9663
301-443-4513
866-615-6464

TTY: 301-443-8431
E-mail: nimhinfo@nih.gov
www.www.nimh.nih.gov

Francis E Collins, PhD, Director

A component of the National Institute of Health, the NIMH conducts and supports research that seeks to understand, treat and prevent mental illness. The Institute's Information Resources and Inquiries Branch (IRIB) responds to information requests from the lay public, clinicians and the scientific community with a variety of publications on subjects such as basic behavioral research, neuroscience of mental health, rural mental, children's mental disorders, schizophrenia, paranoia, depression, bipolar disorder, learning disabilities, Alzheimer's disease, panic, obsessive compulsive and other anxiety disorders. A publication list is available upon request.

2076 National Institutes of Mental Health Division of Intramural Research Programs (DIRP)
10 Center Drive
Room 4N222 MSC 1381
Bethesda, MD 20892-1
301-496-3501
Fax: 301-480-8348
E-mail: contactNIMH@mail.nih.gov
www.intramural.nimh.nih.gov

Susan G. Amara Ph.D., Scientific Director
Barry B. Kaplan, Ph.D., Associate Director for Fellowshi
Marie Schwartz, Scientific Management Analyst

The Division of Intramural Research Programs (DIRP) at the National Institute of Mental Health (NIMH) is the internal research division of the NIMH. NIMH DIRP scientists conduct research ranging from studies into mechanisms of normal brain function, conducted at the behavioral, systems, cellular, and molecular levels, to clinical investigations into the diagnosis, treatment and prevention of mental illness. Major disease entities studied throughout the lifespan include mood disorders and anxiety, schizophrenia, obsessive-compulsive disorder, attention deficit hyperactivity disorder, and pediatric autoimmune neuropsychiatric disorders.

2077 National Center for HIV, STD and TB Prevention
Centers For Disease Control and Prevention
1600 Clifton Road
NE Mailstop E-10
Atlanta, GA 30333
404-639-3311
800-232-4636
TTY: 888-232-6348
E-mail: cdcinfo@cdc.gov
www.cdc.gov

Robert Delaney, Plant Manager

CDC's mission is to collaborate to create the expertise, information, and tools that people and communities need to protect their health - through health promotion, prevention of disease, injury and disability, aand prepaedness for new health threats and diseases.

2078 National Institute of Alcohol Abuse and Alcoholism: Treatment Research Branch
5635 Fishers Lane
MSC 9304
Bethesda, MD 20892-1

301-443-3860
E-mail: niaaaweb-r@exchange.nih.gov.
www.niaaa.nih.gov/

Dr. George Koob, Director
Mr. Keith Lamirande, Resource Management, Director
Dr. Vivian Faden, Science Policy and Communication
Dr. Abraham Bautista, Extramural Activities, Director

NIAAA provides leadership in the national effort to reduce alcohol-related problems by conducting and supporting research in a wide range of scientific areas including genetics, neuroscience, epidemiology, health risks and benefits of alcohol consumption, prevention, and treatment.

2079 National Institute of Alcohol Abuse and Alcoholism: Homeless Demonstration and Evaluation Branch
5600 Fishers Lane
Msc 9304
Rockville, MD 20852-1750
301-443-4795
Fax: 301-443-0284
E-mail: niaaaweb-r@exchange.nih.gov

Kenneth Warren, PhD, Acting Director
Andrea G Barhtwell, MD, President
John H Krystal, Chairman

NIAAA provides leadership in the national effort to reduce alcohol-related problems by conducting and supporting research in a wide range of scientific areas including genetics, neuroscience, epidemiology, health risks and benefits of alcohol consumption, prevention, and treatment.

2080 National Institute of Alcohol Abuse and Alcoholism: Office of Policy Analysis
The Alcohol Policy Information System (APIS)
5600 Fishers Lane
Room 16-95
Rockville, MD 20857-1
301-443-3864
E-mail: niaaaweb-r@exchange.nih.gov

Kenneth E Warren, PhD, Acting Director
Andrea G Barhtwell, MD, President
John H Krystal, Chairman

The Alcohol Policy Information System (APIS) is an online resource that provides detailed information on a wide variety of alcohol-related policies in the United States at both State and Federal levels. It features compilations and analyses of alcohol-related statutes and regulations. Designed primarily as a tool for researchers, APIS simplifies the process of ascertaining the state of the law for studies on the effects and effectiveness of alcohol-related policies.

2081 National Institute of Drug Abuse: NIDA
6001 Executive Boulevard
Room 5213
Bethesda, MD 20892-9561
301-443-6245
Fax: 301-443-7397
E-mail: information@nida.nih.gov
www.drugabuse.gov

Glenda Conroy, Director, Management
David Daubert, Deputy Director, Management
Mark Swieter, Ph.D., Acting Director

Covers the areas of drug abuse treatment and prevention research, epidemiology, neuroscience and behavioral research, health services research and AIDS. Seeks to report on advances in the field, identify resources, promote an exchange of information, and improve communications among clinicians, researchers, administrators, and policymakers. Recurring features include synopses of research advances and projects, NIDA news, news of legislative and regulatory developments, and announcements.

2082 National Institute of Mental Health: Schizophrenia Research Branch

6001 Executive Boulevard
Room 8184, MSC 9663
Bethesda, MD 20892-1
301-443-4513
E-mail: nimhinfo@nih.gov
www.www.nimh.nih.gov

Sarah E. Morris, Ph.D., Program Chief
Glenda Conroy, Director
David Daubert, Branch Chief

Information available includes a detailed booklet that provides an overview of schizophrenia and also describes symptoms, causes, and treatments, with information on getting help and coping.

2083 National Institute of Mental Health: Mental Disorders of the Aging
National Institutes of Health

6001 Executive Boulevard
Room 8184, MSC 9663
Bethesda, MD 20892-1
301-443-4513
E-mail: nimhinfo@nih.gov
www.www.nimh.nih.gov

Nora D Volkow, MD, Director
Glenda Conroy, Director
David Daubert, Branch Chief

The Aging Research Consortium was established in January 2002 by NIMH. Its mission is to: Stimulate research on mental health and mental illness to benefit older adults; Maintain an infrastructure to better coordinate aging research throughout the Institute; Provide a linkage to the Institute for researchers, advocates, and the public and advance research training for the study of late life mental disorders.

2084 National Institute of Mental Health: Office of Science Policy, Planning, and Communications
National Institutes of Health

6001 Executive Boulevard
Room 8208 MSC 9667
Bethesda, MD 20892-1
301-443-4513
E-mail: nimhinfo@nih.gov
www.www.nimh.nih.gov

Kevin Quinn, Acting Director
Diane Buckley, Deputy Director, OSPPC
Roy Lane Wheat, Program Specialist
Monica Carter, Management Analyst

Plans and directs a comprehensive strategic agenda for national mental health policy, including science program planning and related policy evaluation, research training and coordination, and technology and information transfer. OSPPC plans and implements portfolio analysis, scientific disease coding, and program evaluations for developing and assessing NIMH strategic plans and portfolio management. OSPPC also creates and implements the Institute's communication efforts, including information dissemina-

tion, media relations activities, and internal communications. The Office proposes and guides science education activities concerned with informing the scientific community and public about mental health issues.

2085 National Institute on Alcohol Abuse and Alcoholism

5635 Fishers Lane
Bethesda, MD 20892-2345
800-729-6686
TDD: 800-487-4889
E-mail: niaaaweb-r@exchange.nih.gov.
www.niaaa.nih.gov/

Dr. George Koob, Director
Mr. Keith Lamirande, Resource Management, Director
Dr. Vivian Faden, Science Policy and Communication
Dr. Abraham Bautista, Extramural Activities, Director

NIAAA's vision is to increase the understanding of normal and abnormal biological functions and behavior relating to alcohol use. Improving the diagnosis, prevention, and treatment of alcohol use disorders. Enhancing the quality of health care.

2086 National Institute on Drug Abuse: Division of Clinical Neurosciences and Behavioral Research

6001 Executive Boulevard
Room 3155, MSC 9593
Bethesda, MD 20892-9593
301-443-4877
Fax: 301-443-6814
E-mail: sgrant@nida.nih.gov
www.drugabuse.gov

Joseph Frascella, Director
Dave Thomas, Deputy Director
Barbara Usher, Special Assistant to the Directo
Carolyn Tucker, Extramural Support Assistant

The Clinical Neuroscience Branch (CNB) advances a clinical research and research training program focused on understanding the neurobiological substrates of drug abuse and addiction processes and on characterizing how abused drugs affect the structure, function, development, and maturation of the human central nervous system. Another major emphasis of this program is on etiological studies examining individual differences in neurobiological, genetic, and neurobehavioral factors that underlie increased risk and/or resilience to drug abuse, addiction, and drug-related disorders, as well as on the neurobiological/neurobehavioral factors involved in the transition from drug use to addiction.

2087 National Institute on Drug Abuse: Office of Science Policy and Communications

6001 Executive Boulevard
Room 5213, MSC 9561
Bethesda, MD 20892-9561
301-443-6245
Fax: 301-443-7397
www.drugabuse.gov

Jack Stein, Ph.D., Director
Carole Andrews, Program Analyst
Holly Buchanan, Program Specialist
Geoffrey Laredo, M.P.A., Program Analysis Officer

The Office of Science Policy and Communications (OSPC) carries out a wide variety of functions in support of the Director, NIDA, and on behalf of the Institute. We're made up of the Office of the Director and the International Program Office, and two branches, the Science Policy Branch and the Public Information and Liaison Branch.

2088 National Institutes of Health: National Center for Research Resources (NCCR)

9000 Rockville Pike
Bethesda, MD 20892
301-435-0888
Fax: 301-480-3558
E-mail: info@ncrr.nih.gov
www.www.nih.gov

Frances E Collins, PhD, Director

The National Center for Research Resources (NCRR), a component of the National Institutes of Health that supports primary research to create and develop critical resources, models, and technologies. NCRR funding also provides biomedical researchers with access to diverse instrumentation, technologies, basic and clinical research facilities, animal models, genetic stocks, biomaterials, and more. These resources enable scientific advances in biomedicine that lead to the development of lifesaving drugs, devices, and therapies.

Year Founded: 1962

2089 National Institutes of Mental Health: Office on AIDS

National Institutes of Health

6001 Executive Boulevard
Room 6225, MSC 9621
Bethesda, MD 20892-1
301-443-4513
www.www.nimh.nih.gov

Nora D Volkow, MD, Director
Glenda Conroy, Director

(1) Plans, directs, coordinates, and supports biomedical and behavioral research designed to develop a better understanding of the biological and behavioral causes of HIV (AIDS virus) infection and more effective mechanisms for the diagnosis, treatment, and prevention of AIDS; (2) analyzes and evaluates National needs and research opportunities to identify areas warranting either increased or decreased program emphasis; and (3) consults and cooperates with voluntary and professional health organizations, as well as other NIH components and Federal agencies, to identify and meet AIDS-related needs.

2090 National Library of Medicine

National Institues of Health

8600 Rockville Pike
Bethesda, MD 20894-1
301-496-2447
888-346-3656
Fax: 301-402-0254
E-mail: custserv@nlm.nih.gov/

Donal A B Lindberg, MD, Director
Philip D Osbourne, Dir, Chief Contracting Officer

The National Library of Medicine (NLM), on the campus of the National Institutes of Health in Bethesda, Maryland, is the world's largest medical library. The Library collects materials and provides information and research services in all areas of biomedicine and health care.

1836 pages

2091 Office of Applied Studies, SA & Mental Health Services

1 Choke Cherry Road
Rockville, MD 20857-1
240-276-2000
Fax: 240-276-2010
www.samhsa.gov

The Office of Applied Studies provides the latest national data on alchohol, tobacco, marijuana and other drug abuse in addition to drug related emergency department epidosdes, medical examiner cases and the nation's substance abuse treatment system.

2092 Office of Disease Prevention & Health Promotion

US Department of Health and Human Services

1101 Wootton Parkway, Suite Ll100
Rockville, MD 20852-1059
240-453-8280
Fax: 240-453-8282
www.odphp.osophs.dhhs.gov

The Office of Disease Prevention and Health Promotion, Office of Public Health and Science, Office of the Secretary, U.S. Department of Health and Human Services, works to strengthen the disease prevention and health promotion priorities of the Department within the collaborative framework of the HHS agencies.

Year Founded: 1976

2093 Office of National Drug Control Policy

Drug Policy Information Clearinghouse

PO Box 6000
Rockville, MD 20849-6000
800-666-3332
Fax: 301-519-5212
www.whitehousedrugpolicy.gov/

R Gil Kerlikowske, Director
David K Mineta, Deputy Director
Bejamin B Tucker, Deputy Director
Marily A Quagliotti, Deputy Director

The goal of the Department of Mental Health is to develop, support, and oversee a comprehensive, community-based, consumer-driven, culturally competent, quality mental health system. This system should be responsive and accessible to children, youths, adults, and their families. It should leverage continuous positive change through its ability to learn and to partner. It should also ensure that mental health providers are accountable to consumers and offer services that promote recovery from mental illness.

2094 Office of Program and Policy Development

National Association of Community Health Centers

7501 Wisconsin Ave
Suite 1100W
Bethesda, MD 20814-4838
301-347-0400
Fax: 301-347-0459
www.nachc.com

Gary Wiltz, MD, Chair of the Board
Tom Van Coverden, President and CEO
Darlene De Mott, Corp Executive Manager
Kathy Bennett, Assoc. Corp Exec Manager

NACHC's mission is to promote the provision of high quality, comprehensive, and affordable health care that is coordinated, culturally and linquistically competent, and community directed for all medically underserved populations.

2095 Office of Science Policy OD/NIH

6705 Rockledge Drive
Rockledge 1, Suite 750
Bethesda, MD 20817
301-496-9838
Fax: 301-402-1759
www.ospp.od.nih.gov

Sarah Carr, Acting Director
Marina Volkov, Ph.D., Acting Director
Jacqueline Corrigan-Curay, J.D., , Acting Director
Marina Volkov, Ph.D., Acting Director

Advises the NIH Director on science policy issues affecting the medical research community; Participates in the development of new policy and program initiatives; Monitors and coordinates agency planning and evaluation activities; Plans and implements a comprehensive science education program and Develops and implements NIH policies and procedures for the safe conduct of recombinant DNA and other biotechnology activities.

2096 President's Committee on Mental Retardation

US DHHS, Administration for Children & Families, PCMR
370 L'Enfatne Promenade SW
Washington, DC 20447-1
202-401-4802
www.www.acf.hhs.gov

Jeannie Chaffin, Director of the Office of Commun
Yolanda J. Butler, Deputy Director of the Office
Lauren Christopher, Chief Energy Program Operations
Seth Hassett, Director of the Division of Stat

The PCMR acts in an advisory capacity to the President and the Secretary of Health and Human Services on matters relating to programs and services for persons with mental retardation. It has adopted several national goals in order to better recognize and uphold the right of all people with mental retardation to enjoy a quality of life that promotes independence, self-determination and participation as productive members of society.

2097 Presidential Commission on Employment of the Disabled

Frances Perkins Building
200 Constitution Avenue, NW
Washington, DC 20210-1
866-633-7365
Fax: 202-693-7888
TTY: 866-633-2365
www.dol.gov/odep

Thomas E. Perez, Secretary of Labor
Rhonda Basha, Chief of Staff
Dylan Orr, Specail Assistant/Advisor
Elena Carr, Acting Executive Officer

The Office of Disability Employment Policy (ODEP) was authorized by Congress in the Department of Labor's FY 2001 appropriation. Recognizing the need for a national policy to ensure that people with disabilities are fully integrated into the 21 st Century workforce, the Secretary of Labor Elaine L. Chao delegated authority and assigned responsibility to the Assistant Secretary for Disability Employment Policy. ODEP is a sub-cabinet level policy agency in the Department of Labor.

2098 Protection and Advocacy Program for the Mentally Ill

US Department of Health and Human Services
1 Choke Cherry Road
Rockville, MD 20857-1
240-276-1310
Fax: 240-276-1320
www.samhsa.gov/index.aspx

Federal formula grant program to protect and advocate the rights of people with mental illnesses who are in residential facilities and to investigate abuse and neglect in such facilities.

2099 Public Health Foundation

1300 L Street NW
Suite 800
Washington, DC 20005-4208
202-218-4400
Fax: 202-218-4409
E-mail: info@phf.org
www.phf.org

Rachel H. Stevens, EDd, RN, Chair
Sue Madden, Chief Operating Officer/Chief Fi
Lois Banks, Director, TRAIN
Margie Beaudry, Senior Associate, Performance Im

A high-performing public health system that protects and promotes health in every community by improving public health infrastructure and performance through innovative solutions and measurable results.

2100 SAMHSA's Fetal Alcohol Spectrum Disorders Center for Excellence (FASD)

2101 Gaither Road
Suite 600
Rockville, MD 20850
866-786-7327
E-mail: fasdcenter@samsa.hhs.gov
www.fascenter.samhsa.gov

Patricia Getty, Contact
Year Founded: 2001

2101 Substance Abuse & Mental Health Services Administration of the US Dept of Health and Human Services

1 Choke Cherry Road
Rockville, MD 20857
240-276-2000
www.samhsa.gov

Pamela Hyde JD, Administrator
Eric Broderick DDS, MPH, Deputy Adminstrator
Kana Enomoto MA, Advisor to the Administrator
Elaine Parry MS, Director of Program Services

SAMHSA's mission is to reduce the impact of substance abuse and mental illness on America's communities. The Agency was established by Congress to target effectively substance abuse and mental health services to the people most in need and to translate research in these areas more effectively and more rapidly into the general health care system. SAMHSA has demonstrated that prevention works, treatment is effective, and people recover from mental and substance use disorders. Behavioral health services improve health statuse and reduce health care costs to society. The Agency's programs are carried out through: the Center for Mental Health Services (CMHS); The Centers for Substance Abuse Prevention and Treatment (CSAP/T); and the Office of Applied Studies.

Year Founded: 1992

2102 Substance Abuse and Mental Health Services Administration: Center for Mental Health Services
SAMHSA
1 Choke Cherry Road
Rockville, MD 20857
240-221-4022
800-487-4889
Fax: 240-221-4021
TDD: 866-889-2647
www.www.samhsa.gov

Pamela S. Hyde, J.D., Administrator
Kana Enomoto, M.A., Principal Deputy Administrator
Marla Hendriksson, M.P.M., Director, Communications
Daryl W. Kade, M.A., SAMHSA, Chief Financial Officer and Dire

Year Founded: 1992

2103 US Department of Health and Human Services: Office of Women's Health
200 Independence Avenue SW
SW Room 712E
Washington, DC 20201
202-690-7650
Fax: 202-205-2631
www.www.womenshealth.gov

Barbara F. James, M.P.H., Acting Director, Division of Pro
Valerie Borden, M.P.A., Acting Director, Division of Str
Lisa Begg, Dr.P.H., R.N., Acting Director, Division of Pol
Frances E. Ashe-Goins, R.N., M.P., Associate Director for Partnersh

The Office on Women's Health (OWH) was established in 1991 within the U.S. Department of Health and Human Services. OWH coordinates the efforts of all the HHS agencies and offices involved in women's health. OWH works to improve the health and well-being of women and girls in the United States through its innovative programs, by educating health professionals, and motivating behavior change in consumers through the dissemination of health information.

State

Alabama

2104 Alabama Department of Human Resources
Center For Communications
Gordon Persons Building, Suite 2104
50 North Ripley Street
Montgomery, AL 36130-1001
334-242-1310
Fax: 334-353-1115
www.www.dhr.alabama.gov

Nancy Jinright, Director

Member of the National Leadership Council. The mission of the Alabama Department of Human Resources is to partner with communities to promote family stability and provide for the safety and self-sufficiency of vulnerable Alabamians.

Year Founded: 1935

2105 Alabama Department of Mental Health and Mental Retardation
100 North Union Street
PO Box 301410
Montgomery, AL 36130-1410
334-242-3454
800-367-0955
Fax: 334-242-0725
E-mail: webmaster@mh.alabama.gov
www.mh.alabama.gov

John Houston, Commissioner
Beth Sievers, Administrative Assistant

State agency charged with providing services to citizens with mental illness, mental retardation and substance abuse disorders.

2106 Alabama Department of Public Health
201 Monroe Street
Montgomery, AL 36104-3735
334-206-5300
800-252-1818
www.adph.org

Donald E Williamson, MD, State Officer

Provides public health related information about the State of Alabama.

2107 Alabama Disabilities Advocacy Program
PO Box 870395
Tuscaloosa, AL 35487-395
205-348-4928
800-826-1675
Fax: 205-348-3909
E-mail: adap@adap.ua.edu
www.adap.net/

Angie Allen, Case Advocate
Nancy Anderson, Sr. Staff Attorney
Patrick Hackney, Sr. Staff Attorney
James Tucker, Director

Federally mandated, statewide, Protection and Advocacy system serving eligible individuals with disabilities in Alabama. ADAP's five programs are: Protection and Advocacy for Persons with Developmental Disabilities, Protection and Advocacy for Individuals with Mental Illness, Protection and Advocacy of Individual Rights, Protection and Advocacy for Assistive Technology and Protection and Advocacy for Beneficiaries of Social Security.

Alaska

2108 Alaska Council on Emergency Medical Services
20321 Middle Road
Eagle River, AK 99577-7931
907-465-3028
E-mail: shelley.owens@alaska.gov
www.dhss.alaska.gov

Shelley K Owens, Public Health Specialist

The mission of the Emergency Medical Services program in Alaska is to reduce both the human suffering and economic loss to society resulting from premature death and disability due to injuries and sudden illness.

2109 Alaska Department of Health & Social Services
350 Main Street, Room 404
PO Box 110601
Juneau, AK 99811-0601
907-465-3030
Fax: 907-465-3068
www.hss.state.ak.us

Tara Horton, Special Assistant
Ward Hurlburt, Chief Medical Officer
William Streve, Deputy Commissioner
Craig Christenson, Deputy Commissioner for Medicaid

The mission of the Alaska Department of Health and Social Services is to promote and protect the health and well being of Alaskans.

2110 Alaska Division of Mental Health and Developmental Disabilities
PO Box 110620
Juneau, AK 99811-620
907-465-3370
Fax: 907-465-2668
E-mail: stacy.toner@alaska.gov
www.dhss.alaska.gov

Stacy Toner, Division Operations Manager

The mission of the Division of Behavioral Health is to manage an integrated and comprehensive behavioral health system based on sound policy, effective practices and partnerships.

2111 Alaska Health and Social Services Division of Behavioral Health
350 Main Street, Room 404
PO Box 110601
Juneau, AK 99811-0601
907-465-3030
Fax: 907-465-3068
E-mail: melissa.stone@alaska.gov
www.dhss.alaska.gov

William J. Streur, Commissioner
Ward Hurlburt, Chief Medical Officer
Clay Butcher, Department Communications Manage
Jason Hooley, Special Assistant

The mission of the Division of Behavioral Health is to manage an integrated and comprehensive behavioral health system based on sound policy, effective practices and partnerships.

2112 Alaska Mental Health Board

431 N Franklin Street
Suite 200
Juneau, AK 99801-1186
907-465-8920
Fax: 907-465-4410
E-mail: kathryn.craft@alaska.gov
www.http://hss.state.ak.us/amhb

Brenda Moore, Chair
Ramona Duby, Vice Chair
J. Kate Burkhart, Executive Director
Teri Tibbett, Advocacy Coordinator

Planning and advocacy body for public mental health services. The board works to ensure that Alaska's mental health program is integrated and comprehensive. It recommends operating and capital budgets for the program. The Governor appoints twelve - sixteen members to the board. At least half the members must be consumers of mental health services or family members. Two members are mental health service providers and one an attorney.

2113 Mental Health Association in Alaska

4045 Lake Otis Parkway
Suite 209
Anchorage, AK 99508-5227
907-563-0880
Fax: 907-563-0881
E-mail: mhaa2@pobox.alaska.net
www.alaska.net/~mhaa/

Virginia L. Hostman, M.S., Chairman
Janet McGillivary, M.Ed., President & CEO
William F. Hostman, B.A., Assistant to the CEO

The Mental Health Association in Alaska (MHAA) is a Division of the National Mental Health Association and is dedicated to the promotion of good mental health, the prevention of mental illness and ongoing improvement in the care and treatment of the mentally ill through advocacy, education, referral, research, legislative input and the monitoring of existing programs.

Arizona

2114 Arizona Department of Health Services

150 North 18th Avenue
Phoenix, AZ 85007
602-542-1025
Fax: 602-542-0883
www.azhds.gov

Will Humble, Director

Promotes and protects the health of Arizona's children and adults. Its mission is to set the standard for personal and community health through direct care, science, public policy, and leadership

2115 Arizona Department of Health Services: Behavioral Health Services

150 N. 18th Avenue
#200
Phoenix, AZ 85007-3238
602-364-4558
Fax: 602-364-4570
www.azdhs.gov/bhs/index.htm

Dr. Laura K Nelson, Deputy Director

Administers Arizona's publicly funded behavioral health service system for individuals, families and communities.

Year Founded: 1986

2116 Northern Arizona Regional Behavioral Health Authority

1300 South Yale Street
Flagstaff, AZ 86001-6328
928-774-7128
877-923-1400
Fax: 928-774-5665
E-mail: info@narbha.org
www.narbha.org

Mary Jo Gregory, FACHE, RN, President and Chief Executive Of
Lindsay Miller, MBA, Chief Information Officer/Chief
Teresa Bertsch, MD, Chief Medical Officer
Michael Kuzmin, Chief Financial Officer

The Northern Arizona Regional Behavioral Health Authority's (NARBHA) mission is to provide solutions that improve the health and healthcare experience of diverse communities. We serve individuals and families across northern Arizona who are eligible for State and federally-funded behavioral health services.

Year Founded: 1967

Arkansas

2117 Arkansas Department of Human Services

Donaghey Plaza
PO Box 1437
Little Rock, AR 72203-1437
501-682-1001
Fax: 501-682-6836
TDD: 501-682-8820
www.humanservices.arkansas.gov

John Selig, DHS Director
Janie Huddleston, Deputy Director
Keesa Smith, Deputy Director
Amy Webb, Director, Communications

The Arkansas Department of Human Services provides Medicaid, mental health and substance abuse resources.

Year Founded: 1977

2118 Arkansas Division of Children & Family Service

700 Main Street
P O Box 1437 Slot S 560
Little Rock, AR 72203-1437
501-682-8770
Fax: 501-682-6968
TDD: 501-682-1442
www.humanservices.arkansas.gov/dcfs/

John Selig, Director
Janie Huddleston, Deputy Director
Keesa Smith, Deputy Director
Amy Webb, Director, Communications

The Arkansas Division of Children's Services is a member of the National Leadership Council and provides information and resources on adoption, daycare and child abuse prevention.

2119 Arkansas Division on Youth Services

700 Main Street
Slot 450
Little Rock, AR 72203-1437

502-682-8654
Fax: 501-682-1351
www.humanservices.arkansas.gov/dys

Michael Sanders, Program Development Manager
Judy Miller, Interstate Compact Coordinator
Justin Rash, Program Administrator
Brett Smith, Education Director

The Division of Youth Services (DYS) provides in a manner consistent with public safety, a system of high quality programs to address the needs of the juveniles who come in contact with, or are at risk of coming into contact with the juvenile justice system.

2120 Mental Health Council of Arkansas

501 Woodlane Drive
Suite 136S
Little Rock, AR 72201-1058
501-372-7062
Fax: 501-372-8039
E-mail: mhca@mhca.org
www.mhca.org

Pamela Christie, Executive Director
Janie Cotton, President

The Mental Health Council of Arkansas is a non-profit organization governed by a board of directors with a representative from each of the 13 participating community mental health centers and their affiliates. The MHCA assists its members to achieve the goal of community based treatment which focuses on the whole person with emphasis on physical, mental and emotional wellness and promotes the comprehensive diagnostic, treatment, and wrap around services provided by the private non-profit community mental health centers of Arkansas. The MHCA is dedicated to improving the overall health and well-being of the citizens and communities of Arkansas.

California

2121 California Department of Alcohol and Drug Programs

PO Box 997413
MS# 2603
Sacramento, CA 95899-7413
916-445-9338
800-879-2772
www.www.adp.ca.gov

Edmund G Brown, Governor
Michael Cunnigham, Acting Director

The California Department of Alcohol and Drug Program's mission is to lead California's strategy to reduce alcohol and other drug problems by developing, administering, and supporting prevention and treatment programs.

2122 California Department of Alcohol and Drug Programs: Resource Center

PO Box 997413
MS# 2603
Sacramento, CA 95899-7413
916-445-9338
800-444-3066
www.www.adp.ca.gov

Edmund G Brown, Governor
Michael Cunnigham, Acting Director

The Resource Center at the California Department of Alcohol and Drug Programs maintains a comprehensive collec-

tion of alcohol, tobacco, and other drug prevention and treatment information. This information is provided to all California residents at no cost through a Clearinghouse, a full-service Library, Internet communication links, and a telephone information and referral system. These services can be accessed by letter, fax, Internet, e-mail, telephone, or in person during the business hours of 8:00 a.m. to 4:30 p.m., Monday through Friday, excluding state holidays.

2123 California Department of Corrections and Rehabilitation

1515 S Street
Suite 502
Sacramento, CA 95811-7243
916-445-1310
Fax: 916-322-2998
www.www.cdcr.ca.gov

Dr Grant Jordon, Chief Psychiatrist
Dr Rob Prentice, Sr Psychologist Supervisor
Kathie Moon, Supervising Psych Social Worker

Our mission is founded on delivering a balance of quality and cost-effective health care in a safe, secure correctional setting.

2124 California Department of Education: Healthy Kids, Healthy California

313 West Winston Avenue
Room 176
Hayward, CA 94544-2720
510-670-4581
888-318-8188
Fax: 510-670-4582
www.californiahealthykids.org

Deborah Wood, Executive Director
Angela Amarillas, Program Manager

The California Healthy Kids Resource Center was established to assist schools in promoting health literacy. Health literacy is the capacity of an individual to obtain, interpret, and understand basic health information and services and the competence to use such information and services in ways that are health enhancing.

2125 California Hispanic Commission on Alcohol Drug Abuse

2101 Capitol Avenue
Sacramento, CA 95816-5720
916-443-5473
Fax: 916-443-1732
www.chcada.org

James Hernandez, Executive Director

Services can consist of developing Latino-based agencies, program management, consultation related to proposal development, Board of Directors training, program planning, and information dissemination. Populations or groups served include Latino alcohol and drug service agencies, groups and/or individuals planning to initiate services to Latinos, other AOD agencies with a commitment to serve the Latino community, and County Alcohol and Drug Program offices.

Year Founded: 1975

2126 California Institute for Mental Health

2125 19th Street
2nd Floor
Sacramento, CA 95818-1673

916-556-3480
Fax: 916-556-3483
E-mail: sgoodwin@cimh.org
www.cimh.org

Mark Refowitz, Chairman
Sandra Naylor Goodwin, PhD, M, President and CEO
Doretha Williams-Flournoy, MS, Deputy Director, Chief Operating
Michelle Elder, Chief Financial Officer

Promoting excellence in mental health services through training, technical asistances, research and policy development.

Colorado

2127 Colorado Department of Health Care Policy and Financing
1570 Grant Street
Denver, CO 80203-1818
303-866-2993
800-221-3943
Fax: 303-866-3552
E-mail: Jane.Wilson@state.co.us
www.www.colorado.gov/hcpf?

Sue Birch, Executive Director
Kady Lanoha, Chief of Startegy

The Department of Health Care Policy and Financing manages the Colorado Medicaid Community Mental Health Services program. the program provides mental health care to medicaid clients in Colorado, through Behavioral Health Organization contracts.

2128 Colorado Department of Human Services (CDHS)
1575 Sherman Street
Denver, CO 80203-1702
303-866-5700
Fax: 303-866-4047
E-mail: cdhs.communications@state.co.us
www.www.colorado.gov

Nikki Hatch, Deputy Exec Director, Co-Chair

CDHS oversees the state's 64 county departments of social/human services, the state's public mental health system, Colorado's system of services for people with developmental disabilities, the state's juvenile corrections system and all state and veterans' nursing homes, through more than 5, 000 employees and thousands of community-based service providers. Colorado is a state-supervised, county-administered system for the traditional social services, including programs such as public assistance and child welfare services.

2129 Colorado Department of Human Services: Alcohol and Drug Abuse Division
4055 S. Lowell Blvd.
Denver, CO 80236-3120
303-866-7480
Fax: 303-866-7481
www.www.colorado.gov

Roxy Huber, Executive Director

The Alcohol and Drug Abuse Division (ADAD) of the Colorado Department of Human Services was established by state law in 1971 to: promote healthy, drug-free lifestyles; reduce alcohol and other drug abuse and to reduce abuse-associated illnesses and deaths.

2130 Colorado Medical Assistance Program Information Center
Department of Health Care Policy and Financing
1570 Grant Street
Denver, CO 80203-1818
303-866-2993
E-mail: customerservice@hcpf.state.co.us
www.www.colorado.gov

Susan Birch, Executive Director
Laurel Karabatsos, Director, Medicaid Program
Christopher Underwood, Director, State Programs

Provides numerous resources for policymakers, health care consumers, providers, and all citizens of Colorado.

2131 Colorado Traumatic Brain Injury Trust Fund Program
1575 Sherman Street
4th Floor
Denver, CO 80203-1702
303-866-4085
Fax: 303-866-4905
www.www.colorado.gov

Nancy Smith, Board Chair
Holly Batal, MD, Board Member
Deborah Boyle, Board Member
Susan Charlifue, PhD, Board Member

The TBI Trust Fund will strive to support all people in Colorado with traumatic brain injury through services, research and education.

2132 El Paso County Human Services
1675 W. Garden of the Gods
Colorado Springs, CO 80907-1409
719-636-0000
www.dhs.elpasoco.com

Richard Bengtsson, Executive Director
Rebecca Jacobs, Employment & Family Support Dire
Shirley Rhodus, Child Welfare Administrator
Jennifer Brown, Media Contact

The mission of the El Paso County Department of Human Services is to strengthen families, assure safety, promote self-sufficiency, eliminate poverty, and improve the quality of life in our community. They aim to keep families together and help them to become self sufficient and enable them to work closely with community organizations to stretch the safety net they provide even further.

Connecticut

2133 Connecticut Department of Mental Health and Addiction Services
410 Capitol Avenue
P O Box 341431
Hartford, CT 06134-1431
860-418-7000
800-446-7348
TDD: 860-418-6707
E-mail: dmhas.gov
www.www.ct.gov

Pat Rehmer, Commissioner
Paul Di Leo, Deputy Commissioner
William Quinn, Director, Audit Division
Sabrina Trocchi, Chief of Staff

The mission of the Department of Mental Health and Addiction Services is to improve the quality of life of the people of Connecticut by providing an integrated network of comprehensive, effective and efficient mental health and addiction services that foster self-sufficiency, dignity and respect.

2134 Connecticut Department of Children and Families

505 Hudson Street
Hartford, CT 06106-7107
860-550-6300
866-637-4737
E-mail: commissioner.dcf@ct.gov
www.state.ct.us/dcf/

Joette Katz, Commissioner

The mission of the Department of Children and Families is to protect children, improve child and family well-being and support and preserve families. These efforts are accomplished by respecting and working within individual cultures and communities in Connecticut, and in partnership with others. Member of the National Leadership Council

Delaware

2135 Delaware Department of Health & Social Services

1901 North Dupont Highway
Main Building
New Castle, DE 19720
302-255-9040
Fax: 302-255-4429
www.dhss.delaware.gov

Rita M Landgraf, Secretary
Henry Smith III, Deputy Secretary

The mission of the Delaware Department of Health and Social Services is to improve the quality of life for Delaware's citizens by promoting health and well-being, fostering self-sufficiency, and protecting vulnerable populations.

2136 Delaware Division of Child Mental Health Services

1825 Faulkland Road
Wilmington, DE 19805-1121
302-633-2571
Fax: 302-633-5118
E-mail: cmh.dscyf@state.de.us

Susan Cycyk, Executive Director

The Division of Child Mental Health Services (DCMHS) is part of the Delaware Department of Services for Children, Youth and Their Families. Its primary responsibility is to provide and manage a range of services for children who have experienced abandonment, abuse, adjudication, mental illness, neglect, or substance abuse. Its services include prevention, early intervention, assessment, treatment, permanency, and after care.

2137 Delaware Division of Family Services

1825 Faulkland Road
Wilmington, DE 19805-1195
302-663-2665
E-mail: info.dscyf@state.de.us
www.state.de.us/kids/fs/fs.shtml

Jennifer Ranji, Cabinet Secretary
Rodney Grittingham, Deputy Director

The Division of Family Services is mandated by law to investigate complaints about child abuse and neglect. Since 1875, state agencies have been balancing the children's right of safety and the parent's right to choose what is good for the family. The Adoption and Safe Families Act of 1997 clearly puts the focus on the protection, safety and permanency plan of children as the first priority. Services provided are child oriented and family focused.

Year Founded: 1983

District of Columbia

2138 DC Commission on Mental Health Services

64 New York Avenue, NE
4th Floor
Washington, DC 20002-3329
202-673-7440
888-793-4357
www.dmh.dc.gov/dmh/site/default.asp

Stephen T Baron, Director, Mental Health

Regulates the District's mental health system for adults, children and youth, and their families, and provides mental health services directly through the Community Service Agency (for community-based consumers of mental health services) and St. Elizabeths Hospital.

2139 DC Department of Human Services

64 New York Avenue NE
6th Floor
Washington, DC 20032-2601
202-671-4200
Fax: 202-671-4326
E-mail: dhs@dc.gov
www.dhs.dc.gov/dhs

David A Berns, Director

The Department of Human Services provides protection, intervention and social services to meet the needs of vulnerable adults and families to help reduce risk and promote self sufficiency.

2140 Health & Medicine Counsel of Washington DDNC Digestive Disease National Coalition

507 Capital Court NE
Suite 200
Washington, DC 20002-7705
202-544-7497
Fax: 202-546-7105
www.ddnc.org

Dale Dirks, Administrator
Linda Aukett, Chair

The Digestive Disease National Coalition (DDNC) is an advocacy organization comprised of the major national voluntary and professional societies concerned with digestive diseases. The DDNC focuses on improving public policy related to digestive diseases and increasing public awareness with respect to the many diseases of the digestive system. The DDNC was founded in 1978 and is based in Washington D.C.

Year Founded: 1978

Florida

2141 Florida Department Health and Human Services: Substance Abuse Program
Department of Children and Families
1317 Winewood Boulevard
Building 1 Suite 207
Tallahassee, FL 32399-6570
850-487-1111
Fax: 850-922-2993
www.www.myflfamilies.com

Paul Keith, President
David Wilkins, Secretary
Gerald Peter Digre, Deputy Secretary
Suzanne Vitale, Asst. Deputy Secretary

The Substance Abuse Program Office is dedicated to the development of a comprehensive system of prevention, emergency/detoxification, and treatment services for individuals and families at risk of or affected by substance abuse; to promote their safety, well-being, and self-sufficiency.

2142 Florida Department of Children and Families
1317 Winewood Boulevard
Building 1, Room 202
Tallahassee, FL 32399-6570
850-487-1111
Fax: 850-922-2993
www.www.myflfamilies.com

Esther Jacobo, Interim Secretary
Gerald Peter Dilge, Deputy Secretary
Suzanne Vitale, Asst Deputy Secretary
John Cooper, Asst Secretary for Operations

Provides rules, regulations, monitoring of fifteen district mental health program offices and mental health providers throughout the state.

2143 Florida Department of Health and Human Services
2585 Merchants Row Boulevard
Tallahassee, FL 32399-1
850-245-4444
www.www.floridahealth.gov

Dr Steve Harris, Interim State Surgeon General
Kimberly A Berfield, Deputy Secretary

The mission of the Florida Department of Health and Human Services is to promote and protect the health and safety of all people in Florida through the delivery of quality public health services and the promotion of health care standards.

Year Founded: 1996

2144 Florida Department of Mental Health and Rehabilitative Services
Department of Children and Families
1317 Winewood Boulevard
Building 6
Tallahassee, FL 32399-6570
850-487-1111
Fax: 850-922-2993
www.www.myflfamilies.com

Paul Keith, President

The Mental Health Program Office is committed to focusing its resources to meet the needs of people who cannot otherwise access mental health care.

2145 Florida Medicaid State Plan
2727 Mahan Drive
Tallahassee, FL 32308-5407
888-419-3456
www.ahca.myflorida.com

Elizabeth Dudek, Secretary
Jenn Ungru, Chief of Staff
Molly McKinstry, Deputy Secretary
Justin Senior, Deputy Secretary

Provides information about the Medicare plans, benefits and how to enroll in them. Medicaid is the state and federal partnership that provides health coverage for selected categories of people with low incomes. Its purpose is to improve the health of people who might otherwise go without medical care for themselves and their children. Florida implemented the Medicaid program on January 1, 1970, to provide medical services to indigent people. Over the years, the Florida Legislature has authorized Medicaid reimbursement for additional services. A major expansion occurred in 1989, when the United States Congress mandated that states provide all Medicaid services allowable under the Social Security Act to children under the age of 21.

Georgia

2146 Georgia Department of Human Resources
60 Executive Park South, NE
Suite 3-130
Atlanta, GA 30329
404-679-4940
800-359-4663
Fax: 404-656-9655
TDD: 877-204-1194
www.dca.state.ga.us

Clyde L Reese III, Esq, Commissioner
Sharon King, Deputy Commissioner
Marsha Hopkins, Deputy Commissioner

Provides programs that control the spread of disease, enable older people to live at home longer, prevent children from developing lifelong disabilities, train single parents to find and hold jobs, and help people with mental or physical disabilities live and work in their communities.

2147 Georgia Department of Human Resources: Division of Public Health
60 Executive Park South, NE
Atlanta, GA 30329
404-679-4940
800-359-4663
Fax: 404-656-9655
TDD: 877-204-1194
E-mail: gdphinfo@dhr.state.ga.us
www.dca.state.ga.us

C Wade Sellers, MD, Director, District I
David N Westfall, MD, Director, District II
John Kennedy, Director, District III
Michael Brackett, MD, Director, District IV

Our mission is to promote and protect the health of people in Georgia wherever they live, work, and play. We unite with individuals, families, and communities to improve their health and enhance their quality of life.

2148 Georgia Division of Mental Health Developmental Disabilities and Addictive Diseases (MHDDAD)
2 Peachtree Street NW
24th Floor
Atlanta, GA 30303-3141
404-657-2252
www.mhddad.dhr.georgia.gov

Provides treatment and support services to people with mental illnesses and addictive diseases, and support to people with mental retardation and related developmental disabilities. MHDDAD serves people of all ages with the most severe and likely to be long-term conditions. The division also funds evidenced-based prevention services aimed at reducing substance abuse and related problems.

Hawaii

2149 Hawaii Department of Health
1250 Punchbowl Street
Honolulu, HI 96813-2416
808-586-4400
808-586-4444
www.hawaii.gov/health

Loretta Fuddy, Director
Keith Yamamoto, Deputy Director
Gary Gill, Environmental Health
Lynn Fallin, Behavioral Health

The mission of the Department of Health is to protect and improve the health and environment for all people in Hawaii.

Idaho

2150 Department of Health and Welfare: Medicaid Division
450 West State Street
PO Box 83720
Boise, ID 83720-1
208-334-5546
877-456-1233
Fax: 208-334-6558
www.www.healthandwelfare.idaho.gov

Richard Armstrong, Director
Leslie Clement, Deputy Director, Medicaid
David Taylor, Deputy Director, Support Service
Drew Hall, Deputy Director, Family Services

Our mission is to promote and protect the health and safety of all Idahoans. From birth throughout life, we can help enrich and protect the lives of the people of our state.

2151 Idaho Bureau of Maternal and Child Health
PO Box 83720
Boise, ID 83720-3
208-332-6910
www.healthandwelfare.idaho.gov/

Zsolt H. B Koppanyi, Author

Our mission is to promote and protect the health and safety of all Idahoans. From birth throughout life, we can help enrich and protect the lives of the people of our state.

2152 Idaho Department of Health & Welfare
PO Box 83720
Boise, ID 83720-3
208-332-6910
www.healthandwelfare.idaho.gov

Richard Armstrong, Director
Leslie Clement, Seputy Director

Our mission is to promote and protect the health and safety of all Idahoans. From birth throughout life, we can help enrich and protect the lives of the people of our state.

2153 Idaho Department of Health and Welfare: Family and Child Services
PO Box 83720
Boise, ID 83720-3
208-334-6800
www.healthandwelfare.idaho.gov/

Richard Armstrong, Director
Leslie Clement, Deputy Director

Our mission is to promote and protect the health and safety of all Idahoans. From birth throughout life, we can help enrich and protect the lives of the people of our state.

2154 Idaho Mental Health Center
PO Box 83720
Boise, ID 83720-3
208-332-6910
www.healthandwelfare.idaho.gov/

Richard Armstrong, Director
Leslie Clement, Deputy Director

The Idaho Department of Health and Welfare's programs and services are designed to help people live healthy and be productive, strengthening individuals, families and communities. From birth throughout life, we help people improve their lives.

Illinois

2155 Illinois Alcoholism and Drug Dependency Association
937 S 2nd Street
Springfield, IL 62704-2701
217-528-7335
Fax: 217-528-7340
E-mail: iadda@iadda.org
www.iadda.org

Bruce Suardini, Chairman
Eric Foster, Chief Operating Officer
Pel Thomas, Business Manager
Mary Jo Davies, External Program Manager

The IADD Association works hard to educate the general public about the disease of addiction, sharing the message that addiction can be prevented. It can be treated and people can recover from it. It is done through comprehensive media campaigns, community forums, town hall meetings, and letter writing efforts.

2156 Illinois Department of Alcoholism and Substance Abuse
401 South Clinton Street
Chicago, IL 60607-3224
312-793-2354
800-843-6154
Fax: 312-814-1436
TTY: 312-793-2354
E-mail: dhsa48@dhs.state.il.us
www.www.dhs.state.il.us

Michelle Saddler, Secretary
Grace Hong Duffin, Chief of Staff

Tom Green, Director
Mary Lisa Sullivan, General Counsel

DASA consists of three operational Bureau's designed to reflect our mission and planning goals and objectives. Primary responsibilities are to develop, maintain, monitor and evaluate a statewide treatment delivery system designed to provide screening, assessment, customer-treatment matching, referral, intervention, treatment and continuing care services for indigents alcohol and drug abuse and dependency problems. These services are provided by numerous community-based substance abuse treatment organizations contracted by DASA according to the needs of various communities and populations.

Year Founded: 1997

2157 Illinois Department of Children and Family Services

100 W Randolph Street
Suite 6-200
Chicago, IL 60601-3208
312-814-6800
Fax: 312-814-1436
TDD: 312-814-8783
www.www.state.il.us/dcfs

Richard H Calica, Acting Director

The Illinois Department of Children and Family Services provides child welfare services in Illinois. It is also the nation's largest state child welfare agency to earn accreditation from the Council on Accreditation for Children and Family Services (COA). The Department's organization includes the Divisions of Child Protection, Placement Permanency, Field Operations, Guardian & Advocacy, Clinical Practice & Professional Development, Service Intervention, Budget & Finance, Planning & Performance Management, and Communications.

2158 Illinois Department of Health and Human Services

401 South Clinton Street
Chicago, IL 60607-3800
800-843-6154
TTY: 312-793-2354
www.www.dhs.state.il.us/

Michelle R B Saddler, Secretary
Grace Hong Duffin, Chief Of Staff

DHS serves Illinois citizens through seven main programs: Welfare programs, including temporary assistance for needy families, Food Stamps, and child care; Alcoholism and substance abuse treatment and prevention services; Developmental disabilities; Health services for pregnant women and mothers, infants, children, and adolescents; Prevention services for domestic violence and at-risk youth; Mental health and Rehabilitation services.

Year Founded: 1997

2159 Illinois Department of Healthcare and Family Services

201 S Grand Avenue E
Springfield, IL 62763-1
217-782-1200
Fax: 217-782-5672
www.www2.illinois.gov/hfs

Julie Hamos, Director
Sharron Matthews, Assistant Director

Bradley Hart, Inspector General
Amy Delcomyn, Project Mangement Officer

The Illinois Department of Healthcare and Family Services, formerly the Department of Public Aid, is the state agency dedicated to improving the lives of Illinois' families through health care coverage, child support enforcement and energy assistance.

2160 Illinois Department of Human Services: Office of Mental Health

160 N LaSalle
10th Floor
Chicago, IL 60601-3124
312-793-2800
www.www.dhs.state.il.us

Michelle R B Saddler, Secretary
Grace Hong Duffin, Chief of Staff

Works to improve the lives of persons with mental illness by integrating state operated services, community based programs, and other support services to create an effective and responsive treatment and care network. Management office which plans, organizes, and controls the activities of the organization, but does not offer services to the public.

2161 Illinois Department of Mental Health and Developmental Disabilities

100 South Grand Avenue
2nd Floor
Springfield, IL 62765-1
217-524-7065
800-843-6154
TTY: 217-557-2134
www.dhs.state.il.us/mhdd/dd/

Michelle R B Saddler, Secretary
Grace Hong Duffin, Chief of Staff

Our mission is to provide a full array of quality, outcome-based, person- and community-centered services and supports for individuals with developmental disabilities and their families in Illinois.

2162 Illinois Department of Public Health: Division of Food, Drugs and Dairies/FDD

535 W Jefferson Street
Springfield, IL 62761-1
217-782-4977
Fax: 217-782-3987
TTY: 800-547-0466
www.www.idph.state.il.us

Julie Hamos, Director
Sharron Matthews, Assistant Director
Bradley Hart, Inspector General
Carolyn Williams-Meza, Chief Admin Officer

The mission of the Illinois Department of Public Health is to promote the health of the people of Illinois through the prevention and control of disease and injury.

2163 Mental Health Association in Illinois

70 E Lake Street
Suite 900
Chicago, IL 60601-5995
312-368-9070
Fax: 312-368-0283
www.mhai.org

Joyce Gallagher, President
Ray Connor, Co-Vice President

Laura Zimmerman, Co-Vice President
Phillip Hall, Assistant Treasurer, Chief Finan

Works to promote mental health, prevent mental illnesses, and improve the care and treatment of persons suffering from mental and emotional problems. An affiliate of the National Mental Health Association, MHAI is Illinois' only statewide, non-profit, non-governmental advocacy organization concerned with the entire spectrum of mental and emotional disorders.

Year Founded: 1909

Indiana

2164 Indiana Department of Public Welfare Division of Family Independence: Food Stamps/Medicaid/Training
Family and Social Services Administration
402 W Washington Street
PO Box 7083
Indianapolis, IN 46207-7083
317-232-4946
800-901-1133
Fax: 317-233-4693
www.in.gov/fssa

Michael A Gargano, Secretary
Susie Howard, Chief of Staff
Paul Bowling, Chief Financial Officer
Lisa Hughes, Executive Assistant

The mission of the Division of Family Independence is to strengthenfamilies and children through temporary assistance to needy families, food stamps, housing, child care, foster care, adoption, energy assistance, homeless services, and job programs.

2165 Indiana Family & Social Services Administration
402 W Washington Street
PO Box 7083
Indianapolis, IN 46207-7083
317-233-4454
800-901-1133
Fax: 317-233-4693
www.in.gov/fssa

Michael A Gargano, Secretary
Susie Howard, Chief of Staff
Paul Bowling, Chief Financial Officer
Lisa Hughes, Executive Assistant

The mission of the Indiana Department of Family and Social Services is to strengthen families and children through temporary assistance to needy families, food stamps, housing, child care, foster care, adoption, energy assistance, homeless services, and job programs.

2166 Indiana Family And Social Services Administration
402 W Washington Street
PO Box 7083
Indianapolis, IN 46207-7083
317-233-4454
800-901-1133
Fax: 317-233-4693
www.in.gov/fssa

Michael A Gargano, Secretary
Susie Howard, Chief of Staff

Paul Bowling, Chief Financial Officer
Lisa Hughes, Executive Assistant

The mission of the Indiana Bureau of Family Protection is to strengthen families and children through temporary assistance to needy families, food stamps, housing, child care, foster care, adoption, energy assistance, homeless services, and job programs.

2167 Indiana Family and Social Services Administration: Division of Mental Health
402 W Washington Street
Suite W-353
Indianapolis, IN 46204-2779
317-233-4319
800-901-1133
Fax: 317-233-3472
www.www.in.gov/fssa/dmha/2688.htm

Michael A Gargano, Secretary
Susie Howard, Chief of Staff
Paul Bowling, Chief Financial Officer
Lisa Hughes, Executive Assistant

The mission of the Indiana Family and Social Services Administration Division of Mental Health is to strengthening families and children through temporary assistance to needy families, food stamps, housing, child care, foster care, adoption, energy assistance, homeless services, and job programs.

2168 The Indiana Consortium for Mental Health Services Research (ICMHSR)
Institute for Social Research Indiana University
1022 East Third Street
Bloomington, IN 47401-3779
812-855-3841
Fax: 812-856-5713
E-mail: acapshew@indiana.edu
www.indiana.edu/~icmhsr/

Bernice A Pescosolido Ph.D, Director, Indiana Consortium for
Alex Capshew, Administrative Operations Manage
Jack K. Martin, Director, Karl F. Schuessler Ins
Mary Hannah, Production & Dissemination Manag

The Indiana Consortium for Mental Health Services Research (ICMHSR) focuses on developing high quality scholarly and applied research projects on mental health and related services for people with severe mental disorders. A major commitment of the ICMHSR is to use research to foster public awareness and improve public policy and decision-making regarding these devastating illnesses.

Iowa

2169 Iowa Department Human Services
1305 East Walnut
Des Moines, IA 50319-114
515-281-6899
E-mail: contactdhs@dhs.state.ia.us
www.dhs.state.ia.us

Charles M Palmer, Director

The Mission of the Iowa Department of Human Services is to help individuals and families achieve safe, stable, self-sufficient, and healthy lives, thereby contributing to the economic growth of the state. We do this by keeping a customer focus, striving for excellence, sound stewardship of state resources, maximizing the use of federal funding and leveraging opportunities, and by working with our public and private partners to achieve results.

2170 Iowa Department of Public Health
321 E 12th Street
Des Moines, IA 50319-75
515-281-7689
866-227-9878
www.idph.state.ia.us

Marcia Spangler, Division Director

Under the direction of the director, the Iowa Department of Public Health exercises general supervision of the state's public health; promotes public hygiene and sanitation; does health promotion activities, prepares for and responds to bioemergency situations; and, unless otherwise provided, enforces laws on public health.

2171 Iowa Department of Public Health: Division of Substance Abuse
321 12th Street
Des Moines, IA 50319-1002
515-281-4417
www.idph.state.ia.us/bh

Kathy Stone, Division Director

The Office of Substance Abuse Prevention/Staff of the Office of Substance Abuse Prevention provides the following services: technical assistance to individuals, groups, and contracted agencies and organizations; Coordinate and collaborate with multiple state agencies and organizations for assessment, planning, and implementation of statewide prevention initiatives; and Coordinate, train, and monitor funding to local community-based organizations for alcohol, tobacco, and other drug prevention services.

2172 Iowa Division of Mental Health & Developmental Disabilities: Department of Human Services
1305 E Walnut Street
Des Moines, IA 50319
515-281-7277
Fax: 515-242-6036
E-mail: contactdhs@dhs.state.ia.us
www.dhs.state.ia.us

Jeanne Nesbit, Director

The Division of Mental Health and Developmental Disabilities (MH/DD) is the agency designated as the state mental health authority by the Governor of Iowa. The Division: provides program support services for persons with mental illness, mental retardation and developmental disabilities; plans for state services; works with counties in the development and implementation of their services plans; develops policy for the state mental health institutes and the state resource centers for persons with developmental disabilities; provides consultation and technical assistance; and, provides accreditation for providers of MH/DD services.

Kansas

2173 Kansas Council on Developmental Disabilities Kansas Department of Social and Rehabilitation Services
915 SW Harrison Street
Room 141
Topeka, KS 66612
785-296-2608
888-369-4777

TTY: 785-296-1491
www.www.dcf.ks.gov

Phyllis Gilmore, Secretary

The Kansas Department of Social and Rehabilitation Services was established in 1973 as an umbrella agency to over see social services and state institutions. With amission to protect children and promote adult self sufficiency, SRS serves over 500, 000 Kansans today.

12 pages

Kentucky

2174 Kentucky Cabinet for Health and Human Services
275 East Main Street
1e-B
Frankfort, KY 40621-1
502-564-5497
Fax: 502-564-9523
E-mail: nancy.ovesen@ky.gov
www.chfs.ky.gov/

Steve Beshear, Governor
Jerry Abramson, Lt Governor
Allison Lundergan-Grimes, Secretary of State
Adam Edelen, State Auditor

The goal of the Cabinet for Health and Family Services is to provide the finest health care possible for people in our state facilities; To provide the best preventative services through our public health programs; To provide the most outstanding service for our families and children; To protect and prevent the abuse of children, elders and people with disabilities and To build quality programs across-the-board; and by doing all of these things.

2175 Kentucky Department of Mental Health and Mental Retardation
C/O The Commissioner's Office
100 Fair Oaks Lane 4E-B
Frankfort, KY 40621-1
502-564-4527
Fax: 502-564-5478
TTY: 502-564-5777
www.chfs.ky.gov/mhmr/

Bruce Harper, Commissioner
Mark Farrow, Commissioner

Our mission is to provide leadership, in partnership with others, to prevent disability, build resilience in individuals and their communities, and facilitate recovery for people whose lives have been affected by mental illness, mental retardation or other developmental disability, substance abuse or an acquired brain injury.

2176 Kentucky Justice Cabinet: Department of Juvenile Justice
1025 Capital Center Drive
Frankfort, KY 40601-8205
502-573-2738
www.djj.ky.gov/

Hasan Davis, Acting Commissioner
Sheree Smith Jones, Deputy Commissioner
Diana McGuire, Acting Deputy Commissioner

The Kentucky Department of Juvenile Justice's mission is to improve public safety by providing balanced and comprehensive services that hold youth accountable, and to provide the opportunity for youth to develop into productive, responsible citizens.

Louisiana

2177 Louisiana Commission on Law Enforcement and Administration (LCLE)
602 North Fifth Street
Room 1230
Baton Rouge, LA 70802
225-342-1500
www.cole.state.la.us/

Joey Watson, Executive Director
Robert Mehrtens, Deputy Director
Tyler Downing, Confidential Assistant
Hope Davis, Human Resources

Lastest news and information on LCLE programs, resources, job openings, and general agency information on a monthly basis and for an in-depth review of our criminal justice programs.

2178 Louisiana Department of Health and Hospitals: Office of Mental Health
Bienville Building
628 N 4th Street
Baton Rouge, LA 70802-5342
225-342-9500
Fax: 225-342-5568
www.www.dhh.louisiana.gov

Bruce D Greenstein, Secretary

The Mission of the Office of Mental Health (OMH) is to perform the functions of the state which provide or lead to treatment, rehabilitation and follow-up care for individuals in Louisiana with mental and emotional disorders. OMH administers and/or monitors community-based services, public or private, to assure active quality care in the most cost-effective manner in the least restrictive environment for all persons with mental and emotional disorders.

2179 Louisiana Department of Health and Hospitals: Louisiana Office for Addictive Disorders
628 N 4th Street
PO Box 2790, Bin 18
Baton Rouge, LA 70821-2790
225-342-9500
Fax: 225-342-5568
E-mail: lelsie.deville@la.gov
www.new.dhh.louisiana.gov

Bruce D Greenstein, Secretary

It is the philosophy of this agency that treatment and prevention services should be of high quality and easily accessible to all citizens of the state. The Office for Addictive Disorders offers comprehensive treatment and prevention services through ten Regional/District Offices throughout the state.

Maine

2180 Maine Department Health and Human Services Children's Behavioral Health Services
2 Anthony Avenue
Augusta, ME 04333-11
207-624-7900
888-568-1112
Fax: 207-287-5282

TTY: 207-606-0215
www.www.maine.gov/dhhs/ocfs/cbhs/

Julia Cabral, Juvenile Program Manager
Rebecca Thompson-Greaves, Director, Collateral Services

Children's Behavioral Health Services (CBHS), a branch of the Department of Health and Human Services (DHHS) has a long tradition of advocacy for children with special needs. Once known as the Bureau of Children's with Special Needs (BCSN), this part of the Department became known as Children's Services in 1995. In a continuing effort to meet the diverse and growing needs of Maine families, Children's Behavioral Health Services (CBHS) is going through a further transition. Most services formerly provided directly through the Department are now delivered through contracted community agencies.

2181 Maine Office of Substance Abuse: Information and Resource Center
295 Water Street
Suite 200
Augusta, ME 04330
207-621-8118
800-499-0027
Fax: 207-621-8362
TTY: 800-606-0215
E-mail: osa.ircosa@maine.gov
www.www.masap.org

Pat Kimball, President
Peter McCorison, Vice President
Ruth E. Blauer, Executive Director
Catherine Ryder, Secretary

Provides Maine's citizens with alcohol, tobacco and other drug information, resources and research for prevention, education and treatment.

Maryland

2182 Centers for Medicare and Medicaid Services: Office of Financial Management/OFM
7500 Security Boulevard
Baltimore, MD 21244-1849
410-786-3000
www.www.cms.gov

Deborah Taylor, Director and Chief Financial Off
George Mills, Jr, Deputy Director
Maria Montilla, Director and Deputy Chief Financ
Janet Loftus, Director, Division of Accounting

OFM has overall reponsibility for the fiscal integrity of CMS' programs.

2183 Maryland Alcohol and Drug Abuse Administration
201 West Preston Street
55 Wade Avenue, Room 216
Baltimore, MD 21201
410-767-6500
877-463-3464
Fax: 410-402-8601
www.adaa.dhmh.maryland.gov/

Joshua M Sharfstein, MD, Secretary

The Alcohol and Drug Abuse Administration (ADAA) is the single state agency responsible for the provision, coordination, and regulation of the statewide network of substance abuse prevention, intervention and treatment services. It serves as the initial point of contact for technical assistance and regulatory interpretation for all Maryland Department of Health and Mental Hygiene (DHMH) prevention and certified treatment programs.

2184 Maryland Department of Health and Mental Hygiene
201 West Preston Street
Baltimore, MD 21201-2301
410-767-6500
877-463-3464
E-mail: webadministrator@dhmh.state.md.us
www.dhmh.maryland.gov

Joshua M Sharfstein, MD, Secretary

Provides information on a variety of services including mental health and substance abuse, health plans and providers, nutrition and maternal care, environmental health and developmental disabilities.

Massachusetts

2185 Massachusetts Department of Mental Health
25 Staniford Street
11th Floor
Boston, MA 02114
617-573-1600
800-221-0053
TTY: 617-727-9842
www.mass.gov/dmh/

Dr Judy Ann Bigby, Secretary
Marilyn Chase, Asst Secretary, Youth, Families
Christine Griffin, Asst Secretary, Disability
Stacey Monahan, Chief of Staff

The Massachusetts Department of Mental Health provides clinical, rehabilitative and supportive services for adults with serious mental illness, and children and adolescents with serious mental illness or serious emotional disturbance.

2186 Massachusetts Department of Public Health
1000 Washington Street
Suite 310
Boston, MA 02118-5002
617-790-4000
800-495-0086
Fax: 617-790-4128
TTY: 617-624-6001
www.masspartnership.com

John Auerbach, Commissioner, Public Health

Our mission, to serve all the people in the Commonwealth, particularly the under served, and to promote healthy people, healthy families, healthy communities and healthy environments through compassionate care, education and prevention. Your health is our concern.

2187 Massachusetts Department of Public Health: Bureau of Substance Abuse Services
1000 Washington Street
Suite 310
Boston, MA 02118-5002
617-790-4000
800-495-0086
Fax: 617-790-4128
TTY: 617-536-5872
www.masspartnership.com

John Auerbach, Commissioner, Public Health

The Bureau of Substance Abuse Services oversees the substance abuse prevention and treatment services in the Commonwealth. Responsibilities include: licensing programs and counselors; funding and monitoring prevention and treatment services; providing access to treatment for the indigent and uninsured; developing and implementing policies and programs; and, tracking substance abuse trends in the state.

2188 Massachusetts Department of Transitional Assistance
Massachusetts Department of Health and Human Services
600 Washington Street
Boston, MA 02111-1751
617-348-8500
www.mass.gov/dta/

Julia Kehoe, Commissioner, Transistional

The mission of the Department of Transitional Assistance is to serve the Commonwealth's most vulnerable families and individuals with dignity and respect, ensuring those eligible for our services have access to those services in an accurate, timely and culturally sensitive manner and in a way that promotes client's independence and long term self-sufficiency.

2189 Massachusetts Executive Office of Public Safety
1 Ashburton Place
Suite 2133
Boston, MA 02108-1504
617-727-7775
Fax: 617-727-4764
E-mail: eopsinfo@state.ma.us
www.www.mass.gov/eopss/

Dr Jusy Ann Bigby, Secretary
Marilyn Chase, Assistant Secretary
Christine Griffin, Assistant Secretary
Stacey Monahan, Chief of Staff

Plans and manages public safety efforts by supporting, supervising and providing planning and guidance to a variety of state agencies.

Michigan

2190 Michigan Department of Community Health
Department of Mental Health
Capitol View Building
201 Townsend Street
Lansing, MI 48913-1
517-373-3740
800-649-3777
E-mail: mccurtisj@michigan.gov
www.michigan.gov/mdch/

Nick Lyon, Deputy Director
Angela Minicuci, Public Information Officer
Matthew Davis, M.D., Chief Medical Executive
Melanie Brim, Public Health Administration, De

Provides information on drug control and substance abuse treatment policies.

2191 Michigan Department of Human Services
235 S Grand Ave
PO Box 30037
Lansing, MI 48909-7537
517-373-2305
Fax: 517-335-6101

TTY: 517-373-8071
www.michigan.gov/dhs/

The Department of Human Services (DHS) is Michigan's public assistance, child and family welfare agency. DHS directs the operations of public assistance and service programs through a network of over 100 county department of human service offices around the state.

2192 National Council on Alcoholism and Drug Dependence: Greater Detroit Area
2400 East McNichols
Detroit, MI 48212
313-868-1340
Fax: 313-865-8951
E-mail: info@ncadd-detroit.org
www.ncadd-detroit.org/

Benjamin Jones, President, CEO
Don Denault, Chief Financial Officer
Linda Woodward, Director of Treatment
James Boyce, Jr, Service Leader

The National Council on Alcoholism and Drug Dependence-Greater Detroit Area is a voluntary, non-profit agency committed to improving health through providing substance abuse prevention, education, training, treatment and advocacy for the metropolitan Detroit area.

Minnesota

2193 Department of Human Services: Chemical Health Division
PO Box 64977
Saint Paul, MN 55164-977
651-431-2460
800-366-5411
Fax: 651-431-7449
www.mn.gov/dhs/

Lucinda Jesson, Commissioner
Anne Barry, Deputy Commissioner
Charles Johnson, CFO, Chief Operating Officer
Loren Colman, Asst Commissioner

The Chemical Health Division is the state alcohol and drug authority responsible for defining a statewide response to drug and alcohol abuse. This includes providing basic information on chemical health. It also includes planning a broad-based community service system, evaluating the effectiveness of various chemical dependency services, and funding innovative programs to promote reduction of alcohol and other drug problems and their effects on individuals, families and society

2194 Lake Area Youth Services Bureau
244 North Lake Street
Forest Lake, MN 55025-2517
651-464-3685
Fax: 651-464-3687
E-mail: Jeanne.Walz@ysblakesarea.org
www.web.ysblakesarea.org

Jeanne Walz, Executive Director
Matt Howard, Community Justice Program Mgr
Aaron Lynch, Community Justice Case Manager
Kari Lyn Wampler, Youth, Family Therapist

Provides enrichment programs and intervention support to youth and families. Available on FaceBook and Twitter

Year Founded: 1976

2195 Minnesota Department of Human Services
444 Lafayette Road
Saint Paul, MN 55155-3899
651-431-3515
800-366-5411
Fax: 651-431-7476
www.mn.gov/dhs/

Lucinda Jesson, Commissioner
Anne Barry, Deputy Commissioner
Charles Johnson, CFO, Chief Operating Officer
Loren Colman, Assistant Commissioner

The Minnesota Department of Human Services helps people meet their basic needs by providing or administering health care coverage, economic assistance, and a variety of services for children, people with disabilities and older Minnesotans.

Mississippi

2196 Mississippi Alcohol Safety Education Program
1 Research Blvd
Suite 103
Starkville, MS 39759
662-325-7127
Fax: 662-325-7966
www.www.ssrc.msstate.edu

Alicia Falls, Administrative Assistant I
Angela Robertson, SSRC Interim Director and Resear
Anne Buffington, Technical Writer
Jennifer Alberson, Service Leader

MASEP is the statewide program for first-time offenders convicted of driving under the influence of alcohol or another substance which has impaired one's ability to operate a motor vehicle.

2197 Mississippi Department Mental Health Mental Retardation Services
1101 Robert E Lee Building
239 N. Lamar Street
Jackson, MS 39201-1328
601-359-1288
877-210-8513
Fax: 601-359-6295
TDD: 601-359-6230

Diana Mikula, Director

Has the primary responsibility for the development and implementation of services to meet the needs of individuals with mental retardation/developmental disabilities. This public service delivery system is comprised of five state-operated comprehensive regional centers for individuals with mental retardation/developmental disabilities, a state-operated facility for youth who require specialized treatment and have mental retardation/developmental disabilities, 15 regional community mental health/mental retardation centers, and other nonprofit community agencies/organizations that provide community services.

2198 Mississippi Department of Human Services
750 North State Street
Jackson, MS 39202-3033
601-359-4500
800-345-6347
www.www.mdhs.state.ms.us

Cathy Sykes, Director

The mission of the Department of Human Services is to provide services for people in need by optimizing all available resources to sustain the family unit and to encourage traditional family values thereby promoting self-sufficiency and personal responsibility for all Mississippians.

2199 Mississippi Department of Mental Health: Division of Alcohol and Drug Abuse

239 N Lamar Street
1101 Robert F Lee Building
Jackson, MS 39201
601-359-1288
877-210-8513
Fax: 601-359-6295
TDD: 601-359-6230
www.www.dmh.ms.gov

Dr. Jim Herzog, Chair
Sampat Shivangi, M.D., Vice Chair

The Division of Alcohol and Drug Abuse Services is responsible for establishing, maintaining, monitoring and evaluating a statewide system of alcohol and drug abuse services, including prevention, treatment and rehabilitation. The division has designed a system of services for alcohol and drug abuse prevention and treatment reflecting its philosophy that alcohol and drug abuse is a treatable and preventable illness.

2200 Mississippi Department of Mental Health: Division of Medicaid

239 N Lamar Street
1101 Robert F Lee Building
Jackson, MS 39201
601-359-1288
877-210-8513
Fax: 601-359-6295
TDD: 601-359-6230
www.www.dmh.ms.gov

Dr. Jim Herzog, Chair
Sampat Shivangi, M.D., Vice Chair

Medicaid is a national health care program. It helps pay for medical services for low-income people. For those eligible for full Medicaid services, Medicaid is paid to providers of health care. Providers are doctors, hospitals and pharmacists who take Medicaid. We strive to provide financial assistance for the provision of quality health services to our beneficiaries with professionalism, integrity, compassion and commitment. We are advocates for, and accountable to the people we serve.

2201 Mississippi Department of Rehabilitation Services: Office of Vocational Rehabilitation (OVR)

1281 Highway 51
PO Box 1698
Madison, MS 39110
601-853-5100
800-443-1000
www.www.mdrs.ms.gov

Jack Virden, Chairman
Anita Naik, Office Director???
Chris Howard, Deputy Director, Financial
Tommy Browning, Office Director???, Administrati

The Office of Vocational Rehabilitation (OVR) provides services designed to improve economic opportunities for individuals with physical and mental disabilities through employment. Work related services are individualized and may include but are not limited to: counseling, job development, job training, job placement, supported employment, transition services and employability skills training program. OVR has a network of 17 community rehabilitation centers (Allied Enterprises) located throughout the state, which provide vocational assessment, job training and actual work experience for individuals with disabilities. Thousands of Mississippians are successfully employed each year through the teamwork at OVR.

Missouri

2202 Missouri Department Health & Senior Services

912 Wildwood
PO Box 570
Jefferson City, MO 65102-570
573-751-6400
Fax: 573-751-6010
E-mail: info@health.mo.gov
www.health.mo.gov/

Gail Vasterling, Director
Margaret T Donnelly, Director
Kathy Branson, Deputy Director
Jennifer Stilabower, General Counsel

The Missouri Department of Health and Senior Services provides information on a variety of topics including senior services and health, current news and public notices, laws and regulations, and statistical reports.

2203 Missouri Department of Mental Health

1706 E Elm Street
P O Box 687
Jefferson City, MO 65102-687
573-751-4122
800-364-9687
Fax: 573-751-8224
TTY: 573-526-1201
E-mail: dbhmail@dmh.mo.gov
www.dmh.mo.gov/

Keith Schafer, Director
Jan Heckemeyer, Deputy Director
Bob Bax, Director, Finance
Rikki Wright, General Counsel

State law provides three principal missions for the department: (1) the prevention of mental disorders, developmental disabilities, substance abuse, and compulsive gambling; (2) the treatment, habilitation, and rehabilitation of Missourians who have those conditions; and (3) the improvement of public understanding and attitudes about mental disorders, developmental disabilities, substance abuse, and compulsive gambling.

2204 Missouri Department of Public Safety

301 W. High Street
PO Box 36
Jefferson City, MO 65102
573-751-2764
Fax: 573-526-3898
E-mail: dpsinfo@dps.mo.gov
www.www.dps.mo.gov

Jerry Lee, Director
Andrea Spillars, Deputy Director, Gen Counsel
Tracy McGinnis, General Counsel
Chris Pickering, Homeland Security Coordinator

The Office of the Director is the Department of Public Safety's central administrative unit. Our office administers federal and state funds in grants for juvenile justice, victims' assistance, law enforcement, and narcotics control. Other programs in the Director's Office provide support services and resources to assist local law enforcement agencies and to promote crime prevention.

2205 Missouri Department of Social Services
221 West High Street
P O Box 1527
Jefferson City, MO 65102-1527
573-751-4815
Fax: 573-751-3203
TDD: 800-735-2966
www.dss.mo.gov/

Brian Kinkade, Interim Director

A true measure of a society is the extent of its concern for those less fortunate-its intent of keeping families together, preventing abuse and neglect, and encouraging self-sufficiency and independence. In Missouri, programs dealing with these concerns are administered by the state Department of Social Services.

2206 Missouri Department of Social Services: Medical Services Division
615 Howerton Court
P O Box 6500
Jefferson City, MO 65102-6500
573-751-3425
800-735-2966
Fax: 573-751-6564
www.dss.mo.gov/mhd/

Brian Kinkade, Interim Director

The purpose of the Division of Medical Services is to purchase and monitor health care services for low income and vulnerable citizens of the State of Missouri. The agency assures quality health care through development of service delivery systems, standards setting and enforcement, and education of providers and recipients. We are fiscally accountable for maximum and appropriate utilization of resources

2207 Missouri Division of Alcohol and Drug Abuse
P O Box 687
1706 E Elm Street
Jefferson City, MO 65101-4130
573-751-4942
800-575-7480
E-mail: dbhmail@dmh.mo.gov
www.dmh.mo.gov/mentalillness/

Brian Kinkade, Interim Director

The Division provides funding for prevention, outpatient, residential, and detoxification services to community-based programs that work with communities to develop and implement comprehensive coordinated plans. The Division provides technical assistance to these agencies and operates a certification program that sets standards for treatment programs, qualified professionals, and alcohol and drug related educational programs.

2208 Missouri Division of Comprehensive Psychiatric Service
PO Box 687
1706 E Elm Street
Jefferson City, MO 65101-4130

573-751-8017
E-mail: cpsmail@dmh.mo.gov
www.dmh.missouri.gov/cps/cpsindex.htm

Vicky Davidson, Executive Director
Sherrie Hanks, Office Manager
Bernard Simons, Division Director
Mary Luebbert, Administrative Assistant

The division is committed to serving four target populations: persons with serious and persistent mental illness (SMI); persons suffering from acute psychiatric conditions; children and youth with serious emotional disturbances (SED) and forensic clients. In addition, CPS has identified four priority groups within the target populations: (1) individuals in crisis, (2) people who are homeless, (3) those recently discharged from inpatient care and (4) substantial users of public funds. These target populations currently constitute the majority of clientele whom the Division serves both in inpatient and ambulatory settings.

2209 Missouri Division of Mental Retardation and Developmental Disabilities
1706 E Elm Street
PO Box 687
Jefferson City, MO 65102-687
573-751-8676
E-mail: mrddmail@dmh.mo.gov
www.dmh.missouri.gov/mrdd/mrddindex.htm

Vicky Davidson, Executive Director
Sherrie Hanks, Office Manager
Bernard Simons, Division Director
Mary Luebbert, Administrative Assistant

The Division of Mental Retardation and Developmental Disabilities (MRDD), established in 1974, serves a population that has developmental disabilities such as mental retardation, cerebral palsy, head injuries, autism, epilepsy, and certain learning disabilities. Such conditions must have occurred before age 22, with the expectation that they will continue. To be eligible for services from the Division, persons with these disabilities must be substantially limited in their ability to function independently.

Montana

2210 Montana Department of Health and Human Services: Child & Family Services Division
Cogswell Building
1400 Broadway
Helena, MT 59601-5231
406-444-5900
www.dphhs.mt.gov/

The Child and Family Services Division (CFSD) is a part of the Montana Department of Public Health and Human Services. Its mission is to keep Montana's children safe and families strong. The division provides state and federally mandated protective services to children who are abused, neglected, or abandoned. This includes receiving and investigating reports of child abuse and neglect, working to prevent domestic violence, helping families to stay together or reunite, and finding placements in foster or adoptive homes.

2211 Montana Department of Human & Community Services
111 N Jackson Street, 5th Floor
PO Box 202925
Helena, MT 59601-4168

406-444-5902
Fax: 406-444-2547
TTY: 406-444-1421
www.dphhs.mt.gov/

Jamie Palagi, Division Adminstrator
Kathe Quittenton, Public Aid Bureau
Jim Nolan, Human Services Management
Vacant , Early Childhood Services

The mission of the Montana Department of Human &
Community Services is to promote job preparation and
work as a means to help needy families become self-sufficient.

**2212 Montana Department of Public Health &
Human Services: Addictive and Mental
Disorders**
555 Fuller Avenue
PO Box 202905
Helena, MT 59601-3394
406-444-3964
www.dphhs.mt.gov/

Lou Thompson, Administrator
Joan Cassidy, Chemical Dependency Chief
E Lee Simes, Medical Director
Deb Matteucci, Behavioral Health

The mission of the Addictive and Mental Disorders Division (AMDD) of the Montana Department of Public Health
and Human Services is to implement and improve an appropriate statewide system of prevention, treatment, care,
and rehabilitation for Montanans with mental disorders or
addictions to drugs or alcohol.

**2213 Montana Department of Public Health and
Human Services: Montana Vocational
Rehabilitation Programs**
Disability Services Division
111 North Last Chance Gulch
Suite 4c
Helena, MT 59601-4520
406-444-2590
877-296-1197
Fax: 406-444-3632
www.dphhs.mt.gov/

Jim Marks, Program Director
Clay Calton, Budget Analyst
Barbara Kriskovich, Grant Project Director

The mission of the Disability Services Division (DSD) of
the Montana Department of Public Health and Human Services is to provide services that help Montanans with disabilities to live, work and fully participate in their
communities.

Nebraska

**2214 Nebraska Department of Health and Human
Services (NHHS)**
301 Centennial Mall South
PO Box 95026
Lincoln, NE 68509-5026
402-471-3121
E-mail: dhhs.helpline@nebraska.gov
www.dhhs.ne.gov

Kerry Winterer, Chief Executive Officer
Eric Henrichsen, Information Systems

Kathle Osterman, Director, Communications
Matt Clough, Director, Operations

The mission of the NHHS is to help people live better lives
through effective health and human services.

**2215 Nebraska Health & Human Services: Medicaid
and Managed Care Division**
Department of Finance & Support
PO Box 95026
Lincoln, NE 68509-5026
402-471-3121
www.hhs.state.ne.us

Vivianne Chaumont, Director
Dr Alan Nissen, Medical Director
Ruth Vineyard, Medicaid Initiatives
Catherine Gekas-Steeby, Eligibility Administrator

The Finance and Support agency aligns human resources,
financial resources, and information needs for the Nebraska
Health and Human Services System and is the designated
Title XIX (Medicaid) agency responsible for provider en-
rollment activities.

**2216 Nebraska Health and Human Services Division:
Department of Mental Health**
P O Box 95026
Lincoln, NE 68509-5026
402-471-7824
www.hhs.state.ne.us

Jim Harvey, Behavioral Health Housing Manage
Blaine Shaffer, PhD, Chief Clinical Officer

Mental health services are designed for individuals and
their families who have a serious and persistent mental illness that can create lifetime disabilities, and in some cases
make the individuals dangerous to themselves or others.
Services are also designed for people experiencing acute,
serious mental illnesses, which in some cases may cause a
life threatening event such as suicide attempts. In addition,
services are provided for children and to their families.

2217 Nebraska Mental Health Centers
4545 South 86th Street
Lincoln, NE 68526-9227
402-483-6990
888-210-8064
Fax: 402-483-7045
E-mail: drness@nmhc-clinics.com
www.www.nmhc-clinics.com/?

Jill Zlome McPherson, Owner, Executive Director
Dr Lee Zlomke, Clinical Director
Lisa Logsden, Psy.D., Staff Psychologist

We are a primary mental health care center that is truly
committed to being of service to the Lincoln/Lancaster
community and Greater Nebraska.

Nevada

**2218 Nevada Department of Health and Human
Services**
4126 Technology Way
Room 100
Carson City, NV 89706-2013
775-684-4000
E-mail: nvdhs@dhhs.nv.gov
www.dhhs.nv.gov

Mike Willden, Director
Ellen Crecelius, Fiscal Services, Deputy Director
Amber Joiner, Programs, Deputy Director
Kareen Masters, Administrative Services, Deputy

The Department of Health and Human Services (DHHS) promotes the health and well-being of Nevadans through the delivery or facilitation of essential services to ensure families are strengthened, public health is protected, and individuals achieve their highest level of self-sufficiency.

2219 Nevada Division of Mental Health & Developmental Services

4126 Technology Way
2nd Floor
Carson City, NV 89706-2027
775-684-5943
Fax: 775-684-5966
E-mail: mhdswebmaster@mhds.nv.gov
www.mhds.state.nv.us

Richard Whitley, Acting Administrator
Jane Gruner, Deputy Adminstrator
Tracey Green, MD, Northen Medical Director
Karen Hayes, Office Manager

The Nevada Division of Mental Health provides a full array of clinical services to over 24, 000 consumers each year. Services include: crisis intervention, hospital care, medication clinic, outpatient counseling, residential support and other mental health services targeted to individuals with serious mental illness.

2220 Nevada Employment Training & Rehabilitation Department

500 East Third Street
Carson City, NV 89713-1
775-684-3849
Fax: 775-684-3850
TTY: 775-687-5353
www.nvdetr.org/

Larry Mosley, Director

The Department of Employment, Training and Rehabilitation (DETR) is comprised of four divisions with numerous bureaus programs, and services housed in offices throughout Nevada to provide citizens the state's premier source of employment, training, and rehabilitative programs.

2221 Northern Nevada Adult Mental Health Services

480 Galletti Way
Sparks, NV 89431-5573
775-688-2001
Fax: 775-688-2192
www.mhds.state.nv.us

Richard Whitely, Acting Administrator
Jane Gruner, Deputy Administrator
Tracey Green, MD, Northern Medical Director

The mission of Northern Nevada Adult Mental Health Services is to provide psychiatric treatment and rehabilitation services in the least restrictive setting to support personal recovery and enhance quality of life.

2222 Southern Nevada Adult Mental Health Services

6161 W Charleston Boulevard
Las Vegas, NV 89146-1148
702-486-6000
www.mhds.state.nv.us

Richard Whitley, Acting Administrator
Jane Gruner, Deputy Administrator
Tracey Green, MD, Northern Medical Director

State operated community mental health center. Provides inpatient and outpatient psychiatric services.

New Hampshire

2223 New Hampshire Department of Health & Human Services: Bureau of Community Health Services

29 Hazen Drive
Concord, NH 03301-6503
603-271-4638
800-852-3345
Fax: 603-271-8705
TDD: 800-735-2964
www.www.dhhs.state.nh.us/dphs/bchs/index.htm

The Bureau of Community Health Services oversees grants to community-based agencies for medical and preventive health services, sets policy, provides technical assistance and education, and carries out quality assurance activities in its programmatic areas of expertise.

2224 New Hampshire Department of Health and Human Services: Bureau of Developmental Services

105 Pleasant Street
Concord, NH 03301-3852
603-271-5034
800-852-3345
Fax: 603-271-5166
TDD: 800-735-2964
www.www.dhhs.state.nh.us/dcbcs/bds/index.htm

The NH developmental services system offers its consumers with developmental disabilities and acquired brain disorders a wide range of supports and services within their own communities. BDS is comprised of a main office in Concord and 12 designated non-profit and specialized service agencies that represent specific geographic regions of NH; the community agencies are commonly referred to as Area Agencies. All direct services and supports to individuals and families are provided in accordance with contractual agreements between BDS and the Area Agencies.

2225 New Hampshire Department of Health and Human Services: Bureau of Behavioral Health

105 Pleasant Street
Concord, NH 03301-3852
603-271-5000
800-852-3345
Fax: 603-271-5058
TDD: 800-735-2964
www.www.dhhs.state.nh.us/dcbcs/bbh/index.htm

The Bureau of Behavioral Health (BBH) seeks to promote respect, recovery, and full community inclusion for adults, including older adults, who experience a mental illness and children with an emotional disturbance. By law and rule, BBH is mandated to ensure the provision of efficient and effective services to those citizens who are most severely and persistently disabled by mental, emotional, and behavioral dysfunction. To this end, BBH has apportioned the entire state into community mental health regions. Each of the ten regions has a BBH contracted Community Mental Health Center and many regions have Peer Support Agencies.

New Jersey

2226 Juvenile Justice Commission

1001 Spruce Street
Suite 202
Trenton, NJ 08638-3957
609-292-1400
Fax: 609-943-4611
E-mail: commission@njjjc.org
www.www.nj.gov/lps/jjc/index.html

Kevin M. Brown, Executive Director
Felix Mickens, Deputy Executive Director
Keith Poujol, Director, Administration
Robert Montalbano, Deputy Executive Dir., Programs

The Juvenile Justice Commission (JJC) has three primary responsibilities: the care and custody of juvenile offenders committed to the agency by the courts, the support of local efforts to plan for and provide services to at-risk and court-involved youth through County Youth Services Commissions and the state Incentive Program, and the supervision of youth on aftercare/parole.

2227 New Jersey Department of Human Services
Capital Place One
P O Box 700
222 S Warren Street
Trenton, NJ 08608-2306
609-292-3717
Fax: 609-292-3824
www.www.state.nj.us/humanservices/

Jennifer Velez, Esq, Commissioner

The New Jersey Department of Human Services (DHS) is the state's social services agency, serving more than one million of New Jersey 's most vulnerable citizens, or about one of every eight New Jersey residents. Through the work of DHS and its 13 major divisions, individuals and families in need are able to keep their lives on track, their families together, a roof over their heads, and their health protected. Human Services offers individuals and families the breathing room they need in order to find permanent solutions to otherwise daunting problems.

2228 New Jersey Division of Mental Health Services

PO Box 700
PO Box 727
Trenton, NJ 08625
800-382-6717
www.www.state.nj.us/humanservices/dmhs/

Jennifer Velez, Esq, Commissioner

The Division of Mental Health Services (DMHS) serves adults with serious and persistent mental illnesses. Central to the Division's mission is the fact that these individuals are entitled to dignified and meaningful lives. With an operating budget of $588, 377, 000 for FY 2005 and 5, 700 employees, services are available to anyone in the state who feels they need help with a mental health problem.

New Mexico

2229 New Mexico Behavioral Health Collaborative

37 Plaza La Prensa
PO Box 2348
Santa Fe, NM 87507-2348
505-827-6250
Fax: 505-827-3185

E-mail: deborah.fickling@state.nm.us
www.www.bhc.state.nm.us

Linda Roebuck, Chief Executive Officer

At the heart of the Collaborative's vision is the expectation that the lives of individuals with mental illness and substance use disorders (customers) will improve, that customers and family members will have an equal voice in the decisions that affect them and their loved ones, and that those most affected by mental illness and substance abuse can recover to lead full, meaningful lives within their communities. To achieve this will require a paradigm shift not only within the service delivery culture but also within the existing customer/family member networks.

2230 New Mexico Department of Health

1190 S St. Francis Drive
PO Box 26110
Santa Fe, NM 87505-4173
505-827-2613
www.nmhealth.org

Alfredo Vigil, Manager

The mission of the New Mexico Department of Health is to promote health and sound health policy, prevent disease and disability, improve health services systems and assure that essential public health functions and safety net services are available to New Mexicans.

2231 New Mexico Department of Human Services

PO Box 2348
Santa Fe, NM 87504-2348
505-827-7750
Fax: 505-827-6286
E-mail: eckert@state.nm.us
www.state.nm.us/hsd/

Sidone Squier, Secretary
Lisa Medina Lujan, Constituent Services
Matt Kennicott, Communications Director
Betina McCracken, Public Records Custodian

The Department strives to provide New Mexicans access to support and services so that they may move toward self-sufficiency.

2232 New Mexico Health & Environment Department

1190 St. Francis Drive
Suite N4050
Santa Fe, NM 87505-4173
800-219-6157
www.nmenv.state.nm.us/

Elaine Olah, Administrative Services Division

Our mission is to provide the highest quality of life throughout the state by promoting a safe, clean and productive environment.

2233 New Mexico Kids, Parents and Families Office of Child Development: Children, Youth and Families Department

760 Motel Blvd
Suite C
Las Cruces, NM 88007-4169
505-827-7946
Fax: 505-476-0490
E-mail: dmhaggard@cyfd.state.nm.us
www.newmexicokids.org/Family/

Dan Haggard, Director

The Children, Youth and Families Department Office of Child Development (OCD) works collaboratively with the State Department of Education, Department of Health, Department of Labor and higher education and community programs to establish a five-year plan for Early Care, Education and Family Support Professional Development. The New Mexico Professional Development Initiative supports OCD's legislative mandate to articulate and implement training and licensure requirements for individuals working in all recognized settings with children from birth to age eight.

New York

2234 New York State Office of Mental Health
44 Holland Avenue
Albany, NY 12229-1
518-474-5554
800-597-8481
www.www.omh.ny.gov

Michael Hogan, Director

Promoting the mental health of all New Yorkers with a particular focus on providing hope and recovery for adults with serious mental illness and children with serious emotional disturbances.

North Carolina

2235 North Carolina Division of Mental Health
325 North Salisbury Street
Raleigh, NC 27603-1388
919-733-7011
Fax: 919-508-0951
E-mail: contactdmh@ncmail.net
www.www.ncdhhs.gov/mhddsas/

Courtney Cantrell, Acting Director
Jim Jarrard, Deputy Director
Diana Simmons, Human Resources Manager
Ureh N. Lekwauwa, Chief, Clinical Policy

North Carolina will provide people with, or at risk of, mental illness, developmental disabilities and substance problems and their families the necessary prevention, intervention, treatment, services and supports they need to live successfully in communities of their choice.

2236 North Carolina Division of Social Services
820 S. Boylan Avenue
Dorothea Dix Campus, McBryde Building
Raleigh, NC 27603
919-527-6335
Fax: 919-334-1018
www.www.ncdhhs.gov/dss/

Sherry S Bradsher, Director
Laketha Miller, Controller
Emery Edwards Miliken, General Counsel

The North Carolina Dept of Health and Human Services, in collaboration with its partners, protects the health and safety of all North Carolinians and provides essential human services.

2237 North Carolina Substance Abuse Professional Certification Board (NCSAPCB)
PO Box 10126
Raleigh, NC 27605-126

919-832-0975
Fax: 919-833-5743
www.ncsapcb.org

Anna Misenheimer, Executive Director
Barden Culbreth, Associate Director
Katie Faulkner, Associate
Matt Musselwhite, Controller

Provides guidelines for the certification of professionals in the substance abuse field of human services.

North Dakota

2238 North Dakota Department of Human Services Division of Mental Health and Substance Abuse Services
1237 West Divide Avenue
Suite 1C
Bismarck, ND 58501-1208
701-328-8920
800-755-2719
Fax: 701-328-8969
E-mail: dhsmhsas@nd.gov
www.nd.gov/dhs/services/mentalhealth

Steve Jordan, Director
Jim Jarrard, Deputy Director
Diana Simmons, Human Resources Manager
Jesse Sowa, Support, Clinical Policy

Provides leadership for the planning, development and oversight of a system of care for children, adults and families with severe emotional disorders, mental illness and/or substance abuse issues. Mental health and substance abuse services are delivered through eight Regional Human Services Centers and the North Dakota State Hospital in Jamestown.

Ohio

2239 Ohio Department of Mental Health
30 East Broad Street
8th Floor
Columbus, OH 43215-3430
614-466-2596
877-275-6364
TTY: 614-752-9696
E-mail: questions@mha.ohio.gov
www.www.mha.ohio.gov

Tracy J Plouk, Director
Mark A Hurst, MD, Medical Director
James Lapczynski, Administration Assistant Directo
Angie Bergefurd, Community Assistant Director

Ensures high quality mental health care is available to all Ohioans, particularly individuals with severe mental illness.

Oklahoma

2240 Oklahoma Department of Human Services
2400 North Lincoln Blvd
Oklahoma City, OK 73105
405-521-3646
800-522-3511
www.okdhs.org

Diane Haser-Bennett, Director

The mission of the Oklahoma Department of Human Services is to help individuals and families in need help themselves lead safer, healthier, more independent and productive lives.

2241 Oklahoma Department of Mental Health and Substance Abuse Service (ODMHSAS)
1200 NE 13th Street
PO Box 53277
Oklahoma City, OK 73152-3277
405-522-3908
800-522-9054
Fax: 405-522-3650
TDD: 405-522-3851
www.www.ok.gov

Vacant , Director

State agency responsible for mental health, substance abuse, and domestic violence and sexual assault services.

2242 Oklahoma Healthcare Authority
2401 N W 23rd Street
Suite 1A
Oklahoma City, OK 73107-3400
405-522-7300
www.www.okhca.org

Charles Ed McFall, Chairman
Tony Armstrong, Vice Chairman

Provides health and medical policy information to Medicaid consumers and providers, administers SoonerCare and other health related programs.

2243 Oklahoma Mental Health Consumer Council
3200 NW 48th
Suite 102
Oklahoma City, OK 73112-5911
405-604-6975
888-424-1305
E-mail: consumercouncil@okmhcc.org
www.omhcc.org

Becky Tallent, Executive Director

2244 Oklahoma Office of Juvenile Affairs
3812 North Santa Fe
Suite 400
Oklahoma City, OK 73118-8500
918-530-2800
Fax: 918-530-2890
www.ok.gov/oja/

T. Keith Wilson, Executive Director
James Adams, Chief of Staff
Jeff Gifford, Division Director, Support Servi
Jim Goble, Division Administrator, Juvenile

State agency charged with delivery of programs and services to delinquent youth. Services include delinquency prevention, diversion, counseling in both community and secure residential programs. OJA provides counseling services with counselors, social workers and psychologists, as well as contracted service providers.

Year Founded: 1995

Oregon

2245 Marion County Health Department
3180 Center Street North East
Suite 2100
Salem, OR 97301

503-588-5357
Fax: 503-364-6552
E-mail: health@co.marion.or.us
www.co.marion.or.us

Jeff White, Chief Financial Officer
Laurie Steel, Treasurer

The Marion County Health Department fosters wellness, monitors health trends, and responds to community health needs.

2246 Oregon Department of Human Resources: Division of Health Services
800 NE Oregon Street
Portland, OR 97232-2162
971-673-1555
Fax: 971-673-1562
TTY: 971-673-0372
www.oregonindependentcontractors.com

Stephanie Hoskins, Chief Executive Officer
Jerry Waybrant, Deputy Asst Director
Sandy Dugan, Operations Support Manager

Health Services administers low-income medical programs, and mental health and substance abuse services. It provides public health services such as monitoring drinking-water quality and communicable-disease outbreaks, inspecting restaurants and promoting healthy behaviors.

2247 Oregon Health Policy and Research: Policy and Analysis Unit
1225 Ferry Street Se
1st Floor
Salem, OR 97301-4278
503-373-1824
www.oregon.gov/

Facilitates collaborative health services and research and policy analysis on issues affecting the Oregon Health Plan population and works to effectively communicate timely, quality results of health services research and analysis in the interest of informing health policy.

Pennsylvania

2248 Pennsylvania Department of Public Welfare and Mental Health Services
PO Box 2675
Harrisburg, PA 17105-2675
717-787-6443
800-932-0582
www.www.dpw.state.pa.us/foradults/mentalhealthservices

Beverly D Mackereth, Secretary

The Department of Public Welfare is charged with numerous program areas that include all children, youth and family concerns, mental health, mental retardation, income maintenance, medical assistance and social program issues in the Commonwealth. They also license assisted living facilities and day care centers.

Rhode Island

2249 Rhode Island Council on Alcoholism and Other Drug Dependence
500 Prospect Street
Suite 202
Pawtucket, RI 02860-6260

401-725-0410
Fax: 401-725-0768
E-mail: info@ricaodd.org
www.www.ricaodd.org

Heather Cabral, Director of Community Housing
Athena Sirignano, Administrative Assistant
Stephanie Coolbaugh, Housing Coordinator
Nicholas Sousa, Case Manager - Veterans

The Rhode Island Council on Alcoholism and Other Drug Dependence is a private, non-profit corporation whose mission is to help individuals, youth and families who are troubled with alcohol, tobacco and other drug dependence.

Year Founded: 1969

2250 Rhode Island Division of Substance Abuse
14 Harrington Road
Cranston, RI 02920-3080
401-462-4680
Fax: 401-462-6078
www.mhrh.state.ri.us

Craig Stenning, Executive Director

Substance Abuse Treatment and Prevention Services (SATPS) is responsible for planning, coordinating and administering a comprehensive statewide system of substance abuse, treatment and prevention activities. SATPS develops, supports and advocates for high quality, accessible, comprehensive and clinically appropriate substance abuse prevention and treatment services in order to decrease the negative effects of alcohol, tobacco and other drug use in Rhode Island, and improve the overall behavioral health of Rhode Islanders.

2251 State of Rhode Island Department of Mental Health, Retardation and Hospitals
Division of Behavioral Healthcare Services
14 Harrington Road
Cranston, RI 02920-3080
401-462-2339
Fax: 401-462-1564
www.mhrh.state.ri.us/

Craig S Stenning, Executive Director

Our overall mission will focus on the unique needs and goals of individuals who experience a mental illness, an emotional disturbance, and/or a substance abuse or addiction problem and to prevent, whenever possible, these from ever occurring.

South Carolina

2252 Mental Health Association in South Carolina
1823 Gadsden Street
Columbia, SC 29201-2344
803-779-5363
800-375-9894
Fax: 803-929-6147
E-mail: mha@mha-sc.org
www.mha-sc.org

Joy Jay, Executive Director
Natasha M. Scott, Clinical Director
Anita T. Baker, Shelter Plus Housing Director
Greta Swink, Financial Administrator

The Mental Health Association in South Carolina believes in a healthy society in which all people are accorded respect, dignity and the opportunity to achieve their full potential free from stigma and prejudice. The MHASC is

dedicated to preventing mental disorders through research and achieving victory over mental illnesses through systems and individual advocacy, education and unmet service development.

2253 South Carolina Department of Alcohol and Other Drug Abuse Services
2414 Bull street
PO Box 8268
Columbia, SC 29201
803-896-5555
Fax: 803-896-5557
E-mail: btooney@daodas.sc.gov
www.www.daodas.state.sc.us

Bob Toomey, Director
Kaitlin Blanco-Silva, Project manager
Lillian Roberson, Manager, Division of Operations
Lachelle Frederick, Administrative Coordinator

DAODAS is the cabinet-level department responsible for ensuring the availability of comprehensive alcohol and other drug abuse services for the citizens of South Carolina.

Year Founded: 1957

2254 South Carolina Department of Mental Health
2414 Bull Street
Columbia, SC 29202
803-898-8319
TTY: 864-297-5130
www.www.state.sc.us

John H Magill, Executive Director

The administrative offices of the South Carolina Department of Mental Health are located in Columbia and provide support services including long-range planning, performance and clinical standards, evaluation and quality assurance, personnel management, communications, information resource management, legal counsel, financial, and procurement. In addition, the central office administers services for the hearing impaired; children, adolescents and their families; people with developmental disabilities; those needing alcohol and drug treatment; the elderly; and patients who need long-term care.

2255 South Carolina Department of Social Services
1535 Confederate Avenue Extension
P O Box 1520
Columbia, SC 29202-1520
803-898-7601
www.dss.sc.gov

Kathleen Hayes, State Director

The mission of the South Carolina Department of Social Services is to ensure the safety and health of children and adults who cannot protect themselves, and to assist those in need of food assistance and temporary financial assistance while transitioning into employment.

South Dakota

2256 South Dakota Department of Social Services
Office of Medical Services
700 Governors Drive
Pierre, SD 57501-2291
605-773-3165
Fax: 605-773-4950
E-mail: Medical@STATE.SD.US
www.www.dss.sd.gov

Dan Siebersma, Director

The South Dakota Office of Medical Services covers medical care provided to low income people who meet eligibility standards either under Medicaid (Title XIX) or the Children's Health Insurance Program (CHIP). These programs are financed jointly by state and federal government and are managed by the SD Department of Social Services.

2257 South Dakota Human Services Center

3515 Broadway Avenue
PO Box 7600
Yankton, SD 57078-7600
605-668-3100
800-273-8255
Fax: 605-668-3460
www.www.dss.sd.gov/behavioralhealthservices/hsc

Ric Compton, Administator

To provide persons who are mentally ill or chemically dependent with effective, individualized professional treatment that enables them to achieve their highest level of personal independence in the most therapeutic environment.

Tennessee

2258 Bureau of TennCare: State of Tennessee

310 Great Circle Road
Nashville, TN 37243-1700
800-342-3145
E-mail: Tenn.Care@tn.gov
www.state.tn.us/tenncare/

Darin Gordon, Deputy Commissioner

On January 1, 1994, Tennessee began a new health care reform program called TennCare. This program, which required no new taxes, essentially replaced the Medicaid program in Tennessee. TennCare was designed as a managed care model. It extended coverage to uninsured and uninsurable persons who were not eligible for Medicaid.

2259 Council for Alcohol & Drug Abuse Services (CADAS)

207 Spears Avenue
Chattanooga, TN 37405
423-756-7644
877-282-2327
Fax: 423-756-7646
TTY: 423-752-0352
E-mail: info@cadas.org
www.cadas.org

Paul Fuchcar MEd, EdD, Executive Director

Welcome to CADAS, founded in 1964. The CADAS mission is to deliver the highest quality treatment, prevention, and educational services to the chemically dependent, their families, and the community at large.

Year Founded: 1964

2260 Memphis Alcohol and Drug Council

1430 Poplar Avenue
Memphis, TN 38104-2901
901-274-0056
E-mail: info @madcinc.org
www.www.madcinc.org

Catherine Bailey, Director

Provides referrals, alcohol and other drug prevention, intervention and treatment services. Also, regional and county school prevention coordination, and a clearinghouse for Shelby County including national data search and materials distribution.

2261 Middle Tennessee Mental Health Institute

221 Stewarts Ferry Pike
Nashville, TN 37214-3325
615-902-7400
Fax: 615-902-7571
www.state.tn.us

Robert Micinski, CEO

TDMHDD operates 5 Regional Mental Health Institutes (RMHIs). Lakeshore Mental Health Institute (Knoxville), Moccasin Bend Mental Health Institute (Chattanooga) and Memphis Mental Health Institute provide in-patient psychiatric services for adults; Middle Tennessee Mental Health Institute (Nashville) and Western Mental Health Institute (Bolivar) provide in-patient psychiatric services for both adults and children/youth. Most RMHI admissions are on an emergency involuntary basis, with a variety of court-ordered inpatient evaluation and treatment services also provided. The RMHIs provide psychiatric services based upon the demonstrated and emerging best practices of each clinical discipline.

2262 Tennessee Commission on Children and Youth

502 Deaderick St., 9th Fl.
Andrew Jackson Bldg
Nashville, TN 37243-0800
615-741-2633
E-mail: linda.oneal@state.tn.us
www.www.tennessee.gov/tccy/

Linda O'Neal, Executive Director
Pat Wade, Program Director

2263 Tennessee Department of Health

710 James Robertson Parkway
Andrew Johnson Tower
Nashville, TN 37243-3400
615-741-3111
E-mail: TN.health@state.tn.us
www.www.health.state.tn.us

Suzanne Hayes, Director

Provides information on a wide variety of topics including community services, health maintenance organizations, immunizations and alcohol and drug services.

2264 Tennessee Department of Human Services

400 Deaderick Street
15th Floor
Nashville, TN 37243-1403
615-313-4700
Fax: 615-741-1791
E-mail: Human-Services.Webmaster@state.tn.us
www.www.tn.gov

Gina Lodge, Commissioner

Provides information about available programs and services, such as family assistance and child support, community programs, and rehabilitation services.

Texas

2265 Harris County Mental Health: Mental Retardation Authority

7011 Southwest Freeway
Houston, TX 77074-2007

713-970-7000
www.mhmraharris.org

MHMRA of Harris County is one of the largest mental health centers in the United States, serving more than 30,000 persons in the Houston metropolitan area who suffer from mental illness and/or mental retardation. We serve the 'priority population' - adults who are diagnosed with severe and persistent mental illness, children with serious

2266 Mental Health Association of Greater Dallas

624 North Good-Latimer
200
Dallas, TX 75204-5818
214-871-2420
Fax: 214-954-0611
E-mail: tvaughn@mhadallas.org
www.mhadallas.org

Matt Roberts, President
Sarah Bayley, Development Director
Janie Metzinger, Public Policy Director
Ricardo Aguilar, Director of Consumer Programs

To lead, coordinate and involve the community in improving mental health by advocating for improved care and treatment of people with mental illness.

2267 Texas Commission on Alcohol and Drug Abuse
Texas Department of State Health Services

909 West 45th Street
Austin, TX 78751-2803
512-206-5000
E-mail: contact@tcada.state.tx.us
www.tcada.state.tx.us/

The Department of State Health Services promotes optimal health for individuals and communities while providing effective health, mental health and substance abuse services to Texans.

2268 Texas Department of Family and Protective Services

701 West 51st Street
PO Box 149030
Austin, TX 78714-9030
512-438-4800
800-720-7777
www.www.dfps.state.tx.us

Christina Martin, Chairman
Imogen Sherman Papadopoulos, Vice Chairman
Traci Henderson, Chief Financial Officer
Jennifer Sims, Chief Operating Officer(interim)

The mission of the Texas Department of Family and Protective Services (DFPS) is to protect the unprotected _ children, elderly, and people with disabilities _ from abuse, neglect, and exploitation.

Utah

2269 Utah Department of Health

288 North 1460 West
Cannon Health Building
Salt Lake Cty, UT 84116-3231
801-538-6003
www.health.utah.gov

W David Patton, PhD, Executive Director
Robert T Rolfs, MD, MPH, Deputy Director
Michael Hales, MPA, Deputy Director, Medicaid Health
Wu Xu, PhD, Director, Center for Health Data

Oversees and regulates health care services for children, seniors, the mentally ill, substance abusers, and all residents of Utah.

2270 Utah Department of Health: Health Care Financing Box 143101
Salt Lake City, UT 84114-3101

801-538-6406
www.health.utah.gov/medicaid

Provides information and assistance on Utah Medicaid programs including eligibility and additional contact info and links for administrators of the program.

2271 Utah Department of Human Services

195 North 1950 West
Salt Lake City, UT 84116
801-538-4171
800-662-3722
Fax: 801-538-4016
E-mail: dirdhs@utah.gov
www.dhs.utah.gov

Ann S Williamson, Executive Director
Jennifer Evans, Chief Financial Officer
Mark Brasher, Deputy Director
Lana Stohl, Deputy Director

Provides services for the elderly, substance abusers, people with disabilities, ed children, youthful offenders, mentally ill and others.ple with disabilities,

2272 Utah Department of Human Services: Division of Substance Abuse And Mental Health

195 North 1950 West
Salt Lake City, UT 84116
801-538-4171
Fax: 801-538-9892
E-mail: dsamh@utah.gov
www.www.dsamh.utah.gov

Douglas P Thomas, Director
Paula Bell, Vice Chair

The Utah State Division of Substance Abuse and Mental Health Division is the agency responsible for ensuring that substance abuse and mental health prevention and treatment services are available statewide. The Division also acts as a resource by providing general information, research, and statistics to the public regarding substances of abuse and mental health services.

2273 Utah Division of Substance Abuse and Mental Health

195 North 1950 West
Salt Lake City, UT 84116
801-538-4171
Fax: 801-538-9892
E-mail: dsamh@utah.gov
www.www.dsamh.utah.gov

Douglas P Thomas, Director

The Utah Division of Mental Health is the State agency responsible for ensuring that prevention and treatment services for subsatnce abuse and mental health are available statewide.

Virginia

2274 Virginia Department of Behavioral Health and Developmental Services (DBHDS)
PO Box 1797
Richmond, VA 23218-1797
804-786-3921
800-451-5544
Fax: 804-371-6638
TDD: 804-371-8977
www.www.dbhds.virginia.gov

Chris Foca, Director, Administrative services
Ken Gunn, Director, Budget and Financial Re
Neila Gunter, Director, Human Resources
John Pezzoli, Acting Commisioner

DMHMRSAS provides leadership and service to improve Virginia's system of quality treatment, habilitation, and prevention services for individuals and their families whose lives are affected by mental illness, mental retardation, or substance use disorders.

2275 Virginia Department of Medical Assistance Services
600 East Broad Street
Richmond, VA 23219-1832
804-786-7933
TDD: 800-343-0634
E-mail: info@dmas.virginia.gov
www.www.dmas.virginia.gov

Patrick Finnerty, Director

DMAS is the agency that administers Medicaid and the State Childrens Health Insurance Program (CHIP) in the State of Virginia.

2276 Virginia Department of Social Services
801 East Main Street
Richmond, VA 23219-2901
804-726-7000
800-552-3431
TDD: 800-828-1120
TTY: 800-828-1120
E-mail: citizen.services@dss.virginia.gov
www.www.dss.virginia.gov

Margaret Ross Schultze, Commisioner

Promotes self-reliance, prevention, and protection by serving as a catalyst for healthy families and communities.

2277 Virginia Office of the Secretary of Health and Human Resources
Patrick Henry Building
1111 East Broad Street
Richmond, VA 23219-1934
804-786-2211
Fax: 804-371-6984
www.hhr.virginia.gov/

The DHHR administers programs that benefit the citizens of West Virginia.

West Virginia

2278 West Virginia Bureau for Behavioral Health and Health Facilities
West Virginia Department of Health and Human Resources
350 Capitol Street
Room 350
Charleston, WV 25301-1757
304-356-4811
Fax: 304-558-1008
E-mail: obhs@wvdhhr.org
www.www.dhhr.wv.gov/bhhf/

John E Bianconi, Commissioner

We ensure that positive meaningful opportunities are available for persons with mental illness, chemical dependency, developmental disabilities and those at risk. We provide support for individuals, families, and communities in assisting persons to achieve their potential and to gain greater control over the direction of their future.

2279 West Virginia Department of Health & Human Resources (DHHR)
350 Capitol Street
Room 730
Charleston, WV 25301-1757
304-558-2974
Fax: 304-558-4194
www.wvdhhr.org/default.asp

The DHHR administers programs that benefit the citizens of West Virginia.

2280 West Virginia Department of Welfare Bureau for Children and Families
West Virginia Department of Health & Human Resources
350 Capitol Street
Room 730
Charleston, WV 25301-1757
304-558-4069
Fax: 304-558-4623
www.wvdhhr.org/bcf/family_assistance/fs.asp

The Bureau for Children and Families provides an accessible, integrated, comprehensive quality service system for West Virginia's children, families and adults to help them achieve.

Wisconsin

2281 Dane County Mental Health Center
625 West Washington Avenue
Madison, WI 53703-2637
608-280-2700
Fax: 608-280-2707
E-mail: webmaster@mhcdc.org
www.www.journeymhc.org

James Christiansen, Chair
William Greer, President/CEO
Karen Milner, M.D., Medical Director
Lynn A. Brady, M.P.A., Chief Operating Officer

The mission of the Mental Health Center of Dane County, Inc. is to provide individuals and families with high quality, community based, recovery oriented, mental health, substance abuse, and advocacy services that respect cultural differences and foster hope, strength, and self determination. We will give priority to individuals and families with high needs and low resources.

2282 University of Wisconsin Center for Health Policy and Program Evaluation
610 Walnut Street
Suite 760
Madison, WI 53726-2336
608-263-6294
Fax: 608-262-6404
E-mail: UWPHI@med.wisc.edu
www.uwphi.pophealth.wisc.edu/

Karen Timberlake, JD, Director
Alison Bergum, MPA, Associate Researcher, Evidence L
Brooke Blaalid, SD SPFSIG, Evaluator/Trainer
Jenny Buechner, BS, Research Specialist

The Institute serves as a focal point for applied public health and health policy within the University of Wisconsin-Madison School of Medicine and Public Health as well as a bridge to public health and health policy practitioners in the state. We strive to: address a broad range of real world problems of importance to government, business, providers and the public; and catalyze partnerships of inquiry between researchers and users of research and break down barriers between the academic community and public and private policy makers.

2283 Wisconsin Department of Health and Family Services
1 West Wilson Street
Madison, WI 53703-3445
608-266-1865
TTY: 608-267-7371
www.www.dhs.wisconsin.gov

Cremear Mims, Manager

The Wisconsin Department of Health and Family Services administers a wide range of services to clients in the community and at state institutions.

Wyoming

2284 Wyoming Department of Family Services
2300 Capitol Avenue
Hathaway Building, 3rd Floor
Cheyenne, WY 82002-1
307-777-7561
Fax: 307-777-7747
www.dfsweb.state.wy.us

Steve Corsi, Psy.D, Director
Chris Smith, DFS Human Resources Manager
Tony Lewis, Communications Officer, Sr Busine
Nichole Anderson, Policy Analyst

The mission of the Wyoming Department of Family Services is to have Families assume more responsibility for raising their own children. Communities will assume more responsibility for their own families. The Department of Family Services will facilitate both.

Professional & Support Services

Accreditation & Quality Assurance

2286 American Board of Examiners in Clinical Social Work
241 Humphrey Street
Shetland Park
Marblehead, MA 01945
781-639-5270
800-694-5285
Fax: 781-639-5278
E-mail: abe@abecsw.org
www.www.abecsw.org

Bob Booth, CEO
Robert Booth, Executive Director
Michael Brooks MSW BCD, Business Development, Policy Dir

Clinical Social Work certifying and standard setting organization. ABE's no cost online and CD ROM directories (both searchable/sortable) are sources used by the healthcare industry nationwide for network development and referrals. They contain verified information about the education, training, experience and practice specialties of over 11, 000 Board Certified Diplomates in Clinical Social Work (BCD). Visit our website for the directory, employment resources, continuing education and other services.

2287 American Board of Examiners of Clinical Social Work Regional Offices
645 Broadway
Suite C
Sonoma, CA 95476
707-938-5833
888-279-9378
Fax: 781-639-5278
E-mail: abe@abecsw.org
www.abecsw.org

Yvette Colon, PhD, BCD, President
Robert Booth, Executive Director
Carolyn Messner, DSW, BCD, Vice President
Bob Booth, Chief Executive Officer

Sets national practice standards, issues an advance-practice credential, and publishes reference information about its board-certified clinicians.

Year Founded: 1987

2288 Brain Imaging Handbook
WW Norton & Company
500 5th Avenue
New York, NY 10110-54
212-354-5500
800-233-4830
Fax: 212-869-0856
E-mail: npb@wwnorton.com
www.books.wwnorton.com/

J. Douglas Bremner, Author

The past 10 years have seen an explosion in the use of brain imaging technologies to aid treatment of medical as well as mental health conditions. MRI, CT scans, and PET scans are now common. This book is the first quick reference to these technologies, rich in illustrations and including discussions of which techniques are best used in particular instances of care.

224 pages

2289 CARF International
6951 East SouthPoint Road
Tucson, AZ 85756-9407
520-325-1044
888-281-6531
Fax: 520-318-1129
TTY: 888-281-6531
www.carf.org

Brian J Boon, PhD, President/CEO
Cindy L Johnson, CPA, Chief Resource and Strategic Dev
Leslie Ellis-Lang, Managing Director
Amanda Birch, Administrator of Operations

CARF assists organizations to improve the quality of their services, to demonstrate value, and to meet internationally recognized organizational and practice standards.

Year Founded: 1966

2290 Cenaps Corporation
13194 Spring Hill Drive
Spring Hill, FL 34609
352-596-8000
Fax: 352-596-8002
E-mail: info@cenaps.com
www.cenaps.com

Tresa Watson, Business Manager

CENAPS is an acronym for the Center for Applied Sciences. They are a private training firm committed to providing advanced clinical skills training for the addiction and behavioral health fields.

2291 CompHealth Credentialing
6440 South Millrock Drive
Suite 175
Salt Lake City, UT 84121
801-930-3000
800-453-3030
Fax: 801-930-4517
E-mail: info@comphealth.com
www.comphealth.com

Assists in analyzing the total costs involved in credentialing verifications, including some items frequently overlooked; assesses and/or develops a provider application to meet accreditation standards; can assess current credentialing files; can assist in developing policy and procedures for the verification process.

2292 Consumer Satisfaction Team
1210 Stanbridge Street
Suite 600
Norristown, PA 19401-5300
610-270-3685
Fax: 610-270-9155
E-mail: watsons@cstmont
www.cstmont.com

Sue Soriano, President
Tim Tunner, Vice President
Molly Frantz, Treasurer
Dr Romani George, Secretary

The central role of CST is to provide the Montgomery County Office of MH/MR/DD with information about satisfaction with the mental health services that adults are receiving and make recommendations for change.

2293 Council on Social Work Education
1701 Duke Street
Suite 200
Alexandria, VA 22314-3457
703-683-8080
Fax: 703-683-8099
E-mail: info@cswe.org
www.cswe.org

Barbara W Shank, Chairman
Darla Spence Coffey, PhD, MSW, President and Chief Executive Of
Alejandro Garcia, Vice Chair/Secretary
Armin H Leopold, Director, Finance and Administrat

A national association that preserves and enhances the quality of social work education for the purpose of promoting the goals of individual and community well being and social justice. Pursues this mission through setting and maintaining policy and program standards, accrediting bachelors and masters degree programs in social work, promoting research and faculty development, and advocating for social work education.

Year Founded: 1952

2294 Healtheast Behavioral Care
559 Capitol Boulevard
Saint Paul, MN 55103-2101
651-232-2228
www.healtheast.org

Robert Beck, President/CEO
Robert D. Gill, VP Finance/CFO
Robert J. Beck, VP Medical Affairs

Assessment and referral for: Psychiatric, Inpatient, Chemical Dependancy.

2295 Joint Commission on Accreditation of Healthcare Organizations
1 Renaissance Boulevard
Oakbrook Terrace, IL 60181-4294
630-792-5000
Fax: 630-792-5617
E-mail: customerservice@jcaho.org
www.jointcommission.org

Mark Chassin, President
Mark Angood, VP/Chief Patient Safety Officer

The Joint Commission evaluates and accredits nearly 20,000 health care organizations and programs in the United States. An independent, not-for-profit organization, the Joint Commission is the nation's predominant standards-setting and accrediting body in health care. The Joint Commission has developed state-of-the-art, professionally-based standards and evaluated the compliance of health care organizations against these benchmarks.

Year Founded: 1951

2296 Lanstat Incorporated
4663 Mason Street
Port Townsend, WA 98368
425-334-3124
800-672-3166
Fax: 425-334-3124
E-mail: info@lanstat.com
www.lanstat.com

Landon Kimbrough, President
Sherry Kimbrough, VP/Co-Founder

Provides quality technical assistance to behavioral health treatment agencies nationawide, including tribal and goverment agencies.

2297 Med Advantage
11301 Corporate Boulevard
Suite 300
Orlando, FL 32817-1445
407-282-5131
Fax: 407-282-9240
E-mail: info@med-advantage.com
www.www.med-advantage.com

John Witty, Owner

Fully accredited by URAC and certified in all 11 elements by NCQA, Med Advantage is one of the oldest credentials verification organizations in the country. Over the past eight years, they have developed sophisticated computer systems and one of the largest data warehouses of medical providers in the nation, containing information on over 900, 000 healthcare providers. Their system is continually updated from primary source data required to meet the standards of the URAC, NCQA and JCAHO.

2298 Mertech
PO Box 787
Norwell, MA 02061-787
781-659-0701
888-794-7447
Fax: 781-659-2049
E-mail: kwoodman@mertech.org
www.mertech.org

John Kopacz, Founder

A business development organization that specializes in helping clients capitalize on business opportunities in an efficient and effective manner to meet their goals and objectives. They have three business units: Mertech Health Care Consultants, Mertech Personal Health Improvement Program and Managed Care Information Systems.

2299 National Board for Certified Counselors
3 Terrace Way
Greensboro, NC 27403-3670
336-547-0607
Fax: 336-547-0017
E-mail: nbcc@nbcc.org
www.nbcc.org

Joseph D. Wehrman, Chairman
Thomas Clawson, President/CEO
Brandon Hunt, Vice Chair
Kylie P. Dotson-Blake, Secretary

National voluntary certification board for counselors. Certified counselors have met minimum criteria. Referral lists can be provided to consumers.

Year Founded: 1982

2300 National Register of Health Service Providers in Psychology
1200 New York Ave NW
Ste 800
Washington, DC 20005
202-783-7663
Fax: 202-347-0550
www.nationalregister.org

Raymond A. Follen, President/Chairman
Glenace E. Edwall, Vice President/Vice-Chair

Erica H. Wise, Secretary
William A. Hancur, Treasurer

Nonprofit credentialing organization for psychologists; evaluates education, training, and experience of licensed psychologists. Committed to advancing psychology as a profession and improving the delivery of health services to the public.

Year Founded: 1974

2301 SUPRA Management
2424 Edenborn Avenue
Suite 660
Metairie, LA 70001-6465
504-837-5557

Associations

2302 Academy of Psychosomatic Medicine
5272 River Road
Suite 630
Bethesda, MD 20816-1453
301-718-6520
Fax: 301-656-0989
E-mail: apm@apm.org
www.apm.org

Linda L.M Worley, MD, FAPM, President
James Vrac, Executive Director
Steven A Epstein, MD, FAPM, Vice President
Robert Boland, MD, FAPM, Treasurer

Represents psychiatrists dedicated to the advancement of medical science, education, and healthcare for persons with comorbid psychiatric and general medical conditions and provides national and international leadership in the furtherance of those goals.

2303 Agency for Healthcare Research & Quality
Office of Communications and Knowledge Transfer
540 Gaither Road
Suite 2000
Rockville, MD 20850-6649
301-427-1364
Fax: 301-427-1364
E-mail: info@ahrq.gov
www.www.ahrq.gov

Jeffrey Toven, Chief Operating Officer
Richard Kronick, PhD, Director
Boyce Ginieczki, PhD, Acting Deputy Director

The Agency for Healthcare Research and Quality's (AHRQ) mission is to improve the quality, safety, efficiency, and effectiveness of health care for all Americans. Information from AHRQ's research helps people make more informed decisions and improve the quality of healthcare services.

Year Founded: 1989

2304 Alliance for Children and Families
11700 W Lake Park Drive
Milwaukee, WI 53224-3021
414-359-1040
800-221-3726
Fax: 414-359-1074
E-mail: pgoldberg@alliance1.org
www.www.alliance1.org

Dennis Richardson, Chair
Susan Dreyfus, President/CEO
Polina Makievsky, Senior Vice President of Knowled

National membership association representing more than three hundred forty private, nonprofit child and family-serving organizations. It's mission is to strengthen members' capacity to serve and advocate for children, families and communities.

2305 American Academy of Addiction Psychiatry (AAAP)
400 Massasoit Avenue
Suite 307 - 2nd Floor
East Providence, RI 02914-4800
401-524-3076
Fax: 401-272-0922
E-mail: info@aaap.org
www.aaap.org

Kathryn Cates-Wessel, Executive Director
Isabel Vieira, Director, Education
Franc Lemirehal MD, Director, Grants Administration
Laura F. McNicholas MD, PhD, Head, Research Section

Professional membership organization with approximately 1, 000 members in the United States and around the world. The membership consists of psychiatrists who work with addiction in their practices, faculty at various academic institutions.

2306 American Academy of Child & Adolescent Psychiatry
3615 Wisconsin Avenue NW
Washington, DC 20016-3007
202-966-7300
Fax: 202-966-2891
E-mail: communications@aacap.org
www.www.aacap.org

Paramjit T. Joshi, M.D., President
Aradhana Sood, M.D., Secretary
David G. Fassler, M.D., Treasurer

Provides information on childhood psychiatric disorders.

2307 American Academy of Clinical Psychiatrists
PO Box 458
Glastonbury, CT 06033-458
860-633-6023
Fax: 866-668-9858
E-mail: aacp@cox.net
www.aacp.com

Donald W Black MD, President
Richard Baton, Vice President
James Wilcox DO, PhD, Secretary/Treasurer

Practicing board-eligible or board-certified psychiatrists. Promotes the scientific practice of psychiatric medicine. Conducts educational and teaching research. Publications: Annals of Clinical Psychiatry, quarterly journal. Clinical Psychiatry Quarterly, newsletter. Annual conference and exhibits in fall.

Year Founded: 1975

2308 American Academy of Medical Administrators
330 N Wabash Avenue
Suite 2000
Chicago, IL 60611
312-321-6815
Fax: 312-673-6705

E-mail: info@aameda.org
www.aameda.org

Eric Conde, MSA, CFAAMA, Chairman
Thomas Draper, MBA, FAACVPR, , Treasurer
Maj (Retired Bonds, MA, BS, CFAAMA, Vice Chair
Susan Eget, Director, Communications

Their mission is to advance Academy member and the field of healthcare management, and promote excellence and integrity in healthcare delivery and leadership.

Year Founded: 1957

2309 American Academy of Psychiatry and the Law (AAPL)

One Regency Drive
PO Box 30
Bloomfield, CT 06002-30
860-242-5450
800-331-1389
Fax: 860-286-0787
E-mail: office@aapl.org
www.aapl.org

Robert Weinstock, MD, President
Jacquelyn T Coleman, C.A.E, Executive Director
Richard L Frierson, MD, Vice President
Emily A Keram, MD, Vice President

Seeks to exchange ideas and experience in areas where psychiatry and the law overlap and develop standards of practice in the relationship of psychiatry to the law and encourage the development of training programs for psychiatrists in this area. Publications: Journal of the American Academy of Psychiatry and the Law, quarterly. Scholarly articles on forensic psychiatry. Newsletter of the American Academy of Psychiatry and Law, quarterly. Membership Directory, annual.

Year Founded: 1969

2310 American Academy of Psychoanalysis and Dynamic Psychiatry

One Regency Drive
PO Box 30
Bloomfield, CT 06002-30
888-691-8281
Fax: 860-286-0787
E-mail: info@aapdp.org
www.aapsa.org

Michael Blumenfield, MD, President
Jacquelyn T Coleman CAE, Executive Director
Eugenio M Rothe, MD, Treasurer
Eugene Della Badia, D.O, Secretary

Founded in 1956 to provide an open forum for psychoanalysts to discuss relevant and responsible views of human behavior and to exchange ideas with colleagues and other social behavioral scientists. Aims to develop better communication among psychoanalysts and psychodynamic psychiatrists in other disiplines in science and the humanities. Meetings of the Academy provide a forum for inquiry into the phenomena of individual and interpersonal behavior. Advocates an acceptance of all relevant and responsible psychoanalytic views of human behavior, rather than adherence to one particular doctrine.

Year Founded: 1956

2311 American Association for Marriage and Family Therapy

PO Box 2276
Bellingham, VA 98227
360-733-1753
888-553-1228
Fax: 703-838-9805
E-mail: central@aamft.org
www.wamft.org

Kim Gilliland, President
Kirk Roberts, Executive Director
Robin Gray, Treasurer
Susan Arneson, Secretary

The professional association for the field of marriage and family therapy. They represent the professional interests of more than 23, 000 marriage and family therapists throughout the United States, Canada and abroad. They facilitate research, theory development and education. They develop standards for graduate education and training, clinical supervision, professional ethics and the clinical practice of marriage and family therapy. They host an annual national training conference each fall as well as a week-long series of continuing education institutes in the summer.

2312 American Association of Community Psychiatrists (AACP)

PO Box 570218
Dallas, TX 75357-218
972-613-0985
Fax: 972-613-5532
E-mail: frda1@airmail.net
www.www.communitypsychiatry.org/

Anita Everett MD, DFAFA, President
Annelle Primm, Vice President
Francis Bell, Administrative Director

The mission of AACP is to inspire, empower and equip Community Psychiatrists to promote and provide quality care and to integrate practice with policies that improve the well being of individuals and communities.

2313 American Association of Chairs of Departments of Psychiatry (AACDP)

AACDP C/O Lucille Meinsler #319
1594 Cumberland Street
Lebanon, PA 17042-4532
717-270-1673
E-mail: aacdp@verizon.net
www.aacdp.org

Laura Roberts MD, MA, President
Stuart Munro MD, President-Elect
David Baron DO, Secretary/Treasurer
Leighton Huey MD, Advocacy Task Force

Represents the leaders of departments of psychiatry in all the medical schools in the United States and Canada. They are committed to promotion of excellence in psychiatric education, research and clinical care. They are also committed to advocating for health policy to create appropriate and affordable psychiatric care for all.

2314 American Association of Children's Residential Centers

11700 W Lake Park Drive
Milwaukee, WI 53224-3021
877-332-2272
Fax: 877-362-2272

E-mail: ksisson@aacrc-dc.org
www.aacrc-dc.org

Christopher Bellonci, M.D., President
Laurah Currey, Treasurer
Mary Hollie, Secretary
Okpara Rice, President Elect

Funded by the Mental Health Community Support Program. The purpose of the association is to share information about services, providers and ways to cope with mental illnesses. Available services include referrals, professional seminars, support groups and a variety of publications.

2315 American Association of Directors of Psychiatric Residency Training
1594 Cumberland Street
Lebanon, PA 17042-4532
717-270-1673
E-mail: aadprt@verizon.net
www.aadprt.org

Lucille Meinsler, Administrative Director
Lucille Meinsler, Administrative Manager

To better meet the nation's mental healthcare needs, the mission of the American Association of Directors of Psychiatric Residency Training is to promote excellence in education and training of future psychiatrists.

2316 American Association of Geriatric Psychiatry (AAGP)
7910 Woodmont Avenue
Suite 1050
Bethesda, MD 20814-3004
301-654-7850
Fax: 301-654-4137
E-mail: main@aagponline.org
www.aagponline.org

Susan K. Schultz, MD, President
Christine deVries, Chief Executive Officer/Executiv
Denise Disque, Office Manager/Executive Assista
Kate McDuffie, Director, Communications & Marke

Members are psychiatrists interested in promoting better mental health care for the elderly. Maintains placement service and speakers' bureau. Publications: AAGP Membership Directory, annual. Geriatric Psychiatry News, bimonthly newsletter. Growing Older and Wiser, covers consumer and general public information. Annual meeting and exhibits in February or March.

Year Founded: 1978

2317 American Association of Healthcare Consultants
5938 N Drake Avenue
Chicago, IL 60659-3203
888-350-2242
Fax: 773-463-3552
E-mail: info@aahcmail.org
www.www.consultprism.com/aahc.htm

Billy Adkisson, Chairman

Serve as the preeminent credentialing, professional, and practice development organization for the healthcare consulting profession; to advance the knowledge, quality, and standards of practice for consulting to management in the healthcare industry; and to enhance the understanding and image of the healthcare consulting profession and Member Firms among its various publics.

Year Founded: 1949

2318 American Association of Homes and Services for the Aging
2519 Connecticut Avenue NW
Washington, DC 20008-1520
202-783-2242
Fax: 202-783-2255
E-mail: info@LeadingAge.org
www.aahsa.org

William L Minnix Jr, President and Chief Executive Of
Katrinka Smith Sloan, COO/SVP Member Services
Bruce Rosenthal, Vice President, Corporate Partne
Lea Chambers-Johnson, Assistant to the Preside

An association committed to advancing the vision of healthy, affordable, ethical long term care for America. The association represents 5, 600 million driven, not-for-profit nursing homes, continuing care facilities and community care retirement facilities and community service organizations.

2319 American Association of Pastoral Counselors
9504A Lee Highway
Fairfax, VA 22031-2303
703-385-6967
Fax: 703-352-7725
E-mail: info@aapc.org
www.aapc.org

Alice M. Graham, Ph.D., President
Pamela Holliman, Ph.D., Vice President
Douglas M. Ronsheim, Executive Director
William Manseau, Secretary

Organized in 1963 to promote and support the ministry of pastoral counseling within religious communities and the field of mental health in the United States and Canada.

Year Founded: 1963

2320 American Association of Pharmaceutical Scientists
2107 Wilson Boulevard
Suite 700
Arlington, VA 22201-3042
703-243-2800
Fax: 703-243-9650
www.aaps.org

Karen Habucky, President
John Lisack, Executive Director

The American Association of Pharmaceutical Scientists will be the premier organization of all scientists dedicated to the discovery, development and manufacture of pharmaceutical products and therapies through advances in science and technology.

2321 American Association of Retired Persons
601 E Street NW
Washington, DC 20049-2
202-434-2277
888-687-2277
Fax: 202-434-7599
TTY: 877-434-7598
www.aarp.org

A Barry Rand, CEO
Erik Olsen, President

AARP is a non profit membership organization of persons 50 and older dedicated to addressing their needs and interests.

2322 American Association on Intellectual and Developmental Disabilities (AAIDD)
501 3rd Street NW
Suite 200
Washington, DC 20001
202-387-1968
800-424-3688
Fax: 202-387-2193
E-mail: anam@aaidd.org
www.aaidd.org

Danielle Webber, MSW, Manager, Educational Programs
Jason Epstein, Communications Coordinator
Kathleen McLane, Director, Publications Program
Michael Winfield, Coordinator, Publications Progra

AAIDD promotes progressive policies, sound research, effective practices and universal human rights for people with intellectual and developmental disabilities.

2323 American Board of Professional Psychology (ABPP)
600 Market Street
Suite 300
Chapel Hill, NC 27516
919-537-8031
Fax: 919-537-8034
E-mail: office@abpp.org
www.abpp.org

Randy K. Otto, PhD, ABPP, President
David R. Cox, PhD, ABPP, Executive Officer
Nancy O. McDonald, Assistant Executive Officer
Jerry Sweet, PhD, ABPP, Treasurer

The mission is to increase consumer protection through the examination and certification of psychologists who demonstrate competence in approved specialty areas in professional psychology

2324 American Board of Psychiatry and Neurology (ABPN)
2150 E Lake Cook Road
Suite 900
Buffalo Grove, IL 60089-1875
847-229-6500
Fax: 847-229-6600
www.abpn.com

Burton Reifler, President
Patricia Coyle, Vice President

ABPN is a nonprofit organization that promotes excellence in the practice of psychiatry and neurology through lifelong certification including compentency testing processes.

2325 American College Health Association
1362 Mellon Road
Suite 180
Hanover m, MD 21076
410-859-1500
Fax: 410-859-1510
www.acha.org

Pat Ketcham, PhD, CHES, FA, President
Keith Anderson, PhD, FACHA, Vice President
Charley Bradley, BPS, RNBC, FA, Treasurer

Principal advocate and leadership organization for college and university health. Provides advocacy, education, communications, products and services as well as promotes research and culturally competent practices to enhance its members' ability to advance the health of all students and the campus community.
Year Founded: 1920

2326 American College of Health Care Administrators (ACHCA)
1321 Duke Street
Suite 400
Alexandria, VA 22314
202-536-5120
Fax: 888-874-1585
E-mail: wodonnell@achca.org
www.achca.org

Marianna Kern Grachek, MSN, CNH, President & CEO
Becky Reisinger, Director, Membership and Busines
Whitney O'Donnell, Coordinator, Member Services
Chelsea Whitman-Rush, Coordinator, Member and Chapter

A non-profit professional membership association which provides superior educataional programming, professional certification, and career development opportunities for its members. Available on Facebook.
Year Founded: 1962

2327 American College of Healthcare Executives
One N Franklin Street
Suite 1700
Chicago, IL 60606-3529
312-424-2800
Fax: 312-424-0023
E-mail: contact@ache.org
www.ache.org

Christine M. Candio, Chairman
Deborah J. Bowen, FACHE, President and CEO
Thomas C Dolan, President, CEO

International professional society of nearly 30, 000 healthcare executives. ACHE is known for its prestigious credentialing and educational programs. ACHE is also known for its journal, Journal of Healthcare Management, and magazine, Healthcare Executive, as well as ground-breaking research and career development programs. Through its efforts, ACHE works toward its goal of improving the health status of society by advancing healthcare management excellence.

2328 American College of Mental Health Administration (ACMHA)
7804 Loma del Norte Road NE
Albuquerque, NM 87109-5419
505-822-5038
E-mail: executive.director@acmha.org
www.acmha.org

Colette Croze, MSW, President
Kris Ericson, PhD, Executive Director
Christopher Wilkins, Sr., MHA, Treasurer
Steve Scoggin, PsyD, LPC, Secretary

Advancing the field of mental health and substance abuse administration and to promote the continuing education of clinical professionals in the areas of administration and policy. Publication: ACMHA Newsletter, quarterly. Annual Santa Fe Summit, conference.
Year Founded: 1979

2329 American College of Osteopathic Neurologists & Psychiatrists
142 E. Ontario St.
Suite 200
Chicago, IL 60611-2864
312-202-8000
800-062- 177
Fax: 312-202-8200
E-mail: acn-aconp@msn.com
www.osteopathic.org

Norman E. Vinn, DO, President
Adrienne White-Faines, MPA, Executive Director and CEO

Purpose is to promote the art and science of osteopathic medicine in the fields of neurology and psychiatry; to maintain and further elevate the highest standards of proficiency and training among osteopathic neurologists and psychiatrists; to stimulate original research and investigation in neurology and psychiatry; and to collect and disseminate the results of such work for the benefit of the members of the college, the public, the profession at large, and the ultimate benefit of all humanity.

2330 American College of Psychiatrists
122 S. Michigan Ave
Suite 1360
Chicago, IL 60603-6185
312-662-1020
Fax: 312-662-1025
E-mail: angel@acpsych.org
www.acpsych.org

Maureen Shick, Executive Director
Angel Waszak, Administrative Assistant

Nonprofit honorary association of psychiatrists who, through excellence in their chosen fields, have been recognized for thier significant contributions to the profession. The society's goal is to promote and support the highest standards in psychiatry through education, research and clinical practice.

Year Founded: 1963

2331 American College of Psychoanalysts (ACPA)
PO Box 570218
Dallas, TX 75357-218
972-613-0985
www.acopsa.org

Ralph H. Beaumont, III, M.D., President
Barbara Young, M.D., Secretary, General Counsel
Mervin S. Stewart, M.D., Treasurer

Honorary, scientific and professional organization for physician psycholanalysts. Goal is to contribute to the leadership and support high standards in the practice of psychoanalysis, and understanding the relationship between mind and brain.

2332 American Counseling Association
5999 Stevenson Avenue
Alexandria, VA 22304-3304
703-823-9800
800-347-6647
Fax: 703-823-0252
E-mail: webmaster@counseling.org
www.counseling.org

Richard Yep, CAE, Executive Director
Dr Don W Locke, President
Dr Bradley T Erford, President Elect

ACA serves professional counselors in the US and abroad. Provides a variety of programs and services that support the personal, professional and program development goals of its members. ACA works to provide quality services to the variety of clients who use their services in college, community agencies, in mental health, rehabilitation and related settings. Offers a large catalog of books, manuals and programs for the professional counselor.

Year Founded: 1952

2333 American Counseling Association (ACA)
5999 Stevenson Avenue
Alexandria, VA 22304-3304
703-823-9800
800-347-6647
Fax: 703-823-0252
E-mail: webmaster@counseling.org
www.counseling.org

Richard Yep, Executive Director

A not-for-profit, professional and educational organization that is dedicated to the growth and enhancement of the counseling profession.

Year Founded: 1952

2334 American Geriatrics Society
40 Fulton Street
18th Floor
New York, NY 10038
212-308-1414
Fax: 212-832-8646
E-mail: info@americangeriatrics.org
www.americageriatrics.org

Cathy Alessi, MD, AGSF, President
Nancy Lundebjerg, Deputy EVP, COO
Marianna Drootin, Associate Director
Melissa Fisher, Director of Development

Nationwide, nonprofit association of geriatric health care professionals, research scientists and other concerned individuals dedicated to improving the health, independence and quality of life for all older people. Pivotal force in shaping attitudes, policies and practices regarding health care for older people.

Year Founded: 1942

2335 American Group Psychotherapy Association
25 E 21st Street
6th Floor
New York, NY 10010-6207
212-477-2677
877-668-2472
E-mail: info@agpa.org
www.agpa.org

Les R. Greene, President
Marsha S. Block, CAE, CFRE, Chief Executive Officer
Angela Stephens, CAE, Professional Development Directo
Diane C. Feirman, CAE, Public Affairs Director

Interdisciplinary community that has been enhancing practice, theory and research of group therapy for over 50 years. Provides support to enhance your work as a mental health care professional, or your life as a member of a therapeutic group.

Year Founded: 1942

2336 American Health Care Association
1201 L Street NW
Washington, DC 20005-4046
202-842-4444
Fax: 202-842-3860
www.www.ahcancal.org

Bruse Yarwood, President

Nonprofit federation of affiliated state health organizations, together representing nearly 12, 000 nonprofit and for profit assisted living, nursing facility, developmentally disabled and subacute care providers that care for more than 1.5 million elderly and disabled individuals nationally. AHCA represents the long term care community at large — to government, business leaders and the general public. It also serves as a force for change within the long term care field, providing information, education, and administrative tools that enhance quality at every level.

2337 American Health Information Management Association
233 N Michigan Avenue
21st Floor
Chicago, IL 60601-5809
312-233-1100
Fax: 312-233-1090
E-mail: info@ahima.org
www.ahima.org

Linda Kloss, Executive Director
Linda L Kloss CAE, CEO

Dynamic professional association that represents more than 46, 000 specially educated health information management professionals who work throughout the healthcare industry. Health information management professionals serve the health care industry and the public by managing, analyzing and utilizing data vital for patient care and making it accessible to healthcare providers when it is needed most.

2338 American Humane Association
1400 16th Street, NorthWest
Suite 360
Washington, DC 20036
303-792-9900
800-227-4645
Fax: 303-792-5333
E-mail: info@americanhumane.org
www.americanhumane.org

John Payne, Chair
Robert R Ganzert, PhD, President and Chief Executive Of
Clifford Rose, Chief Financial Officer
Audrey Lang, Chief of Staff

Leader in developing programs, policies and services to prevent the abuse and neglect of children, while strengthening families and communities and enhancing social service systems.

Year Founded: 1877

2339 American Medical Association
330 N. Wabash Ave.
Chicago, IL 60611-5885
312-464-5000
800-621-8335
Fax: 312-464-4184
www.ama-assn.org

James L Madara, MD, CEO, Executive Vice President
Bernard L Hengesbaugh, Chief Operating Officer

Denise M. Hagerty, Senior Vice President & Chief Fi
Craig Ethridge, Group Vice President & Chief Inf

Speaks out in issues important to patients and the nation's health. AMA policy on such issues is decided through its democratic policy making process, in the AMA House of Delegates, which meets twice a year. The House is comprised of physician delegates representing every state; nearly 100 national medical specialty societies, federal service agents, including the Surgeon General of the US; and 6 sections representing hospital and clinic staffs, resident physicians, medical students, young physicians, medical schools and international medical graduates. The AMA's envisioned future is to be a part of the professional life of every physician and an essential force for progress in improving the nation's health.

Year Founded: 1847

2340 American Medical Directors Association
11000 Broken Land Parkway
Suite 400
Columbia, MD 21044-3532
410-740-9743
800-876-2632
Fax: 410-740-4572
E-mail: webmaster@amda.com
www.www.amda.com

Matthew S Wayne, MD, President
Leonard Gelman. MD, Vice President
Milta O Little, Secretary

Professional association of medical directors and physicians practicing in the long-term care continuum, dedicated to excellence in patient care by providing education, advocacy and professional development.

2341 American Medical Group Association
One Prince Street
Alexandria, VA 22314
703-838-0033
Fax: 703-548-1890
E-mail: roconnor@amga.org
www.amga.org

Donald W. Fisher, Ph.D., President/CEO

The American Medical Group Association (AMGA) is a 501(c)(6) trade association representing medical groups, health systems and other organized systems of care, including some of the nation's largest, most prestigious integrated delivery systems. AMGA is a leading voice in advocating for efficient, team-based, and accountable care. AMGA members encompass all models of organized systmes of care in the healthcare industry. MOre than 150, 000 physicians practice in AMGA member organizations, providing healthcare services for 120 million patients (approximately 1 in 3 Americans). AMGA's mission is to support its members in enhancing population health and care for patients through integrated systems of care.

Year Founded: 1950

2342 American Medical Informatics Association
4720 Montgomery Lane
Suite 500
Bethesda, MD 20814-6052
301-657-1291
Fax: 301-657-1296
E-mail: mail@amia.org
www.amia.org

Blackford Middleton, MD, MPH, MS, Chairman
Karen Greenwood, Executive Vice President & COO
Ross D. Martin, MD, MHA, Vice President of Policy and Dev
Susanna Aguirre, Policy and Development Specialis

Nonprofit membership organization of individuals, institutions and corporations dedicated to developing and using information technologies to improve health care. Our members include physicians, nurses, computer and information scientists, biomedical engineers, medical librarians, academic researchers and educators. Holds an annual syposium, 2 congresses, prints a journal and maintains a resource center.

Year Founded: 1988

2343 American Mental Health Counselors Association (AMHCA)

801 N Fairfax Street
Suite 304
Alexandria, VA 22314-1775
703-548-6002
800-326-2642
Fax: 703-548-4775
E-mail: vmoore@amhca.org
www.amhca.org

Judith Bertenthal-Smith, President
Joel E. Miller, Executive Director & CEO
James K. Finley, Associate Executive Director & D
Linda Morano, Manager for Membership & Member

Professional counselors employed in mental health services and students. Aims to deliver quality mental health services to children, youth, adults, families and organizations and to improve the availability and quality of services through licensure and certification, training standards and consumer advocacy. Publishes an Advocate Newsletter, Journal of Mental Health Counseling, quarterly, Mental Health Brights, brochures. Annual National Conference.

2344 American Neuropsychiatric Association

700 Ackerman Road
Suite 625
Columbus, OH 43202-4505
614-447-2077
Fax: 614-263-4366
E-mail: anpa@osu.edu
www.www.anpaonline.org

Sandy Bornstein, Executive Director
C. Edward Coffey, Treasurer

An association of professionals in neuropsychiatry and clinical neurosciences. Their mission is to promote neuroscience for the benefit of people. They work together in a collegial fashion to provide a forum for learning and provide excellent, scientific and compassionate care. They hold their annual scientific meeting in the early spring.

Year Founded: 1988

2345 American Nurses Association

8515 Georgia Avenue
Suite 400
Silver Spring, MD 20910-3492
301-628-5000
800-274-4262
Fax: 301-628-5001
E-mail: webmaster@ana.org
www.nursingworld.org

Karen Daley, PhD, RN, FAAN, President
Marla J. Weston, PhD, RN, FAAN, Chief Executive Officer
Cindy R. Balkstra, MS, RN, CNS-, First Vice President
Jennifer S. Mensik, PhD, RN, NEA-B, Second Vice President

A full-service professional organization representing the nation's 2.7 million registered nurses through its 54 constituent members associations. The ANA advances the nursing profession by fostering high standards of nursing practice, promoting the economic and general welfare of nurses in the workplace, projecting a positive and realistic view of nursing, and by lobbying the Congress and regulatory agencies on health care issues affecting nurses and the public.

2346 American Pharmacists Association

2215 Constitution Avenue NW
Washington, DC 20037
202-628-4410
800-237-2742
Fax: 202-783-2351
E-mail: feedback@pharmacist.com
www.pharmacist.com

Joseph J. Janela, Chief Financial Officer
Elizabeth K. Keyes, Chief Operating Officer
Stacie Maass, Senior Vice President, Pharmacy
Thomas E. Menighan, Chief Executive Officer

National professional society of pharmacists, formerly the American Pharmaceutical Association. Our members include practicing pharmacists, pharmaceutical students, pharmacy scientists, pharmacy technicians, and others interested in advancing the profession. Provides professional information and education for pharmacists and advocates for improved health of the American public through the provision of comprehensive pharmaceutical care.

Year Founded: 1852

2347 American Psychiatric Association (APA)

1000 Wilson Boulevard
Suite 1825
Arlington, VA 22209-3924
703-907-7300
888-35 -7924
Fax: 703-907-1085
E-mail: apa@psych.org
www.www.psychiatry.org

Margaret Cawley Dewar, Director
Ardell Lockerman, Sr Governance Specialist

The American Psychiatric Association is a medical specialty society comprised of over 35, 000 members who work together to ensure appropriate care and effective treatment for all persons with mental disorders, including mental retardation and substance-related disorders.

Year Founded: 1844

2348 American Psychiatric Nurses Association

3141 Fairview Park Drive
Suite 625
Falls Church, VA 22042
571-533-1919
855-863-2762
Fax: 855-883-2762
E-mail: clement.1@osu.edu
www.apna.org

Nick Croce, Executive Director
Karla Lewis, Director of Finance & Administra

Lisa Deffenbaugh Nguyen, MS, Director of Operations
Patricia Federinko, Membership Manager

Provides leadership to promote the psychiatric-mental health nursing profession, improve mental health care for culturally diverse individuals, families, groups and communities and shape health policy for the delivery of mental health services.

2349 American Psychiatric Publishing

1000 Wilson Boulevard
Suite 1825
Arlington, VA 22209-3924
703-907-7300
888-357-7924
Fax: 703-907-1085
E-mail: apa@psych.org
www.psych.org

Tara L Burkholder, Marketing
Joan Lang, Treasurer
Year Founded: 1844

2350 American Psychoanalytic Association (APsaA)

309 E 49th Street
New York, NY 10017-1601
212-752-0450
Fax: 212-593-0571
E-mail: info@apsa.com
www.apsa.org

Dean K. Stein, Executive Director
Tina Faison, Administrative Assistant to Exec
Carolyn Gatto, Scientific Program & Meetings Di
Michael Candela, Meetings & Exhibits Coordinator

Professional Membership Organization with approximately 3, 500 members nationwide, with 43 Affiliate Societies and 29 Training Institutes. Seeks to establish and maintain standards for the training of psychoanalysts and for the practice of psychoanalysis, fosters the integration of psychoanalysis with other disciplines (psychiatry, psychology, social work), and encourages research. Publications include: Journal of the Psychoanalyst (JAPA), American Psychoanalyst, a quarterly newsletter; Ethics Case Book; and Roster. Twice a year the organization sponsors scientific meetings and exhibits.

2351 American Psychologial Association: Division of Family Psychology

750 1st Street NE
Washington, DC 20002-4242
202-336-5500
800-374-2721
Fax: 202-336-5518
TDD: 202-336-6123
TTY: 202-336-6123
E-mail: webmaster@apa.org
www.apa.org

Nadine Kaslow, PhD, President
Norman B Anderson, Chief Executive Officer and Exec
Jennifer F Kelly, Secretary
Bonnie Markham, PhD, PsyD, Treasurer

A division of the American Psychological Association. Psychologists intersted in research, teaching, evaluation, and public interest initiatives in family psychology. Seeks to promote human welfare through the development, dissemination, and application of knowledge about the dynamics, structure, and functioning of the family. Conducts research and specialized education programs.

2352 American Psychological Association

750 1st Street NE
Washington, DC 20002-4242
202-336-5500
800-374-2721
Fax: 202-336-5518
TDD: 202-336-6123
TTY: 202-336-6123
www.apa.org

Nadine Kaslow, PhD, President
Norman B Anderson, Chief Executive Officer and Exec
Jennifer F Kelly, Secretary
Bonnie Markham, PhD, PsyD, Treasurer

Scientific and professional society of psychologists. Students participate as affiliates. Works to advance psychology as a science, as a profession, and as means of promoting human welfare. Annual convention.

2353 American Psychological Association: Applied Experimental and Engineering Psychology

750 First Street NE
Washington, DC 20002-4242
202-336-6013
Fax: 202-336-5518
www.apa.org

Frank A Drews, President
Scott Shappell, Secretary-Treasurer

A division of the American Psychological Association. Individuals whose principal fields of study, research, or work are within the area of applied experimental and engineering psychology. Promotes research on psychological factors in the design and use of environments and systems within which human beings work and live.

2354 American Psychology- Law Society (AP-LS)
AP-LS Central Office

750 First St. NE
Washington, DC 20002-4242
202-336-5500
TDD: 202-336-6123
TTY: 202-336-6123
E-mail: div41apa@comcast.net
www.ap-ls.org

Jennifer Skeem, President
Eve Brank, Treasurer
Jeremy Blumenthal, Secretary

A division of the American Psychological Association. It is an interdisciplinary organization devoted to the scholarship, practice and public service in psychology and law. Their goals include advancing the contributions of psychology to the understanding of law and legal institutions through basic and applied research; promoting the education of psychologists in matters of law and education of legal personnel in matters of psychology.

2355 American Psychosomatic Society

6728 Old McLean Village Drive
McLean, VA 22101-3906
703-556-9222
Fax: 703-556-8729
E-mail: info@psychosomatic.org
www.psychosomatic.org

Karen L. Weihs, MD, President
George K. Degnon, CAE, Executive Director
Laura E. Degnon, CAE, Associate Executive Director
Urs Markus Nater, PhD, Secretary-Treasurer

A worldwide community of scholars and clinicians dedicated to the scientific understanding of the interaction of mind, brain, body and social context in promoting health and contributing to the pathogenesis, course and treatment of disease. Holds an annual meeting in a different location each year.

Year Founded: 1942

2356 American Society for Adolescent Psychiatry (ASAP)

PO Box 570218
Dallas, TX 75357-218
972-613-0985
Fax: 972-613-5532
E-mail: info@adolpsych.org
www.adolpsych.org

Frances Bell, Executive Director
Mohan Nair, President

Psychiatrists concerned with the behavior of adolescents. Provides for the exchange of psychiatric knowledge, encourages the development of adequate standards and training facilities and stimulates research in the psychopathology and treatment of adolescents. Publications: Adolescent Psychiatry, annual journal. American Society for Adolescent Psychiatry Newsletter, quarterly. ASAP Membership Directory, biennial. Journal of Youth and Adolescence, bimonthly. Annual conference. Workshops.

Year Founded: 1967

2357 American Society for Clinical Pharmacology & Therapeutics

528 N Washington Street
Alexandria, VA 22314-2314
703-836-6981
Fax: 703-836-5223
E-mail: info@ascpt.org
www.ascpt.org

Sharon J. Swan, CAE, Chief Executive Officer
Judy E. Dalie, Director, Education and Meetings
Natalie Ngo, Publications Manager
Lisa Williamson, Director of Member Services

Over 1, 900 professionals whose primary interest is to promote and advance the science of human pharmacology and theraputics. Most of the members are physicians or other doctoral scientists. Other members are pharmacists, nurses, research coordinators, fellows in training and other professionals.

Year Founded: 1900

2358 American Society of Addiction Medicine

4601 N Park Avenue
Upper Arcade #101
Chevy Chase, MD 20815-4520
301-656-3920
Fax: 301-656-3815
E-mail: email@asam.org
www.asam.org

Stuart Gitlow, MD, MPH, MBA, , President
Penny S. Mills, MBA, Executive Vice President / CEO
Arlene C. Deverman, CAE, Vice President, Professional Development
Carolyn C. Lanham, CAE, Chief Operating Officer

Increase access to and improve the quality of addictions treatment. Educate physicians, medical and osteopathic, and the public.

2359 American Society of Consultant Pharmacists

1321 Duke Street
Alexandria, VA 22314-3507
703-739-1300
800-355-2727
Fax: 703-739-1321
E-mail: info@ascp.com
www.ascp.com

Sean M. Jeffery, Chairman of the Board
Jeffrey C. Delafuente, President
Jan Allen, Secretary/Treasurer
Jessilyn Dechevalier, Educational Affairs

International professional association that provides leadership, education, advocacy and resources to advance the practice of senior care pharmacy. Consultant pharmacists specializing in senior care pharmacy practice are essential participants in the health care system, ensuring that their patients medications are the most appropriate, effective, the safest possible and are used correctly. They identify, resolve and prevent medication related problems that may interfere with the goals of therapy.

Year Founded: 1969

2360 American Society of Group Psychotherapy & Psychodrama

301 N Harrison Street
Suite 508
Princeton, NJ 08540-3512
609-737-8500
Fax: 609-737-8510
E-mail: asgpp@asgpp.org
www.asgpp.org

Dave Moran, ASGPP, President
Eduardo Garcia, Executive Director
Sue Barnum, Secretary

Fosters national and international cooperation among all concerned with the theory and practice of psychodrama, sociometry, and group psychotherapy. Promotes research and fruitful application and publication of the findings. Maintains a code of professional standards.

Year Founded: 1942

2361 American Society of Health System Pharmacists

7272 Wisconsin Avenue
Bethesda, MD 20814-4836
301-657-3000
Fax: 301-664-8877
E-mail: Custserv@ashp.org
www.ashp.org

Gerald Meyer, Chairman of the Board
Paul W. Abramowitz, CEO

Thirty thousand member national professional association that represents pharmacists who practice in hospitals, health maintenance organizations, long-term care facilities, ambulatory care, home care and other components of health care systems. ASHP helps people make the best use of their medications, advances and supports the professional practice of pharmacists in hospitals and health systems and serves as their collective voice on issues related to medication use and public health.

2362 American Society of Psychoanalytic Physicians (ASPP)
13528 Wisteria Drive
Germantown, MD 20874-1049
301-540-3197
E-mail: cfcotter@aspp.net
www.aspp.net

Christine Cotter, Executive Director

An organization of physicians established for non-profit education, scientific, and professional purposes. Its objective is to futher the study of psyhcoanalytic methods for the treatment and prevention of emotional disorders and mental illnesses. The Society provides scientific meetings to foster its aims and to share information, namely research, evaluation of treatment, dissemination of information, and to publish and recognize achievement and provide professional opportunities among its members.

Year Founded: 1985

2363 American Society on Aging
575 Market St.
Suite 2100
San Francisco, CA 94105-2869
415-974-9600
800-537-9728
Fax: 415-974-0300
E-mail: info@asaging.org
www.asaging.org

Ken Dychtwald, President and CEO
Robert Lowe, Director Of Operations

Nonprofit organization committed to enhancing the knowledge and skills of those working with older adults and their families. They produce educational programs, publications, conferences and workshops.

Year Founded: 1954

2364 Annie E Casey Foundation
701 St. Paul Street
Baltimore, MD 21202-2311
410-547-6600
Fax: 410-547-6624
E-mail: webmail@aecf.org
www.aecf.org

Patrick McCarthy, President and Chief Executive Of
Teresa Markowitz, Vice President, Center for Syste
Ryan Chao, Vice President, Civic Sites and
Debra Joy P,rez, Vice President, Research, Evalua

Working to build better futures for disadvantaged children and their families in the US. The primary mission of the Foundation is to foster policies, human service reforms and community supports that more effectively meet the needs of today's vulnerable children and families.

Year Founded: 1948

2365 Association for Academic Psychiatry (AAP)
562 S. Hillcrest Avenue
#147
Elmhurst, IL 60126
770-222-2265
Fax: 866-884-6103
E-mail: lhedrick@academicpsychiatry.org
www.academicpsychiatry.org

Carole Berney MA, Administrative Director
Joan Anzia, President

Focuses on education in psychiatry at every level from beginning of medical school through lifelong learning for psychiatrists and other physicians. It seeks to help psychiatrists who are interested in careers in academic psychiatry develop the skills and knowledge in teaching, research and career development that they must have to succeed. The Association provides a forum for members to exchange ideas on teaching techniques, curriculum, and other issues to work together to solve problems. It works with other professional organizations on mutual interests and objectives through committee liaison and collaborative programs.

2366 Association for Ambulatory Behavioral Healthcare
247 Douglas Avenue
Portsmouth, VA 23707-1520
757-673-3741
Fax: 757-966-7734
E-mail: mickey@aabh.org
www.www.aabh.org/?

Christopher McGowan, President

Powerful forum for people engaged in providing mental health services. Promoting the evolution of flexible models of responsive cost-effective ambulatory behavioral healthcare.

2367 Association for Applied Psychophysiology & Biofeedback
10200 W 44th Avenue
Suite 304
Wheat Ridge, CO 80033-2840
303-422-8436
800-477-8892
Fax: 303-422-8894
E-mail: info@aapb.org
www.www.aapb.org/

David Stumph, Executive Director
Monta Greenfield, Associate Director

Their purpose is to advance the development, dissemination, and utilization of knowledge about applied psychophysiology and biofeedback to improve health and the quality of life through research, education and practice.

Year Founded: 1969

2368 Association for Behavior Analysis
550 W. Centre Avenue
Portage, MI 49024
269-492-9310
Fax: 269-492-9316
E-mail: mail@abainternational.org
www.abainternational.org

Janet Twyman, President
Maria E Malott PhD, Executive Director

Their purpose is to develop, enhance and support the growth and vitality of behavior analysis through research, education and practice.

Year Founded: 1974

2369 Association for Behavioral and Cognitive Therapies
305 Seventh Avenue
16th Floor
New York, NY 10001-6008

212-647-1890
Fax: 212-647-1865
E-mail: mebrown@abct.org
www.www.abct.org

Mary Jane Eimer, Executive Director
Mary Ellen Brown, Director of Education and Meetin
David Teisler, Director of Communications
Lisa Yarde, Membership Services Manager

Professional, interdisciplinary organization that is concerned with the application of behavioral and cognitive sciences to understanding human behavior, developing interventions to enhance the human condition and promoting the appropriate utilization of these interventions.

2370 Association for Birth Psychology

PO Box 150966
Lakewood, CO 80215
707-887-2838
Fax: 707-887-2838
E-mail: consultant@birthpsychology.com
www.birthpsychology.com

Maureen Wolfe, Executive Director
David Chamberlain, Treasurer/Website Editor

Obstetricians, pediatricians, midwives, nurses, psychotherapists, psychologists, counselors, social workers, sociologists, and others interested in birth psychology, a developing discipline concerned with the experience of birth and the correlation between the birth process and personality development. Seeks to promote communication among professionals in the field; encourage commentary, research and theory from different points of view; establish birth psychology as an autonomous science of human behavior; develop guidelines and give direction to the field. Annual conference, regional meetings, workshops.

2371 Association for Child Psychoanalysis (ACP)

7820 Enchanted Hills Blvd
#A-233
Rio Rancho, NM 87144
505-771-0372
E-mail: childanalysis@comcast.net
www.childanalysis.org

Anita Schmukler, D.O., President
Tricia Hall, Administrator

An international not-for-profit organization in which all members are highly trained child and adolescent psychoanalysts. Provides a forum for the interchange of ideas and clinical experience in order to advance the psychological treatment and understanding of children and adolescents and their families.

2372 Association for Hospital Medical Education

109 Brush Creek Road
Irwin, PA 15642-9504
724-864-7321
866-617-4780
Fax: 724-864-6153
E-mail: info@ahme.org
www.ahme.org

Carrie Eckart, MBA, President and Board Chairman
Kimball Mohn, MD, Executive Director
Margie Kleppick, Association Staff Manager
Sandi Parsons, Director of Association and Meet

National, nonprofit professional association involved in the continuum of medical education — undergraduate, graduate, and continuing medical education. More than 600 members represent hundreds of teaching hospitals, academic medical centers and consortia nationwide. Promotes improvement in medical education to meet health care needs, serves as a forum and resource for medical education information, advocates the value of medical education in health care.

Year Founded: 1956

2373 Association for Humanistic Psychology

14B Beach Road
PO Box 1190
Tiburon, CA 94920
310-692-0495
Fax: 415-435-1654
E-mail: ahpoffice@aol.com
www.ahpweb.org

Carroy U Ferguson, Co-President
Leland Bagget, Co-President
M.A. Bjarkman, Treasurer

Enhances the quality of human experience and to advance the evolution of human consciousness.

Year Founded: 1962

2374 Association for Pre- & Perinatal Psychology and Health

PO Box 150966
Lakewood, CO 80215
707-887-2838
Fax: 707-887-2838
E-mail: consultant@birthpsychology.com
www.birthpsychology.com

Maureen Wolfe, Executive Director
David Chamberlain, Treasurer/Website Editor

Forum for individuals from diverse backgrounds and disciplines interested in psychological dimensions of prenatal and perinatal experiences. Typically, this includes childbirth educators, birth assistants, doulas, midwives, obstetricians, nurses, social workers, perinatologists, pediatricians, psychologists, counselors researchers and teachers at all levels. All who share these interests are welcome to join. Quarterly journal published.

Year Founded: 1983

2375 Association for Psychoanalytic Medicine (APM)

41 Union Square West
Rm. 402
New York, NY 10003
718-548-6088
Fax: 212-866-4817
E-mail: gsagi@mac.com
www.theapm.org

Marvin Wasserman, President
Juliette Meyer, Ph.D, Secretary
David Gutman, M.D., Treasurer

A non-profit organization that is a component society of both the American Psychoanalytic Association and the International Psychoanalytic Association.

Year Founded: 1945

2376 Association for Psychological Science (APS)

1133 15th Street NW
Suite 1000
Washington, DC 20005
202-293-9300
Fax: 202-293-9350

E-mail: akraut@psychologicalscience.org
www.psychologicalscience.org

Elizabeth A. Phelps, President
Alan G. Kraut, Executive Director
G□n R. Semin, Secretary
Roberta L. Klatzky, Treasurer

The APS (previously the American Psychological Society) is a nonprofit organization dedicated to the advancement of scientific psychology and its representation at the national and international levels. The Association's mission is to promote, protect, and advance the interests of scientifically oriented psychology in research, application, teaching and the improvement of human welfare. Available on Facebook and Twitter.

Year Founded: 1988

2377 Association for Psychological Type
2415 Westwood Ave.
Suite B
Richmond, VA 23230
804-523-2907
800-847-9943
Fax: 804-288-3551
E-mail: info@aptinternational.org
www.aptinternational.org

Susan Nash, President
Jane Kise, President

Individuals involved in organizational development, religion, management, education and counseling, and who are interested in psychological type, the Myers-Briggs Type Indicator, and the works of Carl G Jung. Purpose is to share ideas related to the uses of MBTI and the application of personality type theory in any area; promotes research, development, and education in the field. Sponsors seminars, conferences, and training sessions on the use of psychological type.

2378 Association for Women in Psychology
Florida International University
DM 212
University Park
Miami, FL 33199-1
305-348-2408
Fax: 305-348-3143
E-mail: awp@fiu.edu
www.awpsych.org

Suzanna Rose PhD, Director

Nonprofit scientific and educational organization committed to encouraging feminist psychological research, theory and activism. They are an organization with a history of affirming and celebrating differences, deepening challenges, and experiencing growth as feminists.

Year Founded: 1969

2379 Association for the Advancement of Psychology
PO Box 38129
Colorado Springs, CO 80937-8129
800-869-6595
Fax: 719-520-0375
E-mail: Krivard@AAPNet.org
www.AAPNet.org

Stephen M Pfeiffer PhD, Executive Officer
Karen Rivard, Administrator

Promotes the interests of all psychologists before public and governmental bodies. AAP's fundamental mission is

the support of candidates for the US Congress who are sympathetic to psychology's concerns, through electioneering activities.

Year Founded: 1974

2380 Association of Black Psychologists
7119 Allentown Road
Suite 203
Ft. Washington, DC 20744
301-449-3082
Fax: 301-449-3084
E-mail: abpsi_office@abpsi.org
www.abpsi.org

Taasogle Daryl Rowe, Ph.D., President
Satira Streeter, Ph.D., Secretary
Carolyn Moore, Ph.D, Treasurer

Members are professional psychologists and others in associated disciplines. Aims to: enhance the psychological well-being of black people in America; define mental health in consonance with newly established psychological concepts and standards, develop policies for local, state, and national decision making that have impact on the mental health of the black community; support established black sister organizations and aid in the development of new, independent black institutions to enhance the psychological educational, cultural, and economic situation. Offers training and information on AIDS. Conducts seminars, workshops and research. Periodic conference, annual convention.

Year Founded: 1968

2381 Association of State and Provincial Psychology Boards
PO Box 3079
Peachtree City, GA 30269
678-216-1175
Fax: 678-216-1176
E-mail: aspbb@asppb.org
www.asppb.org

Fred Mill n, President
Stephen T. DeMers, Ed.D., Chief Executive Officer
Carol Webb, Ph.D., ABPP, Chief Operating Officer
Mark Russell, CPA, Financial Officer

ASPPB is the association of psychology licensing boards in the United States and Canada. They create the Examination for Professional Practice in Psychology which is used in licensing boards to assess candidates for licensure and certification. They also publish training materials for training programs and for students preparing to enter the profession

Year Founded: 1961

2382 Association of the Advancement of Gestalt Therapy
PO Box 42221
Portland, OR 97242
971-238-2248
Fax: 212-202-3974
E-mail: info@aagt.org
www.aagt.org

Peter Philippson, President
Sylvie Falschlunger, Administrative Assistant

Dynamic, inclusive, energetic nonprofit organization committed to the advancement of theory, philosophy, practice and research in Gestalt Therapy and its various applications. This includes but is not limited to personal growth, mental health, education, organization and systems development, political and social development and change, and the fine and performing arts. Their international member base includes psychiatrists, psychologists, social workers, teachers, academics, artists, writers, organizational consultants, political and social analysts, activists and students.

2383 Bazelon Center for Mental Health Law

1101 15th Street NW
Suite 1212
Washington, DC 20005-5002
202-467-5730
Fax: 202-223-0409
TDD: 202-467-4232
E-mail: communications @ bazelon.org
www.bazelon.org

Robert Berstein, President and CEO
Ira Burnim, Director
Jennifer Mathis, Deputy Director
Emily Read, Senior Staff Attorney

Provides technical support to lawyers and advocates on legal issues affecting children and adults with mental disabilities. Website has extensive legal advocacy resources and an online book store with handbooks, manuals and other publications.

Year Founded: 1972

2384 Behavioral Health Systems

2 Metroplex Drive
Suite 500
Birmingham, AL 35209-6827
205-879-1150
800-245-1150
Fax: 205-879-1178
E-mail: generalwebsite@bhs-inc.com
www.behavioralhealthsystems.com

Deborah L Stephens, Founder, Chairman & CEO
Kyle Strange, Executive Vice President & MCO
William M Patterson, M.D., Medical Director
Pat Friedley, Executive Vice President & CQO

Provides behavioral health services to business and industry which are high quality and state of the art, cost effective and accountable, uniformly accessible over a broad geographic area and care continuum, and managed within a least restrictive treatment approach.

2385 CG Jung Foundation for Analytical Psychology

28 E 39th Street
New York, NY 10016-2587
212-697-6430
Fax: 212-953-3989
E-mail: info@cgjungny.org
www.www.cgjungny.org

David Rottman, President
Joenine Roberts, Vice President
Rollin Bush, Treasurer
Anne Ortelee, Secretary

Analysts who follow the precepts of Carl G Jung, a Swiss psychologist, and any other persons interested in analytical psychology. Sponsors public lectures, films, continuing education, courses and professional seminars. Operates book service which provides publications on analytical psychology and related topics, and lectures on audio cassettes. Publishes journal, Quadrant.

Year Founded: 1962

2386 California Psychological Association

1231 I Street
Suite 204
Sacramento, CA 95814-2933
916-286-7979
Fax: 916-286-7971
E-mail: membership@cpapsych.org
www.cpapsych.org

Robert deMayo, Ph.D., ABPP, President
Jo Linder-Crow PhD, Chief Executive Officer
Patricia VanWoerkom, Director Administration & Direct
April Fernando, Ph.D., Secretary

A non-profit professional association for licensed psychologists and others affiliated with the delivery of psychological services.

Year Founded: 1948

2387 Center for Applications of Psychological Type

2815 NW 13th Street
Suite 401
Gainesville, FL 32609-2878
352-375-0160
800-777-2278
Fax: 352-378-0503
E-mail: customerservice@capt.org
www.capt.org

Nonprofit organization founded to conduct research and develop applications of the Myers-Briggs Type Indicator for the constructive use of differences. The MBTI is based on CG Jung's theory of psychological types. CAPT provides training for users of the MBTI and the Murphy-Meisgeier Type Indicator for Children, publishes and distributes books and resource materials, and maintains the Isabel Briggs Myers memorial library and the MBTI Bibliography. The MBTI is used in counseling individuals and families, to understand differences in learning styles, and for improving leadership and teamwork in organizations.

Year Founded: 1975

2388 Children's Health Council

650 Clark Way
Palo Alto, CA 94304-2340
650-326-5530
Fax: 650-688-3676
E-mail: info@chconline.org
www.chconline.org

Andrew P Valentine, Chair
James Otieno, Vice-Chair
Carol M Roccuzzo, MBA, CHC, Director of Operations & Human R
Chris Harris, MEd, Director of CHC Schools & Head o

Working to make a measurable difference in the lives of children who face severe or complex behavioral and developmental challenges by providing interdisciplinary educational, assessment and treatment services and professional training.

2389 Christian Association for Psychological Studies

PO Box 365
Batavia, IL 60510-0365
630-639-9478
Fax: 630-454-3799

E-mail: info@caps.net
www.caps.net

Stephen P Greggo, Psy.D., Chair
Sally Schwer Canning, Ph.D., Vice Chair
Rod Marshall, Ed.S., Treasurer
Julia P Grimm, Ph.D., Secretary

Psychologists, marriage and family therapists, social workers, educators, physicians, nurses, ministers, researchers,
pastoral counselors, and rehabilitation workers and others
professionally engaged in the fields of psychology, counseling, psychiatry, pastoring and related areas. Association
is based upon a genuine commitment to superior clinical,
pastoral and scientific enterprise in the theoretical and applied social sciences and theology, assuming persons in
helping professions will be guided to professional and
personal growth and a greater contribution to others in this
way.

Year Founded: 1956

2390 Clinical Social Work Federation

PO Box 10
Garrisonville, VA 22463
703-340-1456
855-279-2669
Fax: 703-269-0707
E-mail: nfscswlo@aol.com
www.www.clinicalsocialworkassociation.org

Stephanie Hadley, LCSW, President
Michael Rose, Ph.D., LCSW, Treasurer
Angela Oddone, LCSW, Secretary

A confederation of 31 state societies for clinical social
work. The state societies are formed as voluntary associations for the purpose of promoting the highest standards of
professional education and clinical practice. Each society
is active with legislative advocacy and lobbying efforts for
adequate and appropriate mental health services and coverage at their state and national levels of government.

2391 Commission on Accreditation of Rehabilitation Facilities

6951East Southpoint Road
Tucson, AZ 85756-9407
520-325-1044
888-281-6531
Fax: 520-318-1129
TTY: 888-281-6531
www.carf.org

Brian J Boon PhD, President/CEO
Amanda E Birch, Administrator of Operations

Promotes the quality, value and optimal outcomes through
a consultative accreditation process that centers on enhancing the lives of the people served.

Year Founded: 1966

2392 Commonwealth Fund

One E 75th Street
New York, NY 10021-2692
212-606-3800
Fax: 212-606-3500
E-mail: cmwf@cmwf.org
www.www.commonwealthfund.org

James R. Tallon, Jr., Chairman
David Blumenthal, President
John E. Craig, Executive Vice President and Chi
Donald Moulds, Executive Vice President for Pro

Private foundation that supports independent research on
health and social issues and make grants to improve health
care practice and policy.

2393 Community Action Partnership

1140 Connecticut Avenue
Suite 1210
Washington, DC 20036
202-265-7546
Fax: 202-265-5048
E-mail: info@communityactionpartnership.com
www.communityactionpartnership.com

Thomas Tenorio, CCAP, Chair
Joyce J Dorsey, 1st Vice Chair
Dalitso S Sulamoyo, CCAP, 2nd Vice Chair
Peter Kilde, 3rd Vice Chair

The national organization representing the interests of the
1, 000 Community Action Agencies working to fight poverty at the local level.

Year Founded: 1971

2394 Community Anti-Drug Coalitions of America

625 Slaters Lane
Suite 300
Alexandria, VA 22314-1176
703-706-0560
800-542-2322
Fax: 703-706-0565
E-mail: info@cadca.org
www.www.cadca.org

Arthur T. Dean, Chairman & CEO
Celeste Brown, Office Manager
Jasmine Carrasco, Youth Programs Associate
Na'Denna Colbert, Membership Manager

With more than five thousand members across the country,
CADCA is working to build and strengthen the capacity of
community coalitions to create safe, healthy, and drug free
communities. CADCA supports its members with technical
assistance and training, public policy, media and marketing,
conferences and special events.

Year Founded: 1992

2395 Corporate Counseling Associates

475 Park Avenue South
Fifth Floor
New York, NY 10016-6901
212-686-6827
800-833-8707
Fax: 212-686-6511
E-mail: info@corporatecounseling.com
www.www.ccainc.com

Robert Levy, President
Thomas Diamante, PhD, Principal
Georgia Critsimilios, LCSW, Senior Vice President
Russell Correa, EdM, Director

Customized, integrated workplace solutions designed to enhance business performance by enriching employee
productivity.

Year Founded: 1984

2396 Council on Social Work Education

1701 Duke Street
Suite 200
Alexandria, VA 22314-3457

703-683-8080
Fax: 703-683-8099
E-mail: info@cswe.org
www.cswe.org

Julia M. Watkins PhD, Executive Director
Nicole Demarco, Executive Assistant To Exec. Dir

A national association that preserves and enhances the quality of social work education for the purpose of promoting the goals of individual and community well being and social justice. Pursues this mission through setting and maintaining policy and program standards, accrediting bachelors and masters degree programs in social work, promoting research and faculty development, and advocating for social work education.

Year Founded: 1952

2397 Developmental Disabilities Nurses Association

PO Box 536489
Orlando, FL 32853-6489
407-835-0642
800-888-6733
Fax: 407-426-7440
www.ddna.org

Kathy Brown, President
Wendy Herbers, RN, CDDN, QDD, Vice-President
Richanne Cunningham, RN, QMRP, , Secretary
Karen Hill, RN, BSN, CDDN, Treasurer

National nonprofit professional association for nurses working with individuals with developmental disabilities. Publishes a quarterly newsletter.

Year Founded: 1992

2398 Division of Independent Practice of the American Psychological Association (APADIP)

919 W Marshall Avenue
Phoenix, AZ 85013-1734
602-246-6219
Fax: 602-246-6577
E-mail: div42apa@cox.net
www.division42.org

Gordon I Herz PhD, President
Gerald Koocher PhD, Treasurer
June W J Ching PhD, President-Elect

Members of the American Psychological Association engaged in independent practice. Works to ensure that the needs and concerns of independent psychology practitioners are considered by the APA. Gathers and disseminates information on legislation affecting the practice of psychology, managed care, and other developments in the health care industries, office management, malpractice risk and insurance, hospital management. Offers continuing professional and educational programs. Semiannual convention, with board meeting.

2399 Employee Assistance Professionals Association

EAPA Exchange
4350 North Fairfax Drive
Suite 740
Arlington, VA 22203
703-387-1000
Fax: 703-522-4585
E-mail: ceo@eap-association.org
www.eapassn.org

Jill Royer, President
Linda Dismuke, Acting Secretary

International association of approximately 5, 000 members who are primarily employee assistance professionals as well as individuals in related fields such as human resources, chemical dependency treatment, mental health treatment, managed behavioral health care, counseling and benefits administration. Hosts annual EAP conference.

Year Founded: 1971

2400 Employee Assistance Society of North America

2001 Jefferson Davis Highway
Suite 1004
Arlington, VA 22202-3617
703-416-0060
Fax: 703-416-0014
E-mail: easnamember@ardel.com
www.www.easna.org

George Martin, President
Judith Plotkin, MSW, Vice President
Bob Mc Lean, Executive Director
Patrick Gagne, Treasurer

International group of professional leaders with competencies in such specialties as workplace and family wellness, employee benefits and organizational development. Maintains accreditation program, membership services and professional training opportunities, promotes high standards of employee assistance programs.

Year Founded: 1985

2401 Gerontoligical Society of America

1220 L Street NW
Suite 901
Washington, DC 20005-1503
202-842-1275
Fax: 202-842-1150
E-mail: geron@geron.org
www.geron.org

Patricia Walker, Executive Director
Linda Krogh Harootyan, Interim Executive Director

Nonprofit professional organization with more than 5000 members in the field of aging. GSA provides researchers, educators, practitioners and policy makers with opportunities to understand, advance, integrate and use basic and applied research on aging to improve the quality of life as one ages.

2402 Gorski-Cenaps Corporation Training & Consultation

13194 Spring Hill Drive
Spring Hill, FL 34609
352-596-8000
Fax: 352-596-8002
E-mail: tresa@cenaps.com
www.cenaps.com

Tresa Watson, Manager
Tresa Watson, Business Manager

Cenaps provides advanced clinical skills training for the addiction behavioral health and mental health fields. Their focus is recovery and relapse prevention.

2403 Group for the Advancement of Psychiatry

PO Box 570218
Dallas, TX 75357-218
972-613-0985
Fax: 972-613-5532

E-mail: frad1@airmail.net
www.ourgap.org

Frances Roton, Executive Director

An organization of nationally respected psychiatrists dedicated to shaping psychiatric thinking, public programs and clinical practice in mental health. Meets twice a year at the Renaissance Westchester Hotel in White Plains, NY.

Year Founded: 1946

2404 Institute of HeartMath

14700 W Park Avenue
Boulder Creek, CA 95006-9318
831-338-8700
800-711-6221
Fax: 831-338-8504
E-mail: info@heartmath.org
www.heartmath.org

Katherine Floriano, Chairwoman
Sara Childre, President and CEO
Rollin McCraty, Ph.D., Executive Vice President and Dir
Brian Kabaker, Chief Financial Officer and Dire

Nonprofit research and education on stress, emotional physiology and heart-brain interactions. Purpose is to reduce stress, school violence, improve mental and emotional attitudes, promote harmony within facilities and communities, improve academic performance and improve workplace health and performance. Research facility provides psychometric assessments for both individual and organizational assessment as well as autonomic assessments for physiological assessment and diagnostic purposes. Education initiative currently developing curriculum for rehabilitation of incarcerated teen felons in drug and alcohol recovery program.

Year Founded: 1991

2405 Institute on Psychiatric Services: American Psychiatric Association

1000 Wilson Boulevard
Suite 1825
Arlington, VA 22209-3924
703-907-7300
888-35 -7924
E-mail: apa@psych.org
www.psych.org

Carol Robinowitz, President

Open to employees of all psychiatric and related health and educational facilities. Includes lectures by experts in the field and workshops and accredited courses on problems, programs and trends. Offers on-site Job Bank, which lists opportunities for mental health professionals. Organized scientific exhibits. Publications: Psychiatric Services, monthly journal. Annual Institute on Psychiatric Services conference and exhibits in October, Chicago, IL.

2406 International Center for the Study of Psychiatry And Psychology (ISCPP)

1036 Park Avenue
Suite 1B
New York, NY 10028-971
212-861-7400
E-mail: djriccio@aol.com
www.icspp.org

Peter Breggin, Founder/Director Emeritus
Dominick Riccio PhD, Executive Director

Nonprofit research and educational network whose focus is the critical study of the mental health movement. ICSPP is completely independent and their funding consists solely of individual membership dues. Fosters prevention and treatment of mental and emotional disorders. Promotes alternatives to administering psychiatric drugs to children.

2407 International Society for Developmental Psychobiology

8181 Tezel Road
#10269
San Antonio, TX 78250-3092
830-796-9393
866-377-4416
Fax: 830-796-9394
E-mail: isdp@isdpcentraloffice.org
www.isdp.org

Pamela Hunt, President
Hawley Montgomery-Downs, Conference Coordinator
Susan Swithers, Program Director
Gale Kleven, Treasurer

Members are research scientists in the field of developmental psychobiology and biology and psychology students. Promotes research in the field of developmental psychobiology, the study of the brain and brain behavior throughout the life span and in relation to other biological proccesses. Stimulates communication and interaction among scientists in the field. Provides the editorship for the journal, Development Psychobiology. Bestows awards. Compiles statistics. Annual conference.

2408 International Society of Political Psychology
Moynihan Institute of Global Affairs

126 Ward Street
Suite 1213
Columbus, NC 28722
828-894-5422
Fax: 315-443-9085
E-mail: ispp@maxwell.syr.edu
www.http://ispp.org

Stanley Feldman, President
Severine Bennett, Executive Director

Facilitates communication across disciplinary, geographic and political boundaries among scholars, concerned individuals in government and public posts, the communication media and elsewhere who have a scientific interest in the relationship between politics and psychological processes. ISPP seeks to advance the quality of scholarship in political psychology and to increase the usefulness of work in political psychology.

2409 International Transactional Analysis Association (ITAA)

2843 Hopyard Road
Suite 155
Pleasanton, CA 94588
925-600-8110
Fax: 925-600-8112
E-mail: info@itaa-net.org
www.www.itaaworld.org

Ken Fogleman, Manager
Lee Beer, Webmaster

A non-profit educational organization with members in over 65 countries. Its purpose is to advance the theory, methods and principles of transactional analysis.

2410 Jean Piaget Society: Society for the Study of Knowledge and Development (JPSSSKD)
Department Of Psychology
Clark University
950 Main St
Worcester, MA 01610-1400
508-793-7250
Fax: 508-793-7265
E-mail: webmaster@piaget.org
www.piaget.org

Nancy Budwig, President
Ashley Maynard, Treasurer

Scholars, teachers, and researchers interested in exploring the nature of the developmental construction of human knowledge. Purpose is to further research on knowledge and development, especially in relation to the work of Jean Piaget, a Swiss developmentalist noted for his work in child psychology, the study of human development, and the origin and growth of human knowledge. Conducts small meetings and programs.

2411 Med Advantage
11301 Corporate Boulevard
Suite 300
Orlando, FL 32817-1445
407-282-5131
Fax: 407-282-9240
E-mail: info@med-advantage.com
www.www.med-advantage.com/

John Witty, Owner

Fully accredited by URAC and certified in all 11 elements by NCQA, Med Advantage is one of the oldest credentials verification organizations in the country. Over the past eight years, they have developed sophisticated computer systems and one of the largest data warehouses of medical providers in the nation, containing information on over 900,000 healthcare providers. Their system is continually updated from primary source data required to meet the standards of the URAC, NCQA and JCAHO.

2412 Medical Group Management Association
104 Inverness Terrace E
Englewood, CO 80112-5313
303-799-1111
877-275-6462
Fax: 303-643-9599
E-mail: service@mgma.com
www.mgma.com

William Jessee, CEO
Steve Hellebush, COO

The national membership association providing information networking and professional development for the individuals who manage and lead medical group practices.

Year Founded: 1926

2413 Mental Health Corporations of America
1876-A Eider Court
Tallahassee, FL 32308-4537
850-942-4900
Fax: 850-942-0560
E-mail: heveyd@mhca.com
www.mhca.com

Chris Wyre MBA, Chairman
Dale Shreve, President & CEO

Tara Boyter, Director, Communications & Membe
Glenda Deal, Director, Conference Services &

Membership in MHCA is by invitation only. It is the organization's intent to include in its network only the highest quality behavioral healthcare organizations in the country. Their alliance is designed to strengthen members' competitive position, enhance their leadership capabilities and facilitate their strategic networking opportunities.

2414 Mental Health Materials Center (MHMC)
PO Box 304
Bronxville, NY 10708-304
914-337-6596
Fax: 914-779-0161

Alex Sareyan, President

Professionals of mental health and health education, seeking to stimulate the development of wider, more effective channels of communication between health educators and the public. Provides consulting services to nonprofit organizations on the implementation of their publishing operations in areas related to mental health and health. Publications: Study on Suicide Training Manual. Survival Manual for Medical Students. Books, booklets and pamphlets. Annual Meeting in New York City.

2415 National Academy of Neuropsychology (NAN)
7555 E Hampden Ave
Ste 525
Denver, CO 80231-4836
303-691-3694
Fax: 303-691-5983
E-mail: office@nanonline.org
www.nanonline.org

Daniel Allen, Ph.D., President
Laurie Ryan, Ph.D., Treasurer
Donna Broshek, Ph.D., Secretary

Clinical neuropsychologists and others interested in brain-behavior relationships. Works to preserve and advance knowledge regarding the assessment and remediation of neuropsychological disorders. Promotes the development of neuropsychology as a science and profession; develops standard of practice and training guidelines for the field; fosters communication between members, represents the professional interests of members, serves as an information resource, facilitates the exchange of information among related organizations. Offers continuing education programs, conducts research.

Year Founded: 1975

2416 National Association For Children's Behavioral Health
1025 Connecticut Avenue NW
Suite 1012
Washington, DC 20036-5417
202-857-9735
Fax: 202-362-5145
www.www.nacbh.org

Beth Chadwick, President
Joy Midman, Executive Director

To promote the availability and delivery of appropriate and relevant services to children and adolescents with, or at risk of, serious emotional disturbances and their families. Advocate for the full array of mental health and related services necessary, the development and use of assessment and outcome tools based on functional as well as clinical indicators, and the elimination of categorial funding barriers.

2417 National Association for Advancement of Psychoanalysis

80 Eighth Avenue
Suite 1501
New York, NY 10011-5126
212-741-0515
Fax: 212-366-4347
E-mail: NAAP@NAAP.org
www.naap.org

Doughlas F. Maxwell, President
Margery Quackenbush, Executive Director
Kirsty Cardinale, NAAP News Editor
Lucinda Antrim, Secretary

Year Founded: 1972

2418 National Association for the Advancement of Psychoanalysis
NAAP News, E-Bulletin

80 Eighth Avenue
Suite 1501
New York, NY 10011-5126
212-741-0515
Fax: 212-366-4347
E-mail: NAAP@NAAP.org
www.naap.org

Margery Quackenbush, Executive Director
Douglas F. Maxwell, President
Kirsty Cardinale, NAAP News Editor

Certified psychoanalysts disseminating psychoanalytic principles to the medical-psychiatric profession and the general community. Conducts scientific meetings. Supports research programs, sponsors public educational lectures. Publications: NAAP News, Quarterly; Registry of Psycho-analysts, Annual, E-Bulletin, Online Publication

Year Founded: 1972

2419 National Association of Addiction Treatment Providers

11380 ProsperityFarms Road
Suite 209A
Palm BeachGardens, FL 33410
561-429-4527
Fax: 561-429-4650
E-mail: rhunsicker@naatp.org
www.naatp.org

Michael E. Walsh, MS, CAP, BRI I, President/CEO

The mission of the National Association of Addiction Treatment Providers (NAATP) is to promote, assist and en-hance the delivery of ethical, effective, research-based treatment for alcoholism and other drug addictions. Pro-vides members and the public with accurate, responsible in-formation and other resources related to the treatment of these diseases, advocates for increased access to and avail-ability of quality treatment for those who suffer from alco-holism and other drug addictions; works in partnership with other organizations and individuals that share NAATP's mission and goals.

Year Founded: 1978

2420 National Association of Community Health Centers

7501 Wisconsin Ave
Suite 1100W
Bethesda, MD 20814
301-347-0400
Fax: 301-347-0459
www.nachc.com

Tom Van Coverdan, President/CEO
Dave Taylor, Chief Operating Officer
Darline DeMott, Corporate Executive Manager
Kathy Bennett, Associate Corporate Executive Ma

A non-profit organization whose mission is to enhance and expand access to quality, community-responsive health care for America's medically underserved and uninsured. A major source for information, data, research and advo-cacy on key issues affecting community-based health cen-ters and the delivery of health care. Provides education, training, technical assistance and leadership development to health center staff, boards and others to promote excel-lence and cost-effectiveness in health delivery practice and community board governance. Builds partnerships and linkages that stimulate public and private sector investment in the delivery of quality health care services to medically underserved communities.

Year Founded: 1971

2421 National Association of Nouthetic Counselors

2825 Lexington Road
Louisville, KY 40280
502-410-5526
Fax: 317-337-9199
E-mail: info@nanc.org
www.nanc.org

Heath Lambert, Executive Director
Randy Patten, Director of Training & Advanceme
Jim Patten, Conference Director
Amber Komatsu, Membership Services Coordinator

NANC is a fellowship of Christian counselors and laymen who have banded together to promote excellence in biblical counseling. NANC was founded in 1975 in service to Christ to address several needs in the counseling community.

Year Founded: 1975

2422 National Association of Psychiatric Health Systems

900 17th Street NW
Suite 420
Washington, DC 20006-2507
202-393-6700
Fax: 202-783-6041
E-mail: naphs@naphs.org
www.naphs.org

Mark Covall, CEO
Kathleen McCann, Director of Quality
Maria Merlie, Director of Administration
Caroline Scott, Administrative Assistant

Advocates for behavioral health and represents provider systems that are committed to the delivery of responsive, accountable, and clinically effective treatment and preven-tion programs for children, adolescents, adults and older adults with mental and substance abuse disorders.

Year Founded: 1933

2423 National Association of School Psychologists (NASP)
4340 East West Highway
Suite 402
Bethesda, MD 20814-4468
301-657-0270
Fax: 301-657-0275
E-mail: sgorin@naspweb.org
www.nasponline.org

Sally Baas, President
Susan Gorin, Executive Director
Laura Benson, Chief Operating Officer
Katie Britton, Manager, Special Projects

School psychologists who serve the mental health and educational needs of all children and youth. Encourages and provides opportunites for professional growth of individual members. Informs the public on the services and practice of school psychology, and advances the standards of the profession. Operates national school psychologist certification system. Sponsers children's services.

2424 National Association of Social Workers
750 First Street NE
Suite 700
Washington, DC 20002-4241
202-408-8600
800-638-8799
Fax: 202-336-8313
www.socialworkers.org

Jeane W. Anastas, PhD, LMSW, President
E. Jane Middleton, DSW, MSW, Vice President
Jacqueline Durham, MSW, LCSW, Secretary
Mary L. McCarthy, PhD, LMSW, Treasurer

Works to enhance the professional growth and development of its members, to create and maintain professional standards, and to advance sound social policies.

2425 National Association of State Mental Health Program Directors (NASMHPD)
66 Canal Center Plaza
Suite 302
Alexandria, VA 22314-1568
703-739-9333
Fax: 703-548-9517
E-mail: roy.praschil@nasmhpd.org
www.nasmhpd.org

Robert W Glover, Executive Director
Shina Animasahun, Network Manager
Stuart Gordon, JD, Director/Policy & Healthcare Ref
Kelle Masten, Program Associate

State commissioners in charge of state mental disability programs for children and youth, aged, legal services, forensic services and adult services. Promotes state government agencies to deliver services to mentally disabled persons and fosters the exchange of scientific and program information in the administration of public mental health programs. Publications: Children and Youth Update, periodic. Federal Agencies, periodic newsletter. State Report, periodic newsletter.

2426 National Business Coalition Forum on Health (NBCH)
1015 18th Street NW
Suite 730
Washington, DC 20036-5207

202-775-9300
Fax: 202-775-1569
E-mail: awebber@nbch.org
www.www.nbch.org

Brian Klepper, Chief Executive Officer
Susan Dorsey, Vice President of Education
Sara Hanlon, Vice President of Member Support
Maria Cornejo, Director of Operations

A national, non-profit membership organization of employer-based coalitions. Dedicated to value-based purchasing of health care services through the collective action of public and private purchasers. NCBH seeks to accelerate the nations progress towards safe, efficient, high quality health care and the improved health status of the American population.

2427 National Coalition for the Homeless
2201 P Street NW
Washington, DC 20037-1033
202-462-4822
E-mail: info@nationalhomeless.org
www.www.nationalhomeless.org

Jerry Jones, Executive Director
Michael Stoops, Director of Community Organizing
Megan Hustings, Director of Operations
Brian Parks, Director of National Service Pro

A national network of people who are currenlty experiencing or have experienced homelessness, activists and advocates, community-based and faith-based service providers, and others commiited to ending homelessness.

Year Founded: 1984

2428 National Committee for Quality Assurance
1100 13th Street NW
Suite 1000
Washington, DC 20005-4285
202-955-3500
Fax: 202-955-3599
www.ncqa.org

Margaret E O'Kane, President
Tom Fluegel, Chief Operating Officer
Patricia Barrett, Vice President, Product Developm
Mary Barton, Vice President, Performance Meas

A non-profit organization whose mission is to improve health care quality everywhere and to transform health care quality through measurement, transparency and accountability.

2429 National Council of Juvenile and Family Court Judges
PO Box 8970
Reno, NV 89507-8970
775-784-6012
Fax: 775-784-6628
E-mail: staff@ncjfcj.org
www.ncjfcj.org

David Stucki, President
Mari Kay Bickett, JD, Chief ExecutiveOfficer
Cheryl Dailey, CPA, CMA, CFE, , Chief Financial Officer
Cheryl Davidek, Chief Administrative Officer

Their mission is to improve courts and systems practice and raise awareness of the core issues that touch the lives of many of our nation's childrens and families.

Year Founded: 1937

2430 National Council on Aging
1901 L Street NW
4th Floor
Washington, DC 20036-3540
202-479-1200
Fax: 202-479-0735
E-mail: info@ncoa.org
www.ncoa.org

Richard Browdie, Chair
James Firman, EdD, President and CEO
Andrew Greene, Secretary & Treasurer
Jay Greenberg, ScD, CEO, NCOA Services, LLC

NCOA is a nonprofit service and advocacy organization. NCOA is a ntional voice for millions of older adults, especially those that are vulnerable and disadvantaged and the community organizations that serve them. It brings together non profit organizations, businesses, and government to develop creative solutions that improve the lives of older adults.

Year Founded: 1950

2431 National Mental Health Association
2000 N Beauregard Street
6th Floor
Alexandria, VA 22311-1748
703-684-7722
800-969-6642
Fax: 703-684-5968
TTY: 800-433-5959
www.mentalhealthamerica.net

David Shern, CEO
Kate Gaston, VP Afiliate Services

Dedicated to improving treatments, understanding and services for adults and children with mental health needs. Working to win political support for funding for school mental health programs. Provides information about a wide range of disorders.

Year Founded: 1909

2432 National Nurses Association
1767 Business Center Drive
Suite 150
Reston, VA 20190-5332
703-438-3000
877-662-6253
E-mail: info@nationalnurses.org
www.nationalnurses.org

Laurie Campbell PhD, Executive Director

Purpose is to help enhance the personal development as well as economic well being of its members. They provide services and benefits meaningful to the unique demands of the nursing professional.

Year Founded: 1984

2433 National Pharmaceutical Council
1717 Pennsylvania Ave., NW
Suite 800
Washington, DC 20006
202-827-2100
Fax: 202-827-0314
E-mail: info@npcnow.com
www.www.npcnow.org/?

Dan Leonard, MA, President
Patricia L. Adams, VP, Business Operations & Extern

Robert W. Dubois, MD, PhD, Chief Science Officer
Melissa Baulkwill, Director, Administration

NPC sponsors a variety of research and education projects aimed at demonstrating that the appropriate use of pharmaceuticals improves both patient treatment outcomes and the cost effective delivery of overall health care services.

2434 National Psychological Association for Psychoanalysis (NPAP)
40 West 13th Street
New York, NY 10011-7802
212-924-7440
Fax: 212-989-7543
E-mail: info@npap.org
www.npap.org

Carl Weinberg, President
Rosaleen Horn, Vice President
Ann Rose Simon, Treasurer
Penny Rosen, Corresponding Secretary

Professional society for practicing psychoanalysts. Conducts training program leading to certification in psychoanalysis. Offers information and private referral service for the public. Operates speakers' bureau. Publications: National Psychological Association for Psychoanalysis-Bulletin, biennial. National Psychological Association for Psychoanalysis-News and Reviews, semiannual. Psychoanalytic Review, bimonthly journal.

Year Founded: 1948

2435 National Register of Health Service Providers in Psychology
1200 New York Avenue NW
Suite 800
Washington, DC 20005-3873
202-783-7663
Fax: 202-347-0550
www.nationalregister.org

Raymond A Folen, PhD, President/Chair
Andrew P Boucher, Assistant Director
Julia Bernstein, Membership Coordinator
Deanne Canieso, Communications Coordinator, MPH,

Psychologists who are licensed or certified by a state/provincial board of examiners of psychology and who have met council criteria as health service providers in psychology.

Year Founded: 1974

2436 National Treatment Alternative for Safe Communities
1500 N Halsted
Chicago, IL 60642-2517
312-376-0950
Fax: 312-376-5889
E-mail: information@tasc-il.org
www.tasc-il.org

Marcia J. Lipetz, PhD, Chair
Cecil V. Curtwright, Vice Chair / Secretary
Andreason Brown, Chief Financial Officer
Lancert A. Foster, CPA, Treasurer

TASC is a not-for-profit organization that provides behavioral health recovery management services for individuals with substance abuse and mental health disorders. They provide direct services, design model programs and build collaborative networks between public systems and community-based human service providers. TASC's purpose is to see that under-served populations gain access to the services they need for health and self-sufficiency, while also ensuring that public and private resources are used most efficiently.

2437 North American Society of Adlerian Psychology (NASAP)

NASAP
429 E. Dupont Road
Suite 276
Fort Wayne, IN 46825
260-267-8807
Fax: 260-818-2098
E-mail: info@alfrdadler.org
www.alfredadler.org

Richard Watts, President
Susan Belangee, Vice President
Michele Frey, Secretary
Susan (Zsuzs Burak, Treasurer

NASAP is a professional organization for couselors, educators, psychologists, parent educators, business professionals, researchers and others who are interested in Adler's Individual Psychology. Membership includes journals, newsletters, conferences and training.

Year Founded: 1952

2438 Pharmaceutical Care Management Association

601 Pennsylvania Avenue NW
7th Floor
Washington, DC 20004-2601
202-756-7210
Fax: 202-207-3623
E-mail: info@pcmanet.org
www.pcmanet.org

Dirk McMahon, Chairman
Mark Merritt, President & Chief Executive Offi
Kristin Bass, Senior Vice President, Federal A
Timothy Brogan, Assistant Vice President, Public

A national association representing Pharmacy Benefit Managers. They are dedicated to enhancing the proven tools and techniques that PBMs have pioneered in the marketplace and working to lower the cost of prescription drugs for more than 200 million Americans.

2439 Physicians for a National Health Program

29 E Madison
Suite 602
Chicago, IL 60602-4406
312-782-6006
Fax: 312-782-6007
E-mail: info@pnhp.org
www.pnhp.org

Andrew D Coates, MD, FACP, President
Quentin D Young, MD, MACP, National Coordinator
Claudia M Fegan, MD, CHCQM, FACP, Treasurer
Gordon Schiff, MD, Secretary

A single issue organization advocating a universal, comprehensive Single-Payer National Health Program.

Year Founded: 1987

2440 Professional Risk Management Services

The Psychiatrists' Program
1401 Wilson Boulevard
Suite 700
Arlington, VA 22209-2434
800-245-3333
www.www.prms.com

Stephen Sills, CEO
Deriny Rodriguez, JD, COO

PRMS, Inc. specializes in medical professional liability insurance programs and claims and risk management services - on a bundled and unbundled basis for individual healthcare providers, group practices, facilities, associations, and organizations.

2441 Psychiatric Society of Informatics American Association for Technology in Psychiatry

PO Box 11
Bronx, NY 10464-11
718-502-9469
E-mail: aatp@techpsych.org
www.techpsych.org

Robert Kennedy, Executive Director
Carlyle Chan, Secretary
Naakesh Dewan, President

Year Founded: 1995

2442 Psychohistory Forum

627 Dakota Trail
Franklin Lakes, NJ 07417-1043
201-891-7486
E-mail: pelovitz@aol.com
www.cliospsyche.org

Paul H Elovitz PhD, Editor

Psychologists, psychiatrists, psychotherapists, social workers, historians, psychohistorians and others having a scholarly interest in the integration of depth psychology and history. Aids individuals in psychohistorical research. Holds lecture series. Publications: Clio's Psyche: Understanding the Why of Current Events and History, quarterly journal. Immigrant Experience: Personal Narrative and Psychological Analysis, monograph. Periodic Meeting.

Year Founded: 1994

2443 Psychology of Religion

Doctoral Program in Clinical Psychology
750 First Street NE
Washington, DC 20002-4242
202-336-6013
Fax: 202-218-3599
E-mail: division@apa.org
www.www.apa.org/about/division/div36.aspx

Elizabeth Hall, President
Gina Magyar-Russell, Secretary

A division of the American Psychologial Association. Seeks to encourage and accelerate research, theory, and practice in the psychology of religion and related areas. Facilitates the dissemination of data on religious and allied issues and on the integration of these data with current psychological research, theory and practice.

2444 Psychonomic Society

2785 E. Posse Court
Green Valley, AZ 85614

520-232-3117
Fax: 520-232-3117
E-mail: secretary-treasurer@psychonomic.org
www.psychonomic.org

Gavin Wilson, Manager
Roger Mellgren, Convention Manager

Persons qualified to conduct and supervise scientific research in psychology or allied sciences; members must hold a PhD degree or its equivalent and must have published significant research other than doctoral dissertation. Promotes the communication of scientific research in psychology and allied sciences.

Year Founded: 1959

2445 Rapid Psychler Press
2014 Holland Ave
Suite 374
Port Huron, MI 48060-1994
519-667-2335
888-779-2453
Fax: 519-675-0610
E-mail: rapid@psychler.com
www.psychler.com

David Robinson, Publisher

Produces books and presentation media for educating mental health professionals. Products cover a wide range of learning needs. Where possible, humor is incorporated as an educational aid to enhance learning and retention.

2446 Risk and Insurance Management Society
1065 Avenue Of The Americas
13th Floor
New York, NY 10018
212-286-9292
Fax: 212-986-9716
www.rims.org

Carolyn Snow, President
Mary Roth, Executive Director
Richard Roberts, Vice President
Aurea Hernando, Executive Assistant

2447 Screening for Mental Health
1 Washington Street
Suite 304
Wellesley Hills, MA 02481-1706
781-239-0071
Fax: 781-431-7447
E-mail: smhinfo@mentalhealthscreening.org
www.mentalhealthscreening.org

Douglas George Jacobs, M.D., President & Medical Director

Nonprofit organization devoted to assisting people with undiagnosed, untreated mental illness connect with local treatment resources via national screening programs for depression, anxiety, eating disorders and alcohol problems.

2448 Sigmund Freud Archives (SFA)
16 Channing Place
c/o Harold P Blum, MD
Cambridge, MA 02138
516-621-6850
E-mail: aok@kris.org
www.www.freudarchives.org

Deanna Holtzman, President
Anton O. Kris, Executive Director
John M. Ross, Secretary/Treasurer

Psychoanalysts interested in the preservation and collection of scientific and personal writings of Sigmund Freud. Assists in research on Freud's life and work and the evolution of psychoanalytic thought. Collects and classifies all documents, papers, publications, personal correspondence and historical data written by, to, and on Freud. Transmits all materials collected to the Library of Congress. Annual meeting in New York City.

Year Founded: 1951

2449 Society for Pediatric Psychology (SPP)
Citadel
PO Box 3968
Lawrence, KS 66046
785-856-0713
Fax: 785-856-0759
E-mail: APAdiv54@gmail.com
www.www.apadivisions.org/division-54/index.aspx

Lori Stark, President
Christina Adams, Secretary

Dedicated to research and practice addressing the relationship between children's physical, cognitive, social, and emotional functioning and their physical well-being, including maintenance of health, promotion of positive health behaviors, and treatment of chronic and serious medical conditions. A division of the APA. Bimonthly Journal, Newletter three times a year.

2450 Society for Personality Assessment
6109H Arlington Boulevard
Falls Church, VA 22044-2708
703-534-4772
Fax: 703-564-6905
E-mail: manager@spaonline.org
www.personality.org

Ronald J Ganellen, Ph.D., President
Giselle Hass, PsyD, Secretary
John McNulty, Ph.D., Treasurer
Robert Bornstein, PhD, President-Elect

International professional trade association for psychologists, behavioral scientists, anthropologists, and psychiatrists. Promotes the study, research development and application of personality assessment.

2451 Society for Psychophysiological Research
2424 American Lane
Madison, WI 53704-3102
608-443-2470
Fax: 608-443-2474
E-mail: homeoffice@scmhr.org
www.scmhr.org

Lisa Nelson, Manager
Karen Quigley, Treasurer

Founded in 1960, the Society for Psychophysiological Research is an international scientific society. The purpose of the society is to foster research on the interrelationship between physiological and phychological aspects of behavior.

2452 Society for Women's Health Research (SWHR)
1025 Connecticut Avenue NW
Suite 601
Washington, DC 20036-5447

202-223-8224
Fax: 202-833-3472
E-mail: info@swhr.org
www.www.womenshealthresearch.org

Susan Alpert, PhD, MD, Chair
Phyllis Greenberger, MSW, President & CEO
Mary V. Hornig, COO & CFO
Yonas G. Weldemariam, MBA, Director of Finance

The nation's only not-for-profit organization whose sole mission is to improve the health of women through research. Founded in 1990, The SWHR advocates increased funding for research on women's health, encourages the study of sex differences that may affect the prevention, diagnosis and treatment of disease, and promotes the inclusion of women in medical research studies.

Year Founded: 1990

2453 Society for the Advancement of Social Psychology (SASP)

630 Convention Tower
Buffalo, NY 14202
301-405-5921
Fax: 301-314-9566
E-mail: info@sesp.org
www.sesp.org

Garold Stasser, Secretary
Charles Stangor, Executive Officer

Social psychologists and students in social psychology. Advances social psychology as a profession by facilitating communication among social psychologists and improving dissemination and utilization of social psychological knowledge. Annual meeting every October.

2454 Society for the Psychological Study of Social Issues (SPSSI)

208 I Street NE
Washington, DC 20002-4340
202-675-6956
877-310-7778
Fax: 202-675-6902
E-mail: spssi@spssi.org
www.www.spssi.org

Susan Dudley, Executive Director
Anila Balkissoon, Administrative & Awards Coordina
Brad Sickels, Administrative Assistant
Gabriel Twose, Policy Director

An international group of over 3, 500 psychologists, allied scientists, students, and others who share a common interest in research on the psychological aspects of important social issues. The Society seeks to bring theory and practice into focus on human problems of the group, the community, and nations as well as the increasingly important problems that have no national boundaries.

2455 Society of Behavioral Medicine

555 East Wells Street
Suite 1100
Milwaukee, WI 53202-3823
414-918-3156
Fax: 414-276-3349
E-mail: info@sbm.org
www.sbm.org

Dawn K Wilson, PhD, President
Michael A Diefenbach, PhD, Secretary/Treasurer
Lisa M Klesges, PhD, President-Elect

A non-profit organization is a scientific forum for over 3, 000 behavioral and biomedical researchers and clinicians to study the interactions of behavior, physiological and biochemical states, and morbidity and mortality. SBM provides an interactive network for education and collaboration on common research, clinical and public policy concerns related to prevention, diagnosis and treatment, rehabilitation, and health promotion.

Year Founded: 1978

2456 Society of Multivariate Experimental Psychology (SMEP)
University of Virginia

102 Gilmer Hall
Department of Psychology
Charlottesville, VA 22903
804-924-0656
E-mail: shrout@psych.nyu.edu
www.smep.org

Steve West, President
Wayne Velicer, President-Elect

An organization of researchers interested in multivariate quantitative methods and their application to substantive problems in psychology. Membership is limited to 65 regular active members. SMEP oversees the publication of a research journal which publishes research articles on multivariate methodology and its use in psychological research. Annual meeting held every October.

Year Founded: 1960

2457 Society of Teachers of Family Medicine

11400 Tomahawk Creek Parkway
Suite 540
Leawood, KS 66211-2681
913-906-6000
800-274-2237
Fax: 913-906-6096
E-mail: stmoffice@stfm.org
www.stfm.org

Stacy Brungardt, Executive Director
Tom Vansaghi, PhD, Chief Development Officer
Dana Greco, CAE, Chief Financial Officer
Priscilla Noland, Senior Meeting Planner

Mulitdisciplinary, medical organization that offers numerous faculty development opportunities for individuals involved in family medicine education. STFM publishes a monthly journal, hosts a web site, distributes books, coordinates CME conferences devoted to family medicine teaching and research and other activities designed to improve teaching skills of family medicine educators.

2458 United States Psychiatric Rehabilitation Organization (USPRA)

1760 Old Meadow Road
Suite 500
McLean, VA 22102
703-442-2078
Fax: 703-506-3266
E-mail: info@uspra.org
www.uspra.org

Lisa Razzano, PhD, CPRP, Chair
Tom Gibson, Interim Chief Executive Officer
Casey Goldberg, Chief Staff Officer, Certificati
Cherilyn Cepriano, CAE, JD, , Vice President, Public Policy

The USPRA, formerly IAPSRS, is an organization of psychosocial rehabilitation agencies, practitioners, and interested organizations and individuals dedicated to promoting, supporting and strengthening community-oriented rehabilitation services and resources for persons with psychiatric disabilities.

Year Founded: 1975

2459 Wellness Councils of America

17002 Marcy St.
Suite 140
Omaha, NE 68118
402-827-3590
Fax: 402-827-3594
E-mail: wellworkplace@welcoa.org
www.welcoa.org

Stephen M. LaCagnin, Chairman
Ryan Picarella, MS, SPHR, President
David Hunnicutt, PhD, CEO
Brittanie Leffelman, MS, Vice President of Operations

A national non-profit membership organization dedicated to promoting healthier life styles for all Americans, especially through health promotion initiatives at the worksite. They publish a number of source books, a monthly newsletter, an extensive line of brochures and conducts numerous training seminars.

Year Founded: 1987

2460 WorldatWork

14040 N Northsight Boulevard
Scottsdale, AZ 85260-3627
877-951-9191
480-951-9191
Fax: 866-816-2962
E-mail: customerrelations@worldatwork.org
www.worldatwork.org

Anne Ruddy, President
Marcia Rhodes, Media Relations

A not-for-profit professional association dedicated to knowledge leadership in compensation, benefits and total rewards. Focuses on human resources disciplines associated with attracting, retaining and motivating employees. Provides education programs, a monthly magazine, online information resources, surveys, publications, conferences, research and networking opportunities.

Year Founded: 1955

Books

2461 A Family-Centered Approach to People with Mental Retardation
AAMR
444 N Capitol Street NW
Suite 846
Washington, DC 20001-1569
202-637-0475
800-424-3688
Fax: 202-637-0585
E-mail: dcroser@aaidd.org

Linda Leal, Author
Paul Aitken, Director Finance/Administration
Bruce Appelgren, Director Of Publications

Outlines key principles relevant to a family-centered approach to mental retardation and identifies four components to family-centered practice. *$12.95*

53 pages ISBN 0-940898-59-4

2462 A History of Nursing in the Field of Mental Retardation
AAMR
444 N Capitol Street NW
Suite 846
Washington, DC 20001-1569
202-637-0475
800-424-3688
Fax: 202-637-0585
E-mail: dcroser@aamr.org

Wendy M. Nehring, Author
Gary N. Siperstein, Author

For nursing scholars and anyone interested in the history of the treatment of people with mental retardation. *$19.95*

205 pages ISBN 0-940898-68-3

2463 A Primer on Rational Emotive Behavior Therapy
Research Press
PO Box 7866
Champaign, IL 61826-9177
217-352-3273
800-519-2707
Fax: 217-352-1221
E-mail: rp@researchpress.com
www.researchpress.com

Dr Windy Dryden, Author
Dr Raymond DiGiuseppe, Author
Michael Neenan, Author

This concise, systematic guide addresses recent developments in the theory and practice of Rational Emotive Behavior Therapy (REBT). The authors discuss rational versus irrational thinking, the ABC framework, the three basic musts that interfere wtih rational thinking and behavior, two basic biological tendencies, two fundamental human disturbances, and the theory of change in REBT. A detailed case example that includes verbatim dialogue between therapist and client illustrates the 18-step REBT treatment sequence. An appendix by Albert Ellis examines the special features of REBT. *$13.95*

136 pages ISBN 0-878224-78-5

2464 A Research Agenda for DSM-V
American Psychiatric Publishing, Inc.
1000 Wilson Boulevard
Suite 1825
Arlington, VA 22209-3901
703-907-7322
800-368-5777
Fax: 703-907-1091
E-mail: appi@psych.org
www.appi.org

Michael B First, M.D, Editor
David J. Kupfer, M.D, Editor
Darrel Regier, M.D., M.P.H., Editor

In the ongoing quest to improve our psychiatric diagnostic system, we are now searching for new approaches to understanding the etiological and pathophysiological mechanisms that can improve the validity of our diagnoses and the consequent power of our preventative and treatment interventions-venturing beyond the current DSM paradigm and DSM-IV framework. This volume represents a far-reaching attempt to stimulate research and discussion in the field in preparation for the start of the DSM-V process, still several years away, and to integrate information from a wide variety of sources and technologies. Copyright 2002. *$38.95*

336 pages Year Founded: 2002 ISBN 0-890422-92-3

2465 Adaptive Behavior and Its Measurement Implications for the Field of Mental Retardation
AAMR
444 N Capitol Street NW
Suite 846
Washington, DC 20001-1569
202-637-0475
800-424-3688
Fax: 202-637-0585
E-mail: dcroser@aamr.org

Robert L. Schalock, Editor

Integrates the concept of adaptive behavior more fully into the AAMR definition of mental retardation.

227 pages ISBN 0-940898-64-0

2466 Addressing the Specific needs of Women with Co-Occuring Disorders in the Criminal Justice System
Policy Research Associates
345 Delaware Avenue
Delmar, NY 12054-1905
518-439-7415
800-444-7415
Fax: 518-439-7612
E-mail: pra@prainc.com
www.prainc.com

Henry Steadman, President

Brochure emphasizes the need for gender specific programs to meet the management needs of female offenders. For law enforcement and justice administrators.

2467 Advances in Projective Drawing Interpetation
Charles C Thomas Publisher Ltd.
2600 S 1st Street
Springfield, IL 62704-4730
217-789-8980
800-258-8980
Fax: 217-789-9130
E-mail: books@ccthomas.com
www.ccthomas.com

Michael P Thomas, President

Exceptional contributors were chosen for their pertinence, range and inventiveness. This outstanding book assembles the progress in the science and in the clinical art of projective drawings as we enter the twenty-first century. Copyright 1997. *$80.95*

476 pages ISBN 0-398067-43-0

2468 Advancing DSM: Dilemmas in Psychiatric Diagnosis
American Psychiatric Publishing, Inc.
1000 Wilson Boulevard
Suite 1825
Arlington, VA 22209-3901
703-907-7322
800-368-5777
Fax: 703-907-1091

E-mail: appi@psych.org
www.appi.org

Katharine A Phillips, M.D, Editor
Michael B First, M.D, Editor
Harold Alan Pincus, M.D, Editor

Presents case studies from leading clinicians and researchers that illuminate the need for a revamped system. Each chapter presents a diagnostic dilemma from clinical practice that is intriguing, controversial, unresolved and remarkable in its theoretical and scientific complexity. Chapter by chapter, Advancing DSM raises important questions about the nature of diagnosis under the current DSM system and recommends broad changes. Copyright 2002. *$41.95*

264 pages Year Founded: 2003 ISBN 0-890422-93-1

2469 Adverse Effects of Psychotropic Drugs
Gilford Press
72 Spring Street
New York, NY 10012-4019
212-431-9800
Fax: 212-966-6708

John M. Kane, Editor
Jeffrey A. Lieberman, Editor
$63.00

2470 Agility in Health Care
John Wiley & Sons
111 River Street
Hoboken, NJ 07030-5773
201-748-6000
Fax: 210-748-6088
www.wiley.com
$42.95

250 pages ISBN 0-787942-11-1

2471 American Psychiatric Glossary
American Psychiatric Publishing, Inc.
1000 Wilson Boulevard
Suite 1825
Arlington, VA 22209-3901
703-907-7322
800-368-5777
Fax: 703-907-1091
E-mail: appi@psych.org
www.appi.org

Robert E Hales MD, Editor-in-Chief
Ron McMillen, Chief Executive Officer
John McDuffie, Editorial Director

Hardcover. Paperback also available. Copyright 1994. *$28.50*

224 pages ISBN 0-880485-26-4

2472 American Psychiatric Publishing Textbook of Clinical Psychiatry
American Psychiatric Publishing, Inc.
1000 Wilson Boulevard
Suite 1825
Arlington, VA 22209-3901
703-907-7322
800-368-5777
Fax: 703-907-1091
E-mail: appi@psych.org
www.appi.org

Robert E Hales MD, Editor-in-Chief
Ron McMillen, Chief Executive Officer
John McDuffie, Editorial Director

This densely informative textbook comprises 40 scholarly, authoritative chapters by an astonishing 89 experts and combines junior and senior authors alike to enhance the rich diversity and quality of clinical perspectives. Copyright 2002. *$239.00*

1776 pages ISBN 1-585620-32-7

2473 Americans with Disabilities Act and the Emerging Workforce
AAMR
444 N Capitol Street NW
Suite 846
Washington, DC 20001-1569
202-637-0475
800-424-3688
Fax: 202-637-0585
E-mail: dcroser@aamr.org

David L. Braddock, Author
Peter David Blanck, Author

Presents an empirical investigation of ADA issues and their effect on the employment of people with disabilities. Filled with legal cases, court opinions, charts, and tables. *$39.95*

303 pages ISBN 0-940898-52-7

2474 Assesing Problem Behaviors
AAMR
444 N Capitol Street NW
Suite 846
Washington, DC 20001-1569
202-637-0475
800-424-3688
Fax: 202-637-0585
E-mail: dcroser@aamr.org

Mary Ann Demchak, Author
Karen W. Bossert, Author

Shows how to conduct a functional assessment, to link assessment results to interventions, and gives an example of completed fuctional analysis. *$21.95*

44 pages ISBN 0-940898-39-X

2475 Basic Personal Counseling: Training Manual for Counslers
Charles C Thomas Publisher Ltd.
2600 S 1st Street
Springfield, IL 62704-4730
217-789-8980
800-258-8980
Fax: 217-789-9130
E-mail: books@ccthomas.com
www.ccthomas.com

David Geldard, Author

Contents: Becoming a Counselor; The Counseling Relationship; An Overview of Skills Training; Attending to the Client and the Use of Minimal Responses; Reflection of Feeling; Reflection of Content and Feeling; The Seeing, Hearing, and Feeling Modes; Asking Questions; Summarizing; Exploring Options; Reframing; Confrontation; Challenging Self-Destructive Beliefs; Termination; Procedure of the Counseling Experience; The Immediacy of the Counseling Experience; The Human Personality as it Emerges in the Counseling Experience; The Angry Client; Loss and Grief Counseling; The Suicidal Client; Arrangement of the

Counseling Room; Keeping Records of Counseling Sessions; Confidentiality; Supervision and Ongoing Training; and The Counselor's Own Well-Being. Copyright 1989. *$42.95*

214 pages Year Founded: 1989 ISBN 0-398055-40-8

2476 Best of AAMR: Families and Mental Retardation
AAMR
444 N Capitol Street NW
Suite 846
Washington, DC 20001-1569
202-637-0475
800-424-3688
Fax: 202-637-0585
E-mail: dcroser@aamr.org

Jan B. Blacher, Author
Bruce L. Baker, Author

Provides a comprehensive look at families and mental retardation in the 20th century through the eyes of some of its most respected researchers and service providers. *$59.95*

382 pages ISBN 0-940898-76-4

2477 Boundaries and Boundary Violations in Psychoanalysis
American Psychiatric Publishing, Inc.
1000 Wilson Boulevard
Suite 1825
Arlington, VA 22209-3901
703-907-7322
800-368-5777
Fax: 703-907-1091
E-mail: appi@psych.org
www.appi.org

Glen O Gabbard, M.D, Author
Eva P Lester, M.D, Author
John McDuffie, Editorial Director

Copyright 2002.

240 pages Year Founded: 2003 ISBN 1-585620-98-X

2478 Brain Calipers: Descriptive Psychopathology and the Mental Status Examination, Second Edition
Rapid Psychler Press
2014 Holland Ave
Suite 374
Port Huron, MI 48060-1994
519-667-2335
888-779-2453
Fax: 519-675-0610
E-mail: rapid@psychler.com
www.psychler.com

David Robinson, Publisher

$34.95

ISBN 1-894328-02-7

2479 Breakthroughs in Antipsychotic Medications: A Guide for Consumers, Families, and Clinicians
WW Norton & Company
500 5th Avenue
New York, NY 10110-54
212-354-5500
800-233-4830
Fax: 212-869-0856

E-mail: admalmud@wwnorton.com
www.books.wwnorton.com/

Ronald J. Diamond, Author
Ruth Ross, Author
Patricia L. Scheifler, Author
Peter J. Weiden, Author

Gives patients and their families needed information about the pros and cons of switching medications, possible side effects. Copyright 1999. *$22.95*

208 pages ISBN 0-393703-03-7

2480 Brief Coaching for Lasting Solutions
WW Norton & Company
500 5th Avenue
New York, NY 10110-54
212-354-5500
800-233-4830
Fax: 212-869-0856
E-mail: npb@wwnorton.com
www.books.wwnorton.com/

Insoo Kim Berg, Author
Peter Szab¢, Author

Successful coaching is about finding solutions and optimizing clients' lives. Insoo Kim Berg, one of the founders of solution-focused psychotherapy, collaborates with Peter Szabo in order to show how to help clients achieve their goals by applying their therapeutic approach to coaching.

264 pages ISBN 0-393704-72-6

2481 Brief Therapy and Managed Care
Joh Wiley & Sons
111 River Street
Hoboken, NJ 07030-5774
201-748-6000
Fax: 201-748-6088
www.wiley.com

Provides focused, time-sensitive treatment to your patients. Pratical guidelines on psychotherapy that are conscientiously managed, appropriate, and sensitive to a client's needs. *$40.95*

443 pages ISBN 0-787900-77-X

2482 Brief Therapy with Intimidating Cases
Jossey-Bass Publishers
111 River Street
Hoboken, NJ 07030-5774
201-748-6000
800-956-7739
Fax: 201-748-6088
E-mail: info@wiley.com
www.as.wiley.com

Richard Fisch, Author
Karin Schlanger, Author

This hands-on guide shows you how to apply the proven principles of brief therapy to a range of complex psychological problems once thought to be treatable only through long-term therapy or with medication. Learn how to focus on your clients' primary complaint and understand how and in what context the undesired behavior is performed. *$34.95*

192 pages Year Founded: 1998 ISBN 0-787943-64-9

2483 CURRENT Diagnosis & Treatment: Psychiatry
McGraw-Hill Medical Publishing Group
2 Penn Plaza
New York, NY 10121
212-904-2000
Fax: 212-904-6030
www.mhprofessional.com/product/php?isbn=0071422927

Michael H Ebert, Co-Author
Peter T Loosen, Co-Author
Barry Nurcombe, Co-Author
James F Leckman, Co-Author

This second edition is a reference for quickly answering day-to-day questions on psychiatric illness in both adults and children. Comprehensive in scope, and streamlined in coverage, this is a time-saving clinical companion. It reviews essential psychopharmacologic and psychotherapeutic approaches to the full range of psychiatric disorders. Copyright 2008. *$72.95*

758 pages ISBN 0-071422-92-7

2484 Cambridge Handbook of Psychology, Health and Medicine
Cambridge University Press
32 Avenue of the Americas
New York, NY 10013-2473
212-337-5000
Fax: 212-691-3239
E-mail: customer_service@cambridge.org
www.cambridge.org

Andrew Baum, Editor
Susan Ayers, Editor
Chris McManus, Editor
Stanton Newman, Editor

This important text collates international and interdisciplinary expertise to form a unique encyclopedic handbook to this field that will be valuable to medical practitioners as well as psychologists. Copyright 1997. *$85.00*

678 pages ISBN 0-521436-86-9

2485 Challenging Behavior of Persons with Mental Health Disorders and Severe Developmental Disabilities
AAMR
444 N Capitol Street NW
Suite 846
Washington, DC 20001-1569
202-637-0475
800-424-3688
Fax: 202-637-0585
E-mail: dcroser@aamr.org

Ronald H. Hanson, Author
Norman A. Wiesler, Editor

Provides a valuable compendium of the current knowledge base and empirically tested treatments for individuals with severe developmental disabilities, especially when problematic patterns of behavior are evident. *$39.95*

278 pages ISBN 0-940898-66-7

2486 Changing Health Care Marketplace
John Wiley & Sons
111 River Street
Hoboken, NJ 07030-5774
201-748-6000
Fax: 201-748-6088
www.wiley.com

$35.95

366 pages ISBN 0-787902-52-7

2487 Clinical Dimensions of Anticipatory Mourning
Research Press
PO Box 7866
Champaign, IL 61826-9177
217-352-3273
800-519-2707
Fax: 217-352-1221
E-mail: rp@researchpress.com
www.researchpress.com

Russell Pense, VP Marketing

Dr. Therese Rando is joined by 17 contributing authors to present the most comprehensive resource available on the perspectives, issues, interventions, and changing views associated with anticipatory mourning. *$29.95*

616 pages ISBN 0-878223-80-0

2488 Clinical Integration
Jossey-Bass Publishers
111 River Street
Hoboken, NJ 07030-5774
201-748-6000
800-956-7739
Fax: 201-748-6088
E-mail: info@wiley.com
www.as.wiley.com

Mary Tonges, Editor

Learn how to create information systems that can support care coordination and management across delivery sites, develop a case management model program for multi-provider systems, and more. *$41.95*

239 pages Year Founded: 1998 ISBN 0-787940-39-9

2489 Cognitive Therapy in Practice
WW Norton & Company
500 5th Avenue
New York, NY 10110-54
212-354-5500
800-233-4830
Fax: 212-869-0856
E-mail: npd@wwnorton.com
www.books.wwnorton.com/

Jacqueline B Persons, Author

Basic text for graduate studies in psychotherapy, psycholgy nursing social work and counseling. *$29.00*

224 pages Year Founded: 1989 ISBN 0-393700-77-1

2490 Collaborative Therapy with Multi-Stressed Families
Guilford Press
72 Spring Street
New York, NY 10012-4068
212-431-9800
800-365-7006
Fax: 212-966-6708
E-mail: info@guilford.com

William C. Madsen, Author

Written with a clear and fresh style, this is a guide to working in collaboration with clients, therapists and agencies. Experienced and beginning clinicians will appreciate a progressive approach to intricate problems. Copyrigt 1999. *$31.50*

388 pages ISBN 1-572304-90-1

2491 Communicating in Relationships: A Guide for Couples and Professionals
Research Press
PO Box 7866
Champaign, IL 61826-9177
217-352-3273
800-519-2707
Fax: 217-352-1221
E-mail: rp@researchpress.com
www.researchpress.com

Russell Pense, VP Marketing

Addresses the behavioral, affective and cognitive aspects of communicating in relationships. The book can be used by couples as a self-help guide, by professionals as an adjunct to therapy, or as a supplementary text for related college courses. Numerous readings are interspersed with 44 exercises that provide a hands-on approach to learning. The authors outline 18 steps for developing communication skills and describe procedures for integrating the skills into relationships. *$29.95*

280 pages ISBN 0-878223-42-8

2492 Community-Based Instructional Support
AAMR
444 N Capitol Street NW
Suite 846
Washington, DC 20001-1569
202-637-0475
800-424-3688
Fax: 202-637-0585
E-mail: dcroser@aamr.org

David Wesley Test, Author
Fred Spooner, Author

Offers practical guidelines for applying instructional strategies for adults who are learning community-based tasks. *$12.95*

34 pages ISBN 0-940898-43-8

2493 Comprehensive Textbook of Geriatric Psychiatry
WW Norton & Company
500 5th Avenue
New York, NY 10110-54
212-354-5500
800-233-4830
Fax: 212-869-0856
E-mail: npb@wwnorton.com
www.books.wwnorton.com/

George T. Grossberg, Editor
Lissy F. Jarvik, Editor
Barnett S. Meyers, Editor
Joel Sadavoy, Editor

Sponsored by the American Association for Geriatric Psychiatry (AAGP), this invaluable reference covers the entire range of geriatric psychiatry, including: the ageing process; psychiatric disorders of the elderly; princpiles of diagnosis and treatment; medical-legal, ethical, and financial issues.

1352 pages ISBN 0-393704-26-2

2494 Computerization of Behavioral Healthcare
Jossey-Bass Publishers
111 River Street
Hoboken, NJ 07030-5774

201-748-6000
800-956-7739
Fax: 201-748-6088
E-mail: info@wiley.com
www.as.wiley.com

Tom Trabin, Author

How computers and networked interactive information systems can help to contain costs, improve clinical outcomes, make your organizations more competitive using practical guidelines. Copyright 1996. *$27.95*

284 pages Year Founded: 1996 ISBN 0-787902-21-7

2495 Concise Guide to Marriage and Family Therapy
American Psychiatric Publishing, Inc.
1000 Wilson Boulevard
Suite 1825
Arlington, VA 22209-3901
703-907-7322
800-368-5777
Fax: 703-907-1091
E-mail: appi@psych.org
www.appi.org

Robert E Hales MD, Editor-in-Chief
Ron McMillen, Chief Executive Officer
John McDuffie, Editorial Director

Developed for use in the clinical setting, presents the core knowledge in the field in a single quick-reference volume. With brief, to-the-point guidance and step-by-step protocols, it's an invaluable resource for the busy clinician. Copyright 2002. *$29.95*

240 pages ISBN 1-585620-77-7

2496 Concise Guide to Psychiatry and Law for Clinicians
American Psychiatric Publishing, Inc.
1000 Wilson Boulevard
Suite 1825
Arlington, VA 22209-3901
703-907-7322
800-368-5777
Fax: 703-907-1091
E-mail: appi@psych.org
www.appi.org

Robert E Hales MD, Editor-in-Chief
Ron McMillen, Chief Executive Officer
John McDuffie, Editorial Director

Practical information for psychiatrists in understanding legal regulations, legal decisions and present managed care applications. Copyright 1998. *$29.95*

296 pages ISBN 0-880483-29-6

2497 Concise Guide to Psychopharmacology
American Psychiatric Publishing, Inc.
1000 Wilson Boulevard
Suite 1825
Arlington, VA 22209-3901
703-907-7322
800-368-5777
Fax: 703-907-1091
E-mail: appi@psych.org
www.appi.org

Lauren B Marangell, M.D, Author
James M Martinez, M.D, Author
John McDuffie, Editorial Director

Packed with practical information that is easy to access via detailed tables and charts, this pocket-sized volume (it literally fits into a lab coat or jacket pocket) is designed to be immediately useful for students, residents and clinicians working in a variety of treatment settings, such as inpatient psychiatry units, outpatient clinics, consultation-liaison services and private offices. Copyright 2002. *$29.95*

260 pages Year Founded: 2006 ISBN 1-585620-75-0

2498 Consent Handbook for Self-Advocates and Support Staff
AAMR
444 N Capitol Street NW
Suite 846
Washington, DC 20001-1569
202-637-0475
800-424-3688
Fax: 202-637-0585
E-mail: dcroser@aamr.org

Cathy Ficker Terrill, Author, Editor

Offers options for self-advocates and those for people who cannot consent on their own. *$14.95*

36 pages ISBN 0-904898-69-1

2499 Countertransference Issues in Psychiatric Treatment
American Psychiatric Publishing, Inc.
1000 Wilson Boulevard
Suite 1825
Arlington, VA 22209-3901
703-907-7322
800-368-5777
Fax: 703-907-1091
E-mail: appi@psych.org
www.appi.org

Glen O Gabbard, M.D, Editor
Ron McMillen, Chief Executive Officer
John McDuffie, Editorial Director

Overview of countertransference: theory and technique. Copyright 1999. *$37.50*

144 pages Year Founded: 1999 ISBN 0-880489-59-6

2500 Crisis: Prevention and Response in the Community
AAMR
444 N Capitol Street NW
Suite 846
Washington, DC 20001-1569
202-637-0475
800-424-3688
Fax: 202-637-0585
E-mail: dcroser@aamr.org

Ronald Halton Hanson, Author
Norman Anthony Wieseler, Editor

Provides a look at crisis services for people with developmental disabilities and how they impact the surrounding community. *$49.95*

240 pages ISBN 0-940898-74-8

2501 Cross-Cultural Perspectives on Quality of Life
AAMR
444 N Capitol Street NW
Suite 846
Washington, DC 20001-1569

202-637-0475
800-424-3688
Fax: 202-637-0585
E-mail: dcroser@aamr.org

Robert L. Schalock, Author
Kenneth D. Keith, Editor

Provides a ground-breaking global outlook on qual-
ity-of-life issues for people with mental retardation. *$47.95*

380 pages ISBN 0-940898-70-5

**2502 Cruel Compassion: Psychiatric Control of
Society's Unwanted**
John Wiley & Sons
605 3rd Avenue
New York, NY 10158-180
212-850-6301
E-mail: info@wiley.com

Thomas Szasz, Author

Demonstrates that the main problem that faces mental
health policy makers today is adult dependency. A sobering
look at some of our most cherished notions about our humane treatment of society's unwanted, and perhaps more
importantly, about ourselves as a compassionate and democratic people. Copyright 1994. *$19.95*

184 pages ISBN 0-471010-12-X

**2503 Culture & Psychotherapy: A Guide to Clinical
Practice**
American Psychiatric Publishing, Inc.
1000 Wilson Boulevard
Suite 1825
Arlington, VA 22209-3901
703-907-7322
800-368-5777
Fax: 703-907-1091
E-mail: appi@psych.org
www.appi.org

Wen-Shing Tseng, M.D, Editor
Jon Streltzer, M.D, Editor
John McDuffie, Editorial Director

Case presentations, analysis, special issues and populations
are covered. Copyright 2001. *$51.50*

320 pages Year Founded: 2001 ISBN 0-880489-55-3

**2504 Cutting-Edge Medicine: What Psychiatrists
Need to Know**
American Psychiatric Publishing, Inc.
1000 Wilson Boulevard
Suite 1825
Arlington, VA 22209-3901
703-907-7322
800-368-5777
Fax: 703-907-1091
E-mail: appi@psych.org
www.appi.org

Nada L Stotland, M.D., M.P.H, Editor
Ron McMillen, Chief Executive Officer
John McDuffie, Editorial Director

Offers a comprehensive overview of recent developments
in cardiovascular illness, gastrointestinal disorders, trans-
plant medicine, and premenstrual mood disorders. Copyright 2003. *$36.95*

164 pages Year Founded: 2002 ISBN 1-585620-72-6

2505 Cybermedicine
John Wiley & Sons
111 River Street
Hoboken, NJ 07030-5774
201-748-6000
Fax: 201-748-6088
www.wiley.com

A passionate plea for the use of computers for initial diagnosis and assessment, treatment decisions, and for
self-care, research, prevention, and above all, patient empowerment. *$25.00*

235 pages ISBN 0-787903-43-4

2506 DRG Handbook
Dorland Health
1500 Walnut Street
Suite 1000
Philadelphia, PA 19102-3512
215-875-1212
800-784-2332
Fax: 215-735-3966
E-mail: info@dorlandhealth.com
www.dorlandhealth.com

Diagnosis-related groups are the building blocks of hospital
reimbursement under the Medicare Prospective Payment
System. Also provides the ability to forecast and manage
information at DRG-specific levels using comparison
groups of like hospitals, a critical tool for both providers
and payers. Copyright 1998. *$399.00*

1 per year ISBN 1-573721-39-5

**2507 DSM: IV Diagnostic & Statistical Manual of
Mental Disorders**
American Psychiatric Publishing, Inc.
1000 Wilson Boulevard
Suite 1825
Arlington, VA 22209-3901
703-907-7322
800-368-5777
Fax: 703-907-1091
E-mail: appi@psych.org
www.appi.org

Robert E Hales MD, Editor-in-Chief
Ron McMillen, Chief Executive Officer
John McDuffie, Editorial Director

Focuses on clinical, research and educational findings.
Practical and useful for clinicians and researchers of many
orientations. Leatherbound. Hardcover and paperback also
available. Copyright 1994. *$75.00*

991 pages Year Founded: 2013 ISBN 0-890420-64-5

2508 DSM: IV Personality Disorders
Rapid Psychler Press
2014 Holland Ave
Suite 374
Port Huron, MI 48060-1994
519-667-2335
888-779-2453
Fax: 519-675-0610
E-mail: rapid@psychler.com
www.psychler.com

David Robinson, Publisher

$9.95

ISBN 1-894328-23-x

2509 Designing Positive Behavior Support Plans
AAMR
444 N Capitol Street NW
Suite 846
Washington, DC 20001-1569
202-637-0475
800-424-3688
Fax: 202-637-0585
E-mail: dcroser@aamr.org

Provides a conceptual framework for understanding, designing, and evaluating positive behavior support plans.
$21.95

43 pages ISBN 0-940898-55-1

2510 Developing Mind: Toward a Neurobiology of Interpersonal Experience
Guilford Press
72 Spring Street
New York, NY 10012-4068
212-431-9800
800-365-7006
Fax: 212-966-6708
E-mail: info@guilford.com

Daniel J. Siegel, MD, Author

Concise research results as to the origins of our behavior based on cognitive neuroscience.

2511 Disability at the Dawn of the 21st Century and the State of the States
AAMR
444 N Capitol Street NW
Suite 846
Washington, DC 20001-1569
202-637-0475
800-424-3688
Fax: 202-637-0585
E-mail: dcroser@aamr.org

Consumate source book on the analysis of financing services and supports for people with developmental disabilities in the United States. A detailed state-by-state analysis of public financial support for persons with MR/DD, mental illness, and physical disabilities.

512 pages ISBN 0-940898-85-3

2512 Diversity in Psychotherapy: The Politics of Race, Ethnicity, and Gender
Praeger
2727 Palisade Avenue
Suite 4H
Bronx, NY 10463-1020
718-796-0971
Fax: 718-796-0971
www.vd6@columbia.edu

Victor De La De La Cancela, Author
Jean Lau Chin, Author
Yvonne M. Jenkins, Author

This challenging and insightful work wrestles with difficult treatment problems confronting both culturally and socially oppressed clients and psychotherapists. Case studies offer highly valuable resource material and insights into challenging perpsectives on behavioral health services. Copyright 1993. *$49.95*

224 pages ISBN 0-275941-80-9

2513 Doing What Comes Naturally: Dispelling Myths and Fallacies About Sexuality and People with Developmental Disabilities
High Tide Press
Ste 2n
2081 Calistoga Dr
New Lenox, IL 60451-4833
815-206-2054
888-487-7377
E-mail: managing.editor@hightidepress.com

Orieda Horn Anderson, Author
Jennifer Luvert, Author

Uncovers misconceptions about adults whose sexual needs vary greatly, and yet are often treated as children or non-sexual people. Includes heartwarming success stories from adults Mrs. Anderson has supported, as well as suggestions for teaching and a guide to sexual incident reporting. *$19.95*

127 pages ISBN 1-892696-13-4

2514 Dynamic Psychotherapy: An Introductory Approach
American Psychiatric Publishing, Inc.
1000 Wilson Boulevard
Suite 1825
Arlington, VA 22209-3901
703-907-7322
800-368-5777
Fax: 703-907-1091
E-mail: appi@psych.org
www.appi.org

Robert E Hales MD, Editor-in-Chief
Ron McMillen, Chief Executive Officer
John McDuffie, Editorial Director

Principles and techniques. Copyright 1990. *$33.50*

229 pages

2515 Electroconvulsive Therapy: A Guide
Madison Institute of Medicine
7617 Mineral Point Road
Suite 300
Madison, WI 53717-1623
608-827-2470
E-mail: mim@miminc.org
www.factsforhealth.org

Margarett Baudhuin, Manager

ECT is an extremely effective method of treatment for severe depression that does not respond to medication. This guidebook explains what ECT is and how it is used today to help patients overcome depression and other serious, treatment resistant psychiatric disorders. *$5.95*

19 pages

2516 Embarking on a New Century: Mental Retardation at the end of the Twentieth Century
AAMR
444 N Capitol Street NW
Suite 846
Washington, DC 20001-1569
202-637-0475
800-424-3688
Fax: 202-637-0585
E-mail: dcroser@aamr.org

This volume of 18 essays summarizes major public policy and service delivery advancements from 1975 to 2000. These changes can be summarized as a siginificant shift in many areas — from services to supports; from passive to active consumer roles; from normalization to quality. *$29.97*

265 pages

2517 Emergencies in Mental Health Practice
Guilford Press
72 Spring Street
New York, NY 10012-4068
212-431-9800
800-365-7006
Fax: 212-966-6708
E-mail: info@guilford.com

Phillip M. Kleespies PhD, Editor

Focusing on acute clinical situations in which there is an imminent risk of serious harm or death to self or others, this practical resource helps clinicians evaluate and manage a wide range of mental health emergencies. The volume provides guidelines for interviewing with suicidal patients, potentially violent patients, vulnerable victims of violence, as well as patients facing life-and-death medical decisions, with careful attention to risk management and forensic issues. *$24.95*

450 pages ISBN 1-572305-51-7

2518 Essential Guide to Psychiatric Drugs
St. Martin's Press
175 5th Avenue
New York, NY 10010-7848
212-674-5151
Fax: 212-674-3179
E-mail: webmaster@stmartins.com

Jack M. Gorman, Author

Information not found in other drug references. Lists many common drugs and not so common side effects, including drug interaction and the individual's reaction, including sexual side effects. Expert but nontechnical narrative. Copyright 1998. *$6.99*

448 pages ISBN 0-312954-58-1

2519 Essentials of Clinical Psychiatry: Based on the American Psychiatric Press Textbook of Psychiatry
American Psychiatric Publishing, Inc.
1000 Wilson Boulevard
Suite 1825
Arlington, VA 22209-3901
703-907-7322
800-368-5777
Fax: 703-907-1091
E-mail: appi@psych.org
www.appi.org

Robert E Hales MD, Editor-in-Chief
Ron McMillen, Chief Executive Officer
John McDuffie, Editorial Director

51 distinguished experts have created a compelling reference reflecting a biopsychosocial approach to patient treatment that is at once exciting and accessible. Copyright 1999. *$77.00*

1032 pages ISBN 0-880488-48-4

2520 Ethical Way
John Wiley & Sons
111 River Street
Hoboken, NJ 07030-5774
201-748-6000
Fax: 201-748-6088
www.wiley.com

Leads you through a maze of ethical principles and crucial issues confronting mental health professionals. *$38.95*

254 pages ISBN 0-787907-41-X

2521 Evidence-Based Mental Health Practice: A Textbook
WW Norton & Company
500 5th Avenue
New York, NY 10110-54
212-354-5500
800-233-4830
Fax: 212-869-0856
E-mail: npb@wwnorton.com
www.books.wwnorton.com/

Robert E. Drake, Editor
David W. Lynde, Editor
Matthew R. Merrens, Editor

The specific term evidence-based medicine was introduced in 1990 to refer to a systematic approach to helping doctors to apply scientific evidence to decision-making at the point of contact with a specific consumer. As support for evidence-based medicine grows in mental health, the need to clarify its fundamental principles also increases. An essential primer for all practititioners and students who are grappling with the new age of evidence-based practice.

528 pages ISBN 0-393704-43-2

2522 Executive Guide to Case Management Strategies
John Wiley & Sons
111 River Street
Hoboken, NJ 07030-5774
201-748-6000
Fax: 201-748-6088
www.wiley.com

A guide to plan, organize, develop, improve and help case management programs reach their full potential in the clinical and financial management of care. *$58.00*

160 pages ISBN 1-556481-28-4

2523 Family Approach to Psychiatric Disorders
American Psychiatric Publishing, Inc.
1000 Wilson Boulevard
Suite 1825
Arlington, VA 22209-3901
703-907-7322
800-368-5777
Fax: 703-907-1091
E-mail: appi@psych.org
www.appi.org

Richard A Perlmutter, M.D., Author
Ron McMillen, Chief Executive Officer
John McDuffie, Editorial Director

Examines how treatment can and should involve the family of the patient. Copyright 1996. *$67.50*

406 pages Year Founded: 1996

2524 Family Stress, Coping, and Social Support
Charles C Thomas Publisher Ltd.
2600 S 1st Street
Springfield, IL 62704-4730
217-789-8980
800-258-8980
Fax: 217-789-9130
E-mail: books@ccthomas.com
www.ccthomas.com

Michael P Thomas, President

Copyright 1982. *$48.95*

294 pages   ISSN 0-398-06275-7ISBN 0-398046-92-1

2525 Family Therapy Progress Notes Planner
John Wiley & Sons
10475 Crosspoint Boulevard
Indianapolis, IN 46256-3386
317-572-3000
Fax: 317-572-4000
E-mail: consumers@wiley.com
www.wiley.com

Arthur E. Jongsma, Jr., Author
David J Berghuis, MA, LLP, Author

Extends the line into the growing field of family therapy. Included is critical information about HIPAA guidelines, which greatly impact the privacy status of patient progress notes. Helps mental health practitioners reduce the amount of time spent on paperwork by providing a full menu of pre-written progress notes that can be easily and quickly adapted to fit a particular patient need or treatment situation. *$ 49.95*

352 pages   ISBN 0-471484-43-1

2526 Fifty Ways to Avoid Malpractice: A Guidebook for Mental Health Professionals
Professional Resource Press
PO Box 3197
Sarasota, FL 34230-3197
941-343-9601
800-443-3364
Fax: 941-343-9201
E-mail: orders@prpress.com
www.prpress.com

Laurie Girsch, Managing Editor

Offers straightforward guidance on providing legally safe and ethically appropriate services to your clients. Copyright 1988. *$ 18.95*

158 pages   ISBN 0-943158-54-0

2527 First Therapy Session
John Wiley & Sons
111 River Street
Hoboken, NJ 07030-5774
201-748-6000
Fax: 201-748-6088
www.wiley.com

Presents an effective, straightforward approach for conducting first therapy sessions, showing step-by-step, how to identify client problems and help solve them within families. *$27.95*

ISBN 1-555421-94-6

2528 Five-HTP: The Natural Way to Overcome Depression, Obesity, and Insomnia
Bantam Doubleday Dell Publishing
1745 Broadway
New York, NY 10019-4343
212-782-9000

Jeff Rechtzigel, Publisher

An authorative and comprehensive guide to realizing the health benefits of 5-HTP. Explains how this natural amino acid can safely and effectively regulate low serotonin levels, which have been linked to depression, obesity, insomnia, migraines, and anxiety. 5-HTP is also a powerful antioxidant that can protect the body from free-radical damage, reducing the risk of serious illnesses such as cancer. Copyright 1999. *$11.95*

304 pages   ISBN 0-553379-46-1

2529 Flawless Consulting
Jossey-Bass Publishers
111 River Street
Hoboken, NJ 07030-5774
201-748-6000
800-956-7739
Fax: 201-748-6088
E-mail: info@wiley.com
www.as.wiley.com

Peter Block, Author

This book offers advice on what to say and what to do in specific situations to see your recommendations through. *$39.95*

214 pages   ISBN 0-893840-52-1

2530 Forgiveness: Theory, Research and Practice
Guilford Press
72 Spring Street
New York, NY 10012-4068
212-431-9800
800-365-7006
Fax: 212-966-6708
E-mail: info@guilford.com

Michael E. McCullough Phd, Editor
Kenneth I. Pargament PhD, Editor
Carl E. Thoresen Phd, Editor

Scholarly, up-to-date examination of forgiveness ranges many disiplines for mental health professionals. Copyright 2000. *$ 35.00*

334 pages   ISBN 1-572305-10-X

2531 Foundations of Mental Health Counseling 4th Edition
Charles C Thomas Publisher Ltd.
2600 S 1st Street
Springfield, IL 62704-4730
217-789-8980
800-258-8980
Fax: 217-789-9130
E-mail: books@ccthomas.com
www.ccthomas.com

Artis J. Palmo, Author
William J. Weikel, Author
David P. Borsos, Author

The importance of mental health counseling has grown, including the array of mental health issues that arise in an uncertain and fragile world. This fourth edition expands the information in the previous editions by updating the positive changes in the field of mental health counseling including the recognition of licensed professional counselors by managed care organizations and insurance companies. This book continues to be the most up-to-date resource in the field of mental health counseling and is a must read for anyone working or aspiring to work as a mental health counselor. *$87.95*

508 pages Year Founded: 2011 ISBN 0-398086-35-0

2532 Fundamentals of Psychiatric Treatment Planning
American Psychiatric Publishing, Inc.
1000 Wilson Boulevard
Suite 1825
Arlington, VA 22209-3901
703-907-7322
800-368-5777
Fax: 703-907-1091
E-mail: appi@psych.org
www.appi.org

James A Kennedy, M.D., Author
Ron McMillen, Chief Executive Officer
John McDuffie, Editorial Director

Professional discussion of important basics. Copyright 2002. *$49.00*

350 pages Year Founded: 2003 ISBN 1-585620-61-0

2533 Group Involvement Training
NewHarbinger Publications
5674 Shattuck Avenue
Oakland, CA 94609-1662
510-652-0215
800-748-6273
Fax: 510-652-5472
E-mail: customerservice@newharbinger.com
www.newharbinger.com

Matthew McKay, Owner

This book shows how training chronically ill mental patients in a series of structured group tasks can be used to treat the symptoms of apathy, withdrawl, poor interpersonal skills, helplessness, and the inability to structure leisure time constructively. Copyright 1988. *$24.95*

160 pages ISBN 0-934986-65-7

2534 Guide to Possibility Land: Fifty One Methods for Doing Brief, Respectful Therapy
WW Norton & Company
500 5th Avenue
New York, NY 10110-54
212-354-5500
Fax: 212-869-0856
E-mail: admalmud@wwnorton.com
www.books.wwnorton.com/

Sandy Beadle, Author
Bill O'Hanlon, Author

The creator of Possibility therapy, William O'Hanlon, outlines acknowledging patient's experience and opinions about their lives while seeing that possibilites for change are explored and underlined. Copyright 1999. *$13.00*

94 pages ISBN 0-393702-97-9

2535 Guide to Treatments That Work
Oxford University Press/Oxford Reference
198 Madison Avenue
New York, NY 10016-4308
212-726-6400
800-451-7556

Peter E. Nathan, Author
Jack M. Gorman, Author

A systematic review of various treatments currently in use for virtually all of the recognized mental disorders. Copyright 1997. *$75.00*

784 pages ISBN 0-195102-27-4

2536 Handbook on Quality of Life for Human Service Practitioners
AAMR
444 N Capitol Street NW
Suite 846
Washington, DC 20001-1569
202-637-0475
800-424-3688
Fax: 202-637-0585
E-mail: dcroser@aamr.org

Robert L. Schalock, Author
Miguel Angel Verdugo, Author

Revolutionary generic model for quality of life that integrates core domains and indicators with a cross-cultural systems prespective that can be used in all human services. *$59.95*

430 pages ISBN 0-940898-77-2

2537 Health Insurance Answer Book
Garner Consulting
630 North Rosemead Blvd
Suite 300
Pasadena, CA 91107
626-351-2300
Fax: 626-351-2331
E-mail: info@garnerconsulting.com
www.garnerconsulting.com

Gerti Reagan Garner, President
John C Garner, Chief Executive Officer
Carl Isaacs, Principal
Araceli Sandoval, Associate

This easy-to-use guide will help you manage a cost effective health insurance plan and ensure that your decisions are in compliance with constantly changing health care legislation. Offers instant access to information on everything from HMOs, PPOs, COBRA, HIPPA, OBRA anad flexible benefits to plan rating, funding, cost containment, and administration. *$290.00*

1100 pages ISBN 0-735582-18-7

2538 Helper's Journey: Working with People Facing Grief, Loss, and Life-Threatening Illness
Research Press
PO Box 7866
Champaign, IL 61826-9177
217-352-3273
800-519-2707
Fax: 217-352-1221
E-mail: rp@researchpress.com
www.researchpress.com

Dr Dale G Larson, Author

Written for both professional and volunteer caregivers, this unique manual provides exercises, activities and specific strategies for more successful caregiving, increased personal growth and effective stress management. The author explores the theory and practice of helping. He includes numerous case examples and verbatim disclosures of fellow caregivers that powerfully convey the joys and sorrows of the helper's journey. Cited as a 'Book of the Year' by the American Journal of Nursing. *$21.95*

292 pages ISBN 0-878223-44-4

2539 High Impact Consulting
Jossey-Bass Publishers
111 River Street
Hoboken, NJ 07030-5774
201-748-6000
800-956-7739
Fax: 201-748-6088
E-mail: info@wiley.com
www.as.wiley.com

Robert H Schaffer, Author

Offers a new model for consulting services that shows how to produce short-term successes and use them as a springboard to larger accomplishments and, ultimately, to organization-wide continuous improvement. Also includes specific guidance to assist clients in analyzing their situation, identifying their real needs, and choosing an appropriate consultant. *$26.00*

288 pages Year Founded: 2002 ISBN 0-787903-41-8

2540 Home Maintenance for Residential Service Providers
High Tide Press
Ste 2n
2081 Calistoga Dr
New Lenox, IL 60451-4833
815-206-2054
888-487-7377
E-mail: managing.editor@hightidepress.com

Nathan Cohen, Author

What happens when a human service organization becomes a large, commercial landlord, not unlike a real estate firm or condominium management company? Property management for homes supporting persons with disabilities requires a unique blend of human services and physical plant expertise. Provides detailed checklists for all house systems, fixtures and furnishings. Includes a discussion of maintaining an attractive residence that blends with the neighborhood. *$10.95*

43 pages ISBN 0-965374-46-7

2541 How to Partner with Managed Care
John Wiley & Sons
605 3rd Avenue
New York, NY 10158-180
212-850-6301
E-mail: info@wiley.com

Charles H. Browning, Author
Beverly J Browning, Author

A Do It Yourself Kit for Building Working Relationships & Getting Steady Referrals. Copyright 1996.

358 pages

2542 Improving Clinical Practice
John Wiley & Sons
111 River Street
Hoboken, NJ 07030-5774
201-748-6000
Fax: 201-748-6088
www.wiley.com

Enhance your organization's clinical decision making, and ultimately improve the quality of patient care. *$41.95*

342 pages ISBN 0-787900-93-1

2543 Improving Therapeutic Communication
Jossey-Bass Publishers
111 River Street
Hoboken, NJ 07030-5774
201-748-6000
800-956-7739
Fax: 201-748-6088
E-mail: info@wiley.com
www.as.wiley.com

D. Corydon Hammond, Author
Dean H Hepworth, Author
Veon G Smith, Author

Improve your communication technique with this definitive guide for counselors, therapists, and caseworkers. Focuses on the four basic skills that facilitate communication in therapy: empathy, respect, authenticity, and confrontation. *$62.95*

400 pages Year Founded: 2002 ISBN 0-875893-08-2

2544 In Search of Solutions: A New Direction in Psychotherapy
WW Norton & Company
500 5th Avenue
New York, NY 10110-54
212-354-5500
800-233-4830
Fax: 212-869-0856
E-mail: npb@wwnorton.com
www.books.wwnorton.com/

Bill O'Hanlon, Author
Michele Weiner-Davis, Author

O'Hanlon and Weiner-Davis provide guidelines for clinicians in implementing solution-oriented language and explain how to aviod dead ends. New material bring the reader up to date on advances in this field since the book's original publication in 1989.

ISBN 0-393704-37-8

2545 Increasing Variety in Adult Life
AAMR
501 3rd Street
NW Suite 200
Washington, DC 20001
202-387-1968
800-424-3688
Fax: 202-387-2193
E-mail: dcroser@aamr.org
www.www.aaidd.org

Step-by-step guidelines for implementing the general-case instructional process and shows how the process can be used across a variety of activities. *$12.95*

38 pages ISBN 0-940898-43-2

2546 Independent Practice for the Mental Health Professional
Brunner/Routledge
325 Chestnut Street
Philadelphia, PA 19106-2614
800-821-8312
Fax: 215-269-0363

Ralph H Earle PhD, Author
Dorothy J Barnes MC, Author

An excellent resource for beginning therapists considering private practice or for experienced therapists moving from agency or institutional settings into private practice. Offers practical, down-to-earth suggestions for practice settings, marketing and working with clients. The authors provide worksheets and examples of successful planning for the growth of a practice. *$24.95*

192 pages ISBN 0-876308-38-8

2547 Infanticide: Psychosocial and Legal Perspectives on Mothers Who Kill
American Psychiatric Publishing, Inc.
1000 Wilson Boulevard
Suite 1825
Arlington, VA 22209-3901
703-907-7322
800-368-5777
Fax: 703-907-1091
E-mail: appi@psych.org
www.appi.org

Margaret C Spinelli, M.D., Editor
Ron McMillen, Chief Executive Officer
John McDuffie, Editorial Director

Written to help remedy today's dearth of up-to-date, research-based literature, this unique volume brings together a multidisciplinary group of 17 experts who focus on the psychiatric perspective of this tragic cause of infant death. Balanced perspective on a highly emotional issue will find a wide audience among psychiatric and medical professionals, legal professionals, public health professionals and interested laypersons. Copyright 2002. *$53.50*

296 pages Year Founded: 2003 ISBN 1-585620-97-1

2548 Innovative Approaches for Difficult to Treat Populations
American Psychiatric Publishing, Inc.
1000 Wilson Boulevard
Suite 1825
Arlington, VA 22209-3901
703-907-7322
800-368-5777
Fax: 703-907-1091
E-mail: appi@psych.org
www.appi.org

Scott W Henggeler, Ph.D, Editor
Alberto B Santos, M.D., Editor
John McDuffie, Editorial Director

Alternate methods when the usual approaches are not helpful. Copyright 1997. *$86.95*

552 pages Year Founded: 1997

2549 Insider's Guide to Mental Health Resources Online
Guilford Press
72 Spring Street
New York, NY 10012-4068

212-431-9800
800-365-7006
Fax: 212-966-6708
E-mail: info@guilford.com

John M. Grohol PsyD, Author
John M. Grohol, Author

This guide helps readers take full advantage of Internet and world-wide-web resources in psychology, psychiatric, self-help and patient education. The book explains and evaluates the full range of search tools, newsgroups, databases and describes hundreds of specific disorders, find job listings and network with other professionals, obtain needed articles and books, conduct grant searches and much more. *$ 21.95*

338 pages ISBN 1-572305-49-5

2550 Instant Psychopharmacology
WW Norton & Company
500 5th Avenue
New York, NY 10110-54
212-354-5500
800-233-4830
Fax: 212-869-0856
E-mail: admalmud@wwnorton.com
www.books.wwnorton.com/

Ronald J. Diamond, Author

Revision of the best selling guide to all the new medications. Straightforward book teaches non medical therapists, clients and their families how the five different classes of drugs work, advice on side effects, drug interaction warnings and much more practical information. Copyright 2002. *$18.95*

168 pages ISBN 0-393703-91-6

2551 Integrated Treatment of Psychiatric Disorders
American Psychiatric Publishing, Inc.
1000 Wilson Boulevard
Suite 1825
Arlington, VA 22209-3901
703-907-7322
800-368-5777
Fax: 703-907-1091
E-mail: appi@psych.org
www.appi.org

Jerald Kay, M.D., Editor
Ron McMillen, Chief Executive Officer
John McDuffie, Editorial Director

Psychodynamic therapy and medication. Copyright 2001. *$34.95*

216 pages Year Founded: 2001 ISBN 1-585620-27-0

2552 Integrating Psychotherapy and Pharmacotherapy: Disolving the Mind-Brain Barrier
WW Norton & Company
500 5th Avenue
New York, NY 10110-54
212-354-5500
800-233-4830
Fax: 212-869-0856
E-mail: npb@wwnorton.com
www.books.wwnorton.com/

Drake McFeely, CEO

Will help all mental health clinicians to dissolve their conceptual mind/brain barriers by recognizing the reciprocal influences of psychological and pharmacological interventions. The reader responds to thought-provoking questions and vignettes of problematic cases.

ISBN 0-393704-03-3

2553 Integrative Brief Therapy: Cognitive, Psychodynamic, Humanistic & Neurobehavioral Approaches
Impact Publishers, Inc.
PO Box 6016
Atascadero, CA 93423-6016
805-466-5917
800-246-7228
Fax: 805-466-5919
E-mail: info@impactpublishers.com
www.impactpublishers.com

John Preston, Psy.D., Author

Thorough discussion of the factors that contribute to effectiveness in therapy carefully integrates key elements from diverse theoretical viewpoints. *$27.95*

272 pages Year Founded: 2006 ISBN 1-886230-09-5

2554 International Handbook on Mental Health Policy
Greenwood Publishing Group
88 Post Road W
PO Box 5007
Westport, CT 06881-5007
203-226-3571
Fax: 203-222-1502

Donna R. Kemp, Editor

Major reference book for academics and practitioners that provides a systematic survey and analysis of mental health policies in twenty representative countries. Copyright 1993. *$125.00*

512 pages ISBN 0-313275-67-X

2555 Interpersonal Psychotherapy
American Psychiatric Publishing, Inc.
1000 Wilson Boulevard
Suite 1825
Arlington, VA 22209-3901
703-907-7322
800-368-5777
Fax: 703-907-1091
E-mail: appi@psych.org
www.appi.org

John C Markowitz, M.D, Editor
Ron McMillen, Chief Executive Officer
John McDuffie, Editorial Director

An overview of interpersonal psychotherapy for depression, preventative treatment for depression, bulimia nervosa and HIV positive men and women. Copyright 1998. *$37.50*

184 pages Year Founded: 1998 ISBN 0-880488-36-0

2556 Introduction to Time: Limited Group Psychotherapy
American Psychiatric Publishing, Inc.
1000 Wilson Boulevard
Suite 1825
Arlington, VA 22209-3901

703-907-7322
800-368-5777
Fax: 703-907-1091
E-mail: appi@psych.org
www.appi.org

K Roy MacKenzie, M.D., F.R.C, Author
Ron McMillen, Chief Executive Officer
John McDuffie, Editorial Director

Do more with limited time and sessions. Copyright 1997. *$57.95*

336 pages Year Founded: 1990

2557 Introduction to the Technique of Psychotherapy: Practice Guidelines for Psychotherapists
Charles C Thomas Publisher Ltd.
2600 S 1st Street
Springfield, IL 62704-4730
217-789-8980
800-258-8980
Fax: 217-789-9130
E-mail: books@ccthomas.com
www.ccthomas.com

Samuel I Greenberg, Author

A basic, simply written book, with a minimum of theory, helpful to the beginning therapist. Discuss how to conduct psychotherapy: by having a format in mind, taking a comprehensive history, and a careful, observing examination of the patient. Copyright 1998. *$34.95*

122 pages Year Founded: 1998 ISSN 0-398-06905-0ISBN 0-398069-04-2

2558 Languages of Psychoanalysis
Analytic Press
7625 Empire Drive
Florence, KS 41042-2919
510-547-7860
800-634-7064
Fax: 800-248-4724
E-mail: orders@taylorandfrancis.com
www.www.routledgementalhealth.com/

John E Gedo, Author
John Kerr PhD, Sr Editor

A guide to understanding the full range of human discourse, especially behavioral conflicts and communicational deficits as they impinge upon the transactions of the analytic dyad. Available in hardcover. Copyright 1996. *$39.95*

224 pages ISBN 0-881631-86-8

2559 Leadership and Organizational Excellence
AAMR
444 N Capitol Street NW
Suite 846
Washington, DC 20001-1569
202-637-0475
800-424-3688
Fax: 202-637-0585
E-mail: dcroser@aamr.org

Examines key managerial and organizational strategies that can be used to help ensure high-quality work environments for both staff and service delivery for people with developmental disabilities. *$ 14.95*

33 pages ISBN 0-940898-78-0

2560 Making Money While Making a Difference: Achieving Outcomes for People with Disabilities
High Tide Press
Ste 2n
2081 Calistoga Dr
New Lenox, IL 60451-4833
815-206-2054
888-487-7377
E-mail: managing.editor@hightidepress.com

Diane J Bell, Managing Editor

Unique handbook for corporations and nonprofits alike. The authors guide readers through a step-by-step process for implementing strategic alliances between nonprofit organizations and corporate partners. Learn the tenets of cause related marketing and much more. *$14.95*

231 pages ISBN 0-965374-49-1

2561 Managed Mental Health Care in the Public Sector: a Survival Manual
Brunner/Routledge
325 Chestnut Street
Philadelphia, PA 19106-2614
800-821-8312
Fax: 215-269-0363

Manual for administrators, planners, clinicians and consumers with concepts and strategies to maneuver in public sector managed mental healthcare system. Copyright 1996. *$35.00*

336 pages ISBN 9-057025-37-X

2562 Managing Client Anger: What to Do When a Client is Angry with You
NewHarbinger Publications
5674 Shattuck Avenue
Oakland, CA 94609-1662
510-652-0215
800-748-6273
Fax: 510-652-5472
E-mail: customerservice@newharbinger.com
www.newharbinger.com

Matthew McKay, Owner

Guide to help therapists understand their reactions and make interventions when clients express anger toward them. Copyright 1998. *$49.95*

261 pages ISBN 1-572241-23-3

2563 Manual of Clinical Psychopharmacology
American Psychiatric Publishing, Inc.
1000 Wilson Boulevard
Suite 1825
Arlington, VA 22209-3901
703-907-7322
800-368-5777
Fax: 703-907-1091
E-mail: appi@psych.org
www.appi.org

Alan F Schatzberg, M.D, Author
Jonathan O Cole, M.D., Author
Charles DeBattista, D.M.H., M., Author

Examines the recent changes and standard treatments in psychopharmacology. Copyright 2002. *$63.00*

744 pages Year Founded: 2010 ISBN 0-880488-65-4

2564 Mastering the Kennedy Axis V: New Psychiatric Assessment of Patient Functioning
American Psychiatric Publishing, Inc.
1000 Wilson Boulevard
Suite 1825
Arlington, VA 22209-3901
703-907-7322
800-368-5777
Fax: 703-907-1091
E-mail: appi@psych.org
www.appi.org

James A Kennedy, M.D., Author
Ron McMillen, Chief Executive Officer
John McDuffie, Editorial Director

Professional evaluation methods. Copyright 2002. *$44.00*

294 pages Year Founded: 2003 ISBN 1-585620-62-9

2565 Meditative Therapy Facilitating Inner-Directed Healing
Impact Publishers
PO Box 6016
Atascadero, CA 93423-6016
805-466-5917
800-246-7228
Fax: 805-466-5919
E-mail: info@impactpublishers.com
www.impactpublishers.com

Michael L Emmons, Ph.D., Author
Janet Emmons, M.S., Author

Offers to the professional therapist a full description of the therapeutic procedures that facilitate inner-directed healing and explains the therapist's role in guiding clients' growth psychologically, physiologically and spiritually. Copyright 1999. *$27.95*

230 pages ISBN 1-886230-11-0

2566 Mental Disability Law: Primer, a Comprehensive Introduction
Commission on the Mentally Disabled
1800 M Street NW
Washington, DC 20036-5802
202-331-2240

An updated and expanded version of the 1984 edition provides a comprehensive overview of mental disability law. Part I of the Primer examines the scope of mental disability law, defines the key terms and offers tips on how to provide effective representation for clients. Part II reviews major federal legislative initiatives including the Americans with Disabilities Act. *$15.00*

ISBN 0-897077-98-9

2567 Mental Health Rehabilitation: Disputing Irrational Beliefs
Charles C Thomas Publisher Ltd.
2600 S 1st Street
Springfield, IL 62704-4730
217-789-8980
800-258-8980
Fax: 217-789-9130
E-mail: books@ccthomas.com
www.ccthomas.com

Michael P Thomas, President

Applicable to a wide variety of disciplines involved with therapeutic counseling of people with mental and/or physical disabilities such as rehabilitation counseling, mental health counseling, pastoral counseling, school counseling, clinical social work, clinical and counseling psychology, and behavioral science oriented medical specialities and related health and therapeutic professionals. Copyright 1995. *$36.95*

106 pages ISBN 0-398065-31-4

2568 Mental Health Resources Catalog
Paul H Brookes Company
PO Box 10624
Baltimore, MD 21285-624
410-337-9580
800-638-3775
Fax: 410-337-8539
E-mail: custserv@brookespublishing.com
www.brookespublishing.com

This catalog offers practical resources for mental health professionals serving young children and their families, including school psychologists, teachers and early intervention professionals. FREE.

2 per year

2569 Mental Retardation: Definition, Classification, and Systems of Supports
AAMR
444 N Capitol Street NW
Suite 846
Washington, DC 20001-1569
202-637-0475
800-424-3688
Fax: 202-637-0585
E-mail: dcroser@aamr.org

Danielle Webber, MSW, Manager, Educational Programs
Maria Alfaro, Meetings/Web Manager
Jason Epstein, Communications Coordinator
Kathleen McLane, Director, Publications Program

Presents a complete system to define and diagnose mental retardation, classify and describe strengths and limitations, and plan a supports needs profile. *$79.95*

238 pages ISBN 0-940898-81-0

2570 Metaphor in Psychotherapy: Clinical Applications of Stories and Allegories
Impact Publishers
PO Box 6016
Atascadero, CA 93423-6016
805-466-5917
800-246-7228
Fax: 805-466-5919
E-mail: info@impactpublishers.com
www.impactpublishers.com

Comprehensive resource aids therapists in helping clients change distorted views of the human experience. Dozens of practical therapeutic activities involving metaphor, drama, fantasy, and meditation. Copyright 1998. *$29.95*

320 pages ISBN 1-886230-10-2

2571 Microcounseling
Charles C Thomas Publisher Ltd.
2600 S 1st Street
Springfield, IL 62704-4730
217-789-8980
800-258-8980
Fax: 217-789-9130

E-mail: books@ccthomas.com
www.ccthomas.com

Thomas Daniels, Author
Allen Ivey, Author

Innovations in Interviewing, Counseling, Psychotherapy, and Psychoeducation. Copyright 1978. *$91.95*

296 pages Year Founded: 2007 ISSN 0-398-06175-0ISBN 0-398037-12-4

2572 Natural Supports: A Foundation for Employment
AAMR
444 N Capitol Street NW
Suite 846
Washington, DC 20001-1569
202-637-0475
800-424-3688
Fax: 202-637-0585
E-mail: dcroser@aamr.org

Step-by-step strategy for developing a network of natural supports aimed at promoting the goals and interests of all individuals in the work setting. *$12.95*

34 pages ISBN 0-940898-65-9

2573 Negotiating Managed Care: Manual for Clinicians
American Psychiatric Publishing, Inc.
1000 Wilson Boulevard
Suite 1825
Arlington, VA 22209-3901
703-907-7322
800-368-5777
Fax: 703-907-1091
E-mail: appi@psych.org
www.appi.org

Michael A Fauman, Ph.D., M.D., Author
Ron McMillen, Chief Executive Officer
John McDuffie, Editorial Director

Help for professionals to successfully present a case during clinical review. Copyright 2002. *$26.95*

128 pages Year Founded: 2002 ISBN 1-585620-42-4

2574 Neurobiology of Violence
American Psychiatric Publishing, Inc.
1000 Wilson Boulevard
Suite 1825
Arlington, VA 22209-3901
703-907-7322
800-368-5777
Fax: 703-907-1091
E-mail: appi@psych.org
www.appi.org

Jan Volavka, M.D., Ph.D., Author
Ron McMillen, Chief Executive Officer
John McDuffie, Editorial Director

Important information on the basic science of violence, including genetics, with topics of great practical value to today's clinician, including major mental disorders and violence; alcohol and substance abuse and violence; and psychopharmacological approaches to managing violent behavior. Copyright 2002. *$69.00*

410 pages Year Founded: 2002 ISBN 1-585620-81-5

2575 Neurodevelopment & Adult Psychopathology
Cambridge University Press
40 W 20th Street
New York, NY 10011-4211
212-924-3900
Fax: 212-691-3239
E-mail: marketing@cup.org
www.cup.org

2576 Neurology for Clinical Social Work: Theory and Practice
WW Norton & Company
500 5th Avenue
New York, NY 10110-54
212-354-5500
800-233-4830
Fax: 212-869-0856
E-mail: npb@wwnorton.com
www.books.wwnorton.com/

Bernard D. Beitman, Author
Barton J. Blinder, Author
Michael E. Thase, Author
Debra L. Safer, Author

Social work educators Jeffrey Applegate and Janet Shapiro demystify the explosion of recent research on neurobiology and present it anew with social workers specifically in mind. Abundant case examples show clinicians how to make use of neurobiological concepts in assessment as well as in designing treatment plans and interventions. Community mental health, family service agencies, and child welfare settings are discussed.

ISBN 0-393704-20-3

2577 Neuropsychiatry and Mental Health Services
American Psychiatric Publishing, Inc.
1000 Wilson Boulevard
Arlington, VA 22209-3901
703-907-7322
800-368-5777
Fax: 703-907-1091
E-mail: appi@psych.org
www.appi.org

Fred Ovsiew, M.D., Editor
Ron McMillen, Chief Executive Officer
John McDuffie, Editorial Director

Cognitive therapy practices in conjunction with mental health treatment. Copyright 1999. *$79.95*

420 pages Year Founded: 1999 ISBN 0-880487-30-5

2578 Neuropsychology of Mental Disorders: Practical Guide
Charles C Thomas Publisher Ltd.
2600 S 1st Street
Springfield, IL 62704-4730
217-789-8980
800-258-8980
Fax: 217-789-9130
E-mail: books@ccthomas.com
www.ccthomas.com

Michael P Thomas, President

Discusses the advances in diverse areas such as biology, electrophysiology, genetics, neuroanatomy, pharmacology, psychology, and radiology which are increasingly important for a practical understanding of behavior and its pathology. Copyright 1994. *$70.95*

338 pages ISBN 0-398059-05-5

2579 New Roles for Psychiatrists in Organized Systems of Care
American Psychiatric Publishing, Inc.
1000 Wilson Boulevard
Suite 1825
Arlington, VA 22209-3901
703-907-7322
800-368-5777
Fax: 703-907-1091
E-mail: appi@psych.org
www.appi.org

Jeremy A Lazarus, M.D, Editor
Steven S Sharfstein, M.D, Editor
John McDuffie, Editorial Director

Comprehensive view of opportunities, challenges and roles for psychiatrists who are working for or with new organized systems of care. Discusses the ethical dilemmas for psychiatrists in managed care settings and training and identity of the field as well as historical overviews of health care policy. Copyright 1998. *$50.00*

288 pages Year Founded: 1998 ISBN 0-880487-58-5

2580 Of One Mind: The Logic of Hypnosis, the Practice of Therapy
WW Norton & Company
500 5th Avenue
New York, NY 10110-54
212-354-5500
800-233-4830
Fax: 212-869-0856
E-mail: admalmud@wwnorton.com
www.books.wwnorton.com/

Douglas Flemons, Author

A new approach to an old treatment, the author explains his ideas on connecting with patients in hypno and brief therapies. Copyright 2001. *$30.00*

240 pages ISBN 0-393703-82-7

2581 On Being a Therapist
John Wiley & Sons
111 River Street
Hoboken, NJ 07030-5774
201-748-6000
Fax: 201-748-6088
www.wiley.com

This thoroughly revised and updated edition shows you how to use the insights gained from your clients' experiences to solve your own problems, realize positive change in yourself, and become a better therapist. *$22.00*

320 pages ISBN 1-555425-55-0

2582 On the Counselor's Path: A Guide to Teaching Brief Solution Focused Therapy
NewHarbinger Publications
5674 Shattuck Avenue
Oakland, CA 94609-1662
510-652-0215
800-748-6273
Fax: 510-652-5472
E-mail: customerservice@newharbinger.com
www.newharbinger.com

Matthew McKay, Owner

A teacher's guide for conducting training sessions on solution focused techniques. Copyright 1996. *$24.95*

92 pages ISBN 1-572240-48-2

2583 Opportunities for Daily Choice Making
AAMR
444 N Capitol Street NW
Suite 846
Washington, DC 20001-1569
202-637-0475
800-424-3688
Fax: 202-637-0585
E-mail: dcroser@aamr.org

Provides strategies for increasing choice-making opportunities for people with developmental disabilities. It describes basic principles of choice-making, shows how to teach choice-making skills to the passive learner, describes how to build in multiple choice-making opportunities within daily routines, introduces self-scheduling, and addresses common questions. *$12.95*

48 pages ISBN 0-904898-44-6

2584 Participatory Evaluation for Special Education and Rehabilitation
AAMR
444 N Capitol Street NW
Suite 846
Washington, DC 20001-1569
202-637-0475
800-424-3688
Fax: 202-637-0585
E-mail: dcroser@aamr.org

Nine-step method for identifying and weighing the importance of disparate goals and outcomes. *$31.95*

90 pages ISBN 0-940898-73-X

2585 Person-Centered Foundation for Counseling and Psychotherapy
Charles C Thomas Publisher Ltd.
2600 S 1st Street
Springfield, IL 62704-4730
217-789-8980
800-258-8980
Fax: 217-789-9130
E-mail: books@ccthomas.com
www.ccthomas.com

Angelo V Boy, Author
Gerald J Pine, Author

Focusing on counseling and psychotherapy, its goals are to renew interest in the person-centered approach in the US, make a signigicant contribution to extending person-centered theory and practice, and promote fruitful dialogue and futher development of person-centered theory. Presents: the rationale for an eclectic application of person-centered counseling; the rationale and process for reflecting clients' feelings; the importance of the theory as the foundation for the counseling process; the importance of values and their influence on the counseling relationship; the modern person-centered counselor's role; and the essential characteristics of a person-centered counseling relationship. Copyright 1999.

274 pages Year Founded: 1999 ISSN 0-398-06966-2ISBN 0-398069-64-6

2586 PharmaCoKinetics and Therapeutic Monitering of Psychiatric Drugs
Charles C Thomas Publisher Ltd.
2600 S 1st Street
Springfield, IL 62704-4730
217-789-8980
800-258-8980
Fax: 217-789-9130
E-mail: books@ccthomas.com
www.ccthomas.com

Michael P Thomas, President

$52.95

226 pages ISBN 0-398058-41-5

2587 Positive Bahavior Support for People with Developmental Disabilities: A Research Synthesis
AAMR
444 N Capitol Street NW
Suite 846
Washington, DC 20001-1569
202-637-0475
800-424-3688
Fax: 202-637-0585
E-mail: dcroser@aamr.org

Offers a careful analysis documenting that positive behavioral procedures can produce important change in the behavior and lives of people with disabilities. *$31.95*

128 pages ISBN 0-940898-60-8

2588 Positive Behavior Support Training Curriculum
AAMR
501 3rd Street
NW Suite 200
Washington, DC 20001
202-387-1968
800-424-3688
Fax: 202-387-2193
E-mail: dcroser@aamr.org
www.www.aaidd.org

Dennis H. Reid, Author
Marsha B. Parsons, Author

Designed for training supervisors of direct support staff, as well as direct support professionals themselves in the values and practices of positive behavior support.

2589 Practical Guide to Cognitive Therapy
WW Norton & Company
500 5th Avenue
New York, NY 10110-54
212-354-5500
Fax: 212-869-0856
E-mail: admalmud@wwnorton.com
www.books.wwnorton.com/

Dean Schuyler, Author

Based on highly successful workshops by the author, this book provides a framework to apply cognitive therapy model to office practices. Copyright 1991. *$22.95*

200 pages ISBN 0-393701-05-0

2590 Practical Psychiatric Practice Forms and Protocols for Clinical Use
American Psychological Publishing
1400 K Street NW
Washington, DC 20005-2403
202-682-6262
800-368-5777
Fax: 202-789-2648
E-mail: appi@psych.org
www.appi.org

Katie Duffy, Marketing Assistant

Designed to aid psychiatrists in organizing their work. Provides rating scales, model letters, medication tracking forms, clinical pathology requests and sample invoices. Handouts on disorders and medication are provided for patients and their families. Spiralbound. Copyright 1998. *$47.50*

312 pages ISBN 0-880489-43-X

2591 Practice Guidelines for Extended Psychiatric Residential Care: From Chaos to Collaboration
Charles C Thomas Publisher Ltd.
2600 S 1st Street
Springfield, IL 62704-4730
217-789-8980
800-258-8980
Fax: 217-789-9130
E-mail: books@ccthomas.com
www.ccthomas.com

Michael P Thomas, President
Stanley McCracken, Author/Editor
Joseph Mehr, Author/Editor

Presents a set of practice guidelines that represent state-of-the-art treatments for consumers of extended residential care. Written for line-level staff charged with the day-to-day services: psychiatrists, psychologists, social workers, activity therapists, nurses, and psychiatric technicians who work closely with consumers in residential programs and program administrators who have immediate responsibility for supervising treatment teams. Copyright 1995. *$47.95*

176 pages ISSN 0-398-06536-5ISBN 0-398065-35-7

2592 Primer of Brief Psychotherapy
WW Norton & Company
500 5th Avenue
New York, NY 10110-54
212-354-5500
Fax: 212-869-0856
E-mail: admalmud@wwnorton.com
www.books.wwnorton.com/

John F. Cooper, Author

Positive guide to brief therapy is a task oriented aid with emphasis on the first session and details of procedures afterward. Copyright 1995. *$19.55*

348 pages ISBN 0-393701-89-1

2593 Primer of Supportive Psychotherapy
Analytic Press
7625 Empire Drive
Florence, KS 41042-2919
201-358-9477
800-634-7064
Fax: 800-248-4724

E-mail: orders@taylorandfrancis.com
www.www.routledgementalhealth.com/

Henry Pinsker, Author
John Kerr PhD, Sr Editor

Focuses on the rationale for and techniques of supportive psychotherapy as a form of dyadic intervention distinct from expressive psychotherapies. The realities, ironies, conundrums and opportunities of the therapeutic encounter are vividly portrayed in scores of illustrative dialogues drawn from actual treatments. Among the topics covered are how to provide reassurance in the realistic way, how to handle requests for advice, the role of praise and reinforcement, the appropriate use of reframing techniques and of modeling, negotiating patients' concerns about medication and other collateral forms of treatment. *$45.00*

296 pages Year Founded: 1997 ISBN 0-881632-74-0

2594 Psychiatry in the New Millennium
American Psychiatric Publishing, Inc.
1000 Wilson Boulevard
Suite 1825
22209-3901
703-907-7322
800-368-5777
Fax: 703-907-1091
E-mail: appi@psych.org
www.appi.org

Sidney Weissman, M.D, Editor
Melvin Sabshin, M.D, Editor
Harold Eist, M.D, Editor

Keeping the standards and utilizing advances in diagnosis and treatment. *$66.50*

392 pages Year Founded: 1999 ISBN 0-880489-38-3

2595 Psychoanalysis, Behavior Therapy & the Relational World
American Psychological Association
750 1st St NE
Washington, DC 20002-4242
202-336-5500
Fax: 202-336-5518
www.apa.org

Paul L Wachtel, Author

484 pages

2596 Psychoanalytic Therapy as Health Care Effectiveness and Economics in the 21st Century
Analytic Press
7625 Empire Drive
Florence, KS 41042-2919
201-358-9477
800-634-7064
Fax: 800-248-4724
E-mail: orders@taylorandfrancis.com
www.www.routledgementalhealth.com/

Harriette Kaley, PhD, Editor
Morris Eagle, Ph.D, Editor
David L Wolitzky, Ph.D, Editor

Drawing on a wide range of clinical and empirical evidence, authors argue that contemporary psychoanalytic approaches are applicable to seriously distressed persons in a variety of treatment contexts. Failure to include such long term therapies within health care delivery systems, they conclude, will deprive many patients of help they need, and help from which they can benefit in enduring ways that far transcend the limited treatment goals of managed care. Available in hardcover. *$ 49.95*

312 pages Year Founded: 1999 ISBN 0-881632-02-3

2597 Psychodynamic, Affective, and Behavioral Theories to Psychotherapy
Charles C Thomas Publisher Ltd.
2600 South First Street
Springfield, IL 62704
800-258-8980
Fax: 217-789-9130
E-mail: books@ccthomas.com

Marty Sapp, Author

The goal of this book is to examine three major theories and their approach to psychotherapy psychodynamic, affective, and behavioral which are defined as specific skills that a clinician or student can readily understand. Experiential exercises, glossaries, and examination questions are included in each chapter. This unique and comprehensive book will be of interest to mentalhealth workers, educational therapists, counselors, psychologists, psychiatrists, and students. *$59.95*

242 pages Year Founded: 2010 ISBN 0-398078-95-9

2598 Psychological Aspects of Women's Health Care
American Psychiatric Publishing, Inc.
1000 Wilson Boulevard
Suite 1825
Arlington, VA 22209-3901
703-907-7322
800-368-5777
Fax: 703-907-1091
E-mail: appi@psych.org
www.appi.org

Nada L Stotland, M.D., M.P.H, Editor
Donna E Stewart, M.D., D.Psych, Editor
John McDuffie, Editorial Director

The Interface Between Psychiatry and Obstetrics and Gynecology, Second Edition. Discussion from major leaders in the specialties of psychiatry and obstetrics/gynecology covering every major area of contemporary concern. Issues in pregnancy, gynecology, and general issues such as reproductive choices, breast disorders, violence, lesbian health care, and the male perspective are included. *$77.00*

672 pages Year Founded: 2001 ISBN 0-880488-31-X

2599 Psychologists' Desk Reference
Oxford University Press/Oxford Reference Book Society
198 Madison Avenue
New York, NY 10016-4308
212-726-6400
800-451-7556

Gerald P. Koocher, Editor
John C. Norcross, Editor
Beverly A. Greene, Editor

For the practicing psychologist; easily accessible, current information on almost any topic by some of the leading thinkers and innovators in the field. *$65.00*

840 pages Year Founded: 1998 ISBN 0-195111-86-9

2600 Psychoneuroendocrinology: The Scientific Basis of Clinical Practice
American Psychiatric Publishing, Inc.
1000 Wilson Boulevard
Suite 1825
Arlington, VA 22209-3901
703-907-7322
800-368-5777
Fax: 703-907-1091
E-mail: appi@psych.org
www.appi.org

Owen M Wolkowitz, M.D., Editor
Anthony J Rothschild, M.D, Editor
John McDuffie, Editorial Director

Applications of scientific research.

606 pages Year Founded: 2003 ISBN 0-880488-57-3

2601 Psychopharmacology Desktop Reference
Manisses Communications Group
208 Governor Street
Providence, RI 02906-3246
401-831-6020
800-333-7771
Fax: 401-861-6370
E-mail: manissescs@manisses.com
www.manisses.com

Karienne Stovell, Editor

Covers medications for all types of mental disorders. Provides detailed information on all the latest drugs as well as colored photographs of the different kinds of drugs. Helps you spot side effects and avoid drug interactions. Includes revealing case studies and outcomes data. *$159.00*

ISBN 1-864937-69-1

2602 Psychopharmacology Update
Manisses Communications Group
208 Governor Street
Providence, RI 02906-3246
401-831-6020
800-333-7771
Fax: 401-861-6370
E-mail: manissescs@manisses.com
www.manisses.com

Karienne Stovell, Editor

Offers psychopharmacology advice for general practitioners and nonprescribing professionals in the mental health field. Covers child psychopharmacology and street drugs. Contains case reports. Recurring features include news of research and book reviews. *$147.00*

12 per year ISSN 1068-5308

2603 Psychosocial Aspects of Disability
Charles C Thomas Publisher Ltd.
PO Box 19265
Springfield, IL 62794-9265
217-789-8980
800-258-8980
Fax: 217-789-9130
www.ccthomas.com

George Henderson, Author
Willie V Bryan, Author

This expanded and updated new edition continues the theme of the first and second editions of emphasizing that attitudinal barriers create environmental barriers for persons with disabilities. The new edition is improved as a primary introductory text or a supplemental text for student helping professionals with the addition of chapters on employment, understanding ethnic groups, concepts, theories, therapies, and issues for the twenty-first century. Available in paperback for $55.95. *$75.95*

274 pages Year Founded: 2011 ISBN 0-398074-86-0

2604 Psychotherapist's Duty to Warn or Protect
Charles C Thomas Publisher Ltd.
2600 S 1st Street
Springfield, IL 62704-4730
217-789-8980
800-258-8980
Fax: 217-789-9130
E-mail: books@ccthomas.com
www.ccthomas.com

Michael P Thomas, President

$47.95

194 pages Year Founded: 1989 ISBN 0-398055-46-7

2605 Psychotherapist's Guide to Cost Containment: How to Survive and Thrive in an Age of Managed Care
Sage Publications
2455 Teller Road
Thousand Oaks, CA 91320-2234
805-499-0721
800-818-7243
Fax: 805-499-0871
E-mail: info@sagepub.com
www.sagepub.com

Bernard D Beitman, Author

$23.50

176 pages Year Founded: 1998 ISBN 0-803973-81-0

2606 Psychotherapy Indications and Outcomes
American Psychiatric Publishing, Inc.
1000 Wilson Boulevard
Suite 1825
Arlington, VA 22209-3901
703-907-7322
800-368-5777
Fax: 703-907-1091
E-mail: appi@psych.org
www.appi.org

David S Janowsky, M.D., Editor
Ron McMillen, Chief Executive Officer
John McDuffie, Editorial Director

Clinical approaches to different symptoms. *$66.50*

432 pages Year Founded: 1999 ISBN 0-880487-61-5

2607 Psychotropic Drug Information Handbook
Lexicomp Inc.
1100 Terex Road
Hudson, OH 44236-4438
330-650-6506
800-837-5394
Fax: 330-650-6506
www.lexi.com

Steven Kerscher, Owner

Concise handbook, designed to fit into your lab coat, is a current and portable psychotropic drug reference with 150

drugs and 35 herbal monographs. Perfect companion to Drug Information Handbook for Psychiatry. *$38.75*

1 per year ISBN 1-591951-15-1

2608 Psychotropic Drugs: Fast Facts
WW Norton & Company
500 5th Avenue
New York, NY 10110-54
212-354-5500
800-233-4830
Fax: 212-869-0856
E-mail: npb@wwnorton.com
www.books.wwnorton.com/

Sidney H. Kennedy, Author
Jerrold S. Maxmen, Author
Roger S. McIntyre, Author

Now in its third edition, Psychotropic Drugs: Fast Facts continues to present valuable information in a clear and accessible format. The book organizaes and presents data clinicians need to choose the right treatment for common psychiatric problems and to anticipate and deal with problems that arise in treatment.

ISBN 0-393703-01-0

2609 Quality of Life: Volume II
AAMR
444 N Capitol Street NW
Suite 846
Washington, DC 20001-1569
202-637-0475
800-424-3688
Fax: 202-637-0585
E-mail: dcroser@aamr.org

Focuses on how the concepts and research on quality of life can be applied to people with mental retardation. *$19.95*

267 pages ISBN 0-940898-41-1

2610 Questions of Competence
Cambridge University Press
40 W 20th Street
New York, NY 10011-4211
212-924-3900
Fax: 212-691-3239
E-mail: marketing@cup.org
www.cup.org

2611 Reaching Out in Family Therapy: Home Based, School, and Community Interventions
Guilford Press
72 Spring Street
New York, NY 10012-4068
212-431-9800
800-365-7006
Fax: 212-966-6708
E-mail: info@guilford.com

Brenna Hafer Bry, Author
Nancy Boyd-Franklin, Author

Practical framework for clinicians using multisystems intervention. *$27.00*

244 pages Year Founded: 2000 ISBN 1-572305-19-3

2612 Recognition and Treatment of Psychiatric Disorders: Psychopharmacology Handbook for Primary Care
American Psychiatric Publishing, Inc.
1000 Wilson Boulevard
Suite 1825
Arlington, VA 22209-3901
703-907-7322
800-368-5777
Fax: 703-907-1091
E-mail: appi@psych.org
www.appi.org

Robert E Hales MD, Editor-in-Chief
Ron McMillen, Chief Executive Officer
John McDuffie, Editorial Director

Provides the primary care physician with practical and timely strategies for screening and treating patients who have psychiatric disorders. Includes an overview of the epidemiology, pathophysiology, presentation, diagnostic criteria and screening tests for common psychiatric disorders including anxiety, mood, substance abuse, somatization and eating disorders, as well as insomnia, dementia and schizophrenia. *$35.00*

324 pages

2613 Recognition of Early Psychosis
Cambridge University Press
40 W 20th Street
New York, NY 10011-4211
212-924-3900
Fax: 212-691-3239
E-mail: marketing@cup.org
www.cup.org

2614 Review of Psychiatry
American Psychiatric Publishing, Inc.
1000 Wilson Boulevard
Suite 1825
Arlington, VA 22209-3901
703-907-7322
800-368-5777
Fax: 703-907-1091
E-mail: appi@psych.org
www.appi.org

Robert E Hales MD, Editor-in-Chief
Ron McMillen, Chief Executive Officer
John McDuffie, Editorial Director

Cognitive therapy, repressed memories and obsessive-compulsive disorder across the life cycle. *$59.95*

928 pages Year Founded: 1997 ISBN 0-880484-43-8

2615 Schools for Students with Special Needs
Resources for Children with Special Needs
116 E 16th Street
Fifth Floor
New York City, NY 10003-2112
212-677-4650
Fax: 212-254-4070
E-mail: info@resourcesnyc.org
www.resourcesnyc.org

Rachel Howard, Executive Director

The first complete book listing private day and residential schools for parents, caregivers and professionals seeking schools for students 5 and up with developmental, emotional, physical and learning disabilities in the NYC metro area. More than 400 schools and residential programs that serve children in the elementary through high school grades are listed with contact information, ages and populations served, class sizes and student-teacher ratios, special services and diplomas offered. Includes a 46-page section of Schools for Children with Autism Spectrum Disorders, as well as a guide with a list of websites on autism spectrum disorders. *$25.00*

342 pages

2616 Selecting Effective Treatments: a Comprehensive, Systematic, Guide for Treating Mental Disorders
Jossey-Bass Publishers
111 River Street
Hoboken, NJ 07030-5774
201-748-6000
800-956-7739
Fax: 201-748-6088
E-mail: info@wiley.com
www.as.wiley.com

Linda Seligman, Author
Lourie W Reichenberg, Author

$39.95

609 pages Year Founded: 2014 ISBN 0-787943-07-X

2617 Social Work Dictionary
National Association of Social Workers
750 1st Street NE
Suite 700
Washington, DC 20002-4241
202-408-8600
800-227-3590
Fax: 202-336-8313
E-mail: press@naswdc.org
www.naswpress.org

Robert L Barker, Author

More than 8, 000 terms are defined in this essential tool for understanding the language of social work and related disciplines. The resulting reference is a must for every human services professional. *$34.95*

620 pages Year Founded: 1999 ISBN 0-871012-98-7

2618 Strategic Marketing: How to Achieve Independence and Prosperity in Your Mental Health Practice
Professional Resource Press
PO Box 3197
Sarasota, FL 34230-3197
941-343-9601
800-443-3364
Fax: 941-343-9201
E-mail: orders@prpress.com
www.prpress.com

Laurie Girsch, Managing Editor

Presents ways to reshape your practice to capitalize on new opportunities for success in today's healthcare marketplace. *$21.95*

152 pages Year Founded: 1997 ISBN 1-568870-31-0

2619 Supports Intensity Scale
AAMR
501 3rd Street
NW Suite 200
Washington, DC 20001
202-387-1968
800-424-3688
Fax: 202-387-2193
E-mail: dcroser@aamr.org
www.www.aaidd.org

Designed to help you plan meaningful supports for adults with mental retardation. Consists of a comprehensive scoring system that measures the needs of persons with mental retardation in 57 key life activities based on 7 areas of competence. *$125.00*

128 pages

2620 Surviving & Prospering in the Managed Mental Health Care Marketplace
Professional Resource Press
PO Box 3197
Sarasota, FL 34230-3197
941-343-9601
800-443-3364
Fax: 941-343-9201
E-mail: orders@prpress.com
www.prpress.com

Laurie Girsch, Managing Editor

Includes examples of different managed care models, extensive references, and checklists. Offers examples of the typical steps in providing outpatient treatment in a managed care milieu, and other extremely useful resources. *$14.95*

106 pages Year Founded: 1994 ISBN 1-568870-04-3

2621 Suzie Brown Intervention Maze
High Tide Press
Ste 2n
2081 Calistoga Dr
New Lenox, IL 60451-4833
815-206-2054
888-487-7377
E-mail: managing.editor@hightidepress.com

John Shephard, Author

Suzie Brown, age 25, has severe developmental disabilities. She lives in a staffed house for six adults, where you work as a team. She has major communication difficulties, is prone to self-injurous behavior, and no longer responds to all the usual calming methods. What can you do? This workbook offers a practical blueprint for group decision making. Each option page presents a new scenario and ideas for moving forward. Decision logs keep track of decisions as they are made. The binder format allows for easy photocopying. *$69.99*

72 pages ISBN 1-892696-09-6

2622 Teaching Goal Setting and Decision-Making to Students with Developmental Disabilities
AAMR
444 N Capitol Street NW
Suite 846
Washington, DC 20001-1569
202-637-0475
800-424-3688

Fax: 202-637-0585
E-mail: dcroser@aamr.org

Link four basic steps of goal setting and decision making to twelve instructional principles that engage students in activities. *$12.95*

34 pages ISBN 0-940898-97-7

2623 Teaching Practical Communication Skills
AAMR
444 N Capitol Street NW
Suite 846
Washington, DC 20001-1569
202-637-0475
800-424-3688
Fax: 202-637-0585
E-mail: dcroser@aamr.org

Discusses strategies for teaching students to request their preferences, protest non-preferred activities, and clarify misunderstandings. *$12.95*

30 pages ISBN 0-940898-42-X

2624 Teaching Problem Solving to Students with Mental Retardation
AAMR
501 3rd Street
NW Suite 200
Washington, DC 20001
202-387-1968
800-424-3688
Fax: 202-387-2193
E-mail: dcroser@aamr.org
www.www.aaidd.org

Martin Agran, Author
Michael Wehmeyer, Author

Gives clear teaching strategies for social problem-solving, including role-playing, modeling, and training sequences. *$12.95*

30 pages ISBN 0-940898-62-4

2625 Teaching Students with Severe Disabilities in Inclusive Settings
AAMR
501 3rd Street
NW Suite 200
Washington, DC 20001
202-387-1968
800-424-3688
Fax: 202-387-2193
E-mail: dcroser@aamr.org
www.www.aaidd.org

MaryAnn Demchak, Author

Presents student-specific strategies for teaching students with severe disabilities in inclusive settings. Strategies include how to write IEPs in inclusive settings; effective scheduling; planning for adaptations of objectives; materials, responses, and settings; and anticipating the need for support. *$12.95*

50 pages ISBN 0-940898-49-7

**2626 Textbook of Family and Couples Therapy:
Clinical Applications**
American Psychiatric Publishing, Inc.
1000 Wilson Boulevard
Suite 1825
Arlington, VA 22209-3901
703-907-7322
800-368-5777
Fax: 703-907-1091
E-mail: appi@psych.org
www.appi.org

G Pirooz Sholevar, M.D, Editor
Linda D Schwoeri, Ph.D, Editor
John McDuffie, Editorial Director

Blending theoretical training and up-to-date clinical strategies. It's a must for clinicians who are currently treating
couples and families, a major resource for training future
clinicians in these highly effective therapeutic techniques.
$63.00

968 pages Year Founded: 2003 ISBN 0-880485-18-3

2627 The Annals of Clinical Psychiatry
American Academy of Clinical Psychiatrists
PO Box 458
Glastonbury, CT 06033-458
860-633-6023
Fax: 866-668-9858
E-mail: aacp@cox.net
www.aacp.com

Sanjay Gupta MD, President
John B Reichman MD, Vice President
James Wilcox DO, PhD, Secretary/Treasurer
Donald W Black MD, President-Elect/Author

The journal of the American Academy of Clinical Psychiatrists. The Annals publishes high-quality articles that focus
on the advancement of patient care. Contributions furnish
professionals and students with a continuing medical perspective on their discipline, addressing problems and concerns that arise in clinical practice as well as their potential
solutions. Covers ongoing research and the theories and
techniques used by leading authorities in the field.

**2628 The Role of Companion Animals in Counseling
and Psychology, Discovering Their Use in the
Therapeutic Process**
Charles C Thomas Publisher Ltd.
2600 South First Street
Springfield, IL 62704
800-258-8980
Fax: 217-789-9130
E-mail: books@ccthomas.com

Jane K. Wilkes, Author

The human health benefits derived from relationships with
companion animals has attracted an abundance of scientific
interest and research. However, there is a need for theoretical conceptualizations in order to understand the healinig
benefits of human-animal interactions. The goal of this
book is to seek these answers and the how and why companion animals play a role in counseling and psychology.
In-depth semi-structured interviews were conducted with
three psychologists who use animals in their therapy settings. Replete with informative appendices that will serve
as valuable knowledge, this book is a significant resource
on the subject of animal-assisted therapy for mental health

professionals such as counselors, clinical social workers,
and therapists. *$32.95*

168 pages Year Founded: 2009 ISBN 0-398078-63-8

2629 Theory and Technique of Family Therapy
Charles C Thomas Publisher Ltd.
2600 S 1st Street
Springfield, IL 62704-4730
217-789-8980
800-258-8980
Fax: 217-789-9130
E-mail: books@ccthomas.com
www.ccthomas.com

Michael P Thomas, President
Ramon Garrido Corrales, Author

Contents: The Family as an Interactional System; The
Family as an Intergenerational System; A Model for the
Therapeutic Relationship in Family Theory, The Therapeu-
tic Process and Related Concerns; Therapeutic Intervention
Techniques and Adjuncts; Marital Group and Multiple
Family Therapy; Counseling at Two Critical Stages of
Family Development, Formation and Termination of Mar-
riage. Useful information for students and practitioners of
family therapy, social workers, the clergy, psychiatrists,
psychologists, counselors, and related professionals. *$55.95*

352 pages Year Founded: 1981 ISBN 0-398038-59-7

2630 Thesaurus of Psychological Index Terms
American Psychological Association Database
Department/PsycINFO
750 1st Street NE
Washington, DC 20002-4242
202-336-5500
800-374-2722
Fax: 202-336-5518
TDD: 202-336-6123
E-mail: psycinfo@apa.org
www.apa.org

Norman B Anderson, CEO

Reference to the PsycINFO database vocabulary of over 5,
400 descriptors. Provides standardized working to represent each concept for complete, efficient and precise retrieval of psychological information and is updated
regularly. 9th edition published 2001. *$60.00*

379 pages ISBN 1-557987-75-0

2631 Three Spheres: Psychiatric Interviewing Primer
Rapid Psychler Press
2014 Holland Ave
Suite 374
Port Huron, MI 48060-1994
519-667-2335
888-779-2453
Fax: 519-675-0610
E-mail: rapid@psychler.com
www.psychler.com

David Robinson, Publisher

$16.95

ISBN 0-968032-49-4

2632 Through the Patient's Eyes
Jossey-Bass Publishers
111 River Street
Hoboken, NJ 07030-5774

201-748-6000
800-956-7739
Fax: 201-748-6088
E-mail: info@wiley.com
www.as.wiley.com

Margaret Gerteis, Editor
Thomas Delbanco, Editor
Susan Edgman-Levitan, Editor
Jennifer Daley, Editor

Learn how providers can improve their ability to meet patient's needs and enhance the quality of care by bringing the patient's perspective to the design and delivery of health services. *$36.95*

360 pages Year Founded: 2002 ISBN 7-555425-44-5

2633 Tools of the Trade: A Therapist's Guide to Art Therapy Assessments
Charles C Thomas Publisher Ltd.
PO Box 19265
Springfield, IL 62794-9265
217-789-8980
800-258-8980
Fax: 217-789-9130
www.ccthomas.com

Stephanie L. Brooke, Author

Provides critical reviews of art therapy tests along with some new reviews of assessments and updated research in the field. Comprehensive in the approach to consider reliability and validity evidence provided by test authors. Available in paperback for $35.95. *$53.95*

256 pages Year Founded: 2004 ISBN 0-398075-21-2

2634 Total Quality Management in Mental Health and Mental Retardation
AAMR
444 N Capitol Street NW
Suite 846
Washington, DC 20001-1569
202-637-0475
800-424-3688
Fax: 202-637-0585
E-mail: dcroser@aamr.org

Describes how this leadership philosophy helps an organization identify and achive quality outcomes for all its customers. *$14.95*

64 pages ISBN 0-940898-67-5

2635 Training Behavioral Healthcare Professionals
Jossey-Bass Publishers
350 Sansome Street
5th Floor
San Francisco, CA 94104-1310
800-956-7739

James M. Schuster, Editor
Mark R. Lovell, Editor
Anthony M. Trachta, Editor

Provides text on strategies for training mental health professionals in the skills necessary for providing services in a framework of limited resources. *$46.00*

180 pages Year Founded: 1997 ISBN 0-787907-95-2

2636 Training Families to do a Successful Intervention: A Professional's Guide
Hazelden
15251 Pleasant Valley Road
PO Box 176
Center City, MN 55012-176
651-213-2121
800-328-9000
Fax: 651-213-4590
E-mail: customersupport@hazelden.org
www.hazelden.org

Helps professionals explain basic intervention concepts and give clients step-by-step instructions. *$15.95*

152 pages ISBN 1-562461-16-8

2637 Treatment of Complicated Mourning
Research Press
PO Box 7866
Champaign, IL 61826-9177
217-352-3273
800-519-2707
Fax: 217-352-1221
E-mail: rp@researchpress.com
www.researchpress.com

Dr. Therese Rando, Author

This is the first book to focus specifically on complicated mourning, often referred to as pathological, unresolved or abnormal grief. It provides caregivers with practical therapeutic strategies and specific interventions that are necessary when traditional grief counseling is unsufficient. The author provides critically important information on the prediction, identification, assessment, classification and treatment of complicated mourning. *$39.95*

768 pages ISBN 0-878223-29-0

2638 Treatments of Psychiatric Disorders
American Psychiatric Publishing, Inc.
1000 Wilson Boulevard
Suite 1825
Arlington, VA 22209-3901
703-907-7322
800-368-5777
Fax: 703-907-1091
E-mail: appi@psych.org
www.appi.org

Robert E Hales MD, Editor-in-Chief
Ron McMillen, Chief Executive Officer
John McDuffie, Editorial Director

Examines customary approaches to the major psychiatric disorders. Diagnostic, etiologic and therapeutic issues are clearly addressed by experts on each topic. *$307.00*

2800 pages Year Founded: 1995 ISBN 0-880487-00-3

2639 Using Computers In Educational and Psychological Research
Charles C Thomas Publisher Ltd.
PO Box 19265
Springfield, IL 62794-9265
217-789-8980
800-258-8980
Fax: 217-789-9130
www.ccthomas.com

This book has been designed to assist researchers in the social sciences and education fields who are interested in learning how information technologies can help them successfully navigate the research process. Most researchers are familiar with the use of programs like SPSS to analyze data, but many are not aware of other ways informaiton technologies can support the research process. This book is available in paperback for $44.95. *$69.95*

274 pages Year Founded: 2006 ISBN 0-398076-16-2

2640 Values Clarification for Counselors
harles C Thomas Publisher Ltd.
2600 S 1st Street
Springfield, IL 62704-4730
217-789-8980
800-258-8980
Fax: 217-789-9130
E-mail: books@ccthomas.com
www.ccthomas.com

Michael P Thomas, President

How Counselors, Social Workers, Psychologists, and Other Human Service Workers Can Use Available Techniques. *$24.95*

104 pages Year Founded: 1978 ISBN 0-398038-47-3

2641 What Psychotherapists Should Know About Disability
Guilford Press
72 Spring Street
New York, NY 10012-4068
212-431-9800
800-365-7006
Fax: 212-966-6708
E-mail: info@guilford.com

Rhoda Olkin Phd, Author

Available in alternate formats for people with disabilities, this guide confronts biases and relates the human dimesions of disability. Stereotypes and discomfort can get in the way of even a well intentioned therapist, this helps achieve a clearer professional relationship with clients of special need. *$35.00*

368 pages Year Founded: 1999 ISBN 1-572302-27-5

2642 Where to Start and What to Ask: An Assessment Handbook
WW Norton & Company
500 5th Avenue
New York, NY 10110-54
212-354-5500
800-233-4830
Fax: 212-869-0856
E-mail: npb@wwnorton.com
www.books.wwnorton.com/

Susan Lukas, Author

As a life raft for beginners and their supervisors, provides all the necessary tools for garnering information from clients. Offers a framework for thinking about that information and formulating a thorough assessment, helps neophytes organize their approach to the initial phase of treatment. Copyright 1993.

ISBN 0-393701-52-2

2643 Women's Mental Health Services: Public Health Perspective
Sage Publications
2455 Teller Road
Thousand Oaks, CA 91320-2234

805-499-0721
800-818-7243
Fax: 805-499-0871
E-mail: info@sagepub.com
www.sagepub.com

Bruce Lubotsky Levin, Author
Andrea K Blanch, Author
Ann Jennings, Author

Paperback, hardcover also available. *$29.95*

448 pages Year Founded: 1998 ISBN 0-761905-09-X

2644 Workbook: Mental Retardation
AAMR
444 N Capitol Street NW
Suite 846
Washington, DC 20001-1569
202-637-0475
800-424-3688
Fax: 202-637-0585
E-mail: dcroser@aamr.org

Presents key components from a practical point of view. *$29.95*

64 pages ISBN 0-940898-82-9

2645 Working with the Core Relationship Problem in Psychotherapy
Jossey-Bass Publishers
111 River Street
Hoboken, NJ 07030-5774
201-748-6000
800-956-7739
Fax: 201-748-6088
E-mail: info@wiley.com
www.as.wiley.com

Althea J Horner, Author

Learn to reveal, understand, and use the core relationship problem, which is formed from earliest childhood and creates an image of the self in relation to others so it can aid in understanding the underlying conflict that repeatedly plays out in a client's behavior. *$39.95*

185 pages Year Founded: 1998 ISBN 0-787943-01-0

2646 Writing Behavioral Contracts: A Case Simulation Practice Manual
Research Press
PO Box 7866
Champaign, IL 61826-9177
217-352-3273
800-519-2707
Fax: 217-352-1221
E-mail: rp@researchpress.com
www.researchpress.com

Dr William J DeRiski, Author
Dennis Wiziecki, Marketing

The most difficult aspect of using contingency contracting is designing a contract acceptable to and appropriate for all involved parties. This unusually versatile book improves contract-writing skills through practice with typical cases. Valuable for social workers, mental health professionals and educators. *$11.95*

94 pages ISBN 0-878221-23-9

2647 Writing Psychological Reports: A Guide for Clinicians
Professional Resource Press
PO Box 3197
Sarasota, FL 34230-3197
941-343-9601
800-443-3364
Fax: 941-343-9201
E-mail: orders@prpress.com
www.prpress.com

Greg J Wolber, Author
William F Carne, Author

Presents widely accepted structured format for writing psychological reports. Numerous useful suggestions for experienced clinicians, and qualifies as essential reading for all clinical psychology students. *$21.95*

158 pages Year Founded: 2002 ISBN 1-568870-76-0

Adjustment Disorders

2648 Ambiguous Loss: Learning to Live with Unresolved Grief
Harvard University Press
79 Garden Street
Cambridge, MA 02138-1400
617-495-1000
Fax: 617-495-5898
E-mail: CONTACT_HUP@harvard.edu
www.hup.harvard.edu

William Sisler, President

$22.00

192 pages Year Founded: 1999 ISBN 0-674017-38-2

2649 Attachment and Interaction
Jessica Kingsley
711 3rd Avenue
8th Floor
New York, NY 10017
212-216-7800
Fax: 212-564-7854
www.taylorandfrancis.com

Available in paperback. *$29.95*

238 pages Year Founded: 1998 ISBN 1-853025-86-0

2650 Body Image: Understanding Body Dissatisfaction in Men, Women and Children
Routledge
2727 Palisade Avenue
Suite 4H
Bronx, NY 10463-1020
718-796-0971
Fax: 718-796-0971
E-mail: vdg@columbia.edu

Sarah Grogan, Author

$75.00

264 pages Year Founded: 1998 ISBN 0-415147-84-0

2651 Cognitive Therapy in Practice
WW Norton & Company
500 5th Avenue
New York, NY 10110-54
212-354-5500
800-233-4830
Fax: 212-869-0856
E-mail: npd@wwnorton.com
www.books.wwnorton.com/

Jacqueline B Persons, Author

Basic text for graduate studies in psychotherapy, psycholgy nursing social work and counseling. *$29.00*

224 pages Year Founded: 1989 ISBN 0-393700-77-1

Alcohol/Substance Abuse & Dependence

2652 Addiction Treatment Homework Planner
John Wiley & Sons
10475 Crosspoint Boulevard
Indianapolis, IN 46256-3386
317-572-3000
Fax: 317-572-4000
E-mail: consumers@wiley.com
www.wiley.com

James R Finley, Author
Brenda S Lenz, Author

Helps clients suffering from chemical and nonchemical addictions develop the skills they need to work through problems. *$49.95*

384 pages ISBN 0-471274-59-3

2653 Addiction Treatment Planner
John Wiley & Sons
10475 Crosspoint Boulevard
Indianapolis, IN 46256-3386
317-572-3000
Fax: 317-572-4000
E-mail: consumers@wiley.com
www.wiley.com

Robert R Perkinson, Editor
Arthur E. Jongsma, Jr., Editor

Provides all the elements necessary to quickly and easily develop formal treatment plans that satisfy the demands of HMOs, managed care companies, third-party payers, and state and federal review agencies. *$49.95*

384 pages ISBN 0-471418-14-5

2654 Addictive Behaviors Across the Life Span
Sage Publications
2455 Teller Road
Thousand Oaks, CA 91320-2234
805-499-0721
800-818-7243
Fax: 805-499-0871
E-mail: info@sagepub.com
www.sagepub.com

John S Baer, Author
G Alan Marlatt, Author
Robert J McMahon, Author

Leading scholars, researchers and clinicians in the field of addictive behavior provide and examination of drug dependency from a life span perspective in this authoritative volume. Four general topic areas include: etiology; early intervention; integrated treatment; and policy issues across the life span. Other topics include biopsychosocial perspectives on the intergenerational transmission of alcoholism to children and reducing the risks of addictive behaviors. *$59.95*

358 pages Year Founded: 1993 ISBN 0-803950-78-0

2655 Addictive Thinking: Understanding Self-Deception
Health Communications
292 Fernwood Avenue
Edison, NJ 08837-3839
732-346-0027
Fax: 732-346-0442
www.hcomm.com

Exposes the irrational and contradictory patterns of addictive thinking, and shows how to overcome them and barriers they create; low self-esteem and relapse.

140 pages ISBN 1-568381-38-7

2656 Adolescents, Alcohol and Drugs: A Practical Guide for Those Who Work With Young People
Charles C Thomas Publisher Ltd.
2600 S 1st Street
Springfield, IL 62704-4730
217-789-8980
800-258-8980
Fax: 217-789-9130
E-mail: books@ccthomas.com
www.ccthomas.com

Michael P Thomas, President

$41.95

210 pages Year Founded: 1988 ISBN 0-398053-93-6

2657 American Psychiatric Press Textbook of Substance Abuse Treatment
American Psychiatric Publishing, Inc.
1000 Wilson Boulevard
Suite 1825
Arlington, VA 22209-3901
703-907-7322
800-368-5777
Fax: 703-907-1091
E-mail: appi@psych.org
www.appi.org

Marc Galanter, M.D, Editor
Herbert D. Kleber, M.D, Editor
John McDuffie, Editorial Director

Comprehensive view of basic science and psychology underlying addiction and coverage of all treatment modalities. New topics include the neurobiology of alcoholism, stimulants, marijuana, opiates and hallucinogens, club drugs, and addiction in women. *$95.00*

770 pages Year Founded: 2008 ISBN 0-880488-20-4

2658 An Elephant in the Living Room: Leader's Guide for Helping Children of Alcoholics
Hazelden
15251 Pleasant Valley Road
PO Box 176
Center City, MN 55012-176
651-213-2121
800-328-9000
Fax: 651-213-4590
www.hazelden.org

Marion H Typpo PhD, Co-Author
Jill M Hastings PhD, Co-Author

Practical guidance for education and health professionals who help young people cope with a family member's chemical dependency. *$9.95*

144 pages ISBN 1-568380-34-8

2659 Assessing Substance Abusers with the Million Clinical Multiaxial Inventory
Charles C Thomas Publisher Ltd.
PO Box 19265
Springfield, IL 62794-9265
217-789-8980
800-258-8980
Fax: 217-789-9130
www.ccthomas.com

The construct validity of a psychological test is assessed by a multitrai-multimethod nomothetic matrix, which means that the psychometric properties of an assessment instrument are studied with a variety of populations and in a variety of settings and weighed against a variety of other measures that purportedly assess the same construct.This concept implies that a test might have strong validity with some populations and weak validity with others, and this is the central theme of this book. Also, the book comes in paperback for only $26.95. *$ 46.95*

164 pages Year Founded: 2005 ISBN 0-398075-91-3

2660 Before It's Too Late: Working with Substance Abuse in the Family
WW Norton & Company
500 5th Avenue
New York, NY 10110-54
212-354-5500
Fax: 212-869-0856
E-mail: admalmud@wwnorton.com
www.books.wwnorton.com/

David C. Treadway, Author

Sometimes, the problem a patient or the family of the patient's root cause to the problem they seek help for, is actually substance abuse. How to present the problem, and step-by-step models for working with families dealing with substance abuse are examined. *$ 23.95*

224 pages Year Founded: 1989 ISBN 0-393700-68-2

2661 Behind Bars: Substance Abuse and America's Prison Population
Center on Addiction at Columbia University
633 3rd Avenue
19th Floor
New York, NY 10017-8155
212-841-5200
Fax: 212-956-8020
www.casacolumbia.org

William H Foster, CEO

Results of a three year study of American prisons and the reason drugs are responsible for the booming prison population and escalating costs. *$25.00*

Year Founded: 1998

2662 Blaming the Brain: The Truth About Drugs and Mental Health
Free Press
866 3rd Avenue
New York, NY 10022-6221
212-744-0379
800-323-7445
www.freepeople.com

Erin Legg, Manager

Exposes weaknesses inherent in the scientific arguments supporting the theory that biochemical imbalances are the main cause of mental illness. It discusses how the accidental discovery of mood-altering drugs stimulated an interest in psychopharmacology. *$25.00*

320 pages Year Founded: 1998 ISBN 0-684849-64-X

2663 Building Bridges: States Respond to Substance Abuse and Welfare Reform
Center on Addiction at Columbia University
633 3rd Avenue
19th Floor
New York, NY 10017-8155
212-841-5200
Fax: 212-956-8020
www.casacolumbia.org

William H Foster, CEO

Prepared in partnership with the American Public Human Services Association, this two year study among the front line workers in the nation's welfare offices, job training programs and substance abuse agencies reveals what they find works and does not work in helping clients. *$15.00*

Year Founded: 1999

2664 CASAWORKS for Families: Promising Approach to Welfare Reform and Substance-Abusing Women
Center on Addiction at Columbia University
633 3rd Avenue
19th Floor
New York, NY 10017-8155
212-841-5200
Fax: 212-956-8020
www.casacolumbia.org

William H Foster, CEO

Designed for TANF recipients, this promising approach to welfare reform is used in 11 cities and nine states. *$5.00*

Year Founded: 2001

2665 Clinician's Guide to the Personality Profiles of Alcohol and Drug Abusers: Typological Descriptions Using the MMPI
Charles C Thomas Publisher Ltd.
2600 S 1st Street
Springfield, IL 62704-4730
217-789-8980
800-258-8980
Fax: 217-789-9130
E-mail: books@ccthomas.com
www.ccthomas.com

Michael P Thomas, President
Dennis M Eshbaugh, Author
Michael A Murphy, Author

$39.95

156 pages Year Founded: 1993 ISSN 0-399-06463-6ISBN 0-398058-85-7

2666 Critical Incidents: Ethical Issues in Substance Abuse Prevention and Treatment
Hazelden
15251 Pleasant Valley Road
PO Box 176
Center City, MN 55012-176

651-213-2121
800-328-9000
Fax: 651-213-4590
www.hazelden.org

Two hundred critical situations for health care professionals to sharpen their decision-making skills about everyday ethical dilemmas that arise in their field. *$17.95*

276 pages ISBN 0-938475-03-7

2667 Dangerous Liaisons: Substance Abuse and Sex
Center on Addiction at Columbia University
633 3rd Avenue
19th Floor
New York, NY 10017-8155
212-841-5200
Fax: 212-956-8020
www.casacolumbia.org

William H Foster, CEO

An intensive report on the dangerous and sometimes life-threatening connection between alcohol, drug abuse and sexual activity. Parents, guidance professionals and others will find this useful. *$22.00*

170 pages Year Founded: 1999

2668 Determinants of Substance Abuse: Biological, Psychological, and Environmental Factors
Kluwer Academic/Plenum Publishers
233 Spring Street
New York, NY 10013-1522
212-242-1490

Mark Galizio, Editor
Stephen A. Maisto, Editor

Hardcover. *$90.00*

443 pages Year Founded: 1985 ISBN 0-306418-73-8

2669 Drug Information for Teens: Health Tips About the Physical and Mental Effects of Substance Abuse
Omnigraphics
615 Giswold
Detroit, MI 48226-3900
313-961-1340
Fax: 313-961-1383
E-mail: info@omnigraphics.com
www.omnigraphics.com

Provides students with facts about drug use, abuse, and addiction. It describes the physical and mental effects of alcohol, tobacco, marijuana, ecstasy, inhalants and many other drugs and chemicals that are often abused. It includes information about the process that leads from casual use to addiction and offers suggestions for resisting peer pressure and helping friends stay drug free.

452 pages ISBN 0-780804-44-9

2670 Ethics for Addiction Professionals
Hazelden
15251 Pleasant Valley Road
PO Box 176
Center City, MN 55012-176
651-213-2121
800-328-9000
Fax: 651-213-4590
www.hazelden.org

The first on ethics written by and for addiction professionals that addresses complex issues such as patient confidentiality versus mandatory reporting, clinician relapse, personal and social relationships with clients and other important related issues. *$14.95*

60 pages ISBN 0-894864-54-8

2671 Hispanic Substance Abuse
Charles C Thomas Publisher Ltd.
2600 S 1st Street
Springfield, IL 62704-4730
217-789-8980
800-258-8980
Fax: 217-789-9130
E-mail: books@ccthomas.com
www.ccthomas.com

Michael P Thomas, President

Addresses the concerns of students and professionals who work with Hispanics. Brings together current research on this problem by well-known experts in the fields of alcohol and drug abuse. Useful for scholars and researchers, practitioners in the human services, and the general public. There is shown the extent of substance abuse problems in Hispanic communities, the differences between the Hispanic subgroups and the casual factors that are involved. There are detailed strategies for prevention and the necessary approaches to treatment. *$57.95*

258 pages Year Founded: 1993 ISSN 0-398-06274-9ISBN 0-398058-49-0

2672 Jail Detainees with Co-Occurring Mental Health and Substance Use Disorders
Policy Research Associates
345 Delaware Avenue
Delmar, NY 12054-1905
518-439-7415
800-444-7415
Fax: 518-439-7612
E-mail: pra@prainc.com
www.prainc.com

Henry Steadman, President

Brief report that discusses the issue of keeping federal benefits for jail detainees.

2673 Love First: A New Approach to Intervention for Alcoholism and Drug Addiction
Hazelden
15245 Pleasant Valley Road
PO Box 11-CO 3
Center City, MN 55012-9640
651-257-4010
800-257-7810
Fax: 651-213-4394
www.hazelden.org

Mark Mishek, CEO

A straightforward, simple and practical resource written specifically for families seeking to help a loved one struggling with substance addiction.

280 pages ISBN 1-568385-21-8

2674 Malignant Neglect: Substance Abuse and America's Schools
Center on Addiction at Columbia University
633 3rd Avenue
19th Floor
New York, NY 10017-8155
212-841-5200
Fax: 212-956-8020
www.casacolumbia.org

William H Foster, CEO

Six years of exhaustive research of focus groups, schools, parents and professionals. Findings of the costs of drug abuse in dollars, student behavior, truancy and more. *$22.00*

117 pages Year Founded: 2001

2675 Missed Opportunity: National Survey of Primary Care Physicians and Patients on Substance Abuse
Center on Addiction at Columbia University
633 3rd Avenue
19th Floor
New York, NY 10017-8155
212-841-5200
Fax: 212-956-8020
www.casacolumbia.org

William H Foster, CEO

Findings and recomendations based on a CASA report that revealed 94% of primary care physicians fail to diagnose symptoms of alcohol abuse in adult patients, and 41% of pediatricians missed a diagnosis of drug abuse when presented with a classic description of a teenage patient with these symptoms. The report also sheds light on the fact that many physicians feel unprepared to diagnose substance abuse and have little confidence in the effectiveness of treatments available. *$22.00*

Year Founded: 2000

2676 Motivational Interviewing: Prepare People to Change Addictive Behavior
Hazelden
15251 Pleasant Valley Road
PO Box 176
Center City, MN 55012-176
651-213-2121
800-328-9000
Fax: 651-213-4590
www.hazelden.org

William K Miller, Co-Author
Stephen Rollnick, Co-Author

A key resource for clinical psychologists, social workers and chemical dependency counselors for mastering interviewing skills and working with resistant clients. *$21.95*

348 pages ISBN 0-898624-69-X

2677 Narrative Means to Sober Ends: Treating Addiction and Its Aftermath
Guilford Press
72 Spring Street
New York, NY 10012-4068
212-431-9800
800-365-7006
Fax: 212-966-6708
E-mail: info@guilford.com

Jonathan Diamond, Author

This eloquently written volume illuminates the devastating power of addiction and describes an array of innovative approaches to facilitating clients' recovery. Demonstrated are creative ways to help clients explore their relationship to drugs and alcohol, take the first steps toward sobriety and develop meaningful ways of living without addiction. *$37.95*

386 pages ISBN 1-572305-66-5

2678 No Place to Hide: Substance Abuse in Mid-Size Cities and Rural America
Center on Addiction at Columbia University
633 3rd Avenue
19th Floor
New York, NY 10017-8155
212-841-5200
Fax: 212-956-8020
www.casacolumbia.org

William H Foster, CEO

Surprisingly to some, young people in smaller cities and rural areas are more likely to use many forms of illegal substances. Tobacco use is also higher away from the major cities. The findings on other statistics of drugs and rural adolescent and teenager use are included. *$10.00*

Year Founded: 2000

2679 No Safe Haven: Children of Substance-Abusing Parents
Center on Addiction at Columbia University
633 3rd Avenue
19th Floor
New York, NY 10017-8155
212-841-5200
Fax: 212-956-8020
www.casacolumbia.org

William H Foster, CEO
Peggy Macchetto, Author
Susan Foster, Author

Comprehensive report with shattering facts and figures reveals the impact of substance abuse on parenting skills and child neglect. The number of children affected by their parent's substance abuse driven behavior has more than doubled in the last ten years, greater than the rise in children's overall population. This report calls for a reworking of the child welfare system, and provides guidelines to when the child should be permanently remove from the home. *$22.00*

Year Founded: 1999

2680 Non Medical Marijuana: Rite of Passage or Russian Roulette?
Center on Addiction at Columbia University
633 3rd Avenue
19th Floor
New York, NY 10017-8155
212-841-5200
Fax: 212-956-8020
www.casacolumbia.org

William H Foster, CEO

The most recent numbers available find that more teens from 19 years old and younger enter treatment for marijuana abuse than for any other drug, including alcohol. Many teens also have a problem with secondary drugs.

This report released by CASA at Columbia University, concludes that non medical marijuana is indeed a dangerous substance. *$20.00*

Year Founded: 1999

2681 Perfect Daughters
Health Communications
292 Fernwood Avenue
Edison, NJ 08837-3839
732-346-0027
Fax: 732-346-0442
www.hcomm.com

Identifies what differentiates the adult daughters of alcoholics from other women. Adult daughters of alcoholics operate from a base of harsh and limiting views of themselves and the world. Having learned that they must function perfectly in order to avoid unpleasant situations, these women often assume responsibility for the failures of others. They are drawn to chemically dependent men and are more likely to become addicted themselves. This book collects the thoughts, feelings and experience of twelve hundred perfect daughters, offering readers an opportunity to explore their own life's dynamics and thereby heal and grow.

350 pages ISBN 1-558749-52-7

2682 Principles of Addiction Medicine
American Society of Addiction Medicine
4601 N Park Avenue
Suite 101, Upper Arcade
Chevy Chase, MD 20815-4519
301-656-3920
800-844-8948
Fax: 301-656-3815
E-mail: email@asam.com
www.asam.org

Eileen McGrath, Executive VP

Textbook on the basic and clinical science of prevention and treatment of alcohol, nicotine, and other drug dependencies and addictions. *$155.00*

1338 pages ISBN 1-880425-04-0

2683 Proven Youth Development Model that Prevents Substance Abuse and Builds Communities
Center on Addiction at Columbia University
633 3rd Avenue
19th Floor
New York, NY 10017-8155
212-841-5200
Fax: 212-956-8020
www.casacolumbia.org

William H Foster, CEO

How-to manual developed with nine years of research. The program is a collaboration of local school, law enforcement, social service and health teams to help high risk youth between the ages of 8 - 13 years old and their families prevent substance abuse and violent behavior. Used in 23 urban and rural communities in 11 states and the District of Columbia. *$50.00*

79 pages Year Founded: 2001

2684 Psychological Theories of Drinking and Alcoholism
Guilford Press
72 Spring Street
New York, NY 10012-4068
212-431-9800
800-365-7006
Fax: 212-966-6708
E-mail: info@guilford.com

Howard T. Blane, Editor
Kenneth E. Leonard, Editor

Multidisciplinary approach discusses biological, pharmacological and social factors that influence drinking and alcoholism. Contributors review established and emerging approaches that guide research into the psychological processes influencing drinking and alcoholism. *$47.95*

467 pages Year Founded: 1999 ISBN 1-572304-10-3

2685 Relapse Prevention Maintenance: Strategies in the Treatment of Addictive Behaviors
Guilford Press
72 Spring Street
New York, NY 10012-4068
212-431-9800
800-365-7006
Fax: 212-966-6708
E-mail: info@guilford.com

G. Alan Marlatt PhD, Editor
Dennis M. Donovan PhD, Editor

Research on relapse prevention to problem drinking, smoking, substance abuse, eating disorders and compulsive gambling. Analyzes factors that may lead to relapse and offers practical techniques for maintaining treatment gains. *$55.00*

416 pages Year Founded: 1985 ISBN 0-898620-09-0

2686 Relapse Prevention Maintenance: Strategies in the Treatment of Addictive Behaviors
Guilford Press
72 Spring Street
New York, NY 10012-4068
212-431-9800
800-365-7006
Fax: 212-966-6708
E-mail: info@guilford.com

G. Alan Marlatt PhD, Editor
Dennis M. Donovan PhD, Editor

Research on relapse prevention to problem drinking, smoking, substance abuse, eating disorders and compulsive gambling. Analyzes factors that may lead to relapse and offers practical techniques for maintaining treatment gains. *$55.00*

416 pages Year Founded: 1985 ISBN 0-898620-09-0

2687 So Help Me God: Substance Abuse, Religion and Spirituality
Center on Addiction at Columbia University
633 3rd Avenue
19th Floor
New York, NY 10017-8155
212-841-5200
Fax: 212-956-8020
www.casacolumbia.org

William H Foster, CEO

Results of a 2 year study, finding that spirituality has enormous power to potentially lower the risks of substance abuse. When this is combined with professional treatment, an individual's religion helps greatly with recovery. *$10.00*

Year Founded: 2001

2688 Solutions Step by Step: Substance Abuse Treatment Manual
WW Norton & Company
500 5th Avenue
New York, NY 10110-54
212-354-5500
Fax: 212-869-0856
E-mail: admalmud@wwnorton.com
www.books.wwnorton.com/

Insoo Kim Berg, Author
Norman H. Reuss, Author

Quick tips, questions and examples focusing on successes that can be experienced helping substance abusers help themselves. *$ 25.00*

192 pages Year Founded: 1997 ISSN 70251-0

2689 Substance Abuse and Learning Disabilities: Peas in a Pod or Apples and Oranges?
Center on Addiction at Columbia University
633 3rd Avenue
19th Floor
New York, NY 10017-8155
212-841-5200
Fax: 212-956-8020
www.casacolumbia.org

William H Foster, CEO

Report originating from a conference in 1999 sponsored by CASA, the relationship between learning disabilities that are not addressed, and possible substance abuse by these same children is examined. Attention Deficit/Hyperactivity Disorder and Conduct Disorder and the link to substance abuse is also considered. *$10.00*

2690 Substance Abuse: A Comprehensive Textbook
Lippincott Williams & Wilkins
PO Box 1600
Hagerstown, MD 21741-1600
301-714-2300
800-638-3030
Fax: 301-824-7390
www.lww.com

$162.00

956 pages Year Founded: 1997 ISBN 0-683181-79-3

2691 Teens and Alcohol: Gallup Youth Survey Major Issues and Trends
Mason Crest Publishers
450 Parkway Drive
Suite D
Broomall, PA 19008-4017
866-627-2665
Fax: 610-543-3878
E-mail: gbrffr@masoncrest.com
www.masoncrest.com

Eighty-seven percent of high school seniors have tried alcohol and, according to a Gallup Youth Survey, 27 percent of teenagers say it is very easy for them to get alcoholic beverages. Alcohol is a contributor to the three leading causes of death for teens and young adults: automobile crashes, homicide and suicides.

112 pages ISBN 1-590847-23-7

2692 Therapeutic Communities for Addictions: Reading in Theory, Research, and Practice
Charles C Thomas Publisher Ltd.
2600 S 1st Street
Springfield, IL 62704-4730
217-789-8980
800-258-8980
Fax: 217-789-9130
E-mail: books@ccthomas.com
www.ccthomas.com

Michael P Thomas, President
James T Ziegenfuss Jr, Author

Contents: The Therapeutic Community (TC) for Substance Abuse; Democratic TCs or Programmatic TCs or Both?; Motivational Aspects of Heroin Addicts in TCs; A Sociological View of the TC; Psychodynamics of TCs for Treatment of Heroin Addicts; Britain and the Psychoanalytic Tradition in TCs; TC Research; Outcomes of Drug Abuse Treatment; 12-Year Follow-up Outcomes, College Training in a TC; Client Evaluations of TCs and Retention; Side Bets and Secondary Adjustments; Measuring Program Implementation; The TC Looking Ahead; TCs within Prisons; Uses and Abuses of Power and Authority. *$51.95*

282 pages Year Founded: 1986 ISBN 0-398052-06-9

2693 Treating Substance Abuse: Part 1
American Counseling Association
5999 Stevenson Avenue
Alexandria, VA 22304-3304
703-823-9800
800-422-2648
Fax: 703-823-0252
TDD: 703-823-6862
E-mail: webmaster@counseling.org
www.counseling.org

Richard Yep, Executive Director

The first of a two-volume set presents up-to-date findings on the treatment of alcoholism and addiction to cocaine, caffeine, hallucinogens, and marijuana. Techniques and case examples are offered from a variety of approaches, including motivational enhancement therapy, marriage and family therapy as well as cognitive-behavioral. *$26.95*

280 pages ISBN 1-886330-48-4

2694 Treating Substance Abuse: Part 2
American Counseling Association
5999 Stevenson Avenue
Alexandria, VA 22304-3304
703-823-9800
800-422-2648
Fax: 703-823-0252
E-mail: webmaster@counseling.org
www.counseling.org

Richard Yep, Executive Director

For treating select populations of substance-abusing clients, including those with disabilities, psychiatric disorders, schizophrenia and major depression. Also serves adolescents, older adults, pregnant women and clients whose addictions affect their ability to function in the workplace. *$29.95*

311 pages ISBN 1-886330-49-2

2695 Treating the Alcoholic: Developmental Model of Recovery
John Wiley & Sons
605 3rd Avenue
New York, NY 10158-180
212-850-6301
E-mail: info@wiley.com

376 pages Year Founded: 1985

2696 Under the Rug: Substance Abuse and the Mature Woman
Center on Addiction at Columbia University
633 3rd Avenue
19th Floor
New York, NY 10017-8155
212-841-5200
Fax: 212-956-8020
www.casacolumbia.org

William H Foster, CEO

Discusses the fact that millions of mature women are robbed of a healthy and longer lifespan due to a substance abuse problem that they discreetly hide. Their reluctance to get help costs them and the health systems billions. *$25.00*

Year Founded: 1998

2697 Understanding Psychiatric Medications in the Treatment of Chemical Dependency and Dual Diagnoses
Charles C Thomas Publisher Ltd.
2600 S 1st Street
Springfield, IL 62704-4730
217-789-8980
800-258-8980
Fax: 217-789-9130
E-mail: books@ccthomas.com
www.ccthomas.com

Michael P Thomas, President

Designed to address coexisting chemical dependency and psychiatric disorder (dual diagnoses) and specifically to focus on the appropriate role of psychotropic medications in the treatment of dual diagnonsis patients. The text presents a comprehensive overview of psychiatric medication treatment for dual diagnoses that speaks to a broad professional audience while being sensitive to the values and beliefs of the chemical dependents. *$39.95*

134 pages Year Founded: 1995 ISSN 0-398-05964-0ISBN 0-398059-63-2

2698 Your Drug May Be Your Problem: How and Why to Stop Taking Pyschiatric Medications
Perseus Books Group
550 Central Avenue
Boulder, CO 80301
800-386-5656
Fax: 720-406-7336
E-mail: westview.orders@perseusbooks.com
www.perseusbooksgroup.com

In a very short time, a doctor may prescribe a drug which an individual may take for months, years, even the rest of their lives. This book provides up-to-date, descriptions of the pros and cons of taking psychiatric medication, dangers involved, and explains a safe method of withdrawl if needed. *$17.00*

288 pages Year Founded: 2000 ISBN 0-738203-48-3

Anxiety Disorders

2699 Anxiety Disorders: A Scientific Approach for Selecting the Most Effective Treatment
Professional Resource Press
PO Box 3197
Sarasota, FL 34230-3197
941-343-9601
800-443-3364
Fax: 941-343-9201
E-mail: orders@prpress.com
www.prpress.com

Laurie Girsch, Managing Editor

Presents descriptive and empirical information on the differential diagnosis of DSM-IV and DSM-III-R categories of anxiety disorders. Explicit decision rules are provided for developing treatment plans based on both scientific research and clinical judgement. *$14.95*

114 pages Year Founded: 1994 ISBN 1-568870-00-0

2700 Applied Relaxation Training in the Treatment of PTSD and Other Anxiety Disorders
New Harbinger Publications
5674 Shattuck Avenue
Oakland, CA 94609-1662
510-652-0215
800-748-6273
Fax: 510-652-5472
E-mail: customerservice@newharbinger.com
www.newharbinger.com

Matthew McKay, Owner

Comes with a one hundred five minute video tape and a 52 page paperback manual. *$100.00*

Year Founded: 1998 ISBN 1-889287-08-3

2701 Assimilation, Rational Thinking, and Suppression in the Treatment of PTSD and Other Anxiety Disorders
New Harbinger Publications
5674 Shattuck Avenue
Oakland, CA 94609-1662
510-652-0215
800-748-6273
Fax: 510-652-5472
E-mail: customerservice@newharbinger.com
www.newharbinger.com

Matthew McKay, Owner

Comes with two videotapes and a ninety four page paperback manual. *$150.00*

Year Founded: 1998 ISBN 1-889287-06-7

2702 Body Remembers: Psychophysiology of Trauma and Trauma Treatment
WW Norton & Company
500 5th Avenue
New York, NY 10110-54
212-354-5500
Fax: 212-869-0856
E-mail: admalmud@wwnorton.com
www.books.wwnorton.com/

Babette Rothschild, Author

Unites traditional verbal therapy and body oriented therapies for Post Traumatic Stress Disorder patients, as memories sometimes present in a physical disorder. *$30.00*

224 pages Year Founded: 2000 ISSN 70327-4

2703 Brief Therapy for Post Traumatic Stress Disorder
John Wiley & Sons
605 3rd Avenue
New York, NY 10158-180
212-850-6301
E-mail: info@wiley.com

Stephen Bisbey, Author
Lori Beth Bisbey, Author

Discusses a new and exciting treatment technique that has proven to be more effective than the widely used direct theraputic exposure technique. Fills the growing need for a step by step practical treatment manual for PTSD using Traumatic Incident Reduction. It is an ideal companion to training workshops.

192 pages Year Founded: 1998

2704 Client's Manual for the Cognitive Behavioral Treatment of Anxiety Disorders
New Harbinger Publications
5674 Shattuck Avenue
Oakland, CA 94609-1662
510-652-0215
800-748-6273
Fax: 510-652-5472
E-mail: customerservice@newharbinger.com
www.newharbinger.com

Matthew McKay, Owner

$10.00

106 pages Year Founded: 1994 ISBN 1-889287-99-7

2705 Cognitive Processing Therapy for Rape Victims
Sage Publications
2455 Teller Road
Thousand Oaks, CA 91320-2234
805-499-0721
800-818-7243
Fax: 805-499-0871
E-mail: info@sagepub.com
www.sagepub.com

Blaise R Simqu, CEO

Information regarding the assessment and treatment of rape victims. Discusses disorders that result from rape and add to a victim's suffering such as post traumatic stress, depression, poor self-esteem, interpersonal difficulties and sexual dysfunction. *$46.00*

192 pages Year Founded: 1993 ISBN 0-803949-01-4

2706 Cognitive Therapy
American Psychiatric Publishing, Inc.
1000 Wilson Boulevard
Suite 1825
Arlington, VA 22209-3901
703-907-7322
800-368-5777
Fax: 703-907-1091
E-mail: appi@psych.org
www.appi.org

Jesse H Wright, M.D., Ph.D, Editor
Michael E Thase, M.D., Editor
John McDuffie, Editorial Director

Cognitive therapy for anxiety, substance abuse, personality, eating and mental disorders. *$37.50*

174 pages Year Founded: 1997 ISBN 0-880484-45-4

2707 Cognitive Therapy in Practice
WW Norton & Company
500 5th Avenue
New York, NY 10110-54
212-354-5500
800-233-4830
Fax: 212-869-0856
E-mail: npd@wwnorton.com
www.books.wwnorton.com

Drake McFeely, CEO

Basic text for graduate studies in psychotherapy, psychology nursing social work and counseling. *$29.00*

224 pages Year Founded: 1923 ISBN 0-393700-77-1

2708 Concise Guide to Brief Dynamic Psychotherapy
American Psychiatric Publishing, Inc.
1000 Wilson Boulevard
Suite 1825
Arlington, VA 22209-3901
703-907-7322
800-368-5777
Fax: 703-907-1091
E-mail: appi@psych.org
www.appi.org

Robert E Hales, M.D., M.B.A., Editor-in-Chief
Ron McMillen, Chief Executive Officer
John McDuffie, Editorial Director
Rebecca D. Rinehart, Publisher

Seven brief psychodynamic therapy models including supportive, time - limited, interpersonal, time - limited dynamic, short term dynamic for post traumatic stress disorder and brief dynamic for substance abuse. *$21.00*

224 pages Year Founded: 1997 ISBN 0-880483-46-6

2709 Current Treatments of Obsessive-Compulsive Disorder
American Psychiatric Publishing, Inc.
1000 Wilson Boulevard
Suite 1825
Arlington, VA 22209-3901
703-907-7322
800-368-5777
Fax: 703-907-1091
E-mail: appi@psych.org
www.appi.org

Robert E Hales, M.D., M.B.A., Editor-in-Chief
Ron McMillen, Chief Executive Officer
John McDuffie, Editorial Director
Rebecca D. Rinehart, Publisher

Helps clinicians better match treatment approaches with each patients unique needs.

Year Founded: 01 ISBN 0-880487-79-8

2710 Does Stress Damage the Brain? Understanding Trauma-Related Disorders from a Mind-Body Perspective
WW Norton & Company
500 5th Avenue
New York, NY 10110-54

212-354-5500
800-233-4830
Fax: 212-869-0856
E-mail: npb@wwnorton.com
www.books.wwnorton.com

Drake McFeely, CEO

Shows that extreme stress may result in lasting damage to the brain, especially a part of the brain involved in memory. This new neurobiological understanding of the relation between cognitive problems and trauma has many important implications for both self-understanding of trauma survivors and for the treatment of the effects of trauma.

Year Founded: 1923 ISBN 0-393704-74-2

2711 Effective Treatments for PTSD: Practice Guidelines from the International Society for Traumatic Stress Studies
Guilford Press
72 Spring Street
New York, NY 10012-4068
212-431-9800
800-365-7006
Fax: 212-966-6708
E-mail: info@guilford.com
www.www.guilford.com

Bob Matloff, President
Seymour Weingarten, Editor-in-Chief

Developed under the auspices of the PTSD Treatment Guidelines Task Force of the International Society for Traumatic Stress Studies, this comprehensive volume brings together leading authorities on psychological trauma to offer best practice guidelines for the treatment of PTSD. Approaches covered include acute interventions, cognitive-behavior therapy, pharmacotherapy, EMDR, group therapy, psychodynamic therapy, impatient treatment, psychosocial rehabilitation, hypnosis, creative therapies, marital and family treatment. *$42.00*

388 pages Year Founded: 1973 ISBN 1-572305-84-3

2712 Even from a Broken Web: Brief, Respectful Solution Oriented Therapy for Sexual Abuse and Trauma
WW Norton & Company
500 5th Avenue
New York, NY 10110-54
212-354-5500
800-233-4830
Fax: 212-869-0856
E-mail: npb@wwnorton.com
www.books.wwnorton.com

Drake McFeely, CEO

Recent years have shown more people than ever coming to therapy with the after affects of sexual abuse. The authors provide therapists solution oriented treatment that considers a person's inner healing abilities. This method is less traumatic and disruptive to the patient's life than traditional therapies. *$16.95*

208 pages Year Founded: 1923 ISBN 0-393703-94-0

2713 Eye Movement Desensitization and Reprocessing: Basic Principles, Protocols, and Procedures
Guilford Press
72 Spring Street
New York, NY 10012-4068
212-431-9800
800-365-7006
Fax: 212-966-6708
E-mail: info@guilford.com
www.www.guilford.com

Bob Matloff, President
Seymour Weingarten, Editor-in-Chief

Reviews research and development, discusses theoretical constructs and possible underlying mechanisms, and presents protocols and procedures for treatment of adults and children with a range of presenting complaints. Material is applicable for victims of sexual abuse, crime, combat and phobias. *$45.00*

398 pages Year Founded: 1973 ISBN 0-898629-60-8

2714 Gender Differences in Mood and Anxiety Disorders: From Bench to Bedside
American Psychiatric Publishing, Inc.
1000 Wilson Boulevard
Suite 1825
Arlington, VA 22209-3901
703-907-7322
800-368-5777
Fax: 703-907-1091
E-mail: appi@psych.org
www.appi.org

Robert E Hales, M.D., M.B.A., Editor-in-Chief
Ron McMillen, Chief Executive Officer
John McDuffie, Editorial Director
Rebecca D. Rinehart, Publisher

Gender differences in neuroimaging. Discusses women, stress and depression, sex differences in hypothalamic-pituitary-adrenal axis regulation, modulation of anxiety by reproductive hormones. Questions if hormone replacement and oral contraceptive therapy induce or treat mood symptoms. *$37.50*

224 pages Year Founded: 1999 ISBN 0-880489-58-8

2715 Generalized Anxiety Disorder: Diagnosis, Treatment and Its Relationship to Other Anxiety Disorders
American Psychiatric Publishing, Inc.
1000 Wilson Boulevard
Suite 1825
Arlington, VA 22209-3901
703-907-7322
800-368-5777
Fax: 703-907-1091
E-mail: appi@psych.org
www.appi.org

Robert E Hales, M.D., M.B.A., Editor-in-Chief
Ron McMillen, Chief Executive Officer
John McDuffie, Editorial Director
Rebecca D. Rinehart, Publisher

Historical introduction, diagnosis, classification and differential diagnosis. Relationship with depression, panic and OCD. Treatments. *$74.95*

96 pages Year Founded: 1998 ISBN 1-853176-59-1

2716 Group Treatments for Post-Traumatic Stress Disorder
Brunner/Routledge
7625 Empire Drive
Florence, KY 41042-2919
800-634-7064
Fax: 215-269-0363
E-mail: orders@taylorandfrancis.com
www.www.routledgementalhealth.com

Contains contributions from renowned PTSD experts who provide group treatment to trauma survivors. It reviews the state-of-the-art applications of group therapy for such survivors of trauma as rape victims, combat veterans, adult survivors of childhood abuse, motor vehicle accident survivors, survivors of disaster, homicide witnesses and disaster relief workers. *$34.95*

216 pages ISBN 0-876309-83-X

2717 Integrative Treatment of Anxiety Disorders
American Psychiatric Publishing, Inc.
1000 Wilson Boulevard
Suite 1825
Arlington, VA 22209-3901
703-907-7322
800-368-5777
Fax: 703-907-1091
E-mail: appi@psych.org
www.appi.org

Robert E Hales, M.D., M.B.A., Editor-in-Chief
Ron McMillen, Chief Executive Officer
John McDuffie, Editorial Director
Rebecca D. Rinehart, Publisher

Up-to-date look at combined pharmacotherapy and cognitive behavioral therapy in the treatment of anxiety disorders. *$41.50*

320 pages Year Founded: 1995 ISBN 0-880487-15-1

2718 Life After Trauma: Workbook for Healing
Guilford Press
72 Spring Street
New York, NY 10012-4068
212-431-9800
800-365-7006
Fax: 212-966-6708
E-mail: info@guilford.com
www.www.guilford.com

Bob Matloff, President
Seymour Weingarten, Editor-in-Chief

Useful exercises for clinicians and trauma survivors, very empowering. *$17.95*

352 pages Year Founded: 1973 ISBN 1-572302-39-9

2719 Long-Term Treatments of Anxiety Disorders
American Psychiatric Publishing, Inc.
1000 Wilson Boulevard
Suite 1825
Arlington, VA 22209-3901
703-907-7322
800-368-5777
Fax: 703-907-1091
E-mail: appi@psych.org
www.appi.org

Robert E Hales, M.D., M.B.A., Editor-in-Chief
Ron McMillen, Chief Executive Officer

John McDuffie, Editorial Director
Rebecca D. Rinehart, Publisher

Treatment of anxiety disorders encapsulating important advances made over the past two decades. *$56.00*

464 pages Year Founded: 1996 ISBN 0-880486-56-2

2720 Memory, Trauma and the Law
WW Norton & Company
500 5th Avenue
New York, NY 10110-54
212-354-5500
800-233-4830
Fax: 212-869-0856
E-mail: admalmud@wwnorton.com
www.books.wwnorton.com

Drake McFeely, CEO

Professionals need to be informed of memory in the legal context to avoid malpractice liability suits. Recovered memory research, trauma treatment and the controversy of false memory in some cases are covered. *$100.00*

960 pages Year Founded: 1923 ISSN 70254-5

2721 Obsessive-Compulsive Disorder: Contemporary Issues in Treatment
Lawrence Erlbaum Associates
10 Industrial Avenue
Mahwah, NJ 07430-2253
201-825-3200
800-926-6577
Fax: 201-236-0072
E-mail: orders@erlbaum.com
www.erlbaum.com

Hardcover.

Year Founded: 00 ISBN 0-805828-37-0

2722 Obsessive-Compulsive and Related Disorders in Adults: a Comprehensive Clinical Guide
Cambridge University Press
100 Gold Street
2nd Floor
New York, NY 10038
212-924-3900
Fax: 212-691-3239
E-mail: marketing@cup.org
www.www.nyc.gov

The author challenges the current implicit models used in alcohol problem prevention and demonstrates an ecological perspective of the community as a complex adaptive systems composed of interacting subsystems. This volume represents a new and sensible approach to the prevention of alcohol dependence and alcohol-related problems. *$65.00*

380 pages Year Founded: 1999 ISBN 0-521559-75-8

2723 Overcoming Agoraphobia and Panic Disorder
New Harbinger Publications
5674 Shattuck Avenue
Oakland, CA 94609-1662
510-652-0215
800-748-6273
Fax: 510-652-5472
E-mail: customerservice@newharbinger.com
www.newharbinger.com

Matthew McKay, Owner
Patrick Fanning , Co-Founder

A twelve to sixteen session treatment. *$11.95*

88 pages Year Founded: 1973 ISBN 1-572241-46-2

2724 Overcoming Obsessive-Compulsive Disorder
New Harbinger Publications
5674 Shattuck Avenue
Oakland, CA 94609-1662
510-652-0215
800-748-6273
Fax: 510-652-5472
E-mail: customerservice@newharbinger.com
www.newharbinger.com

Matthew McKay, Owner
Patrick Fanning, Co-Founder

A fourteen session treatment. *$11.95*

72 pages Year Founded: 1973 ISBN 1-572241-29-2

2725 Overcoming Post-Traumatic Stress Disorder
New Harbinger Publications
5674 Shattuck Avenue
Oakland, CA 94609-1662
510-652-0215
800-748-6273
Fax: 510-652-5472
E-mail: customerservice@newharbinger.com
www.newharbinger.com

Matthew McKay, Owner
Patrick Fanning, Co-Founder

An eleven to twenty four session treatment. *$11.95*

95 pages Year Founded: 1973 ISBN 1-572241-47-0

2726 Overcoming Specific Phobia
New Harbinger Publications
5674 Shattuck Avenue
Oakland, CA 94609-1662
510-652-0215
800-748-6273
Fax: 510-652-5472
E-mail: customerservice@newharbinger.com
www.newharbinger.com

Matthew McKay, Owner
Patrick Fanning, Co-Founder

$9.95

72 pages Year Founded: 1973 ISBN 1-572241-15-2

2727 Panic Disorder: Clinical Diagnosis, Management and Mechanisms
American Psychiatric Publishing, Inc.
1000 Wilson Boulevard
Suite 1825
Arlington, VA 22209-3901
703-907-7322
800-368-5777
Fax: 703-907-1091
E-mail: appi@psych.org
www.appi.org

Robert E Hales, M.D., M.B.A., Editor-in-Chief
Ron McMillen, Chief Executive Officer
John McDuffie, Editorial Director
Rebecca D. Rinehart, Publisher

Novel and important new discoveries for biological research together with up to date information for the diagnosis and treatment for the practicing clinician. *$75.00*

264 pages Year Founded: 1998 ISBN 1-853175-18-8

2728 Panic Disorder: Theory, Research and Therapy
John Wiley & Sons
111 River Street
Hoboken, NJ 07030-5774
201-748-6000
Fax: 201-748-6088
E-mail: info@wiley.com
www.www.wiley.com

Stephen M. Smith, President and Chief Executive Officer
Ellis E. Cousens, Executive Vice President
John Kritzmacher, Executive Vice President
MJ O'Leary, Senior Vice President, Human Resources

364 pages Year Founded: 1807

2729 Phobias: Handbook of Theory, Reseach and Treatment
John Wiley & Sons
111 River Street
Hoboken, NJ 07030-5774
201-748-6000
Fax: 201-748-6088
E-mail: info@wiley.com
www.www.wiley.com

Stephen M. Smith, President and Chief Executive Officer
Ellis E. Cousens, Executive Vice President
John Kritzmacher, Executive Vice President
MJ O'Leary, Senior Vice President, Human Resources

Provides an up-to-date summary of current knowledge of phobias. Psychological treatments available for specific phobias have been refined considerably in recent years. This extensive handbook acknowledges these treatments and includes the description and nature of prevalent phobias, details of symptoms, prevalence rates, individual case histories, and a brief review of of our knowledge of the etiology of phobias.

364 pages Year Founded: 1807

2730 Post Traumatic Stress Disorder
New Harbinger Publications
5674 Shattuck Avenue
Oakland, CA 94609-1662
510-652-0215
800-748-6273
Fax: 510-652-5472
E-mail: customerservice@newharbinger.com
www.newharbinger.com

Matthew McKay, Owner
Patrick Fanning, Co-Founder

Includes techniques for managing flashbacks, anxiety attacks, nightmares, insomnia, and dissociation; working through layers of pain; and handling survivor guilt, secondary wounding, low self esteem, victim thinking, anger, and depression. *$49.95*

384 pages Year Founded: 1973 ISBN 1-879237-68-7

2731 Post Traumatic Stress Disorder: Complete Treatment Guide
200 E Joppa Road
PO Box 436
Brooklandville, MD 21022-0436
410-825-8888
888-825-8249
Fax: 410-560-0134
E-mail: sidran@sidran.org
www.sidran.org

Esther Giller, President and Director
Sheila Sidran Giller, Secretary/Treasurer
J. G. Goellner, Director Emeritus
Tracy Howard, Book Sales/Office Manager

For clinicians who want to work more effectively with trauma survivors, this textbook provides a step by step description of PTSD treatment strategies. Includes chapters on definitions, diagnostic criteria and the biochemistry of PTSD. Reflects a generalized 'ideal' structure of the healing process. Includes cognitive and behavioral techniques for managing flashbacks, anxiety attacks, sleep disturbances and dissociation; a comprehensive program for working through deeper layers of pain; plus PTSD related problems such as survivor guilt, secondary wounding, low self esteem, victim thinking, anger and depression. Presents trauma issues clearly for both general audiences and trauma professionals. *$49.95*

345 pages Year Founded: 1986

2732 Post Traumatic Stress Disorders in Children and Adolescents Handbook
WW Norton & Company
500 5th Avenue
New York, NY 10110-54
212-354-5500
800-233-4830
Fax: 212-869-0856
E-mail: npb@wwnorton.com
www.books.wwnorton.com

Drake McFeely, CEO

The 15 chapters gathered here address different aspects of childhood and adolescent trauma-some consider a distinct therapeutic situation (abuse and neglect), others pertain to standard clinical procedure (assessment), and still others focus on complex research issues (neurobiology and genetics of PSTD).

Year Founded: 1923 ISBN 0-393704-12-2

2733 Practice Guideline for the Treatment of Patients with Panic Disorder
American Psychiatric Publishing, Inc.
1000 Wilson Boulevard
Suite 1825
Arlington, VA 22209-3901
703-907-7322
800-368-5777
Fax: 703-907-1091
E-mail: appi@psych.org
www.appi.org

Robert E Hales, M.D., M.B.A., Editor-in-Chief
Ron McMillen, Chief Executive Officer
John McDuffie, Editorial Director
Rebecca D. Rinehart, Publisher

Summarizes data, evaluation of the patient for coexisting mental disorders and issues specific to the treatment of panic disorders in children and adolescents. *$22.50*

160 pages Year Founded: 1998 ISBN 0-890423-11-3

2734 Rebuilding Shattered Lives: Responsible Treatment of Complex Post-Traumatic and Dissociative Disorders
John Wiley & Sons
111 River Street
Hoboken, NJ 07030-5774

201-748-6000
Fax: 201-748-6088
E-mail: info@wiley.com
www.www.wiley.com

Stephen M. Smith, President and Chief Executive Officer
Ellis E. Cousens, Executive Vice President
John Kritzmacher, Executive Vice President
MJ O'Leary, Senior Vice President, Human Resources

The most up-to-date, integrative and emperically sound account of trauma theory and practice availible. Based on more than a decade of clinical research and treatment experience at the Harvard Medical School, this comprehensive and nontechnical text offers a stage oriented approach to understanding and treating complex and difficult traumatized patients, integrating modern trauma theory with traditional theraputic interventions. *$47.50*

364 pages Year Founded: 1807 ISBN 0-471247-32-4

2735 Remembering Trauma: Psychotherapist's Guide to Memory & Illusion
John Wiley & Sons
111 River Street
Hoboken, NJ 07030-5774
201-748-6000
Fax: 201-748-6088
E-mail: info@wiley.com
www.www.wiley.com

Stephen M. Smith, President and Chief Executive Of
Ellis E. Cousens, Executive Vice President, Chief
John Kritzmacher, Executive Vice President, Chief
MJ O'Leary, Senior Vice President, Human Res

364 pages Year Founded: 1807

2736 Shy Children, Phobic Adults: Nature and Treatment of Social Phobia
American Psychiatric Publishing, Inc.
1000 Wilson Boulevard
Suite 1825
Arlington, VA 22209-3901
703-907-7322
800-368-5777
Fax: 703-907-1091
E-mail: appi@psych.org
www.appi.org

Robert E Hales, M.D., M.B.A., Editor-in-Chief
Ron McMillen, Chief Executive Officer
John McDuffie, Editorial Director
Rebecca D. Rinehart, Publisher

Describes the similiarities and differences in the syndrome across all ages. Draws from the clinical, social and developmental literatures, as well as from extensive clinical experience. Illustrates the impact of developmental stage on phenomenology, diagnoses and assessment and treatment of social phobia. *$39.95*

321 pages Year Founded: 1998 ISBN 1-557984-61-1

2737 Social Phobia: Clinical and Research Perspectives
American Psychiatric Publishing, Inc.
1000 Wilson Boulevard
Suite 1825
Arlington, VA 22209-3901
703-907-7322
800-368-5777
Fax: 703-907-1091

E-mail: appi@psych.org
www.appi.org

Robert E Hales, M.D., M.B.A., Editor-in-Chief
Ron McMillen, Chief Executive Officer
John McDuffie, Editorial Director
Rebeccaa DD. Rinehart, Publisher

Comprehensive and practice guide for mental health professionals who encounter individuals with social phobia. *$48.00*

384 pages Year Founded: 1995 ISBN 0-880486-53-8

2738 Standing in the Spaces: Essays on Clinical Process, Trauma, and Dissociation
Analytic Press
7625 Empire Drive
Florence, KY 41042-2919
800-634-7064
Fax: 215-269-0363
E-mail: orders@taylorandfrancis.com
www.www.routledgementalhealth.com

Paul E Stepansky PhD, Managing Director
John Kerr PhD, Sr Editor

Bromberg's essays are delightfully unpredictable, as they strive to keep the reader continually abreast of how words can and cannot capture the subtle shifts in relatedness that characterize the clinical process. Radiating clinical wisdom infused with compassion and wit, Standing in the Spaces, is a classic destined to be read and reread by anlysts and therapists for decades to come. *$55.00*

376 pages Year Founded: 1998 ISBN 0-881632-46-5

2739 The Body Remembers Casebook: Unifying Methods and Models in the Treatment of Trauma and PTSD
WW Norton & Company
500 5th Avenue
New York, NY 10110-54
212-354-5500
800-233-4830
Fax: 212-869-0856
E-mail: npb@wwnorton.com
www.books.wwnorton.com

Drake McFeely, CEO

Emphasizes the importance of tailoring every trauma therapy to the particular needs of each individual client. Each varied and complex case is approached with a combination of methods ranging from traditional psychodynamic approaches and applications of attachment theory to innovative trauma methods including EMDR and Levine's SIBAM model.

Year Founded: 1923 ISBN 0-393704-00-9

2740 The Body Remembers: The Psychphysiology of Trauma and Trauma Treatment
WW Norton & Company
500 5th Avenue
New York, NY 10110-54
212-354-5500
800-233-4830
Fax: 212-869-0856
E-mail: npb@wwnorton.com
www.books.wwnorton.com

Drake McFeely, CEO

There is tremendous value in understanding the psychophysiology of trauma and knowing what to do about its manifestations. This book illuminates psychophysiology, casting light on the impact of trauma on the body and the phenomenon of somatic memory. Presents principles and non-touch techniques for giving the body its due.

Year Founded: 1923 ISBN 0-393703-27-4

2741 The Pathology of Man: A Study of Human Evil
Charles C Thomas Publisher Ltd.
PO Box 19265
Springfield, IL 62794-9265
217-789-8980
800-258-8980
Fax: 217-789-9130
www.ccthomas.com

Charles C Thomas, Publisher

Deals with a topic that is both timely and of enduring importance. Expected to be a unique and important contribution that responds to the concerns of students and professionals in a wide range of diciplines. A comprehensive and solid study of the multi-casual nature of phonomenon that, until now, has been treated almost exclusively in terms of religion, myth, symbolism, moral philosophy, and ethics. Available in paperback for $53.95.
$73.95

376 pages Year Founded: 1927 ISBN 0-398075-57-3

2742 The Trauma Spectrum: Hidden Wounds and Human Resiliency
WW Norton & Company
500 5th Avenue
New York, NY 10110-54
212-354-5500
800-233-4830
Fax: 212-869-0856
E-mail: npb@wwnorton.com
www.books.wwnorton.com

Drake McFeely, CEO

Scaer, a neurologist with over 30 years experience working with car accident victims, extends the conceptual and practical horizons of trauma treatment, redefining trauma as a continuum of variably negative life events occuring over a lifespan-including 'little traumas' such as car accidents, risky medical interventions, childhood abuse and neglect, and social discrimination and poverty-that shape every aspect of our existence.

Year Founded: 1923 ISBN 0-393704-66-1

2743 Transforming Trauma: EMDR
WW Norton & Company
500 5th Avenue
New York, NY 10110-54
212-354-5500
Fax: 212-869-0856
E-mail: admalmud@wwnorton.com
www.books.wwnorton.com

Drake McFeely, CEO

Has helped thousands of people dealing with abuse histories or recent traumatic events. The author has a unique perspective, as she is both a client of EMDR and a therapist. *$14.95*

288 pages Year Founded: 1923 ISSN 31757-9

2744 Trauma Response
WW Norton & Company
500 5th Avenue
New York, NY 10110-54
212-354-5500
Fax: 212-869-0856
E-mail: admalmud@wwnorton.com
www.books.wwnorton.com

Drake McFeely, CEO

Different causes of psychological trauma and modes of recovery. *$22.36*

240 pages Year Founded: 1923

2745 Treating Anxiety Disorders
Jossey-Bass Publishers
111 River Street
Hoboken, NJ 07030-5774
201-748-6000
Fax: 201-748-6088
www.www.wiley.com

Stephen M. Smith, President and Chief Executive Of
Ellis E. Cousens, Executive Vice President, Chief
John Kritzmacher, Executive Vice President, Chief
MJ O'Leary, Senior Vice President, Human Res
$30.95

288 pages Year Founded: 1999 ISBN 0-787903-16-7

2746 Treating Anxiety Disorders with a Cognitive
New Harbinger Publications
5674 Shattuck Avenue
Oakland, CA 94609-1662
510-652-0215
800-748-6273
Fax: 510-652-5472
E-mail: customerservice@newharbinger.com
www.newharbinger.com

Matthew McKay, Owner
Patrick Fanning, Co-Founder

Behavioral Exposure Based Approach and the Eye Movement Technique comes with a fifty eight minute videotape and a fifty one page paperback manual. *$100.00*

Year Founded: 1973 ISBN 1-889287-02-4

2747 Treating Panic Disorder and Agoraphobia: A Step by Step Clinical Guide
New Harbinger Publications
5674 Shattuck Avenue
Oakland, CA 94609-1662
510-652-0215
800-748-6273
Fax: 510-652-5472
E-mail: customerservice@newharbinger.com
www.newharbinger.com

Matthew McKay, Owner
Patrick Fanning, Co-Founder

Treatment program covering breath control training, changing automatic thoughts and underlying beliefs. *$49.95*

296 pages Year Founded: 1973 ISBN 1-572240-84-9

2748 Treatment of Obsessive Compulsive Disorder
Guilford Press
72 Spring Street
New York, NY 10012-4068

212-431-9800
800-365-7006
Fax: 212-966-6708
E-mail: info@guilford.com
www.www.guilford.com

Bob Matloff, President
Seymour Weingarten, Editor-in-Chief

Provides everything the mental health professional needs for working with clients who suffer from obsessions and compulsions. Supplies background by describing in detail up-to-date clinically relevant information and a step-by-step guide for conducting behavioral treatment. *$39.95*

224 pages   Year Founded: 1973 ISBN 0-898621-84-4

ADHD

2749   ADHD in Adolesents: Diagnosis and Treatment
Guilford Press
72 Spring Street
New York, NY 10012-4068
212-431-9800
800-365-7006
Fax: 212-966-6708
E-mail: info@guilford.com
www.www.guilford.com

Bob Matloff, President
Seymour Weingarten, Editor-in-Chief

Practical reference with a down to earth approach to diagnosing and treatment of ADHD in adolesents. A structured intervention program with guidelines to using educational, psycholgical and medical components to help patients. Many reproducible handouts, checklists and rating scales. *$24.95*

461 pages   Year Founded: 1973 ISBN 1-572305-45-2

2750   ADHD in Adulthood: Guide to Current Theory, Diagnosis and Treatment
Johns Hopkins University Press
2715 North Charles Street
Baltimore, MD 21218-4363
410-516-6900
800-537-5487
Fax: 410-516-6998
E-mail: webmaster@jhupress.jhu.edu
www.www.press.jhu.edu

William Brody, President

Discusses how ADHD manifests itself in adult life and answers popular questions posed by physicians and by adults with ADHD. Provides health professionals with a practical approach for treatment and diagnosis in adult ADHD patients. *$49.95*

392 pages   Year Founded: 1878 ISBN 0-801861-41-1

2751   All About ADHD: Complete Practical Guide for Classroom Teachers
ADD WareHouse
300 NW 70th Avenue
Suite 102
Plantation, FL 33317-2360
954-792-8100
800-233-9273
Fax: 954-792-8545
E-mail: websales@addwarehouse.com
www.addwarehouse.com

Harvey C Parker, Owner

Brings together both the art and science of effective teaching for students with ADHD using the Parallel Teaching Model as the base for blending behavior management and teaching, particularly in regular classroom settings. Real-life examples are used throughout the book and are intended to help you design strategies for you own classrooms to help your students be the best they can be. *$17.00*

175 pages   Year Founded: 1990

2752   Attention Deficit Disorder ADHD and ADD Syndromes
Pro-Ed Publications
8700 Shoal Creek Boulevard
Austin, TX 78757-6897
512-451-3246
800-897-3202
Fax: 512-451-8542
E-mail: info@proedinc.com
www.www.proedinc.com

Donald D Hammill, Owner

This book enters its third edition with even more complete explanations of how ADHD and ADD interfere with: classroom learning, behavior at home, job performance, and social skills development. *$19.00*

216 pages   Year Founded: 1998 ISBN 0-890797-42-0

2753   Attention Deficit Disorder and Learning Disabilities: Realities, Myths and Controversial Treatments
ADD WareHouse
300 NW 70th Avenue
Suite 102
Plantation, FL 33317-2360
954-792-8100
800-233-9273
Fax: 954-792-8545
E-mail: websales@addwarehouse.com
www.addwarehouse.com

Harvey C Parker, Owner

Designed to help parents and professionals recognize symptoms of learning disabilities and attentional disorders. Covers in detail conventional treatments that have been scientifically validated plus more controversial methods of treatment such as orthomolecular therapies, amino acid supplementation, dietary interventions, EEG biofeedback, cognitive therapy and visual training. *$13.00*

240 pages   Year Founded: 1990

2754   Attention Deficit/Hyperactivity Disorder
American Psychiatric Publishing, Inc.
1000 Wilson Boulevard
Suite 1825
Arlington, VA 22209-3901
703-907-7322
800-368-5777
Fax: 703-907-1091
E-mail: appi@psych.org
www.appi.org

Robert E Hales, M.D., M.B.A., Editor-in-Chief
Ron McMillen, Chief Executive Officer
John McDuffie, Editorial Director
Rebecca D. Rinehart, Publisher

Clinical Guide to Diagnosis and Treatment for Health and Mental Health Professionals making the proper diagnosis, and treatment strategies. *$29.95*

298 pages Year Founded: 1999 ISBN 0-880489-40-5

2755 Attention-Deficit Hyperactivity Disorder: A Handbook for Diagnosis and Treatment
Guilford Press
72 Spring Street
New York, NY 10012-4068
212-431-9800
800-365-7006
Fax: 212-966-6708
E-mail: info@guilford.com
www.www.guilford.com

Bob Matloff, President
Seymour Weingarten, Editor-in-Chief

This second edition incorporates the latest finding on the nature, diagnosis, assessment and treatment of ADHD. Includes select chapters by seasoned colleagues covering their respective areas of expertise and providing clear guidelines for practice in clinical, school and community settings. *$56.95*

602 pages Year Founded: 1973 ISBN 1-572302-75-5

2756 Attention-Deficit/Hyperactivity Disorder in the Classroom
Pro-Ed Publications
8700 Shoal Creek Boulevard
Austin, TX 78757-6897
512-451-3246
800-897-3202
Fax: 512-451-8542
E-mail: info@proedinc.com
www.www.proedinc.com

Donald D Hammill, Owner

Provides educators with a complete guide on how to deal effectively with students with attention deficits in their classroom. Emphasizes practical applications for teachers to use that will facilitate the success of students, both academically and socially, in a school setting. *$29.00*

291 pages Year Founded: 1998 ISBN 0-890796-65-3

2757 Family Therapy for ADHD: Treating Children, Adolescents and Adults
Guilford Press
72 Spring Street
New York, NY 10012-4068
212-431-9800
800-365-7006
Fax: 212-966-6708
E-mail: info@guilford.com
www.www.guilford.com

Bob Matloff, President
Seymour Weingarten, Editor-in-Chief

ADHD affects the entire family. This book helps the clinician evaluate its impact on marital dynamics, parent/sibling/child relationships and the complex treatment of ADHD in a larger context. Includes session by session plans and clinical material. *$32.95*

270 pages Year Founded: 1973 ISBN 1-572304-38-3

2758 How to Operate an ADHD Clinic or Subspecialty Practice
ADD WareHouse
300 NW 70th Avenue
Suite 102
Plantation, FL 33317-2360
954-792-8100
800-233-9273
Fax: 954-792-8545
E-mail: websales@addwarehouse.com
www.addwarehouse.com

Harvey C Parker, Owner

This book goes beyond academic discussions of ADHD and gets down to how to establish and manage an ADHD practice. In addition to practice guidelines and suggestions, this guide presents a compendium of clinic forms and letters, interview formats, sample reports, tricks of the trade and resource listings, all of which will help you develop or refine your clinic/counseling operation. *$65.00*

325 pages Year Founded: 1990

2759 Medications for Attention Disorders and Related Medical Problems: A Comprehensive Handbook
ADD WareHouse
300 NW 70th Avenue
Suite 102
Plantation, FL 33317-2360
954-792-8100
800-233-9273
Fax: 954-792-8545
E-mail: websales@addwarehouse.com
www.addwarehouse.com

Harvey C Parker, Owner

ADHD and ADD are medical conditions and often medical intervention is regarded by most experts as an essential component of the multimodal program for the treatment of these disorders. This text presents a comprehensive look at medications and their use in attention disorders. *$37.00*

420 pages Year Founded: 1990

2760 Parenting a Child With Attention Deficit/Hyperactivity Disorder
Pro-Ed Publications
8700 Shoal Creek Boulevard
Austin, TX 78757-6897
512-451-3246
800-897-3202
Fax: 512-451-8542
E-mail: info@proedinc.com
www.www.proedinc.com

Donald D Hammill, Owner

Offers proven parenting approaches for helping children between the ages of 5-11 years improve their behavior. *$29.00*

150 pages Year Founded: 1999 ISBN 0-890797-91-9

2761 Pretenders: Gifted People Who Have Difficulty Learning
High Tide Press
2081 Calistoga Dr
Suite 2N
New Lenox, IL 60451-4833
815-717-3780
888-487-7377

Fax: 815-717-3783
E-mail: managing.editor@hightidepress.com
www.www.hightidepress.com

Monica Regan, Managing Editor

Profiles of 8 adults with dyslexia and/or ADD with whom the author has worked. Informative, fascinating, at times heartbreaking, but ultimately inspiring. *$24.50*

177 pages ISBN 1-892696-06-1

Autism Spectrum Disorders

2762 Asperger Syndrome Diagnostic Scale (ASDS)
Pro-Ed
8700 Shoal Creek Boulevard
Austin, TX 78757-6897
512-451-3246
800-897-3202
Fax: 512-451-8542
E-mail: feedback@proedinc.com
www.www.proedinc.com

Donald D Hammill, Owner
Stacey Bock
Richard Simpson

The ASDS is a quick, easy-to-use rating scale that helps determine whether a child has Asperger Syndrome. Anyone who knows the child or youth well can complete the scale. Parents, teachers, siblings, paraeducators, speech-language pathologists, psychologists, psyciatrists and other professionals can answer the 50 yes/no items in 10 to 15 minutes. *$100.00*

2763 Asperger Syndrome: a Practical Guide for Teachers
ADD WareHouse
300 NW 70th Avenue
Suite 102
Plantation, FL 33317-2360
954-792-8100
800-233-9273
Fax: 954-792-8545
E-mail: websales@addwarehouse.com
www.addwarehouse.com

Harvey C Parker, Owner

A clear and concise guide to effective classroom practice for teachers and support assistants working with children with Asperger Syndrome in school. The authors explain characteristics of children with Asperger Syndrome, discuss methods of assessment and offer practical strategies for effective classroom interventions. *$24.95*

90 pages Year Founded: 1990

2764 Children and Youth with Asperger Syndrome
Program Development Associates
32 Court St
21st Floor
Brooklyn, NY 11201
315-452-0643
800-876-1710
Fax: 718-488-8642
E-mail: info@disabilitytraining.com
www.disabilitytraining.com

Classroom teachers now get special information to accommodate students with Asperger Syndrome, who display symptoms similar to, but milder than, autism. Strategies include research-based instructional, behavioral and environmental modifications. *$35.95*

200 pages Year Founded: 1997

Cognitive Disorders

2765 Cognitive Therapy in Practice
WW Norton & Company
500 5th Avenue
New York, NY 10110-54
212-354-5500
800-233-4830
Fax: 212-869-0856
E-mail: npd@wwnorton.com
www.books.wwnorton.com

Drake McFeely, CEO

Basic text for graduate studies in psychotherapy, psycholgy nursing social work and counseling. *$29.00*

224 pages Year Founded: 1923 ISBN 0-393700-77-1

2766 Geriatric Mental Health Care: A Treatment Guide for Health Professionals
Guilford Press
72 Spring Street
New York, NY 10012-4068
212-431-9800
800-365-7006
Fax: 212-966-6708
E-mail: info@guilford.com
www.www.guilford.com

Bob Matloff, President
Seymour Weingarten, Editor-in-Chief

Designed for mental health practitioners and primary care providers without advanced training in geriatric psychiatry. Covers depression, anxiety, the dementias, psychosis, mania, sleep disturbances, personality and pain disorders, adapting principles, sexuality, elder issues, alcohol and substance abuse, suicide risk, consultation, legal and ethic issues, exercise and much more. *$39.00*

347 pages Year Founded: 1973 ISBN 1-572305-92-4

2767 Guidelines for the Treatment of Patients with Alzheimer's Disease and Other Dementias of Late Life
American Psychiatric Publishing, Inc.
1000 Wilson Boulevard
Suite 1825
Arlington, VA 22209-3901
703-907-7322
800-368-5777
Fax: 703-907-1091
E-mail: appi@psych.org
www.appi.org

Robert E Hales, M.D., M.B.A., Editor-in-Chief
Ron McMillen, Chief Executive Officer
John McDuffie, Editorial Director
Rebecca D. Rinehart, Publisher

Diagnosis and treatment strategies. *$22.50*

40 pages Year Founded: 1995 ISBN 0-890423-04-0

2768 Loss of Self: Family Resource for the Care of Alzheimer's Disease and Related Disorders
WW Norton & Company
500 5th Avenue
New York, NY 10110-54
212-354-2907
Fax: 212-869-0856
E-mail: admalmud@wwnorton.com
www.books.wwnorton.com

Drake McFeely, CEO

How to help a relative and also meet a family's own needs during the long and tragic period of care involved with Alzheimer's Disease. Challenges are more than medical and can be emotional, involve family conflict, sexuality, abuse, and eventually, dealing with death. As well as the emotional challenges, the latest treatments, drugs and diagnosis information, plus causes and preventative measures are included. *$27.95*

432 pages Year Founded: 1923 ISBN 0-393050-16-5

2769 Neurobiology of Primary Dementia
American Psychiatric Publishing, Inc.
1000 Wilson Boulevard
Suite 1825
Arlington, VA 22209-3901
703-907-7322
800-368-5777
Fax: 703-907-1091
E-mail: appi@psych.org
www.appi.org

Robert E Hales, M.D., M.B.A., Editor-in-Chief
Ron McMillen, Chief Executive Officer
John McDuffie, Editorial Director
Rebecca D. Rinehart, Publisher

Study of aging and Alzheimer's. Contains investigations of the basic neurobiologic aspects of the etiology of dementia, clear discussions of the diagnostic process with regard to imaging and other laboratory tests, psychopharmacologic treatment and genetic counseling. *$61.50*

440 pages Year Founded: 1998 ISBN 0-880489-15-4

2770 Strange Behavior Tales of Evolutionary Neurology
WW Norton & Company
500 5th Avenue
New York, NY 10110-54
212-354-5500
800-233-4830
Fax: 212-869-0856
E-mail: webmaster@wwnorton.com
www.books.wwnorton.com

Drake McFeely, CEO

Both educational and entertaining, the author presents an array of people with unusual problems who have one thing in common, brain disorder. Carefully constructed, this book outlines the functioning of the brain and evolution of language skills. *$13.95*

256 pages Year Founded: 1923 ISBN 0-393321-84-3

2771 The New Handbook of Cognitive Therapy Techniques
WW Norton & Company
500 5th Avenue
New York, NY 10110-54

212-354-5500
800-233-4830
Fax: 212-869-0856
E-mail: npb@wwnorton.com
www.books.wwnorton.com

Drake McFeely, CEO

Describes, explains, and demonstrates over a hundred cognitive therapy techniques, offering for each the theorretical basis, a thumbnail description of the method, case examples, and resources for further information.

Year Founded: 1923 ISBN 0-393703-13-4

2772 Treating Complex Cases: The Cognitive Behavioral Therapy Approach
John Wiley & Sons
111 River Street
Hoboken, NJ 07030-5774
201-748-6000
Fax: 201-748-6088
E-mail: info@wiley.com
www.www.wiley.com

Stephen M. Smith, President and Chief Executive Officer
Ellis E. Cousens, Executive Vice President
John Kritzmacher, Executive Vice President
MJ O'Leary, Senior Vice President, Human Resources

This book brings together some of the most experiences and expert cognitive behavioral therapists to share their specialist experience of formulation and treatment of complex problems such as co-morbidity, psychotic conditions, and chronic conditions. The experienced clinician will find: evidence-based approaches to assessment and formulation of complex cases; a wide range of problems not restricted to disorder categories, including anger, low self-esteem, abuse and shame; a concern with the realities of clinical practice which involves complex cases that do not fit into simple case conceptualisations or diagnostic categories. Copyright 2000. *$80.00*

364 pages Year Founded: 1807 ISBN 0-471978-39-8

Conduct Disorder

2773 Behavioral Risk Management
Jossey-Bass Publishers
111 River Street
Hoboken, NJ 07030-5774
201-748-6000
Fax: 201-748-6088
E-mail: info@wiley.com
www.www.wiley.com

Stephen M. Smith, President and Chief Executive Officer
Ellis E. Cousens, Executive Vice President
John Kritzmacher, Executive Vice President
MJ O'Leary, Senior Vice President

Learn to identify potential mental health and behavioral problems on the job and apply effective intervention strategies for behavioral risk. *$41.95*

364 pages Year Founded: 1807 ISBN 0-787902-20-9

2774 Beyond Behavior Modification: Cognitive-Behavioral Approach to Behavior Management in the School
Pro-Ed Publications
8700 Shoal Creek Boulevard
Austin, TX 78757-6897

512-451-3246
800-897-3202
Fax: 512-451-8542
E-mail: info@proedinc.com
www.www.proedinc.com

Donald D Hammill, Owner

Focuses on traditional behavior modification, and presents a social learning theory approach. *$39.00*

643 pages Year Founded: 1995 ISBN 0-890796-63-7

2775 Inclusion Strategies for Students with Learning and Behavior Problems
Pro-Ed Publications
8700 Shoal Creek Boulevard
Austin, TX 78757-6897
512-451-3246
800-897-3202
Fax: 512-451-8542
E-mail: info@proedinc.com
www.www.proedinc.com

Donald D Hammill, Owner

Provides the components necessary to implement successful inclusion by presenting the experience of those directly impacted by inclusion: an individual with a disability; parents of a student with a disbility; teachers who implement inclusion; and researchers of best practices. Integrates theory and practice in an easy, how-to manner. *$36.00*

416 pages Year Founded: 1997 ISBN 0-890796-98-X

2776 Outrageous Behavior Mood: Handbook of Strategic Interventions for Managing Impossible Students
Pro-Ed Publications
8700 Shoal Creek Boulevard
Austin, TX 78757-6897
512-451-3246
800-897-3202
Fax: 512-451-8542
E-mail: info@proedinc.com
www.www.proedinc.com

Donald D Hammill, Owner

This handbook is for educators who have had success in managing difficult students. Introduces such methods as planned confusion, disruptive word pictures, unconscious suggestion, double-bind predictions, off the wall interpretations, and even some straight faced paradoxical assignments. *$26.00*

154 pages Year Founded: 1999 ISBN 0-890798-17-6

Dissociative Disorders

2777 Dissociative Identity Disorder: Diagnosis, Clinical Features, and Treatment of Multiple Personality
John Wiley & Sons
111 River Street
Hoboken, NJ 07030-5774
201-748-6000, Fax: 201-748-6088
E-mail: info@wiley.com
www.www.wiley.com

Stephen M. Smith, President and Chief Executive Officer
Ellis E. Cousens, Executive Vice President
John Kritzmacher, Executive Vice President
MJ O'Leary, Senior Vice President, Human Resources

Comprehensive and interesting, this account of the history of MPD dispells many myths and presents new insight into the treatment of MPD. Perfect for sexual abuse clinics, child abuse agencies, correctional facilities and clinicians of all fields. *$64.50*

364 pages Year Founded: 1807 ISBN 0-471132-65-9

2778 Rebuilding Shattered Lives: Responsible Treatment of Complex Post-Traumatic and Dissociative Disorders
John Wiley & Sons
111 River Street
Hoboken, NJ 07030-5774
201-748-6000, Fax: 201-748-6088
E-mail: info@wiley.com
www.www.wiley.com

Stephen M. Smith, President and Chief Executive Officer
Ellis E. Cousens, Executive Vice President
John Kritzmacher, Executive Vice President
MJ O'Leary, Senior Vice President, Human Resources

The most up-to-date, integrative and emperically sound account of trauma theory and practice availible. Based on more than a decade of clinical research and treatment experience at the Harvard Medical School, this comprehensive and nontechnical text offers a stage oriented approach to understanding and treating complex and difficult traumatized patients, integrating modern trauma theory with traditional theraputic interventions. *$47.50*

364 pages Year Founded: 1807 ISBN 0-471247-32-4

Eating Disorders

2779 Biting The Hand That Starves You: Inspiring Resistance to Anorexia/Bulimia
WW Norton & Company
500 5th Avenue
New York, NY 10110-54
212-354-5500
800-233-4830
Fax: 212-869-0856
E-mail: npb@wwnorton.com
www.books.wwnorton.com

Drake McFeely, CEO

Details a unique way of thinking and speaking about anorexia/bulimia (a/b), by having conversations with insiders in which the problem is viewed as an external influence rather than a part of the person. Coercion is sidestepped in favor of practices that are collaborative, accountable, and spirit-nurturing.

Year Founded: 1923 ISBN 0-393703-37-1

2780 Drug Therpay and Eating Disorders
Mason Crest Publishers
370 Reed Road
Suite 302
Broomall, PA 19008-4017
610-543-6200
866-627-2665
Fax: 610-543-3878
E-mail: dtaylor@masoncrest.com
www.masoncrest.com

Provides a clear, concise account of the history, symptoms, and current treatment of anorexia nervosa and bulimia nervosa. It is estimated the eating disorders affect five million Americans each year, and many more millions among other nations.

ISBN 1-590845-65-X

2781 Handbook of Treatment for Eating Disorders
Guilford Press
72 Spring Street
New York, NY 10012-4068
212-431-9800
800-365-7006
Fax: 212-966-6708
E-mail: info@guilford.com
www.www.guilford.com

Bob Matloff, President
Seymour Weingarten, Editor-in-Chief

Includes coverage of binge eating and examines pharmacological as well as therapeutic approaches to eating disorders. Presents cognitive behavioral, psychoeducational, interpersonal, family, feminist, group and psychodynamic approaches, as well as the basics of pharmacological management. Features strategies for handling sexual abuse, substance abuse, concurrent medical conditions, personality disorder, prepubertal eating disorders and patients who refuse therapy. *$56.95*

540 pages Year Founded: 1973 ISBN 1-572301-86-4

2782 Interpersonal Psychotherapy
American Psychiatric Publishing, Inc.
1000 Wilson Boulevard
Suite 1825
Arlington, VA 22209-3901
703-907-7322
800-368-5777
Fax: 703-907-1091
E-mail: appi@psych.org
www.appi.org

Robert E Hales, M.D., M.B.A., Editor-in-Chief
Ron McMillen, Chief Executive Officer
John McDuffie, Editorial Director
Rebecca D. Rinehart, Publisher

An overview of interpersonal psychotherapy for depression, preventative treatment for depression, bulimia nervosa and HIV positive men and women. *$26.00*

156 pages Year Founded: 1998 ISBN 0-880488-36-0

2783 Sexual Abuse and Eating Disorders
200 E Joppa Road
PO Box 436
Brooklandville, MD 21022-0436
410-825-8888
888-825-8249
Fax: 410-560-0134
E-mail: sidran@sidran.org
www.sidran.org

EstherGiller, President and Director
Sheila Sidran Giller, Secretary/Treasurer
J. G.Goellnerÿ, Director Emeritus
Tracy Howard, Book Sales/Office Manager

This is the first book to explore the complex relationship between sexual abuse and eating disorders. Sexual abuse is both an extreme boundary violation and a disruption of attachment and bonding; victims of such abuse are likely to exhibit symptoms of self injury, including eating disorders. This volume is a discussion of the many ways that sexual abuse and eating disorders are related, also has accounts by

a survivor of both. Investigates the prevalence of sexual abuse amoung individuals with eating disorders. Also examines how a history of sexual violence can serve as a predictor of subsequent problems with food. Looks at related social factors, reviews trauma based theories, more controversial territory and discusses delayed memory versus false memory. *$34.95*

345 pages Year Founded: 1986

Gender Identification Disorder

2784 Gender Loving Care
WW Norton & Company
500 5th Avenue
New York, NY 10110-54
212-354-5500
Fax: 212-869-0856
E-mail: admalmud@wwnorton.com
www.books.wwnorton.com

Drake McFeely, CEO

Understanding and treating gender identity disorder, especially transexuals, who may feel stuck in the wrong-sexed body. *$ 25.00*

196 pages Year Founded: 1923 ISBN 0-393703-40-5

2785 Homosexuality and American Psychiatry: The Politics of Diagnosis
Princeton University Press
41 William Street
Princeton, NJ 08540-5237
609-258-4900
800-777-4726
Fax: 609-258-6305
www.press.princeton.edu

Fred Appel, Executive Editor
Al Bertrand, Assistant Director
Eric Crahan, Senior Editor
Seth Ditchik, Executive Editor

$18.00

249 pages Year Founded: 1905 ISBN 0-691028-37-0

2786 Principles and Practice of Sex Therapy
Guilford Press
72 Spring Street
New York, NY 10012-4068
212-431-9800
800-365-7006
Fax: 212-966-6708
E-mail: info@guilford.com
www.www.guilford.com

Bob Matloff, President
Seymour Weingarten, Editor-in-Chief

Many new developments in theory, diagnosis and treatment of sexual disorders have occured in the past decade. The authors set clear guidlines for assessment and treatment with fresh clinical material. A text for professionals and students in a wide range of mental health fields; sexual disorders, male and female, paraphilias, gender identity disorders, vasoactive drugs and more are covered. *$50.00*

518 pages Year Founded: 1973 ISBN 1-572305-74-6

2787 Psychoanalytic Therapy & the Gay Man
Analytic Press
7625 Empire Drive
Florence, KY 41042-2919

800-634-7064
Fax: 215-269-0363
E-mail: orders@taylorandfrancis.com
www.www.routledgementalhealth.com

Paul E Stepansky PhD, Managing Director
John Kerr PhD, Sr Editor

Explores of the subjectivities of gay men in psychoanalytic psychotherapy. It is a vitally human testament to the richly varied inner experiences of gay men. Offers that sexual identity, which encompass a spectrum of possibilities for any gay man, must be addressed in an atmosphere of honest encounter that allows not only for exploration of conflict and dissasociation but also for restitutive conformation of the patient's right to be himself. Available in hardcover. *$55.00*

384 pages Year Founded: 1998 ISBN 0-881632-08-2

Impulse Control Disorders

2788 Abusive Personality: Violence and Control in Intimate Relationships
Guilford Press
72 Spring Street
New York, NY 10012-4068
212-431-9800
800-365-7006
Fax: 212-966-6708
E-mail: info@guilford.com
www.www.guilford.com

Bob Matloff, President
Seymour Weingarten, Editor-in-Chief

A study of domestic violence, especially male perpetrators. *$26.95*

214 pages Year Founded: 1973 ISBN 1-572303-70-0

2789 Coping With Self-Mutilation: a Helping Book for Teens Who Hurt Themselves
Rosen Publishing Group
29 E 21st Street
New York, NY 10010-6209
212-777-3017
800-237-9932
Fax: 888-436-4643
E-mail: info@rosenpub.com
www.rosenpublishing.com

Roger Rosen, President

Examines the reasons for this phenomenon, and ways one might seek help. *$17.95*

Year Founded: 1950 ISBN 0-823925-59-5

2790 Dealing with Anger Problems: Rational-Emotive Therapeutic Interventions
Professional Resource Press
PO Box 3197
Sarasota, FL 34230-3197
941-343-9601
800-443-3364
Fax: 941-343-9201
E-mail: cs.prpress@gmail.com
www.prpress.com

Laurie Girsch, Managing Editor

Demonstrates ways to apply rational-emotive therapy techniques to help your clients control their anger. Offers step-by-step anger control treatment program that includes a variety of cognitive, emotive, and behavioral homework assignments, and procedures for modifying behaviors and facilitating change. *$11.95*

68 pages Year Founded: 1980 ISBN 0-943158-59-1

2791 Domestic Violence 2000: Integrated Skills Program for Men
WW Norton & Company
500 5th Avenue
New York, NY 10110-54
212-354-5500
Fax: 212-869-0856
E-mail: admalmud@wwnorton.com
www.books.wwnorton.com

Drake McFeely, CEO

Various theories are examined to deal with this difficult social problem. For group classes. *$23.20*

224 pages Year Founded: 1923 ISSN 70314-2

2792 Sex Murder and Sex Aggression: Phenomenology Psychopathology, Psychodynamics and Prognosis
Charles C Thomas Publisher Ltd.
2600 S 1st Street
Springfield, IL 62704-4730
217-789-8980
800-258-8980
Fax: 217-789-9130
E-mail: books@ccthomas.com
www.ccthomas.com

Michael P Thomas, President
Charles CThomas, Publisher

By Eugene Revitch, Robert Wood Johnson School of Medicine, Piscataway, New Jersey, and Louis B Schlesinger, New Jersey Medical School, Newark. With a foreword by Robert R Hazelwood. Contents: The Place of Gynocide and Sexual Aggression in the Classification of Crime; Catathymic Gynocide; Compulsive Gynocide; Psychodynamics, Psychopathology and Differential Diagnosis; Prognostic Considerations. *$43.95*

152 pages Year Founded: 1927 ISSN 0-398-06346-X
ISBN 0-398055-56-4

2793 Teaching Behavioral Self Control to Students
Pro-Ed Publications
8700 Shoal Creek Boulevard
Austin, TX 78757-6897
512-451-3246
800-897-3202
Fax: 512-451-8542
E-mail: info@proedinc.com
www.www.proedinc.com

Donald D Hammill, Owner

Demonstrates how teachers, counselors and parents can help children of all ages and ability levels to modify their own behavior. Clear step-by-step methods describe how common childhood problems can be solved by helping children become more responsible and independent. *$21.00*

122 pages Year Founded: 1995 ISBN 0-890796-17-3

Mood Disorders

2794 Active Treatment of Depression
WW Norton & Company
500 5th Avenue
New York, NY 10110-54
212-354-5500
Fax: 212-869-0856
E-mail: admalmud@wwnorton.com
www.books.wwnorton.com

Drake McFeely, CEO

A candid discussion on depression and effective, hopeful therapy strategies. *$35.00*

272 pages Year Founded: 1923 ISSN 70322-3

2795 Antidepressant Fact Book: What Your Doctor Won't Tell You About Prozac, Zoloft, Paxil, Celexa and Luvox
Perseus Books Group
2465 Central Avenue
Boulder, CO 80301
303-444-3541
800-386-5656
Fax: 720-406-7336
E-mail: westview.orders@perseusbooks.com
www.perseusbooksgroup.com

David Steinberger, President & CEO

What antidepressants will and won't treat, documented side and withdrawl effects, plus what parents need to know about teenagers and antidepressants. The author has been a medical expert in many court cases invloving the use and misuse of psychoactive drugs. *$13.00*

240 pages Year Founded: 2001 ISBN 0-738204-51-X

2796 Cognitive Therapy of Depression
Guilford Press
72 Spring Street
New York, NY 10012-4068
212-431-9800
800-365-7006
Fax: 212-966-6708
E-mail: info@guilford.com
www.www.guilford.com

Bob Matloff, President
Seymour Weingarten, Editor-in-Chief

Shows how psychotherapists can effectively treat depressive disorders. Case examples illustrate a wide range of strategies and techniques. Chapter topics include the role of emotions in cognitive therapy, application of behavioral techniques and cognitive therapy and antidepressant medications. Hardcover. Paperback also available. *$ 46.95*

425 pages Year Founded: 1973 ISBN 0-898620-00-7

2797 Concise Guide to Mood Disorders
American Psychiatric Publishing, Inc.
1000 Wilson Boulevard
Suite 1825
Arlington, VA 22209-3901
703-907-7322
800-368-5777
Fax: 703-907-1091
E-mail: appi@psych.org
www.appi.org

Robert E Hales, M.D., M.B.A., Editor-in-Chief
Ron McMillen, Chief Executive Officer
John McDuffie, Editorial Director
Rebecca D. Rinehart, Publisher

Designed for daily use in the clinical setting, the Concise Guide to Mood Disorders is a fingertip library of the latest information, easy to understand and quick to access. This practical reference summarizes everything a clinician needs to know to diagnose and treat unipolar and bipolar mood disorders. *$29.95*

320 pages Year Founded: 2002 ISBN 1-585620-56-4

2798 Concise Guide to Women's Mental Health
American Psychiatric Publishing, Inc.
1000 Wilson Boulevard
Suite 1825
Arlington, VA 22209-3901
703-907-7322
800-368-5777
Fax: 703-907-1091
E-mail: appi@psych.org
www.appi.org

Robert E Hales, M.D., M.B.A., Editor-in-Chief
Ron McMillen, Chief Executive Officer
John McDuffie, Editorial Director
Rebecca D. Rinehart, Publisher

Examines the biological, psychological, and sociocultural factors that influence a woman's mental health and often contribute to psychiatric disorders. Supplies clinicians with important information on gender related differences on differential diagnosis, case formulation and treatment planning. Topics include premenstrual dysphoric disorder, hormonal contraception and effects on mood, psychiatric disorders in pregnancy, postpartum psychiatric disorders and perimenopause and menopause. *$21.95*

187 pages Year Founded: 1997 ISBN 0-880483-43-1

2799 Depression in Context: Strategies for Guided Action
WW Norton & Company
500 5th Avenue
New York, NY 10110-54
212-354-5500
Fax: 212-869-0856
E-mail: admalmud@wwnorton.com
www.books.wwnorton.com

Drake McFeely, CEO

Description of Behavioral Activation, a new treatment for Depression. *$32.00*

224 pages Year Founded: 1923 ISSN 70350-9

2800 Evaluation and Treatment of Postpartum Emotional Disorders
Professional Resource Press
PO Box 3197
Sarasota, FL 34230-3197
941-343-9601
800-443-3364
Fax: 941-343-9201
E-mail: cs.prpress@gmail.com
www.prpress.com

Laurie Girsch, Managing Editor

Teaches how to recognize and treat postpartum emotional disorders. Procedures for clinical assessment, psychotherapeutic interventions, and medical - psychiatric treatments are described. *$ 13.95*

110 pages Year Founded: 1980 ISBN 1-568870-24-8

2801 Handbook of Depression
Guilford Press
72 Spring Street
New York, NY 10012-4068
212-431-9800
800-365-7006
Fax: 212-966-6708
E-mail: info@guilford.com
www.www.guilford.com

Bob Matloff, President
Seymour Weingarten, Editor-in-Chief

Brings together well-known authorities who address the need for a comprehensive review of the most current information available on depression. Surveys current theories and treatment models, covering both what the MD and non-MD needs to know. *$65.00*

628 pages Year Founded: 1973 ISBN 0-898628-41-5

2802 Postpartum Mood Disorders
American Psychiatric Publishing, Inc.
1000 Wilson Boulevard
Suite 1825
Arlington, VA 22209-3901
703-907-7322
800-368-5777
Fax: 703-907-1091
E-mail: appi@psych.org
www.appi.org

Robert E Hales, M.D., M.B.A., Editor-in-Chief
Ron McMillen, Chief Executive Officer
John McDuffie, Editorial Director
Rebecca D. Rinehart, Publisher

$38.50

280 pages Year Founded: 1999 ISBN 0-880489-29-4

2803 Scientific Foundations of Cognitive Theory and Therapy of Depression
John Wiley & Sons
111 River Street
Hoboken, NJ 07030-5774
201-748-6000
Fax: 201-748-6088
E-mail: info@wiley.com
www.www.wiley.com

Stephen M. Smith, President and Chief Executive Officer
Ellis E. Cousens, Executive Vice President
John Kritzmacher, Executive Vice President
MJ O'Leary, Senior Vice President, Human Resources

A synthesis of decades of research and practice, this semminal book presents and critically evaluates this scientific and emprical status of co author Aaron Beck's revised cognitive theory and therapy of depression. The authors explore the evolution of cognitive theory and therapy of depression and discuss the future directions for the treatment of depression.

364 pages Year Founded: 1807

2804 Symptoms of Depression
John Wiley & Sons
111 River Street
Hoboken, NJ 07030-5774
201-748-6000
Fax: 201-748-6088
E-mail: info@wiley.com
www.www.wiley.com

Stephen M. Smith, President and Chief Executive Officer
Ellis E. Cousens, Executive Vice President
John Kritzmacher, Executive Vice President
MJ O'Leary, Senior Vice President, Human Resources

364 pages Year Founded: 1807

2805 Treating Depressed Children: A Therapeutic Manual of Proven Cognitive Behavioral Techniques
New Harbinger Publications
5674 Shattuck Avenue
Oakland, CA 94609-1662
510-652-0215
800-748-6273
Fax: 510-652-5472
E-mail: customerservice@newharbinger.com
www.newharbinger.com

Matthew McKay, Owner
Patrick Fanning, Co-Founder

A full twelve session treatment program incorporates cartoons and role playing games to help children recognize emotions, change negative thoughts, gain confidence and learn crucial interpersonal skills. *$49.95*

160 pages Year Founded: 1973 ISBN 1-572240-61-X

2806 Treating Depression
Jossey-Bass Publishers
111 River Street
Hoboken, NJ 07030-5774
201-748-6000
Fax: 201-748-6088
E-mail: info@wiley.com
www.www.wiley.com

Stephen M. Smith, President and Chief Executive Officer
Ellis E. Cousens, Executive Vice President
John Kritzmacher, Executive Vice President
MJ O'Leary, Senior Vice President, Human Resources

$27.95

364 pages Year Founded: 1807 ISBN 0-787915-85-8

2807 Treatment of Recurrent Depression
American Psychiatric Publishing, Inc.
1000 Wilson Boulevard
Suite 1825
Arlington, VA 22209-3901
703-907-7322
800-368-5777
Fax: 703-907-1091
E-mail: appi@psych.org
www.appi.org

Robert E Hales, M.D., M.B.A., Editor-in-Chief
Ron McMillen, Chief Executive Officer
John McDuffie, Editorial Director
Rebecca D. Rinehart, Publisher

Five topics covered are, Lifetime Impact of Gender on Recurrent Major Depressive Disorder in Women, Treatment Stategies, Prevention of Recurrences in Bipolar Patients, Potential Applications and Updated Recommendations. *$29.95*

208 pages Year Founded: 2001 ISBN 1-585620-25-4

Personality Disorders

401

2808 Biological Basis of Personality
Charles C Thomas Publisher Ltd.
2600 S 1st Street
Springfield, IL 62704-4730
217-789-8980
800-258-8980
Fax: 217-789-9130
E-mail: books@ccthomas.com
www.ccthomas.com

Michael P Thomas, President
Charles CThomas, Publisher

$70.95

420 pages Year Founded: 1927 ISBN 0-398005-38-9

2809 Biology of Personality Disorders
American Psychiatric Publishing, Inc.
1000 Wilson Boulevard
Suite 1825
Arlington, VA 22209-3901
703-907-7322
800-368-5777
Fax: 703-907-1091
E-mail: appi@psych.org
www.appi.org

Robert E Hales, M.D., M.B.A., Editor-in-Chief
Ron McMillen, Chief Executive Officer
John McDuffie, Editorial Director
Rebecca D. Rinehart, Publisher

Content topics include neurotransmitter function in personality disorders, new biological researcher strategies for personality disorders, the genetics psychobiology of the seven - factor model of personality disorders, and significance of biological research for a biopsychosocial model of personality disorders. *$25.00*

166 pages Year Founded: 1998 ISBN 0-880488-35-2

2810 Borderline Personality Disorder: A Therapist Guide to Taking Control
WW Norton & Company
500 5th Avenue
New York, NY 10110-54
212-354-5500
800-233-4830
Fax: 212-869-0856
E-mail: npb@wwnorton.com
www.books.wwnorton.com

Drake McFeely, CEO

From identification to relapse prevention, this guide helps therapists manage a patient's treatment for the rather complex problem of Borderline Personality Disorder, an often difficult and sometimes life threatening condition. *$27.50*

224 pages Year Founded: 1923 ISBN 0-393703-52-5

2811 Borderline Personality Disorder: Tailoring the Psychotherapy to the Patient
American Psychiatric Publishing, Inc.
1000 Wilson Boulevard
Suite 1825
Arlington, VA 22209-3901
703-907-7322
800-368-5777
Fax: 703-907-1091
E-mail: appi@psych.org
www.appi.org

Robert E Hales, M.D., M.B.A., Editor-in-Chief
Ron McMillen, Chief Executive Officer
John McDuffie, Editorial Director
Rebecca D. Rinehart, Publisher

$34.00

256 pages Year Founded: 1996 ISBN 0-880486-89-9

2812 Cognitive Therapy for Personality Disorders: a Schema-Focused Approach
Professional Resource Press
PO Box 3197
Sarasota, FL 34230-3197
941-343-9601
800-443-3364
Fax: 941-343-9201
E-mail: cs.prpress@gmail.com
www.prpress.com

Laurie Girsch, Managing Editor

A guide to treating the most difficult cases in your practice: personality disorders and other chronic, self - defeating problems. Contains rationale, theory, practical applications, and active cognitive behavioral techniques. *$13.95*

96 pages Year Founded: 1980 ISBN 1-568870-47-7

2813 Cognitive Therapy of Personality Disorders
Guilford Press
72 Spring Street
New York, NY 10012-4068
212-431-9800
800-365-7006
Fax: 212-966-6708
E-mail: info@guilford.com
www.www.guilford.com

Bob Matloff, President
Seymour Weingarten, Editor-in-Chief

Focuses on the use of cognitive therapy to treat people with personality disorders who do not usually engage in therapy. Emanates the research and practical experience of Beck and his associates and is the first to focus specifically on this diverse and clinically demanding population. Case vignettes are used throughout. *$43.00*

396 pages Year Founded: 1973 ISBN 0-989624-34-7

2814 Dealing With the Problem of Low Self-Esteem: Common Characteristics and Treatment
Charles C Thomas Publisher Ltd.
2600 S 1st Street
Springfield, IL 62704-4730
217-789-8980
800-258-8980
Fax: 217-789-9130
E-mail: books@ccthomas.com
www.ccthomas.com

Michael P Thomas, President
Charles CThomas, Publisher

Considers the practice of psychotherapy from the self-esteem perspective. Describes the common characteristics of low self-esteem that are manifested in clients with diverse problems; focuses on the functions the therapist performs in addressing these characteristics. The third is to consider the modalities of treatment through which the therapist delivers these therapeutic functions. *$ 48.95*

228 pages Year Founded: 1927 ISSN 0-398-05951-9ISBN 0-398059-36-5

2815 Disorders of Personality: DSM-IV and Beyond
John Wiley & Sons
111 River Street
Hoboken, NJ 07030-5774
201-748-6000
Fax: 201-748-6088
E-mail: info@wiley.com
www.www.wiley.com

Stephen M. Smith, President and Chief Executive Of
Ellis E. Cousens, Executive Vice President, Chief
John Kritzmacher, Executive Vice President, Chief
MJ O'Leary, Senior Vice President, Human Res

Clarifies the distinctions between the vast array of personality disorders and helps clinicians make accurate diagnoses; thoroughly updated to incorporate the recent change in
the DSM - IV. Guides the clinicians throught the intricate
maze of personality disorders, with special attention on
changes in their conceptualization over the last decade.
DSM-V due out in 2013 *$85.00*

364 pages Year Founded: 1807 ISBN 0-471011-86-X

2816 Group Exercises for Enhancing Social Skills &
Self-Esteem
Professional Resource Press
PO Box 3197
Sarasota, FL 34230-3197
941-343-9601
800-443-3364
Fax: 941-343-9201
E-mail: cs.prpress@gmail.com
www.prpress.com

Laurie Girsch, Managing Editor

Includes exercises for enhancing self-esteem utilizing
proven social, emotional, and cognitive skill-building techniques. These exercises are useful in therapeutic,
psychoeducational, and recreational settings. *$24.95*

150 pages Year Founded: 1980 ISBN 1-568870-20-5

2817 Personality Characteristics of the Personality
Disordered
John Wiley & Sons
111 River Street
Hoboken, NJ 07030-5774
201-748-6000
Fax: 201-748-6088
E-mail: info@wiley.com
www.www.wiley.com

Stephen M. Smith, President and Chief Executive Officer
Ellis E. Cousens, Executive Vice President
John Kritzmacher, Executive Vice President
MJ O'Leary, Senior Vice President, Human Resources
364 pages Year Founded: 1807

2818 Personality Disorders and Culture: Clinical and
Conceptual Interactions
John Wiley & Sons
111 River Street
Hoboken, NJ 07030-5774
201-748-6000
Fax: 201-748-6088
E-mail: info@wiley.com
www.www.wiley.com

Stephen M. Smith, President and Chief Executive Officer
Ellis E. Cousens, Executive Vice President

John Kritzmacher, Executive Vice President
MJ O'Leary, Senior Vice President, Human Resources

Discusses two of the most timely and complex areas in
mental health, personality disorders and the impact of cultural variables. Treading on the timeless nature - nurture
debate, it suggests that social variables have a dramatic impact on the definition, development, and manifestation of
personality disorders.

364 pages Year Founded: 1807

2819 Personality and Stress: Individual Differences
in the Stress Process
John Wiley & Sons
111 River Street
Hoboken, NJ 07030-5774
201-748-6000
Fax: 201-748-6088
E-mail: info@wiley.com
www.www.wiley.com

Stephen M. Smith, President and Chief Executive Officer
Ellis E. Cousens, Executive Vice President
John Kritzmacher, Executive Vice President
MJ O'Leary, Senior Vice President, Human Resources
364 pages Year Founded: 1807

2820 Psychotherapy for Borderline Personality
John Wiley & Sons
111 River Street
Hoboken, NJ 07030-5774
201-748-6000
Fax: 201-748-6088
E-mail: info@wiley.com
www.www.wiley.com

Stephen M. Smith, President and Chief Executive Officer
Ellis E. Cousens, Executive Vice President
John Kritzmacher, Executive Vice President
MJ O'Leary, Senior Vice President, Human Resources

Based on the work of a research team, this manual offers
techniques and strategies for treating patients with Borderline Personality Disorder using Transference Focused Psychology. Provides therapists with an overall strategy for
treating BPD patients and helpful tactics for working with
individual patients on a session by session basis.

364 pages Year Founded: 1807

2821 Role of Sexual Abuse in the Etiology of
Borderline Personality Disorder
200 E Joppa Road
PO Box 436
Brooklandville, MD 21022-0436
410-825-8888
888-825-8249
Fax: 410-560-0134
E-mail: sidran@sidran.org
www.sidran.org

EstherGiller, President and Director
Sheila Sidran Giller, Secretary/Treasurer
J. G.Goellnerÿ, Director Emeritus
Tracy Howard, Book Sales/Office Manager

Presenting the latest generation of research findings about
the impact of traumatic abuse on the development of BPD.
This book focuses on the theoretical basis of BPD, including topics such as childhood factors associated with the development, the relationship of child sexual abuse to
dissociation and self mutilation, severity of childhood

abuse, borderline symptoms and family environment. Twenty six contributors cover every aspect of BPD as it relates to childhood sexual abuse. *$42.00*

345 pages Year Founded: 1986

2822 Shorter Term Treatments for Borderline Personality Disorders
NewHarbinger Publications
5674 Shattuck Avenue
Oakland, CA 94609-1662
510-652-0215
800-748-6273
Fax: 510-652-5472
E-mail: customerservice@newharbinger.com
www.newharbinger.com

Matthew McKay, Owner
Patrick Fanning, Co-Founder

This guide offers approaches designed to help clients stabilize emotions, decrease vulnerability and work toward a more adaptive day to day functioning. *$49.95*

184 pages Year Founded: 1973 ISBN 1-572240-92-X

Psychosomatic (Somatizing) Disorders

2823 Anatomy of a Psychiatric Illness: Healing the Mind and the Brain
American Psychiatric Publishing, Inc.
1000 Wilson Boulevard
Suite 1825
Arlington, VA 22209-3901
703-907-7322
800-368-5777
Fax: 703-907-1091
E-mail: appi@psych.org
www.appi.org

Robert E Hales, M.D., M.B.A., Editor-in-Chief
Ron McMillen, Chief Executive Officer
John McDuffie, Editorial Director
Rebecca D. Rinehart, Publisher

$22.95

232 pages Year Founded: 1993

2824 Concise Guide to Neuropsychiatry and Behavioral Neurology
American Psychiatric Publishing, Inc.
1000 Wilson Boulevard
Suite 1825
Arlington, VA 22209-3901
703-907-7322
800-368-5777
Fax: 703-907-1091
E-mail: appi@psych.org
www.appi.org

Robert E Hales, M.D., M.B.A., Editor-in-Chief
Ron McMillen, Chief Executive Officer
John McDuffie, Editorial Director
Rebecca D. Rinehart, Publisher

Provides brief synopsis of the major neuropsychiatric and neurobehavioral syndromes, discusses their clinical assessment, and provides guidelines for management. *$21.00*

368 pages Year Founded: 1995 ISBN 0-880483-43-1

2825 Concise Guide to Psychodynamic Psychotherapy: Principles and Techniques in the Era of Managed Care
American Psychiatric Publishing, Inc.
1000 Wilson Boulevard
Suite 1825
Arlington, VA 22209-3901
703-907-7322
800-368-5777
Fax: 703-907-1091
E-mail: appi@psych.org
www.appi.org

Robert E Hales, M.D., M.B.A., Editor-in-Chief
Ron McMillen, Chief Executive Officer
John McDuffie, Editorial Director
Rebecca D. Rinehart, Publisher

Thoroughly updated coverage of all the major principles and important issues in psychodynamic psychotherapy and issues not commonly addressed in the standard training curriculum, including the office setting, suicidal and dangerous patients, and what to do when the therapist makes an error. *$21.00*

272 pages Year Founded: 1998 ISBN 0-880483-47-4

2826 Manual of Panic: Focused Psychodynamic Psychotherapy
American Psychiatric Publishing, Inc.
1000 Wilson Boulevard
Suite 1825
Arlington, VA 22209-3901
703-907-7322
800-368-5777
Fax: 703-907-1091
E-mail: appi@psych.org
www.appi.org

Robert E Hales, M.D., M.B.A., Editor-in-Chief
Ron McMillen, Chief Executive Officer
John McDuffie, Editorial Director
Rebecca D. Rinehart, Publisher

A psychodynamic formulation applicable to many or most patients with Axis 1 panic disorders. *$28.00*

112 pages Year Founded: 1997 ISBN 0-880488-71-9

2827 Munchausen Syndrome by Proxy: Issues in Diagnosis and Treatment
Lexington Books
4501 Forbes Boulevard
Suite 200
Lanham, MD 20706-4346
301-459-3365
www.nbooks.com

AV Levin, Editor
MS Sheridan, Editor

Reference/Resource material for professionals.

Year Founded: 1995

2828 Somatization, Physical Symptoms and Psychological Illness
American Psychiatric Publishing, Inc.
1000 Wilson Boulevard
Suite 1825
Arlington, VA 22209-3901
703-907-7322
800-368-5777
Fax: 703-907-1091

E-mail: appi@psych.org
www.appi.org

Robert E Hales, M.D., M.B.A., Editor-in-Chief
Ron McMillen, Chief Executive Officer
John McDuffie, Editorial Director
Rebecca D. Rinehart, Publisher

$99.95

351 pages Year Founded: 1990 ISBN 0-632028-39-4

2829 Somatoform Dissociation: Phenomena, Measurement, and Theoretical Issues
WW Norton & Company
500 5th Avenue
New York, NY 10110-54
212-354-5500
800-233-4830
Fax: 212-869-0856
E-mail: npb@wwnorton.com
www.books.wwnorton.com

Drake McFeely, CEO

In this first North Americacn edition of his work, Nijenhuis expands upon his theory of somatoform dissociation by providing two new chapters-one on dissociation and the re-call of sexual abuse and a second on the phycometric characteristics of the Traumatic Experiences Checklist (TEC).

Year Founded: 1923 ISBN 0-393704-60-2

2830 Somatoform and Factitious Disorders
American Psychiatric Publishing, Inc.
1000 Wilson Boulevard
Suite 1825
Arlington, VA 22209-3901
703-907-7322
800-368-5777
Fax: 703-907-1091
E-mail: appi@psych.org
www.appi.org

Robert E Hales, M.D., M.B.A., Editor-in-Chief
Ron McMillen, Chief Executive Officer
John McDuffie, Editorial Director
Rebecca D. Rinehart, Publisher

Consise yet thorough, this book covers Factitious disorders, Somatization disorder, Conversion disorder, Hypochondriasis and Body dysmorphic disorder. Explores the latest on these conditions and emphasises the need for further research to improve patient treament and understanding. *$29.95*

208 pages Year Founded: 2001 ISBN 1-585620-29-7

Schizophrenia

2831 Behavioral High-Risk Paradigm in Psychopathology
Springer-Verlag New York
175 5th Avenue
New York, NY 10010-7703
212-477-8200
800-777-4643
Fax: 212-473-6272
E-mail: custserv@springer-ny.com
www.www.springer.com

Derk Haank, CEO
Martin Moss, COO
Ulrich Vest, CFO

Examines both traditional clinical research on psychopathology and psychophysiological research on psychopathology, with an emphasis on risk for schizophrenia and for mood disorders. Complementing treatments of risk for psychopathology in other sources which emphasize either genetic factors or large-scale psychosocial factors, chapters focus on research in specific areas of each disorder. Hardcover. *$98.00*

304 pages Year Founded: 1842 ISBN 0-387945-04-0

2832 Cognitive Therapy for Delusions, Voices, and Paranoia
John Wiley & Sons
111 River Street
Hoboken, NJ 07030-5774
201-748-6000
Fax: 201-748-6088
E-mail: info@wiley.com
www.www.wiley.com

Stephen M. Smith, President and Chief Executive Officer
Ellis E. Cousens, Executive Vice President
John Kritzmacher, Executive Vice President
MJ O'Leary, Senior Vice President, Human Resources

A cognitive view of delusions and voices. The practice of therapy and the problem of engagement.

364 pages Year Founded: 1807

2833 Delusional Beliefs
John Wiley & Sons
111 River Street
Hoboken, NJ 07030-5774
201-748-6000
Fax: 201-748-6088
E-mail: info@wiley.com
www.www.wiley.com

Stephen M. Smith, President and Chief Executive Officer
Ellis E. Cousens, Executive Vice President
John Kritzmacher, Executive Vice President
MJ O'Leary, Senior Vice President, Human Resources

Unique collection of ideas and empirical data provided by leading experts in a variety of disciplines. Each offers perspectives on questions such as: What criteria should be used to identify, describe and classify delusions? How can delusional individuals be identified? What distinguishes delusions from normal beliefs? *$95.00*

364 pages Year Founded: 1807 ISBN 0-471836-35-4

2834 Families Coping with Schizophrenia: Practitioner's Guide to Family Groups
John Wiley & Sons
111 River Street
Hoboken, NJ 07030-5774
201-748-6000
Fax: 201-748-6088
E-mail: info@wiley.com
www.www.wiley.com

Stephen M. Smith, President and Chief Executive Officer
Ellis E. Cousens, Executive Vice President
John Kritzmacher, Executive Vice President
MJ O'Leary, Senior Vice President, Human Resources

364 pages Year Founded: 1807

2835 Practice Guideline for the Treatment of Patients with Schizophrenia
American Psychiatric Publishing, Inc.
1000 Wilson Boulevard
Suite 1825
Arlington, VA 22209-3901
703-907-7322
800-368-5777
Fax: 703-907-1091
E-mail: appi@psych.org
www.appi.org

Robert E Hales, M.D., M.B.A., Editor-in-Chief
Ron McMillen, Chief Executive Officer
John McDuffie, Editorial Director
Rebecca D. Rinehart, Publisher

$22.00

146 pages Year Founded: 1997

2836 Schizophrenia Revealed: From Nuerons to Social Interactions
WW Norton & Company
500 5th Avenue
New York, NY 10110-54
212-354-5500
800-233-4830
Fax: 212-869-0856
E-mail: admalmud@wwnorton.com
www.books.wwnorton.com

Drake McFeely, CEO

Helps explain some of the former mysteries of Schizophrenia that are now possible to study through advances in neuroscience. *$ 10.80*

Year Founded: 1923 ISBN 0-398704-48-1

Sexual Disorders

2837 Assessing Sex Offenders: Problems and Pitfalls
Charles C Thomas Publisher Ltd.
PO Box 19265
Springfield, IL 62794-9265
217-789-8980
800-258-8980
Fax: 217-789-9130
www.ccthomas.com

Charles CThomas, Publisher

This book reviews the scientific evidence relevant to assessing the recidivism risk of sex offenders. Too often, the issues detailed in these chapters have been overlooked and/or misinterpreted. As a result, the likelihood of psychologists misusing and abusing scientific data when assessing sex offenders whould not be underestimated. The text identifies numerous instances of such misuse and abuse. Paperback is available for $41.95. *$61.95*

266 pages Year Founded: 1927 ISBN 0-398075-02-6

2838 Cognitive Therapy in Practice
WW Norton & Company
500 5th Avenue
New York, NY 10110-54
212-354-5500
800-233-4830
Fax: 212-869-0856
E-mail: npd@wwnorton.com
www.books.wwnorton.com

Drake McFeely, CEO

Basic text for graduate studies in psychotherapy, psycholgy nursing social work and counseling. *$29.00*

224 pages Year Founded: 1923 ISBN 0-393700-77-1

2839 Erectile Dysfunction: Integrating Couple Therapy, Sex Therapy and Medical Treatment
WW Norton & Company
500 5th Avenue
New York, NY 10110-54
212-354-5500
Fax: 212-869-0856
E-mail: admalmud@wwnorton.com
www.books.wwnorton.com

Drake McFeely, CEO

Helpful to marriage and couple therapists, very up to date and encompassing, with simple and professional writing. *$30.00*

208 pages Year Founded: 1923 ISSN 70330-4

2840 Hypoactive Sexual Desire: Integrating Sex and Couple Therapy
WW Norton & Company
500 5th Avenue
New York, NY 10110-54
212-354-5500
Fax: 212-869-0856
E-mail: admalmud@wwnorton.com
www.books.wwnorton.com

Drake McFeely, CEO

Discussion of treating the couple, not the individual with lack of desire, the authors include distinguishing between organic and psychogenic problems plus how to combine relational and sex therapy. Although lack of desire is one of the most common problems couples face, it is one of the most challenging to treat. *$30.00*

288 pages Year Founded: 1923 ISSN 70344-4

Pediatric & Adolescent Issues

2841 Adolescents in Psychiatric Hospitals: A Psychodynamic Approach to Evaluation and Treatment
harles C Thomas Publisher Ltd.
2600 S 1st Street
Springfield, IL 62704-4730
217-789-8980
800-258-8980
Fax: 217-789-9130
E-mail: books@ccthomas.com
www.ccthomas.com

Michael P Thomas, President
Charles CThomas, Publisher

A short history of adolescent inpatient psychiatry and its clinical methods, and a month-long, running account of the morning meetings of a typical inpatient ward. For trainees in child and adolescent psychiatry, nurses, social workers, administrators, and psychologists working in the field of adolescent inpatient psychiatry. *$32.95*

208 pages Year Founded: 1927 ISBN 0-398068-60-7

2842 Adolescents, Alcohol and Drugs: A Practical Guide for Those Who Work With Young People
Charles C Thomas Publisher Ltd.
2600 S 1st Street
Springfield, IL 62704-4730
217-789-8980
800-258-8980
Fax: 217-789-9130
E-mail: books@ccthomas.com
www.ccthomas.com

Michael P Thomas, President
Charles CThomas, Publisher

$41.95

210 pages Year Founded: 1927 ISBN 0-398053-93-6

2843 Adolescents, Alcohol and Substance Abuse: Reaching Teens through Brief Interventions
Guilford Press
72 Spring Street
New York, NY 10012-4019
212-431-9800
800-365-7006
Fax: 212-966-6708
E-mail: info@guilford.com
www.www.guilford.com

Bob Matloff, President
Seymour Weingarten, Editor-in-Chief

Reviews a range of empirically supported approachs to dealing with the growing problems of substance use and abuse among young people. While admission to specialized treatment programs is relatively rare in today's health care climate, there are many opportunities for brief interventions. Brief interventions also allow the clinician to work with the teen on his or her home turf, emphasize autonomy and personal responsibility, and can be used across the full range of teens who are engangAing in health risk-behavior.

350 pages Year Founded: 1973 ISBN 1-572306-58-0

2844 Adolesent in Family Therapy: Breaking the Cycle of Conflict and Control
Guilford Press
72 Spring Street
New York, NY 10012-4068
212-431-9800
800-365-7006
Fax: 212-966-6708
E-mail: info@guilford.com
www.www.guilford.com

Bob Matloff, President
Seymour Weingarten, Editor-in-Chief

Family relationships that are troubled can be catalysts for change. A guide to treating a wide range of parent/adolesent problems with straightforward advice.
$19.95

336 pages Year Founded: 1973 ISBN 1-572305-88-6

2845 At-Risk Youth in Crises
Pro-Ed Publications
8700 Shoal Creek Boulevard
Austin, TX 78757-6897
512-451-3246
800-897-3202
Fax: 512-451-8542

E-mail: info@proedinc.com
www.www.proedinc.com

Donald D Hammill, Owner

This edition has updated material in the chapters covering divorce, loss, abuse, severe depression and suicide. *$31.00*

268 pages Year Founded: 1994 ISBN 0-890795-74-6

2846 Attachment, Trauma and Healing: Understanding and Treating Attachment Disorder in Children and Families
200 E Joppa Road
PO Box 436
Brooklandville, MD 21022-0436
410-825-8888
888-825-8249
Fax: 410-560-0134
E-mail: sidran@sidran.org
www.sidran.org

Esther Giller, President and Director
Sheila Sidran Giller, Secretary/Treasurer
J. G. Goellner, Director Emeritus
Tracy Howard, Book Sales/Office Manager

An in depth look at the causes of attachment disorder, explains the normal development of attachment, examines the research in this area and present treatment plans. Numerous appendices include a sample intake packet, two brief day in the life accounts of children with attachment disorder, assessment guides, treatment plans and references. *$34.95*

345 pages Year Founded: 1986

2847 Basic Child Psychiatry
American Psychiatric Publishing, Inc.
1000 Wilson Boulevard
Suite 1825
Arlington, VA 22209-3901
703-907-7322
800-368-5777
Fax: 703-907-1091
E-mail: appi@psych.org
www.appi.org

Robert E Hales, M.D., M.B.A., Editor-in-Chief
Ron McMillen, Chief Executive Officer
John McDuffie, Editorial Director
Rebecca D. Rinehart, Publisher

$46.95

416 pages Year Founded: 1995 ISBN 0-632037-72-5

2848 Behavior Modification for Exceptional Children and Youth
Pro-Ed Publications
8700 Shoal Creek Boulevard
Austin, TX 78757-6897
512-451-3246
800-897-3202
Fax: 512-451-8542
E-mail: info@proedinc.com
www.www.proedinc.com

Donald D Hammill, Owner

An authoritative textbook for courses in behavior modification. Serves as a practical, comprehensive reference work for clinicians working with people with disabilities and behavior problems. *$37.00*

296 pages Year Founded: 1993 ISBN 1-563720-42-6

2849 Behavior Rating Profile
Pro-Ed Publications
8700 Shoal Creek Boulevard
Austin, TX 78757-6897
512-451-3246
800-897-3202
Fax: 512-451-8542
E-mail: info@proedinc.com
www.www.proedinc.com

Donald D Hammill, Owner

Provides different evaluations of a student's behavior at home, at school, and in interpersonal relationships from the varied perpsectives of parents, teachers, peers, and the target students themselves. Identifies students whose behavior is perceived to be deviant, the settings in which behavior problems are prominent, and the persons whose perceptions of student's behavior are different from those of other respondents. *$194.00*

Year Founded: 1990

2850 Behavioral Approach to Assessment of Youth with Emotional/Behavioral Disorders
Pro-Ed Publications
8700 Shoal Creek Boulevard
Austin, TX 78757-6897
512-451-3246
800-897-3202
Fax: 512-451-8542
E-mail: info@proedinc.com
www.www.proedinc.com

Donald D Hammill, Owner

This new book addresses one of the most challenging aspects of special education: evaluating students referred for suspected emotional/behavioral disorders. Geared to the practical needs and concerns of school-based practitioners, including special education teachers, school psychologists and social workers. *$44.00*

729 pages Year Founded: 1996 ISBN 0-890796-25-4

2851 Brief Therapy for Adolescent Depression
Professional Resource Press
PO Box 3197
Sarasota, FL 34230-3197
941-343-9601
800-443-3364
Fax: 941-343-9201
E-mail: cs.prpress@gmail.com
www.prpress.com

Laurie Girsch, Managing Editor

Useful book for practicing clinicians and advanced students interested in building new skills for working with depressed young people. Written from the perspective that adaptations of cognitive therapy are necessary when working with adolescents both because of the difference in thinking (relative verses absolute) between adults and adolescents, and because adolescents are deeply embedded in their families of origin and effective treatment rarely can be conducted without intervening with the family. Includes detailed clinical vignettes to illustrate key principles and techniques of this treatment model. *$13.95*

112 pages Year Founded: 1980 ISBN 1-568870-28-0

2852 Candor, Connection and Enterprise in Adolesent Therapy
WW Norton & Company
500 5th Avenue
New York, NY 10110-54
212-354-5500
Fax: 212-869-0856
E-mail: admalmud@wwnorton.com
www.books.wwnorton.com

Drake McFeely, CEO

Suggestions and troubleshooting for therapists dealing with uncooperative adolesent patients. Avoiding the appearence of trying too hard, dialouges that seem to go nowhere, and gaining the faith of a child who may not appreciate efforts on their behalf. *$35.00*

208 pages Year Founded: 1923 ISSN 70356-8

2853 Child Friendly Therapy: Biophysical Innovations for Children and Families
WW Norton & Company
500 5th Avenue
New York, NY 10110-54
212-354-5500
Fax: 212-869-0856
E-mail: admalmud@wwnorton.com
www.books.wwnorton.com

Drake McFeely, CEO

Family centered treatment for children. Suggestions and case studies, therapy room set up and session structure, multi sensory skill building leading to a fresh understanding of often misunderstood children. Family members can be incorporated to work as a team to help with therapy. *$32.00*

256 pages Year Founded: 1923 ISSN 70355-X

2854 Child Psychiatry
American Psychiatric Publishing, Inc.
1000 Wilson Boulevard
Suite 1825
Arlington, VA 22209-3901
703-907-7322
800-368-5777
Fax: 703-907-1091
E-mail: appi@psych.org
www.appi.org

Robert E Hales, M.D., M.B.A., Editor-in-Chief
Ron McMillen, Chief Executive Officer
John McDuffie, Editorial Director
Rebecca D. Rinehart, Publisher

Provides the essential facts and concepts for everyone involved in child psychiatry, the book includes 200 questions and answers for trainees approaching professional examinations. *$46.95*

336 pages Year Founded: 1987 ISBN 0-632038-85-3

2855 Child Psychopharmacology
American Psychiatric Publishing, Inc.
1000 Wilson Boulevard
Suite 1825
Arlington, VA 22209-3901
703-907-7322
800-368-5777
Fax: 703-907-1091
E-mail: appi@psych.org
www.appi.org

Robert E Hales, M.D., M.B.A., Editor-in-Chief
Ron McMillen, Chief Executive Officer
John McDuffie, Editorial Director
Rebecca D. Rinehart, Publisher

Includes: Tic disorders and obsessive-compulsive disorder; Attention-deficit/hyperactivity disorder; Children and adolescents with psychotic disorders; Affective disorders in children and adolescents; Anxiety disorders; Eating disorders. *$26.00*

200 pages ISBN 0-880488-33-6

2856 Child and Adolescent Mental Health Consultation in Hospitals, Schools and Courts
American Psychiatric Publishing, Inc.
1000 Wilson Boulevard
Suite 1825
Arlington, VA 22209-3901
703-907-7322
800-368-5777
Fax: 703-907-1091
E-mail: appi@psych.org
www.appi.org

Robert E Hales, M.D., M.B.A., Editor-in-Chief
Ron McMillen, Chief Executive Officer
John McDuffie, Editorial Director
Rebecca D. Rinehart, Publisher

Leading experts present a practical guide for mental health professionals. *$38.50*

316 pages Year Founded: 1993 ISBN 0-880484-18-7

2857 Child and Adolescent Psychiatry: Modern Approaches
American Psychiatric Publishing, Inc.
1000 Wilson Boulevard
Suite 1825
Arlington, VA 22209-3901
703-907-7322
800-368-5777
Fax: 703-907-1091
E-mail: appi@psych.org
www.appi.org

Robert E Hales, M.D., M.B.A., Editor-in-Chief
Ron McMillen, Chief Executive Officer
John McDuffie, Editorial Director
Rebecca D. Rinehart, Publisher

ISBN 0-632028-21-1

2858 Child-Centered Counseling and Psychotherapy
Charles C Thomas Publisher Ltd.
2600 S 1st Street
Springfield, IL 62704-4730
217-789-8980
800-258-8980
Fax: 217-789-9130
E-mail: books@ccthomas.com
www.ccthomas.com

Michael P Thomas, President
Charles C Thomas, Publisher

Topics include an introduction to child-centered counseling, counseling as a three-phase process, applying the reflective process, phase three alternatives, counseling through play, consultation, and professional issues. It represents the status of child-centered counseling which also indentifies ideas which can influence its future. *$62.95*

262 pages Year Founded: 1927 ISSN 0-398-06522-5
ISBN 0-398065-21-7

2859 Childhood Behavior Disorders: Applied Research and Educational Practice
Pro-Ed Publications
8700 Shoal Creek Boulevard
Austin, TX 78757-6897
512-451-3246
800-897-3202
Fax: 512-451-8542
E-mail: info@proedinc.com
www.www.proedinc.com

Donald D Hammill, Owner

Provides the balance of theory, research and practical relevance needed by students in graduate and undergraduate introductory courses, as well as practicing teachers and other professionals. *$ 39.00*

550 pages Year Founded: 1998 ISBN 0-890797-19-6

2860 Childhood Disorders
Brunner/Routledge
7625 Empire Drive
Florence, KY 41042-2919
800-634-7064
Fax: 215-269-0363
E-mail: orders@taylorandfrancis.com
www.www.routledgementalhealth.com

Provides an up-to-date summary of the current information about the psychological disorders of childhood as well as their causes, nature and course. Together with discussion and evaluation of the major models that guide psychological thinking about the disorders. Gives detailed consideration of the criteria used to make the diagnoses, a presentation of the latest research findings on the nature of the disorder and an overview of the methods used and evaluations conducted for the treatment of the disorders. *$26.95*

240 pages ISBN 0-863776-09-4

2861 Children in Therapy: Using the Family as a Resource
WW Norton & Company
500 5th Avenue
New York, NY 10110-54
212-354-5500
800-233-4830
Fax: 212-869-0856
E-mail: npb@wwnorton.com
www.books.wwnorton.com

Drake McFeely, CEO

This anthology presents theoretical perspectives of five different competency-based approaches: solution-oriented brief therapy, narrative therapy, collaborative language systems therapy, internal family systems therapy, and emotionally focused family therapy.

Year Founded: 1923 ISBN 0-393704-85-8

2862 Childs Work/Childs Play
303 Crossways Park Dr
Woodbury, NY 11797-2099
800-962-1141
Fax: 800-262-1886
E-mail: info@childswork.com
www.childswork.com

Catalog of books, games, toys and workbooks relating to child development issues such as recognizing emotions, handling uncertainty, bullies, ADD, shyness, conflicts and other things that children may need some help navigating.

2863 Clinical & Forensic Interviewing of Children & Families
Jerome M Sattler
PO Box 3557
La Mesa, CA 91944-1060
619-460-3667
Fax: 619-460-2489
www.sattlerpublisher.com

2864 Clinical Application of Projective Drawings
Charles C Thomas Publisher Ltd.
2600 S 1st Street
Springfield, IL 62704-4730
217-789-8980
800-258-8980
Fax: 217-789-9130
E-mail: books@ccthomas.com
www.ccthomas.com

Michael P Thomas, President
Charles C Thomas, Publisher

On its way to becoming the classic in the field of projective drawings, this book provides a grounding in fundamentals and goes on to consider differential diagnosis, appraisal of psychological resources as treatment potentials and projective drawing usage in therapy. *$65.95*

688 pages Year Founded: 1927 ISBN 0-398007-68-3

2865 Clinical Child Documentation Sourcebook
John Wiley & Sons
111 River Street
Hoboken, NJ 07030-5774
201-748-6000
Fax: 201-748-6088
E-mail: info@wiley.com
www.www.wiley.com

Stephen M. Smith, President and Chief Executive Officer
Ellis E. Cousens, Executive Vice President
John Kritzmacher, Executive Vice President
MJ O'Leary, Senior Vice President, Human Resources

This easy to use resource offers child psychologists and therapists a full array of forms, inventories, checklists, client handouts, and clinical records essential to a successful practice in either and organizational or clinical setting. *$49.95*

364 pages Year Founded: 1807 ISBN 0-471291-11-0

2866 Concise Guide to Child and Adolescent Psychiatry
American Psychiatric Publishing, Inc.
1000 Wilson Boulevard
Suite 1825
Arlington, VA 22209-3901
703-907-7322
800-368-5777
Fax: 703-907-1091
E-mail: appi@psych.org
www.appi.org

Robert E Hales, M.D., M.B.A., Editor-in-Chief
Ron McMillen, Chief Executive Officer

John McDuffie, Editorial Director
Rebecca D. Rinehart, Publisher

Topics include evaluation and treatment planning, axis I disorders usually first diagnosed in infancy, childhood or adolescence, attention deficit and disruptive behavior disorders, developmental disorders, special clinical circumstances, psychopharmacology, and psychosocial treatments. *$21.95*

400 pages Year Founded: 1998 ISBN 0-880489-05-7

2867 Counseling Children with Special Needs
American Psychiatric Publishing, Inc.
1000 Wilson Boulevard
Suite 1825
Arlington, VA 22209-3901
703-907-7322
800-368-5777
Fax: 703-907-1091
E-mail: appi@psych.org
www.appi.org

Robert E Hales, M.D., M.B.A., Editor-in-Chief
Ron McMillen, Chief Executive Officer
John McDuffie, Editorial Director
Rebecca D. Rinehart, Publisher
$29.95

224 pages Year Founded: 1997 ISBN 0-632041-51-

2868 Creative Therapy with Children and Adolescents
Impact Publishers
PO Box 6016
Atascadero, CA 93423-6016
805-466-5917
800-246-7228
Fax: 805-466-5919
E-mail: info@impactpublishers.com
www.impactpublishers.com

Encourages creativity in therapy, assists therapists in talking with children to facilitate change. From simple ideas to fresh innovations, the activities are to be used as tools to supplement a variety of therapeutic approaches, and can be tailored to each child's needs. *$21.95*

192 pages Year Founded: 1999 ISBN 1-886230-19-6

2869 Defiant Teens
Guilford Press
72 Spring Street
New York, NY 10012-4068
212-431-9800
800-365-7006
Fax: 212-966-6708
E-mail: info@guilford.com
www.www.guilford.com

Bob Matloff, President
Seymour Weingarten, Editor-in-Chief

Guidelines for best practices in working with families and their teenaged children.

250 pages Year Founded: 1973 ISBN 1-572304-40-5

2870 Developmental Therapy/Developmental Teaching
Pro-Ed Publications
8700 Shoal Creek Boulevard
Austin, TX 78757-6897

512-451-3246
800-897-3202
Fax: 512-451-8542
E-mail: info@proedinc.com
www.www.proedinc.com

Donald D Hammill, Owner

Provides extensive applications for teachers, counselors, parents and other adults concerned about the behavior and emotional stability of children and teens. The focus is on helping children and youth to cope effectively with the stresses of comtemporary life, with an emphasis on the positive effects adults can have on students when they adjust strategies to the social emotional needs of children. *$41.00*

398 pages Year Founded: 1996 ISBN 0-890796-64-5

2871 Drug Information for Teens: Health Tips About the Physical and Mental Effects of Substance Abuse
Omnigraphics
615 Giswold
Detroit, MI 48226-3900
313-961-1340
Fax: 313-961-1383
E-mail: info@omnigraphics.com
www.omnigraphics.com

Provides students with facts about drug use, abuse, and addiction. It describes the physical and mental effects of alcohol, tobacco, marijuana, ecstasy, inhalants and many other drugs and chemicals that are often abused. It includes information about the process that leads from casual use to addiction and offers suggestions for resisting peer pressure and helping friends stay drug free.

452 pages ISBN 0-780804-44-9

2872 Effective Discipline
Pro-Ed Publications
8700 Shoal Creek Boulevard
Austin, TX 78757-6897
512-451-3246
800-897-3202
Fax: 512-451-8542
E-mail: info@proedinc.com
www.www.proedinc.com

Donald D Hammill, Owner

Designed to provide principals, counselors, teachers, and college students preparing to become educators with information about research-based techniques that reduce or eliminate school behavior problems. Provides the knowledge to prevent discipline problems, identify specific behaviors that disrupt the environment, match interventions with behavioral infractions, implement a variety of intervention tactics, and evaluate the effectiveness of the intervention program. *$28.00*

220 pages Year Founded: 1993 ISBN 0-890795-79-7

2873 Empowering Adolescent Girls
WW Norton & Company
500 5th Avenue
New York, NY 10110-54
212-354-5500
Fax: 212-869-0856
E-mail: admalmud@wwnorton.com
www.books.wwnorton.com

Drake McFeely, CEO

Strategies and activities for professionals who work with adolesent girls (teachers, counselors, therapists) to offer support and encouagement through the Go Girls program. *$32.00*

256 pages Year Founded: 1923 ISSN 70347-9

2874 Enhancing Social Competence in Young Students
Pro-Ed Publications
8700 Shoal Creek Boulevard
Austin, TX 78757-6897
512-451-3246
800-897-3202
Fax: 512-451-8542
E-mail: info@proedinc.com
www.www.proedinc.com

Donald D Hammill, Owner

Addresses conceptual and practical issues of providing social competence-enhancing interventions for young students in schools, based on research findings. Summarizes recent advances in social skills programming for at-risk students and prevention interventions for all students. Discussions of developmental issues of childhood maladjustment, intervention strategies, implementation issues and assessment/evaluation issues are provided. *$28.00*

281 pages Year Founded: 1995 ISBN 0-890796-20-3

2875 Group Therapy With Children and Adolescents
American Psychiatric Publishing, Inc.
1000 Wilson Boulevard
Suite 1825
Arlington, VA 22209-3901
703-907-7322
800-368-5777
Fax: 703-907-1091
E-mail: appi@psych.org
www.appi.org

Robert E Hales, M.D., M.B.A., Editor-in-Chief
Ron McMillen, Chief Executive Officer
John McDuffie, Editorial Director
Rebecca D. Rinehart, Publisher

Explores a major treatment modality often used with adult populations and rarely considered for child and adolescent treatments. With contributions from international experts, this book looks at the effectiveness of treatment and cost of group therapy as it applies to this particular age group. *$52.00*

400 pages ISBN 0-880484-06-3

2876 Handbook of Child Behavior in Therapy and in the Psychiatric Setting
John Wiley & Sons
111 River Street
Hoboken, NJ 07030-5774
201-748-6000
Fax: 201-748-6088
E-mail: info@wiley.com
www.www.wiley.com

Stephen M. Smith, President and Chief Executive Officer
Ellis E. Cousens, Executive Vice President
John Kritzmacher, Executive Vice President
MJ O'Leary, Senior Vice President, Human Resources

364 pages Year Founded: 1807

2877 Handbook of Infant Mental Health
Guilford Press
72 Spring Street
New York, NY 10012-4068
212-431-9800
800-365-7006
Fax: 212-966-6708
E-mail: info@guilford.com
www.www.guilford.com

Bob Matloff, President
Seymour Weingarten, Editor-in-Chief

Included are chapters on neurobiology, diagnostic issues, parental mental health issues and family dynamics. *$60.00*

588 pages Year Founded: 1973 ISBN 1-572305-15-0

2878 Handbook of Parent Training: Parents as Co-Therapists for Children's Behavior Problems
John Wiley & Sons
111 River Street
Hoboken, NJ 07030-5774
201-748-6000
Fax: 201-748-6088
E-mail: info@wiley.com
www.www.wiley.com

Stephen M. Smith, President and Chief Executive Officer
Ellis E. Cousens, Executive Vice President
John Kritzmacher, Executive Vice President
MJ O'Leary, Senior Vice President, Human Resources

This completely revised handbook shows professionals who work with troubled children how to teach parents to become co-therapists. It presents various techniques and behavior modification skills that will help parents to better relate, communicate, and respond to their child. Updates are provided on such problems as noncompliance, ADHD, and conduct disorder, and a new section on special needs parents which includes adolescent mothers, aggressive parents, substance abusing parents, and more.

364 pages Year Founded: 1807

2879 Handbook of Psychiatric Practice in the Juvenile Court
American Psychiatric Publishing, Inc.
1000 Wilson Boulevard
Suite 1825
Arlington, VA 22209-3901
703-907-7322
800-368-5777
Fax: 703-907-1091
E-mail: appi@psych.org
www.appi.org

Robert E Hales, M.D., M.B.A., Editor-in-Chief
Ron McMillen, Chief Executive Officer
John McDuffie, Editorial Director
Rebecca D. Rinehart, Publisher

Examines the role that psychiatrists and other mental health professionals are asked to play when children, adolescents, and their families end up in court. *$12.95*

198 pages ISBN 0-890422-33-8

2880 Helping Parents, Youth, and Teachers Understand Medications for Behavioral and Emotional Problems
American Psychiatric Publishing, Inc.
1000 Wilson Boulevard
Suite 1825
Arlington, VA 22209-3901
703-907-7322
800-368-5777
Fax: 703-907-1091
E-mail: appi@psych.org
www.appi.org

Robert E Hales, M.D., M.B.A., Editor-in-Chief
Ron McMillen, Chief Executive Officer
John McDuffie, Editorial Director
Rebecca D. Rinehart, Publisher

Valuable resource for anyone involved in evaluating psychiatric disturbances in children and adolescents. Provides a compilation of information sheets to help promote the dialogue between the patient's family, caregivers, and the treating physician. *$39.95*

196 pages Year Founded: 1999 ISBN 0-880487-94-1

2881 How to Teach Social Skills
Pro-Ed Publications
8700 Shoal Creek Boulevard
Austin, TX 78757-6897
512-451-3246
800-897-3202
Fax: 512-451-8542
E-mail: info@proedinc.com
www.www.proedinc.com

Donald D Hammill, Owner

$8.00

ISBN 0-890797-61-7

2882 In the Long Run... Longitudinal Studies of Psychopathology in Children
American Psychiatric Publishing, Inc.
1000 Wilson Boulevard
Suite 1825
Arlington, VA 22209-3901
703-907-7322
800-368-5777
Fax: 703-907-1091
E-mail: appi@psych.org
www.appi.org

Robert E Hales, M.D., M.B.A., Editor-in-Chief
Ron McMillen, Chief Executive Officer
John McDuffie, Editorial Director
Rebecca D. Rinehart, Publisher

$29.95

224 pages Year Founded: 1999 ISBN 0-873182-11-1

2883 Infants, Toddlers and Families: Framework for Support and Intervention
Guilford Press
72 Spring Street
Department 4E
New York, NY 10012-4019
212-431-9800
Fax: 212-966-6708
E-mail: exam@guilford.com
www.www.guilford.com

Bob Matloff, President
Seymour Weingarten, Editor-in-Chief

Examines the complex development in a child's first 3 years of life. Instead of preaching or judging, this book acknowledges the challenges facing all families, especially vulnerable ones, and offers straightforward advice. *$28.95*

204 pages Year Founded: 1973 ISBN 1-572304-87-1

2884 Interventions for Students with Emotional Disorders
Pro-Ed Publications
8700 Shoal Creek Boulevard
Austin, TX 78757-6897
512-451-3246
800-897-3202
Fax: 512-451-8542
E-mail: info@proedinc.com
www.www.proedinc.com

Donald D Hammill, Owner

This graduate textbook for special education students advocates an eclectic approach toward teaching children with social adjustment problems. Provides how-to information for implementing various techniques to successfully enhance positive sociobehavioral development in children with emotional disorders. *$36.00*

212 pages Year Founded: 1991 ISBN 0-890792-96-8

2885 Interviewing Children and Adolesents: Skills and Strategies for Effective DSM-IV Diagnosis
Guilford Press
72 Spring Street
New York, NY 10012-4068
212-431-9800
800-365-7006
Fax: 212-966-6708
E-mail: info@guilford.com
www.www.guilford.com

Bob Matloff, President
Seymour Weingarten, Editor-in-Chief

Guide to developmentally appropriate interviewing. *$45.00*

482 pages Year Founded: 1973 ISBN 1-572305-01-0

2886 Interviewing the Sexually Abused Child
American Psychiatric Publishing, Inc.
1000 Wilson Boulevard
Suite 1825
Arlington, VA 22209-3901
703-907-7322
800-368-5777
Fax: 703-907-1091
E-mail: appi@psych.org
www.appi.org

Robert E Hales, M.D., M.B.A., Editor-in-Chief
Ron McMillen, Chief Executive Officer
John McDuffie, Editorial Director
Rebecca D. Rinehart, Publisher

A guide for mental health professionals who need to know if a child has been sexually abused. Presents guidelines on the structure of the interview and covers the use of free play, toys, and play materials by focusing on the investigate interview of the suspected victim. *$15.00*

80 pages Year Founded: 1993 ISBN 0-880486-12-0

2887 Learning Disorders and Disorders of the Self in Children and Adolesents
WW Norton & Company
500 5th Avenue
New York, NY 10110-54
212-354-5500
Fax: 212-869-0856
E-mail: admalmud@wwnorton.com
www.books.wwnorton.com

Drake McFeely, CEO

Clinicians who work with learning disabled children need to understand the complex, integrated framework of learning and self image problems. Specific problems and treatments are discussed. *$32.00*

332 pages Year Founded: 1923 ISSN 70377-0

2888 Living on the Razor's Edge: Solution-Oriented Brief Family Therapy with Self-Harming Adolesents
WW Norton & Company
500 5th Avenue
New York, NY 10110-54
212-354-5500
Fax: 212-869-0856
E-mail: admalmud@wwnorton.com
www.books.wwnorton.com

Drake McFeely, CEO

Research supported stategies and a therapy model for self harming adolesents and their families to devlop a closer and more meaningful relationships. *$25.60*

320 pages Year Founded: 1923 ISSN 70335-5

2889 Making the Grade: Guide to School Drug Prevention Programs
Drug Strategies
1616 P Street NW
Washington, DC 20036-1434
202-289-9070
Fax: 202-414-6199
E-mail: dspoilcy@aol.com

Mathea Falco, President

Updated and expanded from the 1996 original, this guide to drug prevention programs in America helps parents and educators make informed decisions with often limited budgets. *$14.95*

2890 Manual of Clinical Child and Adolescent Psychiatry
American Psychiatric Publishing, Inc.
1000 Wilson Boulevard
Suite 1825
Arlington, VA 22209-3901
703-907-7322
800-368-5777
Fax: 703-907-1091
E-mail: appi@psych.org
www.appi.org

Robert E Hales, M.D., M.B.A., Editor-in-Chief
Ron McMillen, Chief Executive Officer
John McDuffie, Editorial Director
Rebecca D. Rinehart, Publisher

Addresses current issues such as cost containment, insurance complications, and legal and ethical issues, as well as neuropsychology, alcohol, and substance abuse, and mental retardation and genetics. *$42.50*

528 pages ISBN 0-880485-28-0

2891 Myth of Maturity: What Teenagers Need from Parents to Become Adults
WW Norton & Company
500 5th Avenue
New York, NY 10110-54
212-354-5500
Fax: 212-869-0856
E-mail: admalmud@wwnorton.com
www.books.wwnorton.com

Drake McFeely, CEO

Debunking outdated and misguided ideas about maturity, the author discusses the amount of support teens need from their parents, what is too much for independence, or not enough. *$24.95*

256 pages Year Founded: 1923 ISBN 0-393049-42-6

2892 Narrative Therapies with Children and Adolescents
Guilford Press
72 Spring Street
New York, NY 10012-4068
212-431-9800
800-365-7006
Fax: 212-966-6708
E-mail: info@guilford.com
www.www.guilford.com

Bob Matloff, President
Seymour Weingarten, Editor-in-Chief

Many renowned, creative contributors collaborate to bring this professional resource to the shelf. Transcripts of case examples, using many different methods and mediums are shown to engage children of different perspectives and ages. This book can serve as a text for child/adolescent psychotherapy, or is a useful guide for mental health professionals. *$39.95*

469 pages Year Founded: 1973 ISBN 1-572302-53-4

2893 National Survey of American Attitudes on Substance Abuse VI: Teens
Center on Addiction at Columbia University
633 3rd Avenue
19th Floor
New York, NY 10017-6706
212-841-5200
800-662-4357
Fax: 212-956-8020
www.casacolumbia.org

Jeffrey B. Lane, Chairman
Joseph A. Califano, Jr., Founder and Chairman Emeritus
Samuel A. Ball, Ph.D., President and Chief Executive Of
Susan P. Brown, Vice President and Director of F

Results of the sixth annual CASA National Survey of teens 12 - 17 years old reveals that parents that are more involved with their children's activities and have house rules and expectations can greatly influence teen behavior choices. Other statistics about availability of illegal substances and who may use them. *$22.00*

Year Founded: 1992

2894 No-Talk Therapy for Children and Adolescents
WW Norton & Company
500 5th Avenue
New York, NY 10110-54
212-354-5500
Fax: 212-869-0856
E-mail: admalmud@wwnorton.com
www.books.wwnorton.com

Drake McFeely, CEO

Creative approach to treatment of young people who cannot respond to conversation based therapy. Seemingly sullen patients can be helped to find a voice of their own. *$27.00*

288 pages Year Founded: 1923 ISSN 70286-3

2895 Ordinary Families, Special Children: Systems Approach to Childhood Disability
Guilford Press
72 Spring Street
New York, NY 10012-4068
212-431-9800
800-365-7006
Fax: 212-966-6708
E-mail: info@guilford.com
www.www.guilford.com

Bob Matloff, President
Seymour Weingarten, Editor-in-Chief

Families, including siblings and grandparents are impacted by the special needs of a child's disability. The authors explore personal accounts that shape a family's response to childhood disability and how they come to adapt these unique needs to a satisfactory lifestyle. Available in hardcover and paperback. *$35.00*

324 pages Year Founded: 1973 ISBN 1-572301-55-4

2896 Outcomes for Children and Youth with Emotional and Behavioral Disorders and their Families
Pro-Ed Publications
8700 Shoal Creek Boulevard
Austin, TX 78757-6897
512-451-3246
800-897-3202
Fax: 512-451-8542
E-mail: info@proedinc.com
www.www.proedinc.com

Donald D Hammill, Owner

This new book addresses one of the most challenging aspects of serving children and youth with emotional and behavioral disorders-evaluating the outcomes of the services you've provided. Also includes information on such topics as: child and family outcomes, system level anaylsis, case study analysis, cost analysis, cultural diversity, managed care, and consumer satisfaction. *$44.00*

730 pages Year Founded: 1998 ISBN 0-890797-50-1

2897 PTSD in Children and Adolesents
American Psychiatric Publishing, Inc.
1000 Wilson Boulevard
Suite 1825
Arlington, VA 22209-3901
703-907-7322
800-368-5777
Fax: 703-907-1091

E-mail: appi@psych.org
www.appi.org

Robert E Hales, M.D., M.B.A., Editor-in-Chief
Ron McMillen, Chief Executive Officer
John McDuffie, Editorial Director
Rebecca D. Rinehart, Publisher

Mental health and other professionals who work with Post Traumatic Stress Disorder and the young people who suffer from it will find discussions of evaluation, biological treatment strategies, the need for an integrated approach to juvenile offenders who suffer from PTSD and more. *$29.95*

208 pages Year Founded: 2001

2898 Pediatric Psychopharmacology: Fast Facts
WW Norton & Company
500 5th Avenue
New York, NY 10110-54
212-354-2907
800-233-4830
Fax: 212-869-0856
E-mail: npb@wwnorton.com
www.books.wwnorton.com

Drake McFeely, CEO

This new title in the Fast Facts series, full of up-to-date and authoritative infomration, is a critical resource for all health care professionals, including psychiatrists, prescribing psychologists, psychotherapists, pediatricians, family practice physicians, pediatric neurologists, nurse practitioners, and allied mental health professionals. Clear explanations of clinical directions for the prescriber and nonprescriber alike.

Year Founded: 1923 ISBN 0-393704-61-0

2899 Play Therapy with Children in Crisis: Individual, Group and Family Treatment
Guilford Press
72 Spring Street
New York, NY 10012-4068
212-431-9800
800-365-7006
Fax: 212-966-6708
E-mail: info@guilford.com
www.www.guilford.com

Bob Matloff, President
Seymour Weingarten, Editor-in-Chief

$45.00

506 pages Year Founded: 1973 ISBN 1-572304-85-5

2900 Post Traumatic Stress Disorders in Children and Adolescents Handbook
WW Norton & Company
500 5th Avenue
New York, NY 10110-54
212-354-2907
800-233-4830
Fax: 212-869-0856
E-mail: npb@wwnorton.com
www.books.wwnorton.com

Drake McFeely, CEO

The 15 chapters gathered here address different aspects of childhood and adolescent trauma-some consider a distinct therapeutic situation (abuse and neglect), others pertain to standard clinical procedure (assessment), and still others

focus on complex research issues (neurobiology and genetics of PSTD).

Year Founded: 1923 ISBN 0-393704-12-2

2901 Power and Compassion: Working with Difficult Adolesents and Abused Parents
Guilford Press
72 Spring Street
New York, NY 10012-4068
212-431-9800
800-365-7006
Fax: 212-966-6708
E-mail: info@guilford.com
www.www.guilford.com

Bob Matloff, President
Seymour Weingarten, Editor-in-Chief

Useful as a supplemental text, or for mental health professionals dealing with aggressive teenagers and their parents. Pragmatic guide to help demoralized parents be more understanding, but more decisive. *$16.95*

196 pages Year Founded: 1973 ISBN 1-572304-70-7

2902 Practical Charts for Managing Behavior
Pro-Ed Publications
8700 Shoal Creek Boulevard
Austin, TX 78757-6897
512-451-3246
800-897-3202
Fax: 512-451-8542
E-mail: info@proedinc.com
www.www.proedinc.com

Donald D Hammill, Owner

$29.00

160 pages Year Founded: 1998 ISBN 0-890797-36-6

2903 Proven Youth Development Model that Prevents Substance Abuse and Builds Communities
Center on Addiction at Columbia University
633 3rd Avenue
19th Floor
New York, NY 10017-6706
212-841-5200
800-662-4357
Fax: 212-956-8020
www.casacolumbia.org

Jeffrey B. Lane, Chairman
Joseph A. Califano, Jr., Founder and Chairman Emeritus
Samuel A. Ball, Ph.D., President and Chief Executive Of
Susan P. Brown, Vice President and Director of F

How-to manual developed with nine years of research. The program is a collaboration of local school, law enforcement, social service and health teams to help high risk youth between the ages of 8 - 13 years old and their families prevent substance abuse and violent behavior. Used in 23 urban and rural communities in 11 states and the District of Columbia. *$50.00*

79 pages Year Founded: 1992

2904 Psychological Examination of the Child
John Wiley & Sons
111 River Street
Hoboken, NJ 07030-5774

201-748-6000
Fax: 201-748-6088
E-mail: info@wiley.com
www.www.wiley.com

279 pages Year Founded: 1991

2905 Psychotherapies with Children and Adolescents
American Psychiatric Publishing, Inc.
1000 Wilson Boulevard
Suite 1825
Arlington, VA 22209-3901
703-907-7322
800-368-5777
Fax: 703-907-1091
E-mail: appi@psych.org
www.appi.org

Robert E Hales, M.D., M.B.A., Editor-in-Chief
Ron McMillen, Chief Executive Officer
John McDuffie, Editorial Director
Rebecca D. Rinehart, Publisher

Illustrated with case histories and demonstrates how psychoanalytic techniques can be modified to meet the therapeutic needs of children and adolescents in specific clinical situations. *$47.50*

346 pages ISBN 0-880484-06-3

2906 Safe Schools/Safe Students: Guide to Violence Prevention Stategies
Drug Strategies
770 Broadway
New York, NY 10003
212-206-4400
Fax: 202-414-6199
E-mail: dspoilcy@aol.com
www.www.aol.com

Tim Armstrong, Chairman and Chief Executive Off
Curtis Brown, Executive Vice President and Chi
Karen Dykstra, Executive Vice President and Chi

Practical assistance in rating over 84 violence prevention programs for classroom use, helps examine school policies and possible changes for student protection. *$14.95*

Year Founded: 1985

2907 Severe Stress and Mental Disturbance in Children
American Psychiatric Publishing, Inc.
1000 Wilson Boulevard
Suite 1825
Arlington, VA 22209-3901
703-907-7322
800-368-5777
Fax: 703-907-1091
E-mail: appi@psych.org
www.appi.org

Robert E Hales, M.D., M.B.A., Editor-in-Chief
Ron McMillen, Chief Executive Officer
John McDuffie, Editorial Director
Rebecca D. Rinehart, Publisher

Uniquely blends current research and clinical data on the effects of severe stress on children. Each chapter is written by international experts in their field. *$69.95*

708 pages ISBN 0-880486-57-0

2908 Structured Adolescent Pscyhotherapy Groups
Professional Resource Press
PO Box 3197
Sarasota, FL 34230-3197
941-343-9601
800-443-3364
Fax: 941-343-9201
E-mail: cs.prpress@gmail.com
www.prpress.com

Laurie Girsch, Managing Editor

Provides specific techniques for use in the beginning, middle, and end phase of time-limited structured psychotherapy groups. Offers concrete suggestions for working with hard to reach and difficult adolescents, providing feedback to parents, and dealing with administrative, legal, and ethical issues. Examples of pre/post evaluation forms, therapy contracts, evaluation feedback letters, parent response forms, therapist rating scales, co-therapist rating forms, problem identification forms, supervision and session records, client and patient handouts, and specific group exercises. Solidly anchored to research on the curative factors in group therapy, this book includes empirical data, references, theoretical formulations and examples of group sessions. *$19.95*

164 pages Year Founded: 1980 ISBN 0-943158-74-5

2909 Teaching Buddy Skills to Preschoolers
AAIDD
501 3rd Street NW
Suite 200
Washington, DC 20001
202-387-1968
800-424-3688
Fax: 202-387-2193
E-mail: anam@aaidd.org
www.aaidd.org

Margaret A. Nygren, EdD, Executive Director & CEO
Danielle Webber, MSW, Manager
Kathleen McLane, Director
Paul D. Aitken, CPA, Director

Shows how the rewards of social interactions must outweigh the costs to encouraging friendships between pre-schoolers with and without disabilities. *$12.95*

40 pages ISBN 0-940898-45-4

2910 Textbook of Child and Adolescent Psychiatry
American Psychiatric Publishing, Inc.
1000 Wilson Boulevard
Suite 1825
Arlington, VA 22209-3901
703-907-7322
800-368-5777
Fax: 703-907-1091
E-mail: appi@psych.org
www.appi.org

Robert E Hales, M.D., M.B.A., Editor-in-Chief
Ron McMillen, Chief Executive Officer
John McDuffie, Editorial Director
Rebecca D. Rinehart, Publisher

Includes chapter on changes in DSM-IV classification and discusses the latest research and treatment advances in the areas of epidemiology, fenetics, developmental neurobiology, and combined treatments. A special section covers essential issues such as HIV and AIDS, gender identity disorders, physical and sexual abuse, and substance abuse, for the child and adolescent psychiatrist. *$140.00*

960 pages ISBN 1-882103-03-3

2911 Textbook of Pediatric Neuropsychiatry
American Psychiatric Publishing, Inc.
1000 Wilson Boulevard
Suite 1825
Arlington, VA 22209-3901
703-907-7322
800-368-5777
Fax: 703-907-1091
E-mail: appi@psych.org
www.appi.org

Robert E Hales, M.D., M.B.A., Editor-in-Chief
Ron McMillen, Chief Executive Officer
John McDuffie, Editorial Director
Rebecca D. Rinehart, Publisher

Comprehensive textbook on pediatric medicine. *$175.00*

1632 pages Year Founded: 1998 ISBN 0-880487-66-6

2912 The Special Education Consultant Teacher
Charles C Thomas Publisher Ltd.
PO Box 19265
Springfield, IL 62794-9265
217-789-8980
800-258-8980
Fax: 217-789-9130
www.ccthomas.com

Michael P Thomas, President
Charles C Thomas, Publisher

This book is intended for special education teachers and other professionals providing special education services with information, guidelines and suggestions relating to the role and responsibilities of the special education consultant teacher. Available in paperback for $ 45.95. *$67.95*

330 pages Year Founded: 1927 ISBN 0-398075-10-7

2913 Through the Eyes of a Child
WW Norton & Company
500 5th Avenue
New York, NY 10110-54
212-354-2907
800-233-4830
Fax: 212-869-0856
E-mail: npb@wwnorton.com
www.books.wwnorton.com

Drake McFeely, CEO

Comprehensive and helpful, this book helps therapists work with children and parents in the application of EMDR with children. *$ 37.00*

288 pages Year Founded: 1923 ISSN 70287-1ISBN 0-393702-87-1

2914 Transition Matters From School to Independence: a Guide & Directory of Services for Children & Youth with Disabilities & Special Needs in the Metro New York Area
Resources for Children with Special Needs
116 E 16th Street
5th Floor
New York, NY 10003-2164
212-677-4650
Fax: 212-254-4070

E-mail: info@resourcesnyc.org
www.resourcesnyc.org

Ellen Miller-Wachtel, Chairman
Shon E. Glusky, President
Rachel Howard, Executive Director
Stephen Stern, Director

Youth with disabilities need special guidance when moving from school to adult life. Transition Matters covers every aspect of moving from high school to the world of postsecondary education, job training, employment and idependent living. This guide for parents, caregivers and educators presents a wealth of information about the transition process, and lists 1, 000 agencies and organizations that provide services for youth 14 and up. It explains entitlements and options and helps families navigate systems and procedures. *$15.00*

500 pages Year Founded: 1983 ISBN 0-967836-56-5

2915 Treating Depressed Children: A Therapeutic Manual of Proven Cognitive Behavior Techniques
NewHarbinger Publications
5674 Shattuck Avenue
Oakland, CA 94609-1662
510-652-0215
800-748-6273
Fax: 510-652-5472
E-mail: customerservice@newharbinger.com
www.newharbinger.com

Matthew McKay, Owner
Patrick Fanning, Co-Founder

Program incorporating cartoons and role playing games to help children recognize emotions, change negative thoughts, gain confidence, and learn interpersonal skills. *$49.94*

160 pages Year Founded: 1973 ISBN 1-572240-61-

2916 Treating the Aftermath of Sexual Abuse: a Handbook for Working with Children in Care
Child Welfare League of America
440 First Street NW
Third Floor
Washington, DC 20001-2028
202-638-2952
Fax: 202-638-4004
www.cwla.org

A handbook for working with children in care who have been sexually abused. The authors review the impact of sexual abuse on a child's physical and emotional development and describe the effect of abuse on basic life experiences. Paperback. *$18.95*

176 pages Year Founded: 1998 ISBN 0-878686-93-2

2917 Treating the Tough Adolesent: Family Based Step by Step Guide
Guilford Press
72 Spring Street
New York, NY 10012-4068
212-431-9800
800-365-7006
Fax: 212-966-6708
E-mail: info@guilford.com
www.www.guilford.com

Bob Matloff, President
Seymour Weingarten, Editor-in-Chief

Model for effective family therapy, with reproducible hand-outs. *$35.00*

320 pages Year Founded: 1973 ISBN 1-572304-22-7

2918 Troubled Teens: Multidimensional Family Therapy
WW Norton & Company
500 5th Avenue
New York, NY 10110-54
212-354-2907
Fax: 212-869-0856
E-mail: admalmud@wwnorton.com
www.books.wwnorton.com

Drake McFeely, CEO

Based on 17 years of research, this treatment manual is for therapists who work with youth referred for substance abuse and behavior counseling. Treatment involves drug counseling, family and individual sessions and interventions. People or systems of influence outside the family are also considered. *$35.00*

320 pages Year Founded: 1923 ISBN 0-393703-40-1

2919 Understanding and Teaching Emotionally Disturbed Children and Adolescents
Pro-Ed Publications
8700 Shoal Creek Boulevard
Austin, TX 78757-6897
512-451-3246
800-897-3202
Fax: 512-451-8542
E-mail: info@proedinc.com
www.www.proedinc.com

Donald D Hammill, Owner

Shows how diverse theoretical perspectives translate into practice by exploring forms of therapy and types of interventions currently employed with children and adolescents. *$41.00*

620 pages Year Founded: 1993 ISBN 0-890795-75-4

2920 Ups & Downs: How to Beat the Blues and Teen Depression
Price Stern Sloan Publishing
375 Hudson Street
New York, NY 10014-3657
212-366-2000
Fax: 212-366-2933
www.penguingroup.com

John Makinson, Chairman and Chief Executive Off
Coram Williams, Chief Financial Officer
David Shanks, Chief Executive Officer
Susan Peterson Kennedy, President

This book discusses how to recognize depression in teens and what to do about it. Informal, yet informative, using quotes and case studies representing typical young people who are dealing with mood swings, eating disorders and problems at school or at home. The book also demystifies therapy and advises readers on how to seek help, particularly if they, or their friends, have suicidal thoughts. Reading level ages nine to twelve. *$4.99*

90 pages Year Founded: 1938 ISBN 0-843174-50-1

2921 Working with Self-Harming Adolescents: A Collaborative, Strengths-Based Therapy Approach
WW Norton & Company
500 5th Avenue
New York, NY 10110-54
212-354-2907
800-233-4830
Fax: 212-869-0856
E-mail: npb@wwnorton.com
www.books.wwnorton.com

Drake McFeely, CEO

A unique approach to this illness combines flexability, compassion, and candor. His integration of the family in these treatments demonstrates the complex interplay between self-harming teens and their parents, peers, communities, and culture. Originally published in hardcover as Living on the Razor's Edge.

Year Founded: 1923 ISBN 0-393704-99-8

2922 Youth Violence: Prevention, Intervention, and Social Policy
American Psychiatric Publishing, Inc.
1000 Wilson Boulevard
Suite 1825
Arlington, VA 22209-3901
703-907-7322
800-368-5777
Fax: 703-907-1091
E-mail: appi@psych.org
www.appi.org

Robert E Hales, M.D., M.B.A., Editor-in-Chief
Ron McMillen, Chief Executive Officer
John McDuffie, Editorial Director
Rebecca D. Rinehart, Publisher

Based on more than a decade of clinical research and treatment experience, this comprehensive and non-technical book offers a stage-oriented approach to understanding and treating complex and difficult traumatized patients, integrating modern trauma theory with traditional therapeutic interventions. *$48.50*

336 pages Year Founded: 1998 ISBN 0-880488-09-3

Suicide

2923 A Woman Doctor's Guide to Depression
Hyperion
237 Park Avenue
New York, NY 10017
www.hyperionbooks.com

Mitch Albom, Author
Lauren Groff, Author
Caroline Kennedy, Author
Jamie Oliver, Author

Includes information on what depression feels like and how it affects daily life, women's unique risks of developing depression throughout the life cycle from puberty to menopause and current treatment strategies and their risks and benefits, preventive measures and warning signs. *$9.95*

176 pages Year Founded: 1997 ISBN 0-786881-46-1

2924 Antidepressant Fact Book: What Your Doctor Won't Tell You About Prozac, Zoloft, Paxil, Celexa and Luvox
Perseus Books Group
2465 Central Avenue
Boulder, CO 80301
303-444-3541
800-386-5656
Fax: 720-406-7336
E-mail: westview.orders@perseusbooks.com
www.perseusbooksgroup.com

David Steinberger, President & CEO

What antidepressants will and won't treat, documented side and withdrawl effects, plus what parents need to know about teenagers and antidepressants. The author has been a medical expert in many court cases involving the use and misuse of psychoactive drugs. *$13.00*

240 pages Year Founded: 2001 ISBN 0-738204-51-X

2925 Assessment and Prediction of Suicide
Guilford Press
72 Spring Street
New York, NY 10012-4068
212-431-9800
800-365-7006
Fax: 212-966-6708
E-mail: info@guilford.com
www.www.guilford.com

Bob Matloff, President
Seymour Weingarten, Editor-in-Chief

Comprehensive reference volume that includes contributions from top suicide experts of the current knowledge in the field of suicide. Covers concepts and theories, methods and quantification, in-depth case histories, specific single predictors applied to the case histories and comorbidity. *$90.00*

697 pages Year Founded: 1973 ISBN 0-898627-91-5

2926 Comprehensive Textbook of Suicidology
Guilford Press
72 Spring Street
New York, NY 10012-4068
212-431-9800
800-365-7006
Fax: 212-966-6708
E-mail: info@guilford.com
www.www.guilford.com

Bob Matloff, President
Seymour Weingarten, Editor-in-Chief

This volume presents an authoritative overview of current scientific knowledge about suicide and suicide prevention. Multidisciplinary and comprehensive in scope, the book provides a solid foundation in theory, research and clinical applications. Topics covered include the classification and prevalence of suicidal behaviors, psychiatric and medical factors, ethical and legal issues in intervention as well as the social, cultural and gender context of suicide. *$70.00*

650 pages Year Founded: 1973 ISBN 1-572305-41-X

2927 Interpersonal Psychotherapy
American Psychiatric Publishing, Inc.
1000 Wilson Boulevard
Suite 1825
Arlington, VA 22209-3901
703-907-7322
800-368-5777
Fax: 703-907-1091
E-mail: appi@psych.org
www.appi.org

Robert E Hales, M.D., M.B.A., Editor-in-Chief
Ron McMillen, Chief Executive Officer
John McDuffie, Editorial Director
Rebecca D. Rinehart, Publisher

An overview of interpersonal psychotherapy for depression, preventative treatment for depression, bulimia nervosa and HIV positive men and women. *$26.00*

156 pages Year Founded: 1998 ISBN 0-880488-36-0

2928 Practical Art of Suicide Assessment: A Guide for Mental Health Professionals and Substance Abuse Counselors
John Wiley & Sons
111 River Street
Hoboken, NJ 07030-5774
201-748-6000
Fax: 201-748-6088
E-mail: info@wiley.com
www.www.wiley.com

Lou Peragallo, Manager

Covers the critical elements of suicide assessment, from risk factor analysis to evaluating clients with borderline personality disorders or psychotic process.

316 pages ISBN 0-471237-61-2

2929 Suicide From a Psychological Prespective
Charles C Thomas Publisher Ltd.
2600 S 1st Street
Springfield, IL 62704-4730
217-789-8980
800-258-8980
Fax: 217-789-9130
E-mail: books@ccthomas.com
www.ccthomas.com

Michael P Thomas, President
Charles C Thomas, Publisher

$39.95

142 pages Year Founded: 1927 ISBN 0-398057-09-5

2930 Teens and Suicide
Mason Crest Publishers
370 Reed Road
Suite 302
Broomall, PA 19008-4017
866-627-2665
Fax: 610-543-3878
www.masoncrest.com

Suicide is the third-leading cause of death among adolescents in the United States; in a recent study by The Gallup Organization, 47 percent of teenagers between the ages of 13 and 17 said they know someone who has tried to take their own lives. This volume examines the cause of teen-age suicide and explores such issues as teens and guns as well as suicide rates among minorities.

2931 Treatment of Suicidal Patients in Managed Care
American Psychiatric Publishing, Inc.
1000 Wilson Boulevard
Suite 1825
Arlington, VA 22209-3901
703-907-7322
800-368-5777
Fax: 703-907-1091
E-mail: appi@psych.org
www.appi.org

Robert E Hales, M.D., M.B.A., Editor-in-Chief
Ron McMillen, Chief Executive Officer
John McDuffie, Editorial Director
Rebecca D. Rinehart, Publisher

Suicide is an all too common cause of death and preventable, but the managed care concerns of cost control with rapid diagnosis and treatment of depression puts the clinician in a dilemma. This book guides the professional with advice on knowing who to contact, and getting more of what is needed from the patient's managed care provider. *$39.00*

240 pages Year Founded: 2001 ISBN 0-880488-28-x

Conferences & Meetings

2932 AAIDD Annual Meeting
501 3rd Street NW
Suite 200
Washington, DC 20001
202-387-1968
800-424-3688
Fax: 202-387-2193
E-mail: anam@aaidd.org
www.aaidd.org

Margaret A. Nygren, EdD, Executive Director & CEO
Danielle Webber, MSW, Manager
Kathleen McLane, Director
Paul D. Aitken, CPA, Director

AAIDD promotes progressive policies, sound research, effective practices and universal human rights for people with intellectual and developmental disabilities.

1 per year

2933 AAMA Annual Conference
American Academy of Medical Administrators
330 N Wabash Ave
Suite 2000
Chicago, IL 60611
312-321-6815
Fax: 312-673-6705
E-mail: info@aameda.org
www.aameda.org

Mrs. Linda Larin, MBA, FACCA, FAC, Chairman
Dr. Robert McKenney, PhD, FAAMA, Vice Chairman
Kevin Baliozian, Executive Director
Jennifer Schap, Program Coordinator

Learn the newest trends in healthcare administration; focus on your area of specialty or broaden your knowledge; become energized with new information and contacts in your field; and return to your organization ready to implement new ideas anad face new challenges.

Year Founded: 1999

2934 AMA's Annual Medical Communications Conference
American Medical Association
330 North Wabash Ave
Suite 39300
Chicago, IL 60611-5885
312-464-5000
800-262-3211
Fax: 312-464-4184
www.ama-assn.org

James L. Madara, MD, Chief Executive Officer & Execut
Bernard L. Hengesbaugh, Chief Operating Officer
Denise M. Hagerty, Senior Vice President & Chief Fi
Robert W. Davis, Senior Vice President

Provides hands-on communications training and hear from top-level medical communicators, government leaders and national journalists

Year Founded: 1847

2935 ASHA Annual Convention
American Speech-Language-Hearing Association
2200 Research Blvd
Rockville, MD 20850-3289
301-269-5700
800-638-8255
Fax: 301-296-8580
TTY: 301-296-5650
E-mail: convention@asha.org
www.asha.org

Perry F. Flynn, MEd, CCC-SLP, Co-Chair
Wayne A. Foster, PhD, CCC-SLP/A, Co-Chair
Elizabeth S. McCrea, PhD, CCC-SLP, President
Barbara K. Cone, PhD, CCC-A, Vice President for Academic Affa

ASHA is the professional, scientific and credentialing association for 140, 000 members and affiliates who are audiologists, speech-language pathologists and speech, language and hearing scientists.

1 per year Year Founded: 1925

2936 American Academy of Child and Adolescent Psychiatry (AACAP): Annual Meeting
3615 Wisconsin Avenue NW
Washington, DC 20016-3007
202-966-7300
Fax: 202-966-2891
E-mail: communications@aacap.org
www.www.aacap.org

Warren Y.K. Ng, M.D., Chairman
Paramjit T. Joshi, M.D., President
Aradhana Bela Sood, M.D., Secretary
David G. Fassler, M.D., Treasurer

Professional society of physicians who have completed an additional five years of stimulate and advance medical contributions to the knowledge and treatment of psychiatric illnesses of children and adolescents. Annual meeting.

2937 American Academy of Psychiatry & Law Annual Conference
American Academy of Psychiatry & Law
1 Regency Drive
PO Box 30
Bloomfield, CT 06002-30
860-242-5450
800-331-1389

Fax: 860-286-0787
E-mail: execoff@aapl.org
www.aapl.org

Charles Scott, MD, President
Jacquelyn T. Coleman, Executive Director

Year Founded: 1969

2938 American Academy of Psychoanalysis Preliminary Meeting
American Academy of Psychoanalysis and Dynamic Psychiatry
One Regency Drive
PO Box 30
Bloomfield, CT 06002-30
888-691-8281
Fax: 860-286-0787
E-mail: info@aapdp.org
www.aapdp.org

Michael Blumenfield, M.D., President
Jacquelyn T Coleman CAE, Executive Director
Carol Filiaci, Secretary

Annual meeting, Toronto, Canada.

Year Founded: 1956

2939 American Association of Children's Residential Center Annual Conference
American Association of Children's Residential Centers
11700 W Lake Park Drive
Milwaukee, WI 53224-3021
877-332-2272
Fax: 877-362-2272
E-mail: kbehling@alliance1.org
www.aacrc-dc.org

Christiopher Bellonci, M.D., President
William Powers, MHA, MPA, Chief Executive Officer
Joseph Whalen, Executive Director
Laurah Currey, Treasurer

Funded by the Mental Health Community Support Program. The purpose of the association is to share information about services, providers and ways to cope with mental illnesses. Available services include referrals, professional seminars, support groups and a variety of publications.

2940 American Association of Geriatric Psychiatry Annual Meetings
7910 Woodmont Avenue
Suite 1050
Bethesda, MD 20814-3004
301-654-7850
Fax: 301-654-4137
E-mail: main@aagponline.org
www.aagponline.org

David C. Steffens, MD, MHS, President
Christine M. deVries, CEO/Executive Vice President
Denise Disque, Office Manager/Executive Assista
Kate McDuffie, Director, Communications & Marke

Annual Meeting: March, Puerto Rico

Year Founded: 1978

2941 American Association on Intellectual and Developmental Disabilities Annual Meeting
501 3rd Street NW
Suite 200
Washington, DC 20001
202-387-1968
800-424-3688
Fax: 202-387-2193
E-mail: anam@aaidd.org
www.aaidd.org

Margaret A. Nygren, EdD, Executive Director & CEO
Danielle Webber, MSW, Manager
Kathleen McLane, Director
Paul D. Aitken, CPA, Director

Provides the opportunity of networking with old friends and colleagues, and is a wonderful opportunity to welcome students and new disability professionals to our Association. *$445.00*

2942 American Board of Disability Analysts Annual Conference
770 Broadway
New York, NY 10003
212-206-4400
E-mail: americanbd@aol.com
www.www.aol.com

Tim Armstrong, Chairman and Chief Executive Off
Curtis Brown, Executive Vice President and Chi
Karen Dykstra, Executive Vice President and Chi

Year Founded: 1985

2943 American College of Health Care Administrators (ACHCA) Annual Convocation & Exposition
1321 Duke Street
Suite 400
Alexandria, VA 22314
202-536-5120
Fax: 888-874-1585
E-mail: jspence@achca.org
www.achca.org

Marianna Kern Grachek, MSN, CNH, President & CEO
Becky Reisinger, Director, Membership and Busines
Whitney O'Donnell, Coordinator, Member Services
Chelsea Whitman-Rush, Coordinator, Member and Chapter

A non-profit professional membership association which provides superior educataional programming, professional certification, and career development opportunities for its members.

Year Founded: 1966

2944 American College of Healthcare Executives Educational Events
American College of Healthcare Executives
One N Franklin Street
Suite 1700
Chicago, IL 60606-3529
312-424-2800
Fax: 312-424-0023
E-mail: contact@ache.org
www.ache.org

Diana L. Smalley, FACHE, Chairman
Deborah J. Bowen, FACHE, President and CEO

421

2945 American College of Psychiatrists Annual Meeting
122 S. Michigan Ave
Suite 1360
Chicago, IL 60603-6185
312-662-1020
Fax: 312-662-1025
E-mail: angel@acpsych.org
www.acpsych.org

James H. Scully Jr., President
Frank W. Brown, First Vice President
Gail E. Robinson, Second Vice President
Maureen D. Shick, Executive Director

Nonprofit honorary association of psychiatrists who, through excellence in their chosen fields, have been recognized for their significant contributions to the profession. The society's goal is to promote and support the highest standards in psychiatry through education, research and clinical practice. Annual Meeting in February.
Year Founded: 1963

2946 American Group Psychotherapy Association Annual Conference
American Group Psychotherapy Association
25 E 21st Street
6th Floor
New York, NY 10010-6207
212-477-2677
877-668-2472
Fax: 212-979-6627
E-mail: info@agpa.org
www.agpa.org

Les R. Greene, Ph.D., CGP, LF, President
Jeffrey Kleinberg, PhD, CGP, President
Marsha S. Block, CAE, CFRE, CEO
Lise Motherwell, Ph.D., Psy, Treasurer

Educational conference with a changing annual focus. February.
Year Founded: 1942

2947 American Health Care Association Annual Convention
1201 L Street NW
Washington, DC 20005-4046
202-842-4444
Fax: 202-842-3860
E-mail: teyet@ahca.org
www.www.ahcancal.org

Leonard Russ, Chairman
Bruse Yarwood, President

Exhibits and educational workshops from the nonprofit federation of affiliated state health organizations, together representing nearly 12, 000 nonprofit and for profit assisted living, nursing facility, developmentally disabled and sub-acute care providers that care for more than 1.5 million elderly and disabled individuals nationally. AHCA represents the long term care community at large — to government, business leaders and the general public. It also serves as a force for change within the long term care field, providing information, education, and administrative tools that enhance quality at every level.

2948 American Health Information Management Association Annual Exhibition and Conference
233 N Michigan Avenue
21st Floor
Chicago, IL 60601-5809
312-233-1100
800-335-5535
Fax: 312-233-1090
E-mail: info@ahima.org
www.ahima.org

Angela Kennedy, EdD, MBA, RHI, President, Chairman
Cassi Birnbaum, MS. RHIA, CP, President / Chair-Elect
Becky Garris-Perry, Executive Vice President/CFO
Linda Kloss, Executive Director

Exhibits, business and educational conferences of the dynamic professional association that represents more than 46, 000 specially educated health information management professionals who work throughout the healthcare industry. Health information management professionals serve the health care industry and the public by manageing, analyzing and utilizing data vital for patient care and making it accessible to healthcare providers when it is needed most.

2949 American Society of Addiction Medicine
American Society of Addiction Medicine
4601 N Park Avenue
Upper Arcade #101
Chevy Chase, MD 20815-4520
301-656-3920
Fax: 301-656-3815
E-mail: email@asam.org
www.asam.org

Penny S Mills, Executive VP, CEO
Arlene C. Deverman, CAE, VP, Professional Development
Carolyn C. Lanham, CAE, Chief Operating Officer
Kate Volpe, Director, Marketing, Communicati

Goal is to present the most up-to-date information in the addictions field. to attain this goal, program sessions will focus on the latest developments in research and treatment issues and will tanslate them into clinically useful knowledge. Through a mix of symposia, courses, workshops, didactic lectures, and paper and poster presentations based on submitted abstracts, participants will have an opportunity to interact with experts in their field.

2950 Association for Child Psychoanalysis (ACP) Annual Meeting
900 East Pecan Street
Suite 300, PMB 254
Pflugerville, TX 78660
512-551-8769
Fax: 866-534-7555
E-mail: childanalysis65@gmail.com
www.childanalysis.org

Kerry Kelly Novick, President
Anita Schmukler, D.O., President
Barbara Streeter, Treasurer
Tricia Hall, CAE, CMP, Administrator

An international not-for-profit organization in which all members are highly trained child and adolescent psychoanalysts. Provides a forum for the interchange of ideas and clinical experience in order to advance the psychological treatment and understanding of children and adolescents and their families.

2951 Association of Black Psychologists Annual Convention
7119 Allentown Road
Suite 203
Ft Washington, MD 20744
301-449-3082
Fax: 301-449-3084
E-mail: abpsi@abpsi.org
www.abpsi.org

Cheryl Tawede Grills, PhD, President
Tassogle Daryl Rowe, President-Elect
Kevin Washington, Ph.D., President-Elect
Carolyn Moore, Ph.D, Treasurer

Feature presentations, exhibits and workshops held over a four day period focusing on the unique concerns of Black professionals.

2952 California Psychological Association's Annual Convention
1231 I Street
Suite 204
Sacramento, CA 95814-2933
916-286-7979
Fax: 916-286-7971
E-mail: membership@cpapsych.org
www.cpapsych.org

Robert deMayo, PhD, ABPP, President
Stephen Pfeiffer, PhD, President-Elect
Jo Linder-Crow, Ph.D., CEO
Betsy Levine-Proctor, PhD, Treasurer / Chair - Finance Comm

Poster sessions, roundtable discussions, CE sessions, ethics discussions and featured speakers. *$680.00*

2953 Georgia Psychological Society Annual Conference
2200 Century Parkway
Suite 660
Atlanta, GA 30345
404-634-6272
Fax: 404-634-8230
E-mail: blbrowne@valdosta.edu or crtalor@valdosta.edu
www.georgiapsychologicalsociety.org

Jennifer Stapel-Wax, President
Steven Perlow, PhD, President Elect
Mary Gresham, Vice President
Dr. Chuck Talor, Conference, Newsletter's and Jou

Proposals for symposia, papers, posters and workshops on topics in all areas of psychology are invited. Proposals should not exceed 500 words, and each proposal must include a summary that is no longer than 50 words.

2954 NADD Annual Conference & Exhibit Show
National Association for the Dually Diagnosed
132 Fair Street
Kingston, NY 12401-4802
845-331-4336
800-331-5362
Fax: 845-331-4569
E-mail: info@thenadd.org
www.thenadd.org

Daniel Baker, Ph.D., Conference Chairperson, Presiden
Donna McNelis, Ph.D., President
Robert J. Fletcher DSW, CEO
Brian Tallant, Conference Chairperson

2955 National Alliance on Mental Illness
National Alliance on Mental Illness
3803 N. Fairfax Dr.
Suite 100
Arlington, VA 22203
703-524-7600
800-950-6264
Fax: 703-524-9094
TDD: 703-516-7227
E-mail: convention@nami.org
www.nami.org

Kevin B Sullivan, President
Keris Jan Myrick, M.B.A., M.S., , President
Jim Payne, J.D., First Vice President
Linda E. Jensen, Ph.D., R.N., Second Vice President

Join the thousands who will gather to explore strategy and tactics to improve the lives of people who live with mental illnesses.

2956 National Multicultural Conference and Summit
Brakins Consulting & Psychological Svs
13805 60th Avenue North
Phymouth, MN 55446-3583
www.multiculturalsummit.com

Debra Kawahara, Lead Coordinator
Michael Mobley, Programming Coordinator
Julii Green, Keynote Coordinator
Roberta Nutt, Awards Coordinator

The mission is to convene students, practitioners, and scholars in psychology and related fields to inform and inspire multicultural research and practice.

2957 New England Educational Institute
New England Educational Institute
449 Pittsfield Road
Suite 201
Lenox, MA 01240
413-499-1489
Fax: 413-499-6584
E-mail: learn@neei.org
www.neei.org

Designed to meet the educational needs of physicians (psychiatrists, family practitioners, general practitioners), psychologists, nurse practitioners, physician assistants, nurses and other health care professionals. Each half-day will provide practical and clinically relevant information for day-to-day problems. Morning lectures will be followed by panel discussions.

2958 Traumatic Incident Reduction Workshop
E-Productivity-Services.Net
Division of 21st Century Enterprises
13 NW Barry Rd PMB 214
Kansas City, MO 64155-2728
816-468-4945
Fax: 816-468-6656
E-mail: nld@espn.net
www.espn.net

Frank A Gerbode, Subject Developer
Marian Volkman, President
John Durkin, Vice President
Robert H Moore, Board Member

Defines the Conditioned Response Phenomena, establishes a safe environment, analyzes and applies the Unblocking technique to resolve issues relating to emotionally charged persons, places, things and situations, and analyzes and applies Traumatic Incident Reduction (TIR) to resolve known and unknown past traumatic experiences and the unwanted feelings, emotions, sensations, attitutdes and pain associated with them.

2959 YAI/National Institute for People with Disabilities

460 W 34th Street
New York, NY 10001-2382
212-273-6100
866-292-4546
Fax: 212-947-7524
TDD: 212-290-2787
www.yai.org

Bridget Waldron, L.C.S.W., Senior Vice President, Quality E
Marco Damiani, M.A., Executive Vice President, Innova
Paul Smoller, M.A., Executive Vice President, Talent
Kelly Burke-Quinn, Vice President, Business Analysi

Annual conference "Advancing Services Across the Life Span in Intellectual and Developmental Disabilities". A major forum for the exchange of ideas and the introduction of new models and strategies that have a positive impact in the field.

Periodicals & Pamphlets

2960 AAMI Newsletter
Arizona Alliance for the Mentally Ill (NAMI Arizona)

2210 N 7th Street
Phoenix, AZ 85006-1604
602-244-8166
800-626-5022
Fax: 602-244-9264
E-mail: namiaz@namiaz.org
www.namiaz.org

Diane McVicker, President
Cheryl Weiner, Educutive Director

Provides support, education, research, and advocacy for individuals and families affected by mental illness. Reports on legislative updates, conventions, psychiatry/psychological practices, and activities of the alliance. Newsletter with membership. *$10.00*

8 pages 4 per year

2961 AAPL Newsletter
American Academy of Psychiatry and the Law

One Regency Drive
PO Box 30
Bloomfield, CT 06002-30
860-242-5450
800-331-1389
Fax: 860-286-0787
E-mail: office@aapl.org
www.aapl.org

Jacquelyn T. Coleman, Executive Director
Charles Scott, MD, President
Ezra Griffith, MD, Editor

Scholarly articles on forensice psychiatry. *$130.00*

4 per year ISSN 1093-6793

2962 APA Monitor
American Psychological Association

750 1st Street NE
Washington, DC 20002-4242
202-336-5500
800-374-2721
Fax: 202-336-5518
TDD: 202-336-6123
TTY: 202-336-6123
E-mail: letters.monitor@apa.org
www.apa.org

Nadine J. Kaslow, Ph.D., President
Barry S. Anton, Ph.D., President-Elect
Donald N. Bersoff, PhD, JD, Past President
Norman B Anderson, Ph.D., CEO, EVP

Magazine of the American Psychological Association.

12 per year ISSN 1529-4978

2963 ASAP Newsletter
American Society for Adolescent Psychiatry

PO Box 570218
Dallas, TX 75357-218
972-613-0985
Fax: 972-613-5532
E-mail: info@adolpsych.org
www.adolpsych.org

Mohan Nair, President
Gregg Dwyer, President
Sheldon Glass, President-Elect
Gregory P. Barclay, VP

Contains articles about adolescent psychiatry and society news. Recurring features include news of research, a calendar of events, and book reviews. *$10.00*

16-20 pages 4 per year

2964 Advocate: Autism Society of America
Autism Society of America

4340 East-West Hwy
Suite 350
Bethesda, MD 20814-3067
301-657-0881
800-328-8476
Fax: 301-657-0869
E-mail: sbadesch@autism-society.org
www.autism-society.org

Scott Badesch, President, CEO
Jennifer Repella, VP, Programs
John Dabrowski, CFO
Rose Jochum, Director, Programs

Reports news and information of national significance for individuals, families, and professionals dealing with autism. Recurring features include personal features and profiles, research summaries, government updates, book reviews, statistics, news of research, and a calendar of events.

32-36 pages 6 per year ISSN 0047-9101

2965 Alcohol & Drug Abuse Weekly
John Wiley & Sons

111 River Street
Hoboken, NJ 07030-5774
201-748-6000
Fax: 201-748-6088
E-mail: info@wiley.com
www.wiley.com

Stephen M. Smith, President, CEO
MJ O'Leary, SVP, Human Resources
Edward J. Melando, SVP, Corporate Controller
Gary M. Rinck, SVP, General Counsel

48-issue subsrciption offers significant news and analysis of federal and state policy developments. A resource for directors of addiction treatment centers, managed care executives, federal and state policy makers and healthcare consultants. Topics include the latest findings in treatment and prevention; funding and survival issues for providers; the impact of state and federal policy on treatment and prevention; working under managed care; and co-occurring disorders.

8 pages 48 per year Year Founded: 1992 ISSN 1042-1394

2966 Alliance for Children and Families
Insider
1020 19th St. N.W.
Suite 500
Washington, DC 20036-1540
202-429-0400
800-220-1016
Fax: 202-429-0178
E-mail: policy@alliance1.org
www.www.alliance1.org

Susan Dreyfus, CEO, President
Polina Makievsky, SVP, Knowledge, Leadership, and
Robert Cacase, Chief Information Officer
Tracy Wareing, Executive Director

Alliance for Children and Families' tool for providing members with accurate and up-to-date information on current legislation, issues the Alliance is advocating on Capitol Hill, summaries of how proposed bills will affect member organizations and the people they serve, and suggestions for local advocacy efforts.

12 per year

2967 American Academy of Child and Adolescent Psychiatry
AACAP
3615 Wisconsin Avenue NW
Washington, DC 20016-3007
202-966-7300
Fax: 202-966-2891
E-mail: communications@aacap.org
www.aacap.org

Kristin Kroeger-Ptakowski, Director, Sr Deputy Director
Elizabeth DiLauro, Advocacy Manager
Emma Jellen, Policy Coordinator

The American Academy of Child and Adolescent Psychiatry, (AACAP) publishes a newsletter which focuses events within the Academy, child and adolescent psychiatrists, and AACAP members.

36-64 pages 6 per year

2968 American Association of Community Psychiatrists (AACP)
PO Box 570218
Dallas, TX 75357-0218
972-613-0985
972-613-3997
Fax: 972-613-5532
E-mail: frda1@airmail.net
www.www.communitypsychiatry.org

Wesley Sowers MD, President
Anita Everett, M.D., President
Annelle Primm, Vice President
Stephanie Le Melle, M.D., Vice President

Psychiatrists and psychiatry residents practicing in community mental health centers or similar programs that provide care to the mentally ill regardless of their ability to pay. Addresses issues faced by psychiatrists who practice within CMHCs. Publications: AACP Membership Directory, annual. Community Psychiatrist, quarterly newsletter. Annual meeting, in conjunction with American Psychiatric Association in May. Annual meeting, in conjunction with Institute on Hospital and Community in fall.

4 per year

2969 American Institute for Preventive Medicine
American Institute for Preventive Medicine Press
30445 Northwestern Highway
Suite 350
Farmington Hills, MI 48334-3107
248-539-1800
800-345-2476
Fax: 248-539-1808
E-mail: aipm@healthy.net
www.healthylife.com

Don R Powell, Ph.D., President, CEO
Sue Jackson, VP
Elaine Frank, M.Ed., R.D., VP
Jeanette Karwan, Director, Product Development

AIPM is an internationally renowned developer and provider of wellness programs and publications that address both mental and physical health issues. It works with over 11, 500 corporations, hospitals, MCOs, universities, and goverment agencies to reduce health care costs, lower absenteeism, and improve productivity. The Institute has a number of publications that address mental health issues, including stress management, depression, self - esteem, and EAP issues.

Year Founded: 1999

2970 Behavioral Health Management
3800 Lakeside Avenue
Suite 201
Cleveland, OH 44114
216-391-9100
Fax: 216-391-9200
E-mail: info@vendomegrp.com
www.behavioral.net

Richard Peck, Editorial Director
Douglas J Edwards, Managing Editor, Publisher
Kathi Homenick, Director
Judi Zeng, Traffic Manager

Informs decision makers in managed behavioral healthcare organizations, provider groups, and treatment centers of the ever-changing demands of their field. The magazine publishes analyses, editorials, and organizations case studies to give readers the information they need for best practices in a challenging marketplace.

2971 Biology of Sex Differences
Society for Women's Health Research (SWHR)
1025 Connecticut Avenue NW
Suite 601
Washington, DC 20036-5447

202-466-6069
Fax: 202-833-3472
www.bsd-journal.com

Phyllis Greenberger, MSW, President
Mary V. Hornig, VP Finance & Operations
Arthur Arnold, Univ. CA, Editor

Biology of Sex Differences considers manuscripts on all aspects of the effect of sex on biology and disease. It is an online, open access, peer-reviewed journal published in conjunction with BioMed Central.

Year Founded: 1990

2972 Brown University: Child & Adolescent Psychopharmacology Update
John Wiley & Sons
111 River Street
Hoboken, NJ 07030-5774
201-748-6000
Fax: 201-748-6088
E-mail: info@wiley.com
www.wiley.com

Stephen M. Smith, President, CEO
MJ O'Leary, SVP, Human Resources
Edward J. Melando, SVP, Corporate Controller
Gary M. Rinck, SVP, General Counsel

Monthly newsletter that gives information on children and adolescent's unique psychotropic medication needs. Delivers updates on new drugs, their uses, typical doses, side effects and interactions, examines generic vs. name brand drugs, reports on new research and new indications for existing medications. Each issue also includes case studies, references for future reading, industry news notes, abstracts of current research and a patient psychotropic medication handout. *$190.00*

12 per year Year Founded: 1992 ISSN 1527-8395

2973 Brown University: Digest of Addiction Theory and Application (DATA)
John Wiley & Sons
111 River Street
Hoboken, NJ 07030-5774
201-748-6000
Fax: 201-748-6088
E-mail: info@wiley.com
www.wiley.com

Stephen M. Smith, President, CEO
MJ O'Leary, SVP, Human Resources
Edward J. Melando, SVP, Corporate Controller
Gary M. Rinck, SVP, General Counsel

Monthly synopsis of critical research developments in the treatment and prevention of alcoholism and drug abuse, including dozens of research abstracts chosen from over 75 medical journals. *$129.00*

8 pages 12 per year Year Founded: 1992 ISSN 1040-6328

2974 Brown University: Geriatric Psychopharmacology Update
John Wiley & Sons
111 River Street
Hoboken, NJ 07030-5774
201-748-6000
Fax: 201-748-6088
E-mail: info@wiley.com
www.wiley.com

Stephen M. Smith, President, CEO
MJ O'Leary, SVP, Human Resources
Edward J. Melando, SVP, Corporate Controller
Gary M. Rinck, SVP, General Counsel

This monthly report is an easy way to keep up to date on the newest breakthroughs in geriatric medicine that have an impact on psychiatric practice. *$190.00*

12 per year Year Founded: 1992 ISSN 1529-2584

2975 Brown University: Psychopharmacology Update
John Wiley & Sons
111 River Street
Hoboken, NJ 07030-5774
201-748-6000
Fax: 201-748-6088
E-mail: info@wiley.com
www.wiley.com

Stephen M. Smith, President, CEO
MJ O'Leary, SVP, Human Resources
Edward J. Melando, SVP, Corporate Controller
Gary M. Rinck, SVP, General Counsel

Each issue examines the pros and cons of specific drugs, drug-drug interactions, side effects, street drugs, warning signs, case reports and more. *$199.00*

12 per year Year Founded: 1992 ISSN 1608-5308

2976 Bulletin of Menninger Clinic
Guilford Press
72 Spring Street
New York, NY 10012-4068
212-431-9800
800-288-3950
Fax: 212-966-6708

Bob Matloff, President

Valuable, practical information for clinicans. Recent topical issues have focused on rekindling the psychodynamic vision, treatment of different clinical populations with panic disorder, and treatment of complicated personality disorders in an era of managed care. All in an integrated, psychodynamic approach. *$75.00*

ISSN 0025-9284

2977 Bulletin of Psychological Type
Association for Psychological Type
2415 Westwood Ave.
Suite B
Richmond, VA 23230
804-523-2907
800-847-9943
Fax: 804-288-3551
E-mail: web@aptinternational.org
www.aptinternational.org

Jane Kise, President
Susan Nash, President
Linda Berens, Past President
Maryanne DiMarzo, President-Elect

Provides information on regional, national, and international events to keep professionals up-to-date in the study and application of psychological type theory and the Myers-Briggs Type Indicator. Contains announcements of training workshops; international, national, and regional conferences; and awards, along with articles on issues directly related to type theory.

2978 Capitation Report
National Health Information
PO Box 15429
Atlanta, GA 30333-429
404-607-9500
800-597-6300
Fax: 404-607-0095
www.nhionline.net

NHI publishes specialized, targeted information for health care executives on a variety of topics from capitation to disease management.

2979 Child and Adolescent Psychiatry
American Academy of Child and Adolescent Psychiatry
3615 Wisconsin Avenue NW
Washington, DC 20016-3007
202-966-7300
Fax: 202-966-2891
E-mail: communications@aacap.org
www.www.aacap.org

Robert Hendren, President
William Bernet, Treasurer
Michael Linsky, Assistant Director
David Herzog, Secretary

Journal focusing on today's psychiatric research and treatment of the child and adolescent. *$175.00*

36-64 pages 12 per year ISSN 0890-8567

2980 Clinical Psychiatry News
International Medical News Group
5635 Fishers Lane
Suite 6100
Rockville, MD 20852-1886
240-221-4500
Fax: 240-221-4400
E-mail: aimhoff@frontlinemedcom.com
www.imng.com

Stephen Stoneburn, Chairman
Alan J. Imhoff, President, CEO, Medical News Div
JoAnn Wahl, President, Custom Solutions
Marcy Holeton, President, CEO, Clinical Content

A leading independent newspaper for the Psychiatrist.

2981 Clinical Psychiatry Quarterly
AACP
PO Box 458
Glastonbury, CT 06033-458
860-633-6023
Fax: 866-668-9858
E-mail: aacp@cox.net
www.aacp.com

Donald W. Black, MD, President
Richard Balon, MD, VP
Sanjay Gupta, MD, Immediate Past President
James Wilcox, DO, PhD, Treasurer/Secretary

Informs members of of news and events. Recurring features include letters to the editor, news of research, a calendar of events, reports of meetings, and book reviews.

4 per year

2982 Couples Therapy in Managed Care
Haworth Press
10 Alice Street
Binghamton, NY 13904-1503

607-722-5857
800-429-6784
Fax: 607-722-1424
E-mail: getinfo@haworthpressinc.com
www.haworthpress.com

Provides social workers, psychologists and counselors with an overview of the negative effects of the managed care industry on the quality of marital health care.

ISBN 7-890078-86-6

2983 Current Directions in Psychological Science
Association for Psychological Science
1133 15th Street NW
Suite 1000
Washington, DC 20005
202-293-9300
Fax: 202-293-9350
www.psychologicalscience.org

Linda Bartoshuk, President
Elizabeth A. Phelps, President
Mahzarin R Banaji, President-Elect
Nancy Eisenberg, President-Elect

Current Directions publishes reviews by leading experts covering all of scientific psychology and its applications. Each issue features a diverse mix of reports on various topics such as language, memory and cognition, development, the neural basis of behavior and emotions, various aspects of psychopathology, and theory of mind. The articles keep readers apprised of important developments across subfields. The articles are also written to be accessible to non-experts, making them suited for classroom teaching supplements.

6 per year ISSN 0963-7214

2984 Development & Psychopathology
Cambridge University Press
40 W 20th Street
New York, NY 10011-4211
212-924-3900
Fax: 212-691-3239
E-mail: marketing@cup.org
www.cup.org

This multidisciplinary journal is devoted to the publication of original, empirical, theoretical and review papers which address the interrelationship of normal and pathological development in adults and children. It is intended to serve and intergrate the emerging field of developmental psychopathology which strives to understand patterns of adaptation and maladaptation throughout the lifespan. This journal is of vital interest to psychologists, psychiatrists, social scientists, neuroscientists, pediatricians and researchers. *$66.00*

4 per year ISSN 0954-5794

2985 EAPA Exchange
Employee Assistance Professionals Association
4350 North Fairfax Drive
Suite 740
Arlington, VA 22203
703-387-1000
Fax: 703-522-4585
E-mail: admanager@eapassn.org
www.www.eapassn.org

Steven Haught, President
Lucy Henry, President-Elect

Pam Ruster, Treasurer, Secretary
John Maynard, CEO

2986 ETR Associates
Health Education, Research, Training Curriculum
4 Carbonero Way
Scotts Valley, CA 95066-4200
831-438-4060
800-321-4407
Fax: 831-438-4284
E-mail: support@etr.freshdesk.com
www.etr.org

John Henry Ledwith, National Sales Director
Pamela Anderson, PhD, Senior Reasearch Associate
Eric Blanke, BS, Director, Solutions
Erin Cassidy-Eagle, PhD, Director, Research

Publishes a complete line of innovative materials covering the full spectrum of health education topics, including maternal/child health, HIV/STD prevention, risk and injury prevention, self esteem, fitness and nutrition, college health, and wellness education, engaging in both extensive training and research endeavors and a comprehensive K-12 health curriculum.

2987 Elsevier
Customer Support Department
1600 John F Kennedy Boulevard
Suite 1800
Philadelphia, PA 19103-2879
212-633-3730
888-437-4636
Fax: 212-633-3680
E-mail: newsroom@elsevier.com
www.elsevier.com

Youngsuk (Y.S.) Chi, Chairman
Mark Seeley, SVP, General Counsel
David Ruth, SVP, Global Communications
Adriaan Roosen, EVP, Operations

ISSN 0165-3806

2988 Employee Benefits Journal
International Foundation of Employee Benefit Plans
18700 W. Bluemound Rd.
PO Box 69
Brookfield, WI 53045
414-786-6700
888-334-3327
Fax: 414-786-8670
E-mail: marybr@ifebp.org
www.ifebp.org

Kenneth R. Boyd, President, Chairman
Richard Lyall, Past President
Thomas T. Holsman, President-Elect
Regina C. Reardon, Treasurer

Contains articles on all aspects of employee benefits and related topics. *$70.00*

32-48 pages 4 per year   ISSN 0361-4050

2989 Exceptional Parent
416 Main Street
Johnstown, PA 15901
814-361-3860
Fax: 814-361-3861
E-mail: HMaher@eparent.com
www.eparent.com

Joseph M Valenzano, Jr., President, Publisher, CEO
James McGinnis, VP of Operations, CEO
Rick Rader, MD, Editor-in-Chief
Hamilton Maher, Director of Circulation & Busine

Magazine for parents and professionals involved in the care and development of children and young adults with special needs, including physical disabilities, developmental disabilities, mental retardation, autism, epilepsy, learning disabilities, hearing/vision impairments, emotional problems, and chronic illnesses. *$36.00*

12 per year

2990 Focal Point: Research, Policy and Practice in Children's Mental Health
Regional Research Institue-Portland State University
PO Box 751
Portland, OR 97207-0751
503-725-3000
800-547-8887
Fax: 503-725-4882
E-mail: rtcpubs@pdx.edu
www.rtc.pdx.edu

Janet Walker, Editor

Features information on research, interventions, organizations, strategies, and conferences to aid families that have children with emotional, mental, and/or behavioral disorders.

24 pages

2991 From the Couch
Behavioral Health Record Section-AMRA
919 N Michigan Avenue
Suite 1400
Chicago, IL 60611-1692
312-787-2672
Fax: 312-787-5926

From the couch, the newsletter for the Behavioral Health Record section of the American Medical Record Association, covers aspects of the medical records industry that pertain to mental health records.

4 per year

2992 Frontiers of Health Services Management
American College of Healthcare Executives
1 N Franklin Street
Suite 1700
Chicago, IL 60606-3529
312-424-2800
Fax: 312-424-0023
E-mail: contact@ache.org
www.ache.org

Christine M. Candio, RN, FACHE, Chairman
Richard D. Cordova, FACHE, Chairman-Elect
Diana L. Smalley, FACHE, Immediate Past Chairman
Deborah J. Bowen, FACHE, President, CEO

Enhanced by special access to today's healthcare leaders. Frontiers provides you with the cutting edge insight you want. Each quarterly issue engages you in a vigorous debate on a hot healthcare topic. One stimulating article leads the debate, followed by commentaries and perspectives from recognized experts. Unique combination of opinion, practice and research stimulate you to develop new management strategies. *$70.00*

4 per year   ISSN 0748-8157

2993 General Hospital Psychiatry: Psychiatry, Medicine and Primary Care
Elsevier
1600 John F Kennedy Boulevard
Suite 1800
Philadelphia, PA 19103-2879
314-447-8070
888-615-4500
E-mail: newsroom@elsevier.com
www.elsevier.com

Youngsuk (Y.S.) Chi, Chairman
Mark Seeley, SVP, General Counsel
David Ruth, SVP, Global Communications
Adriaan Roosen, EVP, Operations

Journal that explores the linkages and interfaces between psychiatry, medicine and primary care. As a peer-reviewed journal, it provides a forum for communication among professionals with clinical, academic and research interests in psychiatry's essential function in the mainstream of medicine. *$195.00*

84 pages 6 per year ISSN 01638343

2994 Geriatrics
Advanstar Communications
7500 Old Oak Boulevard
Cleveland, OH 44130-3343
440-243-8100
Fax: 440-891-2740
E-mail: arossetti@advanstar.com
www.act-europe.org

David Briemer, Sales Manager
Rich Ehrlich, Associate Publisher

Peer-reviewed clinical journal for primary care physicians who care for patients age 50 and older.

100 pages 12 per year

2995 Group Practice Journal
Amerian Medical Group Association
One Prince Street
Alexandria, VA 22314-3318
703-838-0033
Fax: 703-548-1890
E-mail: roconnor@amga.org
www.amga.org

Donald W. Fisher, Ph.D., CAE, President, CEO
Clyde L. Woody Morris, C.P.A., CFO
April L. Noland, Assistant to the President and C
Michael J. Pomeroy, C.P.A., Senior Assistant to the CFO

Penned by healthcare professionals, articles in the Group Practice Journal give a view from the trenches of modern medicine on a wide variety of topics, including innovative disease management and clinical best practices. Readers look to the publication to learn strategies and solutions from peers in the profession, healthcare thought leaders, and industry experts.

10 per year

2996 Harvard Mental Health Letter
Harvard Health Publications
10 Shattuck Street
2nf Floor
Boston, MA 02115-6030
617-432-4714
E-mail: mental_health@hms.harvard.edu
www.www.health.harvard.edu

Anthony Komaroff, Owner

Delivers information on current thinking and debate on mental health issues that concern professionals and layment a like. In the ever-changing and complex field of mental health care, the newsletter has become a trusted source for psychiatrists, psychologists, social workers and therapists of all kinds. *$59.00*

8 pages 12 per year Year Founded: 1983 ISSN 08843783

2997 Harvard Review of Psychiatry
Taylor and Francis
01650 Toebben Drive
Independence, KY 41051
800-634-7064
Fax: 800-248-4724

An authoritative source for scholarly reviews and perspectives on important topics in psychiatry. Founded by the Harvard Medical School's Department of Psyatiatry, the Harvard Review of Psychiatry features review papares that summarize and synthesize the key literature in a scholarly and clinically relevant manner. *$185.00*

6 per year

2998 Health & Social Work
National Association of Social Workers
750 1st Street NE
Suite 700
Washington, DC 20002-4241
202-408-8600
Fax: 202-336-8312
E-mail: press@naswdc.org
www.naswpress.org

Elvira Craig De Silva, President
Cheryl Y. Bradley, Publisher
Sharon Fletcher, Publications Marketing Manager
Kiera White, Marketing Coordinator

Articles cover research, policy, specialized servies, quality assurance, inservice training and other topics that affect the delivery of health care services. *$125.00*

2999 Health Data Management
Faulkner & Gray
11 Penn Plaza
New York, NY 10001-2006
212-967-7000
Fax: 212-239-4993
www.www.healthdatamanagement.com

Gary Baldwin, Editorial Director
Greg Gillespie, Editor-in-Chief
Joe Goedert, News Editor

3000 International Drug Therapy Newsletter
Lippincott Williams & Wilkins
351 W Camden Street
Baltimore, MD 21201-2436
410-528-4000
800-882-0483
Fax: 410-528-4414
E-mail: korourke@lww.com
www.lww.com

J Arnold Anthony, Operations

Newsletter that focuses on psychotropic drugs, discussing individual drugs, their effectiveness, and history. Examines illnesses and the drugs used to treat them, studies done on various drugs, their chemical make-up, and new developments and changes in drugs. *$149.00*

8 pages   ISSN 0020-6571

3001   International Journal of Neuropsychopharmacology
Cambridge University Press
40 W 20th Street
New York, NY 10011-4211
212-924-3900
Fax: 212-691-3239
E-mail: marketing@cup.org
www.cup.org

3002   International Journal of Aging and Human Developments
Baywood Publishing Company
26 Austin Avenue
Box 337
Amityville, NY 11701-3052
631-691-1270
800-638-7819
Fax: 631-691-1770
E-mail: info@baywood.com
www.baywood.com

Stuart Cohen, Owner

$218.00

8 per year   Year Founded: 1973   ISSN 0091-4150

3003   International Journal of Health Services
Baywood Publishing Company
26 Austin Avenue
Box 337
Amityville, NY 11701-3052
631-691-1270
800-638-7819
Fax: 631-691-1770
E-mail: info@baywood.com
www.baywood.com

Stuart Cohen, Owner

$160.00

4 per year   Year Founded: 1970

3004   International Journal of Psychiatry in Medicine
Baywood Publishing Company
26 Austin Avenue
Box 337
Amityville, NY 11701-3052
631-691-1270
800-638-7819
Fax: 631-691-1770
E-mail: info@baywood.com
www.baywood.com

Stuart Cohen, Owner

$160.00

4 per year   Year Founded: 1970   ISSN 0091274

3005   Journal of AHIMA
American Health Information Management Association
233 N Michigan Avenue
21st Floor
Chicago, IL 60601-5809
312-233-1100
Fax: 312-233-1090
E-mail: info@ahima.org
www.ahima.org

Angela Kennedy, EdD, MBA, RHI, President, Chairman
Cassi Birnbaum, MS. RHIA, CP, President / Chair-Elect
Jennifer McManis, RHIT, Speaker of the House
Lynne Thomas Gordon, CEO

Monthly magazine with articles, news and event annoucements from the nonprofit federation of affiliated state health organizations, together representing nearly 12,000 nonprofit and for profit assisted living, nursing facility, developmentally disabled and subacute care providers that care for more than 1.5 million elderly and disabled individuals nationally.

3006   Journal of American Health Information Management Association
American Health Information Management Association
233 N Michigan Avenue
21st Floor
Chicago, IL 60601-5809
312-233-1100
Fax: 312-233-1090
E-mail: info@ahima.org
www.ahima.org

Angela Kennedy, EdD, MBA, RHI, President, Chairman
Cassi Birnbaum, MS. RHIA, CP, President / Chair-Elect
Jennifer McManis, RHIT, Speaker of the House
Lynne Thomas Gordon, CEO

3007   Journal of American Medical Information Association
Hanley & Befus
4720 Montgomery Lane
Suite 500
Bethesda, MD 20814
301-657-1291
Fax: 301-657-1296
E-mail: mail@amia.org
www.www.amia.org

Karen Greenwood, EVP, COO
Ross D. Martin, MD, MHA, Vice President of Policy and Dev
Jeffrey Williamson, M.Ed, Vice President, Education and Ac
Pesha Rubinstein, MPH, CCMEP, Director of Education

3008   Journal of Drug Education
Baywood Publishing Company
26 Austin Avenue
Box 337
Amityville, NY 11701-3052
631-691-2048
800-638-7819
Fax: 631-691-1770
E-mail: info@baywood.com
www.baywood.com

Stuart Cohen, Owner

$160.00

4 per year   Year Founded: 1970

3009 Journal of Education Psychology
American Psychological Association
750 1st Street NE
Washington, DC 20002-4242
202-336-5500
800-374-2721
Fax: 202-336-5500
TDD: 202-336-6123
TTY: 202-336-6123
E-mail: order@apa.org
www.apa.org

Nadine J. Kaslow, Ph.D., President
Barry S. Anton, Ph.D., President-Elect
Donald N. Bersoff, PhD, JD, Past President
Norman B Anderson, Ph.D., CEO, EVP

$102.00

4 per year   ISSN 0022-0663

3010 Journal of Emotional and Behavioral Disorders
Pro-Ed Publications
8700 Shoal Creek Boulevard
Austin, TX 78757-6897
512-451-3246
800-897-3202
Fax: 512-451-8542
E-mail: info@proedinc.com

Donald D Hammill, Owner

An international, multidisciplinary journal featuring articles on research, practice and theory related to individuals with emotional and behavioral disorders and to the professionals who serve them. Presents topics of interest to individuals representing a wide range of disciplines including corrections, psychiatry, mental health, counseling, rehabilitation, education, and psychology. *$39.00*

64 pages 4 per year   ISSN 1063-4266

3011 Journal of Intellectual & Development Disability
Taylor & Francis Publishing
711 3rd Avenue
8th Floor
New York, NY 10017
212-216-7800
800-634-7064
Fax: 212-564-7854
E-mail: orders@taylorandfrancis.com
www.taylorandfrancis.com

3012 Journal of Neuropsychiatry and Clinical Neurosciences
American Neuropsychiatric Association
700 Ackerman Road
Suite 625
Columbus, OH 43202-4505
614-447-2077
E-mail: anpa@osu.edu

Sandy Bornstein, Executive Director
C. Edward Coffey, Treasurer

Official publication of the organization and a benefit of membership. Our mission is to apply neuroscience for the benefit of people. Three core values have been identified for the association: advancing knowledge of brain-behavior relationships, providing a forum for learning, and promoting excellent, scientific and compassionate health care.

3013 Journal of Personality Assessment
Society for Personality Assessment
6109H Arlington Boulevard
Falls Church, VA 22044-2708
703-534-4772
Fax: 703-534-6905
E-mail: manager@spaonline.org
www.personality.org

Ronald J. Ganellen, Ph.D., President
Robert Bornstein, Ph.D., President-Elect
Radhika Krishnamurthy, Psy.D., Past President
John McNulty, Ph.D., Treasurer

Publishes articles dealing with the development, evaluation, refinement and application of personality assessment methods.

102 pages   ISSN 0022-3891

3014 Journal of Positive Behavior Interventions
Pro-Ed Publications
8700 Shoal Creek Boulevard
Austin, TX 78757-6897
512-451-3246
800-897-3202
Fax: 512-451-8542
E-mail: info@proedinc.com

Donald D Hammill, Owner

Deals with principles of positive behavioral support in school, home, and community settings for people with challenges in behavioral adaptation. *$39.00*

64 pages 4 per year   ISSN 1098-3007

3015 Journal of Practical Psychiatry
Williams & Wilkins
351 W Camden Street
Baltimore, MD 21201-2436
410-528-4000
800-882-0483
Fax: 410-528-4414
E-mail: korourke@lww.com
www.lww.com

J Arnold Anthony, Operations

8 pages

3016 Journal of Professional Counseling: Practice, Theory & Research
Texas Counseling Association (TCA)
1204 San Antonio
Suite 201
Austin, TX 78701-1870
512-472-3403
800-580-8144
Fax: 512-472-3756
E-mail: jan@txca.org
www.txca.org

Jan Friese, Executive Director

The Texas Counseling Association is dedicated to providing leadership, advocacy and education to promote the growth and development of the counseling profession and those that are served. *$150.00*

50 pages 2 per year

3017 Journal of the American Medical Informatics Association
American Medical Informatics Association
4720 Montgomery Lane
Suite 500
Bethesda, MD 20814-6052
301-657-1291
Fax: 301-657-1296
E-mail: mail@amia.org
www.amia.org

Karen Greenwood, EVP, COO
Ross D. Martin, MD, MHA, Vice President of Policy and Dev
Jeffrey Williamson, M.Ed, Vice President, Education and Ac
Pesha Rubinstein, MPH, CCMEP, Director of Education

JAMIA is a bi-monthly journal that presents peer-reviewed articles on the spectrum of health care informatics in research, teaching, and application. *$212.00*

3018 Journal of the American Psychiatric Nurses Association
Sage Publications
2455 Teller Road
Thousand Oaks, CA 91320-2234
805-499-0721
800-818-7243
Fax: 800-583-2665
E-mail: journals@sagepub.com
www.sagepub.com

Blaise R Simqu, CEO, President
Tracey A Ozmina, EVP, COO
Chris Hickok, SVP, CFO
Phil Denvir, Global Chief Information Officer

Official Journal of the American Psychiatric Nurses Association *$128.00*

ISSN 1078-3903

3019 Journal of the American Psychoanalytic Association
Analytic Press
101 W Street
Hillsdale, NJ 07642-1421
201-358-9477
800-926-6579
Fax: 201-358-4700
E-mail: TAP@analyticpress.com
www.analyticpress.com

Paul E Stepansky PhD, Managing Director
John Kerr PhD, Sr Editor

JAPA is one of the preeminent psychoanalytic journals. Recognized for the quality of its clinical and theoretical contributions, JAPA is now a major publication source for scientists and humanists whose work elaborates, applies, critiques or impinges on psychoanalysis. Topics include child psychoanalysis and the effectiveness of the intensive treatment of children, boundary violations, problems of memory and false memory syndrome, the concept of working through, the scientific status of psychoanalysis and the relevance or irrevance of infant observation for adult analysis. *$115.00*

300 pages 4 per year Year Founded: 1952 ISSN 0003-0651

3020 Journal of the International Neuropsychological Society
Cambridge University Press
40 W 20th Street
New York, NY 10011-4211
212-924-3900
Fax: 212-691-3239
E-mail: marketing@cup.org
www.cup.org

3021 Key
National Mental Health Consumers Self-Help
1211 Chestnut Street
Lobby 100
Philadelphia, PA 19107-4112
215-751-1810
800-553-4539
Fax: 215-636-6310
TTY: 215-751-9655
E-mail: info@mhselfhelp.org
www.mhselfhelp.org

Violet Phillips, Editor

Provides information for consumers of mental health services/psychiatric survivors on mental health issues, including advocacy and alternative mental health services. *$15.00*

12 pages 4 per year

3022 Mayo Clinic Health Letter
Mayo Clinic
200 1st Street SW
Rochester, MN 55905-2
507-284-2511
E-mail: healthletter@mayo.edu
www.mayoclinic.org

Marilyn Carlson Nelson, Chairman
John H Noseworthy, M.D., President, CEO
Shirley A. Weis, VP, CAO
William C. Rupp, M.D., VP

Helping our subscribers achieve healthier lives by providing useful, easy to understand health information that is timely and of broad interest.

ISSN 0741-6245

3023 Mental & Physical Disability Law Reporter
American Bar Association
1050 Connecticut Ave. N.W.
Suite 400
Washington, DC 20036
202-662-1000
800-285-2221
Fax: 202-662-1032
TTY: 202-662-1012
E-mail: CMPDL@abanet.org
www.abanet.org

James R. Silkenat, President
Robert M. Carlson, Chair, House of Delegates
William C. Hubbard, President-Elect
Lucian T. Pera, Treasurer

Contains bylined articles and summaries of federal and state court opinions and legislative developments addressing persons with mental and physical disabilities.

6 per year Year Founded: 1976 ISSN 0883-7902

3024 Mental Health Law Reporter
Business Publishers Inc.
2222 Sedwick Drive
Suite 101
Durham, NC 27713
301-587-6300
800-223-8720
Fax: 800-508-2592
E-mail: custserv@bpinews.com
www.bpinews.com

Nancy Biglin, Director Marketing

Summary of court cases pertaining to mental health professionals. *$273.00*

12 per year   ISSN 0741-5141

3025 Mental Health Report
Business Publishers Inc.
2222 Sedwick Drive
Suite 101
Durham, NC 27713
301-587-6300
800-223-8720
Fax: 800-508-2592
E-mail: custserv@bpinews.com
www.bpinews.com

Nancy Biglin, Director Marketing

Independent, inside Washington coverage of mental health administration, legislation and regulation, state policy plus research and trends. *$396.00*

26 per year   ISSN 0191-6750

3026 Mentally Disabled and the Law
William S. Hein & Co.
2350 North Forest Rd.
Getzville, NY 14068
716-882-2600
800-828-7571
Fax: 716-883-8100
E-mail: mail@wshein.com
www.wshein.com

William Hein, Chairman
Kevin Marmion, President
Daniel Rosati, SVP
Dick Spinelli, EVP

Offers information on treatment rights, the provider-patient relationship, and the rights of mentally disabled persons in the community. *$80.00*

3027 NAAP Newsletter
National Association for Advancement of Psychoanalysis
80 Eighth Avenue
Suite 1501
New York, NY 10011-5126
212-741-0515
Fax: 212-366-4347
E-mail: NAAP@NAAP.org
www.naap.org

Douglas F. Maxwell, President
Margery Quackenbush, Executive Director
Kirsty Cardinale, NAAP News Editor
Elliott Hom, Art Director

Members: 1400 Institute Members: 40 *$24.00*

16 pages   4x per year

3028 NAMI Advocate
National Alliance for the Mentally Ill
3803 N. Fairfax Dr.
Suite 100
Arlington, VA 22203
703-524-7600
888-999-6264
Fax: 703-524-9094
TDD: 703-516-7227
E-mail: frieda@nami.org
www.nami.org

David Levy, CFO
Lynn Borton, COO
Jean Michel Texier, Chief Information Officer
Katrina Gay, National Director, Communication

Newsletter that provides information on latest research, treatment, and medications for brain disorders. Reviews status major policy and legislation at federal, state, and local levels. Recurring features include interviews, news of research, news of educational opportunities, book reviews, politics, legal issues, and columns titled President's Column, Ask the Doctor, and News You Can Use. Included as NAMI membership benefit.

24-28 pages   24 per year

3029 NAMI Beginnings
National Alliance on Mental Illness
3803 N. Fairfax Dr.
Suite 100
Arlington, VA 22203
703-524-7600
888-999-6264
Fax: 703-524-9094
TDD: 703-516-7227
E-mail: david@nami.org
www.nami.org

David Levy, CFO
Lynn Borton, COO
Jean Michel Texier, Chief Information Officer
Katrina Gay, National Director, Communication

A publication dedicated to the Young Minds of America from the Child and Adolescent Action Center, a free newsletter about children and adolescents living with mental illnesses.

4 per year

3030 NASW News
National Association of Social Works
750 1st Street NE
Suite 700
Washington, DC 20002-4241
202-408-8600
Fax: 202-336-8312
E-mail: press@naswdc.org
www.naswpress.org

Elvira Craig De Silva, President
Cheryl Y. Bradley, Publisher
Sharon Fletcher, Publications Marketing Manager
Kiera White, Marketing Coordinator

3031 Newsletter of the American Psychoanalytic Association
Analytic Press
101 W Street
Hillsdale, NJ 07642-1421

201-358-9477
800-926-6579
Fax: 201-358-4700
E-mail: info@analyticpress.com
www.analyticpress.com

Paul E Stepansky PhD, Managing Director
John Kerr PhD, Sr Editor

A scholarly and clinical resource for all analytic practitioners and students of the field. Articles and essays focused on contemporary social, political and cultural forces as they relate to the practice of psychoanalysis, regular interviews with leading proponents of analysis, essays and reminiscences that chart the evolution of anlaysis in America. The newsletter publishes articles that are rarely if ever found in the journal literature. Sample copies available. *$29.50*

4 per year

3032 North American Society of Adlerian Psychology Newsletter
NASAP
429 E. Dupont Road
#276
Fort Wayne, IN 46825
260-267-8807
Fax: 260-818-2098
E-mail: nasap@msn.com
www.alfredadler.org

Richard Watts, President
Susan Belangee, VP
Steven J. Stein, Past-President
Susan Burak, Treasurer

Relates news and events of the North American Society of Alderian Psychology and regional news of affiliated associations. Recurring features include lists of courses and workshops offered by affiliated associations, reviews of new publications in the field, professional employment opportunities, a calendar of events, and a column titled President's Message. *$20.00*

8 pages 24 per year ISSN 0889-9428

3033 ORTHO Update
American Orthopsychiatric Association
PO Box 202798
Denver, CO 80220
720-708-0187
Fax: 303-366-3471
E-mail: amerortho@aol.com
www.www.aoatoday.com

Mary I. Armstrong, MSW, PhD, President
Deborah Klein Walker, EdD, President-Elect
Donald Wertlieb, PhD, Past President
John Sargent, MD, Treasurer

Intended for members of the Association, who are concerned with the early signs of mental and behavioral disorder and preventive psychiatry. Provides news notes and feature articles on the trends, issues and events that concern mental health, as well as Association news.

6-16 pages 3 per year

3034 Open Minds
Behavioral Health Industry News
163 York Street
Gettysburg, PA 17325-1933
717-334-1329
877-350-6463

Fax: 717-334-0538
E-mail: info@openminds.com
www.openminds.com

Monica Oss, Owner
Casey A. Miller, VP, Administration
Aida Porras, Senior Associate
Jim Jenkins, Senior Associate

Provides information on marketing, financial, and legal trends in the delivery of mental health and chemical dependency benefits and services. Recurring features include interviews, news of research, a calendar of events, job listings, book reviews, notices of publications available, and industry statistics. *$185.00*

12 pages 12 per year ISSN 1043-3880

3035 OpenMinds
Open Minds
163 York Street
Gettysburg, PA 17325-1933
717-334-1329
877-350-6463
Fax: 717-334-0538
E-mail: info@openminds.com
www.openminds.com

Monica Oss, Owner
Casey A. Miller, VP, Administration
Aida Porras, Senior Associate
Jim Jenkins, Senior Associate

Provides information on marketing, financial, and legal trends in the delivery of mental health and chemical dependency benefits and services. Recurring features include interviews, news of research, a calendar of events, job listings, book reviews, notices of publications available, and industry statistics. *$185.00*

12 pages 12 per year ISSN 1043-3880

3036 Perspective on Psychological Science
Association for Psychological Science
1133 15th Street NW
Suite 1000
Washington, DC 20005
202-293-9300
Fax: 202-293-9350
E-mail: akraut@psychologicalscience.org
www.psychologicalscience.org

Linda Bartoshuk, President
Elizabeth A. Phelps, President
Mahzarin R Banaji, President-Elect
Nancy Eisenberg, President-Elect

Perspectives publishes an eclectic mix of provocative reports and articles, including board integrative reviews, overviews of research programs, meta-analysis, theoretical statements, book reviews, and articles on topics such as the philosophy of science, opnion pieces about major issues in the field, autobiographical reflections of senior members in the field, and the occasional humorous essay and sketch.

6 per year Year Founded: 1988 ISSN 1745-6916

3037 Professional Counselor
3201 SW 15th Street
Deerfield Beach, FL 33442-8157
954-360-0909
800-851-9100
Fax: 954-570-8506

E-mail: Gary.Seidler@usjt.com
www.professionalcounselor.com

Robert Ackerman, Editor
Gary Seidler, Executive Consulting Editor
Leah Honarbakhsh, Associate Editor
Lorrie Keip, Director of Continuing Education

The number one publication serving the addictions and mental health fields.

3038 Provider Magazine
American Health Care Association
1201 L Street NW
Washington, DC 20005-4046
202-842-4444
888-656-6669
Fax: 202-842-3860
E-mail: sales@ahca.org
www.www.providermagazine.com

Bruse Yarwood, President
Bill Myers, Senior Editor
Meg LaPorte, Managing Editor
Joanne Erickson, Editor in Chief

Of interest to the professionals who work for the nearly 12,000 nonprofit and for profit assisted living, nursing facility, developmentally disabled and subacute care providers that care for more than 1.5 million elderly and disabled individuals nationally. Provides information, education, and administrative tools that enhance quality at every level.

3039 PsycINFO News
American Psychological Association
750 1st Street NE
Washington, DC 20002-4242
202-336-5500
800-374-2721
Fax: 202-336-5518
TDD: 202-336-6123
TTY: 202-336-6123
E-mail: psycinfo@apa.org
www.apa.org

Nadine J. Kaslow, Ph.D., President
Barry S. Anton, Ph.D., President-Elect
Donald N. Bersoff, PhD, JD, Past President
Norman B Anderson, Ph.D., CEO, EVP

Free newsletter that keeps you up to date on enhancements to PsycINFO products.

4 per year

3040 PsycSCAN Series
American Psychological Association
750 1st Street NE
Washington, DC 20002-4242
202-336-5500
800-374-2721
Fax: 202-336-5518
TDD: 202-336-6123
TTY: 202-336-6123
E-mail: psycinfo@apa.org
www.apa.org

Nadine J. Kaslow, Ph.D., President
Barry S. Anton, Ph.D., President-Elect
Donald N. Bersoff, PhD, JD, Past President
Norman B Anderson, Ph.D., CEO, EVP

Quarterly current awareness print publications in the fields of clinical, developmental, and applied psychology, as well

as learning disorders/mental retardation and behavior analysis and therapy. Contains relevant citations and abstracts from the PsycINFO database. PyscScan: Psychopharmacology is an electronic only publication.

4 per year

3041 Psych Discourse
The Association of Black Psychologists
7119 Allentown Road
Suite 203
Washington, MD 20744
301-449-3082
Fax: 301-449-3084
E-mail: abpsi@abpsi.org
www.abpsi.org

Taasogle Daryl Rowe, Ph.D., President
Kevin Washington, Ph.D., President-Elect
Carolyn Moore, Ph.D., Treasurer
Anisha Lewis, Executive Director

Publishes news of the Association. Recurring features include editorials, news of research, letters to the editor, a calendar of events, and columns titled Social Actions, Chapter News, Publications, and Members in the News. *$110.00*

32-64 pages 12 per year Year Founded: 1969 ISSN 1091-4781

3042 Psychiatric News
American Psychiatric Publishing, Inc.
1000 Wilson Boulevard
Suite 1825
Arlington, VA 22209-3901
703-907-7322
800-368-5777
Fax: 703-907-1091
E-mail: appi@psych.org
www.appi.org

Saul Levin, M.D., M.P.A., CEO, Medical Director
Ron McMillen, Chief Executive Officer
Robert E Hales, M.D., M.B.A., Editor-in-Chief
Rebecca D. Rinehart, Publisher

Psychiatric News is the official newspaper for the American Psychiatric Association. It is published twice a month and mailed to all APA members as a member benefit as well as to about 2, 000 subscribers.

3043 Psychiatric Times
Continuing Medical Education
806 Plaza Three
Jersey City, NJ 07311-1112
949-250-1008
800-993-2632
Fax: 949-250-0445
E-mail: pt@mhsource.com
www.psychiatrictimes.com

John L. Schwartz MD, Founder and Editor Emeritus
Ronald Pies, MD, Editor Emeritus
James L. Knoll, MD, Editor in Chief
George I. Papakostas, M.D., Director, Treatment-Resistant De

Allows you to earn CME credit every month with a clinical article, as well as keeping you up to date on the current news in the field. *$54.95*

12 per year

3044 Psychiatry Drug Alerts
MJ Powers & Company
65 Madison Avenue
Ssite 220
Morristown, NJ 07960-7354
973-889-5398
800-875-0058
E-mail: psych@alertpubs.com

Evelyn Powers, Owner

Discusses drugs used in the psychiatric field, including side effects and risks. *$63.00*

8 pages 12 per year ISSN 0894-4873

3045 Psychiatry Research
Customer Support Department
PO Box 945
New York, NY 10159-945
212-633-3730
888-437-4636
Fax: 212-633-3680
www.elsevier.nl/locate/psychres

ISSN 0165-1781

3046 Psychological Abstracts
PsycINFO/American Psychological Association
750 1st Street NE
Washington, DC 20002-4242
202-336-5500
800-374-2721
Fax: 202-336-5518
TDD: 202-336-6123
TTY: 202-336-6123
E-mail: psycinfo@apa.org
www.apa.org

Nadine J. Kaslow, Ph.D., President
Barry S. Anton, Ph.D., President-Elect
Donald N. Bersoff, PhD, JD, Past President
Norman B Anderson, Ph.D., CEO, EVP

Print index containing citations and abstracts for journal articles, books, and book chapters in psychology and related disciplines. Annual indexes.

12 per year

3047 Psychological Assessment Resources INC
16130 North Florida Avenue
Lutz, FL 33549
813-449-4065
800-331-8378
Fax: 800-725-9329
www.www4.parinc.com

R. Bob Smith III, PhD, Chairman, CEO
Cathy Smith, VP, Community Relations

3048 Psychological Science
Association for Psychological Science
1133 15th Street NW
Suite 1000
Washington, DC 20005
202-293-9300
Fax: 202-293-9350
E-mail: akraut@psychologicalscience.org
www.psychologicalscience.org

Linda Bartoshuk, President
Elizabeth A. Phelps, President

Mahzarin R Banaji, President-Elect
Nancy Eisenberg, President-Elect

The flagship journal of the APS, it publishes cutting edge research articles, short reports, and research reports spanning the entire spectrum of the science of psychology. The Journal is the source for the latest findings in cognitive, social, developmental and health psychology, as well as behavioral neuroscience and biopsychology.

12 per year Year Founded: 1988 ISSN 0956-7976

3049 Psychological Science Agenda
American Psychological Association
750 1st Street NE
Washington, DC 20002-4242
202-336-5500
800-374-2721
Fax: 202-336-5518
TDD: 202-336-6123
TTY: 202-336-6123
E-mail: psycinfo@apa.org
www.apa.org/science/psa/psacover.html

Nadine J. Kaslow, Ph.D., President
Barry S. Anton, Ph.D., President-Elect
Donald N. Bersoff, PhD, JD, Past President
Norman B Anderson, Ph.D., CEO, EVP

This newsletter disseminates information on scientific psychology, including news on activities of the Association and congressional and federal advocacy efforts of the Directorate. Recurring features include reports of meetings, news of research, notices of publications available, interviews, and the columns titled Science Directorate News, On Behalf of Science, Science Briefs, Announcements, and Funding Opportunities.

16-20 pages 6 per year ISSN 1040-404X

3050 Psychological Science in the Public Interest
Association for Psychological Science
1133 15th Street NW
Suite 1000
Washington, DC 20005
202-293-9300
Fax: 202-293-9350
E-mail: akraut@psychologicalscience.org
www.psychologicalscience.org

Linda Bartoshuk, President
Elizabeth A. Phelps, President
Mahzarin R Banaji, President-Elect
Nancy Eisenberg, President-Elect

PSPI is a unique journal featuring comprehensive and compelling views of issues that are of direct relevance to the general public. Reviews are written by teams of award-winning specialists representing a range of viewpoints, and are intended to assess the current state-of-the-science with regard to the topic.

3 per year Year Founded: 1988 ISSN 1529-1006

3051 Psychology Teacher Network Education Directorate
American Psychological Association
750 1st Street NE
Washington, DC 20002-4242
202-336-5500
800-374-2721
Fax: 202-336-5518
TDD: 202-336-6123

TTY: 202-336-6123
E-mail: psycinfo@apa.org
www.apa.org

Nadine J. Kaslow, Ph.D., President
Barry S. Anton, Ph.D., President-Elect
Donald N. Bersoff, PhD, JD, Past President
Norman B Anderson, Ph.D., CEO, EVP

Provides descriptions of experiments and demonstrations aimed at introducing topics as a basis for classroom lectures or discussion. Recurring features include news and announcements of courses, workshops, funding sources, and meetings; reviews of teaching aids; and reports of innovative programs or curricula occurring in schools, interviews and brief reports from prominent psychologists. *$15.00*

16 pages 5 per year

3052 Psychophysiology
Cambridge University Press
40 W 20th Street
New York, NY 10011-4211
212-924-3900
Fax: 212-691-3239
E-mail: marketing@cup.org
www.cup.org

3053 Psychosomatic Medicine
American Psychosomatic Society
6728 Old McLean Village Drive
McLean, VA 22101-3906
703-556-9222
Fax: 703-556-8729
E-mail: info@psychosomatic.org
www.psychosomatic.org

William Lovallo, President
Karen L. Weihs, M.D., President
Mustafa al'Absi, Ph.D., President-Elect
George K. Degnon, CAE, Executive Director

News and event annoucements, examines the scientific understanding of the interrelationships among biological, psychological, social and behavioral factors in human health and disease, and the integration of the fields of science that separately examine each.

3054 Psychotherapy Bulletin
American Psychological Association
750 First Street NE
Washington, DC 20002-4242
202-336-5500
800-374-2721
Fax: 202-336-5518
TDD: 202-336-6123
TTY: 202-336-6123
E-mail: psycinfo@apa.org
www.apa.org

Nadine J. Kaslow, Ph.D., President
Barry S. Anton, Ph.D., President-Elect
Donald N. Bersoff, PhD, JD, Past President
Norman B Anderson, Ph.D., CEO, EVP

Recurring features include letters to the editor, news of research, reports of meetings, news of educational opportunities, committee reports, legislative issues, and columns titled Washington Scene, Finance, Marketing, Professional Liability, Medical Psychology Update, and Substance Abuse. *$8.00*

50 pages 4 per year

3055 Psychotherapy Finances
Managed Care Strategies & Psychotherapy
Finances
14255 U.S. Highway 1
Suite 286
Juno Beach, FL 33408-1612
561-624-1155
800-869-8450
Fax: 561-743-3504
E-mail: john@psyfin.com
www.www.psyfin.com

John Klein, Editor
John Nelander, Managing Editor
Anne Marie Church, Marketing Director
Herbert E. Klein, Publisher

3056 Research and Training for Children's Mental Health-Update
University of South Florida
13301 Bruce B Downs Boulevard
Florida Mental Health Institute
Tampa, FL 33612-3807
813-974-4565

Services and research on children with emotional disorders.

2 per year

3057 Rural Mental Health Journal
NARMH
25 Massachusetts Ave NW
Suite 500
Washington, DC 20001
202-942-4276
E-mail: info@narmh.org
www.narmh.org

Jerry Parker, President
Paul Mackie, President-Elect
Linda Werlein, Past-President
David Weden, Treasurer

Provides a information for rural mental health professionals and advocates.

4 per year

3058 Smooth Sailing
Depression and Related Affective Disorders
Association
600 N Wolfe Street
John Hopkins Hospital Meyer 3-181
Baltimore, MD 21287-5
Fax: 410-614-3241
www.med.jhu.edu/drada/

Outreach to students and parents through schools.

4 per year

3059 Social Work
NASW Press
750 1st Street NE
Suite 700
Washington, DC 20002-4241
202-408-8600
Fax: 202-336-8312
E-mail: press@naswdc.org
www.naswpress.org

Elvira Craig De Silva, President
Cheryl Y. Bradley, Publisher
Sharon Fletcher, Publications Marketing Manager
Kiera White, Marketing Coordinator

3060 Social Work Abstracts
NASW Press
750 1st Street NE
Suite 700
Washington, DC 20002-4241
202-408-8600
Fax: 202-336-8312
E-mail: press@naswdc.org
www.naswpress.org

Elvira Craig De Silva, President
Cheryl Y. Bradley, Publisher
Sharon Fletcher, Publications Marketing Manager
Kiera White, Marketing Coordinator

3061 Social Work Research
NASW Press
750 1st Street NE
Suite 700
Washington, DC 20002-4241
202-408-8600
Fax: 202-336-8312
E-mail: press@naswdc.org
www.naswpress.org

Elvira Craig De Silva, President
Cheryl Y. Bradley, Publisher
Sharon Fletcher, Publications Marketing Manager
Kiera White, Marketing Coordinator

3062 Social Work in Education
NASW Press
750 1st Street NE
Suite 700
Washington, DC 20002-4241
202-408-8600
Fax: 202-336-8312
E-mail: press@naswdc.org
www.naswpress.org

Elvira Craig De Silva, President
Cheryl Y. Bradley, Publisher
Sharon Fletcher, Publications Marketing Manager
Kiera White, Marketing Coordinator

3063 Society for Adolescent Psychiatry Newsletter
PO Box 570218
Dallas, TX 75357-218
972-613-0985
Fax: 972-613-5532
E-mail: info@adolpsych.org
www.adolpsych.org

Mohan Nair, President
Gregg Dwyer, President
Sheldon Glass, President Elect
Gregory P. Barclay, VP

Puts psychiatrists in touch with an informed cross-section
of the profession from all over North America. Dedicated
to education development and advocacy of adolescents and
the adolescent psychiatric field.

3064 The Bulletin
American Society of Psychoanalytic Physicians
13528 Wisteria Drive
Germantown, MD 20874-1049
301-540-3197
E-mail: cfcotter@aspp.net
www.aspp.net

Christine Cotter, Executive Director

The Bulletin of the American Society of Psychoanalustic
Physicians is a professional publication containing articles
by members, meeting speakers and other professionals in
addition to newes about the society. Papers are accepted
based on a peer review process.

15 pages 1 per year

3065 World Federation for Mental Health Newsletter
World Federation for Mental Health
PO Box 807
Occoquania, VA 22125
703-838-7525
Fax: 703-490-6926
E-mail: info@wfmh.com
www.wfmh.com

George Christodoulou, President, Greece
Deborah Wan, Hong Kong, Immediate Past President
Gabriel Ivbijaro, President Elect, U.K.
Gwen Dixon, Office Administrator

World-wide mental health reports. Education and advocacy
on mental health issues. Working to protect the human
rights of those defined as mentally ill.

8 pages 1 per year Year Founded: 1984

Testing & Evaluation

3066 Assessment and Treatment of Anxiety
Disorders in Persons with Mental Retardation
NADD
132 Fair Street
Kingston, NY 12401-4802
845-331-4336
800-331-5362
Fax: 845-331-4569
E-mail: info@thenadd.org
www.thenadd.org

Donna McNelis, Ph.D., President
Dan Baker, Ph.D., VP
Julia Pearce, Secretary
L. Jarrett Barnhill, M.D., Treasurer

Anxiety disorders as a group are the commonest mental
health disorders seen in the general population, as they
probably also are in people with developmental disorders.
This upgraded version of a book first published in 1996 describes issues of diagnosis and treatment of various anxiety
disorders, and includes modalities for staff training in those
conditions. *$19.95*

ISBN 1-572560-01-0

3067 Assessment of Neuropsychiatry and Mental
Health Services
American Psychiatric Publishing, Inc.
1000 Wilson Boulevard
Suite 1825
Arlington, VA 22209-3901

703-907-7322
800-368-5777
Fax: 703-907-1091
E-mail: appi@psych.org
www.appi.org

Ron McMillen, Chief Executive Officer
Robert E. Hales MD, M.B.A, Editor-in-Chief
John McDuffie, Editorial Director, Associate Pu
Rebecca D. Rinehart, Publisher

Examines the importance of an integrated approach to neuropsychiatric conditions and looks at ways to overcome the difficulties in assessing medical disorders in psychiatric populations. Addresses neuropsychiatric disorders and their costs and implications on policy. *$94.00*

448 pages Year Founded: 1999 ISBN 0-880487-30-5

3068 Attention-Deficit/Hyperactivity Disorder Test: a Method for Identifying Individuals with ADHD
Pro.Ed
8700 Shoal Creek Boulevard
Austin, TX 78757-6897
512-451-3246
800-897-3202
Fax: 512-451-8542
E-mail: general@proedinc.com
www.www.proedinc.com

Donald D Hammill, Owner

An effective instrument for identifying and evaluating attention - deficit disorders in persons ages three to twenty-three. Designed for use in schools and clinics, the test is easily completed by teachers, parents and others who are knowledgeable about the referred individual. *$110.00*

Year Founded: 1995

3069 Behavioral and Emotional Rating Scale
Pro.Ed
8700 Shoal Creek Boulevard
Austin, TX 78757-6897
512-451-3246
800-897-3202
Fax: 512-451-8542
E-mail: general@proedinc.com
www.www.proedinc.com

Donald D Hammill, Owner

Helps to measure the personal strengths of children ages five through eighteen. Contains 52 items that measure five aspects of a child's strength: interpersonal strength, involvement with family, intrapersonal strength, school functioning, and affective strength. Provides overall strength score and five subtest scores. Identifies individual behavioral and emotional strengths of children, the areas in which individual strengths need to be developed, and the goals for individual treatment plans. *$165.00*

Year Founded: 1998

3070 Childhood History Form for Attention Disorders
A.D.D. Warehouse
300 NW 70th Avenue
Suite 102
Plantation, FL 33317-2360
954-792-8100
800-233-9273
Fax: 954-792-8545

E-mail: websales@addwarehouse.com
www.addwarehouse.com

Harvey C Parker, Owner

This form is completed by parents prior to a history taking session. It is designed to be used in conjunction with standardized assessment questionaires utilized in the evaluation of attention disorders. 25 per package. *$45.00*

10 pages

3071 Children's Depression Inventory
A.D.D. Warehouse
300 NW 70th Avenue
Suite 102
Plantation, FL 33317-2360
954-792-8100
800-233-9273
Fax: 954-792-8545
E-mail: websales@addwarehouse.com
www.addwarehouse.com

Harvey C Parker, Owner

A self-report, symptom-oriented scale which requires at least a first grade reading level and was designed for school-aged children and adolescents. The CDI has 27 items, each of which consists of three choices. Quickscore form scoring make the inventories easy and economical to administer. The profile contains the following five factors plus a total score normed according to age and sex: negative mood, interpersonal problems, ineffectiveness, anhedonia and negative self-esteem. Contains ten items and provides a general indication of depressive symptoms. *$148.00*

3072 Clinical Evaluations of School Aged Children
Professional Resource Press
PO Box 3197
Sarasota, FL 34230-3197
941-343-9601
800-443-3364
Fax: 941-343-9201
E-mail: cs.prpress@gmail.com
www.prpress.com

Laurie Girsch, Managing Editor

This book delineates the specific symptoms and behaviors associated with each DSM - IV diagnostic syndrome and provides an exceptionally well designed system for communicating diagnostic findings with great clarity when working with parents and professionals from different disciplines. *$34.95*

376 pages Year Founded: 1998 ISBN 1-568870-27-2

3073 Clinical Interview of the Adolescent: From Assessment and Formulation to Treatment Planning
Charles C Thomas Publisher Ltd.
2600 S 1st Street
Springfield, IL 62704-4730
217-789-8980
800-258-8980
Fax: 217-789-9130
E-mail: books@ccthomas.com
www.ccthomas.com

Michael P Thomas, President

This book addresses the process of interviewing troubled and psychologically disturbed adolescents who are seen in hospital settings, schools, courts, clinics, and residential facilities. Interviews with adolescents, younger children or adults should follow a logical, sequential and integrated procedure, accomplishing diagnostic closure and the development of a treatment formulation. The nine chapters cover the theoretical and developmental concerns of adolescence; the initial referral; meeting with parents; the therapist; getting acquainted; getting to the heart of the matter; making order out of disorder; the reasons and rationale for the behavior problems. *$59.95*

234 pages Year Founded: 1997 ISBN 0-398067-79-1

3074 Concise Guide to Assessment and Management of Violent Patients
American Psychiatric Publishing, Inc.
1000 Wilson Boulevard
Suite 1825
Arlington, VA 22209-3901
703-907-7322
800-368-5777
Fax: 703-907-1091
E-mail: appi@psych.org
www.appi.org

Ron McMillen, Chief Executive Officer
Robert E. Hales MD, M.B.A, Editor-in-Chief
John McDuffie, Editorial Director, Associate Pu
Rebecca D. Rinehart, Publisher

Written by an expert on violence, this edition provides current information on psychopharmacology, safety of clinicians and how to deal with threats of violence to the clinician. *$32.95*

180 pages Year Founded: 1996 ISBN 0-880483-44-X

3075 Conducting Insanity Evaluations
Guilford Press
72 Spring Street
New York, NY 10012-4068
212-431-9800
800-365-7006
Fax: 212-966-6708
E-mail: info@guilford.com
www.www.guilford.com

Bob Matloff, President
Seymour Weingarten, Editor-in-Chief

Great resource for both psychologists and lawyers. Covers legal standards and their applications to clinical work. Mental health professionals who evaluate defendants or consult to courts on criminal matters will find this a useful resource. *$50.00*

342 pages Year Founded: 2000 ISBN 1-572305-21-5

3076 Conners' Rating Scales
Pro.Ed
8700 Shoal Creek Boulevard
Austin, TX 78757-6897
512-451-3246
800-897-3202
Fax: 512-451-8542
E-mail: general@proedinc.com
www.www.proedinc.com

Donald D Hammill, Owner

Conner's Rating Scales are a result of 30 years of research on childhood and adolescent psychopathology and problem behavior. This revision adds a number of enhancements to a set of measures that has long been the standard instruments

for the measurement of attention-deficit/hyperactivity disorder in children and adolescents. *$153.00*

Year Founded: 1997

3077 Depression and Anxiety in Youth Scale
Pro.Ed
8700 Shoal Creek Boulevard
Austin, TX 78757-6897
512-451-3246
800-897-3202
Fax: 512-451-8542
E-mail: general@proedinc.com
www.www.proedinc.com

Donald D Hammill, Owner

A unique battery of three norm-referenced scales useful in identifying major depressive disorder and overanxious disorders in children and adolescents. *$150.00*

Year Founded: 1994

3078 Diagnosis and Treatment of Multiple Personality Disorder
Guilford Press
72 Spring Street
New York, NY 10012-4068
212-431-9800
800-365-7006
Fax: 212-966-6708
E-mail: info@guilford.com
www.www.guilford.com

Bob Matloff, President
Seymour Weingarten, Editor-in-Chief

Comprehensive and integrated approach to a complex psychotherapeutic process. From first interview to crisis management to final post-integrative treatment each step is systematically reviewed, with detailed instructions on specific diagnostic and therapeutic techniques and examples of clinical applications. Specially geared to the needs of therapists, novice or expert alike, struggling with their first MPD case. *$48.00*

351 pages Year Founded: 1989 ISBN 0-898621-77-1

3079 Diagnosis and Treatment of Sociopaths and Clients with Sociopathic Traits
NewHarbinger Publications
5674 Shattuck Avenue
Oakland, CA 94609-1662
510-652-0215
800-748-6273
Fax: 800-652-1613
E-mail: customerservice@newharbinger.com
www.newharbinger.com

Matthew McKay, Owner

This text presents a full course of treatment, with special attention to safety issues and other concerns for different client populations in a range of treatment settings. *$49.95*

208 pages Year Founded: 1996 ISBN 1-572240-47-4

3080 Draw a Person: Screening Procedure for Emotional Disturbance
Pro.Ed
8700 Shoal Creek Boulevard
Austin, TX 78757-6897
512-451-3246
800-897-3202

Fax: 512-451-8542
E-mail: general@proedinc.com
www.www.proedinc.com

Donald D Hammill, Owner

Helps identify children and adolescents ages six through
seventeen who have emotional problems and require further evaluation. *$140.00*

Year Founded: 1991

3081 Handbook of Psychological Assessment
John Wiley & Sons
111 River Street
Hoboken, NJ 07030-5774
201-748-6000
Fax: 201-748-6088
E-mail: info@wiley.com
www.wiley.com

Stephen M. Smith, President, CEO
MJ O'Leary, SVP, Human Resources
Edward J. Melando, SVP, Corporate Controller
Gary M. Rinck, SVP, General Counsel

Classic, revised and new psychological tests are all considered for validity and overall reliability in the light of current clinical thought and scientific development. The new
edition has expanded coverage of neuropsychological assessment and reports on assessment and treatment planning
in the age of managed care. *$95.00*

862 pages Year Founded: 1997 ISBN 0-471419-79-6

3082 Harvard Medical School Guide to Suicide Assessment and Intervention
Jossey-Bass Publishers
989 Market Street
San Francisco, CA 94103-1708
415-433-1740
Fax: 415-433-0499
www.leadertoleader.org

Debra Hunter, President

The definitive guide for helping mental health professionals determine the risk for suicide and appropriate treatment
strategies for suicidal or at-risk patients. *$85.00*

736 pages ISBN 0-787943-03-7

3083 Health Watch
28 Maple Avenue
Medford, MA 02155-7118
781-395-5515
800-643-2757
Fax: 781-395-6547
www.healthwatch.cc

Bill Govostes, Owner

On site performer of preventative health screening services
and disease risk management programming. Specializing in
point of care testing, we perform fast and accurate health
screening tests and services to assist in indentifying participant's risk for developing future disease.

Year Founded: 1987

3084 Scale for Assessing Emotional Disturbance
Pro.Ed
8700 Shoal Creek Boulevard
Austin, TX 78757-6897
512-451-3246
800-897-3202

Fax: 512-451-8542
E-mail: general@proedinc.com
www.www.proedinc.com

Donald D Hammill, Owner

Helps you identify children and adolescents who qualify
for the federal special education category Emotional Disturbance. *$100.00*

Year Founded: 1998

3085 Screening for Brain Dysfunction in Psychiatric Patients
Charles C Thomas Publisher Ltd.
2600 S 1st Street
Springfield, IL 62704-4730
217-789-8980
800-258-8980
Fax: 217-789-9130
E-mail: books@ccthomas.com
www.ccthomas.com

Michael P Thomas, President

This book presents how medical diseases can be
misdiagnosed as psychiatric disorders and how clinicians
without extensive training in the neurosciences can do a
competent job of screening psychiatric clients for possible
brain disorders. The research cited in this book, dating back
to the 1890's, establishes beyond a doubt that such
misdiagnoses are more common than most clinicians would
guess. This book focuses on one type of medical condition
that is likely to be misdiagnosed: brain injuries and illnesses. *$36.95*

148 pages Year Founded: 1998 ISBN 0-398069-21-2

3086 Sexual Dysfunction: Guide for Assessment and Treatment
Guilford Press
72 Spring Street
New York, NY 10012-4068
212-431-9800
800-365-7006
Fax: 212-966-6708
E-mail: info@guilford.com
www.www.guilford.com

Bob Matloff, President
Seymour Weingarten, Editor-in-Chief

Designed as a succinct guide to contemporary sex therapy,
this book provides an empirically based overview of the
most common sexual dysfunctions and a step-by-step manual for their assessment and treatment. Provides a
biopsychosocial model of sexual function and dysfunction
and describes the authors' general approach to management
of sexual difficulties. *$25.00*

212 pages Year Founded: 1991 ISBN 0-898622-07-7

3087 Social-Emotional Dimension Scale
Pro.Ed
8700 Shoal Creek Boulevard
Austin, TX 78757-6897
512-451-3246
800-897-3202
Fax: 512-451-8542
E-mail: general@proedinc.com
www.www.proedinc.com

Donald D Hammill, Owner

A rating scale for teachers, counselors, and psychologists to screen age 5 1/2 through 18 1/2 who are at risk for conduct disorders, behavior problems, or emotional disturbance. It assesses physical/fear reaction, depressive reaction, avoidance of peer interaction, avoidance of teacher interaction, aggressive interaction, and inappropriate behaviors.
$149.00

Year Founded: 1986

3088 Test Collection at ETS
Educational Testing Service
660 Rosedale Road
Princeton, NJ 08541-1
609-921-9000
Fax: 609-734-5410
www.www.ets.org

Kurt M Landgraf, CEO

Provides 1, 200 plus tests available in microfiche or downloadable for reaserch.

Training & Recruitment

3089 Ackerman Institute for the Family
936 Broadway
2nd Floor
New York, NY 10010
212-879-4900
Fax: 21- 74- 020
E-mail: ackerman@ackerman.org
www.ackerman.org

Lois Braverman, LCSW, President, CEO
Marcia Sheinberg, LCSW, Director of Training and Clinica
Martha E. Edwards, PhD, Director of the Center for the D
Peter Fraenkel, PhD, Director of the Center for Work

A not-for-profit agency devoted to the treatment and study of families and to the training of family therapists. One of the first training institutions in the United States committed to promoting family functioning and family mental health, Acker is dedicated to helping all families at all stages of family life.

3090 Alfred Adler Institute (AAI)
372 Central Park West
New York, NY 10025
212-254-1048
E-mail: director@alfredadler-ny.org
www.www.aai-ny.org

Ellen Mendel, M.Ed., M.S., M, President, Chair of the Board
Brock Hotaling, BSc, Executive Director
Fredrica Levinson, M.A., C.R.C., Dean of Students
Ellen Mendel, M.Ed., M.S., M, Director, Admissions

Offers training in psychotherapy and analysis to psychiatrists, psychologists, social workers, teachers, clergymen and other related professional persons. Conducts three-year program to provide an understanding of the dynamics of personality and interpersonal relationships and to teach therapeutic methods and techniques. Presents the theory of Individual Psychology as formulated by Alfred Adler. Publications: Journal of Individual Psychology, quarterly. Annual meeting. Semi-annual seminar.

3091 Alliance Behavioral Care: University of Cincinnati Psychiatric Services
222 Piedmont Avenue
Suite 8800
Cincinnati, OH 45219-4231
513-475-8622
800-926-8862
www.alliancebehavioral.com

A regional managed behavioral healthcare organization committed to continuously improving the resources and programs that serve their members and providers. Their goal is to provide resources that improve the well-being of those they serve and to integrate the behavioral healthcare within the overall healthcare systems.

3092 Alliant International University
Los Angeles Campus
1000 South Fremont Avenue, Unit 5
Alhambra, CA 91803-8835
626-270-3300
866-825-5426
TDD: 800-585-5087
E-mail: admissions@alliant.edu
www.alliant.edu

Geoffrey Cox PhD, President

Offers industry-specific training to mid-management and supervisory personnel employed in behavioral healthcare organizations.

3093 Alton Ochsner Medical Foundation, Psychiatry Residency
1514 Jefferson Highway
New Orleans, LA 70121-2429
504-842-3000
Fax: 504-736-4978
E-mail: gme@ochsner.org

Doris Ratcliff, Manager

3094 American Academy of Child and Adolescent Psychiatry
3615 Wisconsin Avenue NW
Washington, DC 20016-3007
202-966-7300
Fax: 202-966-2891
E-mail: communications@aacap.org
www.aacap.org

Laurence Lee Greenhill, President
Robert Hendren, President
William Bernet, Treasurer
Michael Linsky, Assistant Director

A non-profit membership based organization composed of over 7, 500 child and adolescent psychiatrists and other interested physicians. Promotes mentally healthy children, adolescents and families through research, training, advocacy, prevention, comprehensive diagnosis and treatment, peer support and collaboration.

Year Founded: 1953

3095 American College of Healthcare Executives
One N Franklin Street
Suite 1700
Chicago, IL 60606-3529
312-424-2800
Fax: 312-424-0023
E-mail: contact@ache.org
www.ache.org

Christine M. Candio, RN, FACHE, Chairman
Richard D. Cordova, FACHE, Chairman-Elect
Diana L. Smalley, FACHE, Immediate Past Chairman
Deborah J. Bowen, FACHE, President, CEO

International professional society of nearly 30, 000 healthcare executives. ACHE is known for its prestigious credentialing and educational programs. ACHE is also known for its journal, Journal of Healthcare Management, and magazine, Healthcare Executive, as well as ground-breaking research and career development programs. Through its efforts, ACHE works toward its goal of improving the health status of society by advancing healthcare management excellence.

3096 American College of Legal Medicine
1100 E Woodfield Road
Suite 350
Schaumburg, IL 60173-5125
847-969-0283
Fax: 847-517-7229
E-mail: info@aclm.org
www.aclm.org

Thomas R. McLean, MD, MS, JD, FC, President-Elect
Victoria Green, MD, JD, MBA, MH, Past President
Daniel L. Orr, II, DDS PhD JD MD, Treasurer
Charles W. Hinnant, Jr., MD, JD, , Secretary

The mission of ACWHP is to advance women-centered healthcare.

3097 Andrus Children's Center
Julia Dyckman Andrus Memorial
1156 N Broadway
Yonkers, NY 10701-1108
914-965-3700

Tecla Critelli, President/CEO

Vision is to 'give opportunity to youth.' A private, non-profit community agency that provides assessment, treatment, education and preventive services for children and their families in residential, day and other restorative programs. Mission is to serve families, without regard to background or financial status, who have or are at risk for developing behavioral health problems. A highly qualified and caring staff uses established techniques and innovative programs to accomplish these purposes.

3098 Asian Pacific Development Center for Human Development
1537 Alton Street
Aurora, CO 80010
303-923-2920
Fax: 303-388-1172
E-mail: info@apdc.org
www.apdc.org

Christine Wanifuchi, CEO
Eri Asano, Clinic Director
Jinny Kim, Director of Strategic Developmen
Edward McCarthy, Office Coordinator

A community-based non-profit organization that serves the needs of a growing population of Asian American and Pacific Islander residents throughout Colorado. APDC operates a licensed Community Mental Health Clinic and a multicultural Interpreters Bank.

Year Founded: 1980

3099 Behavioral Healthcare Center
464 Commonwealth Street
#147
Belmont, MA 02478
617-393-3935
Fax: 617-393-1808
E-mail: cberney@mah.harvard.edu
www.academicpsychiatry.org

Carole Berney, Administrative Director
Joan Anzia, President

A behavorial health facility providing consultation in psychiatry, psychopharmacology and psychotherapy to primary care physicians and their patients.

3100 Behavioral Medicine and Biofeedback Consultants
150 SW 12th Avenue
Suite 207
Pompano Beach, FL 33069-3238
954-202-6200
E-mail: info@behavioralmedicine.com
www.behavioralmedicine.com

Gary S Traub, Owner, Director

3101 Bowling Green University Psychology Department
Bowling Green State University
Bowling Green, OH 43403-0001
419-372-2531
Fax: 419-372-6013
www.www.bgsu.edu

Sherideen S. Stoll, VP, Finance and Administration,
Steve Krakoff, Associate VP, Capital Planning a
John Ellinger, Chief Information Officer
Bradley Leigh, Executive Director, Business Ope

3102 Brandeis University/Heller School
415 South Street
Waltham, MA 02453-2700
781-736-2000
Fax: 781-736-4416
www.brandeis.edu

Fred M. Lawrence, President
David A. Bunis, Senior Vice President, Chief of
Marianne Cwalina, Senior Vice President for Financ
Ellen de Graffenreid, Senior Vice President for Commun

3103 Brandeis University: Schneider Institute for Health Policy
Brandeis University
415 South Street, Mailstop 035
Waltham, MA 02454-9110
781-736-3900
Fax: 781-736-3905
E-mail: colnon@brandeis.edu
www.sihp.brandeis.edu

Stanley S Wallack, Ph.D., Executive Director

Committed to developing an objective, university-based entity capable of providing research assistance to the Federal government on the major problems it faced in financing and delivering care to the elderly, disabled and poor. Our role has always been to solve complex health care problems, and to link research studies to policy change.

3104 Breining Institute College for the Advanced Study of Addictive Disorders
8894 Greenback Lane
Orangevale, CA 95662-4019
916-987-0662
E-mail: college@breining.edu
www.breininginstitute.net

Kathy Breining, Administrator

The mission of Breining Institute faculty and staff is to ensure a consistent standard of higher education, training, testing and certification of professionals working in the field of addictions.

Year Founded: 1986

3105 California Institute of Behavioral Sciences
701 Welch Road
Suite #B 203
Palo Alto, CA 94304-1705
650-325-1501
E-mail: info@ecibs.net
www.www.ecibs.net

Sanjay Jasuja, Medical Director

Provides the following services for children, adolescents, adults and families on national and international level: Objective testing and comprehensive treatment for ADHD/ADD, depression, manic depressive disorder or Bipolar disorder, anxiety disorders, including obsessive compulsive disorder, panic attacks, phobias, post-traumatic stress disorder, Tourette's syndrome, stuttering, psychopharmacology, stress and anger control, violence and workplace issues, learning and behavior problems, and parenting support groups.

3106 Cambridge Hospital: Department of Psychiatry
1493 Cambridge Street
Cambridge, MA 02139-1047
617-665-1000
E-mail: webmaster@challiance.org
www.www.challiance.org

Jay Burke, MD, MPH, Chairman, Chief of Psychiatry
Joy Curtis, SVP, Human Resources
Elizabeth Cadigan, RN, MSN, Senior Vice President, Patient C
Judith Klickstein, SVP, Information Technology and

3107 Center for Health Policy Studies
10440 Little Patuxent Parkway
10th Floor
Columbia, MD 21044-3561
410-715-9400

3108 College of Health and Human Services: SE Missouri State
901 S National Ave
Springfield, MO 65897-27
417-836-5000
www.missouristate.edu

Dr.Frank Einhellig, Provost
Dr.Chris Craig, Associate Provost, Faculty & Aca
Dr.Rachelle Darabi, Associate Provost for Student De
Dr.Joye Norris, Associate Provost for Access and

3109 College of Southern Idaho
315 Falls Avenue
PO Box 1238
Twin Falls, ID 83303-1238

208-732-6221
800-680-0274
Fax: 208-736-4705
E-mail: info@csi.edu
www.csi.edu

Jerry Beck, President
Dr.Jeff Fox, President
Jerry Gee, Executive VP/CAO
Dr.Todd Schwarz, EVP, CAO

Addiction Studies

3110 Colonial Services Board
1657 Merrimac Trail
Williamsburg, VA 23185-5624
757-220-3200
Fax: 757-229-7173
TDD: 757-253-4377
www.colonialcsb.org

David Coe, Executive Director
Keith German, Director, Administrative Service
Dan Longo, Director, Behavioural Services
Nancy Shackleford, Director, Human Resources

MR and substance abuse

3111 Daniel and Yeager Healthcare Staffing Solutions
6767 Old Madison Pike
Suite 690
Huntsville, AL 35806-2198
256-551-1070
800-955-1919
Fax: 256-551-5075
E-mail: info@dystaffing.com
www.dystaffing.com

Mark Kingsley, VP
Susie Brown, COO
Mike Williams, CFO
Hans Edenfield, Director, Human Resources

Setting the standard for excellence in health care staffing.

3112 Dartmouth Univerisity: Department of Psychiatry
Dartmouth-Hitchcock Medical School
One Medical Center Drive
Lebanon, NH 03756
603-650-7075
Fax: 603-650-5842
www.geiselmed.dartmouth.edu/psych

3113 East Carolina University Department of Psychiatric Medicine
600 Moye Boulevard
Room 4E-98
Greenville, NC 27834-4300
252-744-4440

Joseph B Webster

3114 Emory University School of Medicine, Psychology and Behavior
1440 Clifton Road NE
Atlanta, GA 30322-1053
404-727-5630
Fax: 404-727-0473

3115 Emory University: Psychological Center
36 Eagle Row
Room 270
Atlanta, GA 30322-1122
404-727-7438
Fax: 404-727-0372
E-mail: psych@emory.edu
www.psychology.emory.edu

Harold Gouzoules, Ph.D., Department Chair
Nancy Feng, Research Financial Analyst
Kelly Yates, Program Coordinator
Kate Coblin, Assistant Program Director

Nonprofit community clinic providing low cost counseling and psychological testing services for children and adults.

3116 Fletcher Allen Health Care
111 Colchester Avenue
Burlington, VT 05401-1416
802-847-0000
800-358-1144
www.www.fletcherallen.org

Fletcher Allen Health Care is both a community hospital and, in partnership with the University of Vermont, the state's academic health center. Their mission is to improve the health of the people in the communities they serve by integrating patient care, education and research in a caring environment.

3117 Genesis Learning Center (Devereux)
430 Allied Drive
Nashville, TN 37211-3304
615-832-4222
Fax: 615-832-4577
E-mail: admin@genesislearn.org
www.genesislearn.org

Terance Adams, Executive Director
Chuck Goon, PHR, Human Resource Director

3118 George Washington University
2121 Eye Street, NW
Washington, DC 20052-1
202-994-1000
www.www.gwu.edu

Steven Knapp, President
Steve R. Lerman, Provost, EVP, Academic Affairs
Beth Nolan, SVP, General Counsel
Louis H. Katz, EVP, Treasurer

3119 Haymarket Center, Professional Development
932 W Washington
Chicago, IL 60607-2217
312-226-7984
Fax: 312-226-0047
E-mail: info@hcenter.org
www.hcenter.org

Raymond F. Soucek, President
Donald E. Musil, Executive VP
Dan Lustig, VP, Clinical Services
Leo C. Miller, VP, Support Services

Drug and alcohol treatment programs.

3120 Heartshare Human Services
12 Metro Tech Center
29th Floor
Brooklyn, NY 11201-3858
718-422-4200
E-mail: info@heartshare.org
www.heartshare.org

Ralph A. Subbiondo, Chairman
William R. Guarinello, MS, President/ Ceo
Mia Higgins, Executive VP, Operations, Genera
Evelyn Alvarez, SVP, Developmental Disablilities

A nonprofit human services agency dedicated to improving the lives of people in need of special services and support.

3121 Hillcrest Utica Psychiatric Services
1120 S Utica Street
South Physician Bldg Suite 1000
Tulsa, OK 74104-4012
918-579-8000
www.helmerichwomenscenter.com

Steve Dobbs, CEO

3122 Institute for Behavioral Healthcare
PO Box 5710
Santa Rosa, CA 95402
650-851-8411
800-258-8411
Fax: 707-566-7474
E-mail: staff@iahb.org
www.iahb.org

Gerry Piaget, Ph.D., President
Joan Piaget, Executive Director
Jen Dames, Director, Operations

Non-profit educational organization that is a fully accredited sponsor of continuing education and continuing medical education for mental health, chemical dependency, and substance abuse treatment providers in the United States and Canada. Mission is to provide high-quality training to healthcare professionals as well as to companies and individuals with healthcare-related interests.

3123 Jacobs Institute of Women's Health
950 New Hampshire Avenue
NW, 2nd Floor
Washington, DC 20052
202-994-4184
Fax: 202-296-0025
E-mail: whieditor@gwu.edu
www.jiwh.org

Richard Mauery, MS, MPH, Managing Staff Director
Susan Wood, PhD, Executive Director
Chloe E. Bird, PhD, Editor In Chief
Carol Weisman, PhD, Associate Editor

Working to improve health care for women through research, dialogue and information dissemination. Mission is to identify and study women's health care issues involving the interaction of medical and social systems; facilitate informed dialogue and foster awareness among consumers and providers alike; and promote problem resolution, interdisciplinary coordination and information dissemination at the regional, national and international levels.

3124 John A Burns School of Medicine Department of Psychiatry
651 Ilalo Street
Medical Education Building
Honolulu, HI 96813-2409
808-692-0899
Fax: 808-586-2940

E-mail: inip@hawaii.edu
www.jabsom.hawaii.edu

Naleen Andrade, Chair
Jerris Hedges, MD, MS, MMM, Dean and Professor of
Medicine
Nancy Foster, CFO
A. Roy Magnusson, MD, Associate Dean, Clinical Affairs

Medical School Programs and Residency Programs, general, geriatric, addictive and, child and adolescent.

3125 Langley Porter Psych Institute at UCSF Parnassus Campus

401 Parnassus Avenue
San Francisco, CA 94143-2211
415-476-7500
Fax: 415-502-6361
www.psych.ucsf.edu/lpphc.aspx

Alissa M Peterson
Sam Hawgood, MBBS, Interim Chancellor

3126 Laurelwood Hospital and Counseling Centers

35900 Euclid Avenue
Willoughby, OH 44094-4648
440-953-3000
800-438-4673
Fax: 440-602-3938
www.www.windsorlaurelwood.com

Farshid Afsarifard, Administrator
Leonard Barley, M.D., MBA, Chief Medical Officer
Theodore Parran, M.D., Director, Addiction Medicine
Noah Miller, M.D., Director, Child and Adolescent S

Full-service behavioral healthcare system-(comprehensive outpatient and inpatient services).

3127 Life Science Associates

1 Fenimore Road
Bayport, NY 11705-2115
631-472-2111
Fax: 631-472-8146
E-mail: lifesciassoc@pipeline.com
www.lifesciassoc.home.pipeline.com

Joann Mandriota, President
Frank Mandriota, Vice President

Publishes over fifty computer programs for individuals impaired by head trauma and stroke. Also programs for personal memory care, GSSS (Get sharp stay sharp)

3128 Locumtenens.com

2655 Northwinds Parkway
Alpharetta, GA 30009
800-930-0748
E-mail: customerservice@locumtenens.com
www.locumtenens.com

Shane Jackson, President, COO
Kevin Thill, SVP, Psychiatry
Chris Franklin, EVP
Katie Thill, EVP

Specializing in temporary and permanant placement of psychiatrists. Physicians tell us where and when they want to work and locumtenens.com will find a jop that fits those needs.

3129 MCG Telemedicine Center

1120 15th Street
Augusta, GA 30912-6

706-721-2231
E-mail: mcgdean@gru.edu
www.mcg.edu

Daniel W. Rahn, President
Ricardo Azziz, MD, MPH, MBA, President / Ceo
Susan L. Barcus, FAHP, SVP, Advancement, Chief
Developm
David L. Brond, MBA, MHA, SVP, Communications and
Marketin

3130 MCW Department of Psychiatry and Behavioral Medicine

8701 Watertown Plank Road
Milwaukee, WI 53226-3548
414-955-8296
E-mail: webmaster@mcw.edu
www.www.mcw.edu

John R. Raymond, Sr., President, CEO
Joseph E. Kerschner, MD, Deean, EVP
G. Allen Bolton, Jr., SVP, COO

3131 Market Research Alliance

1109 Spring St
Suite 704
Silver Spring, MD 20910-4032
301-588-8732
Fax: 301-625-3001
E-mail: info@mr-twg.com
www.mr-twg.com

Frank Black Jr., Partner, President
John Marty, Managing Director
Nick Campbell, Member
Tom Bergan, Member

3132 Marsh Foundation

1229 Lincoln Highway
PO Box 150
Van Wert, OH 45891-150
419-238-1695
Fax: 419-238-1747
E-mail: marshfound@embarqmail.com
www.marshfoundation.org

Jeff Grothouse, Executive Secretary/Treasurer
Kim Mullins, P.C.C., Executive Director
Kathleen Davis, L.S.W., Director, Residential Services
Sherry Grone, Activities Coordinator

Nonprofit center serving children and families with special emphasis in juvenile sex offender population. Services include individual therapy, group therapy, case management and diagnostic assessment.

3133 Medical College of Georgia

1120 15th Street
Augusta, GA 30912-5563
706-721-0211
Fax: 706-721-6126
E-mail: info@gru.edu
www.mcghealthinc.com

Daniel W. Rahn, President
Ricardo Azziz, MD, MPH, MBA, President / Ceo
Susan L. Barcus, FAHP, SVP, Advancement, Chief
Developm
David L. Brond, MBA, MHA, SVP, Communications and
Marketin

The mission of the Medical College of Georgia is to improve health and resuce the burden of illness in society by discovering, disseminating, and applying knowledge of human health and disease.

3134 Medical College of Ohio

3000 Arlington Avenue
Toledo, OH 43614-2595
419-383-4000
800-321-8383
Fax: 419-383-6140
E-mail: utmc.webmaster@utoledo.edu
www.utmc.utoledo.edu

Mission is to improve the human condition through the creation, dissemination and application of knowledge using wisdom and compassion as our guides.

3135 Medical College of Pennsylvania

3300 Henry Avenue
Philadelphia, PA 19129-1191
215-842-6000

A tertiary care educational facility that reaches out to a regional referral base for select specialty services while continuing to offer primary and secondary service to the residents of its immediate community.

3136 Medical College of Wisconsin

8701 Watertown Plank Road
Milwaukee, WI 53226-3548
414-955-8296
E-mail: webmaster@mcw.edu
www.mcw.edu

John R. Raymond, Sr., President, CEO
Joseph E. Kerschner, MD, Deean, EVP
G. Allen Bolton, Jr., SVP, COO
Douglas R. Campbell, Finance Executive

3137 Medical Doctor Associates

145 Technology Parkway NW
Norcross, GA 30092-2913
770-246-9191
800-780-3500
Fax: 770-246-0882
www.mdainc.com

Ken Shumard, President
Mike Pretiger, Cfo

Committed to providing the most complete staffing services available to the healthcare industry. The family of services offered by Medical Doctor Associates includes Locum Tenens, Contract, and Permanent Placement staffing for physicians, allied health and rehabilitation staffing, and credentials verification and licensing services.

3138 Medical University of South Carolina Institute of Psychiatry, Psychiatry Access Center

104 Colcock Hall
MSC - 003
Charleston, SC 29425-100
843-792-5050
800-296-0269
Fax: 843-792-4975
www.academicdepartments.musc.edu/musc/

Mark S. Sothmann, Ph.D., Interim President, VP, Academic
Lisa Montgomery, EVP, Finance and Operations
Patrick J. Wamsley, CPA, CFO
Stewart Mixon, COO

3139 Meharry Medical College

1005-David B Todd Boulevard
Nashville, TN 37208-3501
615-327-6000
Fax: 615-321-2932
E-mail: admissions@mmc.edu
www.mmc.edu

A. Cherrie Epps, Ph.D., President, CEO
Saletta Holloway, MSP, SVP, Borad of Trustees Relations
Robert Poole, B.A., SVP, Institutional Advancement
Ivanetta Davis Samuels, J.D., SVP, General Counsel and Corpora

3140 Menninger Clinic

12301 S. Main St.
Houston, TX 77035-6207
713-275-5000
800-351-9058
Fax: 713-275-5107
www.www.menningerclinic.com

Ian Aitken, President, CEO
John M. Oldham, MD, MS, SVP, Chief of Staff
Pam Greene, PhD, RN, SVP, Patient Care Services, Chie
Kenny J. Klein, CPA, SVP, CFO

The international psychiatric center of excellence, restoring hope to each person through innovative programs in treatment, research and education.

3141 Nathan S Kline Institute for Psychiatric Research

140 Old Orangeburg Road
Orangeburg, NY 10962-1157
845-398-5500
Fax: 845-398-5510
E-mail: webmaster@nki.rfmh.org
www.www.rfmh.org/nki/

Bennet L Leventhal, MD, Deputy Director
Donald C. Goff, M.D., Director
Antonio Convit, M.D., Deputy Director
Thomas O. O'Hara, M.B.A., Deputy Director

Research programs in Alzheimers disease, analytical psychopharmacology, basic and clinical neuroimaging, cellular and molecular neurobiology, clinical trial data management, co-occuring disorders and many other mental health studies.

3142 National Association of Alcholism and Drug Abuse Counselors

1001 N. Fairfax Street
Suite 201
Alexandria, VA 22314-1535
703-741-7686
800-548-0497
Fax: 703-741-7698
E-mail: naadac@naadac.org
www.naadac.org

Robert C. Richards, MA, NCAC II, , President
Kirk Bowden, PhD, MAC, LISA, President Elect
Cynthia Moreno Tuohy, NCAC II, , Executive Director
Autumn Kramer, Director, Operations

NAADAC is the only professional membership organization that serves counselors who specialize in addiction treatment. With 14, 000 members and 47 state affiliates representing more than 80, 000 addiction counselors, it is the nation's largest network of alcoholism and drug abuse treatment professionals. Among the organization's national certifacation programs are the National Certified Addiction Counselor and the Masters Addiction Counselor designations.

3143 National Association of School Psychologists

4340 E West Highway
Suite 402
Bethesda, MD 20814-4468
301-657-0270
866-331-6277
Fax: 301-657-0275
www.nasponline.org

Sally Baas, President
Stephen E. Brock, President Elect
Amy R. Smith, Past President
Susan Gorin, Executive Director

3144 New York University Behavioral Health Programs

530 1st Avenue
Suite 7D (at 30th Street)
New York, NY 10016-6402
212-263-7419
Fax: 212-263-7460
www.www.med.nyu.edu/nyubhp/

David Ginsberg, Director
Robert Cancro, MD, Professor of Psychiatry and Chai
Norman Sussman, MD, Clinical Professor of Psychiatry
Virginia Sadock, MD, Clinical Professor of Psychiatry

Outpatient psychiatry group for Tisch Hospital at NYU Medical Center. Our multidisciplinary team of licensed psychiatrists and social workers offers you the most up-to-date and scientifically validated treatments.

3145 Northeastern Ohio Universities College of Medicine

4209 State Route 44
PO Box 95
Rootstown, OH 44272-95
800-686-2511
www.neoucom.edu

Jay A. Gershen, D.D.S., Ph.D., President
John R. Wray, Vice President, Administration a
Daniel Blain, Vice President, Advancement, Pre
Michael A. Wolff, J.D., Senior Development Officer

Mission is to graduate qualified physicians who are passionate about serving their communities. All of our graduates, regardless of specialty, have a solid background in community and public health. NEOUCOM strives to improve the quality of health care throughout northeast Ohio by instilling in each graduate the desire to serve the public and the highest ideals of the medical profession.

3146 Northwestern University Medical School Feinberg School of Medicine

420 East Superior Street
Chicago, IL 60611-3128
312-503-8194
Fax: 312-503-8700
E-mail: clinpsych@northwestern.edu
www.www.feinberg.northwestern.edu

Eric G. Neilson, MD, Dean, VP - Medical Affairs
Eva Erskine, Manager
Jim Baker, Ph.D., Science in Medicine Element Co-C
John X. Thomas, Ph.D., Teamwork & Leadership Thread Cha

The Mental Health Services and Policy Program is a multidisciplinary research/educational program on the development and implementation of outcomes management technology.

3147 Ochester Psychological Service

1924 Copper Oaks Circle
Blue Springs, MO 64015-8300
816-224-6500

Jeffery L Miller PhD, Psychologist/Owner

Offers a full range of outpatient mental health services including individuals, couples and family therapy. Offers psychological testing and evaluation. Adults, adolescents and children served.

3148 PRIMA ADD Corp.

12160 N. Abrams Rd
Suite 615
Dallas, TX 75243-4547
972-386-8599
Fax: 972-386-8597
E-mail: robinbinnig@gmail.com
www.primaadd.com; drbinnig.wordpress.com

Robin Binnig, PhD, Owner

Prima ADD Corp specializes in the diagnosis and treatment of Attention-Deficit/Hyperactivity Disorder (ADHD). We treat children and adults. Services include: psychological assessment (including intellectual, achievement and pesonality testing), counseling, coaching and consultation. We also carry books and CD's concerning ADHD.

3149 Parent Child Center

2001 W Blue Heron Blvd
Riviera Beach, FL 33404-5003
561-841-3500
800-955-8770
Fax: 561-844-3577
TTY: 800-955-8771
E-mail: information@parent-childcenter.org
www.www.gocpg.org

Patrick Mc Namara, President, CEO
Laura Barry, Vice President of Community Serv
Pamela Figoras, Vice President of Child & Family
Laura Morse, Vice President of President of Development

3150 Penn State Hershey Medical Center

500 University Drive
Hershey, PA 17033-2390
717-531-6955
800-731-3032
Fax: 717-531-4077
TTY: 717-531-4395
www.hmc.psu.edu

Harold L Paz, M.D., M.S., CEO, SVP, Dean
Jeff Miller, M.D., Associate Dean for Administratio
Lisa Abbott, M.B.A., S.P.H., Associate Vice President for Human Resources
Sean Young, Chief Marketing Officer

3151 Pepperdine University Graduate School of Education and Psychology

6100 Center Drive
Los Angeles, CA 90045-9200
310-506-4000
800-347-4849

Andrew Benton, President

Offers graduate degree programs designed to prepare psychologists, marriage and family therapists, and mental health practitioners. Many programs accommodate a full-time work schedule with evening and weekend classes available in a trimester schedule. The average class size is 15. There are five educational centers in southern California and three community counseling clinics available to the surrounding community.

3152 Portland University Regional Research Institute for Human Services

1600 Sw 4th Ave
Suite 900
Portland, OR 97201-5521
503-725-4040
Fax: 503-725-4180
www.rri.pdx.edu

Tom Keller, Interim Director
Diane Yatchmenoff, Ph.D., Associate Director
Jennifer Williams, Assistant to the Director

3153 Postgraduate Center for Mental Health

71 W 23rd St
New York, NY 10010-4102
212-576-4168
E-mail: crichards@pgcmh.org
www.pgcmh.org

Jacob Barak, Ph.D., MBA, President, CEO
Marcia B. Holman, L.C.S.W., VP for Ambulatory Operations
Harold Moss, L.M.S.W., MA, VP for Residential Operations
John McMasters, Executive Assistant

Information on mental health.

3154 Pressley Ridge

5500 Corporate Drive
Suite 400
Pittsburgh, PA 15237
412-872-9400
Fax: 412-872-9478
www.pressleyridge.org

Susanna L. Cole, MA, President, CEO
Laurah Currey, MA, LPC, LSW, Chief Operating Officer
Douglas A. Mullins, CPA, CFO
Edward J. Yongo, MBA, Chief Development and External R

Founded in 1832. Provides an array of social services, special education programs, and mental health services for troubled children and their families in Delaware, Maryland, Ohio, Pennsylvania, Virginia, Washngton, DC and West Virginia as well as worldwide.

3155 PsychTemps

2404 Auburn Avenue
Cincinnati, OH 45219-2735
513-651-9500
888-651-8367
Fax: 513-651-9558
E-mail: info@psychpros.com
www.psychtemps.com

Holly Dorna MA LPCC, President/CEO
Timberline Knolls, HR Director
Lauren Kofod, M.D., Member
Paul J. Schwartz, M.D., Member

Specialized recruiting and staffing company that fills temporary, permanent, and temp-to-hire job placement for the behavioral healthcare field.

3156 Psychiatric Associates

2216 W Alto Road
Kokomo, IN 46902
765-453-9338

3157 Psychological Center

135 Oakland Street
Pasadena, CA 91101
626-584-5500

Winston Gooden, Manager

3158 QuadraMed Corporation

12110 Sunset Hills Road
Suite 600
Reston, VA 20190-5852
703-709-2300
800-393-0278
Fax: 703-709-2490
E-mail: boardofdirectors@quadramed.com
www.quadramed.com

Daniel Desaulniers, CA, President, Harris Quebec Public
Jim Dowling, Executive Vice President, Enterprise
Sandi Williams, Executive Vice President, Clinic
Duncan W James, CEO

3159 Skills Unlimited

2060 Ocean Ave
Suite 3
Ronkonkoma, NY 11779-6533
631-580-5319
Fax: 631-580-5394
E-mail: success@skillsunlimited.org
www.skillsunlimited.org

Jeffrey Koppelson, Program Director
Richard Kassnove, Executive Director

SUCCESS provides rehabilitative services to indivduals who are recovering from mental illness. In addition to offering clinical treatment, SUCCESS has a schedule of classes and other services that help to identify and achieve personally meaningful goals in the areas of employment, housing, education, health and socialization. Transportation is generally available free of charge. The program is open Monday through Saturday and has ectended hours two evenings per week.

3160 Southern Illinois University School of Medicine: Department of Psychiatry

PO Box 19620
Springfield, IL 62794-9620
217-545-8000
www.siumed.edu

Stephen M Soltys MD, Pfr/Chair Dpt. of Psychiatry
Philip Pan MD, Division Chief
Connie Poole, Associate Dean for Information Resources
Klamen Debra, MD, MHPE, Associate Dean for Education and

3161 Southern Illinois University School of Medicine
SIU School of Medicine

PO Box 19620
Springfield, IL 62794-9620
217-545-8000
www.siumed.edu

Stephen M Soltys MD, Pfr/Chair Dpt. of Psychiatry
Philip Pan MD, Division Chief
Connie Poole, Associate Dean for Information R

Klamen Debra, MD, MHPE, Associate Dean for Education and

Provides high quality clinical treatment, outstanding teaching and solid efforts in research and community service.

3162 Specialzed Alternatives for Family and Youth (SAFY)

10100 Elida Road
Delphos, OH 45833-9056
419-695-8010
800-532-7239
Fax: 419-695-0004
E-mail: webmaster@safy.org
www.safy.org

Scott Spangler, MSW, President, CEO
Jim Sherman, MA, LPC, SVP, Administrative Services
John Hollenkamp, CPA, VP, Contracts and Procurement
Marc Bloomingdale, M.S., VP, Operations

SAFY's mission is to foster an environment that possibly impacts the lives of youth and their families, whether they are with us an hour or a lifetime.

3163 St. Frnacis Medical Psych-Med Association

2616 Wilmington Road
New Castle, PA 16105-1504
724-652-2323

3164 St. Louis Behavioral Medicine Institute

1129 Macklind Avenue
Saint Louis, MO 63110-1440
314-289-9411
877-245-2688
www.slbmi.com

Ronald B. Margolis, Ph.D., President, CEO
Debbie Milfelt, Manager
Geeta Aatre-Prashar, Psy.D., Psychologist
Gelene Adkins, Ph.D., Psychologist

Offers exceptional quality, result-focused treatment. Have remained true to our commitment of providing excellence in clinical care and customer service. We offer comprehensive treatment plans to meet the individual needs of children, adolescents, adults, older adults, and their families suffering from emotional and behavioral problems.

3165 Stonington Institute

75 Swantown Hill Road
N Stonington, CT 06359-1022
860-535-1010
800-832-1022
Fax: 860-445-3030
E-mail: andrea.keeney@uhsinc.com
www.stoningtoninstitute.com

William A. Aniskovich, M.A., J.D., CEO
Jerome M Schnitt, M.D., Medical Director
Georganna Georgie Koppermann, Director, Business Development a
Andrea Keeney, Director of Admissions

3166 Topeka Institute for Psychoanalysis

PO Box 829
Topeka, KS 66601-829
800-288-3950

A training facility for health care professionals, the Topeka Institute for Psychoanalysis has the tripartite mission of promoting research to expand the knowledge base in its field of expertise; providing didactic education and clinical supervision to trainees; and caring for patients in need of its services through a low-fee clinic.

3167 UCLA Neuropsychiatric Institute and Hospital

760 Westwood Plaza
Los Angeles, CA 90095
310-825-0291
www.www.semel.ucla.edu

Peter Whybrow, Director
Fawzy Fawzy, Associate Director
Mark Wheeler, Media Relations
Alan Han, Director of Development

Multidisciplinary institute of human neurosciences, and is unifying focus of scholarly activity at UCLA in this area. Scientific advances recent decades have shown the value in approaches that cut across traditional academic departments, and which emphasize interdisciplinary collaborations.

3168 UCLA School of Nursing

PO Box 951702
Los Angeles, CA 90095-1702
310-825-3109
Fax: 310-267-0330
E-mail: sonsaff@sonnet.ucla.edu
www.nursing.ucla.edu

Courtney H. Lyder, ND, ScD(Hon), F, Professor, Dean
Rene Dennis, Director Development
Rhonda Flenoy-Younger, Director of Recruitment, Outreac
Mark Covin, Recruitment and Admissions Coord

3169 UCSF Department of Psychiatry, Cultural Competence

3 Regent Street
Livingston, NJ 07039
973-436-5000
973-436-5004
www.reprogenetics.com

Santiago Munne, Founder, Director
Jacques Cohen, Laboratory Director, Embryologis
Kelly Ketterson, Director of Operations
Pere Colls, Laboratory Director

3170 USC School of Medicine

Health Sciences Campuses
Name/Department USC
Los Angeles, CA 90089-1
323-442-1100
www.usc.edu/schools/medicine/

3171 Ulster County Mental Health Department

244 Fair Street
PO Box 1800
Kingston, NY 12402
845-340-3000
Fax: 845-340-4094
E-mail: exec@co.ulster.ny.us
www.co.ulster.ny.us

Marshall Beckman, Executive Director
Mike Hein, Ulster County Executive
Elliott Auerbach, Comptroller
D. Holley Carnright, District Attorney

Responsible for planning, funding and monitoring of community mental health, mental retardation/developmental disability and alcohol and substance abuse services in Ulster County.

3172 Union County Psychiatric Clinic
117 Roosevelt Avenue
Plainfield, NJ 07060-1331
908-756-6870
www.www.ucpcbhc.org

Rosalind Hunt Doctor, President
Gerard Kiely, VP
Richard L. Rodgers, MSW, LCSW, Executive Director
Joseph Daniel, MA, LPC, Associate Executive Director

3173 University Behavioral Healthcare
671 Hoes Lane
Piscataway, NJ 08855
732-235-5900
800-969-5300
Fax: 732-235-4594
www.ubhc.rutgers.edu

Christopher Kosseff, President

3174 University of California Davis Psychiatry and Behavioral Sciences Department
2315 Stockton Boulevard
Sacramento, CA 95817-2201
916-734-2011

Offers opportunities for students and faculty for clinical and research applications in all aspects of psychiatry and behavioral sciences.

3175 University of Cincinnati College of Medical Department of Psychiatry
260 Stelson Street
Suite 3200
Cincinnati, OH 45221
513-558-7700
Fax: 513-558-0187
E-mail: uchealthnews@uc.edu
www.www.psychiatry.uc.edu

Stephen M. Strakowski, MD, Chair
Charles Collins, MD, Senior Vice Chair and Director o
Paul Keck, MD, Executive Vice Chair
Henry A. Nasrallah, MD, Vice Chair of Education and Trai

Researches eating disorders, bipolar disorder, and chemical dependency.

3176 University of Colorado Health Sciences Center
1250 14th Street
Denver, CO 80217
303-556-2400
877-472-2586
E-mail: alumni@uchsc.edu
www.www.ucdenver.edu/pages/ucdwelcomepage.aspx

John C Slocumb

3177 University of Connecticut Health Center
263 Farmington Avenue
Farmington, CT 06030-1
860-679-2000
TDD: 860-679-2242
www.www.uchc.edu

Susan Herbst, President
Frank M. Torti, M.D., M.P.H., Executive VP for health affairs
Elizabeth Bolt, Vice President, Human Resources
Marianne Dess-Santoro, VP, Ambulatory Care

3178 University of Iowa Hospital
200 Hawkins Drive
Iowa City, IA 52242-1007
319-356-1616
800-777-8442
TDD: 319-356-4999
E-mail: uihc-webcomments@uiowa.edu
www.www.uihealthcare.org

Kenneth P. Kates, CEO
Kenneth L. Fisher, CFO
Ann Williamson, PhD, RN, Chief Nursing Officer
Theresa Brennan, MD, Chief Medical Officer

3179 University of Kansas Medical Center
3901 Rainbow Boulevard
Kansas City, KS 66160-1
913-588-5000
TDD: 913-588-7963
E-mail: kusmw@kumc.edu
www.www.kumc.edu

Douglas A. Girod, M.D., Executive Vice Chancellor
Barbara Atkinson, Executive Vice Chancellor
Tim Caboni, Vice Chancellor for Public Affai
David Vranicar, M.B.A., Vice Chancellor for Finance/CFO

An integral and unique component of the University of Kansas and the Kansas Board of Regents system, is composed of the School of Medicine, the School of Nursing, the School of Allied Health, the University of Kansas Hospital, and a Graduate School. KU Medical Center is a complex institution whose basic functions include research, education, patient care, and community service involving multiple constituencies at state and national levels.

3180 University of Kansas School of Medicine
3901 Rainbow Boulevard
Kansas City, KS 66160-1
913-588-5000
TDD: 913-588-7963
E-mail: kusmw@kumc.edu
www.kumc.edu

Douglas A. Girod, M.D., Executive Vice Chancellor
Barbara Atkinson, Executive Vice Chancellor
Tim Caboni, Vice Chancellor for Public Affai
David Vranicar, M.B.A., Vice Chancellor for Finance/CFO

3181 University of Louisville School of Medicine
Abell Administration Center
323 E. Chestnut Street
Louisville, KY 40202
502-562-3000
E-mail: meddean@louisville.edu
www.louisville.edu/medicine

Dean Ganzel, Dean
Wes Allison

Mission is to be a vital component in the University of Louisville's quest to become a premier, nationally recognized metropolitan research university, to excel in the education of physicians and scientists for careers in teching, research, patient care and community service, and to bring the fundamental discoveries of our basic and clinical scientists to the bedside.

3182 University of Maryland Medical Systems
22 S. Greene Street
Baltimore, MD 21201-1023

410-328-2132
800-492-5538
TDD: 800-735-2258
www.umm.edu

Robert A. Chrencik, MBA, CPAÿ, President, CEO
Henry J. Franey, MBAÿ, EVP, CFO
Megan M. Arthur, SVP, General Counsel
Janice J. Eisele, SVP, Development

3183 University of Maryland School of Medicine
655 West Baltimore Street
Baltimore, MD 21201-1509
410-706-3681
E-mail: webmaster@som.umaryland.edu
www.medschool.umaryland.edu

Nancy Ryan Lowitt, Dean/Vp Medical Affairs
E. Albert Reece, MD, PhD, MBA, Dean, VP of Medical Affairs
Richard Pierson III, MD, Senior Associate Dean for Academ
Milford M. Foxwell, Jr., MD, Associate Dean for Admissions

Dedicated to providing excellence in biomedical education, basic and clinical research, quality patient care and service to improve the health of the citizens of Maryland and beyond.

3184 University of Massachusetts Medical Center
55 Lake Avenue N
Worcester, MA 01655-1
508-856-8989
www.www.umassmed.edu

Terence R. Flotte, MD, Dean of School of Medicine, Prov
Michael F. Collins, MD, FACP, Senior Vice President for the He
Mariann M. Manno, MD, Interim Associate Dean for Admis
Aaron Lazare, Administrator

Mission is to serve the people of the commonwealth through national distinction in health sciences, education, research, public service and clinical care.

3185 University of Michigan
500 S. State Street
Ann Arbor, MI 48109
734-764-1817
E-mail: info@umich.edu
www.www.umich.edu

Mary Sue Coleman, President
Martha Pollack, Provost
Sally J. Churchill, VP, Secretary
Jerry A. May, VP, Development

3186 University of Minnesota Fairview Health Systems
2450 Riverside Ave
Minneapolis, MN 55454-1450
612-273-2229
Fax: 612-273-2211
TTY: 612-672-7300
www.fairview.org

Gordon Alexander, President
Rulon F. Stacey, PhD, FACHE, President, CEO
Daniel K. Anderson, President of Fairview Community
Daniel Fromm, SVP, CFO

Mission is to improve the health of the communities we serve. We commit our skills and resources to the benefit of the whole person by providing the finest in healthcare, while addressing the physical, emotional and spiritual needs of individuals and their families. Pledge to support the research and education efforts of our partner, the University of Minnesota, and its tradition of excellence.

3187 University of North Carolina School of Social Work
Behavioral Healthcare Resource Institute
301 Pittsboro Street
Cb # 3550
Chapel Hill, NC 27599-1
919-843-3018
E-mail: bhrinstitute@listserv.unc.edu
www.behavioralhealthcareinstitute.org

3188 University of Pennsylvania Health System
399 S 34th Street
Suite 2002 Penn Tower
Philadelphia, PA 19104-4316
215-662-6995
800-789-PENN

3189 University of South Florida Research Center for Children's Mental Health
13301 Bruce B Downs Boulevard
Tampa, FL 33612-3807
813-974-4565
www.rtckids.fmhi.usf.edu

Robert M. Friedman, Ph.D., Center Director
Albert Duchnowski, Ph.D., Deputy Director
Krista Kutash, Ph.D., Deputy Director
Mary Armstrong, PhD, Center Staff

The center conducts research, synthesized and shared existingknowledge, provided training and consultation, and served as a resource for other researchers, policy makers, administrators in the public system, and organizations representing parents, consumers, advocates, professional societies and practitioners.

3190 University of Texas Medical Branch Managed Care
301 University Boulevard
Galveston, TX 77555-5302
409-772-1506
800-917-8906
Fax: 409-772-6216
E-mail: public.affairs@utmb.edu
www.utmb.edu

David L. Callender, MD, MBA, FA, President
Danny O. Jacobs, MD, MPH, EVP, Provost, Dean
Carolee Carrie King, JD, SVP, General Counsel
David W. Niesel, PhD, VP, Dean

3191 University of Utah Neuropsychiatric
501 Chipeta Way
Salt Lake City, UT 84108-1222
801-583-2500
E-mail: sarah.latta@hsc.utah.edu
www.healthcare.utah.edu/uni

Kristin Fontaine, Manager

Located in the University's Research Park, is a full service 90-bed psychiatric hospital providing mental health and substance abuse treatment. Services include inpatient, day treatment, intensive outpatient, and ooutpatient services for children, adolescents and adults. Confidential assessments, referrals, and intervention education are available.

3192 Wake Forest University
1834 Wake Forest Road
Winston Salem, NC 27106
336-758-5000
Fax: 336-759-6074
E-mail: help.wfu.edu
www.wfu.edu

Nathan O. Hatch, President
Rogan Kersh, Provost
Hof Milam, SVP of Finance and Administratio
James J. Dunn, VP, Chief Investment Officer

3193 West Jefferson Medical Center
1101 Medical Center Boulevard
Marrero, LA 70072-3191
504-347-5511
E-mail: guestservicesweb@wjmc.org
www.wjmc.org

A Gary Muller, CEO

Not-for-profit community hospital on the West Bank of Jefferson Parish. Continues to strengthen its community base while maintaining its mission and values. Dedicated to considerate and respectful quality healthcare, the institution welcomes patient, family, and visitor feedback regarding programs, services, and community needs.

3194 Western Psychiatric Institute and Clinic
3811 Ohara Street
Pittsburgh, PA 15213-2597
412-624-2100
877-624-4100
www.www.upmc.com

Rizwan Parvez

A national leader in the diagnosis, management, and treatment of mental health and addictive disorders. Providing the most comprehensive range of behavioral health services available today, but also shaping tomorrow's behavioral health care through clinical innovation, research, and education.

3195 Wordsworth
3905 Ford Road
Philadelphia, PA 19131-2824
215-643-5400
800-769-0088
E-mail: info@wordsworth.org
www.www.wordsworth.org

Debra Lacks, President, CEO
Amir Malek, CFO
Andrew Gross, Executive Director of Community
Jennifer Nickels, Executive Director of Residentia

The mission of Wordsworth, a not-for-profit institution, is to provide quality education, treatment and care to children and families with special needs.

Year Founded: 1952

3196 Asperger's Diagnostic Assessment with Dr. Tony Attwood
Program Development Associates PO Box 2038 Syracuse, NY 13220-2038
315-452-0643
Fax: 315-452-0710
E-mail: info@disabilitytraining.com
www.disabilitytraining.com

New from acclaimed autism expert Dr. Tony Attwood, this 4-hour DVD set with program guide offers diagnostic characteristics of Asperger's Syndrome in children and adults, patient interviews and impacts on girls. An essential guide for Child Psychologists, Special Ed teachers and Parents. *$129.95*

3197 Cognitive Behavioral Assessment
NewHarbinger Publications
5674 Shattuck Avenue
Oakland, CA 94609-1662
510-652-0215
800-748-6273
Fax: 800-652-1613
E-mail: customerservice@newharbinger.com
www.newharbinger.com

Matthew McKay, Owner

A videotape that guides three clients through PAC (Problem, Antecedents, Consequences) method of cognitive behavioral assessment. *$49.95*

Year Founded: 1996 ISBN 1-572243-15-5

3198 Couples and Infertility - Moving Beyond Loss
Guilford Press
72 Spring Street
New York, NY 10012-4068
212-431-9800
800-365-7006
Fax: 212-966-6708
E-mail: info@guilford.com
www.www.guilford.com

Bob Matloff, President
Seymour Weingarten, Editor-in-Chief

A VHS video explores the biological and resulting psychological and social issues of infertility. *$95.00*

Year Founded: 1995 ISBN 1-572302-86-0

3199 Educating Clients about the Cognitive Model
NewHarbinger Publications
5674 Shattuck Avenue
Oakland, CA 94609-1662
510-652-0215
800-748-6273
Fax: 800-652-1613
E-mail: customerservice@newharbinger.com
www.newharbinger.com

Matthew McKay, Owner

Videotape that helps three clients understand their symptoms as they work toward developing a working contract to begin cognitive restructing. *$49.95*

Year Founded: 1996 ISBN 1-572243-19-8

3200 Gender Differences in Depression: Marital Therapy Approach
Guilford Press
72 Spring Street
New York, NY 10012-4068
212-431-9800
800-365-7006
Fax: 212-966-6708
E-mail: info@guilford.com
www.www.guilford.com

Bob Matloff, President
Seymour Weingarten, Editor-in-Chief

Male-female treatment team is shown working with a markedly depressed couple to improve communication and sense of well being in their marriage. *$85.50*
Year Founded: 1996 ISBN 1-572302-87-9

3201 Group Work for Eating Disorders and Food Issues
American Counseling Association
5999 Stevenson Avenue
Alexandria, VA 22304-3304
703-823-9800
800-347-6647
Fax: 703-823-0252
E-mail: webmaster@counseling.org
www.counseling.org

Cirecie A. West-Olatunji, President
Robert L. Smith, President Elect
Bradley T. Erford, Past President
Richard Yep, Executive Director

A plan for working with high school and college age females who are at risk for eating disorders. This video provides a method for identifying at-risk clients, a session-by-session desciption of the group, exercises and information on additional resources. *$89.95*
Year Founded: 1995 ISSN 79801

3202 Help This Kid's Driving Me Crazy - the Young Child with Attention Deficit Disorder
Pro-Ed Publications
8700 Shoal Creek Boulevard
Austin, TX 78757-6897
512-451-3246
800-897-3202
Fax: 512-451-8542
E-mail: general@proedinc.com
www.www.proedinc.com

Donald D Hammill, Owner

This videotape provides information about the behavior and special needs of young children with ADD and offers suggestions on fostering appropriate behaviors. *$89.00*

3203 I Love You Like Crazy: Being a Parent with Mental Illness
Mental Illness Education Project
25 West Street
Westborough, MA Westb-roug
617-562-1111
800-343-5540
Fax: 617-779-0061
E-mail: info@miepvideos.org
www.miepvideos.org

Christine Ledoux, Executive Director

In this videotape, eight mothers and fathers who have mental illness discuss the challenges they face as parents. Most of these parents have faced enormous obstacles from homelessness, addictions, legal difficulties and hospitalizations, yet have maintained a positive and loving relationship with their children. The tape introduces issues of work, fear, stigma, relationships with children and the rest of the family, with professionals, and with the community at large. Discounted price for families/consumers. *$79.95*
Year Founded: 1999

3204 Inner Health Incorporated
Christopher Alsten, PhD
1260 Lincoln Avenue
San Diego, CA 92103-2322
619-299-7273
800-283-4679
Fax: 619-291-7753
E-mail: sleepenhancement@aol.com

Provides a series of prerecorded therapeutic audio programs for anxiety, insomnia and chemical dependency, both for adults and children. Developed over a 15 year period by a practicing psychiatrist and recording engineer they employ state-of-the-art 3-D sound technologies and the latest relaxation and psychological techniques (but no stimulants). Clients include: US Air Force, US Navy, National Institute of Health, National Institute of Aging and various psychiatric and chemical dependency facilities and companies with shiftworkers.

3205 Know Your Rights: Mental Health Private Practice & the Law
American Counseling Association
5999 Stevenson Avenue
Alexandria, VA 22304-3304
703-823-9800
800-347-6647
Fax: 703-823-0252
E-mail: webmaster@counseling.org
www.counseling.org

Cirecie A. West-Olatunji, President
Robert L. Smith, President Elect
Bradley T. Erford, Past President
Richard Yep, Executive Director

Whether you are in private practice or are thinking about opening your own practice, this forum lead by national experts, offers answers to important questions and provides invaluable information for every practitioner. Helps to orientate practitioners on the legally permissible boundaries, legal liabilities that are seldom known and how to respond in the face of legal action. *$145.00*
ISSN 79062

3206 Life Is Hard: Audio Guide to Healing Emotional Pain
Impact Publishers
PO Box 6016
Atascadero, CA 93423-6016
805-466-5917
800-246-7228
Fax: 805-466-5919
E-mail: info@impactpublishers.com
www.impactpublishers.com

In a very warm and highly personal style, psychologist Preston offers listeners powerful advice — realistic, practical, effective, on dealing with the emotional pain life often inflicts upon us. *$11.95*

Year Founded: 1996 ISBN 0-915166-99-2

3207 Life Passage in the Face of Death, Vol II: Psychological Engagement of the Physically Ill Patient
American Psychiatric Publishing, Inc.
1000 Wilson Boulevard
Suite 1825
Arlington, VA 22209-3901
703-907-7322
800-368-5777
Fax: 703-907-1091
E-mail: appi@psych.org
www.appi.org

Ron McMillen, Chief Executive Officer
Robert E. Hales MD, M.B.A, Editor-in-Chief
John McDuffie, Editorial Director
Rebecca D. Rinehart, Publisher

Ongoing explanation of therapy from a recognized expert. Valuable to clinicians and students alike.

3208 Life Passage in the Face of Death, Volume I: A Brief Psychotherapy
American Psychiatric Publishing, Inc.
1000 Wilson Boulevard
Suite 1825
Arlington, VA 22209-3901
703-907-7322
800-368-5777
Fax: 703-907-1091
E-mail: appi@psych.org
www.appi.org

Ron McMillen, Chief Executive Officer
Robert E. Hales MD, M.B.A, Editor-in-Chief
John McDuffie, Editorial Director, Associate Pu
Rebecca D. Rinehart, Publisher

A senior psychoanalyst demonstrates the extraordinary impact of a very brief dynamic psychotherapy on a patient in a time of crisis — the terminal illness and death of a spouse. We not only meet the patient and observe the therapy, but our understanding is guided by the therapist's ongoing explanation of the process. He vividly illustrates concepts such as transference, clarification, interpretation, insight, denial, isolation and above all the relevance of understanding the past for changing the present. This unique opportunity to see a psychotherapy as it is conducted will be of immense value for all mental health clinicians and trainees.

3209 Medical Aspects of Chemical Dependency The Neurobiology of Addiction
Hazelden
15251 Pleasant Valley Road
PO Box 176
Center City, MN 55012-176
651-213-4200
800-257-7810
Fax: 651-213-4590
E-mail: info@hazelden.org
www.hazelden.org

Mark Mishek, President, CEO of Hazelden Betty
Nick Motu, VP of Marketing and Communicatio
William C. Moyers, VP of Foundation Relations
James A. Blaha, VP of Finance and Administration

This interactive curriculum helps professionals educate clients in treatment and other settings about medical effects of chemical use and abuse. The program includes a video that explains body and brain changes that can occur when using alcohol or other drugs, a workbook that helps clients apply the information from the video to their own situations, a handbook that provides in-depth information on addiction, brain chemistry and the physiological effects of chemical dependency and a pamphlet that answers critical questions clients have about the medical effects of chemical dependency. Total price of $244.70, available to purchase separately. Program value packages available for $395.00, with 25 workbooks, two handbooks, two video and 25 pamphlets. *$225.00*

Year Founded: 2003 ISBN 1-568389-87-6

3210 Mental Illness Education Project
25 West Street
Westborough, MA Westb-roug
617-562-1111
800-343-5540
Fax: 617-779-0061
E-mail: info@miepvideos.org
www.miepvideos.org

Christine Ledoux, Executive Director

Engaged in the production of video-based educational and support materials for the following specific populations: people with psychiatric disabilities; families, mental health professionals, special audiences, and the general public. The Project's videos are designed to be used in hospital, clinical and educational settings, and at home by individuals and families.

3211 Physicians Living with Depression
American Psychiatric Publishing, Inc.
1000 Wilson Boulevard
Suite 1825
Arlington, VA 22209-3901
703-907-7322
800-368-5777
Fax: 703-907-1091
E-mail: appi@psych.org
www.appi.org

Ron McMillen, Chief Executive Officer
Robert E. Hales MD, M.B.A, Editor-in-Chief
John McDuffie, Editorial Director, Associate Pu
Rebecca D. Rinehart, Publisher

Designed to help doctors see the signs of depression in their fellow physicians and to alert psychiatrists to the severity of the illness in their physician patients, the tape contains two fifteen-minute interviews, one with an emergency physician and one with a pediatrician. *$25.00*

ISBN 0-890422-78-8

3212 Rational Emotive Therapy
Research Press
PO Box 7886
Champaign, IL 61826-9177
217-352-3273
800-519-2707
Fax: 217-352-1221
E-mail: rp@researchpress.com
www.researchpress.com

Robert W. Parkinson, Founder
Dennis Wiziecki, Marketing

Dr Albert Ellis, Author
Arnold Goldstein, Author

This video illustrates the basic concepts of Rational Emotive Therapy (RET). It includes demonstrations of RET procedures, informative discussions and unstaged counseling sessions. Viewers will see Albert Ellis and his colleagues help clients overcome such problems as guilt, social anxiety, and jealousy. Also, Dr. Ellis shares his perspectives on the evolution of RET. *$195.00*

3213 Solutions Step by Step - Substance Abuse Treatment Videotape
WW Norton & Company
500 5th Avenue
New York, NY 10110-54
212-354-2907
Fax: 212-869-0856
E-mail: admalmud@wwnorton.com

Drake McFeely, CEO

Quick tips, questions and examples focusing on successes that can be experienced helping substance abusers help themselves. *$ 100.00*

Year Founded: 1997 ISSN 70260-X

3214 Testing Automatic Thoughts with Thought Records
NewHarbinger Publications
5674 Shattuck Avenue
Oakland, CA 94609-1662
510-652-0215
800-748-6273
Fax: 800-652-1613
E-mail: customerservice@newharbinger.com
www.newharbinger.com

Matthew McKay, Owner

Videotape that helps a client explore the hot thoughts that contribute to depression. *$49.95*

ISBN 1-572243-17-1

Web Sites

3215 www.42online.org
Psychologists In Independent Practice - American Psych Assn (APADIP)
E-mail: div42apa@cox.net
www.42online.org

Members of the American Psychological Association engaged in independent practice. Works to ensure that the needs and concerns of independent psychology practitioners are considered by the APA. Gathers and disseminates information on legislation affecting the practice of psychology, managed care, and other developments in the health care industries, office management, malpractice risk and insurance, hospital management. Offers continuing professional and educational programs. Semiannual convention, with board meeting.

3216 www.aacap.org Psychiatry
American Academy of Child and Adolescent Psychiatry
3615 Wisconsin Avenue NW
Washington, DC 20016-3007
202-966-7300
Fax: 202-966-2891

E-mail: communications@aacap.org
www.aacap.org

Kristin Kroeger-Ptakowski, Director, Sr Deputy Director
Elizabeth DiLauro, Advocacy Manager
Emma Jellen, Policy Coordinator

Represents over 6, 000 child and adolescent psychiatrists, brochures availible online which provide concise and up-to-date material on issues ranging from children who suffer from depression and teen suicide to stepfamily problems and child sexual abuse.

3217 www.aan.com
American Academy of Neurology
201 Chicago Avenue
Minneapolis, MN 55415
612-928-6000
800-879-1960
Fax: 612-454-2746
E-mail: memberservices@aan.com
www.www.aan.com

Timothy A. Pedley, MD, FAAN, President
Catherine M. Rydell, CAE, Executive Director, CEO

Provides information for both professionals and the public on neurology subjects, covering Alzheimer's and Parkinson's diseases to stroke and migraine, includes comprehensive fact sheets.

3218 www.aapb.org
Association for Applied Psychophysiology and Biofeedback
10200 West 44th Avenue
Suite 304
Wheat Ridge, CO 80033
303-422-8436
800-477-8892
E-mail: info@aapb.org
www.www.aapb.org

Richard Sherman, PhD, Board of Director, President
Stuart C. Donaldson, PhD, BCB, Board of Directors, President-Elect
Jeffrey Bolek, PhD, Board of Directors, Past-President
Richard Harvey, PhD, Board of Directors, Treasurer

Represents clinicians interested in psychopsysiology or biofeedback, offers links to their mission statement, membership information, research, FAQ about biofeedback, conference listings, and links.

3219 www.abecsw.org
American Board of Examiners in Clinical Social Work
241 Humphrey Street
Marblehead, MA 01945
781-639-5270
800-694-5285
Fax: 781-639-5278
E-mail: abe@abecsw.org
www.www.abecsw.org

Bob Booth, CEO
Robert Booth, Executive Director
Michael Brooks, MSW, BCD, Director of Policy and Business
Kathleen Bodoni, Credentials Manager

Information about the American Board of Examiners, credentialing, and ethics.

3220 www.about.com
About.Com

Network of comprehensive Web sites for over 600 mental health topics.

3221 www.abpsi.org
American Association of Black Psychologists
7119 Allentown Road
Suite 203
Fort Washington, MD 20744
301-449-3082
Fax: 301-449-3084
E-mail: abpsi@abpsi.org
www.www.abpsi.org

Cheryl Tawede Grills, PhD, President
Tassogle Daryl Rowe, President-Elect
Kevin Washington, Ph.D., President-Elect
Carolyn Moore, Ph.D, Treasurer

Includes information about the Association's history and objectives, contact and member information, upcoming events, and publications of interest.

3222 www.ama-assn.org
American Medical Association
330 N. Wabash Ave.
Chicago, IL 60611-5885
800-621-8335
www.www.ama-assn.org

Denise M. Hagerty, SVP, CFO
James L. Madara, MD, EVP, CEO
Robert W. Davis, SVP, Human Resources and Corpora
Leslie M. Stokes, SVP, Physician Engagement

Offers a wide range of medical information and links, full-text abstracts of each journal's current and past articles.

3223 www.apa.org
American Psychological Association
750 First St. NE
Washington, DC 20002-4242
202-336-5500
800-374-2721
Fax: 202-336-5518
TDD: 202-336-6123
TTY: 202-336-6123
E-mail: psycinfo@apa.org
www.www.apa.org

Nadine J. Kaslow, Ph.D., President
Barry S. Anton, Ph.D., President-Elect
Donald N. Bersoff, PhD, JD, Past President
Norman B Anderson, Ph.D., CEO, EVP

Information about journals, press releases, professional and consumer information related to the psychological profession; resources include ethical principles and guidelines, science advocacy, awards and funding programs, testing and assessment information, other on-line and real world resources.

3224 www.apna.org
American Psychiatric Nurses Association
3141 Fairview Park Drive
Suite 625
Falls Church, Vi 22042
571-533-1919
855-863-APNA
Fax: 855-883-APNA
www.www.apna.org

Nicholas Croce Jr., MS, Executive Director
Patricia L. Black, PhD, RN, Associate Executive Director
Karla Lewis, Director, Finance and Administration
Lisa Deffenbaugh Nguyen, MS, Director, Operations

Includes membership information, contact information, organizational information, announcements and related links.

3225 www.appi.org
American Psychiatric Publishing Inc
1000 Wilson Boulevard
Suite 1825
Arlington, VA 22209-3901
703-907-7322
800-368-5777
Fax: 703-907-1091
E-mail: appi@psych.org
www.www.appi.org

Ron McMillen, Chief Executive Officer
Robert E. Hales MD, M.B.A, Editor-in-Chief
John McDuffie, Editorial Director
Rebecca D. Rinehart, Publisher

Informational site about mental disorders, 'Lets Talk Facts' brochure series.

3226 www.apsa.org
American Psychoanalytic Asssociation
309 East 49th Street
New York, NY 10017-1601
212-752-0450
Fax: 212-593-0571
E-mail: info@apsa.org
www.www.apsa.org

Robert L. Pyles, M.D., President
Mark Smaller, Ph.D., President-Elect
William A. Myerson, Ph.D., Treasurer
Ralph E. Fishkin, D.O., Secretary

Includes searchable bibliographic database containing books, reviews and articles of a psychoanalytical orientation, links and member information.

3227 www.askdrlloyd.wordpress.com
Ask Dr Lloyd
www.www.askdrlloyd.wordpress.com

Helps individuals understand mental illnesses and addictions, what treatments and services have been proven scientifically effective, how to manage yourself or help your loved one, and how to beat a mental health system.

3228 www.assc.caltech.edu
Association for the Scientific Study of Consciousness
The Associates of the California Institu
1200 East California Boulevard
Pasadena, CA 91125
626-395-3919
Fax: 626-395-5890
E-mail: caltechassociates@caltech.edu
www.associates.caltech.edu

Catherine Reeves, Executive Director
Paula R. Elliott, Associate Director
Jerri Price-Gaines, Associate Director
Nicola Wilkins-Miller, Assistant Director

Electronic journal dedicated to interdisciplinary exploration on the nature of consciousness and its relationship to the brain, congnitive science, philosophy, psychology, physics, neuroscience, and artificial intelligence.

3229 www.blarg.net/~charlatn/voices
Compilation of Writings by People Suffering from Depression

3230 www.bpso.org
BPSO-Bipolar Significant Others
www.www.bpso.org

3231 www.bpso.org/nomania.htm
How to Avoid a Manic Episode

3232 www.cape.org
Cape Cod Institute
Professional Learning Network, LLC
270 Greenwich Avenue
Greenwich, CT 06830
203-422-0535
888-394-9293
Fax: 203-629-6048
E-mail: institute@cape.org
www.www.cape.org

Offers symposia every summer for keeping mental health professionals up-to-date on the latest developments in psychology, treatment, psychiatry, and mental health, outlines available workshops, links and other relevant information.

3233 www.chadd.org
CHADD
4601 Presidents Drive
Suite 300
Lanham, MD 20706
301-306-7070
800-233-4050
Fax: 301-306-7090
www.www.chadd.org

Ruth Hughes, PhD, CEO
Susan Buningh, MRE, Executive Editor
Christine Hoch, Director of Development
Peg Nichols, Director Communications

National non-profit organization representing children and adults with attention deficit/hyperactivity disorder (AD/HD).

3234 www.cnn.com/Health
CNN Health Section
www.www.cnn.com/Health

Updated with health and mental health-related stories three to four times weekly.

3235 www.compuserve.com
IQuest/Knowledge Index
www.www.compuserve.com

On-line research and database information provider.

3236 www.counselingforloss.com
Counseling for Loss and Life Changes
420 West Main Street
Kent, OH 44240
E-mail: jbissler@counselingforwellness.com
www.www.counselingforloss.com

Jane Vair Bissler, Ph.D., L, Counselor, Teacher, Writer and S

Look under articles for reprints of writings and links.

3237 www.cyberpsych.org
CyberPsych
www.www.cyberpsych.org

Hosts the American Psychoanlyists Foundation, American Association of Suicideology, Society for the Exploration of Psychotherapy Intergration, and Anxiety Disorders Association of America. Also subcategories of the anxiety disorders, as well as general information, including panic disorder, phobias, obsessive compulsive disorder (OCD), social phobia, generalized anxiety disorder, post traumatic stress disorder, and phobias of childhood. Book reviews and links to web pages sharing the topics.

3238 www.goaskalice.columbia.edu
GoAskAlice/Healthwise Columbia University
www.www.goaskalice.columbia.edu

Oriented toward students, information on sexuality, sexual health, general health, alcohol and other drugs, fitness and nutrition, emotional wellbeing and relationships.

3239 www.grieftalk.com/help1.html
Grief Journey
800-TAL-
www.www.grieftalk4u.com

Short readings for clients.

3240 www.healthgate.com/
HealthGate
770-754-4513
www.www.healthgate.com

Max Shapiro, M.D., Doctor
Judith Dennis, M.D., Doctor
Richard Dukes, M.D., Doctor
Steven Richman, M.D., Doctor

On-line reference and database information service, $.75/record.

3241 www.healthtouch.com
Healthtouch Online
3500 Westgate Drive
Suite 504
Durham, NC 27707
919-490-4656
www.www.healthtouchnc.com

Anya Adams, Referral Practitioners
Petra Gustin, Referral Practitioners
Ruth Hamilton, Referral Practitioners
Mara Bishop, Referral Practitioners

Healthtouch Online is a resource that brings together valuable information from trusted health organizations.

3242 www.healthy.net
HealthWorld Online
www.www.healthy.net

Consumer-oriented articles on a wide range of health and mental health topics, including: Welcome Center, QuickN'Dex, Site Search, Free Medline, Health Conditions, Alternative Medicine, Referral Network, Health Columns, Global Calendar, Discussion, Cybrarian, Professional Center, Free Newsletter, Opportunities, Healthy Travel, Homepage, Library, University, Marketplace, Health Clinic, Wellness Center, Fitness Center, News

Room, Association Network, Public Health, Self Care Central, and Nutrition Center.

3243 www.helix.com
GlaxoSmithKline
5 Crescent Drive
Philadelphia, PA 19112
888-825-5249
www.www.gsk.com

Roger Connor, President, Global Manufacturing
Deirdre Connelly, President, North America Pharmac
Abbas Hussain, President, Europe, Japan and EMA
Bill Louv, SVP, Core Business Services

Helix is an Education, Learning and Information exchange. Developed especially for healthcare practitioners by GlaxoSmithKline, HELIX is a premire source of on-line education and professional resources on a range of therapeutic and practice-management issues.

3244 www.human-nature.com/odmh
On-line Dictonary of Mental Health

Global information resource and research tool. It is compiled by Internet mental health resource users for Internet mental health resource users, and covers all the disciplines contributing to our understanding of mental health.

3245 www.infotrieve.com
Infotrieve Medline Services Provider
20 Westport Road
PO Box 7102
Wilton, CT 06897
203-423-2130
Fax: 203-423-2155
E-mail: marketing@infotrieve.com
www.www.infotrieve.com

Kenneth J. Benvenuto, President, CEO
Richard H. Dick Weaver, SVP
Donna Pouliot, VP, Sales
Eileen Green, VP, Finance

Infotrieve is a library services company offering full-service document delivery, databases on the web and a variety of tools to simplify the process of identifying, retrieving and paying for published literature.

3246 www.intelihealth.com
InteliHealth

3247 www.krinfo.com
DataStar/Dialog

Information provider: reference and databases.

3248 www.lollie.com/blue/suicide.html
Comprehensive Approach to Suicide Prevention
E-mail: LollieDotCom@gmail.com
www.www.lollie.com/blue/suicide.html

Readings for anyone contemplating suicide.

3249 www.mayohealth.org/mayo
Mayo Clinic Health Oasis Library
4500 San Pablo Road
Jacksonville, FL 32224
904-953-2000
Fax: 904-953-7329
www.www.mayoclinic.org

John H. Noseworthy, M.D., President
Andy Abril, M.D., Rheumatology, Medical Staff
Michael Albus, M.D., Emergency Medicine
Francisco Alvarez, M.D., Pulmonary Medicine

Healthcare library and resources.

3250 www.med.nyu.edu/Psych/index.html
NYU Department of Psychiatry

General mental health information, screening tests, reference desk, continuing educations in psychiatry program, interactive testing in psychiatry, augmentation of antidepressants, NYU Psychoanalytic Institute, Psychology Internship Program, Internet Mental Health Resources links.

3251 www.medscape.com
WebMD Health Professional Network
825 Eighth Avenue
11th Floor
New York, NY 10019
212-301-6700
E-mail: FirstInitialLastName@webmd.net
www.www.medscape.com

Steven L. Zatz M.D., President
Michael B. Glick, EVP, Co-General Counsel
David J. Schlanger, CEO
Peter Anevski, CFO

Oriented toward physicians and medical topics, but also carries information relevant to the field of psychology and mental health.

3252 www.members.aol.com/dswgriff
Now Is Not Forever: A Survival Guide

Print out a no-suicide contract, do problem solving, and other exercises.

3253 www.mentalhealth.com/p20-grp.html
Manic-Depressive Illness

Click on Bipolar and then arrow down to Booklets.

3254 www.mentalhealth.com/story
How to Help a Person with Depression

Valuable family education.

3255 www.mentalhealthamerica.net
Mental Health America
2000 N. Beauregard Street
6th Floor
Alexandria, VA 22311
703-684-7722
800-969-6642
Fax: 703-684-5968
www.www.mentalhealthamerica.net

David L. Shern, Ph.D., Interim President, CEO
Mike Turner, VP, Development
Dianne Felton, Chief Operating Officer
Julio Abreu, Senior Director of Public Policy

Mental Health America is the nation's largest and oldest community-based network dedicated to helping all Americans live mentally healthier lives. With more than 300 affiliates across the country, Mental Health America touches the lives of millions - advocating for changes in policy; educating the public and providing critical information; & delivering urgently needed programs and services.

3256 www.metanoia.org/suicide/
If You Are Thinking about Suicide...Read This First

www.www.metanoia.org/suicide

Excellent suggestions, information and links for the suicidal.

3257 www.mhsource.com
CME Mental Health InfoSource

Mental health information and education, fully accredited for all medical specialties.

3258 www.mhsource.com/
CME Psychiatric Time

Select articles published online from the Psychiatric Times, topics relevant to all mental health professionals.

3259 www.mindfreedom.org
Support Coalition Human Rights & Psychiatry Home Page
454 Willamette, PO Box 11284
Suite 216
Eugene, OR 97440-3484
541-345-9106
877-MAD-PRID
www.www.mindfreedom.org

Celia Brown, Board President
Thomas E. Wittick, MFI Member
Mary Maddock, Founder, MindFreedom Ireland
Al Galves, PhD, Psychologist, Mental Health Cons

Support Coalition is an independent alliance of several dozen grassroots groups in the USA, Canada, Europe, New Zealand; has used protests, publications, letter-writing, e-mail, workshops, Dendron News, the arts and performances. Led by psychiatric survivors, and open to the public, membership is open to anyone who supports its mission and goals.

3260 www.mirror-mirror.org/eatdis.htm
Mirror, Mirror

Relapse prevention for eating disorders.

3261 www.naphs.org
National Association of Psychiatric Health Systems
900 17th Street NW
Suite 420
Washington, DC 20006-2507
202-393-6700
Fax: 202-783-6041
www.www.naphs.org

Mark J. Covall, President, CEO
Kathleen McCann, RN, PhD, Director, Quality and Regulatory
Nancy Trenti, JD, Director, Congressional Affairs
Carole Szpak, Director, Operations and Communi

The NAPHS advocates for behavioral health and represents provider systems that are committed to the delivery of responsive, accountable and clinically effective prevention, treatment and care for children, adolescents and adults with mental and substance use disorders.

3262 www.naswdc.org/
National Associaton of Social Workers
750 First Street, NE
Suite 700
Washington, DC 20002-4241
202-408-8600
800-742-4089
E-mail: press@naswdc.org
www.www.naswdc.org/

Jeane W. Anastas, PhD, LMSW, President
Darrell P. Wheeler, PhD, ACSW, MP, President-Elect
E. Jane Middleton, DSW, MSW, VP
Mary L. McCarthy, PhD, LMSW, Treasurer

Central resource for clinical social workers, includes information about the federation, a conference and workshop calender, information on how to subscribe to social worker mailing lists, legislative and news updates, links to state agencies and social work societies, and publications.

3263 www.ndmda.org/justmood.htm
Just a Mood...or Something Else

A brochure for teens.

3264 www.nimh.nih.gov
National Institute of Mental Health (NIMH)
6001 Executive Boulevard
Rockville, MD 20852
301-443-4513
866-615-6464
Fax: 301-443-4279
TTY: 866-415-8051
E-mail: NIMHinfo@mail.nih.gov
www.www.nimh.nih.gov

Dianne M. Rausch, Ph.D., Director, Office on AIDS
Gemma Weiblinger, Director, Office of Constituency
Suzanne M. Murrin, Associate Director for Managemen
Pamela Y. Collins, M.D., M.P.H., Director, Office of Rural Mental

The mission of NIMH is to diminish the burden of mental illness through research of the biological, behavioral, clinical, epidemiological, economic, and social science aspects of mental illnesses.

3265 www.nmha.org
National Mental Health Association
2000 N. Beauregard Street
6th Floor
Alexandria, VA 22311
703-684-7722
800-969-6642
Fax: 703-684-5968
www.www.mentalhealthamerica.net

David L. Shern, Ph.D., Interim President, CEO
Mike Turner, VP, Development
Dianne Felton, Chief Operating Officer
Julio Abreu, Senior Director of Public Policy

Dedicated to promoting mental health, preventing mental disorders and achieving victory over mental illness through advocacy, education, research and service. NMHA's collaboration with the National GAINS Center for People with Co-Occuring Disorders in the Justice System has produced the Justice for Juveniles Initiative. This program battles to reform the juvenile justice system so that the inmates mental needs are addressed. Envisions a just, humane and healthy society in which all people are accorded respect, dignity and the opportunity to achieve their full potential free from stigma and prejudice.

3266 www.oclc.org
EPIC
6565 Kilgour Place
Dublin, OH 43017-3395
614-764-6000
800-848-5878
E-mail: oclc@oclc.org
www.www.oclc.org

Skip Prichard, President, CEO
Rick Schwieterman, EVP, CFO, Treasurer
Bruce Crocco, VP, Library Services for the Ame
Lorcan Dempsey, VP, OCLC Research and Chief Stra

On-line reference and database information provider, $40/hour (plus connection fees) and $.75/record.

3267 www.oznet.ksu.edu/library/famlf2/
Family Life Library
24 Umberger Hall
Kansas State University
Manhattan, KS 66506-3402
785-532-5830
Fax: 785-532-7938
E-mail: orderpub@k-state.edu
www.www.oznet.ksu.edu/library/famlf2/

3268 www.pace-custody.org
Professional Academy of Custody Evaluators
Furlong, PA 18925
800-633-7223
Fax: 215-794-3386
www.pace411.com

Dr. Barry Bricklin, Ph.D., Chair, Founding Member
Dr. Gail Elliot, Ph.D., Vice Chair, Founding Member
John J. Hare, Jr., Treasurer, Secretary

Nonprofit corporation and membership organization to acknowledge and strengthen the professionally prepared comprehensive custody evaluation; psychologicals legal knowledge base, assessment procedures, courtroom testimony, provides continuing education courses, conferences, conventions and seminars.

3269 www.paperchase.com
PaperChase
PO Box 54
Hood, VA 22723
781-325-6086
800-722-2075
Fax: 540-948-4841
E-mail: support@paperchase.com
www.www.paperchase.com

Searches may be conducted through a browsable list of topics, search engine recognizes queries made in natural language.

3270 www.parenthoodweb.com
Blended Families
Resolving conflicts.

3271 www.planetpsych.com
Planetpsych.com
E-mail: webmaster@planetpsych.com
www.www.planetpsych.com

Learn about disorders, their treatments and other topics in psychology. Articles are listed under the related topic areas. Ask a therapist a question for free, or view the directory of professionals in your area. If you are a therapist sign up for the directory. Current features, self-help, interactive, and newsletter archives.

3272 www.positive-way.com/step.htm
Stepfamily Information
www.www.positive-way.com/step.htm

Introduction and tips for stepfathers, stepmothers and re-married parents.

3273 www.psych.org
American Psychiatric Association
1000 Wilson Boulevard
Suite 1825
Arlington, VA 22209-3901
703-907-7322
800-368-5777
Fax: 703-907-1091
E-mail: appi@psych.org
www.www.psych.org

Ron McMillen, Chief Executive Officer
Robert E. Hales MD, M.B.A, Editor-in-Chief
John McDuffie, Editorial Director, Associate Pu
Rebecca D. Rinehart, Publisher

A medical specialty society recognized world-wide. Its 40, 500 US and international physicians specializing in the diagnosis and treatment of mental and emotional illness and substance use disorders.

384 pages Year Founded: 1993

3274 www.psychcentral.com
Psych Central
www.psychcentral.com

Personalized one-stop index for psychology, support, and mental health issues, resources, and people on the Internet.

3275 www.psychcrawler.com
American Psychological Association
750 1st Street NE
Washington, DC 20002-4242
202-336-5500
800-374-2721
Fax: 202-336-5518
TDD: 202-336-6123
TTY: 202-336-6123
E-mail: psycinfo@apa.org
www.psycnet.apa.org

Nadine J. Kaslow, Ph.D., President
Barry S. Anton, Ph.D., President-Elect
Donald N. Bersoff, PhD, JD, Past President
Norman B Anderson, Ph.D., CEO, EVP

Indexing the web for the links in psychology.

16 pages

3276 www.psychology.com/therapy.htm
Therapist Directory
800-935-3277
Fax: 847-792-7500
www.therapist.psychology.com

Therapists listed geographically plus answers to frequently asked questions.

3277 www.psycom.net/depression.central.html
Dr. Ivan's Depression Central

Medication-oriented site.

3278 www.recovery-inc.com
Recovery

Describes the organizations approach.

3279 www.reutershealth.com
Reuters Health
www.www.reutershealth.com

Relevant and useful clinical information on mental disorders, news briefs updated daily.

3280 www.save.org
SA/VE - Suicide Awareness/Voices of Education
8120 Penn Ave. S.
Suite 470
Bloomington, MN 55431
952-946-7998
800-273-8255
E-mail: dreidenberg@save.org
www.www.save.org

Daniel J. Reidenberg, PSY.D., ÿFA, Executive Director
Francene Young Rolstad, Business Manager
Linda Mars, Events Coordinator
Jennifer Owens, Program Coordinator

3281 www.schizophrenia.com
Schizophrenia.com
E-mail: szwebmaster@yahoo.com
www.www.schizophrenia.com

Brian Chiko, BSc, Executive Director
J. Megginson Hollister, PhD, Editor
Erin Hawkes, MSc, Writer/Contributor
Marvin Ross, Science Writer - Freelance

Offers basic and in-depth information, discussion and chat.

3282 www.schizophrenia.com/ami
Alliance for the Mentally Ill
E-mail: szwebmaster@yahoo.com
www.www.schizophrenia.com

Brian Chiko, BSc, Executive Director
J. Megginson Hollister, PhD, Editor
Erin Hawkes, MSc, Writer/Contributor
Marvin Ross, Science Writer - Freelance

Information on mental disorders, reducing the stigmatization of them in our society today, and how you can be more active in your local community. Includes articles, press information, media kits, mental disorder diagnostic and treatment information, coping issues, advocacy guides and announcements.

3283 www.schizophrenia.com/newsletter
Schizophrenia.com

Comprehensive psychoeducational site on schizophrenia.

3284 www.shpm.com
Self-Help and Psychology Magazine

General psychology and self-help magazine online, offers informative articles on general well being and psychology topics. Features Author of the Month, Breaking News Stories of the Month, Most Popular Pages, What's Hot, Departments, and Soundoff (articles and opinion page). This online compendium of hundreds of readers and professionals.

3285 www.shpm.com/articles/depress
Placebo Effect Accounts for Fifty Percent of Improvement

3286 www.siop.org
Society for Industrial and Organizational Psychology
440 E Poe Rd
Suite 101
Bowling Green, OH 43402
419-353-0032
Fax: 419-352-2645
E-mail: SIOP@siop.org
www.www.siop.org

Tammy Allen, President
David Nershi, Executive Director
Linda Lentz, Administrative Services Director
Larry Nader, IT Manager

Home to the Industrial-Organizational Pyschologist newsletter, links and resources, member information, contact information for doctoral and master's level program in I/O psychology, and announcements of various events and conferences.

3287 www.stepfamily.org/tensteps.htm
Ten Steps for Steps
310 West 85th St.
Suite 1B
New York, NY 10024
212-877-3244
E-mail: Stepfamily@aol.com
www.www.stepfamily.org

Jeannette Lofas, PhD, LCSW, President

Guidelines for stepfamilies.

3288 www.stepfamilyinfo.org/sitemap.htm
Stepfamily in Formation
310 West 85th St.
Suite 1B
New York, NY 10024
212-877-3244
E-mail: Stepfamily@aol.com
www.www.stepfamily.org

Jeannette Lofas, PhD, LCSW, President

3289 www.usatoday.com
USA Today

'Mental Health' category includes news and in-depth reports.

3290 www.webmd.com
WebMD

Kristy Hammam, SVP, Programming and Content Str
Michael W. Smith, MD, Chief Medical Editor
Brunilda Nazario, MD, Lead Medical Editor
Hansa Bhargava, MD, Medical Editor

3291 www.wingofmadness.com
Wing of Madness: A Depression Guide

Accurate information, advice, support, and personal experiences.

3292 Activities for Adolescents in Therapy
Charles C Thomas Publisher Ltd.
2600 S 1st Street
Springfield, IL 62704-4730
217-789-8980
800-258-8980
Fax: 217-789-9130
E-mail: books@ccthomas.com
www.ccthomas.com

Michael P Thomas, President
Susan T. Dennison, Author
Connie M. Knight, Author
Richar J. Laban, Author

In this practical resource manual, professionals will find more than 100 therapeutic group activities for use in counseling troubled adolescents. This new edition provides specifics on establishing an effective group program while, at the same time, outlining therapeutic activities that can be used in each phase of a therapy group. Step-by-step instructions have been provided for setting up, planning and facilitating adolescent groups with social and emotional problems. The interventions provided have been designed specifically for initial, middle and termination phases of group. $39.95 $46.95

264 pages Year Founded: 1998 ISBN 0-398068-07-0

3293 Activities for Children in Therapy: Guide for Planning and Facilitating Therapy with Troubled Children
Charles C Thomas Publisher Ltd.
2600 S 1st Street
Springfield, IL 62704-4730
217-789-8980
800-258-8980
Fax: 217-789-9130
E-mail: books@ccthomas.com
www.ccthomas.com

Michael P Thomas, President
Susan T. Dennison, Author
Connie M. Knight, Author
Richar J. Laban, Author

Provides the mental health professional with a wide variety of age-appropriate activities which are simultaneously fun and therapeutic for the five-to-twelve-year-old troubled child. Activities have been designed as enjoyable games in the context of therapy. Provides a comprehensive listing of books with other therapeutic intervention ideas, bibliotherapy materials, assessment scales for evaluating youngsters, and a sample child assessment for individual therapy. For professionals who provide counseling to children, such as social workers, psychologists, guidance counselors, speech/language pathologists, and art therapists. $52.95

302 pages Year Founded: 1999 ISBN 0-398069-71-9

3294 Chemical Dependency Treatment Planning Handbook
Charles C Thomas Publisher Ltd.
2600 S 1st Street
Springfield, IL 62704-4730
217-789-8980
800-258-8980
Fax: 217-789-9130

E-mail: books@ccthomas.com
www.ccthomas.com

Michael P Thomas, President
Richar J. Laban, Author
Connie M. Knight, Author
Susan T. Dennison, Author

Provides the entry-level clinician with a broad data base of treatment planning illustrations from which unpretentious treatment plans for the chemically dependent client can be generated. They are simple, largely measurable, and purposefully, with language that is cognizant of comprehension and learning needs of clients. It will be of interest to drug and alcohol counselors. $39.95

174 pages Year Founded: 1997 ISBN 0-398067-76-7

3295 Clinical Manual of Supportive Psychotherapy
American Psychiatric Publishing, Inc.
1000 Wilson Boulevard
Suite 1825
Arlington, VA 22209-3901
703-907-7322
800-368-5777
Fax: 703-907-1091
E-mail: appi@psych.org
www.appi.org

Ron McMillen, Chief Executive Officer
Robert E. Hales MD, M.B.A, Editor-in-Chief
John McDuffie, Editorial Director, Associate Pu
Rebecca D. Rinehart, Publisher

New approaches and ideas for your practice. $101.00

384 pages Year Founded: 1993 ISBN 0-880484-03-9

3296 Concise Guide to Laboratory and Diagnostic Testing in Psychiatry
American Psychiatric Publishing, Inc.
1000 Wilson Boulevard
Suite 1825
Arlington, VA 22209-3901
703-907-7322
800-368-5777
Fax: 703-907-1091
E-mail: appi@psych.org
www.appi.org

Ron McMillen, Chief Executive Officer
Robert E. Hales MD, M.B.A, Editor-in-Chief
John McDuffie, Editorial Director, Associate Pu
Rebecca D. Rinehart, Publisher

Basic strategies for applying laboratory testing and evaluation. $19.50

176 pages Year Founded: 1989 ISBN 0-880483-33-4

3297 Creating and Implementing Your Strategic Plan: Workbook for Public and Nonprofit Organizations
John Wiley & Sons
111 River Street
Hoboken, NJ 07030-5774
201-748-6000
Fax: 201-748-6088
E-mail: info@wiley.com
www.wiley.com

Stephen M. Smith, President, CEO
MJ O'Leary, SVP, Human Resources

Edward J. Melando, SVP, Corporate Controller
Gary M. Rinck, SVP, General Counsel

Step-by-step workbook to conducting strategic planning in public and nonprofit organizations. *$30.00*

Year Founded: 1992 ISBN 0-787967-54-8

3298 Handbook for the Study of Mental Health
Cambridge University Press
40 W 20th Street
New York, NY 10011-4211
212-924-3900
Fax: 212-691-3239
E-mail: marketing@cup.org
www.cup.org

Offers the first comprehensive presentation of the sociology of mental health illness, including original, contemporary contributions by experts in the relevant aspects of the field. Divided into three sections, the chapters cover the general perspectives in the field, the social determinants of mental health and current policy areas affecting mental health services. Designed for classroom use in sociology, social work, human relations, human services and psychology. With its useful definitions, overview of the historical, social and institutional frameworks for understanding mental health and illness, and nontechnical style, the text is suitable for advanced undergraduate or lower level graduate students. *$90.00*

694 pages Year Founded: 1999 ISBN 0-521561-33-7

3299 Handbook of Clinical Psychopharmacology for Therapists
NewHarbinger Publications
5674 Shattuck Avenue
Oakland, CA 94609-1662
510-652-0215
800-748-6273
Fax: 800-652-1613
E-mail: customerservice@newharbinger.com
www.newharbinger.com

Matthew McKay, Owner

This newly revised classic includes updates on new medications, and expanded quick reference section, and new material on bipolar illness, the treatment of psychosis, and the effect of severe trauma. *$55.95*

264 pages Year Founded: 2005 ISBN 1-572240-94-6

3300 Handbook of Constructive Therapies
John Wiley & Sons
111 River Street
Hoboken, NJ 07030-5774
201-748-6000
Fax: 201-748-6088
E-mail: info@wiley.com
www.wiley.com

Stephen M. Smith, President, CEO
MJ O'Leary, SVP, Human Resources
Edward J. Melando, SVP, Corporate Controller
Gary M. Rinck, SVP, General Counsel

Learn techniques that focus on the strengths and resources of your clients and look to where they want to go rather than where they have been. *$64.00*

Year Founded: 1992 ISBN 0-787940-44-5

3301 Handbook of Counseling Psychology
John Wiley & Sons
111 River Street
Hoboken, NJ 07030-5774
201-748-6000
Fax: 201-748-6088
E-mail: info@wiley.com
www.wiley.com

Stephen M. Smith, President, CEO
MJ O'Leary, SVP, Human Resources
Edward J. Melando, SVP, Corporate Controller
Gary M. Rinck, SVP, General Counsel

Provides a cross-disciplinary survey of the entire field and offers analysis of important areas of counseling psychology activity. the book elaborates on future directions for research, highlighting suggestions that may advance knowledge and stimulate further inquiry. Specific advice is presented from the literature in counseling psychology and related disciplines to help improve one's counseling practice. *$ 120.00*

Year Founded: 1992 ISBN 0-471254-58-4

3302 Handbook of Managed Behavioral Healthcare
John Wiley & Sons
111 River Street
Hoboken, NJ 07030-5774
201-748-6000
Fax: 201-748-6088
E-mail: info@wiley.com
www.wiley.com

Stephen M. Smith, President, CEO
MJ O'Leary, SVP, Human Resources
Edward J. Melando, SVP, Corporate Controller
Gary M. Rinck, SVP, General Counsel

A comprehensive curriculum to understanding managed care. *$43.00*

Year Founded: 1992 ISBN 0-787941-53-0

3303 Handbook of Medical Psychiatry
Mosby
11830 Westline Industrial Drive
Saint Louis, MO 63146-3318
314-872-8370
800-325-4177
Fax: 314-432-1380

This large-format handbook covers almost every psychiatric, neurologic and general medical condition capable of causing disturbances in thought, feeling, or behavior and includes almost every psychopharmacologic agent available in America today. *$61.95*

544 pages Year Founded: 1996 ISBN 0-323029-11-6

3304 Handbook of Mental Retardation and Development
Cambridge University Press
32 Avenue of the Americas
New York, NY 10013-2473
212-337- 500
845-353-7500
Fax: 212-691-3239
E-mail: newyork@cambridge.org
www.www.cambridge.org

Jacob A. Burack, Co-Author
Robert M. Hodapp, Co-Author
Edward F. Zigler, Co-Author

This book reviews theoretical and empirical work in the developmental approach to mental retardation. Armed with methods derived from the study of typically developing children, developmentalists have recently learned about the mentally retarded child's own development in a variety of areas. These now encompass many aspects of cognition, language, social and adaptive functioning, as well as of maladaptive behavior and psychopathology. In addition to a focus on individuals with mental retardation themselves, other ecological factors have influenced developmental approaches to mental retardation. Comprised of twenty seven chapters on various aspects of development, this handbook provides a comprehensive guide to understanding mental retardation. *$80.00*

782 pages Year Founded: 1998

3305 Handbook of Psychiatric Education and Faculty Development
American Psychiatric Publishing, Inc.
1000 Wilson Boulevard
Suite 1825
Arlington, VA 22209-3901
703-907-7322
800-368-5777
Fax: 703-907-1091
E-mail: appi@psych.org
www.www.appi.org

Saul Levin, M.D., M.P.A., CEO and Medical Director
Jerald Kay, M.D., Co-Editor
Edward K. Silberman, M.D., Co-Editor
Linda Pessar, M.D., Co-Editor

Putting education to work in the real world. *$68.50*

680 pages Year Founded: 1999 ISBN 0-880487-80-1

3306 Handbook of Psychiatric Practice in the Juvenile Court
American Psychiatric Publishing, Inc.
1000 Wilson Boulevard
Suite 1825
Arlington, VA 22209-3901
703-907-7322
800-368-5777
Fax: 703-907-1091
E-mail: appi@psych.org
www.www.appi.org

Robert E Hales M.D., M.B.A., Editor-in-Chief
Saul Levin, M.D., M.P.A., CEO and Medical Director
John McDuffie, Associate Publisher, Acquisition
Rebecca D. Rinehart, Publisher

How your practice can work with the court system, so your patients can get the help they need. *$27.95*

212 pages Year Founded: 1991 ISBN 0-890422-33-8

3307 Living Skills Recovery Workbook
Elsevier Science
PO Box 28430
Saint Louis, MO 63146-930
314-453-7010
800-545-2522
Fax: 314-453-7095
E-mail: orders@bhusa.com or custserv@bhusa.com
www.store.elsevier.com

Katie Hennessy, Medical Promotions Coordinator

Provides clinicians with the tools necessary to help patients with dual diagnoses acquire basic living skills. Focusing on stress management, time management, activities of daily living, and social skills training, each living skill is taught in relation to how it aids in recovery and relapse prevention for each patient's individual lifestyle and pattern of addiction.

224 pages ISBN 0-750671-18-1

3308 On the Client's Path: A Manual for the Practice of Brief Solution - Focused Therapy
NewHarbinger Publications
5674 Shattuck Avenue
Oakland, CA 94609-1662
510-652-0215
800-748-6273
Fax: 800-652-1613
E-mail: customerservice@newharbinger.com
www.newharbinger.com

Matthew McKay, Owner

Provides everything you need to master the solution - focused model. *$49.95*

157 pages Year Founded: 1995 ISBN 1-572240-21-0

3309 Relaxation & Stress Reduction Workbook
NewHarbinger Publications
5674 Shattuck Avenue
Oakland, CA 94609-1662
510-652-0215
800-748-6273
Fax: 800-652-1613
E-mail: customerservice@newharbinger.com
www.newharbinger.com

Matthew McKay, Owner

Details effective stress reduction methods such as breathing exercises, meditation, visualization, and time management. Widely reccomended by therapists, nurses, and physicians throughout the US, this fourth edition has been substantially revised and updated to reflect current research. Line drawings and charts. *$19.95*

276 pages Year Founded: 2005 ISBN 1-879237-82-2

3310 Skills Training Manual for Treating Borderline Personality Disorder, Companion Workbook
Guilford Press
72 Spring Street
New York, NY 10012-4068
212-431-9800
800-365-7006
Fax: 212-966-6708
E-mail: info@guilford.com
www.www.guilford.com

Bob Matloff, President
Seymour Weingarten, Editor-in-Chief

A vital component in Dr. Linehan's comprehensive treatment program, this step-by-step manual details precisely how to implement the skills training procedures and includes practical pointers on when to use the other treatment strategies described. It includes useful, clear-cut handouts that may be readily photocopied. *$27.95*

180 pages Year Founded: 1993 ISBN 0-898620-34-1

3311 Step Workbook for Adolescent Chemical Dependency Recovery
American Psychiatric Publishing, Inc.
1000 Wilson Boulevard
Suite 1825
Arlington, VA 22209-3901
703-907-7322
800-368-5777
Fax: 703-907-1091
E-mail: appi@psych.org
www.appi.org

Ron McMillen, Chief Executive Officer
Robert E. Hales MD, M.B.A, Editor-in-Chief
John McDuffie, Editorial Director, Associate Pu
Rebecca D. Rinehart, Publisher

Strategies for younger patients in your practice. *$62.00*

72 pages Year Founded: 1990 ISBN 0-882103-00-9

3312 Stress Management Training: Group Leader's Guide
Professional Resource Press
PO Box 3197
Sarasota, FL 34230-3197
941-343-9601
800-443-3364
Fax: 941-343-9201
E-mail: cs.prpress@gmail.com
www.prpress.com

Laurie Girsch, Managing Editor

This practical guide will help you define the concept of stress for group members and teach them various intervention techniques ranging from relaxation training to communication skills. Includes specific exercises, visual aids, stress response index, stress analysis form and surveys for evaluating program effectiveness. *$13.95*

96 pages Year Founded: 1990 ISBN 0-943158-33-8

3313 Stress Owner's Manual: Meaning, Balance and Health in Your Life
Impact Publishers
PO Box 6016
Atascadero, CA 93423-6016
805-466-5917
800-246-7228
Fax: 805-466-5919
E-mail: info@impactpublishers.com
www.impactpublishers.com

Offers specific solutions: maps, checklists and rating scales to help you assess your life; dozens of stress buffer activities to help you deal with stress on the spot; life-changing strategies to prepare you for a lifetime of effective stress management. *$15.95*

224 pages Year Founded: 2003 ISBN 1-886230-54-4

3314 The Comprehensive Directory
Resources For Children with Special Needs
116 E 16th Street
5th Floor
New York, NY 10003-2164
212-677-4650
Fax: 212-254-4070
E-mail: info@resourcesnyc.org
www.resourcesnyc.org

Rachel Howard, Executive Director
Stephen Stern, Director , Finance and Administr

Todd Dorman, Director, Communications and Out
Helen Murphy, Director, Program and Fund Devel

The directory for everyone who needs to find services for children with disabilities and special needs. Designed for parents, caregivers and professionals, it includes more than 2, 500 agencies providing more than 4, 000 services and programs. *$30.00*

1200 pages ISBN 0-967836-51-4

3315 Therapist's Workbook
John Wiley & Sons
111 River Street
Hoboken, NJ 07030-5774
201-748-6000
Fax: 201-748-6088
E-mail: info@wiley.com
www.wiley.com

Stephen M. Smith, President, CEO
MJ O'Leary, SVP, Human Resources
Edward J. Melando, SVP, Corporate Controller
Gary M. Rinck, SVP, General Counsel

This workbook nourishes and challenges counselors, guiding them on a journey of self-reflection and renewal. *$35.00*

Year Founded: 1992 ISBN 0-787945-23-4

3316 Treating Alcohol Dependence: a Coping Skills Training Guide
Guilford Press
72 Spring Street
New York, NY 10012-4068
212-431-9800
800-365-7006
Fax: 212-966-6708
E-mail: info@guilford.com
www.www.guilford.com

Bob Matloff, President
Seymour Weingarten, Editor-in-Chief

Treatment program based on a cognitive-social learning theory of alcohol abuse. Presents a straight-forward treatment strategy that copes with how to stop drinking and provides the training skills to make it possible. *$21.95*

240 pages Year Founded: 1989 ISBN 0-898622-15-8

Directories & Databases

3317 AAHP/Dorland Directory of Health Plans
Dorland Health
1500 Walnut Street
Suite 1000
Philadelphia, PA 19102-3512
215-875-1212
855-CAL- DH1
Fax: 301-287-2535
E-mail: info@dorlandhealth.com
www.dorlandhealth.com

Carol Brault, VP
Yolanda Matthews, Product Manager
Anne Llewellyn, Editor in Chief
Richard Scott, Managing Editor

Paperback, published yearly. *$215.00*

3318 **American Academy of Child and Adolescent Psychiatry - Membership Directory**
3615 Wisconsin Avenue NW
Washington, DC 20016-3007
202-966-7300
800-333-7636
Fax: 202-966-2891
E-mail: communications@aacap.org
www.aacap.org

Robert Hendren, President
Kristin Kroeger-Ptakowski, Director, Sr Deputy Director
Elizabeth DiLauro, Advocacy Manager
Emma Jellen, Policy Coordinator

$30.00

179 pages 2 per year

3319 **American Academy of Psychoanalysis and Dynamic Psychiatry**
American Academy of Psychoanalysis and Dynamic Psychiatry
One Regency Drive
PO Box 30
Bloomfield, CT 06002-30
888-691-8281
Fax: 860-286-0787
E-mail: info@aapdp.org
www.aapsa.org

Michael Blumenfield, MD, President
Sherry Katz-Bearnot, President
Jacquelyn T Coleman CAE, Executive Director
Carol Filiaci, Secretary

The journal of the American Academy of Psychoanalysis and Dynamic Psychiatry. Publishes articles by members and other authors who have a significant contribution to make to the community of scholars or practitioners interested in a psychodynamic understanding of human behavior. *$50.00*

70 pages

3320 **American Network of Community Options and Resources-Directory of Members**
ANCOR
1101 King Street
Suite 380
Alexandria, VA 22314-2962
703-535-7850
Fax: 703-535-7860
E-mail: ancor@ancor.org
www.ancor.org

Barbara Merrill, VP, Public Policy
Renee L Pietrangelo, CEO
Katherine Berland, Director, Government Relations
Tony Yu, Director, Web and I.T.

Covers 650 agencies serving people with mental retardation and other developmental disabilities. *$25.00*

179 pages 1 per year

3321 **American Psychiatric Association-Membership Directory**
Harris Publishing
2500 Westchester Avenue
Suite 400
Purchase, NY 10577-2515

800-326-6600
Fax: 914-641-3501
www.bcharrispub.com

$59.95

816 pages

3322 **American Psychoanalytic Association - Roster**
American Psychological Association
750 1st Street NE
Washington, DC 20002-4242
202-336-5500
800-374-2721
Fax: 202-336-5518
TDD: 202-336-6123
TTY: 202-336-6123
E-mail: webmaster@apa.org
www.apa.org

Nadine J. Kaslow, Ph.D., President
Barry S. Anton, Ph.D., President-Elect
Donald N. Bersoff, PhD, JD, Past President
Norman B Anderson, Ph.D., CEO, EVP

$40.00

194 pages

3323 **Association for Advancement of Behavior Therapy: Membership Directory**
305 Seventh Avenue
16th Floor
New York, NY 10001-6008
212-647-1890
Fax: 212-647-1865
E-mail: mebrown@aabt.org
www.www.abct.org

Mary Jane Eimer, Executive Director
Mary Ellen Brown, Administration/Convention
Rosemary Park, Membership Services

Covers over 4, 500 psychologists, psychiatrists, social workers and other interested in behavior therapy. *$50.00*

240 pages 2 per year

3324 **At Health**
7829 Center Blvd SE
Suite #226
Snoqualmie, WA 98065
425-292-0329
888-284-3258
Fax: 623-322-0498
E-mail: support@athealth.com
www.athealth.com

Providing trustworthy online information, tools, and training that enhance the ability of practitioners to furnish high quality, personalized care to those they serve. For the meantl health consumer, find practitioners, treatment center, learn about disorders and conditions, and about medications being used, news and resources.

3325 **CARF International**
Rehabilitation Accreditation Commission
6951ÿEast Southpoint Road
Tucson, AZ 85756-9407
520-325-1044
888-281-6531
Fax: 520-318-1129
TTY: 888-281-6531
www.carf.org

Brian J. Boon, Ph.D., President/CEO
Amanda E. Birch, Administrator Of Operations
Cindy L. Johnson, CPA, Chief Resource and Strategic Dev
Leslie Ellis-Lang, Managing Director

Covers about three thousand organizations in seven thousand locations offering more than eighteen hundred medical rehabilitation, behavioral health, and employment and community support services that have been accredited by CARF. *$100.00*

200 pages 1 per year Year Founded: 1999

3326 Case Management Resource Guide
Dorland Health
1500 Walnut Street
Suite 1000
Philadelphia, PA 19102-3512
215-875-1212
855-CAL- DH1
Fax: 301-287-2535
E-mail: info@dorlandhealth.com
www.dorlandhealth.com

Carol Brault, VP
Yolanda Matthews, Product Manager
Anne Llewellyn, Editor in Chief
Richard Scott, Managing Editor

In four volumes, over 110, 000 health care facilities and support services are listed, including homecare, rehabilitation, psychiatric and addiction treatment programs, hospices, adult day care and burn and cancer centers.

5, 200 pages 1 per year ISBN 1-880874-84-9

3327 Case Manager Database
Dorland Health
1500 Walnut Street
Suite 1000
Philadelphia, PA 19102-3512
215-875-1212
855-CAL- DH1
Fax: 301-287-2535
E-mail: info@dorlandhealth.com
www.dorlandhealth.com

Carol Brault, VP
Yolanda Matthews, Product Manager
Anne Llewellyn, Editor in Chief
Richard Scott, Managing Editor

Largest database of information on case managers in US, especially of case managers who work for health plans and health insurers. Covers over 15, 000 case managers and includes detailed data such as work setting and clinical specialty, which can be used to carefully target marketing communications. $2500 for full database, other prices available.

3328 Complete Directory for People with Disabilities
Grey House Publishing
4919 Route 22
PO Box 56
Amenia, NY 12501
518-789-8700
800-562-2139
Fax: 518-789-0556
E-mail: books@greyhouse.com
www.greyhouse.com

Richard Gottlieb, President
Leslie Mackenzie, Publisher

This one-stop annual resource provides immediate access to the latest products and services available for people with disabilities, such as Periodicals & Books, Assistive Devices, Employment & Education Programs, Camps and Travel Groups. *$165.00*

1200 pages ISBN 1-592370-07-1

3329 Complete Learning Disabilities Directory
Grey House Publishing
4919 Route 22
PO Box 56
Amenia, NY 12501
518-789-8700
800-562-2139
Fax: 518-789-0556
E-mail: books@greyhouse.com
www.greyhouse.com

Richard Gottlieb, President
Leslie Mackenzie, Publisher

This annual resource includes information about Associations & Organizations, Schools, Colleges & Testing Materials, Government Agencies, Legal Resources and much more. *$195.00*

745 pages ISBN 1-930956-79-7

3330 Complete Mental Health Directory
Grey House Publishing
4919 Route 22
PO Box 56
Amenia, NY 12501
518-789-8700
800-562-2139
Fax: 518-789-0556
E-mail: books@greyhouse.com
www.greyhouse.com

Richard Gottlieb, President
Leslie Mackenzie, Publisher

This bi-annual directory offers understandable descriptions of 25 Mental Health Disorders as well as detailed information on Associations, Media, Support Groups and Mental Health Facilities. *$165.00*

800 pages ISBN 1-592370-46-2

3331 DSM-IV Psychotic Disorders: New Diagnostic Issue
American Psychiatric Publishing, Inc.
1000 Wilson Boulevard
Suite 1825
Arlington, VA 22209-3901
703-907-7322
800-368-5777
Fax: 703-907-1091
E-mail: appi@psych.org
www.appi.org

Ron McMillen, Chief Executive Officer
Robert E. Hales MD, M.B.A, Editor-in-Chief
John McDuffie, Editorial Director, Associate Pu
Rebecca D. Rinehart, Publisher

Updates on clinical findings. *$39.95*

Year Founded: 1995

3332 Detwiler's Directory of Health and Medical Resources
Dorland Health
1500 Walnut Street
Suite 1000
Philadelphia, PA 19102-3512
215-875-1212
855-CAL- DH1
Fax: 301-287-2535
E-mail: info@dorlandhealth.com
www.dorlandhealth.com

Carol Brault, VP
Yolanda Matthews, Product Manager
Anne Llewellyn, Editor in Chief
Richard Scott, Managing Editor

An invaluable guide to healthcare information sources. This directory lists information on over 2, 000 sources of information on the medical and healthcare industry. *$195.00*

1 per year Year Founded: 1999 ISBN 1-880874-57-1

3333 Directory for People with Chronic Illness
Grey House Publishing
4919 Route 22
PO Box 56
Amenia, NY 12501
518-789-8700
800-562-2139
Fax: 518-789-0556
E-mail: books@greyhouse.com
www.greyhouse.com

Richard Gottlieb, President
Leslie Mackenzie, Publisher

This bi-annual resource provides a comprehensive overview of the support services and information resources available for people diagnosed with a chronic illness. Includes 12, 000 entries. *$165.00*

1200 pages ISBN 1-592370-81-0

3334 Directory of Developmental Disabilities Services
Nebraska Health and Human Services System
PO Box 94728
Department of Services
Lincoln, NE 68509-4728
402-471-2851
800-833-7352
Fax: 402-479-5094

Covers agencies and organizations that provide developmental disability services and programs in Nebraska.

28 pages

3335 Directory of Health Care Professionals
Dorland Health
1500 Walnut Street
Suite 1000
Philadelphia, PA 19102-3512
215-875-1212
855-CAL- DH1
Fax: 301-287-2535
E-mail: customer@decisionhealth.com
www.dorlandhealth.com

Carol Brault, VP
Yolanda Matthews, Product Manager
Anne Llewellyn, Editor in Chief
Richard Scott, Managing Editor

Helps you easily locate the key personnel and facilities you want by hospital name, system head-quarters, or job title. Valuable for locating industry professionals, recruiting, networking, and prospecting for industry business. *$299.00*

1 per year Year Founded: 1998 ISBN 1-573721-40-9

3336 Directory of Hospital Personnel
Grey House Publishing
4919 Route 22
PO Box 56
Amenia, NY 12501
518-789-8700
800-562-2139
Fax: 518-789-0556
E-mail: books@greyhouse.com
www.greyhouse.com

Richard Gottlieb, President
Leslie Mackenzie, Publisher

Best annual resource for researching or marketing a product or service to the hospital industry. Includes 6, 000 hospitals and over 80, 000 key contacts. *$275.00*

2400 pages ISBN 1-592370-26-8

3338 Directory of Physician Groups and Networks
Dorland Health
1500 Walnut Street
Suite 1000
Philadelphia, PA 19102-3512
215-875-1212
855-CAL- DH1
Fax: 301-287-2535
E-mail: info@dorlandhealth.com
www.dorlandhealth.com

Carol Brault, VP
Yolanda Matthews, Product Manager
Anne Llewellyn, Editor in Chief
Richard Scott, Managing Editor

Reference tool with over 4, 000 entries covering IPAs, PHOs, large medical group practices with 20 or more physicians, MSOs and PPMCs. Paperback, published yearly. *$345.00*

Year Founded: 1998 ISBN 1-880874-50-4

3339 Dorland's Medical Directory
Dorland Health
1500 Walnut Street
Suite 1000
Philadelphia, PA 19102-3512
215-875-1212
855-CAL- DH1
Fax: 301-287-2535
E-mail: info@dorlandhealth.com
www.dorlandhealth.com

Carol Brault, VP
Yolanda Matthews, Product Manager
Anne Llewellyn, Editor in Chief
Richard Scott, Managing Editor

Contains expanded coverage of healthcare facilities with profiles of 616 group practices, 661 hospitals and 750 rehabilitation, subacute, hospice and long term care facilities. *$699.00*

1 per year ISBN 1-880874-82-2

3340 Drug Information Handbook for Psychiatry
Lexicomp Inc.
1100 Terex Road
Hudson, OH 44236-4438
330-650-6506
800-837-5394
Fax: 330-656-4307
www.lexi.com

Steven Kerscher, Owner
Arvind Subramanian, President, CEO, Wolters Kluwer H
Cheri Palmer, Vice President of Commercial Pro
John Pins, Vice President, Finance, Clinica

Written specifically for mental health professionals. Addresses the fact that mental health patients may be taking additional medication for the treatment of another medical condition in combination with their psychtropic agents. With that in mind, this book contains information on all drugs, not just the psychotropic agents. Specific fields of information contained within the drug monograph include Effects on Mental Status and Effects on Psychiatric Treatment. *$38.75*

1 per year ISBN 1-591951-14-3

3341 HMO & PPO Database & Directory
Dorland Health
1500 Walnut Street
Suite 1000
Philadelphia, PA 19102-3512
215-875-1212
855-CAL- DH1
Fax: 301-287-2535
E-mail: info@dorlandhealth.com
www.dorlandhealth.com

Carol Brault, VP
Yolanda Matthews, Product Manager
Anne Llewellyn, Editor in Chief
Richard Scott, Managing Editor

Delivers comprehensive and current information on senior-level individuals at virtually all US HMOs and PPOs at an affordable price. *$400.00*

3342 HMO/PPO Directory
Grey House Publishing
4919 Route 22
PO Box 56
Amenia, NY 12501
518-789-8700
800-562-2139
Fax: 518-789-0556
E-mail: books@greyhouse.com
www.greyhouse.com

Richard Gottlieb, President
Leslie Mackenzie, Publisher

This annual resource provides detailed information about health maintenance organizations and preferred provider organizations nationwide. *$275.00*

500 pages ISBN 1-592370-22-5

3343 Innovations in Clinical Practice: Source Book -
Volumes 4-20
Professional Resource Press
PO Box 3197
Sarasota, FL 34230-3197
941-343-9601
800-443-3364

Fax: 941-343-9201
E-mail: cs.prpress@gmail.com
www.prpress.com

Laurie Girsch, Managing Editor

Provides a comprehensive source of practical information and applied techniques that can be put to immediate use in your practice. *$64.95*

524 pages Year Founded: 1999

3344 Medical & Healthcare Marketplace Guide
Directory
Dorland Health
1500 Walnut Street
Suite 1000
Philadelphia, PA 19102-3512
215-875-1212
855-CAL- DH1
Fax: 301-287-2535
E-mail: info@dorlandhealth.com
www.dorlandhealth.com

Carol Brault, VP
Yolanda Matthews, Product Manager
Anne Llewellyn, Editor in Chief
Richard Scott, Managing Editor

Contains valuable data on pharmaceutical, medical advice, and clinical and non-clinical healthcare service companies worldwide. *$499.00*

3345 Medical Psychoterapist and Disability Analysts
Americel Board of Medical Psychoterapists &
Psychodiagnosticians
4525 Harding Pike
Nashville, TN 37205
615-327-2984
Fax: 615-327-9235
E-mail: americanbd@aol.com

Official newsletter of the American Board of Medical Psychoterapists and Psychodiagnosticians.

3346 Mental Health Directory
Office of Consumer, Family & Public Information
5600 Fishers Lane, Room 15-99
Center For Mental Health Services
Rockville, MD 20857-1
301-443-2792
Fax: 301-443-5163

Covers hospitals, treatment centers, outpatient clinics, day/night facilities, residential treatment centers for emotionally disturbed children, residential supportive programs such as halfway houses, and mental health centers offering mental health assistance. *$23.00*

468 pages

3347 National Association of Psychiatric Health
Systems: Membership Directory
900 17th Street, NW
Suite 420
Washington, DC 20006
202-393-6700
Fax: 202-783-6041
E-mail: naphs@naphs.org
www.naphs.org

Mark J. Covall, President, CEO, Executive Direct
Carole Szpak, Director Communications and Oper
Nancy Trenti, JD, Director, Congressional Affairs

Kathleen McCann, RN, PhD, Director, Quality and Regulatory

Contact information of professional groups working to coordinate a full spectrum of treatment services, including inpatient, residential, partial hospitalization and outpatient programs as well as prevention and management services. *$32.10*

48 pages 1 per year Year Founded: 1933

3348 National Register of Health Service Providers in Psychology

1200 New York Avenue NW
Suite 800
Washington, DC 20005-3873
202-783-7663
Fax: 202-347-0550
E-mail: andrew@nationalregister.org
www.nationalregister.org

Greg Hurley, Vice President/Vice-Chair
Judy E Hall, CEO
Andrew P. Boucher, Assistant Director
Julia Bernstein, Membership Coordinator

Psychologists who are licensed or certified by a state/provincial board of examiners of psychology and who have met council criteria as health service providers in psychology.

Year Founded: 1974

3349 National Registry of Psychoanalysts
National Association for the Advancement of Psychoanalysis

80 8th Avenue
Suite 1501
New York, NY 10011-5126
212-741-0515
Fax: 212-366-4347
E-mail: dfmaxwell@mac.com
www.naap.org

Douglas Maxwell, President
Margery Quackenburh, Executive Director
Kirsty Cardinale, Editor
Elliott Hom, Art Director

NAAP provides information to the public on psychoanalysis. Publishes quarterly NAAP News, annual Registry of Psychoanalysts. *$ 15.00*

175 pages

3350 Patient Guide to Mental Health Issues: Desk Chart
Lexicomp Inc.

1100 Terex Road
Hudson, OH 44236-4438
330-650-6506
800-837-5394
Fax: 330-656-4307
www.lexi.com

Steven Kerscher, Owner
Arvind Subramanian, President, CEO, Wolters Kluwer H
Cheri Palmer, Vice President of Commercial Pro
John Pins, Vice President, Finance, Clinica

Designed specifically for healthcare professionals dealing with mental health patients. Combines eight of our popular Patient Chart titles into one, convenient desktop presentation. This will assist in explaining the most common mental

health issue to your patients on a level that they will understand. *$38.75*

1 per year ISBN 1-591950-54-6

3351 PsycINFO Database
PsycINFO, American Psychological Association

750 1st Street NE
Washington, DC 20002-4242
202-336-5500
800-374-2721
Fax: 202-336-5518
TDD: 202-336-6123
TTY: 202-336-6123
E-mail: psycinfo@apa.org
www.apa.org

Nadine J. Kaslow, Ph.D., President
Barry S. Anton, Ph.D., President-Elect
Donald N. Bersoff, PhD, JD, Past President
Norman B Anderson, Ph.D., CEO, EVP

PsycINFO is a database that contains citations and summaries of journal articles, book chapters, books, dissertations and technical reports in the field of psychology and the psychological aspects of related disciplines, such as medicine, psychiatry, nursing, sociology, education, pharmacology, physiology, linguistics, anthropology, business and law. Journal coverage, spanning 1887 to present, includes international material from 1, 800 periodicals written in over 30 languages. Current chapter and book coverage includes worldwide English language material published from 1987 to present. Over 75, 000 references are added annually through weekly updates.

52 per year

3352 Rating Scales in Mental Health
Lexicomp Inc.

1100 Terex Road
Hudson, OH 44236-4438
330-650-6506
800-837-5394
Fax: 330-656-4307
www.lexi.com

Steven Kerscher, Owner
Arvind Subramanian, President, CEO, Wolters Kluwer H
Cheri Palmer, Vice President of Commercial Pro
John Pins, Vice President, Finance, Clinica

Ideal for clinicians as well as administrators, this title provides an overview of over 100 recommended rating scales for mental health assessment. This book is also a great tool to assist mental healthcare professionals determine the appropriate psychiatric rating scale when assessing their clients. *$38.75*

1 per year ISBN 1-591950-52-X

3353 Roster: Centers for the Developmentally Disabled
Nebraska Department of Health and Human Services

301 Centennial Mall S
Lincoln, NE 68508-2529
402-471-3121
800-254-4202
Fax: 402-471-0555
TDD: 070-119-99
www.dhhs.ne.gov

Joann Erickson RN, Program Manager

Covers approximately 160 licensed facilities in Nebraska for the developmentally disabled.

40 pages 1 per year

3354 Roster: Health Clinics
Nebraska Department of Health and Human Services
301 Centennial Mall S
Lincoln, NE 68508-2529
402-471-3121
800-254-4202
Fax: 402-471-0555
www.dhhs.ne.gov

Joann Erickson RN, Section Administrator

Covers approximately 90 licensed health clinic facilities in Nebraska.

11 pages 1 per year

3355 Roster: Substance Abuse Treatment Centers
Nebraska Department of Health and Human Services
301 Centennial Mall S
Lincoln, NE 68508-2529
402-471-3121
800-254-4202
Fax: 402-471-0555
www.dhhs.ne.gov

Joann Erickson RN, Program Manager

Covers approximately 56 licensed substance abuse treatment centers in Nebraska.

12 pages 1 per year

Publishers

Books

3356 ABC-CLIO
88 Post Road West
Westport, CT 06880-4208
203-226-3571
Fax: 203-222-1502
E-mail: webmaster@greenwood.com
www.www.abc-clio.com/

Wayne Smith, President

Publisher of reference titles, academic and general interest books, texts, books for librarians and other profesionals, and electronic resources.

3357 Active Parenting Publishers
1220 Kennestone Circle
Suite 130
Marietta, GA 30066-6022
770-429-0565
800-825-0060
Fax: 770-429-0334
E-mail: cservice@activeparenting.com
www.ActiveParenting.com

Michael H Popkin, PhD, Founder and President
Gabrielle Tingley, Art Director, Marketing Departmen
Melody Popkin, Manager of Christian Resources
Cathie Jordet, Accounting Manager, Finance Depar

Delivers quality education programs for parents, children and teachers to schools, hospitals, social service organizations, churches and corporate market. Innovator in the educational market.

Year Founded: 1980

3358 American Psychiatric Publishing (APPI)
1000 Wilson Boulevard
Suite 1825
Arlington, VA 22209-3924
703-907-7322
800-368-5777
Fax: 703-907-1091
E-mail: appi@psych.org
www.appi.org

Saul Levin, M.D., M.P.A, CEO and Medical Director
Robert E Hales, M.D., M.B.A, Editor-in-Chief, Books
Rebecca D Rinehart, Publisher
John McDuffie, Editorial Director

Publisher of books, journals, and multi-media on psychiatry, mental healths and behavioral science. Offers authoratative, up-to-date and affordable information geared toward psychiatrists, other mental health professionals, psychiatric residents, medical students and the general public.

3359 Analytic Press
10 Industrial Avenue
Mahwah, NJ 07430-2253
201-258-2200
Fax: 201-760-3735
www.analyticpress.com

Publishes works of substance and originality that constitute genuine contributions to their respective disciplines and professions.

3360 Brookes Publishing
PO Box 10624
Baltimore, MD 21285-0624
410-337-9580
800-638-3775
Fax: 410-337-8539
E-mail: custserv@brookespublishing.com
www.brookespublishing.com

George Stamathis, Vice-President
Jeffrey D Brookes, President
Melissa A Behm, Executive Vice President

Publishes highly respected resources in early childhood, early interventions, inclusive and special education, developmental disabilities, learning disabilities, communication and language, behavior, and mental health

Year Founded: 1978

3361 Brookline Books/Lumen Editions
34 University Road
Brookline, MA 02445-4533
617-734-6772
Fax: 617-734-3952
www.brooklinebooks.com

Publishes books on learning disabilities, study skills, self-advocacy for the disabled, early childhood intervention, and more, in readable language that reaches beyond the academic community.

3362 Brunner-Routledge Mental Health
270 Madison Avenue
New York, NY 10016-601
212-695-6599
800-634-7064

Maura May, Publisher

The Routledge imprint publishes books and journals on clinical psychology, psychiatry, psychoanalysis, analytical psychology, psychotherapy, counseling, mental health and other professional subjects.

3363 Bull Publishing Company
PO Box 1377
Boulder, CO 80306-1377
303-545-6350
800-676-2855
Fax: 303-545-6354
E-mail: jim.bullpubco@comcast.net
www.bullpub.com

Emily Sewell, Vice President of Operations
Claire Cameron, Director of Marketing

Publisher of books focused on addressing the growing need for sound health information and good advice.

3364 Cambridge University Press
32 Avenue of the Americas
New York, NY 10013-2473
212-337-5000
E-mail: newyork@cambrigde.org
www.www.cambridge.org

Printing and publishing house that is an integral part of the University and has similar charitable objectives in advancing knowledge, education, learning and research.

3365 Castal Harlan
150 East 58th Street
New York, NY 10155

212-644-8600
800-775-1800
Fax: 212-207-8042
E-mail: info@castleharlan.com
www.www.castleharlan.com

Leonard M Harlan, Chairman of the Executive Commun
John K Castle, Chairman, CEO
Howard D Morgan, Co-President
William M Pruellage, Co-President

Provides quality information and entertainment services. Worldwide distributor of books, videos, music and games in all disciplines.

Year Founded: 1987

3366 Charles C Thomas Publishers

2600 South First Street
Springfield, IL 62704
217-789-8980
800-258-8980
Fax: 217-789-9130
E-mail: books@ccthomas.com
www.ccthomas.com

Producing a strong list of specialty titles and textbooks in the biomedical sciences. Also very active in producing books for the behavioral sciences, education and special education, speech language and hearing, as well as rehabilitation and long-term care. One of the largest producers of books in all areas of criminal justice and law enforcement.

Year Founded: 1927

3367 Crossroad Publishing

831 Chestnut Ridge Rd
Spring Valley, NY 10977-6356
212-868-1801
Fax: 212-868-2171
E-mail: ask@crossroadspublishing.com
www.cpcbooks.com

Publishes words of thoughtfulness and hope. A leading independent publishing house.

3368 EBSCO Information Services

10 Estes Street
Ipswich, MA 01938-2106
978-356-6500
800-653-2726
Fax: 978-356-6565
www.www.ebsco.com/

Timothy S Collins, President

EBSCO Publishing offers electronic access to a variety of health data: full text databases containing aggregate journals, access to publishers' electronic journals, and the citational databases produced by the American Psychiatric Association to name just a few. Offers a free, nonobligation, on-line trial.

3369 Family Experiences Productions

PO Box 5879
Austin, TX 78763-5879
512-494-0338
Fax: 512-494-0340
E-mail: todd@fepi.com
www.fepi.com

R Geyer, Executive Producer

Consumers Health videos; available individually, or in large volume (private branded) for health providers to give to patients, professionals, staff. Postpartum Emotions, Parenting Preschoolers, Facing Death (5-tape series) and teen grief English and Spanish.

ISSN 1-930772-00-9

3370 Franklin Electronic Publishers

3 Terri Lane
Suite 6
Burlington, NJ 08016-4907
609-386-2500
800-266-5626
Fax: 609-239-5950
E-mail: service@franklin.com
www.franklin.com

Barry J Lipsky, CEO

Publishes materials for healthcare.

3371 Free Spirit Publishing

217 Fifth Avenue North
Suite 200
Minneapolis, MN 55401-1299
612-338-2068
866-703-7322
Fax: 866-419-5199
www.freespirit.com

Judy Galbraith, Founder

Publisher of learning tools that support young people's social and emotional health. Known for unique understanding of what young adults want and need to know to navigate life successfully.

Year Founded: 1983

3372 Grey House Publishing

4919 Route 22
PO Box 56
Amenia, NY 12501
518-789-8700
800-562-2139
Fax: 518-789-0556
E-mail: books@greyhouse.com
www.greyhouse.com

Richard Gottlieb, President

Publishes over 100 titles including reference directories in the areas of business, education, health, statistics and demographics, as well as educational encyclopedias and business handbooks. All titles offer detailed information in well-organized formats. Many titles available online.

Year Founded: 1981

3373 Guilford Publications

72 Spring Street
New York, NY 10012-4068
212-431-9800
800-365-7006
Fax: 212-966-6708
E-mail: info@guilford.com
www.www.guilford.com/

Bob Matloff, President

Publisher of books, periodicals, software and audiovisual programs in mental health, education, and the social sciences.

Year Founded: 1973

3374 Gurze Books
5145 B Avenida Encinas
Carisbad, CA 92008
760-434-7533
800-756-7533
Fax: 760-434-5476
E-mail: info@gurze.net
www.www.gurzebooks.com

Lindsay Cohn, Co-Owner
Leigh Cohn, Co-Owner

Publishing company that specializes in resources and education on eating disorders. Offers high quality materials on understanding and overcoming eating disorders of all kinds.

Year Founded: 1980

3375 Harper Collins Publishers
10 East 53rd Street
New York, NY 10022-5299
212-207-7000
Fax: 212-207-6964
E-mail: feedback2@harpercollins.com
www.harpercollins.com

Brian Murray, President and CEO
Susan Katz, President/publisher, Harper Colli
Chantal Restivo-Alessi, Chief Digital Officer
Larry Nevins, Executive Vice Preisdent, Operati

A subsidiary of News Corporation, Harper Collins produces literary and commercial fiction, business books, children's books, cookbooks, mystery, romance, reference, religious, healthcare and spiritual books.

Year Founded: 1817

3376 Harvard University Press
79 Garden Street
Cambridge, MA 02138-1400
617-495-2600
800-405-1619
Fax: 617-495-5898
E-mail: contact_hup@harvard.edu
www.www.hup.harvard.edu

William Sisler, President

Publishes material on varied topics including healthcare.

Year Founded: 1913

3377 Hazelden
PO Box 11
Center City, MN 55012-0011
651-213-4200
800-257-7810
Fax: 651-213-4793
E-mail: info@hazelden.org
www.hazelden.org

Mark Mishek, President and CEO, Hazeldon Betty
James A Blaha, VP Finance, Administration/CFO
Marvin D Seppala, MD, Chief Medical Officer
Mark Sheets, Execurive Director, Regional serv

A nonprofit organization that helps people transform their lives by providing the highest quality treatment and continuing care services, education, research, and publishing products available today.

Year Founded: 1949

3378 Health Communications
3201 SouthWest 15th Street
Deerfield Beach, FL 33442-8157
954-360-0909
800-441-5569
Fax: 954-360-0034
www.hcibooks.com

Peter Vegso, CEO

Original publisher of informational pamphlets for the recovery community; publishes inspiration, soul/spirituality, relationships, recovery/healing, women's issues and self-help material.

Year Founded: 1977

3379 High Tide Press
Ste 2N
2081 Calistoga Dr
New Lenox, IL 60451-4833
815-206-2054
800-469-9461
www.www.hightidepress.com/

Art Dykstra, Executive Director
Steve Baker, Director

Provides high quality books, training materials and seminars to people working in the field of human services. Seek to provide the best resources in developmental, mental and learning disabilities, as well as psychology, leadership and management.

3380 Hogrefe Publishing
38 Chauncy Street
Suite 485
Boston, MA 02111
866-823-4726
Fax: 617-354-6875
E-mail: customerservice(at)hogrefe-publishing.com
www.www.hogrefe.com

Publisher of journals and books of all different variety titles including healthcare.

3381 Hope Press
110 Mill Run
Monrovia, CA 91016-1658
626-303-0644
800-321-4039
Fax: 626-358-3520
E-mail: dcomings@mail.earthlink.net
www.hopepress.com

Specializes in the publication of books on Tourette Syndrome, Attention Deficit Hyperactivity Disorder (ADHD, ADD), Conduct Disorder, Oppositional Defiant Disorder and other psychological, psychiatric and behavioral problems.

3382 Hyperion Books
237 Park Avenue
New York, NY 10017
Fax: 212-456-1980
www.hyperionbooks.com

Publishes general-interest fiction and nonfiction books for adults including healthcare titles. Includes the Miramax, ESPN Books, ABC Daytime Press, Hyperion East and Hyperion Audiobooks.

3383 Icarus Films
32 Court Street
21st Floor
Brooklyn, NY 11201
718-488-8900
800-937-4113
Fax: 718-488-8642
E-mail: info@fanlight.com
www.www.icarusfilms.com

Distributor of innovative film and video works on the social issues of our time, with a special focus on healthcare, mental health, profesional ethics, aging and gerontology, disabilites, the workplace, and gender and family issues.

Year Founded: 1978

3384 Impact Publishers
PO Box 6016
Atascadero, CA 93423-6016
805-466-5917
800-246-7228
E-mail: info@impactpublishers.com
www.impactpublishers.com

Produces a select list of psychology and self improvement books and audio-tapes for adults, children, families, organizations, and communities. Written by highly respected psychologists and other human service professionals.

Year Founded: 1970

3385 Jerome M Sattler Publisher
PO Box 1060
La Mesa, CA 91944-1060
619-460-3667
888-815-2898
Fax: 619-460-2489
E-mail: sattlerpublisher@sbcglobal.net
www.sattlerpublisher.com

Publishes books that represent the cutting edge of clinical assessment of children and families. Designed for students in training as well as for practitioners ans clinicians.

3386 John Wiley & Sons
111 River Street
Hoboken, NJ 07030-5774
201-748-6000
Fax: 201-748-6088
E-mail: info@wiley.com
www.wiley.com

Peter B Wiley, Chairman of the Board
Stephen M Smith, President and Chief Executive Of
John Kritzmacher, Executive Vice President and CFO
Ellis E Cousens, Executive Vice President and COO

A global publisher of print and electronic products, specializing in scientific, technical, and medical books and journals professional and consumer books and subscription services; also textbooks and other educational materials for undergraduate and graduate students as well as lifelong learners.

3387 John Wiley & Sons, Inc.
111 River Street
Hoboken, NJ 07030-5774
201-748-6000
Fax: 201-748-6088
E-mail: info@wiley.com
www.wiley.com

Peter B Wiley, Chairman of the Board
Stephen M Smith, President and Chief Executive Of
John Kritzmacher, Executive Vice President and CFO
Ellis E Cousens, Executive Vice President and COO

Jossey-Bass publishes books, periodicals, and other media to inform and inspire those interested in developing themselves, their organizations and their communities. The publications feature the work of some of the world's best-known authors in leadership, business, education, religion and spirituality, parenting, nonprofit, public health and health administration, conflict resolution and relationships.

3388 Johns Hopkins University Press
2715 North Charles Street
Baltimore, MD 21218-4363
410-516-6900
Fax: 410-516-6968
E-mail: webmaster@jhupress.jhu.edu
www.www.press.jhu.edu/

William Brody, President

Publishes 58 scholarly periodicals and more than 200 new books each year. A leading online provider of scholarly journals, bringing more than 250 periodicals to the desktops of 9 million students, scholars, and others worldwide.

Year Founded: 1878

3389 Lexington Books
4501 Forbes Boulevard
Suite 200
Lanham, MD 20706-4346
301-459-3366
800-462-6420
Fax: 301-429-5748
E-mail: pzline@rowman.com
www.lexingtonbooks.com

Julie E Kirsch, Vice President/Publisher
Dave Horvath, Senior Marketing manager
Elaine Schleiffer, Publicity and Advertising

Publisher of specialized new work by established and emerging scholars, including material for the healthcare community.

3390 Lippincott Williams & Wilkins
351 West Camden Street
Baltimore, MD 21201
410-528-4000
Fax: 215-521-8902
www.lww.com

Gordon Macomber, CEO

Publishes specialized publications and software for physicians, nurses, students and specialized clinicians. Products include drug guides, medical journals, nursing journals, medical textbooks and medical pda software.

Year Founded: 1998

3391 Love Publishing
9101 East Kenyon Avenue
Suite 2200
Denver, CO 80237-1854
303-221-7333
Fax: 303-221-7444
E-mail: lpc@lovepublishing.com
www.lovepublishing.com

Stan Love, Owner

Publishes books that offer therapy options to children of all ages, adults, and adolescents.

Year Founded: 1968

3392 Mason Crest Publishers
450 Parkway Drive
Suite D
Broomall, PA 19008-4017
610-543-6200
866-627-2665
Fax: 610-543-3878
www.masoncrest.com

Dan Hilferty, President
Louis Cohen, Principal And Creative Director
Michelle Luke, International Rights and Marketi
Becki Stewart, Business Development

Publishes core-related materials for grades K-12. Current catalog includes many titles for health care and mental health curriculums.

3393 New Harbinger Publications
5674 Shattuck Avenue
Oakland, CA 94609-1662
510-652-0215
800-748-6273
Fax: 800-652-1613
E-mail: customerservice@newharbinger.com
www.newharbinger.com

Matthew McKay, Owner
Patrick Fanning, Co-Founder

Publisher of self-help books that teach the reader skills they could use to significantly improve the quality of their lives.

Year Founded: 1973

3394 New World Library
14 Pamaron Way
Nopvato, CA 94949-6215
415-884-2100
800-972-6657
Fax: 415-884-2199
www.newworldlibrary.com

Marc Allen, CEO

Publishes books and audios that inspire and challenge us to improve the quality of our lives and our world.

3395 New York University Press
838 Broadway
3rd Floor
New York, NY 10003-4812
212-998-2575
800-996-6987
Fax: 212-995-3833
E-mail: information@nyupress.org
www.www.nyupress.org

Steve Maikowski, Director
Eric Zinner, Assistant Director, Editor-In-Chi
Mary Beth Jarrad, Marketing and Sales Director
Monica McCormick, Program Officer

Publishes approximately 100 new books each year, and enjoys a backlist of over 1500 titles that includes health care and academic materials.

Year Founded: 1916

3396 Omnigraphics
155 West Congress
Suite 200
Detroit, MI 48226
313-961-1340
800-234-1340
Fax: 313-961-1383
E-mail: contact@omnigraphics.com
www.omnigraphics.com

Fred Ruffner, Co-Founder
Peter Ruffner, Co-Founder

Quality reference resources for libraries and schools.

Year Founded: 1985

3397 Oxford University Press
2001 Evans Road
Cary, NC 27513-2010
919-677-0977
800-445-9714
Fax: 919-677-2673
E-mail: custserv.us@oup.com
www.www.global.oup.com/

Publishes works that further Oxford University's objective of excellence in research, scholarship, and education, including titles in the health care and mental health field.

Year Founded: 1896

3398 Penguin Group
345 Hudson Street
New York, NY 10014-4592
212-366-2372
Fax: 212-366-2933
E-mail: librariansden@us.penguingroup.com
www.www.penguin.com/

John Makinson, Chairman and Chief Executive
Coram Williams, Chief Financial Officer
David Shanks, Chief Executive Officer
Susan Petersen Kennedy, President

Publishes under a wide range of prominent imprints and trademarks, among them Berkeley Books, Dutton, Grosset & Dunlap, New American Library, Penguin, Philomel, G.P. Putnam's Sons, Riverhead Books, Viking and Frederick Warne. Includes a variety of titles in health care and mental health subjects.

3399 Perseus Books Group
210 American Drive
Jackson, TN 38301
731-423-1973
800-343-4499
Fax: 800-351-5073
E-mail: perseus.orders@perseusbooks.com
www.www.perseusbooksgroup.com/

Chris Wagner, VP

Titles include science, public issues, military history, modern maternity, health care and mental health.

3400 Princeton University Press
41 William Street
Princeton, NJ 08540-5223
609-883-1759
800-777-4726
Fax: 609-258-6305
E-mail: orders@cpfsinc.com
www.www.press.princeton.edu/

Peter Dougherty, Director
Martha Camp, Administrative Assistant to the
Patrick Carroll, Associate Director and Controlle
Brigitta van Rheinberg, Assistant Director, Editor in Ch

Independent publisher with close connection to Princeton Unviersity. Fundamental mission is to disseminate through books, journals, and electronic media, with both academia and society at large on a variety of social issues, including health care and mental health.

3401 Pro-Ed Publications

8700 Shoal Creek Blvd
Austin, TX 78757-6897
512-451-3246
800-897-3202
Fax: 512-451-8542
E-mail: feedback@proedinc.com
www.www.proedinc.com/

Donald D Hammill, Owner

Leading publisher of nationally standardized tests, resource and reference texts, curricular and therapy materials, and professional journals covering: speech, language and hearing; psychology and counseling; special education including developmental disabilities, rehabilitation, and gifted education; early childhood intervention; and occupational and physical therapy.

3402 Professional Resource Press

PO Box 3197
Sarasota, FL 34230-3197
941-343-9601
800-443-3364
Fax: 941-343-9201
E-mail: cs.prpress@gmail.com
www.prpress.com

Laurie Girsch, Managing Editor

Publisher of books, continuing education programs and other applied resources for mental health professionals, including psychologists, psychiatrists, clinical social workers, counselors, OTs, and recreational therapists.

Year Founded: 1980

3403 Rapid Psychler Press

2014 Holland Avenue
Suite 374
Port Huron, MI 48060-1994
888-779-2453
Fax: 888-779-2457
E-mail: rapid@psychler.com
www.psychler.com

Produces textbooks and presentation graphics for use in mental health education (mainly psychiatry). Products are thoroughly researched and clinically oriented. Designed by students, instructors and clinicians.

3404 Research Press Publishers

PO Box-7886
Champaign, IL 61826
217-352-3273
800-519-2707
Fax: 217-352-1221
E-mail: rp@researchpress.com
www.researchpress.com

Publishes books and videos in school counseling, special education, psychology, counseling and therapy, parenting, death and dying, and developmental disabilities.

Year Founded: 1968

3405 Riverside Publishing

3800 Golf Road
Suite 200
Rolling Meadows, IL 60008
630-467-7000
800-323-9540
Fax: 630-467-7192
E-mail: RPC_Customer_Service@hmhco.com
www.riverpub.com

Dedicated to providing society with the finest professional testing products and services available. Division of Houghton Mifflin Company.

Year Founded: 1979

3406 Rowman & Littlefield

4501 Forbes Boulevard
Suite 200
Lanham, MD 20706-4346
301-459-3366
800-462-6420
Fax: 301-429-5748
E-mail: pzline@rowman.com
www.www.rowman.com/JasonAronson

Julie E Kirsch, Vice President/Publisher
Sam Caggiula, Publicity Manager
Candace Johnson, Publicity Assistant

Publisher of highly regarded books in psychotherapy. Dedicated to publishing professional, scholarly works by respected and gifted authors.

3407 Sage Publications

2455 Teller Road
Thousand Oaks, CA 91320-2234
805-499-0721
800-818-7243
Fax: 800-583-2665
E-mail: info@sagepub.com
www.sagepub.com

Sara Miller McCune, Founder, Chairman, Publisher
Blaise R Simqu, President and Chief Executive Off
Chris Hickok, Senior VP and Chief Financial Of
Tracey A Ozmina, Executive VP and Chief Operating

An independent international publisher of journals, books, and electronic media, known for commitment to quality and innovation in scholarly, educational and professional markets.

3408 Sidran Institute

PO Box 436
Brooklandville, MD 21022-0436
410-825-8888
Fax: 410-560-0134
E-mail: sidran@sidran.org
www.sidran.org

Esther Giller, President
Sheila Giller, Secretary/Treasurer
Tracy Howard, Book Sales/Office Manager
Stephanie Muszelik, Accountant

Leader in traumatic stress education and advocacy. Devoted to helping people who have experienced traumatic life events by publishing books and educational materials on traumatic stress and dissociative conditions.

Year Founded: 1986

3409 Simon & Schuster
1230 Avenue of the Americas
New York, NY 10020
212-698-7000
Fax: 856-824-2402
www.simonandschuster.com

Carolyn Reidy, President and Chief Executive Of
Dennis Ealau, Executive VP, Operations and Chie
Elinor Hirschhorn, Executive VP, Chief Digital Offic
Adam Rothberg, Sr VP, Director of Corporate Comm

Leader in the field of general interest publishing, providing consumers worldwide with a diverse range of quality books and multimedia products across a wide variety of genres and formats, including health care and mental health.

Year Founded: 1924

3410 Springer Science and Business Media
233 Spring Street
New York, NY 10013-1578
212-460-1500
Fax: 212-460-1575
E-mail: service-ny@springer.com
www.www.springer.com/

William Curtis, President
Martin Mos, COO

Develops, manages and disseminates knowledge through books, journals and the internet in a variety of subjects, including health care and mental health.

3411 St. Martin's Press
175 Fifth Avenue
New York, NY 10010
212-674-5151
Fax: 212-677-7456
E-mail: permissions@stmartins.com
www.us.macmillan.com

John Sargent, CEO

Publishes 700 titles a year, including those titles in a variety of health care and mental health subjects.

3412 Taylor & Francis Group
711 3rd Avenue
8th Floor
New York, NY 10017
212-216-7800
800-634-7064
Fax: 212-564-7854
E-mail: beverley.acreman@tandf.co.uk
www.taylorandfrancis.com

Kevin Bradley, CEO

Publishes more than 1000 journals and 1800 new books each year with a books backlist in excess of 20, 000 specialty titles. Providers of quality information and knowledge that enable our customers to perform their jobs efficiently, continue their education, and help contribute to the advancement of their chosen markets.

Year Founded: 1936

3413 Therapeutic Resources
PO Box 16814
Cleveland, OH 44116-814
888-331-7114
Fax: 440-331-7118
E-mail: contactus@therapeuticresources.com
www.therapeuticresources.com

Publishers of a variety of titles including ADD/ADHD, Alzheimer/Dimentia, Anger Management, Autism/PDD, Bereavement/Adjustment Disorders, Substance Abuse and more.

3414 Underwood Books
PO Box 1919
Nevada City, CA 95959-1919
800-788-3123
E-mail: contact@underwoodbooks.com
www.underwoodbooks.com

A publisher specializing in fantasy art, science fiction, and self-help/health related titles.

3415 University of California Press
155 Grand Avenue
Suite 400
Oakland, CA 94612-3758
510-883-8232
Fax: 510-836-8910
E-mail: askucp@ucpress.edu
www.ucpress.edu

Alison Mudditÿ, Director

Distinguished university press that enriches lives around the world by advancing scholarships in the humanities, social sciences, and natural sciences.

3416 University of Chicago Press
1427 East 60th Street
Chicago, IL 60637-2902
773-702-7700
E-mail: marketing@press.uchicago.edu
www.www.press.uchicago.edu/

Holds an obligation to disseminate scholarship of the highest standard and to publish serious works that promote education, foster public understanding, and enrich cultural life.

Year Founded: 1891

3417 University of Minnesota Press
111 Third Avenue South
Suite 290
Minneapolis, MN 55401-2520
612-627-1970
Fax: 612-627-1980
E-mail: ump@umn.edu
www.upress.umn.edu

Douglas Armato, Director, Administrative
Susan Doerr, Operations Manager, Administrativ
Daniel Oschner, Production Manager
John Henderson, IT Manager

Publisher of groundbreaking work in social and cultural thought, critical theory, race and ethnic studies, urbanism, feminist criticism, and media studies.

Year Founded: 1925

3418 WW Norton
500 Fifth Avenue
New York, NY 10110
212-354-5500
800-233-4830
Fax: 212-869-0856
www.www.wwnorton.com

Drake McFeely, CEO

Publishing house owned by its employees, and publishes books in fiction, nonfiction, poetry, college, cookbooks, art, and professional subjects, including health care and mental health.

3419 Woodbine House
6510 Bells Mill Road
Bethesda, MD 20817-1636
301-897-3570
800-843-7323
Fax: 301-897-5838
E-mail: info@woodbinehouse.com
www.woodbinehouse.com

Irv Shapell, Owner

Publishes special needs books for parents, children, teachers and professionals.

Year Founded: 1985

Facilities

State

Alabama

3420 Taylor Hardin Secure Medical Facility
100 North Union Street
Montgomery, AL 36130-1410
334-242-3454
800-367-0955
Fax: 334-242-0725
E-mail: webmaster@mh.alabama.gov
www.mh.alabama.gov

Michelle Vilamaa, Staff Development Coordinator
Ella White, Staff Development Administrative

Alaska

3421 Alaska Psychiatric Institute
3700 Piper Street
Anchorage, AK 99508-4677
907-269-7100
Fax: 907-269-7251
www.dhss.alaska.gov/dbh/Pages/api/default.aspx

Ronald Adler, CEO
R Duane Hopson MD, Medical Director

In partnership with individuals, their families and the community, natural network and providers, API's Alaska Recovery Center provides therapeutic services which assist individuals to achieve a personal level of satisfaction and success in their recovery.

Arizona

3422 Arizona State Hospital
2500 East Van Buren
Phoenix, AZ 85008-6079
602-244-1331
Fax: 602-220-6355
www.www.azdhs.gov/azsh

John C Cooper, CEO
M Megan Mitscher LMSW, Admissions & Tribal Liaison

The Arizona State Hospital provides specialized psychiatric services to support people in achieving mental health recovery in a safe and respectful environment.

Year Founded: 1887

Arkansas

3423 Arkansas State Hospital
305 South Palm Street
Little Rock, AR 72205
501-686-9000
Fax: 501-686-9464
E-mail: barbra.brooks@arkansas.gov
www.humanservices.arkansas.gov/dbhs/Pages/ArStateHospi

Steven Henson, Interim Administrator
Steven Domon, MD, Medical Director
April Coe-Hout, MD, Clinical Director
Hillary Hunt, Internship Training Director

The Arkansas State Hospital is a psychiatric inpatient treatment facility for those with mental or emotional disorders which includes 90 beds for acute psychiatric admission; a 60-bed forensic treatment services program which offers assistance to circuit courts throughout the state; a 16-bed adolescent treatment program for youth 13-18; and a program for juvenile sex offenders.

3424 Center for Outcomes and Evidence
Agency for Healthcare Research and Quality
540 Gaither Road
Suite 2000
Rockville, MD 20850
301-427-1104
Fax: 301-427-1520
www.ahrq.gov

Richard Kronick, Ph.D., Director
Boyce Ginieczki, Ph.D., Acting Deputy Director

Formerly the Center for Outcomes and Effectiveness Research. Conducts and supports research and assessment of health care practices, technologies, processes, and systems.

3425 UAMS Psychiatric Research Institute
4301 West Markham
Suite 605
Little Rock, AR 72205
501-660-7559
Fax: 501-660-7542
E-mail: kramerteresal@uams.edu
www.uams.edu

Combining research, education and clinical services into one facility, PRI offers inpatiend and outpatient services, with 40 psychiatric beds, therapy options, and specialized treatment for specific disorders, including: addictive eating, anxiety, deppressive and post-traumatic stress disorders. Research focuses on evidence-based care takes into consideration the education of future medical personnel while relying on research scientists to provide innovative forms of treatment. PRI includes the Center for Addiction Research as well as a methadone clinic.

California

3426 ANKA Behavioral Health
1875 Willow Pass Road
Suite 300
Concord, CA 94520-2527
925-825-4700
Fax: 925-825-2610
E-mail: info@ankabhi.org
www.www.ankabhi.org

Naja W. Boyd, PsyD, Chief Operating Officer
Chris Withrow, Chief Executive Officer
Nzinga Harrison, Chief Medical Officer
Yolanda Braxton, PsyD, VP of Business Development

Offers comprehensive services and programs designed to promote a client's overall wellness and to attain an enhanced quality of life.

3427 Atascadero State Hospital
10333 El Camino Real
Atascadero, CA 93422-5808
805-468-2009
Fax: 805-466-6011
E-mail: craig.dacus@ash.dsh.ca.gov
www.dsh.ca.gov

Craig Dacus, Public Information Officer
Joyce Ladwig, Human Resources Department

A maximum security forensic hosptial, providing inpatient forensic services for adult males who are court committed throughout the State of California. The staff members of Atascadero State Hospital (ASH) proudly serve the people of the State of California by providing protection for the community, expert evaluations for the courts, and state-of-the-science psychiatric recovery services for individuals referred to us from across the state.

Year Founded: 1954

3428 Campobello Chemical Dependency Treatment Services

3250 Guerneville Road
Santa Rosa, CA 95401-4030
707-579-4066
800-806-1833
Fax: 707-579-1603
www.campobello.org

Jim Cody, Executive Director
Kathy Leigh Willis, Executive Director

Innovative chemical dependency treatment center with the belief in the 12 step self-help programs of Alcoholics Anonymous, Narcotics Anonymous and Al-Anon for friends and family.

3429 Changing Echoes

7632 Pool Station Road
Angels Camp, CA 95222-9620
209-785-3666
800-633-7066
Fax: 209-785-5238
www.changingechoes.com

J R Maughan, Executive Director

Established as a social model chemical dependency facility with the intent to render high-quality treatment for affordable prices to men and women who suffer from the disease of addiction.

Year Founded: 1989

3430 Department of Mental Health Vacaville Psychiatric Program

1600 California Drive
PO Box 2297
Vacaville, CA 95696-2297
707-449-6504
Fax: 707-453-7047
www.dsh.ca.gov

Victor Brewer, Executive Director

The mission of Vacaville Psychiatric Program is to provide quality mental health evaluation and treatment to inmate-patients. This is accomplished in a safe and therapeutic environment, and as part of a continuum of care.

3431 Exodus Recovery Center

9808 Venice Blvd.
Suite 700
Culver City, CA 90232
310-945-3350
800-829-3923
Fax: 310-840-7023
E-mail: lezlie@exodusrecovery.com
www.exodusrecoveryinc.com

Luana Murphy, MBA, President /Chief Executive Offic
LeeAnn Skorohod, CHC - CCEP, Senior Vice President of Operati

Lezlie Murch, MA, LPCC, Senior Vice President of Program
Grace Lee, MBA, Vice President of Finance

Mission is that we believe that chemically dependent men and women can achieve freedom from the bondage of drugs and alcohol. Teaching patients and their families that the devastation of addiction can be overcome. Produce personal action plans that can produce a lifetime of recovery.

3432 Family Service Agency

123 W Gutierrez Street
Santa Barbara, CA 93101-3424
805-965-1001
Fax: 805-965-2178
E-mail: hr@fsacares.org
www.fsacares.org

Stephanie Wilson, Co-President
Robert Manning, Co-President
Lisa Brabo, Ph.D., Executive Director
Denise Cicourel, MAOM, Director of Administration

A non-profit human service agency whose programs help people help themselves. FSA services prevent family breakdown, intervene effectively where problems are known to exist and help individuals and families build on existing strengt

Year Founded: 1899

3433 Fremont Hospital
Psychiatric Solutions

39001 Sundale Drive
Fremont, CA 94538-2005
510-796-1100
www.fremonthospital.com

Joey A Jacobs, President/CEO/Chairman

A private, modern 96-bed behavioral healthcare facility that provides services to adolescents (ages 12-17) and adults.

3434 Life Steps Pasos de Vida

1431 Pomeroy Road
Arroyo Grande, CA 93420-5943
805-481-2505
800-530-5433
www.lifestepsfoundation.org

Sue Horowitz, President
Virginia Franco, Founder/CEO
Allen C Haile, Secretary

Develops innovative programs that target underserved populations. Goal is to help participants develop healthy lifestyles free of alcohol and drugs.

3435 Lincoln Child Center

4368 Lincoln Avenue
Oakland, CA 94602-2529
510-531-3111
Fax: 510-530-8083
E-mail: info@lincolncc.org
www.lincolncc.org

Diana Netherton, Chairman
Christine Stoner-Mertz, President/CEO
Peggy Padilla, Chief Administrative Officer
Allison Becwar, Chief Program Officer

Enables vulnerable and emotionally troubled children and their families to lead independent and fulfilling live

3436 Mental Health Association of Orange County

822 Town & Country Road
Orange, CA 92868
714-547-7559
Fax: 717-543-4431
E-mail: mhainfo@mhaoc.org
www.mhaoc.org

Dedicated to improving the quality of life of Orange County residents impacted by mental illness through direct service, advocacy, education and information dissemination.

Year Founded: 1958

3437 Metropolitan State Hospital

11401 Bloomfield Avenue
Norwalk, CA 90650-2015
562-863-7011
Fax: 562-929-3131
TDD: 562-863-1743
www.dsh.ca.gov

Sharon Smith Nevins, Executive Director

The mission of Metropolitan State Hospital is to work in partnership with individuals to assist in their recovery by using rehabilitation services as their tool, thus preparing clients for community living.

Year Founded: 1915

3438 Napa State Hospital

2100 Napa-Vallejo Highway
Napa, CA 94558-6293
707-253-5000
Fax: 707-253-5379
TDD: 707-253-5768
E-mail: nshcontact@dmhnsh.state.ca.us
www.dsh.ca.gov

Jennifer Marshall CTRS, RTC, Chief, Rehabilitation Therapy

Napa State Hospital provides treatment and support to adults with serious mental illness, and assists each individual in achieving his/her highest potential for independence and quality of life, leading to recovery and integrating safely and successfully into society.

3439 New Life Recovery Centers

782 Park Avenue
Suite 1
San Jose, CA 95126-4800
408-297-1182
866-894-6572
Fax: 408-297-7450
www.newliferecoverycenters.com

Kevin Richardson, President
Gary Ruble, Founder

Strives to provide our clients with the very best services available. We value our employees as our greatest asset, while collectively and continuously working to adopt and implement the latest and most effective medical, clinical, and social model treatment modalities.

Year Founded: 2004

3440 Northridge Hospital Medical Center

18300 Roscoe Boulevard
Northridge, CA 91328

818-885-8500
Fax: 818-885-5439
www.northridgehospital.org

Mike Wall, President, CEO

Northridge Hospital Medical Center offers a comprehensive Behavioral Health program for both adults and adolescents. Founded in 1955.

3441 PacifiCare Behavioral Health PO Box 31053 Laguna Hills, CA 92654-1053

800-999-9585
www.www.pbhi.com

Richard J Kelliher PsyD, Clinical Director

Provides behavioral health services to children, adolescents, adults, and seniors.

3442 Patton State Hospital
California Department of Mental Health

3102 E Highland Avenue
Patton, CA 92369
909-425-7000
Fax: 909-425-6169
TDD: 909-862-5730
E-mail: cbarrett@dmhpsh.state.ca.us
www.dsh.ca.gov

Harry Oreol, Executive Director
Nitin Kulkarni, Medical Director
Angela Fiore, Forensic Services Manager
Nancy Verela, Director, Human Resources

Patton State Hospital's mission is to empower forensic and civilly committed individuals to recover from mental illness utilizing Recovery principles and evidenced based practices within a safe, structured, and secure environment.

3443 Phoenix Programs Inc

90 E. Leslie Lane
Columbia, MO 65202-1535
573-442-3830
Fax: 925-778-7412
www.www.phoenixprogramsinc.org

Nelly Roach, President
Brock Bukowsky, Vice President/Treasurer
Deborah Beste, Executive Director
Rhiannon Pearson, Chief Financial Officer

Offers an array of services and programs designed to promote overall wellness while making it possible for all to obtain a higher quality of life.

3444 Presbyterian Intercommunity Hospital Mental Health Center

12401 Washington Boulevard
Whittier, CA 90602-1006
562-698-0811
TDD: 562-696-9267
TTY: 562-696-9267
www.www.pihhealth.org

Kenton Woods, Chair
Rich Atwood, Vice Chair
Efrain Aceves, Secretary
Jane Dicus, Treasurer

Offers an inpatient program for those with a variety of mental disorders.

Year Founded: 1959

3445 Twin Town Treatment Centers
4388 E Katella Avenue
Los Alamitos, CA 90720-3565
562-596-0050
Fax: 562-596-0058
www.twintowntreatmentcenters.com

David Lisonbee, President, CEO
Tiran Davidi-Durian, CFO
Ted Williams, MD, ASAM, Medical Director
Debbie Muehl, CATC II, Supervising Counselor

Mission is to introduce new solutions for people who find
that chemically induced coping no longer works.

Colorado

3446 Centennial Mental Health Center
211 W Main Street
Sterling, CO 80751-3168
970-522-4392
E-mail: webmaster@centennialmhc.org
www.centennialmhc.org

Daniel D Hammond, Manager

A non-profit organization dedicated to providing the highest quality comprehensive mental health services to the rural communities of northeastern Colorado.

3447 Colorado Mental Health Institute at Fort Logan
3520 West Oxford Avenue
Denver, CO 80236-3108
303-866-7066
Fax: 303-866-7048
www.colorado.gov

Keith Lagrenade, CEO

The mission of the Colorado Mental Health Institute at Fort
Logan is to provide the highest quality mental health services to persons of all ages with complex, serious and persistent mental illness within the resources available.

3448 Colorado Mental Health Institute at Pueblo
1600 West 24th Street
Pueblo, CO 81003-1411
303-866-5700
Fax: 719-546-4484
www.www.cdhs.state.co.us

John De Quardo, Administrator

Provides quality mental health services focused on sustaining hope and promoting recovery.

3449 Emily Griffith Center
1724 Gilpin Street
Denver, CO 80218
303-237-6865
Fax: 303-237-6873
www.www.griffithcenters.org

Howard Shiffman, CEO
Beth Miller, Deputy Director/COO
John Smrcka, Program Director

Provides troubled children the environment and opportunities to become healthy, participating and productive members of society.

Connecticut

3450 Daytop Residential Services Division
425 Grant Street
Bridgeport, CT 06610-3222
203-337-9943
Fax: 203-337-9986
www.aptfoundation.org/daytop.htm

David Parachini, Chairperson
Janet Ryan, Vice Chairperson
Peter Loomis, Treasurer
Jay Broderick, Secretary

Long-term substance abuse treatment facility based on the
Therapeutic Community model. Combines current research
and treatment methods with traditional therapeutic community concepts.

Year Founded: 1970

3451 Jewish Family Service
733 Summer Street
Suite 602
Stamford, CT 06901-1035
203-921-4161
www.www.ctjfs.org/

Michael Alexanderÿ, President
Matt Greenberg, CEO
Iris Morrison, Associate Executive Director
Saul Cohen, Vice President

Offers a wide range of innovative programs designed to address contemporary problems and issues through counseling and therapy, crisis intervention, Jewish Family Life
Education, Depression, Aging and senior mental health,
Obsessions and compulsions.

Year Founded: 1978

3452 Klingberg Family Centers
370 Linwood Street
New Britain, CT 06052-1998
860-832-5504
Fax: 860-832-8221
E-mail: lynner@klingberg.org
www.klingberg.org

Lynne V. Roe, Director of Intake

To uphold, preserve and restore families in a therapeutic
environment, valuing the absolute worth of every child,
while adhering to the highest ethical principles in accordance with our Judaeo-Christian heritage.

3453 McCall Foundation
58 High Street
PO Box 806
Torrington, CT 06790-806
860-496-2100
Fax: 860-496-2111
E-mail: mccallfoundation@snet.net
www.www.mccall-foundation.org

D'Arcy Lovetere, President
Roxanne Bachand, Vice President
Marie Wallace, Secretary/Treasurer

Provides outpatient, partial hospital, intensive outpatient,
residential, parenting and prevention programs for substance abusers and/or their family members; and helps to
reduce area substance abuse in the local community. Funding is provided by the United Way.

3454 Mountainside Treatment Center
187 South Canaan Road
Route 7
Canaan, CT 06018-717
860-824-1397
800-762-5433
Fax: 888-749-8752
E-mail: admissions@mountainside.org
www.mountainside.org

Maureen O'Neill Biggs, LPC, LA, Clinical Director
Brittanie Decker, Continuing Care Case Manager
Bruce Dechert, LADC, ICADC, Director, Family Wellness
Susan Watso, CAC, Extended Care Counselor

Program is based on strategies and principles that promote healing and enhance the quality of life. Through the utilization of Motivational Interviewing, Directional Therapy, Gender-Specific Groups, the 12-Step Principles and Adventure Based Initiatives, individuals qwill encounter, confront and experience the challenges of recovery.

Year Founded: 1998

3455 Silver Hill Hospital
208 Valley Road
New Canaan, CT 06840-3899
203-966-1380
800-899-4455
E-mail: info@silverhillhospital.org
www.silverhillhospital.org

Siguard Ackerman, President and Medical Director
Elizabeth Moore, Chief Operating Officer
Ruurd Leegstra, JD, CPA, Chief Financial Officer
Missy Fallon, Chief Development Officer

A nationally recognized, independent, not-for-profit psychiatric hospital that is focused exclusively on providing patients the best possible treatment of psychiatric illnesses and substance use disorders, in the best possible environment.

Year Founded: 1931

3456 Yale University School of Medicine: Child Study Center
230 S Frontage Road
New Haven, CT 06519-1124
203-785-2540
www.www.childstudycenter.yale.edu/index.aspx

Fred R Volkmar, MD, Director

Provides a comprehensive range of in-depth diagnostic and treatment services for children with psychiatric and developmental disorders. These services include specialized developmental evaluations for children ages zero-four, and psychological and psychiatric evaluations for children 5-18. Individualized treatment plans following evaluation make use for a range of theraputic interventions, including psychotherapy, group therapy, family therapy, psycho-pharmacological treatment, parent counseling, consultation and service planning. Immediate access for children needing to be seen within 24 hours and walk-in service is also available.

Florida

3457 Archways-A Bridge To A Brighter Future
919 NE 13th Street
Fort Lauderdale, FL 33304-2009

954-763-2030
Fax: 954-763-9847
E-mail: intake@archways.org
www.archways.org

Andrea Katz, CEO

A not-for-profit, privately-governed organization whose mission is to provide quality comprehensive behavioral health care to individuals and families who are in need of improving their quality of life.

3458 Fairwinds Treatment Center
1569 South Fort Harrison
Clearwater, FL 33756-2004
727-449-0300
800-226-0300
Fax: 727-446-1022
E-mail: fairwinds@fairwindstreatment.com
www.fairwindstreatment.com

Jess Loven, Clinical Director, CAP
Thomas H Lewis, Clinical Director

As a dually licensed psychiatric and substance abuse center, reaches far beyond standard treatment to offer medical services for substance abuse, eating disorders, and emotional/mental health issues.

3459 First Step of Sarasota
4579 Northgate Court
Sarasota, FL 34234
941-366-5333
800-266-6866
Fax: 941-351-5161
E-mail: gethelp@fsos.org
www.www.fsos.org/

Richard Carlson, Chair
Peter Abbott, Vice Chair
Elizabeth LaBoone, Secretary

Provides high quality, affordable substance abuse treatment and recovery programs on Florida's Gulf Coast. Offers a variety of programs including a medical detox, residential and outpatient services for adolescents, adults and families.

Year Founded: 1967

3460 Florida State Hospital
1317 Winewood Blvd.
Building 1, Room 202
Tallahassee, FL 32399-0700
850-487-1111
Fax: 850-922-2993
www.www.myflfamilies.com

Diane James, Administrator

FSH provides person-centered treatment and rehabilitations in order to propel the client toward their personal recovery and to prepare for roles and environments that have personal and social value.

Year Founded: 1876

3461 Gateway Community Services
555 Stockton Street
Jacksonville, FL 32204-2597
904-387-4661
Fax: 904-384-5753
E-mail: info@gatewaycommunity.com
www.gatewaycommunity.com

Candace Hodgkins, Ph.D., LMHC, President/Chief Executive Office

Laura Dale, CFO
Randy Jennings, Sr VP Operations
Dr. Yvonne Kennedy, Senior Vice President of Profess

Provides a full continuum of care that delivers effective treatment and rehabilitation services to individuals suffering from alcoholism, substance abuse and related mental health problems.

3462 Genesis House Recovery Residence

4865 40th Way South
Lake Worth, FL 33461-5301
561-439-4070
800-737-0933
Fax: 561-439-4864
E-mail: info@genesishouse.net
www.genesishouse.net

James Dodge, Founder/CEO
Kathryn Shafer, Clinical Director

Works closely with both local and out of state courts. Provides the suffering person with a safe, secure, professional environment to glean the care, answers and support they so desperately need in their lives.

3463 Manatee Glens

391 6th Avenue W
Bradenton, FL 34205-8820
941-782-4299
Fax: 941-782-4301
E-mail: Sondra.Guffey@manateeglens.org
www.www.manateeglens.org/

Paul M Duck, Chair
Mary Ruiz, CEO/President
Deborah Kostroun, COO
Thomas P Nolan, Vice Chair

Helps families in crisis with mental health and addictions services and supports the community through prevention and recovery.

3464 New Horizons of the Treasure Coast

4500 W Midway Road
Ft Pierce, FL 34981-4823
772-468-5600
888-468-5600
Fax: 772-468-5606
www.nhtcinc.org

John Wolsiefer, Chairman
Garry Wilson, Vice Chair
Robert Zomok, Treasurer
Patricia Austin-Novak, Secretary

To improve the quality of life in the community through the provision of accessible, person-centered behavioral health resources.

Year Founded: 1958

3465 North Florida Evaluation and Treatment Center

1200 NE 55th Boulevard
Gainesville, FL 32641-2759
352-375-8484
Fax: 352-264-8305
www.www.dcf.state.fl.us/facilities/nfetc/

William Baxter, Administrator

Dedicated to serving you while fulfilling our responsibilities for safety, security and a positive, caring environment.

Year Founded: 1976

3466 North Star Centre

9033 Glades Road
Boca Raton, FL 33434-3939
561-361-0500
Fax: 561-479-0384
E-mail: inquiry@northstar-centre.com
www.northstar-centre.com

Ira Kaufman, Executive Director
Randi Katz, Administrative Assistant

A uniquely comprehensive facility dedicated to restoring your sense of emotional and physical well being.

3467 Northeast Florida State Hospital

7487 South State Road 121
MacClenny, FL 32063-5480
904-259-6211
Fax: 904-259-7101
www.www.myflfamilies.com/service-programs/mental-healt

Joe Infantino, Administrator
Rufus Johnson, Evening Administrator

To provide comprehensive mental health treatment services to ensure a timely transition to the community.

Year Founded: 1959

3468 Renaissance Manor

509 Berry Street
Punta Gordaÿ, FL 33950
941-916-9621
Fax: 941-460-5119
www.www.renaissancemanor.org/

Heather Eller, Administrator

Community based assisted living facility with a limited mental health license, specializes in serving adults with neuro-biological disorders and mood disorders along with other special mental health needs. Our not-for-profit organization is a program designed to encourage positive mental health while meeting the various interest of our residents.

3469 Seminole Community Mental Health Center

237 Fernwood Blvd
Fern Park, FL 32730-2116
407-831-2411
Fax: 407-831-0195
E-mail: scmhc@scmhc.com

Jim Berko, Manager

A private, nonprofit organization whose goal is to provide comprehensive, biopsychosocial rehabilitation programming in the areas of mental health and substance abuse.

3470 Starting Place

351 North State Road 7
Suite 200
Plantation, FL 33317
954-327-4060
www.startingplace.org

Dr. Tammy Tucker, Chair
Marsha L. Currant, M.S.W, , CEO

Improves the lives through education, treatment and support services related to substance abuse, mental illness and co-occurring disorders

3471 The Transition House
3800 5th Street
St Cloud, FL 34769
407-892-5700
E-mail: counselor@thetransitionhouse.org
www.thetransitionhouse.org

Thomas Griffin, PhD, Chief Executive Officer
Jennifer R. Dellasanta, ICADC, CAP, Chief Operating
Officer
Jeffrey Wainwright, Director of Work Release Program
Brett ms D'Aoust, MSW, CAP, Executive Director of
Correction

The adress above is the men's house. The address for the
women's house is: 505 N Clyde Street Kissimmee, FL
34741. All other information is the same. Mission is to provide a milieu of comprehensive educational, health, prevention and human services to Central Florida's most
disenfranchised populations.

Year Founded: 1993

Georgia

3472 Central State Hospital
620 Broad Street
Milledgeville, GA 31062-7525
478-445-4128
Fax: 478-445-6034
E-mail: info@centralstatehospital.org
www.dbhdd.georgia.gov

Dan Howell, Regional Hospital Administrator
Kay Brooks, Chief Nurse Executive
Lee Ann Molini, Director of Nursing

3473 Georgia Regional Hospital at Atlanta
Two Peachtree Street, N.W.
24th Floor
Atlanta, GA 30303
404-657-2252
Fax: 404-212-4621
E-mail: grha@dhr.state.ga.us
www.dbhdd.georgia.gov

Susan Trueblood, CEO
Gwen Skinner, Director

Located on 174 Acres in DeKalb County, Georgia Regional
Hospital/Atlanta operates 366 licensed, accredited inpatient
beds in five major program areas: Adult Mental Health,
Adolescent Mental Health, Child Mental Health, Forensic
Services, and Developmental Disabilities. In addition,
GRH/Atlanta also offers inpatient and outpatient Dental
Services and an Outpatient Forensic Evaluation Program
for juveniles and adults. Finally, GRH/Atlanta operates the
Fulton County Collaborative Crisis Service System which
provides mobile crisis and residential services to adults
experiencing mental health problems in Fulton County.

3474 Georgia Regional Hospital at Augusta
3405 Mike Padgett Highwayÿ
Augusta, GA 30906-3897
706-792-7000
Fax: 706-792-7030
E-mail: jdclevel@dhr.state.ga.us
www.www.augustareg.dhr.state.ga.us/homeold.htm

Ben Waker EdD, Contact

3475 Georgia Regional Hospital at Savannah
1915 Eisenhower Drive
Savannah, GA 31406
912-356-2011
Fax: 912-356-2691
www.www.garegionalsavannah.com/

Douglas Osborne, Contact

3476 Southwestern State Hospital
400 Pinetree Boulevard
PO Box 1378
Thomasville, GA 31792-1378
229-227-2850
www.swsh.org

Hillary Hooyou, Manager

Provides extensive behavioral healthcare services in community and hospital settings, including: residential MRDD
services; inpatient, residential and case management psychiatric services; and residential care for dual-diagnosed
persons.

3477 West Central Georgia Regional Hospital
3000 Schatulga Road
Columbus, GA 31907
706-568-5000
E-mail: wcgrh@dhr.state.ga.us
www.dbhdd.georgia.gov/

Mission is to treat customers with respect and dignity while
providing comprehensive, person-centered behavioral
healthcare.

Year Founded: 1974

Idaho

3478 Children of Hope Family Hospital
PO Box 1829
Boise, ID 83701-1829
208-703-8688
E-mail: drharper@afo.net
www.childofhope.org

Rev Anthony R Harper PhD, Founder
Craig Hardesty, M.B.A., Treasurer
Penny Nygaard, Secretary

Illinois

3479 Advocate Ravenswood Hospital Medical Center
3075 Highland Parkway Suite 600
Downers Grove, IL 60515
630-572-9393
Fax: 630-990-4752
www.advocatehealth.com

Kelly Jo Golson, CMO, Public Affairs & Marketing
Linda Williger, Manager, Public Affairs & Market
Vincent Pierri, Manager, Public Affairs & Market
Sarah Scroggins, Coordinator, Public Affairs & Ma

Provides a comprehensive array of services for inpatient
(Adult, Adolescent, Substance Abuse), Partial Hospital, Intensive Outpatient, Psychological Rehabilitation, Emer-
gency-Crisis, Assertive Community Outreach, Case
Management, Program for Deaf and Hard of Hearing at
multiple sites on the Northside of Chicago.

3480 Alexian Brothers Bonaventure House
825 W Wellington Avenue
Chicago, IL 60657-9249

773-327-9921
Fax: 773-327-9113
E-mail: info@abam.org
www.www.alexianbrothershousing.org/

Bart Winters, CEO
Marty Hansen, Director Programs/Services

Offers adult men and women with HIV/AIDS-who are homeless or at-risk for homelessness- a chance to rebuild and reclaim their lives. Bonaventure House has a wide array of on-site supportive services-case management, occupational therapy, recovery, and spiritual care-most residents are able to return to independent life in the community within a 24-month period.

3481 Alton Mental Health Center

4500 College Avenue
Alton, IL 62002-5099
618-474-3273
Fax: 618-474-3967
www.illinois.gov

Susan Shobe, Administrator

3482 Andrew McFarland Mental Health Center

901 Southwind Road
Springfield, IL 62703-5125
217-786-6900
Fax: 217-786-7167

Karen Schweighart, Administrator

3483 Delta Center

1400 Commercial Avenue
Cairo, IL 62914-1978
618-734-3626
Fax: 618-734-1999
TTY: 618-734-1350
E-mail: delta1@midwest.net
www.deltacenter.org

Lisa Tolbert, Executive Director

A non-profit mental health center, substance abuse counseling facility, and also provides various community services to Alexander and Pulaski County, Illinois

3484 FHN Family Counseling Center

421 W Exchange Street
Freeport, IL 61032-4008
815-599-6900
Fax: 815-599-6106
www.www.fhn.org/

Lisa Mahoney, VP

3485 Habilitative Systems

415 S Kilpatrick Avenue
Chicago, IL 60644-4958
773-854-1680
Fax: 773-854-8300
TDD: 773-854-8364
E-mail: hsi@habilitative.org
www.www.habilitative.org

Donald Dew, President
Joyce Wade, VP Finance
Karen Barbee-Dixon, EdD, COO

To provide integrated human services to children, adults, families, and persons with disabling conditions that help them to achieve their highest level of self-sufficiency

Year Founded: 1978

3486 John R Day and Associates

3716 W Brighton Avenue
Peoria, IL 61615-2938
309-692-7755
Fax: 309-692-2262
www.christianpsychological.org

John R Day, Partner
Year Founded: 1974

3487 Keys To Recovery

100 North River Road
Des Plaines, IL 60016-1209
847-298-9355
www.www.reshealth.org

Philip Kolski, Director
Debra Ayanian, Nurse Manager

A leading Alcoholism and Drug Treatment Center in the Midwest, providing innovative and effective Alcoholism and Drug Treatment.

3488 MacNeal Hospital

3249 S. Oak Park Avenue
Berwyn, IL 60402
708-783-9100
888-622-6325
TTY: 708-783-3058
E-mail: inf@macnealfp.com
www.www.macneal.com/

Randall K Mc Givney, Program Director
Davis Yang, Center Director
John Gong, Clinical Faculty
Edward C Foley MD, Director Of Research

The MacNeal Family Practice Residency Program was one of the first family practice programs in the country and the first in Illinois. We have continue a progressive tradition in all aspects of our curriculum. Our program is at the forefront of contemporary family medicine offering diverse academic and clinical opportunites and building on the innovative ideas of our residents.

3489 McHenry County Mental Health Board

620 Dakota Street
Crystal Lake, IL 60012-3732
815-455-2828
Fax: 815-455-2925
www.mc708.org

Sandy Lewis, Executive Director
Robert Lesser, Deputy Director

3490 Pfeiffer Treatment Center and Health Research Institute

3S 721 West Ave
Warrenville, IL 60555-4039
630-505-0300
866-504-6076
Fax: 630-836-0667
E-mail: info@hriptc.org
www.hriptc.org

Scott Filer, MPH, Executive Director
Allen Lewis MD, Medical Director
William Walsh, PhD, Research/Found Dir/Co-Founder

A not-for-profit, outpatient medical facility for children, teens and adults seeking a biochemical assessment and treatment for their symptons caused by a biochemical imbalance, or to support health and promote wellness. PTC physician precribes individualized program of vitamins, minerals, and amino acids to address the patient's unique biochemical needs. Common conditions: anxiety, ADHA, autism spectrum disorder, post traumatic stress syndrome, depression, bipolar disorder, schozophrenia and Alzheimer's disease.

3491 Riveredge Hospital

8311 W Roosevelt
Forest Park, IL 60130-2500
708-771-7000
Fax: 708-209-2280
www.riveredgehospital.com

Carey Carlock, CEO
Lucyna Puszkarska, MD, Medical Director
Sheila Orr, JD, RN, Chief Nursing Officer and Chief
Ginny Trainor, LCSW, CADC, Director of Business
Development

Striving to foster an environment that demonstrates compassion and caring with timely and effective communication through comprehensive behavioral health care services of clinical excellence.

3492 Sonia Shankman Orthogenic School

1365 E 60th Street
Chicago, IL 60637-2890
773-702-1203
Fax: 773-702-1304
www.orthogenicschool.uchicago.edu

Henry J Roth PhD, Executive Director

A coeducational residential treatment program for children and adolescents in need of support for emotional issues which cause the student to act in disruptive ways and experience unfulfilling social and educational experiences

Year Founded: 1915

3493 Stepping Stones Recovery Center

1621 Theodore Street
Joliet, IL 60435-1958
815-744-4555
Fax: 815-744-4670
E-mail: info@steppingstonestreatment.com
www.steppingstonestreatment.com

Pat Fera, President
Pete McLenighan, Executive Director

Dedicated to providing effective treatment for persons suffering from the illness of addiction to alcohol and/or other drugs, even if these persons are unable to pay for the cost of such services.

3494 Way Back Inn-Grateful House

1915 W Roosevelt Road
Braodview, IL 60155-2925
708-344-3301
Fax: 708-344-2944
E-mail: frankl@waybackinn.org
www.waybackinn.org

Frank Lieggi, Executive Director
Anita Pindiur, Clinical Director

Provides a high level clinical treatment program specializing in addressing the needs of men and women suffering from both chemical dependence (Alcohol and Drugs) and also Gambling Dependence.

3495 Wells Center

1300 Lincoln Avenue
Jacksonville, IL 62650-4007
217-243-1871
Fax: 217-243-2278
TDD: 217-243-0470
E-mail: bcarter@wellscenter.org
www.www.wellscenter.org

Bruce Carter, Executive Director

Mission has been to improve the health and welfare of individuals and families affected by the ause of alcohol and other substances and by mental health issues. Dedicates its efforts to providing levels of care and support services in settings approval to the individual needs of the patient.

Year Founded: 1974

3496 White Oaks Companies of Illinois

130 Richard Pryor Place
Peoria, IL 61605-2484
309-671-8960
800-475-0257
E-mail: whiteoaks@fayettecompanies.org
www.whiteoaks.com

Non profit agency offering comprehensive, state-of-the-art chemical dependency services, individually designed for each client.

Indiana

3497 Community Hospital Anderson

1515 N Madison Avenue
Anderson, IN 46011-3457
765-298-4242
www.www.communityanderson.com

Beth Tharp, President/CEO

The mission of Community Hospital is to serve the medical, health and human service needs to the people in Anderson-Madison County and contiguous counties with compassion dignity, repect and excellence. Service, although focused on injury, illness and disease will also embrace prevention, education and alternative systems of health care delivery.

Year Founded: 1962

3498 Crossroad: Fort Wayne's Children's Home

2525 Lake Avenue
Fort Wayne, IN 46805-5457
260-484-4153
800-976-2306
Fax: 260-484-2337
www.crossroad-fwch.org

Patrick T Houlihan, Chair
Randall J. Rider, President/CEO
Kyle Zanker, Chief Development Officer
Beth McNeal, Director of Human Resources

A not-for-profit treatment center for emotionally troubled youth.

Year Founded: 1883

3499 Hamilton Center

620 Eighth Avenue
Terre Haute, IN 47804-2771
812-231-8200
800-742-0787

E-mail: HumanResources@hamiltoncenter.org
www.www.hamiltoncenter.org/

Gaylan Good, CEO
Richard Pittelkow, Vice President
Cary Sparks, Treasurer
Virginia Gilman, Secretary

Provides the full continuum of psychological health and addiction services to children, adolescents, adults and families.

3500 Mental Health America of Indiana

1431 North Delaware Street
Indianapolis, IN 46202
317-638-3501
800-555-6424
Fax: 317-638-3540
E-mail: mha@mentalhealthassociation.com
www.mhai.net

Stephen C McCaffrey JD, President/CEO
Lisa Hutcheson, Med, Vice President for Policy and Pr

A statewide organization, with over sicty local chapters, making it the largest Mental Health Association in the country.

Year Founded: 1915

3501 Parkview Hospital Rehabilitation Center

2200 Randilla Drive
Ft. Wayne, IN 46805-4638
260-373-4000
888-480-5151
E-mail: paulette.fisher@parkview.com
www.parkview.com

Sue Ehinger, CEO

31 bed inpatient rehabilitation unit serving a wide variety of diagnoses. CARF accredited for both comprehensive and B1 programs. Outpatient services are offered at several sites throughout the community.

Year Founded: 1995

3502 Richmond State Hospital

498 NW 18th Street
Richmond, IN 47374-2851
765-966-0511
Fax: 765-935-9504
www.richmondstatehospital.org

Jeff Butler, Superintendent
Terresa Bradburn, Human Resources Director
David Shelford, Assistant Superintendent
Josh Nolan, Clinical Director

A public behavioral health facility operated by the State of Indiana that provides psychiatric and chemical dependency treatment to citizens on a state wide basis.

Iowa

3503 Cherokee Mental Health Institute

1251 W Cedar Loop
Cherokee, IA 51012-1599
712-225-6927
Fax: 712-225-6925
E-mail: rmoller@dhs.state.ia.us
www.dhs.state.ia.us/Consumers/Facilities/Cherokee.

Tony Morris, Manager

3504 Four Seasons Counseling Clinic

2015 West Bay Drive
Muscatine, IA 52761-2228
563-263-3869
Fax: 563-263-3869
www.www.fourseasonscounselingclinic.com/

Ruth Evans, Owner

3505 Independence Mental Health Institute

2277 Iowa Avenue
Independence, IA 50644-9215
319-334-2583
E-mail: tmain@dhs.state.ia.us
www.www.dhs.state.ia.us/Consumers/Facilities/Independe

Bhasker Dave, Manager

3506 Mount Pleasant Mental Health Institute

1200 E Washington Street
Mount Pleasant, IA 52641-1898
319-385-7231
Fax: 319-385-8465
E-mail: karla.sandoval@iowa.gov
www.www.dhs.state.ia.us/Consumers/Facilities/MtPleasan

Karla Sandoval, Contact

Kansas

3507 Prairie View

1901 E First Street
Newton, KS 67114-5010
316-284-6400
800-362-0180
E-mail: info@pvi.org
www.www.prairieview.org/

Dee Donatelli-Reber, Chair
Jessie Kaye, President and CEO
Gary Fast, MD, Medical Director
Dorothy Nickel Friesen, Secretary

A behavioral and mental health facility which consists of the main campus in Newton that consists of outpatient services, a 38-bed inpatient hospital and various other divisions of our organization. Also maintain outpatient offices in Hutchinson, KS; Marion, KS; McPherson, KS; along with two outpatient offices in Wichita, KS.

Year Founded: 1954

3508 Via Christi Research

1100 N St. Francis Street
Suite 300
Wichita, KS 67214-2871
316-291-4774
800-362-0070
Fax: 316-291-7704
www.privia.org

Joe Carrithers, Manager
Joe Carrithers, PhD, Research Operations Director

Provide people with mental health conditions such as depression, suicidal thoughts, schizophrenia or dementia have a unique set of needs. They receive highly skilled, compassionate treatment.

Kentucky

3509 Eastern State Hospital
1351 Newtown Pike
Building 1
Lexington, KY 40511-1277
859-253-1686
E-mail: mjdaniluk@bluegrass.org
www.bluegrass.org

Carolyn Siegel, Chair
David E. Hanna, Interim President & CEO
Dee Werline, Vice President Administration &
Dana Royse, Chief Financial Officer

3510 Our Lady of Bellefonte Hospital
St. Christopher Drive
Ashland, KY 41101
606-833-3333
866-910-6524
Fax: 606-833-3946
www.careyoucantrust.com

Tim O'Toole, Manager

Louisiana

3511 Medical Center of LA: Mental Health Services
1532 Tulane Avenue
New Orleans, LA 70112-2860
504-903-3000

Genaro F Arriola Jr, Contact

3512 New Orleans Adolescent Hospital
210 State Street
New Orleans, LA 70118
504-897-3400
Fax: 504-896-4959
www.dhh.louisiana.gov

Provides a fully integrated hospital and community based
continuum of mental health services for children and adolescents, with serious emotional and behavioral problems,
residing in Louisiana.

3513 River Oaks Hospital
1525 River Oaks Road W
New Orleans, LA 70123-2199
504-734-1740
800-366-1740
Fax: 504-733-7020
E-mail: kim.epperson@uhsinc.com
www.www.riveroakshospital.com/

Evelyn Nolting, CEO

A private psychiatric facility for adults, adolescents and
children.

3514 Southeast Louisiana Hospital
23515 Highway 190
PO Box 3850
Mandeville, LA 70470-3850
985-626-6300
Fax: 985-626-6658
www.dhh.louisiana.gov

Patricia Gonzalez, Facility Director

Maine

3515 Dorthea Dix Psychiatric Center
656 State Street
PO Box 926
Bangor, ME 04402-926
207-941-4000
TTY: 888-774-5290
E-mail: larry.larson@maine.gov
www.www.maine.gov/dhhs

N Lawrence Ventura, Contact

DDPC is a 100 bed psychiatric hospital serving two-thirds
of the State's geographic area that provides services for
people with severe mental illness.

3516 Good Will-Hinckley Homes for Boys and Girls
PO Box 159
Hinckley, ME 04944
207-238-4000
E-mail: info@gwh.org
www.gwh.org

Jack Moore, Chairman
Glenn Cummings, Ed.D, President and Executive Director
Robert Moody, Vice President of Operations
Valerie Cote, Human Resource Generalist

Provides a home for the reception and support of needy
boys and girls who are in needs maintaining and operates a
school for them; attends to the physical, industrial, moral
and spiritual development of those who shall be placed in
its care.

3517 Riverview Psychiatric Center
250 Arsenal Street
11 State House Station
Augusta, ME 04333-0011
207-624-3900
888-261-6684
Fax: 207-287-6123
www.maine.gov/dhhs/riverview/index.shtml

Mary Louise McEwen, Superintendent
William Nelson MD, Medical Director
Lauret Grommett RN, Director of Nursing

Acute care psychiatric hospital owned and operated by the
state of Maine.

3518 Spring Harbor Hospital
123 Andover Road
Westbrook, ME 04092-3850
207-761-2200
866-857-6644
www.www.springharbor.org/

Tracy Hawkins, Chair
Dennis King, Chief Executive Officer
Nancy Hasenfus, M.D., Vice Chair
Anna H Wells, Secretary

Southern Maine's premier provider of inpatient services for
individuals who experience acute mental illness or dual disorders issues.

Maryland

3519 Clifton T Perkins Hospital Center
One Renaissance Boulevard
8450 Dorsey Run Road
Oakbrook Terrace, IL 60181

410-724-3000
800-994-6610
Fax: 630-792-5636
E-mail: complaint@jcaho.org
www.dhmh.maryland.gov

Sheilah Davenport, JD, MS, RN, CEO
Muhammed M Ajanah MD, Clinical Director
Steve Mason, COO

CTPHC is a maximum security facility. The mission of the facilty is to perform timely pretrial evaluations of defendants referred by the judicial circuit of Maryland, provide quality assessment of and treatment for all patients, and provide maximum security custody of patients to ensure public safety.

3520 Eastern Shore Hospital Center

PO Box 800
Cambridge, MD 21613
410-221-2300
888-216-8110
Fax: 410-221-2534
www.dhmh.maryland.gov/eshc/SitePages/Home.aspx

Mary K Noren, Contact

3521 John L. Gildner Regional Institute for Children and Adolescents

201 West Preston Street
Baltimore, MD 21201
410-767-6500
877-463-3464
Fax: 301-309-9004
www.dhmh.state.md.us/jlgrica/

Thomas E. Pukalski, CEO
Claudette Bernstein, Medical Director
Debra K. VanHorn, Director of Comm. Res. & Dev.

John L. Gildner Regional Institute for Children and Adolescents (JLG-RICA) is a community-based, public residential, clinical, and educational facility serving children and adolescents with severe emotional disabilities. The program is designed to provide residential and day treatment for students in grades 5-12. JLG-RICA's goal is to successfully return its students to an appropriate family, community, and academic or vocational setting that will lead to happy and successful lives.

3522 Kennedy Krieger Institute

707 North Broadway
Baltimore, MD 21205-1888
443-923-9200
800-873-3377
TTY: 443-923-2645
E-mail: info@kennedykrieger.org
www.www.kennedykrieger.org/

Gary W Goldstein, CEO

Dedicated to improving the lives of children and adolescents with pediatric developmental disabilities through patient care, special education, research, and professional training.

Year Founded: 1937

3523 RICA: Southern Maryland

9400 Surratts Road
Cheltenham, MD 20623

301-372-1840
Fax: 301-372-1906
www.pgcps.org/~rica/

Mary Sheperd, Contact

3524 Sheppard Pratt at Ellicott City

4100 College Avenue
PO Box 0836
Ellicott City, MD 21041-836
443-364-5500
800-883-3322
Fax: 443-364-5501
www.taylorhealth.com

To provide personal, high quality mental health services for your family, by our family of health care professionals.

Year Founded: 1939

3525 Spring Grove Hospital Center

55 Wade Avenue
Catonsville, MD 21228
410-402-6000
www.www.springgrove.com/

Patrick Sokas, Contact

3526 Springfield Hospital Center

6655 Sykesville Road
Sykesville, MD 21784-7966
410-795-2100
800-333-7564
E-mail: shc_admin@dhmh.state.md.us
www.dhmh.state.md.us

Paula Langmead, CEO
Janice Bowen, COO
Jonathan Book, Clinical Director

A regional psychiatric hospital operated by the State of Maryland, Department of Health and Mental Hygiene, Mental Hygiene Administration.

Year Founded: 1894

Massachusetts

3527 Arbour-Fuller Hospital

200 May Street
S Attleboro, MA 02703-5520
508-761-8500
800-828-3934
Fax: 508-761-4240
TTY: 800-974-6006
E-mail: arbourhealth@mindspring.com
www.www.arbourhealth.com

Robert Mansfield, CEO
Frank Kahr MD, Medical Director
Judith Merel, Director Marketing

Psychiatric hospital providing services to adults, adolescents and adults with developmental disabilities.

3528 Baldpate Hospital

83 Baldpate Road
Georgetown, MA 01833-2303
978-352-2131
Fax: 978-352-6755
www.www.detoxma.com/

Lucille M Batal, President

3529 Concord Family and Adolescent Services
A Division of Justice Resource Institute, Inc
160 Gould Street
Suite 300
Needham, MA 02494-2300
781-559-4900
Fax: 978-263-3088
www.jri.org

Arden O'Connor, Chairperson
Andy Pond, MSW, MAT, President
Gregory Canfield, MSW, Executive Vice President
Deborah Reuman, MBA, Chief Financial Officer

Provides professional residential schools, group home, residence for homeless teens, alternative, therapeutic high school, education and parenting programs for children, adults and families throughout Massachusetts.

3530 First Connections and Healthy Families
A Division of Justice Resource Institute, Inc
160 Gould Street
Suite 300
Needham, MA 02494-2300
781-559-4900
www.jri.org

Arden O'Connor, Chairperson
Andy Pond, MSW, MAT, President
Gregory Canfield, MSW, Executive Vice President
Deborah Reuman, MBA, Chief Financial Officer

First Conneections provides resources, education and support to families with children birth through age three. First Connections is dedicated to providing quality, comprehensive parenting support services to a diverse communities seeking resources to compliment and enrich their parenting experience.

3531 Grip Project
A Division of Justice Resource Institute, Inc
319 Wilder St
Suite 433
Lowell, MA 01852-1926
978-452-4522
www.jri.org

Cindy Powers, Program Director

A by teens, for teens young people's program with residential services as a foundation. Grip serves young people, ages 16-20, who are homeless or aging out of foster-care/group homes and are committed to being independent. There is a separate residence for young women and men, both located in Lowell, MA.

3532 Littleton Group Home
A Division of Justice Resource Institute, Inc
22 King Street
Littleton, MA 01460-1519
978-952-6809
Fax: 978-952-8607
www.jri.org

Timothy Considine, Program Director

Prepares young men, ages 13-18 for independent living by helping them to live respectful, dignified and increasingly responsible lives. The young men participate in after school activities and have daily access to the community.

3533 Meadowridge Pelham Academy
A Division of Justice Resource Institute, Inc
160 Gould Street
Suite 300
Needham, MA 02494-2300
781-559-4900
www.jri.org

Arden O'Connor, Chairperson
Andy Pond, MSW, MAT, President
Gregory Canfield, MSW, Executive Vice President
Deborah Reuman, MBA, Chief Financial Officer

A residential treatment program that focuses on the special challenges of adolescent girls with emotional and behavioral difficulties. The students, between the ages of 12-22, have typically experienced trauma and poor functioning in their personal, educational and/or family life.

3534 Meadowridge Walden Street School
A Division of Justice Resource Institute, Inc
160 Gould Street
Suite 300
Needham, MA 02494-2300
781-559-4900
www.jri.org

Arden O'Connor, Chairperson
Andy Pond, MSW, MAT, President
Gregory Canfield, MSW, Executive Vice President
Deborah Reuman, MBA, Chief Financial Officer

A residential school program that focuses on the challenges and special needs of adolescent females age 12-22 whom are coping with educational, emotional and behavioral difficulties.

3535 Sleep Disorders Unit of Beth Israel Hospital
330 Brookline Avenue
Boston, MA 02215-5400
617-667-7000
Fax: 617-667-1134
www.bidmc.org/

Jean K Matheson MD, Contact

Provides testing and treatment for those with sleep disorders and offers educational workshops, plus support for their families.

3536 The Home for Little Wanderers
271 Huntington Avenue
Boston, MA 02115-4554
617-267-3700
888-466-3321
Fax: 617-267-8142
www.thehome.org

Joan Wallace-Benjamin, President/CEO
Michael L. Pearis, Executive Vice President and Chi
Meredith Bryan, Vice President for Development a
Thomas L. Durling, Vice President for Finance

To ensure the healthy, emotional, mental and social development of children at risk, their families and communities.
Year Founded: 1799

3537 Victor School
A Division of Justice Resource Institute, Inc
160 Gould Street
Suite 300
Needham, MA 02494-2300

781-559-4900
www.jri.org

Arden O'Connor, Chairperson
Andy Pond, MSW, MAT, President
Gregory Canfield, MSW, Executive Vice President
Deborah Reuman, MBA, Chief Financial Officer

A private, co-ed, therapeutic day school for students in grades 8-12 with a school philosophy that children learn when they can. Provides innovative and specialized educational and emotional support and treatment.

3538 Windhorse Integrative Mental Health
211 North Street
Suite 1
Northampton, MA 01060-2386
413-586-0207
877-844-8181
Fax: 413-585-1521
E-mail: admissions@windhorseimh.org
www.windhorseimh.org

Eric Friedland-Kays, MA, Admissions Manager
Jeff Bliss MSW, Director, Admissions/Marketing
Sara Watters MA, LMHC, Director, Clinical Operations

Windhorse is a nonprofit treatment and education organization with a whole person approach to recovery from serious psychiatric distress. Services are tailored in close communication with each client and their family.

Year Founded: 1981

Michigan

3539 Hawthorn Center
234 West Baraga Avenue
Marquette, MI 49855
906-228-2850
Fax: 248-349-6893
www.michigan.gov

Shobhana Joshi, Executive Director

To provide high quality inpatient mental health services to emotionally disturbed children and adolescents.

3540 Samaritan Counseling Center
29887 W Eleventh Mile Road
Farmington Hills, MI 48336
248-474-4701
Fax: 248-474-1518
E-mail: info@samaritancounselingmichigan.com
www.samaritancounselingmichigan.com

Robert A. Martin, Executive Director
Sara Kirsten, B.A., Administrative Manager

Provides professional therapeutic counseling and educational services to all God's people seeking wholeness through emotional and spiritual growth.

Minnesota

3541 River City Mental Health Clinic
1360 Energy Park Drive
Suite 340
Saint Paul, MN 55108
651-646-8985
Fax: 651-646-3959
www.rivercityclinic.com

Doug Jensen, Owner

Psychotherapy and assessment for all ages.

Mississippi

3542 East Mississippi State Hospital
PO Box 4128, W Station
Meridian, MS 39304-4128
601-482-6186
Fax: 601-483-5543
www.www.emsh.state.ms.us

Charles Carlisle, Director

To provide a continuum of behavioral health and long term care services for adults and adolescents in a caring, compassionate environment in which ethical principles guide decision making and resources are used responsibly and creatively.

Year Founded: 1882

3543 Mississippi State Hospital
PO Box 157-A
Whitfield, MS 39193-157
601-351-8018
E-mail: info@msh.state.ms.us
www.msh.state.ms.us

Facilitates improvement in the quality of life for Mississippians who are in need of psychiatric, chemical dependency or nursing home survices by rehabilitating to the least restrictive environment utilizing a reange of psychiatric and medical services that reflect the accepted standard of care and are in compliance with statutory and regulatory guidlelines.

3544 North Mississippi State Hospital
1937 Briar Ridge Road
Tupelo, MS 38804-5963
662-690-4200
Fax: 662-690-4227
TDD: 662-690-4239
E-mail: info@nmsh.state.ms.us
www.nmsh.state.ms.us

Paul Callens, Executive Director

3545 South Mississippi State Hospital
823 Highway 589
Purvis, MS 39475-4194
601-794-0100
Fax: 601-794-0210
www.www.smsh.state.ms.us

Wynona Winfield, Executive Director

Provides the highest quality acute psychiatric care for adults who live in southern Mississippi

Missouri

3546 Northwest Missouri Psychiatric Rehabilitation Center
3505 Frederick Avenue
Saint Joseph, MO 64506-2914
816-387-2300
Fax: 816-387-2329
www.mo.gov

Mary Attebury, Manager

Inpatient care for long-term psychiatric/adult.

3547 Southeast Missouri Mental Health Center
1010 W Columbia Street
Farmington, MO 63640-2902

573-218-6792
Fax: 573-218-6703
E-mail: cynthia.forsythe@dmh.mo.gov
www.www.dmh.mo.gov/smmhc/

Karen Adams, CEO

People shall receive services focusing on strenghts and promoting opportunities beyond the limitations of mental illness.

Nebraska

3548 Norfolk Regional Center
1700 N Victory Road
PO Box 1209
Norfolk, NE 68702-1209
402-370-3400
Fax: 402-370-3194
E-mail: Bill.Gibson@nebraska.gov
www.dhhs.ne.gov

William Gibson, CEO
TyLynne Bauer, Facility Operating Officer

A progressive 120-bed state psychiatric hospital providing specialized psychiatric care to adults.

Nevada

3549 Behavioral Health Options: Sierra Health Services
2724 N Tenaya Way
Las Vegas, NV 89128-424
877-393-6094
www.www.uhcnevada.com

Anthony M Marlon, Chairman/CEO

to manage behavioral health services in the private and public sectors on a national basis, creating value for our customers, including brokers, employers, members, providers and shareholders

3550 Northern Nevada Adult Mental Health Services
480 Galletti Way
Sparks, NV 89431-5564
775-688-2001
Fax: 775-688-2192
www.mhds.nv.gov

David Rosin MD, Contact

3551 Southern Nevada Adult Mental Health Services
6161 W Charleston Boulevard
Las Vegas, NV 89146-1148
702-486-6000
www.mhds.state.nv.us

Anuranjan Bist, Contact

New Hampshire

3552 Hampstead Hospital
218 E Road
Hamptead, NH 03841-5303
603-329-5311
Fax: 603-329-4746
www.hamsteadhospital.com

Phillip Kubiak, Chief Executive Officer
Cynthia Gove, Chief Operating Officer
Scott Ranks, Director Support Services
Lisa Ryan, Human Resources Coordinator

Provides a full range of psychiatric and chemical dependency services for children, adolescents, adults and the elderly.

3553 New Hampshire State Hospital
29 Pleasant Street
Concord, NH 03301-3852
603-271-5300
Fax: 603-271-5395
www.dhhs.state.nh.us

Chester G Batchelder, CEO

A state operated, publicly funded hospital providing a range of specialized psychiatric services. NHH advocates for and provides services that support an individual's recovery.

New Jersey

3554 Ancora Psychiatric Hospital
301 Spring Garden Road
Hammonton, NJ 08037
609-561-1700
Fax: 609-567-7294
E-mail: donna.ingram@dhs.state.nj.us
www.www.state.nj.us

John M. Lubitsky, CEO

Provides quality comprehensive psychiatric, medical and rehabilitative services that encourage maximun patient independence and movement towards community reintegration with an enviroment that is safe and caring.

3555 Ann Klein Forensic Center
Sullivan Way
PO Box 7717
W Trenton, NJ 08628-717
609-633-0900
Fax: 609-633-0971
E-mail: mhs.affc-infoline@dhs.state.nj.us
www.www.state.nj.us/humanservices/dmhs/oshm/akfc/

Glenn Ferguson, Ph.D., CEO

A 200-bed psychiatric hospital serving a unique population that requires a secured environment. The facility provides care and treatment to individuals suffering from mental illness who are also within the legal system.

3556 Greystone Park Psychiatric Hospital
59 Koch Avenue
Morris Plains, NJ 07950
973-538-1800
Fax: 973-993-8782
E-mail: william.lanni@dhs.state.nj.us
www.www.state.nj.us/humanservices/dmhs/oshm/gpph/

Janet Monroe, CEO

A 550 bed psychiattric hospital.

New Mexico

3557 Life Transition Therapy
110 Delgado Street
Santa Fe, NM 87501-2781
505-982-4183
800-547-2574
E-mail: therapy@lifetransitiontherapy.com
www.www.lifetransitiontherapy.com

Ralph Steele, Founder
Ralph Steele, Founder

To eliminate the fear, ignorance and conditioning that fuel racism and social injustice within the individual as well as in relationships, families, communities, and the world at large.

3558 Sequoyah Adolescent Treatment Center
3405 W Pan American Freeway NE
Albuquerque, NM 87107-4786
505-222-0355
www.nmsatc.org

Henry Gardner, Manager

A 36 bed residential treatment center whose purpose is to provide care, treatment, and reintegration into society for adolescents who are violent or who have a history of violence and have a mental disorder and who are amenable to treatment.

New York

3559 Arms Acres
75 Seminary Hill Road
Carmel, NY 10512-1921
845-225-3400
888-227-4641
Fax: 845-698-4046
www.www.armsacres.com

Frederick R Hesse, CEO
Sultan Niazi, CFO
Michele Saari, Health Information Management

A private health care system providing high quality, cost-effective care to those suffering from alcoholism and chemical dependency and to the many whose lives are affected by the diseases of addiction.

3560 Berkshire Farm Center and Services for Youth
13640 State Route 22
Canaan, NY 12029-3506
518-781-4567
Fax: 518-781-0507
E-mail: info@berkshirefarm.org
www.berkshirefarm.org

Mr. Robert A Kandel, Board Chairman
Timothy Giacchetta, President and CEO
Mr. Charles Mott, Chairman Emeritus

Mission is to strengthen children and their families so they can lives safely, independently and productively within their home communities.

3561 Bronx Psychiatric Center
1500 Waters Place
Bronx, NY 10461-2796
718-931-0600
Fax: 718-862-4879
E-mail: bronxpc@omh.state.ny.us
www.www.omh.ny.gov

Pamela Turner, Executive Director
Joseph Battaglia, MD, Clinical Director
Roy Thomas, Deputy Director

A 360 bed facility that has three impatient services and a comprehensive outpatient program.

3562 Brooklyn Children's Center
1819 Bergen Street
Brooklyn, NY 11233-4513
718-221-4500
Fax: 718-221-4581
E-mail: bcc@omh.state.ny.us
www.www.omh.ny.gov

Provides high quality comprehensive individualized mental health treatment services to serious emotionally disturbed children and adolescents in Brooklyn, and to continuously strive to improve the quality of those services.

3563 BryLin Hospitals
1263 Delaware Avenue
Buffalo, NY 14209-2497
716-886-8200
800-727-9546
Fax: 716-886-1986
E-mail: info@brylin.com
www.brylin.com

Eric Pleskow, CEO

Founded in 1955. Provides inpatient psychiatric services for children, adolescents, adults and geriatric patients. Outpatient substance abuse services for adolescents and adults. Outpatient mental health services for adults.

3564 Buffalo Psychiatric Center
400 Forest Avenue
Buffalo, NY 14213-1298
716-885-2261
Fax: 716-885-4852
E-mail: bufflopc@omh.state.ny.us
www.www.omh.ny.gov

Kimberly Karalus, Chief of Outpatient Services
Nancy Johnson, Director of Residential Services

Provides psychiatric quality inpatient, outpatient, residential, vocational, and wellness services to adults with serious mental illnesses

3565 Capital District Psychiatric Center
75 New Scotland Avenue
Albany, NY 12208-3474
518-549-6000
Fax: 518-549-6804
www.www.omh.ny.gov

Lewis Campbell, CEO

Provides inpatient psychiatric treatment and rehabilitation to patients who have been diagnosed with serious and persistenet mental illnesses and for whom brief or short-term treatment in a community hospital mental health unit has been unable to provide sympton stability.

3566 Central New York Psychiatric Center
9005 Old River Road
PO Box 300
Marcy, NY 13403
315-765-3600
Fax: 315-765-3629
E-mail: cnypc@omh.state.ny.us
www.www.omh.ny.gov

A comprehensive mental health service delivery system providing a full range of care and treatment to persons incarcerated in the New York State and county correctional system.

3567 Cornerstone of Rhinebeck
500 Milan Hollow Road
Rhinebeck, NY 12572-2970
845-266-3481
800-266-4410
Fax: 845-266-8335
E-mail: admin@cornerstoneny.com
www.cornerstoneny.com

Eileen Mc Curdy, Senior VP

Provides inpatient chemical dependency treatment and offers a comprehensive range of inpatient and outpatient treatment services for alcohol and substance abuse.

Year Founded: 1974

3568 Creedmoor Psychiatric Center
79-25 Winchester Boulevard
Queens Village, NY 11427-2128
718-464-7500
Fax: 718-264-3636
E-mail: crpc_info@omh.state.ny.us
www.www.omh.ny.gov

William Fisher, MD, Clinical Director
Susan Chin, Deputy Director
John Holmes, Deputy Director
Renee Anderson, Chief Nursing Officer

Provides a continuum of inpatient, outpatient and related psychiatric services with inpatient hospitalization at the main campus and five outpatient sites in the boroughs of Queens.

3569 Elmira Psychiatric Center
100 Washington Street
Elmira, NY 14901-2898
607-737-4711
Fax: 607-737-4722
E-mail: elmirapc@omh.state.ny.us
www.www.omh.ny.gov

Mark Stephany, Manager

Provides a wide array of comprehensive psychiatric services.

3570 Freedom Ranch
Freedom Village USA
5275 Rt. 14, PO Box 24
Lakemont, NY 14857-24
607-243-8126
800-842-8679
Fax: 607-243-5521
E-mail: 77pastor@fvusa.com
www.freedomvillageusa.com

Dr Fletcher Brothers, Founder

An extension of Freedom Village, Freedom Ranch offers a residential program for men 21 and older with substance abuse and emotional problems. Freedom Ranch is a faith-based program seeking to help men become productive members of society.

Year Founded: 1948

3571 Freedom Village USA
Freedom Village USA
5275 Rt. 14, PO Box 24
Lakemont, NY 14857-24
607-243-8126
800-842-8679
Fax: 607-243-5521

E-mail: 77pastor@fvusa.com
www.freedomvillageusa.com

Dr Fletcher Brothers, Founder

A not-for-profit residential campus for troubled teens. Offers a faith-based approach to teenagers in crisis or at risk. Students are required to make a voluntary one-year commitment to the program. Freedom Village has an 80% success rate with troubled teenagers.

3572 Gift of Life Home
Freedom Village USA
5275 Rt. 14, PO Box 24
Lakemont, NY 14857-24
607-243-8126
800-842-8679
Fax: 607-243-5521
E-mail: 77pastor@fvusa.com
www.freedomvillageusa.com

Dr Fletcher Brothers, Founder

An affiliate program of Freedom Village, USA, a residential program for troubled teenagers, the Gift of Life Home offers pregnant girls a safe haven, a place of refuge, where they can come and have their baby while transforming their life as well. Freedom Village is a faith-based alternative to other residential placements.

3573 Greater Binghamton Health Center
425 Robinson Street
Binghamton, NY 13904-1775
607-724-1391
Fax: 607-773-4387
E-mail: binghamton@omh.state.ny.us
www.www.omh.ny.gov

Pamela Vredenburgh, Manager

Provides comprehensive outpatient and inpatient services for adults and children who are seriously mentally ill.

3574 Hope House
573 Livingston Ave.
Albany, NY 12206
518-482-4673
Fax: 518-482-0873
E-mail: information@hopehouseinc.org
www.hopehouseinc.org

Kevin M. Connally, Executive Director
Catherine Dowdell, Executive Assistant
Lynda Tymeson, Director of Program Services
Courtney Lerman, Quality Assurance Manager

Started helping the community in need of education, intervention and treatment for the persons affected by substance abuse.

3575 Hutchings Psychiatric Center
620 Madison Street
Syracuse, NY 13210-2338
315-426-3600
Fax: 315-426-3603
www.www.omh.ny.gov

Colleen Sawyer, Executive Director

A comprehensive, community-based mental health facility providing an integrated network of inpatient and outpatient services for children and adults residing in the Central New York Region.

3576 Kingsboro Psychiatric Center
681 Clarkson Avenue
Brooklyn, NY 11203-2199
718-221-7700
Fax: 718-221-7206
E-mail: kingsboro@omh.state.ny.us
www.www.omh.ny.gov

Mark Lerman, Manager

Provides competent compassionate psychiatric care to people with serious mental illness with a purpose of reintegrating them to the community.

3577 Kirby Forensic Psychiatric Center
600 E 125th Street
New York, NY 10035-6000
646-672-5800
Fax: 646-672-6446
E-mail: kirbypc@omh.state.ny.us
www.www.omh.ny.gov

Steve Rabinowitz, Manager

A maximum security hospital of the New York State Office of Mental Health that provides secure treatment and evaluation for the forensic patients and courts of New York City and Long Island.

Year Founded: 1985

3578 Liberty Resources
1045 James Street
Suite 200
Syracuse, NY 13203
315-425-1004
E-mail: info@liberty-resource.org
www.liberty-resource.org

David Harris, President
Carl M. Coyle, MSW, Chief Executive Officer
Joanna Viggiano, BS, CPA, Chief Financial Officer
Kim Prior, BS, Chief Operating Officer

Provides residential and non-residential services to individuals and families, our present array of services include Mental Health; Mental Retardation and Developmental Disabilities; services for individuals living with HIV/AIDS, families and youth involved in the child welfare system, domestic violence services; services to persons in recovery; and diversified case management services.

Year Founded: 1978

3579 Manhattan Psychiatric Center
600 E 125th Street
New York, NY 10035-6000
646-672-6767
Fax: 646-672-6446
E-mail: mpcinfo@omh.state.ny.us
www.www.omh.ny.gov

Steve Rabinowitz, Manager

Offers inpatient and outpatient treatment for adults with mental illness.

3580 Mid-Hudson Forensic Psychiatric Center
2834 Route 17-M
New Hampton, NY 10958
845-374-8700
Fax: 845-374-8860
E-mail: midhudsonfpc@omh.state.ny.us
www.www.omh.ny.gov

Barbara Daria, Manager

A secure adult psychiatric center that provides a comprehensive program of evaluation, treatment, and rehabilitation for patients admitted by court order.

3581 Mohawk Valley Psychiatric Center
1400 Noyes at York
Utica, NY 13502
315-738-3800
Fax: 315-738-4414
E-mail: mvpc@omh.state.ny.us
www.www.omh.ny.gov

Sarah Rudes, CEO

Provides quality, individualized psychiatric treatment and rehabilitation services that promote recovery.

3582 Nathan S Kline Institute for Psychiatric Research
140 Old Orangeburg Road
Orangeburg, NY 10962-1157
845-398-5500
Fax: 845-398-5510
E-mail: webmaster@nki.rfmh.org
www.www.rfmh.org/nki

Donald C. Goff, MD, Director
Antonio Convit, M.D., Deputy Director
Thomas O. O'Hara, MBA, Deputy Director Administration

Research programs in Alzheimers disease, analytical psychopharmacology, basic and clinical neuroimaging, cellular and molecular neurobiology, clinical trial data management, co-occuring disorders and many other mental health studies.

3583 New York Psychiatric Institute
1051 Riverside Drive
New York, NY 10032-1098
212-543-6283
www.www.nyspi.org/

Jeffrey Lieberman, MD, Chairman
Anke Ehrhardt, PhD, Vice Chair for Academic Affairs
Avalon Lance, MHA, Vice Chair for Administration an
Harold A. Pincus, MD, Vice Chair for Strategic Initiat

3584 Odyssey House
120 Wall Street
New York, NY 10005
212-361-1600
Fax: 212-361-1666
E-mail: info@odysseyhouseinc.org
www.odysseyhouseinc.org

Peter Provet, President & Chief Executive Offi
John Tavolacci, Executive Vice President & Chief
Durga Vallabhaneni, Senior Vice President & Chief Fi
Isobelle Surface, Senior Vice President & Director

Develops innovative treatment models to ensure that our systems take into account current research, utilizing what works most effectively to help these individuals overcome their difficulties and build a stable, producitve, drug-free life.

Year Founded: 1967

3585 Pahl Transitional Apartments
559-565 Sixth Avenue
Troy, NY 12182-2620
518-237-9891
Fax: 518-237-9409

E-mail: michael_kennedy@pahlinc.org
www.pahlinc.org

Michael Kennedy, Clinical Director

A 9-12 month residential, chemical dependency treatment facility for males ages 16-25. The goal for the residents is to learn the skills necessary for long-term recovery and independent living.

3586 Phoenix House
164 West 74th Street
New York, NY 10023-2301
646-505-2000
Fax: 646-721-2164
www.phoenixhouse.org

Alan Hargrove, Program Director
Brian Gillam, Managing Director
Christine Balzano, Program Director
Dan Boylan, Program Director

Reclaims disordered lives, encourages individual responsibility, positive behavior, and personal growth, also strengthens families and communities, and safeguards public health. Also, promotes a drug-free society through prevention, treatment, education and training, research, and advocacy.

3587 Pilgrim Psychiatric Center
998 Crooked Hill Road
West Brentwood, NY 11717-1019
631-761-3500
Fax: 631-761-2600
E-mail: pilgriminfo@omh.state.ny.us
www.www.omh.ny.gov

Dean Wienstock, Manager

Provides excellent, integrated care in evaluation, treatment, crisis intervention, rehabilitation, support, and self help/empowerment service to individuals with serious psychiatric illness.

3588 Queens Children's Psychiatric Center
74-03 Commonwealth Boulevard
Bellerose, NY 11426-1839
718-264-4500
E-mail: queenscpc@omh.state.ny.us
www.www.omh.ny.gov

Keith Little, Executive Director

Serves seriously emotionally disturbed children and adolescents from the ages of 5 through 18 in a range of programs including Inpatient hospitalization, outpatient clinic treatment, intensive case management, homemaker services and community education and consultation services.

3589 Rochester Psychiatric Center
1111 Elmwood Avenue
Rochester, NY 14620-3090
585-241-1200
Fax: 585-241-1424
TTY: 585-241-1982
E-mail: rochesterpc@omh.state.ny.us
www.www.omh.ny.gov

Elizabeth Suhre, R.N., B.S., MBA, Executive Director and Director
Philip Griffin, Director for Quality Improvement
Laurence Guttmacher, M.D., Clinical Director
Christopher Kirisits, R.N., M.S.N., Chief Nursing Officer

Provides quality comprehensive treatment and rehabilitation services to people with psychiatric disabilities working toward recovery.

3590 Rockland Children's Psychiatric Center
2 First Avenue
Orangeburg, NY 10962
845-359-7400
800-597-8481
Fax: 845-680-8900
E-mail: rocklandcpc@omh.state.ny.us
www.www.omh.ny.gov

Josefina M Moneda

A psychiatric hospital exclusively for children and adolescents

3591 Rockland Psychiatric Center
140 Old Orangeburg Road
Orangeburg, NY 10962
845-359-1000
Fax: 845-680-5580
E-mail: rpamz01@omh.state.ny.us
www.www.omh.ny.gov

Provides treatment, rehabilitation, and support to adults 18 and older with severe and complex mental illness.

3592 Sagamore Children's Psychiatric Center
197 Half Hollow Road
Dix Hills, NY 11746-5859
631-370-1700
Fax: 631-370-1714
E-mail: scisdcc@omh.state.ny.us
www.www.omh.ny.gov

Dennis Dubey, Executive Director

Programs for youngsters and their families include inpatient hospitalization, day hospitalization, day treatment, outpatient clinic treatment, mobile mental health team crisis services, information and referral, and community consultation and training.

3593 Samaritan Village
138-02 Queens Blvd
Briarwood, NY 11435-2647
718-206-2000
800-532-4357
www.samaritanvillage.org

Tino Hernandez, President/CEO
Douglas Apple, Executive Vice President and Chi
John Iammatteo, Senior Vice President for Financ
Sheila Greene, Vice President of Communications

Mission is to eliminate the devastating impact of substance abuse on individuals, families and communities by helping addicted men and women take responsibility for their own recovery.

3594 South Beach Psychiatric Center
777 Seaview Avenue
Staten Island, NY 10305-3409
718-667-2300
Fax: 718-667-2344
E-mail: sbcsmss@omh.state.ny.us
www.www.omh.ny.gov

Rosanne Gaylor, MD, Executive Director
Rosanne Gaylor, MD, Director, Clinical Services
Doreen Piazza, R.N.C., MS, Director, Nursing
Titus Mathew, BE, Deputy Director, Administration

Provides intermediate level inpatient services to persons living in western Brooklyn, southern Staten Island, and Manhattan south of 42nd street.

3595 St. Lawrence Psychiatric Center
1 Chimney Point Drive
Ogdensburg, NY 13669-2291
315-541-2001
Fax: 315-541-2041
E-mail: slpcinfo@omh.state.ny.us
www.www.omh.ny.gov

Sam Bastien, Executive Director

3596 Veritas Villa
5 Ridgeview Road
Kerhonkson, NY 12446-1555
845-626-3555
Fax: 845-626-3840
E-mail: info@veritasvilla.com
www.veritasvilla.com

Joseph Stoeckeler, CEO

Inpatient rehabilitation and wellness center

Year Founded: 1957

3597 Western New York Children's Psychiatric Center
1010 E & W Road
W Seneca, NY 14224-3698
716-677-7000
Fax: 716-675-6455
E-mail: westernnewyorkcpc@omh.state.ny.us
www.www.omh.ny.gov

Deborah Shiffner, Manager

Provides high quality, comprehensive behavioral health care services to seriously emotionally disturbed children and adolescents, and to partner with their families throughout the continuum of care.

North Carolina

3598 Broughton Hospital
1000 S Sterling Street
Morganton, NC 28655-3999
828-433-2111
E-mail: BH.Information@NCMail.net
www.www.ncdhhs.gov/dsohf/broughton/

Dr Art Robarge, Interim Hospital Director/CEO

3599 Central Regional Hospital
803 Biggs Drive
Raleigh, NC 27699
919-575-7100
www.www.ncdhhs.gov/dsohf

Dale C. Armstrong, MBA, FACHE, Director
Laura White, Team Leader, Hospitals
Carol Donin, Team Leader, Developmental Cente
Wendi McDaniel, Team Leader, Facility Advocates

Formed by the merger of Dorothea Dix Hospital and John Umstead Hospital. Services include adult psychiatric services, clinical research services, child and adolescent services, medical services, and geropsychiatric services.

3600 Cherry Hospital
201 Stevens Mill Road
Goldsboro, NC 27530-1057

919-731-3411
Fax: 919-731-3788
www.www.ncdhhs.gov

J. Luckey Welsh, Jr., CEO
Nathaniel Carmichael, COO
Jim Mayo, MD, Clinical Director
Scott Mann, MD, Medical Director

North Dakota

3601 North Dakota State Hospital
2605 Circle Drive
Jamestown, ND 58401-6905
701-253-3650
Fax: 701-253-3999
TTY: 701-253-3880
www.nd.gov

Alex Schweitzer, CEO

Ohio

3602 Central Behavioral Healthcare
5965 Renaissance Place
Toledo, OH 43623-4728
419-882-5678
Fax: 419-882-7446
E-mail: info@cbhpsych.com
www.cbhpsych.com

Dennis W. Kogut, PhD, Owner

Provides patients with a broad range of high-quality behavioral healthcare in a professional and personal matter.

Year Founded: 1986

3603 Heartland Behavioral Healthcare
3000 Erie Street S
Massillon, OH 44646-7976
330-833-3135
800-783-9301
Fax: 330-833-6564
TDD: 330-832-9991
www.mha.ohio.gov

Jeffrey L. Sims, CEO
Dr. Emmanuel Nwajei, Chief Clinical Officer
Michael Waggoner, Nurse Executive
John Stocker, Client Rights Specialist

3604 Northcoast Behavioral Healthcare System
PO Box 678003
1756 Sagamore Road
Northfield, OH 44067
330-467-7131
Fax: 330-467-2420
TDD: 330-467-5522
www.www.mha.ohio.gov

Doug Kern, Chief Executive Officer
Michael Emerick, Nurse Executive
Muhammad Momen, M.D., Lead Chief Clinical Officer (CCO
Joi Chapman, Client Rights Specialist

3605 Northcoast Behavioral Healthcare System
PO Box 678003
1756 Sagamore Road
Northfield, OH 44067
330-467-7131
Fax: 330-467-2420

TDD: 330-467-5522
www.www.mha.ohio.gov

Doug Kern, Chief Executive Officer
Michael Emerick, Nurse Executive
Muhammad Momen, M.D., Lead Chief Clinical Officer
(CCO
Joi Chapman, Client Rights Specialist

3606 Twin Valley Behavioral Healthcare
Columbus Campus, 2200 W Broad Street
Columbus, OH 43223
614-752-0333
877-301-8824
Fax: 614-752-0087
TDD: 614-274-7137
www.www.mha.ohio.gov

Veronica Lofton, CEO
Dr. Alan Freeland, Chief Clinical Officer (CCO)
David Blahnik, Chief Operations Officer
Susan Cross, Client Rights Specialist

State operated BHD serving severley mentally ill adults in partnership with the community.

Oklahoma

3607 Griffin Memorial Hospital
900 E Main Street
PO Box 151
Norman, OK 73070-151
405-573-6623
Fax: 405-522-8320
www.www.ok.gov

Don Bowen, Contact

3608 Oklahoma Forensic Center
PO Box 69
Vinita, OK 74301-0069
918-256-7841
Fax: 918-256-4491
www.www.ok.gov/

William Burkett, Contact

3609 Willow Crest Hospital
130 A Street Southwest
Miami, OK 74354-6800
918-542-1836
Fax: 918-542-6060
E-mail: aanthony@willowcresthospital.com
www.willowcresthospital.com

Anne Anthony, CEO

Oregon

3610 Blue Mountain Recovery Center
2600 Westgate
Pendleton, OR 97801-9604
541-276-0810
Fax: 541-278-2209
E-mail: Kerry.Kelly@state.or.us
www.www.oregon.gov

Kerry Kelly, Contact

3611 Oregon State Hospital: Portland
1121 NE 2nd Avenue
Portland, OR 97232-2043

503-731-8620
www.www.oregon.gov

Nena Strickland, Executive Director
Year Founded: 1883

3612 Oregon State Hospital: Salem
2600 Center Street NE
Salem, OR 97301-2682
503-945-2800
www.www.oregon.gov

Pam Dickinson, Manager
Year Founded: 1883

3613 Riverside Center
671 Sw Main
PO Box 2259
Winston, OR 97496-2259
541-679-6129
Fax: 541-679-5285
www.riversidecenter.org

3614 St. Mary's Home for Boys
16535 SW Tualatin Valley Highway
Beaverton, OR 97006-5143
503-649-5651
Fax: 503-649-7405
E-mail: reception@stmaryshomeforboys.org
www.www.stmaryshomeforboys.org

Francis Maher, Executive Director

Founded in 1889 as an orphanage for abandoned and wayward children, today St. Mary's is a private, non-profit organization that offers comprehensive residential, day treatment and mental health services to at-risk boys between the ages of 10 and 17 who are emotionally disturbed and/or disruptive behavior disordered.

Year Founded: 1889

Pennsylvania

3615 MHNet
9606 N. Mopac Expressway
Stonebridge Plaza 1, Suite 600
Austin, TX 78759
888-646-6889
Fax: 724-741-4552
E-mail: edwynl@integra-ease.com
www.www.mhnet.com

Wesley J Brockhoeft, PhD, President/CEO
Peter Harris, MD, Corporate Medical Director
Robert Wilson, CFO
Richard T Wright, SVP Business Development

MHNet is an outgrowth of the Center for Individual and Family Counseling, a multi-disciplinary outpatient treatment clinic with a full spectrum behavioral health organization with national service delivery capability.

Year Founded: 1981

3616 National Mental Health Self-Help Clearinghouse
1211 Chestnut Street
Suite 1207
Philadephia, PA 19107-4103
215-751-1810
800-553-4539

Fax: 215-636-6312
www.mhselfhelp.org

Joseph Rogers, Executive Director
Susan Rogers, Director
Christa Burkett, Technical Assistance Coordinator
Britani Nestel, Program Specialist

A national consumer technical assistance center, has played a major role in the development of the mental health consumer movement.

Year Founded: 1986

3617 Renfrew Center Foundation
475 Spring Lane
Philadelphia, PA 19128-3918
215-482-5353
Fax: 215-482-7390
E-mail: foundation@renfrew.org
www.renfrewcenter.com

Sam Menaged, President

A tax-exempt, nonprofit organization advancing the education, prevention, research, and treatment of eating disorders.

Year Founded: 1985

3618 Torrance State Hospital
PO Box 111
Torrance, PA 15779-111
724-459-4406
www.www.dpw.state.pa.us

Lyle Gardner, Director

3619 Warren State Hospital
33 Main Drive
N Warren, PA 16365-5099
814-726-4219
Fax: 814-726-4447
www.www.dpw.state.pa.us

Charlotte M. Uber, LSW, Chief Executive Officer
Nancy Saullo, HR Director
Susan Cramer, Admissions Coordinator

3620 Wernersville State Hospital
PO Box 300
Wernersville, PA 19565-300
610-678-3411
Fax: 610-670-4101
E-mail: ra-weshemployment@.pa.gov
www.www.dpw.state.pa.us

Andrea Kepler, Chief Executive Officer
Year Founded: 1891

Rhode Island

3621 Butler Hospital
345 Blackstone Boulevard
Providence, RI 02906-4829
401-455-6200
E-mail: info@butler.org
www.butler.org

Patricia Recupero, President

Rhode Island's only private, nonprofit psychiatric and substance abuse hospital for adults, adolescents, children and seniors.

Year Founded: 1844

3622 Gateway Healthcare
249 Roosevelt Avenue
Suite 205
Pawtucket, RI 02860-2134
401-724-8400
E-mail: developmentoffice@gatewayhealth.org
www.gatewayhealth.org

Richard Leclerc, President
Scott W DiChristofero, VP Finance
Stephen Chabot MD, Medical Director
Carolyn Kyle, Senior Vice President of Strateg

To promote resiliency and to assist people in their recovery from mental health, substance abuse, and behavioral and emotional disorder

3623 Groden Center
86 Mount Hope Avenue
Providence, RI 02906-1648
401-274-6310
Fax: 401-421-3280
E-mail: grodencenter@grodencenter.org
www.grodencenter.org

June Groden, President

Groden Center has been providing day and residential treatment and educational services to children and youth who have developmental and behavioral difficulties and their families. By providing a broad range of individualized services in the most normal and least restrictive settings possible, children and youth learn skills that will help them engage in typical experiences and interact more successfully with others. Education and treatment take place in Groden Center classrooms, in the student's homes, and in the community with every effort made to maintain typical family and peer relationships. Call or visit our web site for more information about the Center and the publications and materials we have available.

Year Founded: 1976

South Carolina

3624 CM Tucker Jr Nursing Care Center
2200 Harden Street
Columbia, SC 29203-7107
803-737-5300
www.www.state.sc.us

Laura W. Hughes, RN, BSN, MPH, Facility Director

Provides excellence in resident care in an environment of concern and compassion that is respectful to others, adaptive to change and accountable for outcome.

Year Founded: 1970

3625 Columbia Counseling Center
900 St. Andrews Road
Columbia, SC 29210-5816
803-731-4708
Fax: 803-798-7607
www.columbiacounselingcenter.com

Darrel G Shaver, President

3626 Earle E Morris Jr Alcohol & Drug Treatment Center
610 Faison Drive
Columbia, SC 29203-3218

803-935-7200
Fax: 803-935-7329
www.scdmh.org

George Mc Connell, Manager

Provides effective treatment of chemical dependence through comprehensive evaluation, safe detoxification, and state-of-the-art treatment servies.

3627 G Werber Bryan Psychiatric Hospital
220 Faison Drive
Columbia, SC 29203-3210
803-935-5761
Fax: 803-935-7110
www.www.state.sc.us

Versie Bellamy RN, MN, Deputy Director
Kimberly B. Rudd, MD, Medical Director
Algie Bryant, RN, MSN, Director of Performance Improvem
Mesa Foard, Director of Information Technolo

A 277 bed short term intensive care facility that serves adult and geriatric patients ages 16 years and older. Provides therapeutic services in a warm and nurturing environment for individuals in crisis.

3628 Patrick B Harris Psychiatric Hospital
130 Highway 252
PO Box 2907
Anderson, SC 29622-2907
864-231-2600
Fax: 864-225-3297
www.patrickbharrispsychiatrichospital.com

John Fletcher, CEO

Provides intensive, short-term, psychiatric diagnostic and treatment services on a 24 hour, emergency voluntary and involuntary basis.

3629 South Carolina State Hospital
2414 Bull Street
Columbia, SC 29202
803-898-8581
www.www.state.sc.us

John H. Magill, State Director

Psychiatric hospital
Year Founded: 1995

3630 William S Hall Psychiatric Institute
1800 Colonial Drive
PO Box 202
Columbia, SC 29203
803-898-1662
www.www.state.sc.us

Angela Forand, Ph.D., , Program Director
Dr. Phyllis Bryant-Mobley, Medical Director
Natasha Davis, RN (Interim), Director of Nursing Services

South Dakota

3631 South Dakota Human Services Center
3515 Broadway Avenue
PO Box 7600
Yankton, SD 57078-7600
605-668-3100
Fax: 605-668-3460
E-mail: infohsc@state.sd.us
www.dss.sd.gov/behavioralhealthservices/hsc/

Doug Dix, Deputy Financial Officer
Laura Schaeffer, Deputy Financial Officer
Amy Iversen-Pollreisz, Deputy Secretary

To provide persons who are mentally ill or chemically dependent with effective, individualized professional treatment that enables them to achieve their highest level of personal independence in the most therapeutic environment.

Tennessee

3632 Cherokee Health Systems
2018 Weestern Avenue
Knoxville, TN 37921-5718
865-934-6734
www.cherokeehealth.com

Tracey Trench, Manager

Uses an integrated model to provide behavioral health and primary care services in a community-based setting.
Year Founded: 1960

3633 Lakeshore Mental Health Institute
5908 Lyons View Drive
Knoxville, TN 37919-7598
865-584-1561
Fax: 865-450-5203
E-mail: OCA.TDMHSAS@tn.gov.
www.www.tn.gov/

Richard L Thomas, CEO

3634 Memphis Mental Health Institute
951 Court Avenue
Memphis, TN 38103-2813
901-577-1800
Fax: 901-577-1434
www.www.tn.gov

Lisa A. Daniel, CEO
Tammy D. Ali-Carr, Psychiatric Hosp. Asst. Supt.
Lori Minor, Nurse Executive
Scott Baymiller, MD, Clinical Director

55 bed acute adult psychiatric facility operated by the State of Tennessee Department of Mental Health & Substance Abuse Services.

3635 Middle Tennessee Mental Health Institute
221 Stewarts Ferry Pike
Nashville, TN 37214-3325
615-902-7400
Fax: 615-902-7571
www.tennessee.gov

Candance Gilligan, Manager

3636 Moccasin Bend Mental Health Institute
100 Moccasin Bend Road
Chattanooga, TN 37405
423-265-2271
Fax: 423-785-3347
www.tennessee.gov

William Ventress, CEO

3637 Western Mental Health Institute
11100 U.S. Highway 64
Bolivar, TN 38008

731-228-2000
E-mail: OCA.TDMHSAS@tn.gov.
www.www.tn.gov/

Roger Pursley, Chief Officer

3638 Woodridge Hospital
403 State of Franklin Road
Johnson City, TN 37604-6034
423-928-7111
800-346-8899
www.msha.com

Kim Moore, Manager
Kim Cudebec, Clinical Director

Texas

3639 Austin State Hospital
4110 Guadalupe Street
Austin, TX 78751-4223
512-452-0381
Fax: 512-419-2812
www.www.dshs.state.tx.us

Carl Schock, CEO

Provides adult psychiatric services, specialty adult services and child and adolescent psychiatric services.

3640 Big Spring State Hospital
1901 N Highway 87
Big Spring, TX 79720-283
432-267-8216
E-mail: edward.moughon@dshs.state.tx.us
www.www.dshs.state.tx.us

Ed Mougon, CEO

A 195-bed psychiatric hospital that provides hospitalization for people 18 years of age and older with psychiatric illnesses in a 57-county area in West Texas and the Texas Panhandle.

Year Founded: 1938

3641 Choices Adolescent Treatment Center
4521 Karnack Hwy
Marshall, TX 75670
903-938-4455
800-638-0880
Fax: 903-938-8906
E-mail: choices@sydcom.net
www.choicestreatment.com

C G Bowman, CEO

Choices residential treatment program focuses on adolescents which abuse substances and addresses related psychiatric disorders.

3642 Dallas Metrocare Services
1380 Riverbend Drive
Dallas, TX 75247
214-743-1200
877-283-2121
Fax: 214-630-3469
E-mail: metrocare@metrocareservices.org
www.metrocareservices.org

Julia P. Noble, Chair
Jill Martinez, Vice Chair
Judy N. Myers, Secretary

North Texas' leading nonprofit dedicated to helping people with mental illness, developmental disabilities, and severe

emotional problems live healthier lives. Provides a comprehensive array of individually-tailored services to help the people we serve toward meaningful and satisfying lives.

Year Founded: 1967

3643 El Paso Psychiatric Center
4615 Alameda Avenue
El Paso, TX 79905-2702
915-532-2202
E-mail: zulema.carrillo@dshs.state.tx.us
www.dshs.state.tx.us

Zulema C. Carrillo, Superintendent
Raul Luna, Chief Nurse Executive
Amber Bechtel, Quality Oversight Director
David Osterhout, Assistant Superintendent

A 74-bed psychiatric hospital that provides hospitalization to the citizens of far West Texas.

3644 Green Oaks Behavioral Healthcare Service
7808 Clodus Fields Drive
Dallas, TX 75251-2206
972-991-9504
800-866-6554
Fax: 972-789-1865
www.greenoakspsych.com

Committed to developing and emulating the latest, most effective clinical practices always, and, in all things, to promote dignity, holding compassion and respect for patients and their families as the absolute standard.

3645 Homeward Bound
233 West 10th Street
Dallas, TX 75208-4524
214-941-3500
Fax: 214-941-3517
E-mail: ddenton@homewardboundinc.org
www.homewardboundinc.org

Jesse Oliver, Board Chair
Douglas W. Denton, MA, LCDC, LCCA, Executive Director
Diana S. Burns, Director of Grants Management
Phil Ray, M.Ed, M.B.A., Information Systems

Offers chemical dependence treatment for the indigent population anad those referred by the criminal justice system, local hospitals and private practitioners.

Year Founded: 1980

3646 Jewish Family and Children's Services
12500 NW Military Highway
Suite 250
San Antonio, TX 78231-1871
210-302-6920
Fax: 210-302-6952
www.jfs-sa.org

Ilene Kramer, President
Marion Bernstein, 1st Vice-President
Scott McLean, 2nd Vice-President
David Scotch, Treasurer

To strengthen community values, promote human dignity and enhance self-sufficiency of individuals and families through social, psychological, health educaitonal and financial support programs.

Year Founded: 1974

3647 Kerrville State Hospital
721 Thompson Drive
Kerrville, TX 78028-5199
830-896-2211
Fax: 830-792-4926
www.www.dshs.state.tx.us

Linda Highsmith, President

provides care for persons with major mental illnesses who
need the safety, structure, and resources of an in-patient
setting

3648 La Hacienda Treatment Center Hunt, TX 78024
800-749-6160
E-mail: info@lahacienda.com
www.lahacienda.com

Provides treatment for alcoholism and other chemical dependencies

Year Founded: 1972

3649 Laurel Ridge Treatment Center
17720 Corporate Woods Drive
San Antonio, TX 78259-3500
210-491-9400
800-624-7975
Fax: 210-491-3550
www.laurelridgetc.com

Dan Thomas, CEO

A psychiatric hospital offering a comprehensive continuum
of behavioral healthcare services including acute programs
for children, adolescents and adults and residential treatment for children and adolescents.

3650 New Horizons Ranch and Center
PO Box 549
Goldthwaite, TX 76844-549
915-938-5518
Fax: 325-938-5665
www.newhorizonsinc.com

Gary Webb, President
Mark Horn, Vice President
JB Morgan, Secretary
Michael Redden, Executive Director

To provide an environment where children, families and
staff are able to heal and grow through caring relationships
and unconditional love and acceptance.

Year Founded: 1971

3651 North Texas State Hospital: Vernon Campus
4730 College Drive
Vernon, TX 76384-4009
940-552-9901
Fax: 940-553-2500
E-mail: jamese.smith@dshs.state.tx.us
www.dshs.state.tx.us

James E Smith, Superintendent
Bill Lowery, Financial Officer
Kim Hays, Assistant to Financial Officer
Sheila Sidlauskas, Director, Quality Management

3652 North Texas State Hospital: Wichita Falls Campus
6515 Lake Road
Wichita Falls, TX 76308-5419
940-692-1220
Fax: 940-689-5538
E-mail: jamese.smith@dshs.state.tx.us
www.www.dshs.state.tx.us

Jim Smith, Administrator

1917 pages

3653 Rio Grande State Center
1401 South Rangerville
Harlingen, TX 78552-7638
956-364-8000
www.dshs.state.tx.us

Maria G Dill, Superintendent

The only public provider south of San Antonio, Texas that
offers healthcare, inpatient mental health services and long
term mental retardation services.

1956 pages

3654 Rusk State Hospital
805 North Dickinson Drive
Rusk, TX 75785
903-683-3421
E-mail: ted.debbs@dshs.state.tx.us
www.www.dshs.state.tx.us

Brenda Slaton, Superintendent
Michelle Foster, Assistant Superintendent
Frances L. Long, Financial Officer
Joe Bates, M.D., Clinical Director

An inpatient hospital providing psychiatric treatment and
care for citizens primarily from the East Texas region.

3655 San Antonio State Hospital
6711 South New Braunfels
Suite 100
San Antonio, TX 78223-3006
210-532-8811
Fax: 210-531-7780
E-mail: robert.arizpe@dshs.state.tx.us
www.dshs.state.tx.us

Bob Arizpe, Superintendent
Valerie Kroll, Assistant to Superintendent
Jessica Gutierrez-Rodriguez, Assistant Superintendent
Glenda Armstrong Huff, Assistant Superintendent

Provides intensive inpatient diagnostic, treatment, rehabilitative, and referral servious for seriously mentally ill persons from South Texas regardless of their financial status.

3656 Shades of Hope Treatment Center
402-A Mulberry Street
Buffalo Gap, TX 79508
800-588-4673
www.shadesofhope.com

Tennie McCarty, Founder/CEO
Carrie Willey, PhD, LPC, Clinical Director
Camela Balcomb, Executive Director
Becky Forrest, Admission Coordinator

A residential and outpatient all-addictions treatment center
specializing in the intensive treatment of eating disorders.

3657 Starlite Recovery Center
230 Mesa Verde Drive East
PO Box 317
Center Point, TX 78010-317
866-220-1626
Fax: 830-634-2532

E-mail: info@starliterecovery.com
www.starliterecovery.com

Amy J. Swetnam, LPC, LCDC, CE, Executive Director
Bryan M. Davis, D.O., MSPH, Medical Director
Shannon Malish, LMSW, Director of Counseling Services
Nancy Kneupper, L.V.N., Director of Nursing

Provides the highest quality of care in a cost-effective manner, insuring that our valued clients receive treatment that will allow them to return to a productive way of life.

3658 Terrell State Hospital
1200 East Brin
Terrell, TX 75160-2938
972-563-6452
www.www.dshs.state.tx.us

Dorothy Floyd, Ph.D., Superintendent
Nancy Drake, Assistant to Superintendent
Mike Verseckes, Financial Officer
Judy Tanner, Assistant to Financial Officer

A 316 bed, Joint Commission accredited and Medicare certified, psychiatric inpatient hospital, that is responsible for providing services for individuals with mental illnesses residing within a 19 county, 12, 052 square mile service region, with a population of over 3 million.

3659 Waco Center for Youth
3501 N 19th Street
Waco, TX 76708-2097
254-756-2171
Fax: 254-745-5398
E-mail: eddie.greenfield@dshs.state.tx.us
www.dshs.state.tx.us

Eddie Greenfield, Executive Director

A psychiatric residential treatment facility that serves teen-agers, ages 13 through 17, with emotional difficulties and/or behavioral problems.

Utah

3660 Copper Hills Youth Center
5899 Rivendell Drive
West Jordan, UT 84081-6500
801-561-3377
800-776-7116
Fax: 801-569-2959
www.www.copperhillsyouthcenter.com

Phil Sheridan, CEO
Daren Woolstenhulme, CFO
Rebekah Schuler, Director of Clinical Services
Dave Anderton, Director of Risk Management

Residential treatment center for boys and girls ages 12-17. Mental health and substance abuse treatment. Also specialized programs for Autism and sexual misconduct

3661 Utah State Hospital
1300 E Center Street
Provo, UT 84606-3554
801-344-4400
Fax: 801-344-4225
E-mail: jgierisch@utah.gov
www.www.ush.utah.gov

Mark I Payne, Manager

provides excellent care in a safe and respectful environment to promote hope and quality of life for individuals with mental illness

1885 pages

Vermont

3662 Brattleboro Retreat
Anna Marsh Lane
PO Box 803
Brattleboro, VT 05302-803
802-257-7785
Fax: 802-258-3770
www.www.brattlebororetreat.org

Robert E Simpson Jr, President/CEO
John E. Blaha, MBA, Senior Vice President & Chief Fi
Peter Albert, LICSW, Senior Vice President of Governm
Frederick Engstrom, MD, Chief Medical Officer

A not-for-profit health services organization which, above all else, is committed to assisting individuals to improve their health and functioning.

3663 Spring Lake Ranch Therapeutic Community
1169 Spring Lake Road
Cuttingville, VT 05738-4418
802-492-3322
Fax: 802-492-3331
E-mail: info@springlakeranch.org
www.springlakeranch.org

Rachel Stark, Admissions
Ed Oechslie, Executive Director

Offers an alternative therapeutic treatment program for adults with mental illness and/or substance abuse. Our work program and community life help residents grow and recover in the beautiful Green Mountains of Vermont. Our goal is to help people move from hospitalization or period of crisis to an independent life.

Year Founded: 1932

Virginia

3664 Catawba Hospital
5525 Catawba Hospital Drive
Catawba, VA 24070-0200
540-375-4200
800-451-5544
Fax: 540-375-4394
www.www.catawba.dmhmrsas.virginia.gov/

Jack Wood, CEO

To support the continuous process of recovery by providing quality psychiatric services to those individuals entrusted to our care

1909 pages

3665 Central State Hospital
26317 West Washington Street
PO Box 4030
Petersburg, VA 23803-30
804-524-7000
www.csh.dmhmrsas.virginia.gov/default.htm

to provide state of the art mental health care and treatment to forensic and civilly committed patients in need of a structured, secure environment. The major components of the hospital's mission include Evaluation, Treatment, Protection, and Disposition

3666 Commonwealth Center for Children & Adolescents
PO Box 4000
Staunton, VA 24402-4000
540-332-2100
Fax: 540-332-2201
www.ccca.dmhmrsas.virginia.gov

William J Tuell, Contact

CCCA is an acute care mental health facility for minors under the age of 18 years, operated by the State of Virginia, Department of Behavioral Health and Developmental Services.

Year Founded: 1996

3667 Dominion Hospital
2960 Sleepy Hollow Road
Falls Church, VA 22044-2082
703-536-2000
Fax: 703-533-9650
E-mail: Dominion.DLCares@HCAHealthcare.com
www.dominionhospital.com

Trula Minton, CEO

Offers individuals and families hope and help. Treats children, adolescents and adults who suffer from debilitating disorders such as anxiety, panic, depression, delusions, eating disorders, schizophrenia, school refusal, and self-injurious behavior.

3668 Eastern State Hospital
4601 Ironbound Road
Williamsburg, VA 23188-2652
757-253-5161
Fax: 757-253-5065
E-mail: eshinfo@dshs.wa.gov
www.www.esh.dbhds.virginia.gov

David M. Lyon, Director

3669 Northern Virginia Mental Health Institute
3302 Gallows Road
Falls Church, VA 22042-3398
703-207-7100
Fax: 703-207-7160
www.nvmhi.dmhmrsas.virginia.gov

Jim Newton, Facility Director

Actively promoting recovery of individuals with serious mental illness through the use of safe, efficient, and effective treatment

3670 Piedmont Geriatric Hospital
5001 East Patrick Henry Highway
PO Box 427
Burkeville, VA 23922-427
434-767-4401
Fax: 434-767-2346
TDD: 434-767-4454
E-mail: steve.herrick@pgh.dmhmrsas.virginia.gov
www.pgh.dmhmrsas.virginia.gov

Stephen Herrick, Director

A 135-bed psychiatric hospital that provides recovery based MH services to enable the elderly to thrive in the community.

3671 Southern Virginia Mental Health Institute
382 Taylor Drive
Danville, VA 24541-4096
434-799-6220
Fax: 434-773-4241
E-mail: naomi.gibson@dbhds.virginia.gov
www.svmhi.dmhmrsas.virginia.gov

David Lyon, Manager

To be an inpatient mental health service provider within our Regional Service Area that responds to the patient's and area needs.

3672 Southwestern Virginia Mental Health Institute
340 Bagley Circle
Marion, VA 24354-3126
276-783-1200
Fax: 276-783-9712
TDD: 276-783-1365
www.swvmhi.dmhmrsas.virginia.gov

Cynthia Mc Clure, CEO

3673 Western State Hospital
1301 Richmond Avenue
PO Box 2500
Staunton, VA 24402-2500
540-332-8000
Fax: 540-332-8144
TDD: 540-332-8000
www.www.wsh.dbhds.virginia.gov

Jack W Barber, Hospital Director

Year Founded: 1825

Washington

3674 Child Study & Treatment Center
2142 10th Ave West.
Seattle, WA 98119
206-298-9641
800-283-8639
Fax: 206-298-9655
E-mail: ContactCLIP@CLIPadministration.org
www.clipadministration.org

Rick Mehlman, CEO

Treats children from age 5 to 17 who can not be served in less restrictive setting within the community.

3675 Eastern State Hospital
4601 Ironbound Road
PO Box 800 Mail Stop B 32-23
Williamsburg, VA 23188-2652
757-253-5161
Fax: 509-565-4705
E-mail: eshinfo@dshs.wa.gov
www.www.esh.dbhds.virginia.gov

David M. Lyon, Director

Eastern State Hospital is a key partner in assisting adults with psychiatric illness in their recovery through expert inpatient treatment whenever needs exceed community resources.

3676 Ryther Child Center
2400 NE 95th Street
Seattle, WA 98115-2499
206-525-5050
Fax: 206-525-9795
TDD: 800-883-6388
www.ryther.org

Lee Grogg, Executive Director

Offers and develops safe places and opportunities for children, youth and families to heal and grow so that they can reach their highest potential.

West Virginia

3677 Highland Hospital
300 56th Street SE
Charleston, WV 25304-2361
304-926-1600
800-250-3806
Fax: 304-925-1524
www.highlandhosp.com

James H. Dissen, Chairman

Our mission is to identify and respond to mental health needs, and promote physical, social emotional and intellectual well-being.

3678 Mildred Mitchell-Bateman Hospital
1530 Norway Avenue
PO Box 448
Huntington, WV 25709-448
304-525-7801
800-644-9318
E-mail: MMBHospital@wv.gov
www.www.batemanhospital.org

Roy Frasher, Volunteer Services Director

Provides inpatient psychiatric treatment for the adult citizens of southern West Virginia.

3679 Weirton Medical Center
601 Colliers Way
Weirton, WV 26062-5091
304-797-6000
www.weirtonmedical.com

Joseph Endrich, CEO

Weirton Medical Center is a 238 bed, non-profit, acute-care, general community hospital located in the city of Weirton in Brooke County, West Virginia. Weirton Medical Center offers health care services to the residents of West Virginia, Ohio and Pennsylvania.

3680 William R Sharpe, Jr Hospital
936 Sharpe Hospital Road
Weston, WV 26452-8550
304-269-1210
Fax: 304-269-6235
www.www.dhhr.wv.gov

D. Parker Haddix, CEO

1994 pages

Wisconsin

3681 Bellin Psychiatric Center
744 South Webster Avenue
PO Box 23400
Green Bay, WI 54305-3400
920-433-3500
E-mail: Isroet@bellin.org
www.bellin.org/psych

Year Founded: 1907

3682 Mendota Mental Health Institute
301 Troy Drive
Madison, WI 53704-1599

608-301-1000
Fax: 608-301-1358
TDD: 888-241-9442
TTY: 888-241-9442
www.www.dhs.wisconsin.gov

A psychiatric hospital operated by the Wisconsin Department of Health and Family Services, Division of Disability and Elder Services, specializes in serving patients with complex psychiatric conditions, often combined with certain problem behaviors.

1860 pages

3683 Wheaton Franciscan Healthcare: Elmbrook Memorial
19333 W North Avenue
Brookfield, WI 53045-4132
262-785-2000
www.www.mywheaton.org/elmbrook-memorial

3684 Winnebago Mental Health Institute
1300 South Drive
PO Box 9
Winnebago, WI 54985-9
920-235-4910
Fax: 920-237-2043
TDD: 888-241-9438
www.dhfs.wisconsin.gov/mh_winnebago

Winnebago Mental Health Institute (WMHI) serves as a specialized component in a community-based mental health delivery system.

Wyoming

3685 Wyoming State Hospital
831 Highway 150 South
Evanston, WY 82930-5340
307-789-3464
Fax: 307-789-7373

William L Matchinski, Manager

A center for treatment, rehabilitation and recovery.

Clinical Management

Management Companies

3686 ABE American Board of Examiners in Clinical Social Work
27 Congress Street Suite 501
Shetland Park
Salem, MA 01970-5577
978-825-9311
800-694-5285
Fax: 978-740-5395
E-mail: abe@abecsw.org

Robert Booth, CEO
Robert Booth, Executive Director
Leonard Hill MSW BCD, Vice President

The American Board of Examiners in Clinical Social Work (ABE) sets national practice standards, issues an advanced-practice credential, and publishes reference information about its board-certified clinicians

3687 Academy of Managed Care Providers
1945 Palo Verde Avenue
Suite 202
Long Beach, CA 90815-3445
562-682-3559
800-297-2627
Fax: 562-799-3355
E-mail: members@academymcp.org
www.academymcp.org

Dr. John Russell, President
William Adams, Ph.D., Advisory Board Member
Brad Bangerter, Advisory Board Member
Ellen Betts, Ph.D., Advisory Board Member

National organization of clinicans and MCO professionals. Provides many services to members including continuing education, diplomate certification, notification of panel openings and practice opportunities, newsletter, group health insurance and many other benefits.

3688 Action Healthcare Management
6245 N. 24th Parkway
Suite 112
Phoenix, AZ 85016-2029
602-265-0681
800-433-6915
Fax: 602-265-0202
E-mail: jeanr@actionhealthcare.com
www.actionhealthcare.com

Jean Rice, President

Action Healthcare Management has been an independent healthcare management company offering a full range of services that can be tailored to meet your organization's needs-from pre-certification and utilization review, management of high risk pregnancy and workers' compensation cases, to cases involving serious illness, catastrophic injury and cases requiring transplants. AHM works within your budget to assure provision of quality, affordable healthcare, negotiation of provider agreements and cost containment in the structuring of quality utilization management plans. In today's complicated healthcare system, Action Healthcare Management is a partner to both your organization and your insured. We're by your side, every step of the way.

3689 Adanta Group-Behavioral Health Services
130 Southern School Road
Somerset, KY 42501-3152
606-679-4782
Fax: 606-678-5296
TDD: 800-633-5599
TTY: 800-633-5599
E-mail: klworley@adanta.org
www.adanta.org

Jamie Burton, CEO

Adanta is composed of three major divisions which include Human Development Services, Clinical Services and the Regional Prevention Center. While each division is responsible for providing separate and distinct services, each relies on the expertise and resources available within the overall corporation. The three major divisions are made up of many smaller specialized areas, each of which include many professionals, staff and support personnel who take great pride in the quality of their work. Their professional skills, combined with time, energy and caring, have yielded and continue to yield positive results and many success stories across the region.

3690 Adult Learning Systems
1954 S Industrial Highway
Suite A
Ann Arbor, MI 48104-8601
734-668-7447

Sherri Turner, Contact

3691 Alcohol Justice
24 Belvedere Street
San Rafael, CA 94901
415-456-5692
Fax: 415-456-0491
www.alcoholjustice.org

Bruce Lee Livingston, Executive Director
Michael Scippa, Public Affairs Director
Sarah M. Mart, MS, MPH, Director of Research
Karen Kuhn, Administrative Director

3692 Aldrich and Cox
3075 Southwestern Boulevard
Suite 202
Orchard Park, NY 14127-1287
716-675-6300
Fax: 716-675-2098
E-mail: cox@aldrichandcox.com
www.aldrichandcox.com

Herbert C. Cox, Chairman
Charles H. Cox, President
James B. Hood, Jr, Exec. VP/ Secretary
Daniel C. Buser, J.D., CPCU, EVP

Aldrich and Cox provides independent, fee-based Risk Management, Insurance and Employee Benefit Consulting services to a wide range of clientele.

3693 Alliance Behavioral Care
PO Box 19947
Cincinnati, OH 45219-947
513-475-8622
800-926-8862
E-mail: allen.daniels@uc.edu
www.alliancebehavioral.com

Allen Daniels, CEO

Alliance Behavioral Care is a regional managed behavioral healthcare organization located in Cincinnati, Ohio. They are committed to continuously improving the resources and programs that serve their members and providers. Their goal is to provide resources that improve the well-being of those they serve and to integrate the behavioral healthcare within the overall healthcare systems.

3694 Allina Hospitals & Clinics Behavioral Health Services

2925 Chicago Avenue
Minneapolis, MN 55407-1321
612-775-5000
800-877-7878
www.www.allinahealth.org

Penny Ann Wheeler, MD, President, Chief Clinical Office
Duncan P. Gallagher, EVP, Administration, CFO
Christine Bent, SVP, Clinical Service Lines
Kenneth Paulus, CEO

Provides clinically and geographically integrated care delivery. Innovative programs and services across comprehensive continuum of care. Practicing guideline development, outcomes data and quality managment programs to enhance care delivery.

3695 American Managed Behavioral Healthcare Association

1325 G Street, NW
Suite 500
Washington, DC 20005
202-449-7660
Fax: 202-449-7659
E-mail: info@abhw.org
www.www.abhw.org

Pamela Greenberg, MPP, President/CEO
Rebecca Murow Klein, Associate Director, Government A
Tim Murphy, President, CEO, Beacon Health St
Larry Tallman, President, MHN
Year Founded: 1994

3696 Analysis Group

111 Huntington Avenue
Tenth Floor
Boston, MA 02199
617-425-8000
Fax: 617-425-8001
E-mail: agweb@analysisgroup.com
www.analysisgroup.com

Martha Samuelson, President/CEO
Bruce F Deal, Managing Principal
Stephen Cacciola, VP
Brian Ellman, VP

Provides economic, financial, and business strategy consulting to law firms, corporations and government agencies

Year Founded: 1981

3697 Aon Consulting Group

200 East Randolph Street
14th Floor
Chicago, IL 60601-6408
312-381-2738
Fax: 312-701-3100
www.aon.com

Mike Bungert, Chariman, AON Benfield
Gregory C Case, President, CEO

Laurel Meissner, SVP, Global Controller
Christa Davies, EVP, CFO

Aon Corporation is a leading provider of risk management services, insurance and reinsurance brokerage, human capital and management consulting, and specialty insurance underwriting.

3698 Arthur S Shorr and Associates

98 Golden Eye Lane
Port Monmouth, NJ 07758
818-225-7055
800-530-5728
Fax: 732-201-0794
E-mail: expert@hospitalexperts.com
www.arthurshorr.com

Arthur S Shorr, MBA, FACHE, Owner
Nancy Daniels, Senior Consultant-Principal
Tom Bojko, MD, MS, JD, Managing Partner
Debra Petracca, MBA, Executive Director

Consultants to health care providers.

3699 Associated Counseling Services

8 Roberta Drive
Dartmouth, MA 02748-2020
508-992-9376

Douglas Riley, Owner

3700 Barbanell Associates

3629 Sacramento Street
San Francisco, CA 94118-1731
415-929-1155
Fax: 415-929-8485

Harriet Barbanell, Owner

3701 Barry Associates

6807 Knotty Pine Drive
PO Box 3069
Chapel Hill, NC 27515-3069
919-490-8474
Fax: 765-381-1100
E-mail: info@barryonline.com
www.barry-online.com

John S Barry MSW MBA, President

Provides technical assistance services to behavioral health and social service organizations in the areas of performance measurement, survey research, program evaluation, compensation system design and other selected human resource management areas.

3702 Behavioral Health Care

155 Inverness Drive West
Suite 201
Englewood, CO 80112-1411
720-490-4400
877-349-7379
Fax: 720-490-4395
TTY: 855-364-1799
E-mail: bhi@bhicares.org
www.www.bhicares.org

Julie Holtz, Chief Executive Officer
Joe Pastor M.D., Medical Director

BHI is committed to excellence in mental health service delivery. They strive to promote recovery by focusing on the unique needs, strengths and hopes of consumers and families.

3703 Behavioral Health Care Consultants
12 Windham Lane
Beverly, MA 01915-1568
978-921-5968
E-mail: mkatzenstein@bhcconsult.com
www.bhcconsult.com

Michael L Katzenstein, President
Robert A. DeNoble, Staff
Lincoln Williams, Staff

3704 Behavioral Health Management Group
1025 Main Street
Suite 708
Wheeling, WV 26003-2726
304-232-7232
Fax: 304-232-7245
E-mail: user655349@aol.com

William R Coburn, Practice Manager

They offer a wide range of services for men, women, adolescents, and children. The professional staff specializes in mental and emotional disorders, marital and family counseling, group therapy, vocational counseling, alcohol and substance abuse, academic adjustment counseling, psychological testing, biofeedback, and hypnotherapy.

3705 Behavioral Health Services
2925 Chicago Avenue
Minneapolis, MN 55407-1321
612-775-5000
800-877-7878
www.allina.com

Penny Ann Wheeler, MD, President, Chief Clinical Office
Duncan P. Gallagher, EVP, Administration, CFO
Christine Bent, SVP, Clinical Service Lines
Kenneth Paulus, CEO

Provides clinically and geographically integrated delivery system, innovative programs and services across comprehensive continuum of care, practice guidelines development, outcomes data and quality management programs to enhance care delivery systems.

3706 Behavioral Health Systems
2 Metroplex Drive
Suite 500
Birmingham, AL 35209-6827
205-879-1150
800-245-1150
Fax: 205-879-1178
E-mail: generalwebsite@bhs-inc.com
www.behavioralhealthsystems.com

Deborah L. Stephens, Founder, Chairman, CEO
Danny Cooner, President, Safety First
Kyle Strange, Executive Vice President/MCO
Mark Gordon, EVP, Finance and CFO

Provides managed psychiatric and substance abuse and drug testing services to more than 20, 000 employees nationally through a network of 7, 600 providers.

3707 Broward County Health Care Services
115 S Andrews Avenue
Room 302
Fort Lauderdale, FL 33301
954-357-6551
Fax: 954-468-3592
TTY: 800-995-8711

E-mail: civilcitation@broward.org
www.broward.org/healthcare

Bertha Henry, County Administrator
Joni Armstrong Coffey, County Attorney
Evan Lukic, CPA, County Auditor

The Health Care Section of the Community Partnership Division provide mental health, primary health care, and special health care services, as well as funding, Mahogany Project, and the Ryan White Part A Program offices.

3708 Brown Consulting
121 N Erie Street
Toledo, OH 43604-5915
419-241-8547
800-495-6786
Fax: 419-241-8689
E-mail: info@danbrownconsulting.com
www.danbrownconsulting.com

Daniel C Brown, Owner, President
Rhonda Willhight, VP, Operations
Ross Calvin, VP, Consulting
David Galbraith, CFO

Provides a full range of consulting services to behavioral healthcare providers. Has relationships with national, regional and state behavioral healthcare organizations.

Year Founded: 1987

3709 CBCA
10900 Hampshire Avenue S
Bloomington, MN 55438-2384
952-829-3500
800-824-3882
Fax: 952-946-7694
E-mail: info@cbca.com
www.cbca.com

Mary Dixon, Senior VP

Provides total health plan management including 24 hours a day, seven days a week patient access and demand management, care management, behavioral health care management, disease management and disability workers' compensation management, all supported by QualityFIRST clinical decision guidelines. These services are electronically integrated with HRM's national provider networks and electronic claims management. HRM's clients include HMOs, hospital systems, insurance and self-insured plans, workers' compensation and disability plans and Medicare/Medicaid plans throughout the US, Canada and New Zealand.

3710 CIGNA Behavioral Care
11095 Viking Drive
Suite 350
Eden Prairie, MN 55344-7234
952-996-2000
800-334-8925
Fax: 952-996-2579
www.cignabehavioral.com

Keith Dixon, CEO

Provides behavioral care benefit management, EAPs, and work/life programs to consumers through health plans offered by large U.S. employers, national and regional HMOs, Taft-Hartley trusts and disability insurers.

Year Founded: 1974

3711 Cameron and Associates
6100 Lake Forrest Drive
Suite 550
Atlanta, GA 30328-3889
404-843-3399
800-334-6014
Fax: 404-843-3572
www.caiquality.com

William Cameron, Owner

Assists troubled employees and their dependents in resolving personal problems in order to provide their employer a level of acceptable job performance and efficiency, and to provide a safe working environment for all employees.

3712 Carewise
1501 4th Avenue
Suite 700
Seattle, WA 98101-3624
206-749-1100
800-755-2136
Fax: 206-749-1125
www.shps.net

Rishabh Mehrotra, President/CEO
John McCarty, Executive Vice President/CFO

3713 Casey Family Services
127 Church Street
New Haven, CT 06510-2001
203-401-6900
Fax: 203-401-6901
E-mail: info@caseyfamilyservices.org
www.caseyfamilyservices.org

Raymond L Torres, Executive Director
Michael Brennan, Co-Chairman

Year Founded: 1976

3714 Center for the Advancement of Health
2000 Florida Avenue NW
Suite 210
Washington, DC 20009-1231
202-387-2829
Fax: 202-387-2857
E-mail: info@cfah.org
www.cfah.org

Jessie C. Gruman, PhD, President, Founder
David Torresen, VP, Finance and Operations
Dorothy Jeffres, MBA.MSW, MA, Executive Director
Goldie Pyka, Communications Manager

3715 Century Financial Services
23 Maiden Lane
PO Box 98
North Haven, CT 06473
203-239-6364
www.www.centuryfinancialservices.com

William Giovanni, Sr., Director, Operations
Kim Colapietro, Director
William J. Giovanni, Jr., Director, Marketing and Sales
Donella Fields, Collection Manager

3716 Children's Home of the Wyoming Conference, Quality Improvement
1182 Chenango Street
Binghamton, NY 13901-1696
607-772-6904
800-772-6904
Fax: 607-723-2617
E-mail: info@chowc.org
www.chowc.org

Robert K. Chip Houser, President and CEO
Maria Cali, VP, Education
Patricia Giglio, CFO/Chief Admin. Officer
Ann M. MacLaren, CFO

Works with social services, court systems, school systems for children who are at risk, have trouble in the home, or have been abused or abandoned.

3717 ChoiceCare
655 Eden Park Drive, Suite 400
Grand Baldwin Building
Cincinnati, OH 45202-6039
513-241-1400
800-543-7158
Fax: 513-684-7461
www.choicecare.com

3718 College Health IPA
5665 Plaza Drive
Suite 400
Cypress, CA 90630
562-467-5555
800-779-3825
Fax: 562-402-2666
TTY: 800-735-2929
E-mail: info@chipa.com
www.chipa.com

Randy Davis, President/CEO
Kevin Gardiner, VP Of Financial Operations
Brian Wheelan, Executive Vice President for Cor
Dale Seamans, Director, Corporate Communicatio

Culturally sensitive mental health referral service.

3719 College of Dupage
425 Fawell Boulevard
Glen Ellyn, IL 60137-6599
630-942-2800
Fax: 630-942-2947
www.cod.edu

Sunil Chand, President
Robert L. Breuder, President
Thomas J. Glaser, SVP, Administration, Treasurer
Joseph Collins, EVP

3720 College of Southern Idaho
315 Falls Avenue
PO Box 1238
Twin Falls, ID 83303-1238
208-732-6221
800-680-0274
Fax: 208-736-4705
E-mail: info@csi.edu
www.csi.edu

Jerry Beck, President
Dr. Jeff Fox, President
Jerry Gee, Executive VP/CAO
Mike Mason, VP, Administration

3721 Columbia Hospital M/H Services
2201 45th Street
W Palm Beach, FL 33407-2095

561-842-6141
Fax: 561-844-8955
www.columbiahospital.com

Valerie Jackson, CEO
Dana C. Oaks, CEO
Brenda Logan, CNO
Oon Soo Ung, CFO

250-bed acute-care facility with dedicated psychiatry, emergency psychiatry, geriatric psychiatry, inpatient and outpatient psychiatry, and partial day psychiatry units and programs.

3722 ComPsych

455 N City Front Plaza Drive
NBC Tower
Chicago, IL 60611-5322
312-595-4000
800-755-3050
Fax: 312-660-1057
E-mail: mpaskell@compsych.com
www.compsych.com

Richard A Chaifetz, Chairman, CEO

Worlwide leader in guidance resources, including employee assistance programs, managed behavioral health, work-life, legal, financial, and personal convenience services. ComPsych provides services worldwide covering millions of individuals. Clients range from Fortune 100 to smaller public and private concerns, government entities, health plans and Taft-Hartley groups. Guidance Resources transforms traditionally separate services into a seamless integration of information, resources and creative solutions that address personal life challenges and improve workplace productivity and performance.

3723 Comprehensive Care Corporation

3405 W. Martin Luther King Jr. Blvd
Suite 101
Tampa, FL 33607
813-288-4808
Fax: 813-288-4844
E-mail: info@comprehensivecare.com
www.compcare.com

John M Hill, CEO
Robert Landis, Chairman/CFO/Treasurer

Offers a flexible system of services to provide comprehensive, compassionate and cost-effective mental health and substance abuse services to managed care organizations both public and private. CompCare is committed to providing state-of-the-art comprehensive care management services for all levels and phases of behavioral health care.

3724 Consecra Housing Network

1900 Spring Road
Suite 300
Oak Brook, IL 60523-1480
630-766-3570
E-mail: rhodes@consecra.org
www.consecra.org

Tim Rhodes, President/CEO
Susan Sinderson, Vice President
Dave Opitz, Director of Business Development

Provides therapy services in Spanish for children, families and couples. Offers substance abuse treatment and educational groups for men who batter in English and Spanish. Provides comprehensive services to Latina victims of domestic violence and their children in Spanish.

3725 Corphealth

1300 Summit Avenue
6th Floor
Fort Worth, TX 76102-4414
817-333-6400
800-240-8388
E-mail: businessdevelopment@corphealth.com

Patrick Gotcher II, President/CEO
Brae Jacobson, COO
Michael Baker, CFO

3726 Corporate Health Systems

15153 Technology Drive
Suite B
Eden Prairie, MN 55344-2221
952-939-0911
Fax: 952-939-0990
www.corphealthsys.com

Bob Hanalon, President

Benefits consulting firm to partner with clients to find the most flexible and comprehensive benefits packages for their investments.

3727 Counseling Associates

106 Milford Street
Suite 501B
Salisbury, MD 21804
410-546-1692
888-546-1692
Fax: 410-548-9056
E-mail: tim@catherapy.com
www.catherapy.com

Anne Bass Kinlaw, MSW, LCSW, President
Janet Brown, Manager
Joan Guzi, LCPC, Staff
Carol Ireland, LCSW-C, Staff

Provides therapeutic counseling to help individuals lead productive and fulfilled lives.

3728 Counseling Corner

2116 Merrick Avenue
Suite 3008A
Merrick, NY 11566
917-670-6262
E-mail: info@couplesandfamilies.com
www.couplesandfamilies.com

Cari Sans, Founder And Director
Shari D. Siegel, Counsellor

3729 Covenant Home Healthcare

3615 19th Street
Lubbock, TX 79410-1209
806-725-2328
806-725-0000
www.covenanthealth.org

Melinda Clark, CEO

Provides quality home care to patients when hospitalization may be unneccessary, or when the length of stay may be shorter than expected.

3730 Coventry Health Care of Iowa

211 Lake Drive
Newark, DE 19702-3320
302-283-6500
800-752-7242

Al Redmen, CEO

3731 Creative Health Concepts
One Grand Central Place
Suite 2022
New York, NY 10165-2017
212-697-7207
Fax: 212-697-3509
E-mail: info@creativegroupny.com
www.creativegroupny.com

Harry F. Blair, Vice Chairman
Ira N. Gottlieb, President/CEO
Sharon S. Adair, SVP
Dan Pfeiffer, SVP

3732 Cypruss Communications
430 Myrtle Ave
Suite A
Fort Lee, NJ 07024-3913
201-735-7730
800-750-5231
E-mail: peterm@cypruss.com
www.cypruss.com

Peter Miller, VP/CFO

3733 Deloitte and Touche LLP Management Consulting
1700 Market Street
Philadelphia, PA 19103-3984
215-246-2300
Fax: 215-569-2441
www.www.deloitte.com/view/en_US/us/index.htm

Sharon Allen, Chairman
Barry Salzberg, CEO
Punit Renjen, Chairman of the Board, Deloitte
Joe Echevarria, CEO, Deloitte LLP

3734 DeltaMetrics
600 Public Ledger Building
150 S Independence Mall West
Philadelphia, PA 19106-3475
215-399-0988
800-238-2433
Fax: 215-399-0989
www.deltametrics.com

Jack Durell, M.D., President/CEO
John Cacciola, Ph.D., Senior Vice President, Scientifi
Paul Keller, VP, Business Development
Kathleen Geary, Director, Operations

National research, evaluation, and consulting organization dedicated to the improvement of substance abuse and other behavioral health care treatment.

3735 Diversified Group Administrators
6345 Flank Drive
PO Box 6250
Harrisburg, PA 17112-250
717-652-8040
800-877-6490
Fax: 717-652-8328
E-mail: jhoellman@dgatpa.com
www.dgatpa.com

James Hoellman, Contact

3736 Dorenfest Group
455 N Cityfront Plaza Drive
NBC Tower Suite 2725
Chicago, IL 60611-5555
312-464-3000
Fax: 312-467-0541
E-mail: info@dorenfest.com
www.www.dorenfest.com

Sheldon Dorenfest, CEO
Xiao Liu, Manager, Consulting Services
Wei-Tih Cheng, Strategic Advisor
Michael Cohen, Strategic Advisor

3737 Dougherty Management Associates Health Strategies
9 Meriam Street
Suite 4
Lexington, MA 02420-5312
781-863-8003
800-817-7802
Fax: 781-863-1519
E-mail: mail@dmahealth.com
www.dmahealth.com

Richard H. Dougherty, Ph.D., CEO, Owner
Wendy Holt, M.P.P., Principal
D. Russell Lyman, Ph.D., Senior Associate
Lisa Feldman Braude, Ph.D., Senior Associate

Providing the public and private sectors with superior management consulting services to improve healthcare delivery systems and manage complex organizational change.

3738 Dupage County Health Department
111 North County Farm Road
Wheaton, IL 60187-3988
630-682-7400
Fax: 630-462-9261
TDD: 630-932-1447
www.dupagehealth.org

Linda A. Kurzawa, President
Dr. Lanny F. Wilson, VP
Maureen Mc Hugh, Executive Director
Scott J. Cross, Secretary

3739 Echo Management Group
15 Washington Street
PO Box 2150
Conway, NH 03818-2150
603-447-8600
800-635-8209
Fax: 603-447-8680
E-mail: info@echoman.com
www.echoman.com

John Raden, CEO

Provides financial, clinical, and administrative software applications for behavioral health and social service agencies; comprehensive, fully-intergrated Human Service Information System is a powerful management tool that enables agencies to successfully operate their organizations within the stringent guidelines of managed care mandates. Provides implementation planning, training, support and systems consulting services.

3740 Elon Homes for Children
1717 Sharon Road West
Charlotte, NC 28210

704-369-2500
Fax: 704-688-2960
E-mail: info@elonhomes.org
www.elonhomes.org

Dr Frederick Grosse, President/CEO
Andrea Rollins, VP, Administration
Rose Cooper, VP, Institutional Performance
Jane Grosse, VP, Institutional Advancement

Provides over 1, 000 children and families a year in North Carolina an excellent opportunity for safe haven, life skills and education

Year Founded: 1907

3741 Employee Assistance Professionals

1234 Summer Street
Stamford, CT 06905-5558
203-977-2446

3742 Employee Benefit Specialists

PO Box 11657
Pleasanton, CA 94588
888-327-2770
800-229-7683
E-mail: cfankhouser@clickebs.com
www.www.ebsbenefits.com

Alan Curtis, Chairman/CEO
Curtis Fankhouser, President

3743 Employee Network

1040 Vestal Parkway E
Vestal, NY 13850-2354
607-754-1043
800-364-4748
Fax: 607-754-1629
www.eniweb.com

Gene Raymondi, Owner, Founder, CEO
Towhee V. Shupka, President, COO

3744 Entropy Limited

345 South Great Road
Lincoln, MA 01773-4303
781-259-8901
Fax: 781-259-1255
E-mail: clientservices@entropylimited.com
www.entropylimited.com

Ron Christensen, Owner

Uses pattern recognition, statistics, and computer simulation to track past behavior, see current behavior and predict future behavior. Used by insuranch companies and the healthcare industry.

3745 Essi Systems

70 Otis Street
San Francisco, CA 94103-1236
415-252-8224
800-252-3774
Fax: 415-252-5732
E-mail: essi@essisystems.com
www.sesystems.com

Esther Orioli, CEO
Karen Trocki, Research Director

3746 Ethos Consulting

3219 E Camelback Road
Suite 515
Phoenix, AZ 85018-2307

480-296-3801
E-mail: conrad@ethosconsulting.com
www.ethosconsulting.com

Conrad E Prusak, President, Co-Founder
Julie Prusak, CEO, Co-Founder

3747 FCS

1711 Ashley Circle
Suite 6
Bowling Green, KY 42104-5801
502-782-9152
800-783-9152
Fax: 270-782-1055
E-mail: admin@fcspsy.com
www.fcspsy.com

Bob Toth, President, CEO
Brian Browning, VP Of Client Services
Dale Taylor, VP, Client Services
Jason Honshell, VP, Client Services

3748 Findley, Davies and Company

One SeaGate
Suite 2050
Toledo, OH 43604-1525
419-255-1360
Fax: 419-259-5685
www.findleydavies.com

Marc Stockwell, VP, Market Leader

3749 First Consulting Group

1160 West Swedesford Road
Building One, Suite 200
Berwyn, PA 19312
800-345-7672
www.csc.com

Larry Ferguson, CEO
Thomas Watford, COO/CFO

Around the world and across the healthcare spectrum, First Consulting Group is transforming healthcare with better information for better decisions.

3750 Fowler Healthcare Affiliates

2000 Riveredge Parkway
Suite 920
Atlanta, GA 30328-4600
770-635-8758
800-784-9829
Fax: 770-261-6361
www.fowler-consulting.com

Frances J Fowler, Owner, President
Denese Estep, Senior Consultant
Elizabeth Forro, Director
Joanne Judge, Legal Consultant

Developed innovative solutions for managing cost of high cost patients.

3751 GMR Group

755 Business Center Drive
Suite 250
Horsham, PA 19044-3491
215-653-7401
Fax: 215-653-7982
E-mail: webmaster@gmrgroup.com
www.gmrgroup.com

Barron J Ginnetti, CEO
Thomas Bishop, Vice President/COO

Provides strategic and tactical solutions to the marketing and sales challenges their clients face in the managed healthcare environment.

3752 Garner Consulting
630 North Rosemead Blvd
Suite 300
Pasadena, CA 91107-2138
626-351-2300
Fax: 626-351-2331
E-mail: info@garnerconsulting.com
www.garnerconsulting.com

Gerti Reagan Garner, GBA, FL, President
John C. Garner, CEBS, CLU, CFC, CEO
Carl Isaacs, Principal
Zaven K. Kazazian, JD, CBC, Principal

Provides innovative consultation, which produces immediate, bottom line results and long term value.

3753 Gaynor and Associates
100 Whitney Avenue
New Haven, CT 06510-1265
203-865-0865
Fax: 203-865-0093
E-mail: mlg110@columbia.edu

Mark Gaynor LCSW, Principal

Clinical social work provider, EAP services, and clinical practice. Specialty weight management

Year Founded: 1980

3754 Geauga Board of Mental Health, Alcohol and Drug Addiction Services
13244 Ravenna Road
Chardon, OH 44024-9012
440-285-2282
800-750-0750
Fax: 440-285-9617
E-mail: mhrs@geauga.org
www.geauga.org

Jim Adams, Executive Director, CEO
Beth Matthews, Associate Director
Jim Mausser, Finance Manager
Sandy Cohn, Information Coordinator

3755 Glazer Medical Solutions
PO Box 121
Beach Plum Lane
Menemsha, MA 02552
508-645-9635
Fax: 508-645-3212
E-mail: glazermedicalsol@aol.com
www.glazmedsol.com

William M. Glazer, M.D., President/Founder

Glazer Medical Solutions is a national medical education consortium that has facilitated a comprehensive matrix of medical education services since 1994.

3756 HCA Healthcare
1 Park Plaza
Nashville, TN 37203-6527
615-344-9551
www.hcahealthcare.com

Richard M. Bracken, Chairman
Samuel N. Hazen, VP, Operations

R. Milton Johnson, President, CEO
David G. Anderson, SVP, Finance and Treasurer

3757 HPN Worldwide
119 W Vallette Street
Elmhurst, IL 60126-4419
630-941-9030
Fax: 630-941-9064
E-mail: info@hpn.com
www.hpn.com

Bob Gorsky, PhD, Owner
Rick Suray, Staff
Ben Gorsky, Staff
Jennifer Toreja, Staff

Year Founded: 1983

3758 HSP Verified
National Register of Health Service Psychologists
1200 New York Avenue NW
Suite 800
Washington, DC 20005-3893
202-783-7663
Fax: 202-347-0550
www.nationalregister.org

Judy E Hall, CEO
Andrew P. Boucher, Assistant Director
Julia Bernstein, Membership Coordinator
Katie Huppi, Finance and Administration Coord

Offers comprehensive, innovative credential verification services designed to help you find that precious time. It relieves health care providers and management of tedious administrative activities-leaving time and resources to focus on quality health care. Provides valuable information and cultivates alliances between cutting edge health care organizations/plans and qualified health care providers.

3759 Hays Group
1133 20th Street NW
Suite 450
Washington, DC 20036-3452
202-263-4000
E-mail: info@hayscompanies.com

3760 Health Alliance Plan
2850 W Grand Boulevard
Detroit, MI 48202-2692
313-872-8100
800-422-4641
Fax: 313-664-8479
TDD: 800-649-3777
E-mail: msweb1@hap.org
www.www.hap.org

James Connelly, President, CEO
Ronald Berry, Senior Vice President/CFO
Christopher Pike, SVP, COO
Mary Ann Tournoux, SVP, Chief Marketing Officer

3761 Health Capital Consultants
1143 Olivette Executive Pkwy
Saint Louis, MO 63132-3205
314-994-7641
800-394-8258
Fax: 314-991-3435
E-mail: solutions@healthcapital.com
www.healthcapital.com

Robert James Cimasi, MHA, ASA, President, CEO
Todd Zigrang, MBA, MHA, ASA, President
Matthew J. Wagner, MBA, VP
John R. Chwarzinski, MSF, MAE, VP

3762 Health Decisions
409 Plymouth Road
Suite 220
Plymouth, MI 48170-1834
734-451-2230
Fax: 734-451-2835
www.healthdecisions.com

Si Nahra, PhD, Owner, President
Judy L. Mardigian, CEO
Michael Falis, Senior Software Engineer
Tina Pelland, MA, Audit Practice Leader

3763 Health Management Associates
5811 Pelican Bay Boulevard
Suite 500
Naples, FL 34108-2711
239-598-3131
Fax: 239-597-5794
www.hma.com

Gary D Newsome, President, CFO
Kelly E Curry, Chief Financial Officer
Kerry Gillespie, EVP, Operations Finance

3764 HealthPartners
2701 University Avenue SE
Minneapolis, MN 55414-3233
952-967-7992
TTY: 612-627-3584

Mary Brainerd, President/CEO

3765 Healthwise
2601 N Bogus Basin Road
Boise, ID 83702-909
208-345-1161
800-706-9646
Fax: 208-345-1897
www.healthwise.org

Donald W Kemper, MPH, Founder, CEO
Jim Giuffre, MPH, President/COO
Molly Mettler, MSW, SVP
Karen Baker, MHS, SVP

3766 Healthy Companies
2101 Wilson Boulevard
Suite 1002
Arlington, VA 22201-3048
703-351-9901
www.healthycompanies.com

Robert Rosen, Owner, Chairman, CEO
Jim Mathews, Vice Chairman
Tony Rutigliano, President
Eric Sass, COO

3767 HeartMath
14700 W Park Avenue
Boulder Creek, CA 95006-9318
831-338-8500
800-711-6221
Fax: 831-338-8504
E-mail: info@heartmath.org
www.www.heartmath.org

Bruce Cryer, President
Sara Childre, President, CEO
Rollin McCraty, Ph.D., EVP, Director of Research
Brian Kabaker, CFO, Director of Sales and Marke

HeartMath's Freze-Framer Interactive Learning System is an innovative approach to stress relief based on learning to change the heart rhythm pattern and create physiological coherence in the body. The Freeze-Framer has been widely used with clients to help them develop internal awareness, self-recognition and emotional management skills. Clients can learn to prevent stress by becoming aware of when the stress response starts and stopping it in the moment and taking a more active role in preventing stress, managing the emotions associated with stress, creating better health and improving performance.

3768 Helms & Company
1 Pillsbury Street
Suite 200
Concord, NH 03301-3556
603-225-6633
Fax: 603-225-4739
E-mail: info@helmsco.com
www.helmsco.com

J Michael Degnan, President, Co-Founder
Deborah J. White, Senior Consultant, Principal
Susan A. Cambria, Associate
Jeffrey G. White, Associate

They are a New Hampshire based behavioral health management company offering managed behavioral healthcare services, community service programs, and employee assistance programs for health care insurers, members, employers and their employees.

3769 Horizon Behavioral Services
2941 South Lake Vista Drive
Lewisville, TX 75067-3801
972-420-8300
800-931-4646
Fax: 972-420-8252

Mike Saul, President

Provider of national managed care, utilization management and employee assistance programs. Horizon will work in collaboration with HMOs, insurance companies, employers and hospitals to develop seamless, cost-effective managed care services including practitioner panel formation, information system development, utilization management services, EAPs, outcomes measurement systems and sales and marketing functions.

3770 Horizon Mental Health Management
2941 South Lake Vista Drive
Lewisville, TX 75067-3801
972-420-8300
800-931-4646
Fax: 972-420-8383
E-mail: cindy.novak@horizonhealth.com

Johan Smith, VP

Inpatient, outpatient, partial hospitalization and home health psychiatric programs.

3771 Human Behavior Associates
1350 Hayes Street
Suite B-100
Benicia, CA 94510

707-747-0117
800-937-7770
Fax: 707-747-6646
E-mail: corporate@callhba.com
www.callhba.com

James Wallace PhD, President
Yolanda Calderon, Operations Manager

National provider of emploee assistance programs, managed behavioral healthcare services, critical incident stress management services, conflict management, organizational consultation, and substance abuse professional services. Maintains a network of 6500 licensed mental health care providers and 650 hospitals and treatment centers nationwide.

3772 Human Services Research Institute
2336 Massachusetts Avenue
Cambridge, MA 02140
617-876-0426
Fax: 617-492-7401
E-mail: vbradley@hsri.org
www.hsri.org

Valerie Bradley, President
Stephen Leff, Vice President
Virginia Mulkern, Vice President
John Agosta, Vice President

3773 Insurance Management Institute
6 Stafford Court
Mount Holly, NJ 08060-3281
609-267-8998
Fax: 609-267-2472
E-mail: TIMInstitute@aol.com
www.timinstitute.com

Michael C Hill, Management Consultant/Author

3774 Interface EAP
10370 Richmond Avenue
Suite 1100
Houston, TX 77042
713-781-3364
800-324-4327
Fax: 713-784-0425
E-mail: info@ieap.com
www.ieap.com

Fred Newman, CEO
Tina Pace, CFO

3775 Interlink Health Services
4660 Belknap Court
Suite 209
Hillsboro, OR 97124
503-640-2000
800-599-9119
Fax: 503-640-2028
E-mail: administration@interlinkhealth.com
www.interlinkhealth.com

John M. Van Dyke, CEO
Sherrie Simmons, Director of Operations
Jill Miller, Assistant Vice President-Facilit
Elizabeth Grafton, Claims Director

3776 Intermountain Healthcare
36 S State Street
Salt Lake City, UT 84111

801-442-2000
E-mail: contactus@imail.org
www.intermountainhealthcare.org

Charles W. Sorenson, MD, President, CEO
Laura S. Kaiser, Executive Vice President & COO
Greg Poulsen, Senior Vice President & CSO
Bert Zimmerli, Executive Vice President & CFO

3777 Jeri Davis International
PO Box 770534
Memphis, TN 38177-534
901-763-0696
E-mail: jeri@jeridavis.com
www.jeridavis.com

Jeri Davis, Founder/President

3778 KAI Research, Inc.
11300 Rockville Pike
Suite 500
Rockville, MD 20852
301-770-2730
Fax: 301-770-4183
E-mail: kai@kai-research.com
www.kai-research.com

Selma C. Kunitz, Ph D., President
Rene Kozloff, Executive Vice President
Patti Shugarts, Chief Operating Officer

3779 Lake Regional Health System
54 Hospital Drive
Osage Beach, MO 65065
573-348-8000
E-mail: jweber@lakeregional.com
www.lakeregional.com

Michael E. Henze, CEO
Kevin McRoberts, SVP Of Operations
David Halsell, SVP of Financial Services, CFO
Joe Butts, SVP of Facility Services

3780 Lifespan
600 Frederick Street
Santa Cruz, CA 95062
831-469-4900
Fax: 831-469-4950
E-mail: information@lifespancare.com
www.lifespancare.com

Pamela Goodman, President
Becky Peters, CEO
Saundie Isaak, Executive Director
Ute Howland, Lifespan Care Manager

Comprehensive care management for adults who need care.

Year Founded: 1983

3781 MCW Department of Psychiatry and Behavioral Medicine
8701 Watertown Plank Road
Milwaukee, WI 53226
414-955-8990
Fax: 414-955-6299

John R. Raymond, Sr., MD, President/CEO
Joseph Kerschner, MD, Dean/Executive Vice President
G. Allen Bolton, Jr., MPH, MBA, Senior Vice President & COO

3782 MHN
2370 Kerner Blvd.
San Rafael, CA 94901
415-491-7200
800-327-2133
TDD: 800-735-2929
E-mail: mhnfeedback@mhn.com
www.mhn.com

Steven Sell, President/CEO
Juanell Hefner, COO

Provides high-quality, cost-effective behavioral health care
services to the public sector.

3783 MHNet Behavioral Health
9606 N MoPac Expressway
Stonebridge Plaza I, Suite 600
Austin, TX 78759
888-646-6889
Fax: 724-741-4552
www.mhnet.com

Wesley Brockhoeft, President/CEO
Robert Wilson, CFO

Health care management and solutions company providing
employee assistance programs (EAP), work life programs,
managed behavioral health care and consulting services.

3784 Magellan Health Service
6950 Columbia Gateway Drive
Columbia, MD 21046-3308
410-953-1000
800-458-2740
www.magellanhealth.com

Barry M. Smith, Chairman / Chief Executive Offic
Jonathan N. Rubin, Chief Financial Officer
Gary D. Anderson, Chief Information Officer

Provides members with high quality, clinically appropriate,
affordable health care which is tailored to each individual's
needs.

3785 Managed Care Concepts
PO Box 812032
Boca Raton, FL 33481-2032
561-750-2240
800-899-3926
Fax: 561-750-4621
E-mail: info@theemployeeassistanceprogram.com
www.theemployeeassistanceprogram.com

Beth Harrell, Corporate Contacts Director

Provides comprehensive EAP services to large and small
companies in the United States and parts of Canada. Also
provides child/elder care referrals, drug free workplace program services, consultation and training services.

3786 Maniaci Insurance Services
500 Silver Spur Road
Suite 121
Palos Verdes, CA 90275
310-541-4824
866-541-4824
Fax: 310-377-2016
E-mail: mail@maniaciinsurance.com
www.maniaciinsurance.com

Dan Maniaci, Owner
Dan Maniaci, President
Kristy Maniaci, Director Of Operations

3787 McGladery
801 Nicollet Avenue
Suite 1100
Minneapolis, MN 55402
952-835-9930
800-274-3978
Fax: 952-921-7702
www.mcgladrey.com

Joe Adams, Managing Partner and Chief Execu
Mike Kirley, Chief Operating Officer
Doug Opheim, Chief Finance Officer
Bruce Jorth, Chief Risk Officer

3788 McKesson Technology Solutions
5995 Windwrad Parkway
Alphretta, GA 30005
404-338-6000
Fax: 404-338-5112

Patrick J. Blake, Executive Vice President and Gro
Jim Pesce, President, Enterprise Informatio
Patrick Leonard, President, McKesson Business Per
Emad Rizk, MD, President, McKesson Health Solut

3789 Mercer Consulting
200 Clarendon Street
Boston, MA 02116-5026
617-424-3930
Fax: 617-424-3300

M. Michele Burns, Chairman/CEO
Tom Elliott, Chief Operating Officer

**3790 Midwst Center for Personal/Family
Development**
2550 University Avenue W
Suite 435-South
Saint Paul, MN 55114
651-647-1900
Fax: 651-647-1861
E-mail: info@mentalhealthinc.com
www.mentalhealthinc.com

Tim Quesnell, Administrator
Kari Droubic, Manager

3791 Mihalik Group
1300 W Belmont
Suite 500
Chicago, IL 60657
773-929-4276
www.themihalikgroup.com

Gary J. Mihalik, President and CEO
Melinda Orlando, Senior VP Operations
Michael Alcenius, VP, Accreditation Services
Cathie Abrahamsen, Senior Consultant

3792 Milliman, Inc
1301 Fifth Avenue
Suite 3800
Seattle, WA 98101-2646
206-624-7940
Fax: 206-340-1380
E-mail: more.info@milliman.com
www.milliman.com

Jeremy Engdahl-Johnson, Media inquiries

Assist plans and payors in measuring and analyzing their
healthcare costs arising from behavioral health conditions,
identifying specific value opportunities, and designing in-

novative ways to obtain increased quality and value from behavioral health care delivery.

Year Founded: 1947

3793 Murphy-Harpst Children's Centers
740 Fletcher Street
Cedartown, GA 30125
770-748-1500
Fax: 770-749-1094
www.murphyharpst.org

Charles Troutman, Chief Executive Officer
Emily Saltino, Vice President Development
Shirley Richardson, Chief Financial Officer
Tia McKnight, Director of Compliance

3794 NASW-NC
412 Morson Street
Raleigh, NC 27601
919-828-9650
Fax: 919-828-1341
E-mail: membership@naswdc.org
www.naswnc.org

Kathy Boyd, Executive Director
Valerie Arendt, Associate Executive Director
Kay Castillo, Director of Advocacy, Policy & L
Kristen Carter, Office Manager

3795 National Empowerment Center
599 Canal Street
Lawrence, MA 01840
978-685-1494
800-769-3728
Fax: 978-681-6426
www.power2u.org

Daniel B. Fisher, Executive Director
Oryx Cohen, Technical Assistance Center (TAC
Judene Shelley, Director of Special Projects
Leah Harris, Communications and Development D

Consumer/survivor/ex-patient run organization that carries a message of recovery, empowerment, hope and healing to people who have been diagnosed with mental illness.

3796 Oher and Associates
10 Tanglewild Plaza
Suite 100
Chappaqua, NY 10514
917-880-6969
E-mail: joher@oher.net
www.oherandassociates.com

Jim Oher, Founder
Joel Mausner, PhD, Associate
Sheryl Spanier, Associate
Janet Taylor MD, MPH, Associate

3797 Optimum Care Corporation
30011 Ivy Glenn Drive
Suite 219
Laguna Niguel, CA 92677-5018
949-495-1100
Fax: 949-495-4316
www.optimumcare.net

Edward A Johnson, CEO

3798 Options Health Care
240 Corporate Boulevard
Norfolk, VA 23502-4900

757-393-0859
www.valueoptions.com

Barbara B Hill, CEO
Michele Alfano, Chief Operating Officer

Specializes in creating innovative services for a full range of at-risk and administrative services only benefits, including behavioral health programs, customized provider and facility networks, utilization and case management, EAPs and youth services.

3799 PMHCC
123 S Broad Street
23rd Floor
Philadelphia, PA 19109-1029
215-546-0300
Fax: 215-732-1606
E-mail: PMHCCExecOffice@pmhcc.org
www.pmhcc.org

Bernard Borislow, Executive Director
Jay Centifanti, Treasurer

3800 PRO Behavioral Health
7600 E Eastman Avenue
Ste. 500
Denver, CO 80231-4375
303-695-8007
888-687-6755
Fax: 303-695-0100
E-mail: webmaster@probh.com
www.probh.com

Martin Dubin, Senior Vice President
Theodore Wirecki, Chair

A managed behavioral health care company dedicated to containing psychiatric and substance abuse costs while providing high-quality health care. Owned and operated by mental health care professionals, PRO has exclusive, multi-year contracts with HMOs and insurers on both coasts and in the Rocky Mountain region.

3801 PSIMED Corporation
725 Town & Country
Suite 200
Orange, CA 92868-4723
714-689-1544
E-mail: response@arbormed.com
www.psimed-ambs.com

Suzanne Beals, Contact

3802 Paris International Corporation
185 Great Neck Rd
Ste. 305
Great Neck, NY 11021-3352
516-487-2630
Fax: 516-466-6255
E-mail: info@parisintl.com
www.parisint.com

Stuart A. Paris, CIMA, AIF, Founder and President
Robert Testa, Vice President
Michael Paris, AIF
Mark Zigman, Investment Adviser Representativ

3803 Pearson
5601 Green Valley Drive
Bloomington, MN 55437-1187
952-681-3000
800-627-7271

Fax: 952-681-3549
E-mail: pearsonassessments@pearson.com

Robert Whelan, President and Chief Executive Of
Gary Gates, PhD, Senior Vice President, Global Bu
Corey Hoesley, Vice President, Global Operation
Doug Kennedy, Senior Vice President, Finance a

pearson is a publisher of assessment tools and instructional materials in the special needs behavior management, speech, language, and mental health markets. Among their numerous products are the MMPI-2, million inventories, BASC-2, BASC monitor for ADHD, vineland adaptive behavior scales(vineland II) and the Peabody picture vocabulary test (PPVT-4).

3804 Persoma Management

2540 Monroeville Blvd
Monroeville, PA 15146-2329
412-823-5155
Fax: 412-823-8262
www.persoma.com

James Long, President
Richard Heil Jr., Staff Member

3805 Perspectives

20 N Clark Street
Suite 2650
Chicago, IL 60602-5104
312-558-5318
800-866-7556
Fax: 312-558-1570
E-mail: info@perspectivesltd.com
www.perspectivesltd.com

Bernard S. Dyme, President & CEO, Principal
Terry Cahill, Vice President of Sales and Mark
Christopher Kunze, Chief Operations Officer
Maureen Dorgan-Clemens, Vice President of
Organizational

3806 Philadelphia Health Management

260 South Broad Street
18th Floor
Philadelphia, PA 19102-5085
215-985-2500
Fax: 215-985-2550
E-mail: info@phmc.org
www.www.phmc.org

Richard J Cohen, President and Chief Executive Of
Wayne Pendleton, Chief Operating Officer
Marino Puliti, Chief Financial Officer
Tine Hansen-Turton, Chief Strategy Officer

3807 Pinal Gila Behavioral Health Association

2066 W Apache Trail
Suite 116
Apache Junction, AZ 85120-3733
480-982-1317
800-982-1317
Fax: 480-982-7320
E-mail: info@pgbha.org
www.pgbha.org

Sandie Smith, President
Bryan Chambers, Vice President

3808 Porter Novelli

7 World Trade Center
250 Greenwich Street, 36th floor
New York, NY 10007
212-601-8000
Fax: 212-601-8101
E-mail: Darlan.Monterisi@porternovelli.com
www.porternovelli.com

Karen van Bergen, Chief Executive Officer, Senior
Brad MacAfee, President, North America, Senior
John Orme, Senior Partner, President, Asia-
Karen Ovseyevitz, President, Latin America, Senior

3809 Practice Management Resource Group

1564-A Fitzgerald Dr.
#246
Pinole, CA 94564
708-623-8202
Fax: 708-507-2932
E-mail: info@medicalpmrg.com
www.medicalpmrg.com

Ron Rosenberg, President/Founder
Curt Hill, Chief Executive Officer
Donna Connolly, Vice President of Operations

3810 Preferred Mental Health Management

401 E. Douglas
Suite 505
Wichita, KS 67202-3411
316-262-0444
800-819-9571
Fax: 316-262-0003
E-mail: info@pmhm.com
www.pmhm.com

Courtney Ruthven, Owner

Offers managed care services and EAP services.

Year Founded: 1987

3811 ProMetrics CAREeval

480 American Avenue
King of Prussia, PA 19406-4060
610-265-6344
Fax: 610-265-8377
E-mail: admin@prometrics.com
www.prometrics.com

Marc Duey, Owner

A joint venture formed by Father Flanagan's Home (Boys Town), Susquehanna Pathfinders and ProMetrics Consulting. These organizations combine years of experience as service providers and technical resource developers. Provides innovative ways to collect, store and analyze service outcome data to improve the effectiveness of your services.

3812 ProMetrics Consulting & Susquehanna PathFinders

480 American Avenue
King of Prussia, PA 19406-4060
610-265-6344
Fax: 610-265-8377
E-mail: admin@prometrics.com
www.prometrics.com

Marc Duey, Owner

3813 Professional Risk Management Services
1401 Wilson Boulevard
Suite 700
Arlington, VA 22209-2434
703-907-3800
800-245-3333
Fax: 703-276-9530
E-mail: tracy@prms.com
www.prmsva.com

Martin Tracy, CEO
Joseph Detorie, Executive Vice President/CFO

3814 PsycHealth
PO Box 5312
Evanston, IL 60204-5312
847-864-4961
800-753-5456
Fax: 847-864-9930
E-mail: administration@psychealthltd.com
www.psychealthltd.com

Janet O'Brien, Manager

Specialists providing mental health services, managed care and referrals.

Year Founded: 1989

3815 Public Consulting Group
148 State Street
10th Floor
Boston, MA 02109-2589
617-426-2026
800-210-6113
Fax: 617-426-4632
E-mail: info@publicconsultinggroup.com
www.www.publicconsultinggroup.com

Dan Heaney, Chief Financial Officer
Dina Wolfman Baker, Director of Marketing and Commun
Debra V. Clark, Corporate Facilities Director
Grant Blair, Director PCG Education

Year Founded: 1986

3816 Pyrce Healthcare Group
7325 Greenfield Street
River Forest, IL 60305-1256
708-383-7700
Fax: 708-383-7746
E-mail: phg@pyrcehealthcare.com
www.www.pyrcehealthcare.com

Janice M Pyrce, President/Founder

A national consulting firm, founded in 1990, with a focus on behavioral health. The firm specializes in strategic planning, market research, integrated delivery systems, business development, retreat facilitation and management/organizational development. PHG offers significant depth of resources, with direct involvement of experienced senior staff. Clients include hospitals, healthcare systems, academic medical centers, human service agencies, physician/allied practices, professional/trade associations and investor groups. The firm has over 200 organizations with locations in over 40 states.

3817 Quinco Behavioral Health Systems
720 North Marr Road
Columbus, IN 47201-6660
812-314-3400
800-266-2341
Fax: 812-376-4875

E-mail: webmaster@centerstone.org
www.centerstone.org

Robert Williams, CEO

Nonprofit mental health care provider serving south central Indiana. 24 hour crisis line and full continuum of mental health services.

3818 Schafer Consulting
602 Hemlock Road
Coraopolis, PA 15108-9140
724-695-0652
E-mail: ask@schaferconsulting.com
www.schaferconsulting.com

Steve Schafer, Owner

3819 Seelig and Company: Child Welfare and Behavioral Healthcare
140 E 45th Street
19th Floor
New York, NY 10017-7143
212-655-3500
Fax: 212-655-3535
E-mail: rmm@msf-law.com
www.meisterseelig.com

Mark J Seelig, President
Mercedes Medina, Operations Manager
Elizabeth Roe, Billing Manager
Yvette Pe¤a, HR Manager

Year Founded: 1994

3820 Specialized Therapy Associates
83 Summit Avenue
Hackensack, NJ 07601-1262
201-488-6678
Fax: 201-488-6224
E-mail: Information@SpecializedTherapy.com
www.specializedtherapy.com

Dr.Vanessa Gourdine, PsyD, MSN, P, Director
Dr. Cynthia Orosy, Clinical Director
Polina Levit, LPC, Assistant Director
Rick Rothman, MSW, LCSW, Assistant Director

3821 Suburban Research Associates
107 Chesley Drive
Unit 4
Media, PA 19063-1760
610-891-7200
Fax: 610-891-9699
E-mail: mmcnichol@suburbanresearch.com
www.suburbanresearch.com

Nikki Thomas, Marketing Director
Maureen O'Donnell, Sr. Clinical Research Coordnator
Brett Brashers, Clinical Research Coordnator
Ashley Tegler, Clinical Research Coordnator

3822 Supportive Systems
25 Beachway Drive
Suite C
Indianapolis, IN 46224-8506
317-788-4111
800-660-6645
Fax: 317-788-7783
E-mail: staff@supportivesystems.com
www.supportivesystems.com

Pam Ruster, Owner

3823 The Kennion Group Inc
800 Corporate Parkway
Suite 100
Birmingham, AL 35242-2942
205-972-0110
866-241-1682
Fax: 205-969-1199
www.kennion.com

W. Hal Shepherd, President/CEO

3824 The Lewin Group
3130 Fairview Park Drive
Suite 500
Falls Church, VA 22042-4517
703-269-5500
877-227-5042
Fax: 703-269-5501
E-mail: lisa.chimento@lewin.com
www.lewin.com

Lisa Chimento, CEO
Ann Osborn, Vice President
Robert Page, Vice President
Linda Shields, Vice President

The Lewin Group is a national health care and human service policy, research, and consulting firm with more than
40 years' experience delivering objective analyses and strategic counsel to federal, state, and local governments foundations, associations, hospitals and health systems
providers and health plans.

Year Founded: 1970

**3825 Towers Perrin Integrated Heatlh Systems
Consulting**
335 Madison Avenue
New York, NY 10017-4605
212-309-3400
Fax: 212-309-0975
www.towersperrin.com

John Haley, Chief Executive Officer
Julie Gebauer, Managing Director, Talent and Re
Tricia Guinn, Managing Director, Risk and Fina
Gene Wickes, Managing Director, Benefits

Managed behavorial health care consultants specializing in
strategy and operations, clinical effectiveness, actuarial and
reimbursement and human resources for both the provider
and the payer sides.

**3826 Traumatic Incident Reduction Newsletter
Traumatic Incident Reduction Association**
5145 Pontiac Trail
Ann Arbor, MI 48105-9279
734-761-6268
800-499-2751
Fax: 734-663-6861
E-mail: info@tir.org
www.tirbook.org

Victor Volkam, Author

Traumatic Incident Reduction is a brief, person-sentered
treatment for the affects of trauma and loss. This newsletter
offers part of the larger subject of Applied
Metapsychology, which addresses relationship, self-esteem
and well-being issues of all sorts, including traumatic
stress. Additional web site for TIR: www.tir.org.

16 pages 2 per year

3827 United Behavioral Health
425 Market Street
27th Floor
San Francisco, CA 94105-2406
415-547-5000
800-888-2998
www.unitedbehavioralhealth.com

Larry Renfro, CEO
Paul Bleicher, MD, PhD, Chief Executive Officer, Optum L
Stan Dennis, Executive Vice President, Physic
Karen Erickson, Executive Vice President, Chief

**3828 University of North Carolina School of Social
Work, Behavioral Healthcare**
Tate-Turner-Kuralt Building
325 Pittsboro Street Cb#3550
Chapel Hill, NC 27599-3155
919-962-1225
Fax: 919-962-0890
E-mail: ssw@unc.edu
www.http://ssw.unc.edu

Year Founded: 1920

3829 ValueOptions Jacksonville
10199 Southside Blvd
Building 100 Suite 300
Jacksonville, FL 32256-757
800-700-8646
www.valueoptions.com

Heyward R. Donigan, President and Chief Executive Of
Douglas Thompson, M.S., M.B.A., Executive Vice President
and Chi
Kyle A. Raffaniello, Executive Vice President and Chi
Dan Risku, J.D., Executive Vice President and Gen

3830 ValueOptions Norfolk
240 Corporate Blvd
Norfolk, VA 23502-4900
757-459-5100
www.valueoptions.com

Heyward R. Donigan, President and Chief Executive Of
Douglas Thompson, M.S., M.B.A., Executive Vice President
and Chi
Kyle A. Raffaniello, Executive Vice President and Chi
Dan Risku, J.D., Executive Vice President and Gen

Designs and operates innovative administrative and
full-risk services for a wide range of behavioral health and
chemical dependency programs, Medicaid, child welfare
and other human services, and Employee Assistance Programs. Develops collaborative relationships with government agencies, community providers, consumer groups,
health plans, insurers, and others to foster a deeper understanding of the needs of the various populations they serve.
Develops child welfare programs based upon the principles
of managed care.

3831 Vedder Price
222 North LaSalle Street
Chicago, IL 60601-1003
312-609-7500
Fax: 312-609-5005
E-mail: kwendrickx@vedderprice.com
www.vedderprice.com

Michael A. Nemeroff, President and CEO
Robert J. Stucker, Chairman

Dean N. Gerber, Vice Chair
Douglas M. Hambleton, Operating Shareholder

3832 VeriCare
4715 Viewridge Avenue
Suite 110
San Diego, CA 92123
858-454-3610
800-257-8715
Fax: 800-819-1655
E-mail: contactus@vericare.com
www.vericare.com

Cindy Watson, President/CEO
Bennett O. Voit, Chief Financial Officer
Cammile C. Bird, Vice President, Sales and Market
Karim S. Chalhoub, Executive VP of Revenue and Syst

3833 VeriTrak
179 Niblick Road
Suite 149
Paso Robles, CA 93446-4845
800-370-2440
E-mail: support@veritrak.com
www.veritrak.com

3834 Webman Associates
4 Brattle Street
Cambridge, MA 02138-3714
617-864-6769
www.webmanassociates.com

Dorothy Webman, Owner

3835 WellPoint Behavioral Health
9655 Graniteridge Drive
Sixth Floor
San Diego, CA 92123-2674
858-571-8100
800-728-9498

Lori Wright, Manager

Software Companies

3836 ADL Data Systems
9 Skyline Drive
Hawthorne, NY 10532-2100
914-591-1800
Fax: 914-591-1818
E-mail: sales@mail.adldata.com
www.adldata.com

David Pollack, President
Aaron S. Weg, Software Development
Ulysses Fleming, Accounting Solutions
Dorothy Dreiher, Clinical Solutions

The most comprehensive software solution for MH/MRDD and the continuum of care. 38 modules to choose from. Designed to meet all financial, clinical, and administrative needs. For organizations requiring greater flexiblity and processing power. Ask about new Windows-based products utilizing the latest in technology, including bar coding, scanning, etc.

Year Founded: 1977

3837 AHMAC
4600 Linden Ave.
Mechanicsburg, PA 17055

717-730-7189
E-mail: david@hewitsoftware.com
www.hewitsoftware.com

CareManager is a microcomputer based system targeted at small to medium sized HMOs, PPOs and PHOs as well as vertical markets such as Medicaid and managed mental health. Easily customized to meet the needs and requirements of the client.

Year Founded: 1983

3838 Accumedic Computer Systems
11 Grace Avenue
Suite 401
Great Neck, NY 11021-2427
516-466-6800
800-765-9300
Fax: 516-466-6880
E-mail: info@accumedic.com
www.accumedic.com

Mark Kollenscher, President
John Teubner, Vice President

AccudMed EHR, is fully ONC certified. We know the complexities you encounter in your financial and clinical program management. Now you can focus on your mission of improving quality treatment.

3839 Agilent Technologies
5301 Stevens Creek Blvd
Santa Clara, CA 95051-7201
408-345-8886
877-424-4536
Fax: 408-345-8474
E-mail: contact_us@agilent.com
www.agilent.com

William P. (Sullivan, President and Chief Executive Of
Ron Nersesian, Executive Vice President
Henrik Ancher-Jensen, Senior Vice President
Rick Burdsall, Senior Vice President

Clinical measurement and diagnostic solutions for healthcare organizations.

3840 American Medical Software
1180 South State
Route 157
Edwardsville, IL 62025-236
618-692-1300
800-423-8836
Fax: 618-692-1809
E-mail: sales@americanmedical.com
www.americanmedical.com

Practice management software for billing, electronic claims, appointments and electronic medical records.

3841 American Psychiatric Press Reference Library CD-ROM
American Psychiatric Publishing, Inc.
1000 Wilson Boulevard
Suite 1825
Arlington, VA 22209-3901
703-907-7322
800-368-5777
Fax: 703-907-1091
E-mail: appi@psych.org
www.appi.org

Robert E Hales, M.D., M.B.A., Editor-in-Chief
Saul Levin, M.D., M.P.A., CEO and Medical Director
Laura W. Roberts, M.D., Deputy Editor
John W. Barnhill, M.D., Associate Editor

$395.00

Year Founded: 1998

3842 Aries Systems Corporation

200 Sutton Street
North Andover, MA 01845-1656
978-975-7570
Fax: 978-975-3811
E-mail: marketing@edmgr.com
www.www.editorialmanager.com

Lyndon Holmes, President

Provides technical innovations that empower all of the participants in the knowledge retrieval chain: publishers, database developers, librarians.

3843 Askesis Development Group

One Chatham Center
112 Washington Place, Suite 300
Pittsburgh, PA 15219-3458
412-803-2400
Fax: 412-803-2099
E-mail: info@askesis.com
www.askesis.com

Sharon Hicks, President and Chief Executive Of
Bob Teitt, Vice President of Technology and
Beth Rotto, Vice President, Finance and Oper
Nicholas Carosella, MD, Physician Advisor

Askesis Development Group's PsychConsult is a complete informatics solution for behavioral health organizations: inpatient or outpatient behavioral health facilities, managed care organizations, and provider networks. PsychConsult is Windows NT based, and Y2K compliant. ADG development is guided by the PsychConsult Consortium, a collaborative effort of leading institutions in behavioral health.

3844 BOSS Inc

2639 N Downer Avenue
Suite 9
Milwaukee, WI 53211
414-967-9689
800-964-4789
E-mail: bmiller@healthcareboss.com
www.healthcareboss.com

Bob Miller, President

Practice management software that is easy to use and is in more than 29, 000 practices nationally. Outcome management software products for social workers and hospitals. *$1499.00*

Year Founded: 1986

3845 Beaver Creek Software

525 SW 6th Street
Corvallis, OR 97333-4323
541-752-5039
800-895-3344
Fax: 541-752-5221
E-mail: sales@beaverlog.com
www.www.beaverlog.com

Peter Gysegem, Owner

'The THERAPIST' practice management and billing software for Windows operating systems comes in Pro and EZ

versions. The EZ version is powerful yet simple to use and is tailored to needs of smaller offices. The Pro version is designed to handle the complex needs of busy practices. Use Pro to create HIPAA compliant electronic insurance claims. Both versions let you have an unlimited number of providers at no additional cost. *$249.00*

Year Founded: 1989

3846 Behavioral Health Advisor
McKesson Clinical Reference Systems

One Post Street
San Francisco, CA 94104
415-983-8300
800-782-1334
E-mail: consumerproducts@mckesson.com
www.mckesson.com

The Behavioral Health Advisor software program provides consumer health information for more than 600 topics covering pediatric and adult mental illness, disorders and behavioral problems. Includes behavioral health topics from the American Academy of Child and Adolescent Psychiatry. Many Spanish translations available. *$4.75*

Year Founded: 1998

3847 Behaviordata

20863 Stevens Creek Boulevard
Suite 580
Cupertino, CA 95014-2154
408-342-0600
800-627-2673
Fax: 408-342-0617
www.behaviordat.com

Diana Everstine, President
Dr David Nichols, Contact

3848 Bottomline Technologies

325 Corporate Drive
Portsmouth, NH 03801
603-436-0700
800-243-2528
Fax: 603-436-0300
E-mail: info@bottomline.com
www.www.bottomline.com

Robert A. Eberle, President and Chief Executive Of
Kevin M. Donovan, Chief Financial Officer
Karen Brieger, Vice President, Human Resources
Eric Campbell, Senior Vice President, Strategic

Provides software solutions that enable organizations to achieve unprecedented speed, accuracy, functionality and quality in their document processes such as procure-to-pay, order-to-case, manufacturing and healthcare.

Year Founded: 1981

3849 Bull HN Information Systems

285 Billerica Road
Chelmsford, MA 01824
978-294-6000
Fax: 978-244-0085
www.www.bull.us

David W Bradbury, President

Provides solutions and services to key markets, including the public sector, finance, manufacturing, and telecommunications.

3850 CSI Software

3333 Richmond
2nd Floor
Houston, TX 77098-3007
713-942-7779
800-247-3431
Fax: 713-942-7731
E-mail: sales@csisoftwareusa.com
www.csisoftwareusa.com

Frank Mc Duff, VP

CSI Software designs software for the membership industry utilizing the most sophisticated software technologies, coupled with unsurpassed and experience and support.

3851 Center for Health Policy Studies

214 Massachusetts Ave NE
Washington, DC 20002-4999
202-546-4400
E-mail: info@heritage.org
www.heritage.org

Thomas A. Saunders III, Chairman
Richard M. Scaife, Vice Chairman
J. Frederic Rench, Secretary
David S. Addington, Group Vice President, Research

3852 Ceridian Corporation

3311 E Old Shackopee Road
Minneapolis, MN 55425-1640
952-548-5000
800-729-7655
Fax: 952-548-5100
www.ceridian.com

Stuart C. Harvey, Jr., Chairman
David Ossip, Chief Executive Officer
Dave MacKay, President
Lois M. Martin, Executive Vice President and Chi

A computer services and manufacturing company.

Year Founded: 1957

3853 Cincom Systems

55 Merchant Street
Cincinnati, OH 45246-3761
513-612-2769
800-224-6266
Fax: 513-612-2000
E-mail: info@cincom.com
www.www.cincom.com

Thomas M Nies, Founder and CEO

Cincom provides software and service solutions that help our clients create, manage and grow relationships with their customers through adaptive e-business information systems.

3854 Client Management Information System
WilData Systems Group

255 Bradenton Avenue
Dublin, OH 43017-2546
614-734-4719
800-860-4222
Fax: 614-734-1063
E-mail: cmis@wildatainc.com
www.wildatainc.com

A total Electronic Health Records (EHR) solution for behavioral health care organization like mental health centers, substance abuse providers, human service organizations,

and family service agencies. Become 100% paperless by using CMIS in-house or by accessing our web based version called e-CMIS to minimize the up front capital expenditure and ongoing maintenance costs.

3855 CliniSphere version 2.0
Facts and Comparisons

77 Westport Plaza
Suite 450
Saint Louis, MO 63146-3125
317-735-5300
800-223-0554
www.factsandcomparisons.com

Arvind Subramanian, President & CEO
John Pins, Vice President, Finance
Denise Basow, MD, Vice President, General Manager
David A. Del Toro, Vice President and General Manag

Access to all information in a clinical drug reference library, by drug, disease, side-effects; thousands of drugs (prescription, OTC, investigational) all included; contains information from Drug Facts and Comparisons, most definitive and comprehensive source for comparative drug information.

3856 Clinical Nutrition Center

7555 E Hampden Avenue
Suite 301
Denver, CO 80231-4834
303-750-9454
www.clinicalnutritioncenter.com

Ethan Lazarus, M.D., President
Heather Thomas, P.A. -C., Physician Assistant

Our programs are based on the latest development in the field of nutrition, weight loss and weight control, behavior modification.

3857 CoCENTRIX

540 North Tamiami Trail
Sarasota, FL 34236-4823
941-306-4951
Fax: 941-954-2033
E-mail: info@cocentrix.com
www.unicaresys.com

May Ahdab, Ph.D., Chief Executive Officer/Co-Found
Leigh Orlov, President/Co-Founder
Neal Tilghman, Senior Vice President, Product M
Jason Ochipa, CPA, Chief Financial Officer

UNI/CARE's mission is to offer enterprise-based solutions designed to improve clinical recovery outcomes, standardize workflows and maximize revenue cycles within a technical environment, fostering collaboration and informed decision-making. Pro-Filer is a .NETcentric Human Service Enterprise (HSE) platform designed to support the requirements of data processing and use by healthcare organizations providing an array of clinical services. It's viable in a single organization or across a consortium, offering users customized workflows, best practice guides, revenue management tools, and the ability to concurrently meet clinical and financial compliance standards.

Year Founded: 1981

3858 Computer Transition Services

3223 S Loop
Suite 556
Lubbock, TX 79423

806-793-8961
800-687-2874
Fax: 806-793-8968
www.www.ctsinet.com

David Baucum, Owner

Improve the life and business success of clients by providing integrated solutions and professional services to meet their technological and organizational needs.

3859 Cornucopia Software

PO Box 6111
Albany, CA 94706-111
510-528-7000
E-mail: supportstaff@practicemagic.com
www.practicemagic.com

Providers of Practice MAGIC, the billing and practice management software that counts for your psychotherapy practice.

3860 Creative Solutions Unlimited

203 Gilman Street
PO Box 550
Sheffield, IA 50475-550
641-892-4466
800-253-7697
Fax: 641-892-4333
E-mail: mkoch@csumail.com
www.creativesolutionsunlimited.com

Martha Koch, Vp

Reliable, comprehensive, intuitive, fully-integrated clinical software able to manage MDS 2.0 electronic submission, RUGs/PPS, triggers, Quick RAP's, survey reports, QI's, assessments, care plans, Quick Plans, physician orders, CQI, census, and hundreds of reports. Creative Solutions Unlimited provides outstanding toll-free support, training, updates, user groups, newsletters, and continuing education.

Year Founded: 1988

3861 DB Consultants

1259 Cedar Crest Blvd.
Suite 328
Allentown, PA 18103
610-820-0440
Fax: 610-820-7651
E-mail: sales@dbconsultants.com
www.dbconsultants.com

AS/PC includes electronic claims submission. Healtcare professionals rely on AS/PC every day to help them provide quality care.

Year Founded: 1980

3862 DST Output

2600 Sw Blvd
Kansas City, MO 64108-2349
816-221-1234
800-441-7587
E-mail: sales_marketing@dstoutput.com
www.dstoutput.com

Steven J Towle, CEO
Frank Delfer, CTO
Jim Reinert, EVP Business Development

Providing a customer communications solution offering myriad benefits to healthcare payor organizations, including the ability to manage both inbound and outbound communications; ensure document control and content compliance; integrate data from portal entry; distribute data, information, and material to the right place and audience with integrity.

3863 DeltaMetrics

600 Public Ledger Building
150 South Independence Mall West
Philadelphia, PA 19106-3475
215-399-0988
Fax: 215-399-0989
E-mail: mail@deltametrics.com
www.deltametrics.com

Jack Durell, MD, President/CEO
John Cacciola, Ph.D., Senior Vice President & Scientif
Richard Weiss, Ph.D., Director of Research and Evaluat
Kathleen Geary, Director of Operations

DeltaMetrics is now assisting treatment agencies to design and implement programs of Continuous Quality Improvement (CQI) within their systems of care.

3864 Docu Trac

20140 Scholar Drive
Suite 218
Hagerstown, MD 21742-6575
301-766-4130
800-850-8510
Fax: 888-415-7939
E-mail: sales@quicdoc.com
www.www.docutracinc.com

Arnie Schuster, Owner

Offering Quic Doc clinical documentation software, a comprehensive software system designed specifically for behavioral healthcare providers.

Year Founded: 1993

3865 DocuMed

3518 West Liberty Road
Ann Arbor, MI 48103-9013
734-930-9053
800-321-5595
E-mail: info@documed.com
www.www.documed.com

DocuMed 2002 is a comprehensive system for automated documentation of physician/patient encounters in ambulatory settings for solo practitioners or multiple physician groups.

Year Founded: 1988

3866 E Services Group

5115 Pegasus Court
Suite N
Frederick, MD 21704
301-698-1901
Fax: 301-698-1909
E-mail: contactus@esrv.com
www.www.esrv.com

Dave Walsh, Owner

Our primary focus is on finding that perfect marriage of savvy business logic and technologies so that our healthcare IT applications solve the real world business problems of our clients.

3867 EAP Technology Systems

PO Box 1650
Yreka, CA 96097-1650

800-755-6965
Fax: 530-842-4778
E-mail: info@eaptechnology.com
www.eaptechnology.com

Tom Amaral, Ph.D., Founder/President & CEO/Board Me
Roland Alden, Technology Development Director
Bob Watson, Business Strategy Advisor/Board
Wayne Larocque, Business Development/Capital Rai

Provider of technologies that automate work flow and enhance the business value of Employee Assistance Programs.

3868 Echo Group

519 17th Street
Suite 400
Oakland, CA 94612-3461
603-447-8600
800-635-8209
Fax: 603-447-8680
E-mail: info@echoman.com
www.echoman.com

David Allen, Manager

Echo Group has been helping behavioral healthcare organizations to succeed in their missions of healing.

3869 Electronic Healthcare Systems

Ehs One Metroplex Drive
Suite 500
Birmingham, AL 35209
205-871-1031
888-879-7302
Fax: 205-871-1185
E-mail: marketing@ehsmed.com
www.ehsmed.com

EHS develops and markets system solutions to a select group of physicians who are leading the way to clinical excellence and practice efficiency trhough automation.

Year Founded: 1995

3870 Entre Technology Services

1501 14th St W
#201
Billings, MT 59102
406-256-5700
Fax: 406-256-0201
www.entremt.com

Mike Keene, Owner
Ben McClintock, Network Administrator
Veronica Smith, Partner Relations and Customer S
Mike Niles, Senior Systems Engineer

Software applications and website development; off site backup solutions and disaster recovery; managed services; product sales; seminar room and classroom rental; and computer training.

Year Founded: 1984

3871 Experior Corporation

5710 Coventry Lane
Fort Wayne, IN 46804-7141
260-432-2020
800-595-2020
Fax: 260-432-4753
E-mail: sales@experior.com
www.experior.com

J. Richard Presser, President & CEO

Experior provides Innovative Information systems to practice management and ASC marketplace. Out products, SurgeOn and EMS provide scheduling, case costing and billing.

Year Founded: 1978

3872 Family Services of Delaware County

600 North Olive Street
Media, PA 19063-2418
610-566-7540
Fax: 610-566-7677
www.fcsdc.org

Tracy Segal, Director Development

The Where to Turn Database is the most comprehensive listing of Non-Profit Human Service programs in the Delaware County area, the Young Resources Database is a condensed version of the above.

3873 First Data Bank

701 Gateway Blvd.
Suite 600
South San Francisco, CA 94080
650-827-4564
800-633-3453
Fax: 650-588-4003
E-mail: cs@fdbhealth.com
www.firstdatabank.com

Donald M Nielsen, CEO

Provides thousands of drug knowledge base implementations ranging from pharmacy dispensing and claims processing to emerging applications including computerized physician order entry (CPOE), electronic health records (EHR), e-Prescribing and electronic medication administration records (EMAR).

3874 Gelbart and Associates

423 S Pacific Coast Highway
Suite 102
Redondo Beach, CA 90277-3731
310-792-1823
Fax: 310-540-8904
www.www.gelbartandassociates.com

Robert Cutrow, Contact

Comprehensive Psychological and Psychiatric services for individuals, families, couples and groups, treating: anxiety, depression, relationship conflicts and medication management.

3875 Genelco Software Solutions

325 McDonnell Boulevard
Hazelwood, MO 63042-2513
800-548-2040
Fax: 314-593-3517
E-mail: info@genelco.com
www.genelco.com

Offers its flagship software systems in an ASP financial model. An ASP arrangement allows an organization to maintain control over operations without maintaining the software onsite.

3876 HSA-Mental Health

1080 Emeline Avenue
Santa Cruz, CA 95060-1966
831-454-4000
Fax: 831-454-4770
TDD: 831-454-2123

E-mail: info@santacruzhealth.org
www.santacruzhealth.org

Exists to protect and improve the health of the people in Santa Cruz County. Provides programs in environmental health, public health, medical care, substance abuse prevention and treatment, and mental health. Clients are entitled to information on the costs of care and their options for getting health insurance coverage through a variety of programs.

3877 Habilitation Software

204 N Sterling Street
Morganton, NC 28655-3345
828-438-9455
Fax: 828-438-9488
E-mail: info@habsoft.com
www.habsoft.com

Randy Herson, President

Personal Planning System, Windows-based computer program which assists agencies serving people with developmental disabilities with the tasks of person-centered planning; tracks outcomes, services and supports, assists with assesments and quarterly reviews, and maintains a customizable library of training programs. Also includes a census system for agencies which must maintain an exact midnight census, as well as an Accident/Incident system.

3878 Hanover Insurance

440 Lincoln Street
Worcester, MA 01653-0002
508-855-1000
800-853-0456
Fax: 508-853-6332
www.www.hanover.com

Frederick H Eppinger Jr, President and Chief Executive Of
Bruce Bartell, Chief Underwriting Officer - Cha
Mark R. Desrochers, Senior Vice President, President
David Greenfield, Executive Vice President and Chi

Offers hospice programs, rehabilitation groups and mental health services.

3879 Health Probe

5693 Bear Wallow Road
Suite 100
Morgantown, IN 46160-9315
765-346-3332
E-mail: support@healthprobe.com
www.healthprobe.com

EMR created to eliminate the need for paper with electronic medical records.

3880 HealthLine Systems

17085 Camino San Bernardo
San Diego, CA 92127-5709
858-673-1700
800-733-8737
Fax: 858-673-9866
E-mail: cs@healthlinesystems.com
www.healthlinesystems.com

Dan Littrell, CEO

Provide peerless information management solutions and services that maximize the quality and delivery of healthcare.

3881 HealthSoft

PO Box 536489
Orlando, FL 32853-6489
407-648-4857
407-648-4857
Fax: 407-426-7440
E-mail: admin@healthsoftonline.com
www.healthsoftonline.com

CD - ROM and web based software for professionals on mental health nursing and developmental disabilities nursing.

3882 Healthline Systems

17085 Camino San Bernardo
San Diego, CA 92127-5709
858-673-1700
800-254-7347
Fax: 858-673-9866
E-mail: sales@healthlinesystems.com
www.healthlinesystems.com

Dan Littrell, CEO

Provider of Document Management and Physician Credentialing software solutions.

3883 Healthport

120 Bluegrass Valley Parkway
Alpharetta, GA 30005-2204
770-360-1700
800-367-1500
www.healthport.com

Michael J. Labedz, President and Chief Executive Of
Brian M. Grazzini, Chief Financial Officer
Matt Rohs, Vice President and General Manag
Bill Matits, Senior Vice President of Sales

Develops and sells Companion EMR, an electronic medical record system that eliminates paperwork, improves accuracy of information, provides instant access to patient and clinical information, and helps cuts costs while increasing revenue.

3884 Hogan Assessment Systems

2622 East 21st Street
Tulsa, OK 74114-1768
918-293-2300
800-756-0632
Fax: 918-749-0635
www.info.hoganassessments.com

Robert Hogan, President
Aaron Tracy, Chief Operating Officer
Rodney Warrentfeltz, Ph.D., Managing Partner
Ryan Ross, VP of Global Alliances

Focuses on five dimensions of personality including emotional stability, extroversion, likeability, conscientiousness and the degree to which a person needs stimulation.

3885 IBM Global Healthcare Industry

404 Wyman Street
Waltham, MA 02451-1212
781-895-2911
Fax: 617-361-2485
E-mail: tgaffin@us.ibm.com
www.ibm.com/industries/healthcare

IBM has been strategically involved in assisting the healthcare industry in addressing numerous IT challenges. IBM provides clients and partners with the industry's broadest portfolio of technology, services, skills, and insight.

3886 InfoMC
101 W Elm Street
Suite G10
Conshohocken, PA 19428-2075
484-530-0100
Fax: 484-530-0111
E-mail: info@infomc.com
www.infomc.com

JJ Farook, Chairman & CEO
Donald Gravlin, EVP Product Startegy & COO
Rick Jackson, SVP Global Wellness Solutions
Susan Norris, Senior Vice Presodent of Clinica

Develops software solutions for Managed Care organizations, EAP/Work-Life organizations, and Health and Human Services agencies.
Year Founded: 1994

3887 Informix Software
IBM Corporation
1 New Orchard Road
Armonk, NY 10504-1722
914-499-1900
800-426-4968
TTY: 800-426-3383
E-mail: ews@us.ibm.com
www.ibm.com/software

IBM Informix® software includes a comprehensive array of high-performance, stand-alone and integration tools that enable efficient application and Web development, information integration , and database administration.

3888 Inhealth Record Systems
5076 Winters Chapel Road
Atlanta, GA 30360-1832
770-396-4994
800-477-7374
Fax: 770-396-0475
E-mail: sales@inhealth.us
www.inhealthrecords.com

Sue Kay, President

Provides variety of record keeping system products for health care practices and organizations.
Year Founded: 1979

3889 Innovative Data Solutions
386 Newberry Drive
Suite 100
Elk Grove Village, IL 60007-2778
847-923-1926
E-mail: info@idsincp.com
www.idsincp.com

Mark Parianos, President/CEO

Provide effective web based and software solutions for business, small offices and fortune 500 clients.
Year Founded: 1991

3890 Integrated Business Services
736 N Western Ave
125
Lake Forest, IL 60045-1820
847-735-1690
800-451-5478

E-mail: info@medbase200.com
www.www.medbase200.com

Sam Tartamella, Manager

A medical research and information marketing firm providing access to highly selectable medical databases.
Year Founded: 1982

3891 Keane Care
8383 158th Avenue NE
Suite 100
Redmond, WA 98052-3846
425-869-9000
800-426-2675
Fax: 425-307-2220
E-mail: kim_A_Allen@keane.com
www.keanecare.com

Thomas Weitzel, Executive
Jim Ingalls, Director Sales

Develops, markets, and supports a range of clinical and financial software.
Year Founded: 1969

3892 MEDCOM Information Systems
2117 Stonington Avenue
Hoffman Estates, IL 60169-2016
847-885-1553
800-213-2161
Fax: 847-885-1591
E-mail: medcom@emirj.com
www.emirj.com

John Holub, President

Provides a wide variety of products and services to the independent physician clinic as well as the hospital and private clinical laboratories.
Year Founded: 1991

3893 MEDecision
601 Lee Road
Chesterbrook Corporate Center
Wayne, PA 19087-5607
610-540-0202
Fax: 610-540-0270
E-mail: salesinfo@medecision.com
www.medecision.com

Scott A Storrer, CEO

Providing managed care organizations with powerful and flexible care management solutions. MEDecision's tools help managed care organizations improve care management processes and align more closely with their members and providers to improve the quality and cost outcomes of healthcare.
Year Founded: 1988

3894 McKesson HBOC
2700 Snelling Ave N
Roseville, MN 55113-1719
651-697-5900
Fax: 651-697-5910

Chris Bauleke, VP

Our products and services are designed to meet the information needs of all participants in the integrated health system.

3895 MedPLus
4690 Parkway Drive
Mason, OH 45040-8172
513-229-5500
800-444-6235
E-mail: info@medplus.com
www.www.questdiagnostics.com

Richard A Mahoney, President
Thomas R Wagner, CTO
Philip S Present, II, COO

Developer and integrator of clinical connectivity and data management solutions for health care organizations and clinicians.

Year Founded: 1991

3896 Medai
Millenia Park One
4901 Vineland Rd Suite 450
Orlando, FL 32811-7192
321-281-4480
866-422-5156
Fax: 321-281-4499
E-mail: helpdesk@medai.com
www.www.medai.com

Steve Epstein, Owner
Diane Lee, EVP/Co Founder
Swati Abbott, President

Provides solutions for the improvement of healthcare delivery. Utilizing cutting-edge technology, payers are able to predict patients at risk, identify cost drivers for their high-risk population, predict future health plan costs, evaluate patient patterns over time, and improve outcomes.

Year Founded: 1992

3897 Medcomp Software
PO Box 16687
Golden, CO 80402-6010
303-277-0772
Fax: 303-277-9801
E-mail: customerservice@medcompsoftware.com
www.medcompsoftware.com

Developing and designing case management systems for a wide variety of applications.

Year Founded: 1995

3898 Medi-Span
8425 Woodfield Crossing Boulevard
Suite 490
Indianapolis, IN 46240-7300
317-735-5300
855-539-7686
Fax: 317-735-5350
E-mail: medispan-support@wolterskluwer.com
www.medi-span.com

Arvind Subramanian, President & CEO, Wolters Kluwer
John Pins, Vice President, Finance, Clinica
Denise Basow, MD, Vice President, General Manager
David A. Del Toro, Vice President and General Manag

Medi-Span offers a complete line of drug databases, including clinical decision support and disease suite modules, application programming interfaces, and stand-alone PC products.

3899 Medical Records Institute
425 Boylston Street
4th Floor
Boston, MA 02116-3315
617-964-3923
Fax: 617-964-3926
E-mail: peter@medrecinst.com
www.medrecinst.com

Peter Waegemann, CEO

Promote and enhance the journey towards electronic health records, e-health, mobile health, mental health assessment, and related applications of information technologies (IT).

Year Founded: 1983

3900 Medix Systems Consultants
236 E 161st Place
Suite D
S Holland, IL 60473-3374
708-331-1271
Fax: 708-331-1272
E-mail: sales@imsci.com
www.imsci.com

Systems integration and development company committed to client/server multi vendor(open systems) solutions for a diverse vertical market ranging from education and healthcare.

Year Founded: 1987

3901 Mental Health Connections
21 Blossom Street
Lexington, MA 02421-8103
617-510-1318
www.mhc.com

Robert Patterson, MD, Founder/Principal

Developer of medical management software for physicians and research scientists. Their primary product is designed to identify drug interactions based on the mainstream of drug metabolism research.

Year Founded: 1983

3902 Mental Health Outcomes
2941 S Lake Vista Drive
Ste. 100
Lewisville, TX 75067-3801
800-266-4440
Fax: 972-420-8215
E-mail: johan.smith@horizonhealth.com
www.mho-inc.net

Johan Smith, VP Operations/Development

Designs and implements custom outcome measurement systems specifically for behavioral helath programs through its CQI Outcomes Measurement System. This system provides information for a wide range of patient and treatment focused variables for child, adolescent, adult, geriatric and substance abuse programs in the inpatient, partial hospital, residential treatment and outpatient settings.

Year Founded: 1994

3903 Micro Design International
40 Cain Dr.
Brentwood, NY 11717
631-273-4200
800-228-0891

E-mail: sales@mdi.com
www.mdi.com

Martin Legat, President

Provides optical (CD/DVD/MO) storage solutions through innovative achivements, easy-to-use data access, and exceptional service and support.

Year Founded: 1978

3904 Micro Office Systems
3825 Severn Road
Cleveland, OH 44118-1910
216-297-1240
Fax: 216-297-1241
E-mail: info@micro-officesystems.com
www.www.micro-officesystems.com

Norman Efroymson, Chief Executive Officer
Yosef Gold, Manger, PCG Product Group
Michael Post, Integration Solutions/ Chief Sof
Daniel Ostroff, Manager, Data Conversions

Year Founded: 1985

3905 Micromedex
6200 S Syracuse Way
Suite 300
Greenwood Village, CO 80111-4705
303-486-6444
800-525-9083
Fax: 303-486-6450
www.micromedex.com

Roy Martin, Executive Vice President and Chi
Tina Moen, PharmD, Chief Clinical Officer
Jill Sutton, Senior Vice President of Solutio
Brandy O'Connor, Vice President, Sales

A comprehensive suite of alerts, answers, protocols, and interventions directly addresses clinicians need for evidence-based information. This vital information is used to support patient care and improve outcomes.

Year Founded: 1974

3906 Misys Health Care Systems
8529 Six Forks Road
Forum IV
Raleigh, NC 27615-2963
800-877-5678
www.www.allscripts.com

Paul M. Black, Chief Executive Officer and Pres
Rick Poulton, Chief Financial Officer
Dennis Olis, Senior Vice President, Operation
Brian Farley, SVP and General Counsel

Develops and supports software and services for physicians and caregivers.

3907 MphasiS(BPO)
5353 N 16th Street
Suite 400
Phoenix, AZ 85016-3228
602-604-3100
888-604-3100
Fax: 602-604-3115
E-mail: selse@eldocomp.com
www.eldocomp.com

Sally Else, President
Len Miller, Chief Operating Officer
David J Hawkes, Executive Vice President
Hossein Abdollahi, Senior Vice President of Profess

Focused on financial services, logistics and technology verticals and spans across architecture, application development and integration, application management and business process outsourcing, including the operation of large scale customer contact centers.

3908 National Families in Action
PO Box 133136
Atlanta, GA 30333-3136
404-248-9676
Fax: 404-248-1312
E-mail: nfia@nationalfamilies.org
www.nationalfamilies.org

William F. Carter, Chairman of the Board
Sue Rusche, President and Chief Executive Of
Carol S. Reeder, Treasurer
Paula C. Kemp, Secretary

An interactive database of ever-changing names of drugs that people use and abuse for illnesses.

Year Founded: 1977

3909 NetMeeting
Microsoft Corporation
Customer Advocate Center
One Microsoft Way
Redmond, WA 98052-8300
425-882-8080
800-642-7676
Fax: 425-936-7329
www.microsoft.com

Steve Ballmer, CEO

NetMeeting delivers a complete Internet conferencing solution for all Window users with multi-point data conferencing, text chat, whiteboard, and file transfer, as well as point-to-point audio and video.

3910 Netsmart Technologies
570 Metro Place N
Dublin, OH 43017-5317
614-764-0143
800-434-2642
Fax: 614-764-0362
www.ntst.com

Kevin Scalia, Executive Vice President, Corpor
Michael Valentine, Chief Executive Officer
Frances Loshin-Turso, Senior Vice President
Doug Abel, Executive Vice President, Soluti

Offers information systems for mental health, behavioral and public health organizations.

3911 Northwest Analytical
111 SW 5th Avenue
Suite 800
Portland, OR 97204-3606
503-224-7727
888-692-7638
Fax: 503-224-5236
E-mail: nwa@nwasoft.com
www.nwasoft.com

Bob Ward, Chief Executive Officer
Jim Petrusich, Vice President of Sales
T. Olin Nichols, Chief Financial Officer
Louis K. Halvorsen, Chief Technology Officer

Provides comprehensive SPC software tools meeting technically stringent mental health industry requirements.

Year Founded: 1980

3912 OPTAIO-Optimizing Practice Through Assessment, Intervention and Outcome
Harcourt Assessment/PsychCorp
19500 Bulverde Road
San Antonio, TX 78259-3701
210-339-5000
800-622-3231
Fax: 210-339-5046

Mike Cook, Executive

Provides the clinical information necessary for proactive decision making.

3913 Oracle
4150 Network Circle
Santa Clara, CA 95054-1778
650-960-1300
800-633-0925
Fax: 650-786-4557
www.oracle.com

Gregory M Papadopoulos, Executive VP

Provider of healthcare software.

Year Founded: 1982

3914 Oracle Corporation
500 Oracle Parkway
Redwood Shores, CA 94065-1675
650-506-7000
800-392-2999
Fax: 650-506-7200
www.oracle.com

Lawrence J Ellison, Chief Executive Officer
Safra A. Catz, President and Chief Financial Of
Mark Hurd, President
Dorian Daley, Senior Vice President, General C

PeopleSoft provides a range of applications from traditional human resources, payroll and benefits to financials.

Year Founded: 1977

3915 Orion Healthcare Technology
18047 Oak Street
Omaha, NE 68130
402-341-8880
800-324-7966
Fax: 402-341-8911
E-mail: info@orionhealthcare.com
www.myaccucare.com

Bill Allan, Owner

Orion provides technology solutions to meet the ever changing needs of the healthcare industry. To accomodate the behavioral health field, Orion developed the AccuCare software system, a highly integrated and adaptive approach to the clinical practice environment. AccuCare enables clinicians to quickly realize value, effiency and standardization without disrupting their primary focus to provide excellence in health care.

3916 Parrot Software
PO Box 250755
W Bloomfield, MI 48325-755
248-788-3223
800-727-7681
Fax: 248-788-3224

E-mail: support@parrotsoftware.com
www.parrotsoftware.com

Provide 60 different software programs for the remediation of speech, cognitive, language, attention, and memory deficits seen in individuals who have suffered aphasia from stroke or head injury.

Year Founded: 1981

3917 Psychological Assessment Resources
16204 North Florida Avenue
Lutz, FL 33549-8119
813-449-4065
800-331-8378
Fax: 813-961-2196
www.www4.parinc.com

Robert Smith Iii, President

This program produces normative-based interpretive hypotheses based on your client's scores. It produces a profile of T scores, a listing of the associated raw and percentile scores, and interpretive hypotheses for each scale. Although this program is not designed to produce a finished clinical report, it allows you to integrate BRS and SRI data with other sources of information about your client. The report can be generated as a text file for editing.

Year Founded: 1978

3918 Psychological Software Services
3304 W 75th St
Indianapolis, IN 46268
317-257-9672
Fax: 317-257-9674
E-mail: nsc@netdirect.net
www.neuroscience.cnter.com

Comprehensive and easy-to-use multimedia cognitive rehabilitation software. Packages include 64 computerized therapy tasks with modifiable parameters that will accommodate most requirements. Exercises extend from simple attention and executive skills, through multiple modalities of visuospatial and memory skills. For clinical and educational use with head injury, stroke, LD/ADD and other brain compromises. Price range: $260-$2, 500.

Year Founded: 1984

3919 QuadraMed Corporation
12110 Sunset Hills Road
Suite 600
Reston, VA 20190-5852
703-709-2300
800-393-0278
Fax: 703-709-2490
E-mail: boardofdirectors@quadramed.com
www.quadramed.com

Daniel Desaulniers, CA, President, Harris Quebec Public
Jim Dowling, EVP, Enterprise Self-Service Sol
David L. Puckett, EVP, Revenue Cycle & Enterprise
Vicki Wheatley, EVP, Enterprise Master Person In

3920 RCF Information Systems
4200 Colonel Glenn Highway
Suite 100
Beavercreek, OH 45431-1670
937-427-5680
Fax: 937-427-5689
E-mail: administrator@rcfinfo.com
www.rcfinfo.com

Roger Harris, President

Healthcare software.

3921 Raintree Systems

28765 Single Oak Drive
Suite 200
Temecula, CA 92590
951-252-9400
800-333-1033
www.raintreeinc.com

Richard Welty, President/CTO

Provides practice management software for commerical, not-for-profit, government healthcare providers, rehabilitation facilities, and social service agencies.

Year Founded: 1983

3922 SPSS

233 S Wacker Drive
11th Floor
Chicago, IL 60606-6306
312-651-3000
800-543-2185
Fax: 312-651-3668
www.spss.com

Jack Noonan, CEO

Worldwide provider of predictive analytics software and solutions.

Year Founded: 1968

3923 Saner Software

4198 13th ST NW
Garrison, ND 58540
630-762-9440
Fax: 630-562-9443
E-mail: sales@sanersoftware.com
www.sanersoftware.com

John Parkinson, Owner

Develops health practice management software.

Year Founded: 1988

3924 Sanford Health

PO Box M.C
Fargo, ND 58122-1
701-234-2000
800-437-4010
www.www.sanfordhealth.org

Roger Gilbertson, CEO
Craig Hewitt, CIO

MeritCare is able to track your employees' health trends due to a new software program called Occusource.

3925 Stephens Systems Services

267 5th Avenue
Suite 812
New York, NY 10016-7506
212-545-7788
Fax: 212-545-9081
www.stephenssystems.com

Mike Stephens, Owner

Provides healthcare software.

3926 SumTime Software®

1152 Galvez Ct. SE
Los Lunas, NM 87031
505-990-8356
888-821-0771
Fax: 505-866-9041
E-mail: sumtime@sumtime.com
www.sumtime.com

Is the practice management solution for health care professionals. We offer the most comprehensive means for preparing billing statements and tracking payments and maintaining records.

3927 SunGard Pentamation

3 West Broad Street
Bethlehem, PA 18018-6799
610-691-3616
866-905-8989
www.pentamation.com

Provides secure and reliable K-12 student information systems, special education management, financial and human resource management software to school districts.

Year Founded: 1992

3928 Synergistic Office Solutions (SOS Software)

17445 E Apshawa Road
Clermont, FL 34715-9049
352-242-9100
Fax: 888-609-5514
E-mail: sales@sosoft.com
www.sosoft.com

Seth R Krieger, PhD, President

Produce patient management software for behavioral health service providers, including billing, scheduling and clinical records.

Year Founded: 1985

3929 Thomson ResearchSoft

1500 Spring Garden Street, Fourth Floor
Philadelphia, PA 19130
215-823-6600
800-722-1227
Fax: 215-386-6362
www.scientific.thomsonrueters.com

Software for wherever research is performed worldwide including all leading academic, corporate and government institutions, healthcare.

3930 TriZetto Group

9655 Maroon Circle
Englewood, CO 80112
949-718-4940
800-569-1222
Fax: 949-219-2197
E-mail: salesinfo@trizetto.com
www.trizetto.com

R. Andrew Eckert, CEO
Jude Dieterman, President/COO
Douglas E. Barnett, Chief Financial Officer
John Schaefer, Senior Vice President, Chief Leg

Focuses on the business of healthcare and offers a broad portfolio of technology products and services.

Year Founded: 1997

3931 Turbo-Doc EMR

6480 Pentz Rd.
Suite A
Paradise, CA 95969

530-877-8650
800-977-4868
Fax: 530-877-8621
E-mail: turbodoc@turbodoc.com
www.turbodoc.net

Lyle B Hunt, CEO

An electronic medical record system designed to assist physicians and other health care workers in completing medical record tasks.

3932 Vann Data Services
1801 Dunn Avenue
Daytona Beach, FL 32114-1250
386-310-1702
Fax: 386-238-1454
E-mail: sales@vanndata.com
www.vanndata.com

Janice Huffstickler, President

Healthcare practice software.

Year Founded: 1978

3933 Velocity Healthcare Informatics
8441 Wayzata Boulevard
Suite 105
Minneapolis, MN 55426-1349
800-844-5648
E-mail: info@velocity.com

Ellen B White, President/CEO

Provides outcomes management system.

3934 VersaForm Systems Corporation
2505 Carmel Ave
Suite 210
Brewster, NY 10509
800-448-6975
Fax: 845-207-3067
www.versaform.com

Electronic medical records and practice management.

3935 Virtual Software Systems
PO Box 815
Bethel Park, PA 15102-815
412-835-9417
Fax: 412-835-9419
E-mail: sales@vss3.com
www.vss3.com

Thomas Palmquist, Contact

Easy to use practice management, billing, and scheduling software. *$3500.00*

Information Services

3936 3m Health Information Systems
575 West Murray Boulevard
Salt Lake City, UT 84123-4611
801-265-4400
800-367-2447
Fax: 801-263-3657
www.solutions.3m.com

George W Buckley, CEO

3937 Accumedic Computer Systems
11 Grace Avenue
Suite 401
Great Neck, NY 11021-2427
516-466-6800
800-765-9300
Fax: 516-466-6880
E-mail: info@accumedic.com
www.accumedic.com

Mark Kollenscher, President

Practice management solutions for mental health facilities: scheduling, billing, EMR, HIPAA.

Year Founded: 1977

3938 American Institute for Preventive Medicine
30445 Northwestern Highway
Suite 350
Farmington Hills, MI 48334-3107
248-539-1800
800-345-2476
Fax: 248-539-1808
E-mail: aipm@healthylife.com
www.healthylife.com

Don R. Powell, Ph.D., President and CEO

Year Founded: 1983

3939 American Nurses Foundation: National Communications
8515 Georgia Avenue
Suite 400
Silver Spring, MD 20910-3492
301-628-5000
800-274-4262
Fax: 301-628-5001
E-mail: anf@ana.org
www.nursingworld.org

Karen Daley, PhD, RN, FAAN, President
Marla J. Weston, PhD, RN, FAAN, Chief Executive Officer
Cindy R. Balkstra, MS, RN, CNS-, First Vice President
Jennifer S. Mensik, PhD, RN, NEA-B, Second Vice President

3940 Arbour Health System-Human Resource Institute Hospital
227 Babcock Street
Brookline, MA 02446-6773
617-731-3200
www.www.arbourhealth.com

Gary Gilberti, CEO

3941 Arservices, Limited
5904 Richmond Highway
Suite 550
Alexandria, VA 22303
703-820-9000
Fax: 703-824-6438
E-mail: info@arslimited.com
www.arserviceslimited.com

Jerry (Jay) McCargo, President & CEO
Robert Mortis, Chief Operating Officer
Kevin Batchelor, Chief Financial Officer

3942 Association for Ambulatory Behavioral Healthcare
247 Douglas Ave
Portsmouth, VA 23707-1520
757-673-3741
Fax: 757-966-7734
E-mail: mickey@aabh.org
www.www.aabh.org

Mickey Wright, Executive Director
Christopher McGowan, President

Powerful forum for people engaged in providing mental health services. Promoting the evolution of flexible models of responsive cost-effective ambulatory behavioral healthcare.

3943 Behavioral Intervention Planning: Completing a Functional Behavioral Assessment and Developing a Behavioral Intervention Plan
Pro-Ed Publications
8700 Shoal Creek Boulevard
Austin, TX 78757-6897
512-451-3246
800-897-3202
Fax: 512-451-8542
E-mail: general@proedinc.com
www.www.proedinc.com

Donald D Hammill, Owner

Provides school personnel with all tools necessary to complete a functional behavioral assessment, determine whether a behavior is related to the disability of the student, and develop a behavioral intervention plan. *$22.00*

3944 Breining Institute College for the Advanced Study of Addictive Disorders
8894 Greenback Lane
Orangevale, CA 95662-4019
916-987-0662
Fax: 916-987-9384
E-mail: Suggestions@Breining.edu
www.breininginstitute.net

Kathy Breining, Administrator

3945 Brief Therapy Institute of Denver
7800 S. Elati Street
Suite 230
Littleton, CO 80120
303-426-8757
E-mail: tayers@btid.com
www.btid.com

Marne Wine, Therapist

Our form of psychotherapy emphasizes goals, active participation between therapist and client, client strengths, resources, resiliencies and accountability of the therapy process.

3946 Buckley Productions
238 E Blithedale Avenue
Mill Valley, CA 94941-2083
415-383-2009
877-508-3979
Fax: 415-383-5031
E-mail: buckleypro@aol.com
www.buckleyproductions.com

Richard Buckley, Owner

Alcohol and drug education handbooks, videos, and web-based products for safety sensitive employers, supervisiors and employees who are covered by the Department of Transportaion rules. We provide training materials for Substance Abuse Professional (SAPs) and urine collectors.

3947 CareCounsel
101 Lucas Valley Road
Suite 360
San Rafael, CA 94903
415-472-2366
888-227-3334
Fax: 415-507-1906
E-mail: staff@carecounsel.com
www.carecounsel.com

Lawrence N. Gelb, Founder, President & CEO

3948 Catholic Community Services of Western Washington
100 23rd Avenue S
Seattle, WA 98144-2302
206-328-5696
Fax: 206-324-4835
E-mail: info@ccsww.org
www.ccsww.org

Michael Reichert, President

3949 Center for Creative Living
2635 Walnut St
Denver, CO 80205
303-893-0552
Fax: 303-892-0507
E-mail: cclro@aol.com
www.centerforcreativeliving.com

Diane Braun, Owner

3950 Central Washington Comprehensive M/H
PO Box 959
402 S 4th Ave
Yakima, WA 98902-3546
509-575-4200
800-572-8122
Fax: 509-575-4811
E-mail: www.cwcmh.org

Rick Weaver, CEO

3951 Child Welfare Information Gateway
1250 Maryland Avenue, SW
8th Floor
Washington, DC 20024-2141
703-385-7565
800-394-3366
Fax: 703-385-3206
E-mail: info@childwelfare.gov
www.childwelfare.gov

The clearinghouse serves as a facilitator of information and knowledge exchange; the Children's Bureau and its training and technical assistant network; the child abuse and neglect, child welfare, and adoption communities; and allied agencies and professions.

3952 Cirrus Technology
403 Chris Drive
Building 4 Suite H
Huntsville, AL 35802

256-539-2241
Fax: 256-539-4266
E-mail: info@cirrusti.com
www.cirrusti.com

Jerry T Harris, President/CEO
Larry Waller, Vice President Finance
Judy Dunivant, Accounting Manager
Machisa Gaither, Humnan Resources

3953 Community Solutions
9015 Murray Avenue
Suite 100
Gilroy, CA 90520
408-842-7138
Fax: 408-778-9672
E-mail: cs@communitysolutions.org
www.communitysolutions.org

Greg Sellers, Chair
Janie Mardesich, Vice Chair
Nancy Miller, Secretary
Mike Thompson, Treasurer

3954 Consumer Health Information Corporation
8000 Wespark Drive
Suite 120
McLean, VA 22102-3661
703-734-0650
Fax: 703-734-1459
E-mail: info@consumre-health.com
www.consumer-health.com

Dorothy L Smith, President

Specialists in development of evidence-based patient education programs that increase patient safety & patient adherence.

Year Founded: 1983

3955 Control-O-Fax Corporation
3070 W Airline Highway
Waterloo, IA 50703-9591
319-234-4651
800-553-0070
Fax: 319-236-7332
E-mail: info@controlofax.com
www.controlofax.com

Ken Weber, Manager

3956 DCC/The Dependent Care Connection
500 Nyla Farms
Westport, CT 06880-6270
203-226-2680

3957 Dean Foundation for Health, Research and Education
2711 Allen Boulevard
Suite 300
Middleton, WI 53562-2287
608-250-1393
800-576-8773
www.www.deancare.com

Todd Burchill, Vice President of Strategy, Comm
Carolyn J Ogland, Vice President of Medical Affair
Steve R Caldwell, Vice President of Finance
W Gehren Rall, Vice President of Finance

The Dean Foundation is the non-profit research and education entity of DHS. The Foundation currently encompasses Dean's Educational Services Department, supports community service and health education projects, funds research grants, and conducts its own ancillary research including several outcomes management studies and computer-assisted, voice-activated programs for behavioral medicine.

3958 Dorland Healthcare Information
PO Box 25128
Salt Lake City, UT 84125-128
800-784-2332
Fax: 801-365-2300
E-mail: info@dorlandhealth.com
www.dorlandhealth.com

Carol Brault, Vice President
Yolanda Matthews, Product Manager
David J DeJulio, Account Executive
Anne Llewellyn, Editor in Chief

3959 FOCUS: Family Oriented Counseling Services
PO Box 921
1435 Hauck Drive
Rolla, MO 65401-2586
573-364-7551
800-356-5395
Fax: 573-364-4898
www.rollanet.org

3960 Federation of Families for Children's Mental Health
9605 Medical Center Drive
Suite 280
Rockville, MD 20850-6390
240-403-1901
Fax: 240-403-1909
E-mail: ffcmh@ffcmh.org
www.ffcmh.org

Sandra Spencer, Executive Director
Lizette Albright, Finance Director
Lynda Gargan, Senior Managing Director
Barbara Huff, Social Marketing

National family-run organization dedicated exclusively to children and adolesents with mental health needs and their families. Our voice speaks through our work in policy, training and technical assistance programs. Publishes a quarterly newsletter and sponsors an annual conference and exhibits.

3961 HSA-Mental Health
1080 Emeline Avenue
Santa Cruz, CA 95060-1966
831-454-4000
Fax: 831-454-4770
TDD: 831-454-2123
E-mail: info@santacruzhealth.org
www.santacruzhealth.org

Exists to protect and improve the health of the people in Santa Cruz County. Provides programs in environmental health, public health, medical care, substance abuse prevention and treatment, and mental health. Clients are entitled to information on the costs of care and their options for getting health insurance coverage through a variety of programs.

3962 Hagar and Associates
164 W Hospitality Lane
San Bernardino, CA 92408-3316

903-583-7202
www.hagarandassociates.com

Dennis Hagar, Owner
Matt Hager, Owner

Provides clients with data, from national databases, of outcomes, patient demographics, and benchmark data. Can provide technology and/or automated data connection. Provides support in objective outcomes measurement.

3963 Healthcheck
3954 Youngfield Street
Wheat Ridge, CO 80033-3865
916-556-1880
E-mail: msalvatore@hsf.ca
www.www.healthcheck.org

3964 INMED/MotherNet America
20110 Ashbook Place
Suite 260
Ashburn, VA 20147
703-729-4951
Fax: 703-858-7253
www.inmed.org

Paul c Bosland, Chairman
James R Rutherford, Treasurer
Wendy balter, Secretary
Linda Pfieffer, President

3965 Information Access Technology
1100 E 6600 S
Suite 300
Salt Lake City, UT 84121-7411
801-265-8800
800-574-8801
Fax: 801-265-8880
www.iat-cti.com

David H Rudd, CEO

3966 Lad Lake
PO Box 158
W350 S1401 Waterville Rd
Dousman, WI 53118-9020
262-965-2131
Fax: 262-965-4107
www.ladlake.org

Phil Zweig, President
Hon. Derek Mosley, Vice President
Sara Walker, Treasurer
john Mikkelson, Secretary

3967 Lanstat Incorporated
4663 Mason Street
Port Townsend, WA 98368
425-377-2540
800-672-3166
Fax: 425-334-3124
E-mail: info@lanstat.com
www.lanstat.com

Landon Kimbrough, President
Sherry Kimbrough, VP/Co-Founder

Provides quality technical assistance to behavioral health treatment agencies nationwide, including tribal and government agencies.

3968 Liberty Healthcare Management Group
401 E City Avenue
Suite 820
Bala Cynwyd, PA 19004
610-688-800
800-331-7122
E-mail: liberty@libertyhealth.com
www.www.libertyhealthcare.com

Liberty provides individualized programs and a continuum of services for psychiatric and substance abuse treatment at our centers located throughout the Northeast, Oklahoma and Florida. Liberty's commitment to medical excellence within an environment of results-oriented care is evident in our outstanding record of clinical success.

3969 Managed Care Local Market Overviews
Dorland Health
PO Box 25128
Salt Lake City, UT 84125-128
800-784-2332
Fax: 801-365-2300
E-mail: info@dorlandhealth.com
www.dorlandhealth.com

Carol Brault, Vice President
Yolanada Mathews, Product Manager
David DeJulio, Account Executive
Anne Llewellyn, Editor in Chief

Delivers valuable intelligence on local health and managed care marekts. Each of these 71 reports describes key market participants and competitive environment in one US market, including information on: local trends in events, key players, alliances among MCOs and providers, legislative developments, regulatory development, statistics on Managed Penetration. *$475.00*

3970 Manisses Communication Group
Manisses Communications Group
208 Governor Street
Providence, RI 02906-3246
401-831-6020
Fax: 401-861-6370
www.manisses.com

Fraser Lang, President/Publisher
Paul Newman, Director Of Sales

3971 Medical Data Research
5225 Wiley Post Way
Suite 500
Salt Lake City, UT 84116-2825
801-536-1110

Karen Beckstead, Contact

3972 Medipay
521 SW 11th Avenue
Suite 200
Portland, OR 97205-2620
503-227-6491

3973 Meridian Resource Corporation
1401 Enclave Parkway
Suite 300
Houston, TX 77077-2054
281-597-7000
Fax: 281-597-8880

Paul Ching, CEO

3974 Microsoft Corporation
1 Microsoft Way
Redmond, WA 98052-8300
425-882-8080
800-642-7676
Fax: 425-936-7329
www.microsoft.com

Steve Ballmer, CEO

3975 NASW West Virginia Chapter
750 First Street
Suite 700
Washinton, DC 20002-4241
304-345-6279
800-227-3590
E-mail: naswwv@aol.com
www.naswpress.org

Sam Hickman, Executive Director

3976 National Council on Alcoholism and Drug Dependence
217 Broadway
Suite 712
New York, NY 10007
212-269-7797
80 -22 -255
Fax: 212-269-7510
E-mail: national@ncadd.org
www.ncadd.org

William H Foster, President and CEO
Jayne Restivo, Director of Development
Leah Brock, Director of Affiliate Relations
Paul Warren, Executive Assistant

3977 National Families in Action
PO Box 133136
Atlanta, GA 30333-3136
404-248-9676
E-mail: nfia@nationalfamilies.org
www.nationalfamilies.org

William F Carter, Chairman
Sue Rusche, President/Chief Executive Office
Carol S Reeder, Treasurer
Paula C Kemp, Secretary

3978 National Mental Health Self-Help Clearinghouse
1211 Chestnut Street
Suite 1207
Philadelphia, PA 19107-4103
215-751-1810
800-553-4539
Fax: 215-636-6312
E-mail: info@mhselfhelp.org
www.mhselfhelp.org

Joseph Rogers, Executive Director
Susan Rogers, Director
Christa Burkett, Technical Assistance Coordinator
Britani Nestel, Program Specialist

3979 North Bay Center for Behavioral Medicine
1100 Trancas Street
Suite 244
Napa, CA 94558-2960
707-255-7786
www.behavioralmed.org

Frank Lucchetti, Psychologist

Represents comprehensive assessment and a balanced schedule of medical and/or psychological treatments for individuals with disabilities needing relief from chronic pain, disabling conditions and stress related to depression, anxiety, and unhealthy work, community or family conditions.

3980 On-Line Information Services
PO Box 1489
Winterville, NC 28590-1489
252-758-4141
800-765-8268
TDD: 866-630-6400
www.onlineinfoservices.com

3981 Open Minds
Behavioral Health Industry News
163 York Street
Gettysburg, PA 17325-1933
717-334-0538
877-350-6463
Fax: 717-334-0538
E-mail: openminds@openminds.com
www.openminds.com

Provides information on marketing, financial, and legal trends in the delivery of mental health and chemical dependency benefits and services. Recurring features include interviews, news of research, a calendar of events, job listings, book reviews, notices of publications available, and industry statistics. *$185.00*

12 pages 12 per year ISSN 1043-3880

3982 Optum
Mail Route MN010-S203
6300 Olson Memorial Highway
Golden Valley, MN 55427-4946
763-595-3200
800-788-4863
Fax: 763-595-3333

David Elton, Senior VP

A market leader in providing comprehensive information, education and support services that enhance quality of life through improved health and well-being. Through multiple access points-the telephone, audio tapes, print materials, in-person consultations and the Internet-Optum helps participants address daily living concerns, make appropriate health care decisions, and become more effective managers of their own health and well-being.

3983 Our Town Family Center
4131 E 5th Street
Tucson, AZ 85711
520-323-1706
Fax: 520-323-9077

Sue Eggleston, Executive Director

A general social services agency which focuses on serving children, youth, and their families. We offer low or no cost assistance with counseling, prevention, services for homeless youth and runaways (their families too) mediation, services for at risk youth, residential programs, parent mentoring, and much more. Our Town has made a conscious decision to keep its services focused in Pima County, in order to better serve our community. We are nonprofit, and funded by United Way, private donations, and grants with the state, county and city.

3984 Ovid Online
Ovid Technologies
333 7th Avenue
New York, NY 10001-5004
212-563-3006
800-950-2035
Fax: 212-674-6301
E-mail: sales@ovid.com
www.ovid.com

Karen Abramson, CEO

Online reference and database information provider.
$.50/record

3985 Patient Medical Records
901 Tahoka Road
Brownfield, TX 79316-3817
806-637-2556
800-285-7627

3986 Penelope Price
4281 MacDuff Pl
Dublin, OH 43016-9510
614-793-0165

3987 Physicians' ONLINE
560 White Plains Road
Tarrytown, NY 10591-5113
914-333-5800

3988 Quadramed
12110 Sunset Hills Road
Suite 600
Reston, VA 20190-5852
703-709-2300
800-393-0278
Fax: 703-709-2490
www.quadramed.com

Duncan W James, CEO

3989 SilverPlatter Information
100 River Ridge Drive
Suite 200
Norwood, MA 02062-5041
781-769-2599
Fax: 781-769-8763
www.www.silverplatter.info

3990 Stress Management Research Associates
10609-B Grant Road
Houston, TX 77070-4462
281-890-6395
E-mail: relax@stresscontrol.com
www.stresscontrol.com

Edward Charlesworth, Contact

3991 Supervised Lifestyles
2505 Carmel Ave
Suite 210
Brewster, NY 10509-1122
845-279-5639
888-822-7348
Fax: 845-279-7678
E-mail: sls@slshealth.com

3992 Technical Support Systems
775 E 3300 S
Suite 1
Salt Lake City, UT 84106-4078
801-484-1283
Fax: 801-486-8246
E-mail: wspelius@TssUtah.com
www.tssutah.com

Harry Heightman, Manager
Year Founded: 1984

3993 Traumatic Incident Reduction Association
5145 Pontiac Trail
Ann Arbor, MI 48105-9279
734-761-6268
800-499-2751
Fax: 734-663-6861
E-mail: info@tir.org
www.tir.org

Marian Volkman, President
Margaret Nelson, Vice-President
Frank A Gerbode, Developer of the Subject

Traumatic Incident Reduction is a brief, person-sentered
treatmetn for the affects of all sorts of trauma and loss. It is
part of the larger subject of Applied Metapsychology,
which addresses relationship, self-esteem and well-being
issues of all sorts, including traumatic stress. Additional
web site for TIR: www.tirbook.com

3994 UNISYS Corporation
8008 Westpark Drive
McLean, VA 22102-3109
703-847-2412
www.www.unisys.com

J Edward Coleman, Charman
Quincy Allen, Chuef Marketing And Strategy Off
Dominick Cavuoto, President
Janet B Haugen, Chief Financial Officer

3995 Virginia Beach Community Service Board
289 Independence Blvd
#138
Virginia Beach, VA 23462-5492
757-437-6150

3996 Well Mind Association
1201 Western Ave
Seattle, WA 98101-2936
206-728-9770
800-556-5829
Fax: 206-728-1500
www.speakeasy.net

Well Mind Association distributes information on current
research and promotes alternative therapies for mental illness and related disorders. WMA believes that physical
conditions and treatable biochemical imbalances are the
causes of many mental, emotional and behavioral
problems.

Pharmaceutical Companies

Manufacturers A-Z

3997 Abbott Laboratories
100 Abbott Park Road
Abbott Park, IL 60064-3500
847-937-6100
www.abbott.com

Miles D White, Chief Executive Officer
Wallace C Abbot, Founder

Founded in 1890. Manufactures the following psychological drugs: Cylert, Desoxyn, Depakote, Nembutal, Placidyl, Prosom, Tranxene.

3998 Actavis
400 Interpace Parkway
Parsippany, NJ 07054
862-261-7000
www.www.watson.com

Paul M Bisaro, CEO

Manufactures the following medications: Ferrlecit, Quasense, Androderm, Nicotine Polacrilex Gum USP, Trelstar, Oxycodone and Acetaminophen Tablets USP, Oxytrol.

3999 Astra Zeneca Pharmaceuticals
1800 Concord Pike
PO Box 15437
Wilmington, DE 19850-5437
302-886-3000
Fax: 302-886-3119
www.astrazeneca-us.com

David Brennan, Executive Director, CEO
Simon Lowth, Chief Financial Officer
Tony Zook, EVP, Global Commercial
Martin McKay, President

Full range of products in six therapeutic areas; gastrointestinal, oncology, anesthesia, cardiovascular, central nervous system and respiratory.

4000 Bristol-Myers Squibb
345 Park Avenue
New York, NY 10154-28
212-546-4000
Fax: 212-546-4020
E-mail: info@bsm.com
www.bms.com

Lamberto Andreotti, Chief Executive Officer
Charles Bancroft, EVP, Chief Financial Officer
Brian Daniels MD, Senior Vice President
Sandra Leung, General Counsel, Corp Secretary

Manufactures the following psychological drugs: Avapro, Enfamil, Abilify, Provachol, and Serzone.

4001 Cephalon
41 Moores Road
Frazer, PA 19355-1113
610-344-0200
Fax: 610-738-6590
E-mail: humanresources@cephalon.com
www.cephalon.com

Frank Baldino Jr, CEO
Frank Baldino, Chairman/CEO

Manufactures the following pharmaceuticals: Provigil, Amrix, Fentora, Vivitrol, Trisenox, Nuvigil.

4002 Edgemont Pharmaceuticals, LLC
1250 Capital of Texas
Site 400
Austin, TX 78746
512-550-8555
888-594-4332
Fax: 512-329-2094
E-mail: customerservice@edgemontpharma.com
www.edgemontpharma.com

Douglas A Saltel, President & CEO

Manufactures Fluoxetine 60 mg tablets

4003 Eli Lilly and Company
Lilly Corporate Center
Indianapolis, IN 46285
317-276-2000
www.lilly.com

John C Lechleiter, Chairman, President & CEO
Ralph Alvarez, Executive Chairman
Katherine Baicker, Professor of Health Economics
Sir Winfried Bischoff, Chairman

Manufactures the following psychological drugs: Prozac, Ceclor, Zyprexa, Cialis, Strattera, and Symbyax.

4004 Forest Laboratories
909 Third Avenue
New York, NY 10022-4748
212-421-7850
800-947-5227
Fax: 212-750-9152
www.frx.com

Howard Solomon, Chairman, CEO

Manufactures the following psychological drugs: Lexapro, Benicar, Campral, Celexa, Namenda, Tiazac, and Viibryd.

4005 GlaxoSmithKline
5 Moore Drive
PO Box 13398
Research Triangle Park, NC 27709-3398
888-825-5249
Fax: 919-483-5249
www.gsk.com

JP Garnier, CEO

Manufactures the following psychological drugs: Lamictal, Paxil, Parnate, Zyban.

4006 Janssen
1125 Trenton-Harbourton Road
PO Box 200
Titusville, NJ 08560-1002
609-730-2000
800-526-7736
www.janssen.com

Timothy Cost, Senior VP Corporate Affairs

Janssen markets prescription medications for the treatment of schizophrenia and bipolar disorder. Medications include: Invega and Risperdal.

4007 Jazz Pharmaceuticals plc
3180 Porter Drive
Palo Alto, CA 94304

650-496-3777
Fax: 650-496-3781
www.jazzpharma.com

Bruce C Cozadd, Chairman & CEO
Robert M Myers, President
Matthew Young, SVP & Chief Financial Officer
Russell J Cox, Executive Vice President & Chief

Manufactures the following medications: Xyrem, Prialt, FazaClo, LuvoxCR

4008 Johnson & Johnson

One Johnson & Johnson Plaza
New Brunswick, NJ 08933-1
732-524-0400
www.jnj.com

William C Weldon, CEO

Manufactures the following: Concerta, Haldol, Reminyl, Daktarin, Ertaczo, Levaquin.

4009 King Pharmaceuticals

132 Windsor Road
Tenafly, NJ 07670
423-989-8000
800-776-7637
Fax: 972-9 8-5 09
E-mail: comments@king-pharma.com
www.king-pharma.com

Brian A Markison, CEO
David Robinson, Senior Dir. Corporate Affairs

Manufactures some of the following medications: Sonata, Corgard, Cytomel, Humatin, Levoxyl, Procanbid, and Septra.

4010 Mallinckrodt

675 McDonnell Boulevard
St. Louis, MO 63042-2379
314-654-2000
www.www.mallinckrodt.com

Mark Trudeau, President & CEO
Matthew Harbaugh, Senior Vice President & CFO
Peter Edwards, Senior Vice President & General
Dr. Frank Scholz, Senior Vice President, Global Op

Manufactures the following psychological drugs: Dexe-drine, Methylin, Anafranil and Restoril for insomnia.

4011 Merck & Co.

One Merck Drive
PO Box 100
Whitehouse Station, NJ 08889-0100
908-423-1000
www.merck.com

Kenenth C Frazier, Chair, President & CEO
Willie A Deese, EVP & President
Leslie A Brun, Chairman & CEO

Manufactures the following drugs: Remeron™ and Saphris

4012 Mylan

1000 Mylan Blvd
Canonsburg, PA 15317
724-514-1800
www.mylan.com

Robert J Coury, Chairman & CEO
Heather Bresch, Chief Executive Officer
Rajiv Malik, President
John D Sheehan, Chief Financial Officer

Manufactures the following psychological drugs: Ativan, BuSpar, Clonopin, Tranxene, Valium, Xanax, Xanax XR

4013 Novartis

400 Technology Square
Cambridge, MA 02139-3545
617-871-8000
Fax: 617-871-8911
www.novartis.com

Joerg Reinhardt, Chairman
Ulrich Lehner, Vice Chairman
Enrico Vanni, Vice Chairman
Joseph Jimenez, Chief Executive Officer

Manufactures the following products: Diovan, Glivec, Lamisil, Zometa, Focalin and more.

4014 Noven Pharmaceuticals

Empire State Building
350 Fifth Avenue, 37th Floor
New York, NY 10118
212-682-4420
www.www.noven.com

Kazuhide Nakatomi, Chairman
Takehiko Noda, Vice Chairman
Jeffrey F Eisenberg, Director

Manufactures the following mood disorder drugs: Daytrana, Stravzor, Pexeva, Lithobid

4015 Ortho-McNeil Pharmaceutical

1125 Trenton Harbourton Road
PO Box 200
Titusville, NJ 08560-1002
800-526-7736
www.www.janssenpharmaceuticalsinc.com

Manufactures the following: Elmiron, Modicon, Ortho-Novum, and Terazol 3.

4016 Pfizer

235 E 42nd Street
New York, NY 10017-5703
212-573-2323
800-879-3477
www.pfizer.com

Ian C Read, Chairman & CEO
Frank D Amello, Executive VP & CFO
Rady Johnson, Executive VP & Chief Compliance
Doug Lankler, Executive VP, General Councel

Manufactures the following psychological drugs: Geodon, Halcion, Navane, Navane IM, Neurontin, Reboxetine, Relpax, Sinequan, Vistaril, Xanax, Zoloft.

4017 Purdue

1 Stamford Forum
201 Tresser Boulevard
Stamford, CT 06901-3431
203-588-8000
800-877-5666
Fax: 203-588-8850
www.purduepharma.com

Mark Timney, President & CEO
Stuart D Baker, EVP, Counsel to Board
Edward B Mahony, EVP & CFO
David Long, Senior Vice President

Manufactures the following drugs: Betadine, Betasept, Butrans, Colace, Dilaudid, Dilaudid-HP, Intermezzo, MS

Contin Tablets, Oxycontin, OxyIR, Peri-Colace, Ryzolt, Senokot, SenokotXTRA, Slow-Mag

4018 Roxane Laboratories

1809 Wilson Road
PO Box 16532
Columbus, OH 43216-6532
614-276-4000
800-962-8364
Fax: 614-308-3540
www.www.roxane.com

Manufactures detoxification medication: Dolophine.

4019 Sanofi-Aventis

55 Corporate Drive
Bridgewater, NJ 08807-1265
908-981-5000
800-981-2491
Fax: 908-231-4744
www.www.sanofi.us

Thomas Zerzan, President
Gregory Irace, Senior Vice President
David Meeker, Chief Executive Officer

Manufacturer of medication for cardiovascular disease, thrombosis, oncology, diabetes, central nervous system, internal medicine, and vaccines. Medication includes Wellbutrin, Wellbutrin SR, and Wellbutrin XL.

4020 Sepracor Pharmaceuticals

84 Waterford Drive
Marlborough, MA 01752-7010
508-481-6700
800-586-3782
Fax: 508-357-7491
E-mail: info@sepracor.com
www.www.sunovion.com

Hiroshi Nomura, Vice Chair, EVP, CFO
Anthony Loebel, MD, EVP and Chief Medical Officer
Albert P Parker, EVP, General Councel & Corporate
Richard Russell, EVP and Chief Commercial Officer

Manufactures sleep disorder drug Lunesta, as well as other medications Xopenex, and Brovana.

4021 Shire Richwood

5 Riverwalk
City West Business Campus
Dublin, PA 19087-5649
484-595-8800
Fax: 484-595-8200
www.www.shire.com

Matthew Emmens, Chairman
Flemming Ornskov, Chief Executive Officer
James Bowling, Interim Financial Officer

Manufactures the following psychological drugs: Adderall, DextroStat.

4022 Solvay Pharmaceuticals

901 Sawyer Road
Marietta, GA 30062-2250
770-578-9000
Fax: 770-578-5597
www.www.solvay.com

Jean-Pierre Clamadieu, Chairman & CEO
Karim Hajjar, Chief Fianancial Officer
Michael Defourny, General Manager Communications

Manufactures the following psychological drugs: Klonopin, Lithobid, Lithonate.

4023 Sunovion Pharmaceuticals

84 Waterford Drive
Marlborough, MA 01752
508-481-6700
888-394-7377
Fax: 508-357-7491
E-mail: info@sunovion.com
www.sunovion.com

Hiroshi Nomura, Vice Chair, EVP, CFO
Anthony Loebel, MD, EVP and Chief Medical Officer
Albert P Parker, EVP, General Councel & Corporate
Richard Russell, EVP and Chief Commercial Officer

Manufactures the following drugs: Lunesta, Latuda

4024 Synthon Pharmaceuticals

9000 Development Drive
PO Box 110487
Research Triange, NC 27709-5487
919-493-6006
Fax: 919-493-6104
E-mail: info@synthon.com
www.www.synthon.com

Develops, produces and sells high quality alternatives to innovative medicines. Our products are marketed at the earliest possible opportunity and we sell them at competitive prices.

4025 Takeda Pharmaceuticals North America

One Takeda Parkway
Deerfield, IL 60015-5713
224-554-6500
877-582-5332
Fax: 847-383-3080
E-mail: openpayments@takeda.com
www.www.takeda.us

Shinji Honda, CEO

Manufacturer of Rozerem, Duetact, Amitiza, and Actos.

4026 Valeant Pharmaceuticals International

2150 St. Elzear Blvd.
West Laval
Quebec, CA H7l4A
514-744-6792
800-361-1448
Fax: 514-744-6272
www.valeant.com

J Michael Pearson, Chairman & CEO
G. Mason Morfit, Partner
Dr. Pavel Mirovsky, President & General Manager
Fred Hasan, Partnr & Managing Director

Develops, manufactures and markets pharmaceutical products primarily in the areas of neurology, dermatology and infectious disease.

4027 Validus Pharmaceuticals

119 Cherry Hill Road
Suite 310
Parsippany, NJ 07054
973-265-2777
Fax: 973-265-2770
E-mail: jhunter@validuspharma.com
www.validuspharma.com

James R Hunter, President
Lee Rios, Chief Operating Officer
Richard Post, Vice President - Sales and Marke

Manufactures the following psychological drugs: Marplan, Equetro.

4028 Warner Chilcott
400 Interpace Parkway
Parsippany, NJ 07054
862-261-7488
800-521-8813
Fax: 973-442-3204
E-mail: investor.relations@actavis.com
www.wcrx.com

Manufactures Sarafem

Drugs A-Z

4029 Abilify
Generic: aripiprazole

Used in the treatment of psychotic disorders and bipolar disorder. This product is manufactured by Bristol-Myers Squibb and Otsuka. See manufacturers section for company information.

4030 Adderall/Adderall XR
Generic: amphetamine/dextroamphetamine

Used to manage anxiety disorders and some cases of attention deficit hyperactivity disorder. This product is manufactured by Shire Richwood. See Manufacturers section for company information.

4031 Antabuse
Generic: disulfiram

Used in the treatment of alcohol and substance abuse. This product is manufactured by Wyeth-Ayers. See Manufacturers section for company information.

4032 Aricept
Generic: donepezil

Used in the treatment of Alzheimer's disease. This product is manufactured by and Eisai. See Manufacturers section for company information.

4033 Asenapine
Generic: saphris

Sublingual tablets used in the treatment for schizophreina. Manufactured by Schering-Plough. See Manufacturers section for company information.

4034 Ativan
Generic: lorazepam

Used in the treatment of anxiety and as a preanesthetic medication in adults. This product is manufactured by Wyeth. See Manufacturers section for company information.

4035 Celexa
Generic: citalopram

Used in the treatment of depression. This product is manufactured by Forest Laboratories. See Manufacturers section for company information.

4036 Clozaril
Generic: clozapine

Used in the treatment of severe schizophrenia, and also sold as Clozaril and Fazaclo. This product is manufactured by Novartis. See Manufacturers section for company information.

4037 Cymbalta
Generic: dulozetine

Used in the treatment of depression. Manufactured by Eli Lilly and Company. See Manufacturers section for company information.

4038 Daytrana
Generic: methyphenidate transdermal system

Used in the treatment of ADHD in children 6-17 years old. This product is manufactured by Noven Pharmaceuticals. See Manufacturers section for company information.

4039 Depakote
Generic: valproic acid

Used in the treatment of manic episodes associated with bipolar disorder and mania, and also sold as Depakene. This product is manufactured by Abbott Laboratories. See Manufacturers section for company information.

4040 Desoxyn
Generic: methamphetamine

Used in the treatment of attention deficit hyperactivity disorder. This product is manufactured by Abbott Laboratories. See Manufacturers section for company information.

4041 Desyrel
Generic: trazodone hcl

Used in the treatment of major depressive disorder. This product is manufactured by Labopharm Europe Limited. See manufacturers section for company information.

4042 Dexedrine
Generic: dextroamphetamine

Used in the treatment of attention deficit hyperactivity disorder, and also sold as DextroState, Focalin (by Novartis), Metadate, and Methylin. This product is manufactured by Mallinckrodt. See Manufacturers section for company information.

4043 Effexor
Generic: venlafazine

Used in the treatment of depression and generalized anxiety disorder. This product is manufactured by Wyeth-Ayerst Laboratories. See Manufacturers section for company information.

4044 Elavil
Generic: amitryptiline

Used in the treatment of depression, also sold as Limbitrol (by Valeant). This product is manufactured by Astra Zeneca Pharmaceuticals. See Manufacturers section for company information.

4045 Emsam
Generic: selegiline

Used in the treatment of major depressive disorder. This product is manufactured by Bristol-Myers Squibb. See manufacturers section for company information.

4046 Eskalith
Generic: lithium

Used in the treatment of bipolar disorder. This product is manufactured by GlaxoSmithKline. See Manufacturers section for company information.

4047 Exelon
Generic: rivastigmine

Used in the treatment of Alzheimer's disease. This product is manufactured by Novartis. See Manufacturers section for company information.

4048 FazaClo
Generic: clozapine, USP

Used in the treatment of Schizophrenia. This product is manufactured by Jazz Pharmaceuticals plc. See Manufacturers section for company information.

4049 Fluoxetine Tablets, 60 mg

Used in the treatment of Major Depressive Disorder, Obsessive Compulsive Disorder in adults and pediatrics and Bulimia Nervosa and Panic Disorder is adults. This product is manufactured by Edgemont Pharmaceuticals. See Manufacturers section for company information.

4050 Focalin/Focalin XR
Generic: dexmethylphenidate

Used in the treatment of attention deficit hyperactivity disorder. This product is manufactured by Novartis. See Manufacturers section for company information.

4051 Haldol
Generic: haloperidol

Used in the treatment of Schizophrenia. This product is manufactured by Johnson & Johnson. See manufacturers section for company information.

4052 Intermezzo
Generic: zolpidem

Used in the treatment of insomnia. This product is manufactured by Purdue/Transcept. See Manufacturers section for company information.

4053 Invega
Generic: paliperidone

Used in the treatment of Schizophrenia. This product is manufactured by Janssen. See manufacturers section for company information.

4054 Klonopin
Generic: clonazepam

Used in the treatment of panic attacks/anxiety. This product is manufactured by Hoffman-La Roche. See Manufacturers section for company information.

4055 Lamictal
Generic: lamotrigine

Used in the treatment of bipolar disorder. This product is manufactured by GlaxoSmithKline. See Manufacturers section for company information.

4056 Latuda
Generic: lurasidone hcl

Used in the treatment of schizophrenia. This product is manufactured by Sunovion. See manufacturers section for company information.

4057 Lexapro
Generic: escitalopram

Used in the treatment of depression. This product is manufactured by Forest Laboratories. See Manufacturers section for company information.

4058 Lithobid
Generic: lithium carbonate

Used in the treatment of bipolar disorder and depression. This product is manufactured by Noven Pharmaceuticals. See Manufacturers section for company information.

4059 Lunesta
Generic: eszopiclone

Used in the treatment of insomnia. This product is manufactured by Sunovion Pharmaceuticals. See Manufacturers section for company information.

4060 Namenda
Generic: memantine

Used in the treatment of dementia. This product is manufactured by Forest Pharmaceuticals. See Manufacturers section for company information.

4061 Neurontin
Generic: gabapentin

Used in the treatment of seizures and neuropathic pais. This product is manufactured by Pfizer. See Manufacturers section for company information.

4062 Niravam
Generic: alprazolam

Used in the treatment of anxiety. This product is manufactured by Jazz Pharmaceuticals plc. See Manufacturers section for company information.

4063 Parnate
Generic: tranylcypromine

Used to help manage depression. This product is manufactured by GlaxoSmithKline. See Manufacturers section for company information.

4064 Paxil
Generic: paroxetine hcl

Used in the treatment of depression, and anxiety disorders. This product is manufactured by GlaxoSmithKline. Sold also as Pexeva by Synthon. See Manufacturers section for company information.

4065 Pexeva
Generic: paroxetine mesylate

Used in the treatment of depression, and anxiety disorders. This product is manufactured by Noven Pharmaceuticals. See Manufacturers section for company information.

4066 Pristiq
Generic: Desvenlafaxine

Used in the treatment of depression. Manufacturered by Pfizer. See Manufacturers section for company information.

4067 Prozac
Generic: fluozetine

Used in the treatment of depression and anxiety disorders. This product is manufactured by Eli Lilly and Company. See Manufacturers section for company information.

4068 Relpax
Generic: eletriptan

Used in the treatment of migraines. This product is manufactured by Pfizer. See Manufacturers section for company information.

4069 Remeron
Generic: mirtazapine

Used in the treatment of suicidality and depression. This product is manufactured by Merck & Co. See Manufacturers section for company information.

4070 Restoril
Generic: temazepam

Used in the treatment of insomnia. This product is manufactured by Mallinckrodt Pharmaceuticals Group. See manufacturers section for company information.

4071 Risperdal
Generic: risperidone

Used in the treatment of schizophrenia and other mental illnesses such as psychosis. This product is manufactured by Janssen. See Manufacturers section for company information.

4072 Ritalin
Generic: methylphenidate

Used in the treatment of attention deficit hyperactivity disorders and in some forms of narcolepsy. This product is manufactured by Novartis. See Manufacturers section for company information.

4073 Rozerem
Generic: ramelteon

Used in the treatment of insomnia. This product is manufactured by Takeda Pharmaceuticals. See Manufacturers section for company information.

4074 Saphris
Generic: asenapine

Used in the treatment of Schizophrenia and Bipolar Mania. This product is manufactured by Merck & Co. See Manufacturers section for company information.

4075 Sarafem
Generic: fluoxetine

Used in the treatment of premenstrual dysphoric disorder. This product is manufactured by Warner Chilcott. See Manufacturers section for company information.

4076 Stavzor
Generic: valproic acid

Used in the treatment of bipolar disorder. This product is manufactured by Noven Pharmaceuticals. See Manufacturers section for company information.

4077 Strattera
Generic: atomoxetine

Used in the treatment of attention deficit disorder. This product is manufactured by Eli Lilly & Company. See Manufacturers section for company information.

4078 Valium
Generic: diazepam

Used in the treatment of anxiety. This product is manufactured by Hoffman-La Roche. See Manufacturers section for company information.

4079 Viibryd
Generic: vilazodone HCI

Used in the treatment of depression. This product is manufactured by Forest Pharmacueticals. See manufacturers section for company information.

4080 Vyvanse
Generic: lixdexamfetamine

Used in the treatment of attention deficit hyperactivity disorder. This product is manufactured by Shire Richwood. See Manufacturers section for company information.

4081 Wellbutrin, Wellbutrin SR, Wellbutrin XL
Generic: bupropion

Used in the treatment of depression. This product is manufactured by Sanofi-Aventis. See Manufacturers section for company information.

4082 Xanax
Generic: alprazolam

Used in the treatment of anxiety. This product is manufactured by Pfizer. See Manufacturers section for company information.

4083 Xyrem
Generic: sodium oxybate

Used in the treatment of narcolepsy. This product is manufactured by Jazz Pharmaceuticals. See Manufacturers section for company information.

4084 Zoloft
Generic: sertraline

Used in the treatment of depression and anxiety disorders. This product is manufactured by Pfizer. See Manufacturers section for company information.

4085 Zyban
Generic: bupropion

Used in the treatment of depression. This product is manufactured by GlaxoSmithKline. See Manufacturers section
for company information.

ADHD

Adjustment Disorders

Alcohol/Substance Abuse & Dependence

Anxiety Disorders

Autism Spectrum Disorders

Personality Disorders

Post-Traumatic Stress Disorder

Professional & Support Services

Psychosomatic (Somatizing) Disorders

Schizophrenia

E

Informix Software, 3887

Infotrieve Medline Services Provider, 3245

Inhealth Record Systems, 3888

Inner Health Incorporated, 3204

Inner Life of Children with Special Needs, 637

Innovations in Clinical Practice: Source Book - Volumes 4-20, 3343

Innovative Approaches for Difficult to Treat Populations, 1386, 2548

Innovative Data Solutions, 3889

Inside Recovery: How the Twelve Step Program Can Work for You, 121

Inside a Support Group: Help for Teenage Children of Alcoholics, 122

Insider, 2966

Insider's Guide to Mental Health Resources Online, 2549

Insights in the Dynamic Psychotherapy of Anorexia and Bulimia, 912

Insomnia, 1495

Instant Psychopharmacology, 2550

Institute for Behavioral Healthcare, 3122

Institute for Contemporary Psychotherapy, 1327

Institute for Social Research Indiana University, 2168

Institute of HeartMath, 2404

Institute of Living- Anxiety Disorders Center; Center for Cognitive Behavioral Therapy, 1761

The Institute of Living/Hartford Hospital, 1761

Institute on Psychiatric Services: American Psychiatric Association, 2405

Institute on Violence, Abuse and Trauma at Alliant International University, 1762

Insurance Management Institute, 3773

Integrated Business Services, 3890

Integrated Research Services, 183

Integrated Treatment of Psychiatric Disorders, 2551

Integrating Psychotherapy and Pharmacotherapy: Disolving the Mind-Brain Barrier, 2552

Integrative Brief Therapy: Cognitive, Psychodynamic, Humanistic & Neurobehavioral Approaches, 2553

Integrative Treatment of Anxiety Disorders, 321, 2717

InteliHealth, 3246

Interdesciplinary Council on Development and Learning Disorders, 341

Interdisciplinary Council on Development & Learning Disorders, 1091

Interface EAP, 3774

Interlink Health Services, 3775

Intermezzo, 4052

Intermountain Healthcare, 3776

International Association of Eating Disorders Professionals Foundation, 868

International Center for the Study of Psychiatry And Psychology (ISCPP), 2406

International Critical Incident Stress Foundation, 263, 425, 1314

International Drug Therapy Newsletter, 3000

International Foundation of Employee Benefit Plans, 2988

International Handbook on Mental Health Policy, 2554

International Journal of Aging and Human Developments, 3002

International Journal of Health Services, 3003

International Journal of Neuropsychopharmacology, 3001

International Journal of Psychiatry in Medicine, 3004

International Medical News Group, 2980

International OCD Foundation, 404, 412

International Obsessive Compulsive Disorder Foundation, 264

International Society for Developmental Psychobiology, 2407

International Society for Traumatic Stress Studies, 265, 1279

International Society for the Study of Dissociation, 858

International Society for the Study of Trauma And Dissociation, 826

International Society of Political Psychology, 2408

International Society of Psychiatric-Mental Health Nurses, 1763

International Transactional Analysis Association (ITAA), 2409

Internet Mental Health, 240, 429, 782, 1214, 1268, 1315, 1359, 1429, 1454, 1502, 1547

Interpersonal Psychotherapy, 2555, 2782, 2927

Interventions for Students with Emotional Disorders, 2884

Interview with Dr. Pauline Filipek, 703

Interviewing Children and Adolesents: Skills and Strategies for Effective DSM-IV Diagnosis, 2885

Interviewing the Sexually Abused Child, 1444, 2886

Intl Association for the Study of Pain, 1481

Intl Universities Pr Inc, 1205

Introduction to Depression and Bipolar Disorder, 1122

Introduction to Time: Limited Group Psychotherapy, 2556

Introduction to the Technique of Psychotherapy: Practice Guidelines for Psychotherapists, 2557

Invega, 4053

Iowa Department Human Services, 2169

Iowa Department of Public Health, 2170

Iowa Department of Public Health: Division of Substance Abuse, 2171

Iowa Division of Mental Health & Developmental Disabilities: Department of Human Services, 2172

Iowa Federation of Families for Children's Mental Health, 1884

Is Your Child Hyperactive? Inattentive? Impulsive? Distractible?, 510

It's Not All In Your Head: Now Women Can Discover the Real Causes of their Most Misdiagnosed Health Problems, 322

J

Jacobs Institute of Women's Health, 3123

Jail Detainees with Co-Occurring Mental Health and Substance Use Disorders, 2672

Janssen, 4006

Jason Aronson, 912, 1253, 1338, 1395

Jason Aronson Publishing, 1400

Jason Aronson, Inc.- Rowman Littlefield Imprint, 1354

Jason Aronson-Rowman & Littlefield Publishers, 359

The Jason Foundation, Inc., 1672, 1709

Jazz Pharmaceuticals plc, 4007

Jean Piaget Society: Society for the Study of Knowledge and Development (JPSSSKD), 2410

Jeri Davis International, 3777

Jerome M Sattler, 2863

Jerome M Sattler Publisher, 3385

Jessica Kingsley, 2649

Jessica Kingsley Publishers, 607, 613, 1532

Jewish Alcoholics Chemically Dependent Persons, 237

Jewish Family Service, 3451

Jewish Family Service of Atlantic and Cape May Counties, 1951

Jewish Family Service of Dallas, 2014

Jewish Family Service of San Antonio, 2015

Jewish Family and Children's Services, 1912, 3646

Jim Chandler MD, 1179

Joey and Sam, 638

Joh Wiley & Sons, 2481

John A Burns School of Medicine Department of Psychiatry, 3124

John Hopkins University School of Medicine, 1139

John L. Gildner Regional Institute for Children and Adolescents, 3521

John R Day and Associates, 3486

John Wiley & Sons, 3386, 283, 352, 765, 845, 888, 973, 975, 1079, 1234, 1246, 1300, 1443, 1534, 2470, 2486, 2502, 2505, 2520, 2522, 2525

John Wiley & Sons, Inc., 3387

John Wiley and Sons, 1057

Johns Hopkins University Press, 3388, 649, 759, 1069, 2750

Johnson & Johnson, 4008

Join Together, 235

Join Together Online, 195

Joint Commission on Accreditation of Healthcare Organizations, 2295

Jones & Bartlett, 338

Jones & Bartlett Learning, 1231

Jones and Bartlett Publishers, 277

Jones and Bartlett Publishers, Inc., 1470

Jossey-Bass, 111

Jossey-Bass / John Wiley & Sons, 1407

Jossey-Bass / Wiley & Sons, 102, 103, 118, 123, 124, 127, 128, 141, 1679, 1680

Jossey-Bass Publishers, 148, 889, 920, 2482, 2488, 2494, 2529, 2539, 2543, 2616, 2632, 2635, 2645, 2745, 2773, 2806, 3082

Jossey-Bass/Wiley, 340

Journal of AHIMA, 3005

Journal of American Health Information Management Association, 3006

Journal of American Medical Information Association, 3007

Journal of Anxiety Disorders, 390

Journal of Autism and Developmental Disorders, 684

Journal of Drug Education, 3008

Journal of Education Psychology, 3009

Journal of Emotional and Behavioral Disorders, 3010

Journal of Intellectual & Development Disability, 3011

Journal of Mental Health Research, 27

Journal of Neuropsychiatry and Clinical Neurosciences, 3012

Journal of Personality Assessment, 3013

Journal of Positive Behavior Interventions, 3014

Journal of Practical Psychiatry, 3015

Journal of Professional Counseling: Practice, Theory & Research, 3016

Journal of Substance Abuse Treatment, 178

Journal of the American Medical Informatics Association, 3017

Journal of the American Psychiatric Nurses Association, 3018

Journal of the American Psychoanalytic Association, 3019

Journal of the International Neuropsychological Society, 3020

A Journey Together, 26

Judge Baker Children's Center, 1764

Julia Dyckman Andrus Memorial, 3097

Just a Mood...or Something Else, 3263

Juvenile Justice Commission, 2226

K

KAI Research, Inc., 3778

KY-SPIN, 1890

Kansas Council on Developmental Disabilities Kansas Department of Social and Rehabilitation Services, 2173

Kay Redfield Jamison: Surviving Bipolar Disorder, 1163

Keane Care, 3891

Kennedy Krieger Institute, 3522

The Kennion Group Inc, 3823

Kentucky Alliance for the Mentally Ill, 1891

Kentucky Cabinet for Health and Human Services, 2174

Kentucky Department of Mental Health and Mental Retardation, 2175

Kentucky Justice Cabinet: Department of Juvenile Justice, 2176

Kentucky Partnership for Families and Children, 1892

Kentucky Psychiatric Association, 1893
Kerrville State Hospital, 3647
Key, 3021
Keys To Recovery, 3487
Keys for Networking: Kansas Parent Information & Resource Center, 1887
Keys to Parenting the Child with Autism, 639
Kicking Addictive Habits Once & for All: A Relapse Prevention Guide, Revised, 123
Kid Power Tactics for Dealing with Depression, 1595
KidsHealth, 1539, 1610
KidsPeace, 984
Kidspeace National Centers, 1613
King Pharmaceuticals, 4009
Kingsboro Psychiatric Center, 3576
Kirby Forensic Psychiatric Center, 3577
Kleptomaniacs Anonymous, 1013
Klingberg Family Centers, 3452
Klonopin, 4054
Kluwer Academic/Plenum Publishers, 346, 641, 655, 2668
Knopf Publishing Group, 1678
Know Your Rights: Mental Health Private Practice & the Law, 3205
Kristy and the Secret of Susan, 640

L

LSD: Still With Us After All These Years: Based on the National Institute of Drug Abuse Studies on the Resurgence of Contemporary, 124
La Hacienda Treatment Center, 3648
Lad Lake, 3966
Lake Area Youth Services Bureau, 2194
Lake Regional Health System, 3779
Lakeshore Mental Health Institute, 3633
Lamictal, 4055
Langley Porter Psych Institute at UCSF Parnassus Campus, 3125
Languages of Psychoanalysis, 2558
Lanstat Incorporated, 2296, 3967
Larkin Center, 1878
Latuda, 4056
Laurel Ridge Treatment Center, 3649
Laurelwood Hospital and Counseling Centers, 3126
Lawrence Erlbaum Associates, 897, 2721
Leadership and Organizational Excellence, 2559
Learning Disabilities Association of America, 454, 1765, 537
Learning Disabilities: A Multidisciplinary Journal, 537
Learning Disorders and Disorders of the Self in Children and Adolescents, 2887
Learning and Cognition in Autism, 641
Learning to Slow Down and Pay Attention, 511
Left Alive: After a Suicide Death in the Family, 1681
Legacy of Childhood Trauma: Not Always Who They Seem, 413, 1636
Leslie E. Packer, PhD, 1553
Let Community Employment Be the Goal For Individuals with Autism, 642
Let Me Hear Your Voice, 643
Let's Talk About Depression, 1123
Let's Talk Facts About Obsessive Compulsive Disorder, 323
Let's Talk Facts About Panic Disorder, 391
Let's Talk Facts About Post-Traumatic Stress Disorder, 392, 1308
Let's Talk Facts About Substance Abuse & Addiction, 125
Letting Go, 644
The Lewin Group, 3824
Lewis's Child and Adolescent Psychiatry: A Comprehensive Textbook, 4th Edition, 1596
Lexapro, 4057
Lexicomp Inc., 2607, 3340, 3350, 3352
Lexington Books, 3389, 904, 2827
Liberty Healthcare Management Group, 3968
Liberty Resources, 3578

Life After Trauma: Workbook for Healing, 2718
Life Development Institute, 1766
Life Is Hard: Audio Guide to Healing Emotional Pain, 3206
Life Passage in the Face of Death, Vol II: Psychological Engagement of the Physically Ill Patient, 3207
Life Passage in the Face of Death, Volume I: A Brief Psychotherapy, 3208
Life Science Associates, 3127
Life Steps Pasos de Vida, 3434
Life Transition Therapy, 3557
LifeRing, 238
Lifespan, 3780
Lifespire, 1561, 1767
Light for Life Foundation International, 1673
Lincoln Child Center, 3435
Lippincott Williams & Wilkins, 3390, 1589, 1596, 2690, 3000
Lippincott Williams &Wilkins, 914
Lithium and Manic Depression: A Guide, 1080
Lithobid, 4058
Little City Foundation (LCF), 1879
Littleton Group Home, 3532
Living Skills Recovery Workbook, 126, 3307
Living Sober I, 127
Living Sober II, 128
Living Without Depression & Manic Depression: a Workbook for Maintaining Mood Stability, 1081
Living on the Razor's Edge: Solution-Oriented Brief Family Therapy with Self-Harming Adolescents, 2888
Living with Attention Deficit Disorder: Workbook for Adults with ADD, 512
Living with Depression and Manic Depression, 1164
Locumtenens.com, 3128
Lonely, Sad, and Angry: a Parent's Guide to Depression in Children and Adolescents, 1082
Long-Term Treatments of Anxiety Disorders, 2719
Loss of Self: Family Resource for the Care of Alzheimer's Disease and Related Disorders, 2768
Lost in the Mirror: An Inside Look at Borderline Personality Disorder, 842, 1244
Lost in the Mirror: Women with Multiple Personalities, 1262
Louisiana Commission on Law Enforcement and Administration (LCLE), 2177
Louisiana Department of Health and Hospitals: Louisiana Office for Addictive Disorders, 2179
Louisiana Department of Health and Hospitals: Office of Mental Health, 2178
Louisiana Federation of Families for Children's Mental Health, 1897
Love First: A New Approach to Intervention for Alcoholism and Drug Addiction, 2673
Love Publishing, 3391
Love Publishing Company, 666
Loving Healing Press, 840
Lunesta, 4059

M

M.I.S.S. Foundation/Center for Loss & Trauma, 10
MAAP, 686
MAAP Services, 728
MADD-Mothers Against Drunk Drivers, 196
MADD-Mothers Against Drunk Driving, 239
MBP Expert Services, 1358
MCG Telemedicine Center, 3129
MCW Department of Psychiatry and Behavioral Medicine, 3130, 3781
MEDA, 940
MEDCOM Information Systems, 3892
MEDLINEplus on Sleep Disorders, 1506
MEDecision, 3893
MHN, 3782
MHNet, 3615
MHNet Behavioral Health, 3783
MJ Powers & Company, 3044
MacNeal Hospital, 3488

Macomb County Community Mental Health, 1919
Madison Institute of Medicine, 333, 343, 357, 484, 1064, 1071, 1080, 1130, 2515
A Madman's Journal, 1146, 1695
Magellan Health Service, 3784
Maine Department Health and Human Services Children's Behavioral Health Services, 2180
Maine Office of Substance Abuse: Information and Resource Center, 2181
Major Depression in Children and Adolescents, 1124
Making Money While Making a Difference: Achieving Outcomes for People with Disabilities, 2560
Making Peace with Food, 913
Making the Grade: Guide to School Drug Prevention Programs, 2889
Malignant Neglect: Substance Abuse and America's Schools, 2674
Mallinckrodt, 4010
Managed Care Concepts, 3785
Managed Care Local Market Overviews, 3969
Managed Care Strategies & Psychotherapy Finances, 3055
Managed Mental Health Care in the Public Sector: a Survival Manual, 2561
Management of Autistic Behavior, 645
Management of Bipolar Disorder: Pocketbook, 1083
Management of Countertransference with Borderline Patients, 1245
Management of Depression, 1084
Managing Client Anger: What to Do When a Client is Angry with You, 2562
Managing Social Anxiety: A Cognitive Behavioral Therapy Approach Client Workbook, 324
Managing Traumatic Stress Risk: A Proactive Approach, 325, 1296
Manatee Glens, 3463
Manhattan Psychiatric Center, 3579
Mania: Clinical and Research Perspectives, 1085
Maniaci Insurance Services, 3786
Manic-Depressive Illness, 3253
Manic-Depressive Illness: Bipolar Disorders and Recurrent Depression, 2nd Edition, 1086
Manisses Communication Group, 3970
Manisses Communications Group, 2601, 2602, 3970
Manual of Clinical Child and Adolescent Psychiatry, 2890
Manual of Clinical Psychopharmacology, 2563
Manual of Panic: Focused Psychodynamic Psychotherapy, 2826
Marijuana Anonymous, 197
Marijuana: Escape to Nowhere, 218
Marion County Health Department, 2245
Market Research Alliance, 3131
Marsh Foundation, 3132
Maryland Alcohol and Drug Abuse Administration, 2183
Maryland Department of Health and Mental Hygiene, 2184
Maryland Psychiatric Research Center, 1901
Masculinity and Sexuality: Selected Topics, 1445
Mason Crest Publishers, 3392, 20, 302, 303, 495, 521, 669, 763, 839, 1001, 1009, 1072, 1087, 1239, 1335, 1378, 1473, 2691, 2780, 2930
Massachusetts Behavioral Health Partnership, 1913
Massachusetts Department of Health and Human Services, 2188
Massachusetts Department of Mental Health, 2185
Massachusetts Department of Public Health, 2186
Massachusetts Department of Public Health: Bureau of Substance Abuse Services, 2187
Massachusetts Department of Transitional Assistance, 2188
Massachusetts Executive Office of Public Safety, 2189
The Massachusetts General Hospital Bipolar Clinic/Research Program, 1135, 1180
Massachusetts National Alliance on Mental Illness, 1914

Medcomp Software, 3897
Medical Group Management Association, 2412
Mental Health Association of Colorado, 1841
Micromedex, 3905
National Academy of Neuropsychology (NAN), 2415
PRO Behavioral Health, 3800
TriZetto Group, 3930
University of Colorado Health Sciences Center, 3176
Yellow Ribbon Suicide Prevention Program, 1673

Connecticut

American Academy of Clinical Psychiatrists, 2307
American Academy of Psychiatry & Law Annual Conference, 2937
American Academy of Psychiatry and the Law (AAPL), 2309
American Academy of Psychoanalysis Preliminary Meeting, 2938
American Academy of Psychoanalysis and Dynamic Psychiatry, 2310
Casey Family Services, 3713
Century Financial Services, 3715
Connecticut Department of Mental Health and Addiction Services, 2133
Connecticut Department of Children and Families, 2134
Connecticut National Alliance on Mental Illness, 1843
Gaynor and Associates, 3753
Infoline, 194
Institute of Living- Anxiety Disorders Center; Center for Cognitive Behavioral Therapy, 1761
Purdue, 4017
Stonington Institute, 3165
Thames Valley Programs, 1845
University of Connecticut Health Center, 3177
Women's Support Services, 1846
Yale Mood Disorders Research Program, 1142

Delaware

Astra Zeneca Pharmaceuticals, 3999
Attention Deficit Disorder Association, 450
Coventry Health Care of Iowa, 3730
Delaware Alliance for the Mentally Ill, 1847
Delaware Department of Health & Social Services, 2135
Delaware Division of Child Mental Health Services, 2136
Delaware Division of Family Services, 2137
Mental Health Association of Delaware, 1848
National P.O.L.I.C.E. Suicide Foundation, 1667

District of Columbia

AAIDD Annual Meeting, 2932
ASAA A.W.A.K.E. Network, 1489
Administration for Children and Families, 2061
Administration for Children, Youth and Families, 2062
Administration on Aging, 2063
Administration on Developmental Disabilities US Department of Health & Human Services, 2064
American Academy of Child and Adolescent Psychiatry (AACAP): Annual Meeting, 2936
American Academy of Child & Adolescent Psychiatry, 2306
American Academy of Child and Adolescent Psychiatry, 1556, 1722, 3094, 3094
American Association of Homes and Services for the Aging, 2318
American Association of Retired Persons, 2321
American Association of Suicidology, 1660
American Association on Intellectual and Developmental Disabilities Annual Meeting, 1725, 2322, 2941, 2941
American Health Care Association, 2336

American Health Care Association Annual Convention, 2947
American Humane Association, 2338
American Managed Behavioral Healthcare Association, 3695
American Pharmacists Association, 2346
American Psychologial Association: Division of Family Psychology, 2351
American Psychological Association, 1730, 2352
American Psychological Association: Applied Experimental and Engineering Psychology, 2353
American Psychology- Law Society (AP-LS), 2354
American Public Human Services Association, 77
Association for Behavioral Health and Wellness, 1732
Association for Psychological Science (APS), 2376
Association of Black Psychologists, 2380
Association of Maternal and Child Health Programs (AMCHP), 2066
Bazelon Center for Mental Health Law, 1735, 2383
Caregiver Action Network, 745
Center for the Advancement of Health, 3714
Change for Good Coaching and Counseling, 866
Community Action Partnership, 2393
DC Commission on Mental Health Services, 2138
DC Department of Human Services, 2139
DC Department of Mental Health, 2070
Department of Health and Human Services/OAS, 1851
Equal Employment Opportunity Commission, 2071
Federation of Associations in Behavioral and Brain Sciences, 747
Genetic Alliance, 1756
George Washington University, 3118
Gerontoligical Society of America, 2401
HSP Verified, 3758
Hays Group, 3759
Health & Medicine Counsel of Washington DDNC Digestive Disease National Coalition, 2140
Health Systems and Financing Group, 2073
Health and Human Services Office of Assistant Secretary for Planning & Evaluation, 2074
Human Rights Campaign, 961
Jacobs Institute of Women's Health, 3123
National Association Councils on Developmental Disabilities, 748
National Association For Children's Behavioral Health, 2416
National Association for Rural Mental Health, 1774
National Association of Psychiatric Health Systems, 2422
National Association of Social Workers, 1860, 1963, 2424, 2424
National Association of State Alcohol/Drug Abuse Directors, 88
National Business Coalition Forum on Health (NBCH), 2426
National Center for the Prevention of Youth Suicide, 1665
National Coalition for LGBT Health, 963
National Coalition for the Homeless, 89, 2427
National Committee for Quality Assurance, 2428
National Council Community Behavioral Health, 271
National Council for Behavioral Health, 90, 1779
National Council on Aging, 2430
National Disability Rights Network, Inc., 1780
National Dissemination Center, 800
National Dissemination Center for Children with Disabilities, 458, 1563
National Gay and Lesbian Task Force, 965
National Organization for People of Color Against Suicide, 1666
National Organization on Fetal Alcohol Syndrome, 94
National Pharmaceutical Council, 2433
National Register of Health Service Providers in Psychology, 2300, 2435
National Technical Assistance Center for Children's Mental Health, 1565
Parents and Friends of Lesbians and Gays, 968

Parents, Families and Friends of Lesbians and Gays, 969
Pharmaceutical Care Management Association, 2438
President's Committee on Mental Retardation, 2096
Presidential Commission on Employment of the Disabled, 2097
Psychology of Religion, 2443
Public Health Foundation, 2099
Society for Women's Health Research (SWHR), 2452
Society for the Psychological Study of Social Issues (SPSSI), 2454
US Department of Health and Human Services: Office of Women's Health, 2103
ZERO TO THREE: National Center for Infants, Toddlers, and Families, 1574, 1802

Florida

Alliance for Eating Disorders Awareness, 863
Association for Women in Psychology, 2378
Behavioral Medicine and Biofeedback Consultants, 3100
Best Buddies International (BBI), 1737
Broward County Health Care Services, 3707
Career Assessment & Planning Services, 79, 260, 797, 797, 1218, 1277, 1325, 1366
Cenaps Corporation, 2290
Center for Applications of Psychological Type, 2387
CenterLink, 959
CoCENTRIX, 3857
Columbia Hospital M/H Services, 3721
Comprehensive Care Corporation, 3723
Developmental Disabilities Nurses Association, 2397
Family Network on Disabilities, 1852
Florida Alcohol and Drug Abuse Association, 1853
Florida Department Health and Human Services: Substance Abuse Program, 2141
Florida Department of Children and Families, 2142
Florida Department of Health and Human Services, 2143
Florida Department of Mental Health and Rehabilitative Services, 2144
Florida Federation of Families for Children's Mental Health, 1854
Florida Health Care Association, 1855
Florida Health Information Management Association, 1856
Florida Medicaid State Plan, 2145
Florida National Alliance for the Mentally Ill, 1857
Food Addicts Anonymous, 939
Gorski-Cenaps Corporation Training & Consultation, 2402
Grief Guidance Inc., 1663
Health Management Associates, 3763
HealthSoft, 3881
KidsHealth, 1539, 1610
Managed Care Concepts, 3785
Med Advantage, 2297, 2411
Medai, 3896
Mental Health Association of West Florida, 1858
Mental Health Corporations of America, 2413
NAATP National Association of Addiction Treatment Providers, 86
National Alliance on Mental Illness: Florida, 1859
National Association of Addiction Treatment Providers, 2419
Parent Child Center, 3149
Psychological Assessment Resources, 3917
Research and Training Center for Children's Mental Health, 1568
Synergistic Office Solutions (SOS Software), 3928
The National Coalition for a Healthy america, 882
University of South Florida Research Center for Children's Mental Health, 3189
ValueOptions Jacksonville, 3829
Vann Data Services, 3932
Youth Services International, 1573, 1801

Georgia

Association of State and Provincial Psychology Boards, 2381
Cameron and Associates, 3711
Centers for Disease Control & Prevention, 2069
Centers for Disease Control and Prevention, 1515
DailyStrength: Tourette Syndrome Support Forum, 1540
Emory University School of Medicine, Psychology and Behavior, 3114
Emory University: Psychological Center, 3115
Fowler Healthcare Affiliates, 3750
Georgia Association of Homes and Services for Children, 1861
Georgia Department of Human Resources, 2146
Georgia Department of Human Resources: Division of Public Health, 2147
Georgia Division of Mental Health Developmental Disabilities and Addictive Diseases (MHDDAD), 2148
Georgia Parent Support Network, 1862
Georgia Psychological Society Annual Conference, 2953
Grady Health Systems: Central Fulton CMHC, 1863
Healthport, 3883
Inhealth Record Systems, 3888
Locumtenens.com, 3128
MCG Telemedicine Center, 3129
McKesson Technology Solutions, 3788
Medical College of Georgia, 3133
Medical Doctor Associates, 3137
Murphy-Harpst Children's Centers, 3793
National Alliance on Mental Illness: Georgia, 1864
National Center for HIV, STD and TB Prevention, 2077
National Families in Action, 3908
Solvay Pharmaceuticals, 4022

Hawaii

Hawaii Department of Health, 2149
Hawaii Families As Allies, 1865
John A Burns School of Medicine Department of Psychiatry, 3124
National Alliance on Mental Illness: Hawaii, 1866

Idaho

College of Southern Idaho, 3720, 3109
Department of Health and Welfare: Medicaid Division, 2150
Healthwise, 3765
Idaho Alliance for the Mentally Ill, 1867
Idaho Bureau of Maternal and Child Health, 2151
Idaho Department of Health & Welfare, 2152
Idaho Department of Health and Welfare: Family and Child Services, 2153
Idaho Mental Health Center, 2154
National Alliance on Mental Illness: Idaho, 1868

Illinois

AAMA Annual Conference, 2933
AMA's Annual Medical Communications Conference, 2934
Abbott Laboratories, 3997
Allendale Association, 1869
Alzheimer's Association National Office, 741
American Academy of Dental Sleep Medicine, 1461
American Academy of Medical Administrators, 2308
American Academy of Pediatrics, 1557, 1723
American Academy of Sleep Medicine, 1462
American Association of Healthcare Consultants, 2317
American Board of Psychiatry and Neurology (ABPN), 2324

American College of Healthcare Executives, 2327, 2944, 3095, 3095
American College of Legal Medicine, 3096
American College of Osteopathic Neurologists & Psychiatrists, 2329
American College of Psychiatrists, 2330
American College of Psychiatrists Annual Meeting, 2945
American Health Information Management Association Annual Exhibition and Conference, 2337, 2948
American Medical Association, 2339
American Medical Software, 3840
Aon Consulting Group, 3697
Association for Academic Psychiatry (AAP), 2365
Baby Fold, 1870
Chaddock, 1871
Chicago Child Care Society, 1872
Children's Home Association of Illinois, 1873
Christian Association for Psychological Studies, 2389
Coalition of Illinois Counselors Organization, 1874
College of Dupage, 3719
ComPsych, 3722
Compassionate Friends, Inc, 30
Consecra Housing Network, 3724
Depression & Bi-Polar Support Alliance, 1041
Depressive and Bipolar Support Alliance (DBSA), 1932
Dorenfest Group, 3736
Dupage County Health Department, 3738
Families Anonymous, Inc., 1752
Family Service Association of Greater Elgin Area, 1875
HPN Worldwide, 3757
Haymarket Center, Professional Development, 3119
Human Resources Development Institute, 1876
Illinois Alcoholism and Drug Dependency Association, 1877, 2155
Illinois Department of Alcoholism and Substance Abuse, 2156
Illinois Department of Children and Family Services, 2157
Illinois Department of Health and Human Services, 2158
Illinois Department of Healthcare and Family Services, 2159
Illinois Department of Human Services: Office of Mental Health, 2160
Illinois Department of Mental Health and Developmental Disabilities, 2161
Illinois Department of Public Health: Division of Food, Drugs and Dairies/FDD, 2162
Innovative Data Solutions, 3889
Integrated Business Services, 3890
International Association of Eating Disorders Professionals Foundation, 868
International Society for Traumatic Stress Studies, 265, 1279
Joint Commission on Accreditation of Healthcare Organizations, 2295
Larkin Center, 1878
Little City Foundation (LCF), 1879
MEDCOM Information Systems, 3892
Medix Systems Consultants, 3900
Mental Health Association in Illinois, 2163
Metropolitan Family Services, 1880
Mihalik Group, 3791
National Association of Anorexia Nervosa and Associated Disorders (ANAD), 873
National Commission on Correctional Heath Care, 964
National Treatment Alternative for Safe Communities, 2436
Northwestern University Medical School Feinberg School of Medicine, 3146
One Place for Special Needs, 1615
Perspectives, 3805
Physicians for a National Health Program, 2439
PsycHealth, 3814
Pyrce Healthcare Group, 3816

Rainbows, 34, 1616
Recovery International, 406, 1143, 1720, 1720
S.A.F.E. Alternatives, 1256
SPSS, 3922
Section for Psychiatric and Substance Abuse Services (SPSPAS), 98
Southern Illinois University School of Medicine: Department of Psychiatry, 3160
Southern Illinois University School of Medicine, 3161
Takeda Pharmaceuticals North America, 4025
The Balanced Mind Foundation, 802, 1051
Thresholds, 1795
VOR, 1796
Vedder Price, 3831

Indiana

Eli Lilly and Company, 4003
Experior Corporation, 3871
Health Probe, 3879
Indiana Department of Public Welfare Division of Family Independence: Food Stamps/Medicaid/Training, 2164
Indiana Family & Social Services Administration, 2165
Indiana Family And Social Services Administration, 2166
Indiana Family and Social Services Administration: Division of Mental Health, 2167
Indiana Resource Center for Autism (IRCA), 588, 688, 1882, 1882
Medi-Span, 3898
National Alliance on Mental Illness: Indiana, 1883
North American Society of Adlerian Psychology (NASAP), 2437
Psychiatric Associates, 3156
Psychological Software Services, 3918
Quinco Behavioral Health Systems, 3817
Supportive Systems, 3822
The Indiana Consortium for Mental Health Services Research (ICMHSR), 2168

Iowa

Creative Solutions Unlimited, 3860
Iowa Department Human Services, 2169
Iowa Department of Public Health, 2170
Iowa Department of Public Health: Division of Substance Abuse, 2171
Iowa Division of Mental Health & Developmental Disabilities: Department of Human Services, 2172
Iowa Federation of Families for Children's Mental Health, 1884
National Alliance of Mental Illness Iowa, 1885
National Alliance on Mental Illness: Iowa, 1886
University of Iowa Hospital, 3178

Kansas

Council for Learning Disabilities, 1748
Kansas Council on Developmental Disabilities Kansas Department of Social and Rehabilitation Services, 2173
Keys for Networking: Kansas Parent Information & Resource Center, 1887
National Alliance on Mental Illness: Kansas, 1888
Preferred Mental Health Management, 3810
Society for Pediatric Psychology (SPP), 2449
Society of Teachers of Family Medicine, 2457
Topeka Institute for Psychoanalysis, 3166
University of Kansas Medical Center, 3179
University of Kansas School of Medicine, 3180

Kentucky

Adanta Group-Behavioral Health Services, 3689
Depressed Anonymous, 1144
FCS, 3747
KY-SPIN, 1890

Judge Baker Children's Center, 1764
MEDA, 940
Massachusetts Behavioral Health Partnership, 1913
Massachusetts Department of Mental Health, 2185
Massachusetts Department of Public Health, 2186
Massachusetts Department of Public Health:
  Bureau of Substance Abuse Services, 2187
Massachusetts Department of Transitional
  Assistance, 2188
Massachusetts Executive Office of Public Safety,
  2189
Massachusetts National Alliance on Mental Illness,
  1914
Medical Records Institute, 3899
Mental Health Connections, 3901
Mental Health and Substance Abuse Corporations
  of Massachusetts, 1915
Mental Illness Education Project, Inc., 1770
Mercer Consulting, 3789
Mertech, 2298
Multiservice Eating Disorders Association, 870
National Autism Center, 591
National Empowerment Center, 1781, 3795
New England Center for Children, 595
New England Educational Institute, 2957
Novartis, 4013
Parent Professional Advocacy League, 1916
Public Consulting Group, 3815
SADD: Students Against Destructive Decisions,
  202, 1617
Screening for Mental Health, 2447
Screening for Mental Health, Inc. (SMH), 1669
Sepracor Pharmaceuticals, 4020
Sigmund Freud Archives (SFA), 2448
Sunovion Pharmaceuticals, 4023
University of Massachusetts Medical Center, 3184
Webman Associates, 3834

Michigan

A.I.M. Agoraphics in Motion, 256
Adult Learning Systems, 3690
Association for Behavior Analysis, 2368
Association for Children's Mental Health, 1559
Borgess Behavioral Medicine Services, 1917
Boysville of Michigan, 1918
Common Ground Sanctuary, 1415
DocuMed, 3865
Health Alliance Plan, 3760
Health Decisions, 3762
Kleptomaniacs Anonymous, 1013
Macomb County Community Mental Health, 1919
Michigan Alliance for the Mentally Ill, 1920
Michigan Association for Children with Emotional
  Disorders: MACED, 1921
Michigan Association for Children's Mental
  Health, 1922
Michigan Department of Community Health, 2190
Michigan Department of Human Services, 2191
Mississippi Alliance for the Mentally Ill, 1930
National Council on Alcoholism and Drug
  Dependence: Greater Detroit Area, 91, 2192
Parrot Software, 3916
Rapid Psychler Press, 2445
Southwest Counseling & Development Services,
  1924
The Shulman Center for Compulsive Theft,
  Spending & Hoarding, 997
TransYouth Family Allies, 979
Traumatic Incident Reduction Newsletter, 3826
University of Michigan, 3185
Woodlands Behavioral Healthcare Network, 1925

Minnesota

Allina Hospitals & Clinics Behavioral Health
  Services, 3694
Behavioral Health Services, 3705
CBCA, 3709
CIGNA Behavioral Care, 3710
Ceridian Corporation, 3852
Corporate Health Systems, 3726
Department of Human Services: Chemical Health
  Division, 2193
Emotions Anonymous International Service Center,
  403, 1145, 1750, 1750
HealthPartners, 3764
Healtheast Behavioral Care, 2294
Impulse Control Disorders Clinic, 1010
Lake Area Youth Services Bureau, 2194
McGladery, 3787
McKesson HBOC, 3894
Midwst Center for Personal/Family Development,
  3790
Minnesota Department of Human Services, 2195
NASW Minnesota Chapter, 1926
National Multicultural Conference and Summit,
  2956
North American Training Institute: Division of the
  Minnesota Council on Compulsive Gambling,
  1928
PACER Center, 461
Pacer Center, 1929
Pearson, 3803
Suicide Awareness Voices of Education (SAVE),
  1670
University of Minnesota Fairview Health Systems,
  3186
Velocity Healthcare Informatics, 3933

Mississippi

Mississippi Alcohol Safety Education Program,
  2196
Mississippi Department Mental Health Mental
  Retardation Services, 2197
Mississippi Department of Human Services, 2198
Mississippi Department of Mental Health: Division
  of Alcohol and Drug Abuse, 2199
Mississippi Department of Mental Health: Division
  of Medicaid, 2200
Mississippi Department of Rehabilitation Services:
  Office of Vocational Rehabilitation (OVR), 2201

Missouri

Bereaved Parents of the USA, 29
CliniSphere version 2.0, 3855
College of Health and Human Services: SE
  Missouri State, 3108
DST Output, 3862
Genelco Software Solutions, 3875
Health Capital Consultants, 3761
Lake Regional Health System, 3779
Mallinckrodt, 4010
Missouri Alliance for the Mentally Ill, 1933
Missouri Department Health & Senior Services,
  2202
Missouri Department of Mental Health, 2203
Missouri Department of Public Safety, 2204
Missouri Department of Social Services, 2205
Missouri Department of Social Services: Medical
  Services Division, 2206
Missouri Division of Alcohol and Drug Abuse,
  2207
Missouri Division of Comprehensive Psychiatric
  Service, 2208
Missouri Division of Mental Retardation and
  Developmental Disabilities, 2209
Missouri Institute of Mental Health, 1934
National Share Office, 32
Ochester Psychological Service, 3147
Pathways to Promise, 200
St. Louis Behavioral Medicine Institute, 3164
Traumatic Incident Reduction Workshop, 2958

Montana

Entre Technology Services, 3870
Mental Health Association of Montana, 1936
Montana Department of Health and Human
  Services: Child & Family Services Division,
  2210
Montana Department of Human & Community
  Services, 2211
Montana Department of Public Health & Human
  Services: Addictive and Mental Disorders, 2212
Montana Department of Public Health and Human
  Services: Montana Vocational Rehabilitation
  Programs, 2213
National Alliance on Mental Illness: Montana,
  1937

Nebraska

Department of Health and Human Services
  Division of Public Health, 1938
Mutual of Omaha's Health and Wellness Programs,
  1939
Nebraska Department of Health and Human
  Services (NHHS), 2214
Nebraska Family Support Network, 1942
Nebraska Health & Human Services: Medicaid and
  Managed Care Division, 2215
Nebraska Health and Human Services Division:
  Department of Mental Health, 2216
Nebraska Mental Health Centers, 2217
Orion Healthcare Technology, 3915
Pilot Parents: PP, 1567, 1943
Wellness Councils of America, 2459

Nevada

National Alliance on Mental Illness: Carson City,
  NV, 1944
National Council of Juvenile and Family Court
  Judges, 2429
Nevada Department of Health and Human Services,
  2218
Nevada Division of Mental Health &
  Developmental Services, 2219
Nevada Employment Training & Rehabilitation
  Department, 2220
Nevada Principals' Executive Program, 1945
Northern Nevada Adult Mental Health Services,
  2221
Southern Nevada Adult Mental Health Services,
  2222

New Hampshire

Bottomline Technologies, 3848
Dartmouth Univeristy: Department of Psychiatry,
  3112
Echo Management Group, 3739
Helms & Company, 3768
Monadnock Family Services, 1946
New Hampshire Alliance for the Mentally Ill, 1948
New Hampshire Department of Health & Human
  Services: Bureau of Community Health
  Services, 2223
New Hampshire Department of Health and Human
  Services: Bureau of Developmental Services,
  2224
New Hampshire Department of Health and Human
  Services: Bureau of Behavioral Health, 2225

New Jersey

Actavis, 3998
American Society of Group Psychotherapy &
  Psychodrama, 2360
Arthur S Shorr and Associates, 3698
Asperger Autism Spectrum Education Network,
  574
Association for Children of New Jersey, 1949
Community Resource Council, 1825
Cypruss Communications, 3732
Depression After Delivery, 1043
Disability Rights New Jersey, 1950
Insurance Management Institute, 3773

Generic Drug Appendix

Alprazolam, **Niravam**, 4062
Alprazolam, **Xanax**, 4082
Amitryptiline, **Elavil**, 4044
Amphetamine/dextroamphetamine, **Adderrall**, 4030
Aripiprazole, **Abilify**, 4029
Asenapine, **Saphris**, 4074
Atomoxetine, **Strattera**, 4077
Bupropion, **Wellbutrin**, 4081
Bupropion, **Zyban**, 4085
Citalopram, **Celexa**, 4035
Clonazepam, **Klonopin**, 4054
Clozapine, **Clozaril**, 4036
Clozapine USP, **FazaClo**, 4048
Desvenlafaxine, **Pristiq**, 4066
Dexmethyphenidate, **Focalin**, 4050
Dextroamphetamine, **Dexedrine**, 4042
Diazepam, **Valium**, 4078
Disulfiram, **Antabuse**, 4031
Donepezil, **Aricept**, 4032
Dulozetine, **Cymbalta**, 4037
Eletriptan, **Relpax**, 4068
Escitalopram, **Lexapro**, 4057
Eszopiclone, **Lunesta**, 4059
Fluoxetine, **Prozac**, 4075
Fluoxetine, **Sarafem**, 4067
Fluoxetine Tablets, 60 mg, 4049
Gabapentin, **Neurontin**, 4061
Haloperidol, **Haldol**, 4051

Lamotrigine, **Lamictal**, 4055
Lithium Carbonate, **Lithobid**, 4058
Lithium **Eskalith**, 4046
Lixdexamfetamine, **Vynase**, 4080
Lorazepam, **Ativan**, 4034
Lurasidone hcl, **Latuda**, 4056
Memantine, **Namenda**, 4060
Methamphetamine, **Desoxyn**, 4040
Methylphenidate, **Ritalin**, 4072
Methylphenidate Transdermal System, **Daytrana**, 4038
Mirtazapine, **Remeron**, 4069
Paliperidone, **Invega**, 4053
Paroxetine hcl, **Paxil**, 4064
Paroxetine Mesylate, **Pexeva**, 4065
Ramelteon, **Rozerem**, 4073
Risperidone, **Risperdal**, 4071
Rivastigmine, **Exelon**, 4047
Saphris, **Asenapine**, 4033
Selegiline, **Emsam**, 4045
Sertraline, **Zoloft**, 4084
Sodium Oxybate, **Xyrem**, 4083
Temazepam, **Restoril**, 4070
Tranylcypromine, **Parnate**, 4063
Trazodone hcl, **Desyrel**, 4041
Valproic Acid, **Depakote**, 4039
Valproic Acid, **Stavzor**, 4076
Venlafazine, **Effexor**, 4043
Vilazodone hcl, **Viibryd**, 4079
Zolpidem, **Intermezzo**, 4052

Names in bold represent brand name drugs

2014 Title List

Visit **www.GreyHouse.com** for Product Information, Table of Contents and Sample Pages

General Reference

America's College Museums
American Environmental Leaders: From Colonial Times to the Present
An African Biographical Dictionary
An Encyclopedia of Human Rights in the United States
Constitutional Amendments
Encyclopedia of African-American Writing
Encyclopedia of the Continental Congress
Encyclopedia of Gun Control & Gun Rights
Encyclopedia of Invasions & Conquests
Encyclopedia of Prisoners of War & Internment
Encyclopedia of Religion & Law in America
Encyclopedia of Rural America
Encyclopedia of the United States Cabinet, 1789-2010
Encyclopedia of War Journalism
Encyclopedia of Warrior Peoples & Fighting Groups
From Suffrage to the Senate: America's Political Women
Nations of the World
Political Corruption in America
Speakers of the House of Representatives, 1789-2009
The Environmental Debate: A Documentary History
The Evolution Wars: A Guide to the Debates
The Religious Right: A Reference Handbook
The Value of a Dollar: 1860-2009
The Value of a Dollar: Colonial Era
This is Who We Were: A Companion to the 1940 Census
This is Who We Were: The 1920s
This is Who We Were: The 1950s
This is Who We Were: The 1960s
US Land & Natural Resource Policy
Working Americans 1770-1869 Vol. IX: Revolutionary War to the Civil War
Working Americans 1880-1999 Vol. I: The Working Class
Working Americans 1880-1999 Vol. II: The Middle Class
Working Americans 1880-1999 Vol. III: The Upper Class
Working Americans 1880-1999 Vol. IV: Their Children
Working Americans 1880-2003 Vol. V: At War
Working Americans 1880-2005 Vol. VI: Women at Work
Working Americans 1880-2006 Vol. VII: Social Movements
Working Americans 1880-2007 Vol. VIII: Immigrants
Working Americans 1880-2009 Vol. X: Sports & Recreation
Working Americans 1880-2010 Vol. XI: Inventors & Entrepreneurs
Working Americans 1880-2011 Vol. XII: Our History through Music
Working Americans 1880-2012 Vol. XIII: Education & Educators
World Cultural Leaders of the 20th & 21st Centuries

Business Information

Complete Television, Radio & Cable Industry Directory
Directory of Business Information Resources
Directory of Mail Order Catalogs
Directory of Venture Capital & Private Equity Firms
Environmental Resource Handbook
Food & Beverage Market Place
Grey House Homeland Security Directory
Grey House Performing Arts Directory
Hudson's Washington News Media Contacts Directory
New York State Directory
Sports Market Place Directory

Education Information

Charter School Movement
Comparative Guide to American Elementary & Secondary Schools
Complete Learning Disabilities Directory
Educators Resource Directory
Special Education

Health Information

Comparative Guide to American Hospitals
Complete Directory for Pediatric Disorders
Complete Directory for People with Chronic Illness
Complete Directory for People with Disabilities
Complete Mental Health Directory
Diabetes in America: A Geographic & Demographic Analysis
Directory of Health Care Group Purchasing Organizations
Directory of Hospital Personnel
HMO/PPO Directory
Medical Device Register
Older Americans Information Directory

Statistics & Demographics

America's Top-Rated Cities
America's Top-Rated Small Towns & Cities
America's Top-Rated Smaller Cities
American Tally
Ancestry & Ethnicity in America
Comparative Guide to American Hospitals
Comparative Guide to American Suburbs
Profiles of America
Profiles of... Series – State Handbooks
The Hispanic Databook
Weather America

Financial Ratings Series

TheStreet.com Ratings Guide to Bond & Money Market Mutual Funds
TheStreet.com Ratings Guide to Common Stocks
TheStreet.com Ratings Guide to Exchange-Traded Funds
TheStreet.com Ratings Guide to Stock Mutual Funds
TheStreet.com Ratings Ultimate Guided Tour of Stock Investing
Weiss Ratings Consumer Guides
Weiss Ratings Guide to Banks & Thrifts
Weiss Ratings Guide to Credit Unions
Weiss Ratings Guide to Health Insurers
Weiss Ratings Guide to Life & Annuity Insurers
Weiss Ratings Guide to Property & Casualty Insurers

Bowker's Books In Print® Titles

Books In Print®
Books In Print® Supplement
American Book Publishing Record® Annual
American Book Publishing Record® Monthly
Books Out Loud™
Bowker's Complete Video Directory™
Children's Books In Print®
El-Hi Textbooks & Serials In Print®
Forthcoming Books®
Law Books & Serials In Print™
Medical & Health Care Books In Print™
Publishers, Distributors & Wholesalers of the US™
Subject Guide to Books In Print®
Subject Guide to Children's Books In Print®

Canadian General Reference

Associations Canada
Canadian Almanac & Directory
Canadian Environmental Resource Guide
Canadian Parliamentary Guide
Financial Services Canada
Governments Canada
Health Services Canada
Libraries Canada
Major Canadian Cities
The History of Canada

Grey House Publishing | Salem Press | H.W. Wilson
4919 Route, 22 PO Box 56, Amenia NY 12501-0056

2014 Title List

Visit **www.SalemPress.com** for Product Information, Table of Contents and Sample Pages

Literature

American Ethnic Writers
Critical Insights: Authors
Critical Insights: New Literary Collection Bundles
Critical Insights: Themes
Critical Insights: Works
Critical Survey of Drama
Critical Survey of Graphic Novels: Heroes & Super Heroes
Critical Survey of Graphic Novels: History, Theme & Technique
Critical Survey of Graphic Novels: Independents & Underground Classics
Critical Survey of Graphic Novels: Manga
Critical Survey of Long Fiction
Critical Survey of Mystery & Detective Fiction
Critical Survey of Mythology and Folklore: Heroes and Heroines
Critical Survey of Mythology and Folklore: Love, Sexuality & Desire
Critical Survey of Mythology and Folklore: World Mythology
Critical Survey of Poetry
Critical Survey of Poetry: American Poetry
Critical Survey of Poetry: British, Irish & Commonwealth Poets
Critical Survey of Poetry: European Poets
Critical Survey of Poetry: European Poets
Critical Survey of Poetry: Topical Essays
Critical Survey of Poetry: World Poets
Critical Survey of Science Fiction & Fantasy Literature
Critical Survey of Shakespeare's Sonnets
Critical Survey of Short Fiction
Critical Survey of Short Fiction: American Writers
Critical Survey of Short Fiction: British, Irish & Commonwealth Poets
Critical Survey of Short Fiction: European Writers
Critical Survey of Short Fiction: Topical Essays
Critical Survey of Short Fiction: World Writers
Cyclopedia of Literary Characters
Introduction to Literary Context: American Post-Modernist Novels
Introduction to Literary Context: American Short Fiction
Introduction to Literary Context: English Literature
Introduction to Literary Context: World Literature
Magill's Literary Annual 2014
Magill's Survey of American Literature
Magill's Survey of World Literature
Masterplots
Masterplots II: African American Literature
Masterplots II: Christian Literature
Masterplots II: Drama Series
Masterplots II: Short Story Series
Notable African American Writers
Notable American Novelists
Notable Playwrights
Short Story Writers

Science, Careers & Mathematics

Applied Science
Applied Science: Engineering & Mathematics
Applied Science: Science & Medicine
Applied Science: Technology
Biomes and Ecosystems
Careers in Chemistry
Careers in Communications & Media
Careers in Healthcare
Careers in Hospitality & Tourism
Careers in Law & Criminology
Careers in Physics
Computer Technology Inventors
Contemporary Biographies in Chemistry
Contemporary Biographies in Communications & Media
Contemporary Biographies in Healthcare
Contemporary Biographies in Hospitality & Tourism
Contemporary Biographies in Law & Criminology
Contemporary Biographies in Physics
Earth Science
Earth Science: Earth Materials & Resources
Earth Science: Earth's Surface and History
Earth Science: Physics & Chemistry of the Earth
Earth Science: Weather, Water & Atmosphere
Encyclopedia of Energy
Encyclopedia of Environmental Issues
Encyclopedia of Global Resources
Encyclopedia of Global Warming
Encyclopedia of Mathematics and Society
Encyclopedia of the Ancient World
Forensic Science
Internet Innovators
Introduction to Chemistry
Magill's Encyclopedia of Science: Animal Life
Magill's Encyclopedia of Science: Plant life
Magill's Medical Guide
Notable Natural Disasters
Solar System

Health

Addictions & Substance Abuse
Cancer
Complementary & Alternative Medicine
Genetics & Inherited Conditions
Infectious Diseases & Conditions
Magill's Medical Guide
Psychology & Mental Health
Psychology Basics

Grey House Publishing | Salem Press | H.W. Wilson
4919 Route, 22 PO Box 56, Amenia NY 12501-0056

2014 Title List

Visit **www.SalemPress.com** for Product Information, Table of Contents and Sample Pages

History and Social Science

A 2000s in America
50 States
African American History
Agriculture in History (check)
American First Ladies
American Heroes
American Indian Tribes
American Presidents
American Villains
Ancient Greece
Bill of Rights, The
Cold War, The
Defining Documents: American Revolution 1754-1805
Defining Documents: Civil War 1860-1865
Defining Documents: Emergence of Modern America, 1868-1918
Defining Documents: Exploration & Colonial America 1492-1755
Defining Documents: Manifest Destiny 1803-1860
Defining Documents: Reconstruction, 1865-1880
Defining Documents: The 1920s
Defining Documents: The 1930s
Defining Documents: World War I
Eighties in America
Encyclopedia of American Immigration
Fifties in America
Forties in America
Great Athletes
Great Events from History: 17th Century
Great Events from History: 18th Century
Great Events from History: 19th Century
Great Events from History: 20th Century, 1901-1940
Great Events from History: 20th Century, 1941-1970
Great Events from History: 20th Century, 1971-200
Great Events from History: Ancient World
Great Events from History: Middle Ages
Great Events from History: Modern Scandals
Great Events from History: Renaissance & Early Modern Era
Great Lives from History: 17th Century
Great Lives from History: 18th Century
Great Lives from History: 19th Century
Great Lives from History: 20th Century
Great Lives from History: African Americans
Great Lives from History: Ancient World
Great Lives from History: Asian & Pacific Islander Americans
Great Lives from History: Incredibly Wealthy
Great Lives from History: Inventors & Inventions
Great Lives from History: Jewish Americans
Great Lives from History: Latinos
Great Lives from History: Middle Ages
Great Lives from History: Notorious Lives
Great Lives from History: Renaissance & Early Modern Era
Great Lives from History: Scientists & Science
Historical Encyclopedia of American Business
Immigration in U.S. History
Magill's Guide to Military History
Milestone Documents in African American History
Milestone Documents in American History
Milestone Documents in World History
Milestone Documents of American Leaders
Milestone Documents of World Religions
Musicians & Composers 20th Century
Nineties in America
Seventies in America

Sixties in America
Survey of American Industry and Careers
Thirties in America
Twenties in America
U.S. Court Cases
U.S. Laws, Acts, and Treaties
U.S. Legal System
U.S. Supreme Court
United States at War
USA in Space
Weapons and Warfare
World Conflicts: Asia and the Middle East

Grey House Publishing | Salem Press | H.W. Wilson
4919 Route, 22 PO Box 56, Amenia NY 12501-0056

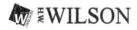
2014 Title List

Visit **www.HwWilsonInPrint.com** for Product Information, Table of Contents and Sample Pages

Current Biography

Current Biography Cumulative Index 1946-2013
Current Biography Magazine
Current Biography Yearbook-2004
Current Biography Yearbook-2005
Current Biography Yearbook-2006
Current Biography Yearbook-2007
Current Biography Yearbook-2008
Current Biography Yearbook-2009
Current Biography Yearbook-2010
Current Biography Yearbook-2011
Current Biography Yearbook-2012
Current Biography Yearbook-2013
Current Biography Yearbook-2014

Core Collections

Senior High Core Collection
Middle & Junior High School Core
Children's Core Collection
Fiction Core Collection
Public Library Core Collection: Nonfiction

Sears List

Sears List of Subject Headings
Sears: Lista de Encabezamientos de Materia

The Reference Shelf

Aging in America
Revisiting Gender
The U.S. National Debate Topic, 2014/2015
Embracing New Paradigms in education
Marijuana Reform
Representative American Speeches 2013-2014
Reality Television
The Business of Food
The Future of U.S. Economic Relations: Mexico, Cuba, and Venezuela
Sports in America
Global Climate Change
Representative American Speeches, 2012-2013
Conspiracy Theories
The Arab Spring
U.S. National Debate Topic: Transportation Infrastructure
Families: Traditional and New Structures
Faith & Science
Representative American Speeches 2011-2012
Social Networking
Dinosaurs
Space Exploration & Development
U.S. Infrastructure
Politics of the Ocean
Representative American Speeches 2010-2011
Robotics
The News and its Future
American Military Presence Overseas
Russia
Graphic Novels and Comic Books
Representative American Speeches 2009-2010

Readers' Guide

Readers Guide to Periodicals Literature
Abridged Readers' Guide to Periodical Literature
Short Story Index

Indexes

Short Story Index
Index to Legal Periodicals & Books

Facts About Series

Facts About the Presidents, Eighth Edition
Facts About China
Facts About the 20th Century
Facts About American Immigration
Facts About World's Languages

Nobel Prize Winners

Nobel Prize Winners, 2002-2013

World Authors

World Authors 2000-2005
World Authors 2006-2013

Famous First Facts

Famous First Facts, Seventh Edition
Famous First Facts About American Politics
Famous First Facts About Sports
Famous First Facts About the Environment
Famous First Facts, International Edition

American Book of Days

The American Book of Days, Fifth Edition
The International Book of Days

Junior Authors & Illustrators

Tenth Book of Junior Authors & Illustrations

Monographs

The Barnhart Dictionary of Etymology
Celebrate the World
Indexing from A to Z
Radical Change: Books for Youth in a Digital Age
The Poetry Break
Guide to the Ancient World

Wilson Chronology

Wilson Chronology of Asia and the Pacific
Wilson Chronology of Human Rights
Wilson Chronology of Ideas
Wilson Chronology of the Arts
Wilson Chronology of the World's Religions
Wilson Chronology of Women's Achievements

Book Review Digest

Book Review Digest, 2014

Grey House Publishing | Salem Press | H.W. Wilson
4919 Route, 22 PO Box 56, Amenia NY 12501-0056